CPT®·PLUS!

A Comprehensive Guide To Current Procedural Terminology

Color Coded

2021

D1223629

PMIC
CODING & COMPLIANCE

ISBN 978-1-57066-566-0 (Coder's Choice® soft cover)
ISBN 978-1-57066-634-6 (Spiral)
ISBN 978-1-57066-635-3 (e-book)

Practice Management Information Corporation
4727 Wilshire Boulevard
Los Angeles, California 90010
1-800-MED-SHOP
http://pmiconline.com/

Printed in China

INTRODUCTION

CPT® PLUS! 2021 is an enhanced CPT® coding resource which includes all official CPT 2021 codes and complete descriptions plus comprehensive CPT coding instructions, full-color anatomical illustrations, a unique color-coding system to help identify CPT codes subject to special coding rules, and a new and improved alphabetic index.

The CPT coding system includes over 9,000 codes and descriptions for reporting medical services, procedures, supplies and materials. Accurate CPT coding provides an efficient method of communicating medical services and procedures among health care providers, health care facilities, and third party payers and enhances the health care provider's control of the reimbursement process.

The CPT coding system is revised annually by the American Medical Association (AMA). Each year hundreds of additions, changes and deletions are made the CPT coding system. These changes become effective on January 1st. CPT is required by federal law for all health insurance claim forms filed with Medicare, Medicaid, CHAMPUS and Federal Employee Health Plans and is accepted or required by all other third party payers.

CPT® PLUS! 2021 provides valuable instructions, coding tips, and other information to help providers maximize reimbursement while minimizing audit liability. Our objective is to make CPT coding faster, easier and more accurate for medical office, healthcare facility and third party payer coding and billing staff, while setting a new standard for CPT coding references.

James B. Davis, Publisher

DISCLAIMER

This publication is designed to offer basic information regarding coding and reporting of medical services, supplies and procedures using the CPT coding system. The information presented is based on a thorough analysis of the CPT coding system and the experience and interpretations of the editors. Though all of the information has been carefully researched and checked for accuracy and completeness, neither the editors nor the publisher accept any responsibility or liability with regard to errors, omissions, misuse or misinterpretation.

CONTENTS

This page intentionally left blank.

CPT CODING FUNDAMENTALS

CPT® is an acronym for Current Procedural Terminology. Physicians' Current Procedural Terminology, Fourth Edition, known as CPT-4 or more commonly CPT, is a systematic listing of codes and descriptions which classify medical services and procedures. CPT codes are used by physicians, hospitals, and other health care professionals, to report specific medical, surgical and diagnostic services and procedures for statistical and third party payment purposes.

The CPT coding system is maintained by the American Medical Association (AMA) and a revised edition of the CPT book is published each fall. The new CPT codes become effective on January 1st of the following year. The revisions in each new edition are prepared by the CPT Editorial Panel with the assistance of physicians representing all specialties of medicine.

A thorough understanding of the CPT coding system is essential in order to provide accurate reporting of medical services and procedures, maximize payments from third parties, minimize denials, rejections and reductions from third parties, and to protect the medical practice from audit liability.

KEY POINTS REGARDING THE CPT CODING SYSTEM

- *CPT codes describe medical procedures, services and supplies.*

- *All CPT codes are five digit codes.*

- *CPT codes are mandated by federal law for Medicare, Medicaid, CHAMPUS and Federal Employee Health Plan (FEHP) reporting and are accepted or required by all other third party payers.*

- *CPT codes are self-definitive, eg. with the exception of CPT codes for unlisted procedures and/or the few CPT codes which include the term specify in the description, each CPT code number represents the universal definition of the service or procedure.*

- *CPT codes are revised and updated annually by the AMA and the revisions become effective each January 1st. Hundreds of CPT codes are added, changed or deleted each year. All health care professionals, third party payers, and health care facilities must maintain copies of the current code books.*

- *Accurate CPT coding provides an efficient method of communicating medical, surgical and diagnostic services and procedures among health care professionals, health care facilities, and third party payers.*

- *Accurate CPT coding enhances the health care provider's control of the reimbursement process.*

STRUCTURE OF THE CPT CODING SYSTEM

The CPT coding system includes over 7,900 codes and definitions for medical services, procedures and diagnostic tests. Each procedure or service is identified by a five digit code, followed by the definition.

*The CPT coding system is divided into eight **SECTIONS**. The eight sections of are:*

Evaluation and Management	99202-99499
Anesthesiology	00100-01999, 99100-99140
Surgery	10004-69990
Radiology (Including Nuclear Medicine & Diagnostic Ultrasound)	70010-79999
Pathology and Laboratory	80047-89398, 0001U-0241U
Medicine (except Anesthesiology)	90281-99199, 99500-99607
Category II Performance Measurement	0001F-9007F
Category III Emerging Technology	0042T-0639T

Each section of the CPT book includes subsections with anatomic, procedural, condition, or descriptor subheadings. The Evaluation and Management (E/M) section is presented first because 1) these codes are used by virtually all health care providers and 2) are the most frequently used CPT codes.

HOW TO USE THE CPT CODING SYSTEM

A provider or coder using the CPT coding system first chooses the name and associated code of the procedure or service which most accurately identifies and describes the service(s) performed. The provider or coder then chooses names and codes for additional services or procedures. If necessary, modifiers are chosen and added to the selected service and procedure codes. All services or procedures coded must also be documented in the patient's medical record.

According to CPT, "The listing of a service or procedure and its code number in a specific section of the CPT book does not restrict its use to a specific specialty group. Any procedure or service in any section of the CPT coding system may be used to designate the services rendered by any qualified physician or other qualified health care professional."

The codes and descriptions listed in the CPT coding system are those that are generally consistent with contemporary medical practice and being performed by health care professionals in clinical practice. Inclusion in the CPT coding system does not represent endorsement by the American Medical Association of any particular diagnostic or therapeutic procedure. In addition, inclusion or exclusion of a procedure does not imply any health insurance coverage or reimbursement policy.

CPT FORMAT AND CONVENTIONS

DESCRIPTIONS

The descriptions associated with CPT codes have been developed by the AMA to provide complete descriptions of medical services and procedures.

Many CPT descriptions include the definition of basic procedures followed by supplemental descriptions for variations or modifications of the basic procedure. In the CPT coding book, the basic procedure description ends with a semicolon (;), followed by the additional description.

If a CPT description includes the same basic procedure as the preceding listing, the basic procedure is not listed. Only the supplemental description is listed, preceded by an indentation. For example:

25100   Arthrotomy, wrist joint; with biopsy

25105   with synovectomy

SYMBOLS

● *A filled BLACK CIRCLE preceding a CPT code indicates that the code is new to this revision of the CPT coding system. A symbol key appears on all left-hand pages.*

▲ *A filled BLACK TRIANGLE preceding a CPT code indicates that there is a revision to the description. Wherever possible, the revised text is identified with underlining.*

( ) *CPT codes enclosed within parenthesis have been deleted from the CPT coding system and should no longer be used.*

+ *A bold plus sign preceding a CPT code indicates that the code is an "add-on" code and must be listed in addition to the main CPT code.*

⊘ *This symbol preceding a CPT code indicates that the code is exempt from the use of modifier 51.*

★ *A star symbol is used to identify codes that may be used to report telemedicine services when appended by modifier 95.*

Note that a CPT code may be preceded by the add-on, star symbol or modifier-51 exempt symbol, in addition to new or changed code symbols.

COLOR CODING

Separate procedure. A procedure or service that is normally performed as an integral component of a total service or procedure. CPT codes identified as separate procedure codes should not be coded in addition to the basic procedure code of which it is considered an integral component.

However, if the procedure or service that is usually designated as a separate procedure is performed independently or is considered to be unrelated or distinct from other procedures or services provided at that time, the separate procedure may be coded by itself. The modifier -59 should be added to the separate procedure code to indicate that the procedure is not considered to be a component of another procedure, but is a distinct, independent procedure.

Unlisted code. Descriptions include the term "unlisted." Use only when a CPT code which specifically describes the service or procedure is unavailable. A report is usually required by third party payers.

Nonspecific code. Descriptions include the term "specify" instructing the coder to include additional information such as the quadrant, the nerve, the muscle, the level of spine, the number of joints, the type of study, the method of dosimetry, the hormone, the receptor, the assay method, the type of kit, the material injected, the type of tests, the number of tests, the doses provided.

CCI comprehensive code. Indicates codes identified as comprehensive codes in the Comprehensive Coding Initiative, revised annually. Per CMS rules, all identifiable component procedures are included in the comprehensive code and should not be billed separately to Medicare.

ITALICIZED AND NON-ITALICIZED TEXT

Italicized text is used throughout this publication to distinguish information authored, contributed or otherwise provided by PMIC.

Non-italicized text is used to distinguish information reproduced verbatim from CPT 2020, published by the American Medical Association.

SECTION OVERVIEWS

Specific guidelines are presented at the beginning of each of the six sections of the CPT coding system. The guidelines define items that are necessary to interpret and report the procedures and services contained in that section. CPT guidelines also provide explanations regarding terms that apply only to a particular section.

REQUESTS TO UPDATE THE CPT CODING SYSTEM

The American Medical Association (AMA) maintains a CPT Editorial Panel that reviews and approves requests for changes to the CPT coding system. Requests to add, delete or revise specific CPT codes should be addressed to:

CPT Editorial Research & Development
American Medical Association
330 North Wabash Ave., Suite 39300
Chicago, Illinois 60611-5885

CPT 2021 AVAILABLE IN ELECTRONIC FORMAT

CPT 2021 codes and descriptions with relative value information are available on CD-ROM or as a download. The data files are available in standard ASCII format and may be imported into your billing and health insurance claims software. CPT Plus! 2021 is also available as a PC resident e-book in PDF format. For more information call (800) 633-7467 or visit http://pmiconline.com.

This page intentionally left blank.

CODING & BILLING ISSUES

Most billing, coding and reporting issues involving the CPT® coding system apply generally to all medical specialties and professions. However, there are some specialty specific issues defined in each section of the CPT coding system that apply only to the specific medical specialty represented.

SUPPORTING DOCUMENTATION

Documentation in the patient's medical report must clearly support the procedures, services and supplies coded on the health insurance claim form. Most medical chart reviewers take the position that if something is not documented in the medical record, then the service or procedure was not performed and therefore is not subject to reimbursement.

If a medical practice is selected for an audit by Medicare or other third party payer, the accuracy and completeness of the documentation of the medical records, or lack thereof, will have a significant impact on the outcome of the audit. The current emphasis on "fraud" and "abuse" by Medicare, Medicaid and private third party payer necessitates a review of documentation by all health care professionals.

SPECIAL MEDICARE CONSIDERATIONS

To satisfy Medicare requirements, there must be sufficient documentation in the medical record to verify the services coded and the level of care required. Section 1833(e) of Title XVIII, Social Security Act requires "available information that documents a claim." If there is no documentation to justify the services or level of care, the claim cannot be considered for Medicare benefits.

If there is insufficient documentation to support claims that have already been paid by Medicare, the reimbursement will be considered an overpayment and a refund will be requested by Medicare. Medicare has the authority to review any information, including medical records, when such information pertains to a Medicare claim.

UNLISTED PROCEDURES OR SERVICES

There are services or procedures performed by health care professionals that are not found in the CPT coding system. These services or procedures may be either new procedures which have not yet been assigned a CPT code or simply a variation of a procedure which precludes using the existing CPT code. Each section of the CPT coding system includes codes for reporting these unlisted procedures.

Unlisted procedure codes should not be coded unless the coder has reviewed the CPT coding system carefully to ensure that a more specific code is not available. If a specific CPT code is not located, check for HCPCS codes that may be reportable.

As a rule, a report needs to be enclosed with the health insurance claim form when reporting unlisted procedure codes. Because unlisted procedure codes are subject to manual medical review, payment is usually slower than for normal processing time.

CPT ADDITIONS, CHANGES, AND DELETIONS

Each year hundreds of codes are added, changed or deleted from the CPT coding system. A summary of these changes is found in Appendix B of the CPT code book, which provides a quick reference for coding review. In addition to the summary, these modifications are identified throughout the CPT code book.

ADDITIONS TO THE CPT CODING SYSTEM

New codes are added to the CPT coding system each year. New CPT codes are identified with a small black circle placed to the left of the code number. Examples of new codes found in CPT 2021 include:

- **30468** Repair of nasal valve collapse with subcutaneous/submucosal lateral wall implant(s)

- **55880** Ablation of malignant prostate tissue, transrectal, with high intensity-focused ultrasound (HIFU), including ultrasound guidance

CHANGES TO CPT CODE DEFINITIONS

Each year the definitions of many CPT codes are revised. CPT codes with changed definitions are identified with a small black triangle placed to the left of the code number. Examples of CPT codes with changed definitions in CPT 2021 include:

▲ **19361**   Breast reconstruction; with latissimus dorsi flap

▲ **33992**   Removal of percutaneous left heart ventricular assist device, arterial or arterial and venous cannula(s), at separate and distinct session from insertion

The only way to determine exactly what part of the definition has been changed is to compare the current changed definition with the definition from the previous edition of the CPT code book.

DELETIONS FROM THE CPT CODING SYSTEM

Each year some CPT codes are deleted. Deleted CPT codes, and references to replacement codes, if there are any, are enclosed within parentheses. Examples of CPT codes deleted from CPT 2021 include:

(**99201**   **deleted 2020 [2021 Edition]. To report, use 99202**)

(**92585**   **deleted 2020 [2021 Edition]. To report, see 92652, 92653**)

NEW SECTIONS AND SUBSECTIONS

New sections and subsections, or renamed sections, are frequently added to the CPT coding system to reflect changes in technology or medical practice and to provide additional code sequences for special purposes.

Prolonged Service With Direct Patient Contact (Except with Office or Other Outpatient Svc)   **99354-99357**
Prolonged Service With or Without Direct Patient Contact on the Date of an Office or Other Outpaient Service   **99417**

CATEGORY II PERFORMANCE MEASUREMENT CODES

Category II, Performance Measurement CPT codes, are designed to facilitate outcomes research. This new section was introduced in the 2005 CPT updates. Category II codes include the letter "F" as the fifth digit of the five digit CPT code. These codes are optional, and are not a substitute for Category I codes.

CATEGORY III EMERGING TECHNOLOGY CODES

Temporary codes for emerging technology, services and procedures designed to permit data collection and assessment of new technologies. All Category III codes include the letter "T" as the fifth digit of the five digit CPT code. The inclusion of a specific service or procedure in this section does not imply or endorse clinical efficacy, safety, or applicability to clinical practice.

STARRED PROCEDURES

The star symbol ★ identifies codes that may be used to report synchronous (real-time) telemedicine services when appended by modifier 59. These procedures involve electronic interactive telecommunications equipment that includes both audio and video.

90791	90837	90951	90960	93268	97802	99202	99214	99242	99253	99310	99409
90792	90838	90952	90961	93270	97803	99203	99215	99243	99254	99354	99417
90832	90845	90954	92227	93271	97804	99204	99231	99244	99255	99355	99495
90833	90846	90955	92228	93272	98960	99205	99232	99245	99307	99406	99496
90834	90847	90957	93228	96040	98961	99212	99233	99251	99308	99407	
90836	90863	90958	93229	96116	98962	99213	99241	99252	99309	99408	

INSTRUCTIONAL NOTES

Notes found in the CPT coding system give instructions for using codes. When selecting a code, look for instructions in the section guidelines for any additional information necessary to code accurately. Also, instructional notes take the form of parenthetical statements and paragraphs, which may appear at the beginning of subsections, headings and subheadings, or above and below the code itself.

DEFINITION OF NEW AND ESTABLISHED PATIENT

Solely to distinguish between new and established patients, professional services are those face-to-face services rendered by physicians and other qualified health care professionals and coded by a specific CPT code(s). A new patient is one who has not received any professional services from the physician/qualified health care professional or another physician/qualified health care professional of the same specialty who belongs to the same group practice, within the past three years. An established patient is one who has received professional services from the physician/qualified health care professional or another physician/qualified health care professional of the same specialty who belongs to the same group practice, within the past three years.

In the instance where a physician/qualified health care professional is on call for or covering for another physician/qualified health care professional, the patient's encounter will be classified as it would have been by the physician/qualified health care professional who is not available.

No distinction is made between new and established patients in the emergency department. Evaluation and Management services in the emergency department category may be coded for any new or established patient who presents for treatment in the emergency department.

PLACE (LOCATION) OF SERVICE

CPT makes specific distinctions for place (location) of service for evaluation and management codes. Place of service may have considerable impact on reimbursement. This list gives CPT code ranges for some specific places of service:

Office or Other Outpatient Services	99202-99215
Hospital Observation Services	99217-99220, 99224-99226
Hospital Inpatient Services	99221-99223, 99231-99239
Emergency Department Services	99281-99288
Nursing Facility Services	99304-99318
Domiciliary, Rest Home, or Custodial Care Services	99324-99337
Domiciliary, Rest Home, or Home Care Plan Oversight Services	99339-99340
Home Services	99341-99350
Inpatient Neonatal and Pediatric Critical Care	99466-99486

PLACE OF SERVICE CODES FOR PROFESSIONAL CLAIMS

Listed below are place of service codes and descriptions. These codes should be used on professional claims to specify the entity where service(s) were rendered. Check with individual payers (e.g., Medicare, Medicaid, other private insurance) for reimbursement policies regarding these codes.

Code	*Place Name*	*Place Description*
01	*Pharmacy*	*A facility or location where drugs and other medically related items and services are sold, dispensed, or otherwise provided directly to patients. (Effective 10/1/03)*
02	*Telehealth*	*The location where health services and health related services are provided or received, through a telecommunicatins system. (Effective 1/1/17)*
03	*School*	*A facility whose primary purpose is education.*
04	*Homeless Shelter*	*A facility or location whose primary purpose is to provide temporary housing to homeless individuals (e.g., emergency shelters, individual or family shelters).*

Code	Place Name	Place Description
05	Indian Health Service Free-standing Facility	A facility or location, owned and operated by the Indian Health Service, which provides diagnostic, therapeutic (surgical and non-surgical), and rehabilitation services to American Indians and Alaska Natives who do not require hospitalization.
06	Indian Health Service Provider-based Facility	A facility or location, owned and operated by the Indian Health Service, which provides diagnostic, therapeutic (surgical and non-surgical), and rehabilitation services rendered by, or under the supervision of, physicians to American Indians and Alaska Natives admitted as inpatients or outpatients.
07	Tribal 638 Free-Standing Facility	A facility or location owned and operated by a federally recognized American Indian or Alaska Native tribe or tribal organization under a 638 agreement, which provides diagnostic, therapeutic (surgical and non-surgical), and rehabilitation services to tribal members who do not require hospitalization.
08	Tribal 638 Provider-based Facility	A facility or location owned and operated by a federally recognized American Indian or Alaska Native tribe or tribal organization under a 638 agreement, which provides diagnostic, therapeutic (surgical and non-surgical), and rehabilitation services to tribal members admitted as inpatients or outpatients
09	Prison-Correctional Facility	A prison, jail, reformatory, work farm, detention center, or any other similar facility maintained by either Federal, State or local authorities for the purpose of confinement or rehabilitation of adult or juvenile criminal offenders. (Effective 7/1/06)
10	Unassigned	N/A
11	Office	Location, other than a hospital, skilled nursing facility (SNF), military treatment facility, community health center, State or local public health clinic, or intermediate care facility (ICF), where the health professional routinely provides health examinations, diagnosis, and treatment of illness or injury on an ambulatory basis.
12	Home	Location, other than a hospital or other facility, where the patient receives care in a private residence.
13	Assisted Living Facility	Congregate residential facility with self-contained living units providing assessment of each resident's needs and on-site support 24 hours a day, 7 days a week, with the capacity to deliver or arrange for services including some health care and other services. (Effective 10/1/03)
14	Group Home	A residence, with shared living areas, where clients receive supervision and other services such as social and/or behavioral services, custodial service, and minimal services (e.g., medication administration). (Effective 10/1/03)
15	Mobile Unit	A facility/unit that moves from place-to-place equipped to provide preventive, screening, diagnostic, and/or treatment services.
16	Temporary Lodging	A short-term accomodation such as a hotel, campground, hostel, cruise ship, or resort where the patient receives care, and which is not identified by any other POS code. (Effective 1/1/08)
17	Walk-in Retail Health Clinic	A walk-in retail health clinic, other than an office, urgent care facility, pharmacy, or independent clinic, which is not described by any other POS code, that is located within a retail operation and provides on an ambulatory basis, preventive and primary care services. (Effective 5/1/10)
18	Place of Employment-Worksite	A location, not described by any other POS code, owned or operated by a public or private entity where the patient is employed, and where a health professional provides on-going or episodic occupational medical, therapeutic or rehabilitative services to the individual. (This code is available for use effective January 1, 2013, but not later than May 1, 2013)
19	Off Campus Outpatient Hospital	A portion of an off-campus hospital provider based department which provides diagnostic, therapeutic (both surgical and nonsurgical), and rehabilitation services to sick or injured persons who do not require hospitalization or institutionalization. (Effective 1/1/2016)

Code	Place Name	Place Description
20	Urgent Care Facility	Location, distinct from a hospital emergency room, an office, or a clinic, whose purpose is to diagnose and treat illness or injury for unscheduled, ambulatory patients seeking immediate medical attention. (Effective 1/1/03)
21	Inpatient Hospital	A facility, other than psychiatric, which primarily provides diagnostic, therapeutic (both surgical and non-surgical), and rehabilitation services by, or under, the supervision of physicians to patients admitted for a variety of medical conditions.
22	On Campus— Outpatient Hospital	A portion of a hospital's main campus which provides diagnostic, therapeutic (both surgical and non-surgical), and rehabilitation services to sick or injured persons who do not require hospitalization or institutionalization. (Description change effective 1/1/16)
23	Emergency Room – Hospital	A portion of a hospital where emergency diagnosis and treatment of illness or injury is provided.
24	Ambulatory Surgical Center	A freestanding facility, other than a physician's office, where surgical and diagnostic services are provided on an ambulatory basis.
25	Birthing Center	A facility, other than a hospital's maternity facilities or a physician's office, which provides a setting for labor, delivery, and immediate post-partum care as well as immediate care of new born infants.
26	Military Treatment Facility	A medical facility operated by one or more of the Uniformed Services. Military Treatment Facility (MTF) also refers to certain former U.S. Public Health Service (USPHS) facilities now designated as Uniformed Service Treatment Facilities (USTF).
27-30	Unassigned	N/A
31	Skilled Nursing Facility	A facility which primarily provides inpatient skilled nursing care and related services to patients who require medical, nursing, or rehabilitative services but does not provide the level of care or treatment available in a hospital.
32	Nursing Facility	A facility which primarily provides to residents skilled nursing care and related services for the rehabilitation of injured, disabled, or sick persons, or, on a regular basis, health-related care services above the level of custodial care to other than mentally retarded individuals.
33	Custodial Care Facility	A facility which provides room, board and other personal assistance services, generally on a long-term basis, and which does not include a medical component.
34	Hospice	A facility, other than a patient's home, in which palliative and supportive care for terminally ill patients and their families are provided.
35-40	Unassigned	N/A
41	Ambulance - Land	A land vehicle specifically designed, equipped and staffed for lifesaving and transporting the sick or injured.
42	Ambulance – Air or Water	An air or water vehicle specifically designed, equipped and staffed for lifesaving and transporting the sick or injured.
43-48	Unassigned	N/A
49	Independent Clinic	A location, not part of a hospital and not described by any other Place of Service code, that is organized and operated to provide preventive, diagnostic, therapeutic, rehabilitative, or palliative services to outpatients only. (effective 10/1/03)
50	Federally Qualified Health Center	A facility located in a medically underserved area that provides Medicare beneficiaries preventive primary medical care under the general direction of a physician.
51	Inpatient Psychiatric Facility	A facility that provides inpatient psychiatric services for the diagnosis and treatment of mental illness on a 24-hour basis, by or under the supervision of a physician.

Code	Place Name	Place Description
52	Psychiatric Facility-Partial Hospitalization	A facility for the diagnosis and treatment of mental illness that provides a planned therapeutic program for patients who do not require full time hospitalization, but who need broader programs than are possible from outpatient visits to a hospital-based or hospital-affiliated facility.
53	Community Mental Health Center	A facility that provides the following services: outpatient services, including specialized outpatient services for children, the elderly, individuals who are chronically ill, and residents of the CMHC's community mental health area who have been discharged from inpatient treatment at a mental health facility; 24-hour a day emergency care services; day treatment, other partial hospitalization services, or psychosocial rehabilitation services; screening for patients being considered for admission to State mental health facilities to determine the appropriateness of such admission; and consultation and education services.
54	Intermediate Care Facility/Individuals with Intellectual Disabilities	A facility which primarily provides health-related care and services above the level of custodial care to individuals with intellectual disabilities but does not provide the level of care or treatment available in a hospital or SNF.
55	Residential Substance Abuse Treatment Facility	A facility which provides treatment for substance (alcohol and drug) abuse to live-in residents who do not require acute medical care. Services include individual and group therapy and counseling, family counseling, laboratory tests, drugs and supplies, psychological testing, and room and board.
56	Psychiatric Resident Treatment Center	A facility or distinct part of a facility for psychiatric care which provides a total 24-hour therapeutically planned and professionally staffed group living and learning environment.
57	Non-residential Substance Abuse Treatment Facility	A location which provides treatment for substance (alcohol and drug) abuse on an ambulatory basis. Services include individual and group therapy and counseling, family counseling, laboratory tests, drugs and supplies, and psychological testing. (Effective 10/1/03)
58	Non-residential Opioid Treatment Facility	A location tht provides treatment for opioid use disorder on an ambulatory basis. Services include methadone and other forms of Medication Assisted Treatment (MAT). (Effective January 1, 2020)
59	Unassigned	N/A
60	Mass Immunization Center	A location where providers administer pneumococcal pneumonia and influenza virus vaccinations and submit these services as electronic media claims, paper claims, or using the roster billing method. This generally takes place in a mass immunization setting, such as, a public health center, pharmacy, or mall but may include a physician office setting.
61	Comprehensive Inpatient Rehabilitation Facility	A facility that provides comprehensive rehabilitation services under the supervision of a physician to inpatients with physical disabilities. Services include physical therapy, occupational therapy, speech pathology, social or psychological services, and orthotics and prosthetics services.
62	Comprehensive Outpatient Rehabilitation Facility	A facility that provides comprehensive rehabilitation services under the supervision of a physician to outpatients with physical disabilities. Services include physical therapy, occupational therapy, and speech pathology services.
63-64	Unassigned	N/A
65	ESRD Treatment Facility	A facility other than a hospital, which provides dialysis treatment, maintenance, and/or training to patients or caregivers on an ambulatory or home-care basis.
66-70	Unassigned	N/A

Code	Place Name	Place Description
71	Public Health Clinic	A facility maintained by either State or local health departments that provide ambulatory primary medical care under the general direction of a physician.
72	Rural Health Clinic	A certified facility which is located in a rural medically underserved area that provides ambulatory primary medical care under the general direction of a physician.
73-80	Unassigned	N/A
81	Independent Laboratory	A laboratory certified to perform diagnostic and/or clinical tests independent of an institution or a physician's office.
82-98	Unassigned	N/A
99	Other Place/Service	Other place of service not identified above.

HOSPITAL CARE

Hospital services frequently cause reimbursement problems for health care professionals. The three most common coding errors are:

- *More than one physician submits an initial hospital care code for the same patient.*

- *Follow-up hospital visits are coded incorrectly.*

- *Concurrent care visits by multiple specialists are coded improperly.*

If more than one physician is involved in the process of hospitalizing a patient, for example, surgeon and internist, the physicians must decide which is going to actually admit the patient and report the admission services on the health insurance claim form. If both do, the first health insurance claim form to arrive will be processed and paid, and the second will be rejected.

There are valid reasons for visiting a patient more than once daily while hospitalized, however, many physicians and even some insurance billers do not know that subsequent hospital visit codes are for "daily" services. When a physician visits the patient twice in one day, providing a brief level of service each time, the physician or insurance biller may incorrectly report two hospital visit services for the same day, instead of a higher level code incorporating both visits.

Reporting multiple hospital visits provided on the same day separately on the health insurance claim form usually results in either the entire claim being returned for clarification, or the second visit being denied as an apparent duplication. Unfortunately, insurance billers who are unclear on the proper coding of same day hospital visits may simply accept the rejection without question and write-off the unpaid visit as uncollectible.

The CPT coding system clearly defines subsequent hospital care as "per day", meaning daily services. If the physician visits the patient twice in one day, providing the equivalent of "brief" services each time, report the service using the appropriate evaluation and management code that defines the cumulative level of service provided.

HOSPITAL DISCHARGE

The CPT codes for hospital discharge services are evaluation and management code 99238 and 99239, defined as Hospital Discharge Day Management. Hospital discharge services include final examination of the patient, discussion of the hospital stay, instructions for continuing care, and preparation of discharge records. Many health insurance companies do not recognize and/or do not reimburse this CPT code.

Options for the use of these codes include the use of one of the other hospital daily services codes from the evaluation and management series 99231-99233 and perhaps using a code that has a higher value than the routine hospital visit.

REFERRAL

A referral is the transfer of the total care or specific portion of care of a patient from one physician to another. A referral is not a request for consultation. If a patient is referred to the physician for total care or a portion of their care, use evaluation and management visit codes, and other CPT codes if appropriate, to report the services provided. If a patient is sent to the physician for a consultation, use evaluation and management consultation codes to report the services provided.

SEPARATE OR MULTIPLE PROCEDURES

It is appropriate to designate multiple procedures that are rendered on the same date by separate entries. For example: if a proctosigmoidoscopy was performed in addition to a hospital visit, the proctosigmoidoscopy would be considered a SEPARATE procedure and listed in addition to the hospital visit on the health insurance claim form. Another example would be individual medical psychotherapy rendered in addition to a brief subsequent hospital service. In this instance, both services would be coded.

SUPPLIES AND MATERIALS SUPPLIED BY THE PHYSICIAN

The CPT coding system includes specific codes for identifying certain supplies and materials provided by the physician. These supply codes are used to report supplies and materials that are not included in the definition of the basic service.

CPT CODES FOR SUPPLIES AND MATERIALS

92310-92371   Supply of spectacles, contact lenses, low vision aids and ocular prosthesis.

95120-95170   Provision of antigens for allergen immunotherapy.

99070   Supplies and materials (except spectacles) provided by the physician.

99071   Educational supplies, such as books, tapes, and pamphlets, provided by the physician for the patient's education at cost to physician.

PURCHASED DIAGNOSTIC SERVICES

It is common for physicians to bill patients and health insurance companies for diagnostic services that were procured or ordered on behalf of the patient but not actually provided by the ordering physician. It is also common for the ordering physician to "mark-up" the fee for the purchased service prior to billing. This is referred to as <u>global</u> <u>billing</u>.

Medical equipment companies, particularly those offering electrocardiography, pulmonary diagnostic equipment, and other diagnostic equipment, have used this global billing concept in the past as a method of selling physicians a new "profit center" for their practice. Some even provided technicians, who were not employees of the practice, to perform the diagnostic tests in the physicians office. OBRA 1987 placed severe restrictions on global billing of certain diagnostic tests as of March 1, 1988.

The Medicare regulations apply to diagnostic tests other than clinical laboratory tests including, but not limited to: EKGs, EEGs, cardiac monitoring, X-rays and ultrasound. Global billing is allowed only when the billing physician personally performs or supervises the diagnostic procedure. To qualify under the supervision definition, the person performing the test must be an employee or the physician or group. Ownership interest in an outside supplier does not meet the supervision requirement.

Billing for purchased services under the new requirement is complicated. The provider must provide the supplier's name, address, provider number and net charge on the health insurance claim form. In addition, a HCPCS Level III modifier must be coded to indicate that the service was purchased. Billing for global services usually will also require a HCPCS Level III modifier to indicate that the service was not purchased. This requirement does not apply to the professional component of these services if provided separately.

Providers should discontinue billing for the technical component of diagnostic services that were not provided or supervised by the provider as defined in this regulation for the following reasons:

1. *The provider is no longer making any profit on these procedures;*

2. *Operating costs are higher due to the increased reporting requirements; and*

3. *Risk of audit liability is increased if these services are not coded properly.*

UNBUNDLING

Unbundling is defined as reporting multiple CPT codes when one CPT code is sufficient. For example, it is considered unbundling if incidental surgical procedures are coded separately, or office visits for uncomplicated follow-up care are separately coded. This practice often happens unintentionally. However, most third-party payers currently have software in place to catch unbundling when it occurs. When physicians continually break out or itemize services in this manner, they often find themselves under close scrutiny and even the focus of an audit by the insurance company. It is most important to know the guidelines to prevent unbundling when coding and billing for services and/or procedures.

MODERATE (CONSCIOUS) SEDATION

Moderate (also known as conscious) sedation is a drug-induced depression of consciousness during which patients respond purposefully to verbal commands, either alone or with light tactile stimulation. No interventions are required to maintain cardiovascular function or a patent airway, and spontaneous ventilation is adequate. For purposes of reporting, intraservice time of moderate sedation is used to select the appropriate moderate sedation codes 99151, 99152, 99153, 99155, 99156, and/or 99157. Moderate sedation is administered in hospitals, outpatient facilities, for example ambulatory surgery centers, and doctors offices to facilitate procedures such as the following:

- *Breast biopsy*
- *Vasectomy*
- *Minor foot surgery*
- *Minor bone fracture repair*
- *Plastic/reconstructive surgery*
- *Dental prosthetic/reconstructive surgery*
- *Endoscopy*

Procedures That Include Moderate (Conscious) Sedation

The summary of CPT codes that include moderate (conscious) sedation has been removed from CPT. The codes that were previously included here have been revised with the removal of the moderate (conscious) sedation symbol. For information/guidance on reporting moderate (conscious) sedation services with codes formerly listed here, please refer to the guidelines for codes 99151, 99152, 99153, 99155, 99156, 99157.

This page intentionally left blank

2021 ADDITIONS, DELETIONS & REVISIONS

Following is a complete list of all additions, deletions and revisions to the CPT coding system. Indicators to the left of each code define the status of the CPT code as follows:

●   Indicates CPT codes that are new to CPT 2021.

▲   Indicates CPT codes that have been revised in CPT 2021.

( )   Indicates CPT codes that have been deleted from CPT 2021.

Evaluation and Management

(99201)   deleted 2020 [2021 edition])

▲ 99202   Office or other outpatient visit for the evaluation and management of a new patient, which requires a medically appropriate history and/or examination and straightforward medical decision making. When using time for code selection, 15-29 minutes of total time is spent on the date of the encounter

▲ 99203   Office or other outpatient visit for the evaluation and management of a new patient, which requires a medically appropriate history and/or examination and low level of medical decision making. When using time for code selection, 30-44 minutes of total time is spent on the date of the encounter.

▲ 99204   Office or other outpatient visit for the evaluation and management of a new patient, which requires a medically appropriate history and/or examination and moderate level of medical decision making. When using time for code selection, 45-59 minutes of total time is spent on the date of the encounter.

▲ 99205   Office or other outpatient visit for the evaluation and management of a new patient, which requires a medically appropriate history and/or examination and high level of medical decision making. When using time for code selection, 60-74 minutes of total time is spent on the date of the encounter.

▲ 99211   Office or other outpatient visit for the evaluation and management of an established patient, that may not require the presence of a physician or other qualified health care professional. Usually, the presenting problem(s) are minimal.

▲ 99212   Office or other outpatient visit for the evaluation and management of an established patient, which requires a medically appropriate history and/or examination and straightforward medical decision making. When using time for code selection, 10-19 minutes of total time is spent on the date of the encounter.

▲ 99213   Office or other outpatient visit for the evaluation and management of an established patient, which requires a medically appropriate history and/or examination and low level of medical decision making. When using time for code selection, 20-29 minutes of total time is spent on the date of the encounter.

▲ 99214   Office or other outpatient visit for the evaluation and management of an established patient, which requires a medically appropriate history and/or examination and moderate level of medical decision making. When using time for code selection, 30-39 minutes of total time is spent on the date of the encounter.

▲ 99215   Office or other outpatient visit for the evaluation and management of an established patient, which requires a medically appropriate history and/or examination and high level of medical decision making. When using time for code selection, 40-54 minutes of total time is spent on the date of the encounter.

▲ +99354   Prolonged service(s) in the outpatient setting requiring direct patient contact beyond the time of the usual service; first hour (List separately in addition to code for outpatient Evaluation and Management or psychotherapy service, except with office or other outpatient services [99202, 99203, 99204, 99205, 99212, 99213, 99214, 99215])

▲ +99355   each additional 30 minutes (List separately in addition to code for prolonged service)

▲ +99356   Prolonged service in the inpatient or observation setting, requiring unit/floor time beyond the usual service; first hour (List separately in addition to code for inpatient or observation Evaluation and Management service)

▲ +99415   Prolonged clinical staff service (the service beyond the highest time in the range of total time of the service) during an evaluation and management service in the office or outpatient setting, direct patient contact with physician supervision; first hour (List separately in addition to code for outpatient Evaluation and Management service)

▲ +99416   each additional 30 minutes (List separately in addition to code for prolonged service)

● +99417   Prolonged office or other outpatient evaluation and management service(s) beyond the minimum required time of the primary procedure which has been selected using total time, requiring total time with or without direct patient contact beyond the usual service, on the date of the primary service, each 15 minutes of total time (List separately in addition to codes 99205, 99215 for office or other outpatient Evaluation and Management services)

▲ 99490   Chronic care management service with the following required elements:

       multiple (two or more) chronic conditions expected to last at least 12 months, or until the death of the patient;,

       chronic conditions place the patient at significant risk of death, acute exacerbation/decompensation, or functional decline;

comprehensive care plan established, implemented, revised, or monitored.;

first 20 minutes of clinical staff time directed by a physician or other qualified health care professional, per calendar month.

● +99439   each additional 20 minutes of clinical staff time directed by a physician or other qualified health care professional, per calendar month (List separately in addition to code for primary procedure)

▲ 99487   Complex chronic care management services, with the following required elements: .

multiple (two or more) chronic conditions expected to last at least 12 months, or until the death of the patient,

chronic conditions place the patient at significant risk of death, acute exacerbation/decompensation, or functional decline,

comprehensive care plan established, implemented, revised, or monitored,

moderate or high complexity medical decision making;

first 60 minutes of clinical staff time directed by a physician or other qualified health care professional, per calendar month.

▲ +99489   each additional 30 minutes of clinical staff time directed by a physician or other qualified health care professional, per calendar month (List separately in addition to code for primary procedure)

Surgery

▲ 11970   Replacement of tissue expander with permanent implant

▲ 11971   Removal of tissue expander(s) without insertion of implant 30468

▲ 19318   Breast Rreduction

  (19324)   deleted 2020 [2021 edition])

▲ 19325   Breast augmentation with implant

▲ 19328   Removal of intact breast implant

▲ 19330   Removal of ruptured breast implant, including implant contents (eg, saline, silicone gel)

▲ 19340   Insertion of breast implant on same day of mastectomy (ie, immediate)

▲ 19342   Insertion or replacement of breast implant on separate day from mastectomy

▲ 19357   Tissue expander placement in breast reconstruction, including subsequent expansion(s)

▲ 19361   Breast reconstruction; with latissimus dorsi flap

▲ 19364   with free flap (eg, fTRAM, DIEP, SIEA, GAP flap)

  (19366   deleted 2020 [2021 edition])

▲ 19367   with single-pedicled transverse rectus abdominis myocutaneous (TRAM) flap

▲ 19368   with single-pedicled transverse rectus abdominis myocutaneous (TRAM) flap, requiring separate microvascular anastomosis (supercharging)

▲ 19369   with bipedicled transverse rectus abdominis myocutaneous (TRAM) flap

▲ 19370   Revision of peri-implant capsule, breast, including capsulotomy, capsulorrhaphy, and/or partial capsulectomy

▲ 19371   Peri-implant capsulectomy, breast, complete, including removal of all intracapsular contents

▲ 19380   Revision of reconstructed breast (eg, significant removal of tissue, re-advancement and/or re-inset of flaps in autologous reconstruction or significant capsular revision combined with soft tissue excision in implant-based reconstruction)

▲ 29822   debridement, limited, 1 or 2 discrete structures (eg, humeral bone, humeral articular cartilage, glenoid bone, glenoid articular cartilage, biceps tendon, biceps anchor complex, labrum, articular capsule, articular side of the rotator cuff, bursal side of the rotator cuff, subacromial bursa, foreign body[ies])

▲ 29823   debridement, extensive, 3 or more discrete structures (eg, humeral bone, humeral articular cartilage, glenoid bone, glenoid articular cartilage, biceps tendon, biceps anchor complex, labrum, articular capsule, articular side of the rotator cuff, bursal side of the rotator cuff, subacromial bursa, foreign body[ies])

● 30468   Repair of nasal valve collapse with subcutaneous/submucosal lateral wall implant(s)

  (32405)   deleted 2020 [2021 edition])

● 32408   Core needle biopsy, lung or mediastinum, percutaneous, including imaging guidance, when performed

● 33741   Transcatheter atrial septostomy (TAS) for congenital cardiac anomalies to create effective atrial flow, including all imaging guidance by the proceduralist, when performed, any method (eg, Rashkind, Sang-Park, balloon, cutting balloon, blade)

● 33745   Transcatheter intracardiac shunt (TIS) creation by stent placement for congenital cardiac anomalies to establish effective intracardiac flow, including all imaging guidance by the proceduralist, when performed, left and right heart diagnostic cardiac catheterization for congenital cardiac anomalies, and target zone angioplasty, when performed (eg, atrial septum, Fontan fenestration, right ventricular outflow tract, Mustard/Senning/Warden baffles); initial intracardiac shunt

● +33746   each additional intracardiac shunt

● 33995   Insertion of ventricular assist device, percutaneous, including radiological supervision and interpretation; right heart, venous access only

▲ 33990   left heart, arterial access only

▲ 33991   left heart, both arterial and venous access, with transseptal puncture

▲ 33992   Removal of percutaneous left heart ventricular assist device, arterial or arterial and venous cannula(s), at separate and distinct session from insertion

● 33997   Removal of percutaneous right heart ventricular assist device, venous cannula, at separate and distinct session from insertion

▲ 33993   Repositioning of percutaneous right or left heart ventricular assist device with imaging guidance at separate and distinct session from insertion

  (49220)   code deleted 20020 [2021 edition])

● 55880   Ablation of malignant prostate tissue, transrectal, with high intensity-focued ultrasound (HIFU), including ultrasound guidance

  (57112)   code deleted 2020 [2021 edition])

● + 57465   Computer-aided mapping of cervix uteri during colposcopy, including optical dynamic spectral imaging and algorithmic quantification of the acetowhitening effect (List separately in addition to code for primary procedure)

  (58293)   code deleted 2020 [2021 edition])

  (61870)   code deleted 2020 [2021 edition])

  (62163)   code deleted 2020 [2021 edition])

  (63180)   code deleted 2020 [2021 edition])

  (63182)   code deleted 2020 [2021 edition])

▲ 64455   plantar common digital nerve(s) (eg, Morton's neuroma)

▲ 64479   transforaminal epidural, with imaging guidance (fluoroscopy or CT), cervical or thoracic, single level

▲ +64480   transforaminal epidural, with imaging guidance (fluoroscopy or CT), cervical or thoracic, each additional level (List separately in addition to code for primary procedure)

▲ 64483   transforaminal epidural, with imaging guidance (fluoroscopy or CT), lumbar or sacral, single level

▲ +64484   transforaminal epidural, with imaging guidance (fluoroscopy or CT), lumbar or sacral, each additional level (List separately in addition to code for primary procedure)

  (69605)   code deleted 2020 [2021 edition])

● 69705   Nasopharyngoscopy, surgical, with dilation of eustachian tube (ie, balloon dilation); unilateral

● 69706   Nasopharyngoscopy, surgical, with dilation of eustachian tube (ie, balloon dilation); bilateral

Radiology

▲ 71250   Computed tomography, thorax, diagnostic; without contrast material

▲ 71260   with contrast material(s)

▲ 71270   without contrast material, followed by contrast material(s) and further sections

● 71271   Computed tomography, thorax, low dose for lung cancer screening, without contrast material(s)

▲ 74425   Urography, antegrade, radiological supervision and interpretation

● 76145   Medical physics dose evaluation for radiation exposure that exceeds institutional review threshold, including report

▲ 76513   anterior segment ultrasound, immersion (water bath) B-scan or high resolution biomicroscopy, unilateral or bilatera

  (76970)   code deleted 2020 [2021 edition])

▲ 78130   Red cell survival study;

  (78135)   code deleted 2020 [2021 edition])

Pathology and Laboratory

● 80143   Acetaminophen

● 80151   Amiodarone

● 80161   Carbamazepine, -10, 11-epoxide

● 80167   Felbamate

● 80181   Flecainide

● 80189   Itraconazone

● 80193   Leflunomide

● 80204   Methotrexate

● 80210   Rufinamide

● 80179   Salicylate

▲ 80415   estradiol response

    This panel must include the following:

    Estradiol, total (82670 x 2 on 3 pooled blood samples)

● 81168   *CCND1/IGH (t(11;14))* (eg, mantle cell lymphoma) translocation analysis, major breakpoint, qualitative and quantitative, if performed

● 81278   *IGH@/BCL2 (t(14;18))* (eg, follicular lymphoma) translocation analysis, major breakpoint region (MBR) and minor cluster region (mcr) breakpoints, qualitative or quantitative

● 81279   *JAK2 (Janus kinase 2)* (eg, myeloproliferative disorder) targeted sequence analysis (eg, exons 12 and 13)

● 81338   *MPL (MPL proto-oncogene, thrombopoietin receptor)* (eg, myeloproliferative disorder) gene analysis; common variants (eg, W515A, W515K, W515L, W515R)

● 81339   sequence analysis, exon 10

● 81191   *NTRK1 (neurotrophic receptor tyrosine kinase 1)* (eg, solid tumors) translocation analysis

● 81192   *NTRK2 (neurotrophic receptor tyrosine kinase 2)* (eg, solid tumors) translocation analysis

● 81193   *NTRK3 (neurotrophic receptor tyrosine kinase 3)* (eg, solid tumors) translocation analysis

● 81194   *NTRK (neurotrophic-tropomyosin receptor tyrosine kinase 1, 2, and 3)* (eg, solid tumors) translocation analysis

● 81347   *SF3B1 (splicing factor [3b] subunit B1)* (eg, myelodysplastic syndrome/acute myeloid leukemia) gene analysis, common variants (eg, A672T, E622D, L833F, R625C, R625L)

● 81348   *SRSF2 (serine and arginine-rich splicing factor 2)* (eg, myelodysplastic syndrome, acute myeloid leukemia) gene analysis, common variants (eg, P95H, P95L)

● 81351   *TP53 (tumor protein 53)* (eg, Li-Fraumeni syndrome) gene analysis; full gene sequence

● 81352   *TP53 (tumor protein 53)* (eg, Li-Fraumeni syndrome) gene analysis; targeted sequence analysis (eg, 4 oncology)

● 81353   *TP53 (tumor protein 53)* (eg, Li-Fraumeni syndrome) gene analysis; known familial variant

● 81357   *U2AF1 (U2 small nuclear RNA auxiliary factor 1)* (eg, myelodysplastic syndrome, acute myeloid leukemia) gene analysis, common variants (eg, S34F, S34Y, Q157R, Q157P)

● 81360   *ZRSR2 (zinc finger CCCH-type, RNA binding motif and serine/arginine-rich 2)* (eg, myelodysplastic syndrome, acute myeloid leukemia) gene analysis, common variant(s) (eg, E65fs, E122fs, R448fs)

▲ 81401   Molecular pathology procedure, Level 2 (eg, 2-10 SNPs, 1 methylated variant, or 1 somatic variant [typically using nonsequencing target variant analysis], or detection of a dynamic mutation disorder/triplet repeat)

▲ 81402   Molecular pathology procedure, Level 3 (eg, >10 SNPs, 2-10 methylated variants, or 2-10 somatic variants [typically using non-sequencing target variant analysis], immunoglobulin and T-cell receptor gene rearrangements, duplication/deletion variants of 1 exon, loss of heterozygosity [LOH], uniparental disomy [UPD])

▲ 81403   Molecular pathology procedure, Level 4 (eg, analysis of single exon by DNA sequence analysis, analysis of >10 amplicons using multiplex PCR in 2 or more independent reactions, mutation scanning or duplication/deletion variants of 2-5 exons)

▲ 81404   Molecular pathology procedure, Level 5 (eg, analysis of 2-5 exons by DNA sequence analysis, mutation scanning or duplication/ deletion variants of 6-10 exons, or characterization of a dynamic mutation disorder/triplet repeat by Southern blot analysis)

▲ 81405   Molecular pathology procedure, Level 6 (eg, analysis of 6-10 exons by DNA sequence analysis, mutation scanning or duplication/deletion variants of 11-25 exons, regionally targeted cytogenomic array analysis)

● 81419   Epilepsy genomic sequence analysis panel, must include analyses for *ALDH7A1, CACNA1A, CDKL5, CHD2, GABRG2, GRIN2A, KCNQ2, MECP2, PCDH19, POLG, PRRT2, SCN1A, SCN1B, SCN2A, SCN8A, SLC2A1, SLC9A6, STXBP1, SYNGAP1, TCF4, TPP1, TSC1, TSC2,* and *ZEB2*

● 81513   Infectious disease, bacterial vaginosis, quantitative realtime amplification of RNA markers for Atopobium vaginae, Gardnerella vaginalis, and Lactobacillus species, utilizing vaginal-fluid specimens, algorithm reported as a positive or negative result for bacterial vaginosis

● 81514   Infectious disease, bacterial vaginosis and vaginitis, quantitative real-time amplification of DNA markers for Gardnerella vaginalis, Atopobium vaginae, Megasphaera type 1, Bacterial Vaginosis Associated Bacteria-2 (BVAB- 2), and Lactobacillus species (L. crispatus and L. jensenii), utilizing vaginal-fluid specimens, algorithm reported as a positive or negative for high likelihood of bacterial vaginosis, includes separate detection of Trichomonas vaginalis and/or Candida species (C. albicans, C. tropicalis, C. parapsilosis, C. dubliniensis), Candida glabrata, Candida krusei, when reported

● 81529   Oncology (cutaneous melanoma), mRNA, gene expression profiling by real-time RT-PCR of 31 genes (28 content and 3 housekeeping), utilizing formalin-fixed paraffinembedded tissue, algorithm reported as recurrence risk, including likelihood of sentinel lymph node metastasis

(81545   code deleted 2020 [2021 edition])

● 81546   Oncology (thyroid), mRNA, gene expression analysis of 10,196 genes, utilizing fine needle aspirate, algorithm reported as a categorical result (eg, benign or suspicious)

● 81554   Pulmonary disease (idiopathic pulmonary fibrosis [IPF]), mRNA, gene expression analysis of 190 genes, utilizing transbronchial biopsies, diagnostic algorithm reported as categorical result (eg, positive or negative for high probability of usual interstitial pneumonia [UIP])

▲ 82075   Alcohol (ethanol); breath

● 82077   Alcohol (ethanol); any specimen except urine and breath, immunoassay (eg, IA, EIA, ELISA, RIA, EMIT, FPIA) and enzymatic methods (eg, alcohol dehydrogenase)

▲ 82670   Estradiol; total

● 82681   Estradiol; free, direct measurement (eg, equilibrium dialysis)

▲ 86318   Immunoassay for infectious agent antibody(ies), qualitative or semiquantitative, single-step method (eg, reagent strip);

● 86328   Immunoassay for infectious agent antibody(ies), qualitative or semiquantitative, single-step method (eg, reagent strip); severe acute respiratory syndrome coronavirus 2 (SARS-CoV-2) (Coronavirus disease [COVID-19])

● 86769   severe acute respiratory syndrome coronavirus 2 (SARS-CoV-2) (Coronavirus disease [COVID-19])

● 87635   Infectious agent detection by nucleic acid (DNA or RNA); severe acute respiratory syndrome coronavirus 2 (SARS-CoV-2) (Coronavirus disease [COVID-19]), amplified probe technique

● 87636   Infectious agent detection by nucleic acid (DNA or RNA); severe acute respiratory syndrome coronavirus 2 (SARS-CoV-2) (Coronavirus disease [COVID-19]) and influenza virus types A and B, multiplex amplified probe technique

● 87637   Infectious agent detection by nucleic acid (DNA or RNA); severe acute respiratory syndrome coronavirus 2 (SARS-CoV-2) (Coronavirus disease [COVID-19]), influenza virus types A and B, and respiratory syncytial virus, multiplex, amplified probe technique

● 87811   severe acute respiratory syndrome coronavirus 2 (SARS-CoV-2) (Coronavirus disease [COVID-19])

(0006U   code deleted 2020 [2021 edition])

(0085U   code deleted 2020 [2021 edition])

(0124U   code deleted 2020 [2021 edition])

(0125U   code deleted 2020 [2021 edition])

(0126U   code deleted 2020 [2021 edition])

(0127U   code deleted 2020 [2021 edition])

(0128U   code deleted 2020 [2021 edition])

● 0139U   Neurology (autism spectrum disorder [ASD]), quantitative measurements of 6 central carbon metabolites (ie, a-ketoglutarate, alanine, lactate, phenylalanine, pyruvate, and succinate), LC-MS/MS, plasma, algorithmic analysis with result reported as negative or positive (with metabolic subtypes of ASD)

● 0140U   Infectious disease (fungi), fungal pathogen identification, DNA (15 fungal targets), blood culture, amplified probe technique, each target reported as detected or not detected

● 0141U   Infectious disease (bacteria and fungi), gram-positive organism identification and drug resistance element detection, DNA (20 gram-positive bacterial targets, 4 resistance genes, 1 pan gram-negative bacterial target, 1 pan Candida target), blood culture, amplified probe technique, each target reported as detected or not detected

● 0142U   Infectious disease (bacteria and fungi), gram-negative bacterial identification and drug resistance element detection, DNA (21 gram-negative bacterial targets, 6 resistance genes, 1 pan gram-positive bacterial target, 1 pan Candida target), amplified probe technique, each target reported as detected or not detected

● 0143U   Drug assay, definitive, 120 or more drugs or metabolites, urine, quantitative liquid chromatography with tandem mass spectrometry (LC-MS/MS) using multiple reaction monitoring (MRM), with drug or metabolite description, comments including sample validation, per date of service (duplicate PLA test)

● 0144U   Drug assay, definitive, 160 or more drugs or metabolites, urine, quantitative liquid chromatography with tandem mass spectrometry (LC-MS/MS) using multiple reaction monitoring (MRM), with drug or metabolite description, comments including sample validation, per date of service

● 0145U   Drug assay, definitive, 65 or more drugs or metabolites, urine, quantitative liquid chromatography with tandem mass spectrometry (LC-MS/MS) using multiple reaction monitoring (MRM), with drug or metabolite description, comments including sample validation, per date of service

● 0146U   Drug assay, definitive, 80 or more drugs or metabolites, urine, by quantitative liquid chromatography with tandem mass spectrometry (LC-MS/MS) using multiple reaction monitoring (MRM), with drug or metabolite description, comments including sample validation, per date of service

● 0147U   Drug assay, definitive, 85 or more drugs or metabolites, urine, quantitative liquid chromatography with tandem mass spectrometry (LC-MS/MS) using multiple reaction monitoring (MRM), with drug or metabolite description, comments including sample validation, per date of service

- 0148U Drug assay, definitive, 100 or more drugs or metabolites, urine, quantitative liquid chromatography with tandem mass spectrometry (LC-MS/MS) using multiple reaction monitoring (MRM), with drug or metabolite description, comments including sample validation, per date of service

- 0149U Drug assay, definitive, 60 or more drugs or metabolites, urine, quantitative liquid chromatography with tandem mass spectrometry (LC-MS/MS) using multiple reaction monitoring (MRM), with drug or metabolite description, comments including sample validation, per date of service

- 0150U Drug assay, definitive, 120 or more drugs or metabolites, urine, quantitative liquid chromatography with tandem mass spectrometry (LC-MS/MS) using multiple reaction monitoring (MRM), with drug or metabolite description, comments including sample validation, per date of service (duplicative PLA Test)

- 0151U Infectious disease (bacterial or viral respiratory tract infection), pathogen specific nucleic acid (DNA or RNA), 33 targets, real-time semi-quantitative PCR, bronchoalveolar lavage, sputum, or endotracheal aspirate, detection of 33 organismal and antibiotic resistance genes with limited semi-quantitative results 3 CPT Changes: An Insider's View 2021

- 0152U Infectious disease (bacteria, fungi, parasites, and DNA viruses), DNA, PCR and next-generation sequencing, plasma, detection of >1,000 potential microbial organisms for significant positive pathogens

- 0153U Oncology (breast), mRNA, gene expression profiling by next-generation sequencing of 101 genes, utilizing formalin-fixed paraffin-embedded tissue, algorithm reported as a triple negative breast cancer clinical subtype(s) with information on immune cell involvement

▲ 0154U Oncology (urothelial cancer), RNA, analysis by real-time RT-PCR of the FGFR3 (fibroblast growth factor receptor 3) gene analysis (ie, p.R248C [c.742C>T], p.S249C [c.746C>G], p.G370C [c.1108G>T], p.Y373C [c.1118A>G], FGFR3-TACC3v1, and FGFR3-TACC3v3), utilizing formalin-fixed paraffin-embedded urothelial cancer tumor tissue, reported as FGFR gene alteration status

▲ 0155U Oncology (breast cancer), DNA, PIK3CA (phosphatidylinositol-4,5- bisphosphate 3-kinase, catalytic subunit alpha) (eg, breast cancer) gene analysis (ie, p.C420R, p.E542K, p.E545A, p.E545D [g.1635G>T only], p.E545G, p.E545K, p.Q546E, p.Q546R, p.H1047L, p.H1047R, p.H1047Y), utilizing formalin-fixed paraffin- embedded breast tumor tissue, reported as PIK3CA gene mutation status

- 0156U Copy number (eg, intellectual disability, dysmorphology), sequence analysis

- +0157U APC (APC regulator of WNT signaling pathway) (eg, familial adenomatosis polyposis [FAP]) mRNA sequence analysis (List separately in addition to code for primary procedure)

- +0158U MLH1 (mutL homolog 1) (eg, hereditary non-polyposis colorectal cancer, Lynch syndrome) mRNA sequence analysis (List separately in addition to code for primary procedure)

- +0159U MSH2 (mutS homolog 2) (eg, hereditary colon cancer, Lynch syndrome) mRNA sequence analysis (List separately in addition to code for primary procedure)

- +0160U MSH6 (mutS homolog 6) (eg, hereditary colon cancer, Lynch syndrome) mRNA sequence analysis (List separately in addition to code for primary procedure)

- +0161U PMS2 (PMS1 homolog 2, mismatch repair system component) (eg, hereditary non-polyposis colorectal cancer, Lynch syndrome) mRNA sequence analysis (List separately in addition to code for primary procedure)

- +0162U Hereditary colon cancer (Lynch syndrome), targeted mRNA sequence analysis panel (MLH1, MSH2, MSH6, PMS2) (List separately in addition to code for primary procedure)

- 0163U Oncology (colorectal) screening, biochemical enzymelinked immunosorbent assay (ELISA) of 3 plasma or serum proteins (teratocarcinoma derived growth factor-1 [TDGF-1, Cripto-1], carcinoembryonic antigen [CEA], extracellular matrix protein [ECM]), with demographic data (age, gender, CRC-screening compliance) using a proprietary algorithm and reported as likelihood of CRC or advanced adenomas

- 0164U Gastroenterology (irritable bowel syndrome [IBS]), immunoassay for anti-CdtB and anti-vinculin antibodies, utilizing plasma, algorithm for elevated or not elevated qualitative results

▲ 0165U Peanut allergen-specifc quantitative assessment of multiple epitopes using enzyme-linked immunosorbent assay (ELISA), blood, individual epitope results and probability of peanut allergy

- 0166U Liver disease, 10 biochemical assays (a2-macroglobulin, haptoglobin, apolipoprotein A1, bilirubin, GGT, ALT, AST, triglycerides, cholesterol, fasting glucose) and biometric and demographic data, utilizing serum, algorithm reported as scores for fibrosis, necroinflammatory activity, and steatosis with a summary interpretation

- 0167U Gonadotropin, chorionic (hCG), immunoassay with direct optical observation, blood

- 0168U Fetal aneuploidy (trisomy 21, 18, and 13) DNA sequence analysis of selected regions using maternal plasma without fetal fraction cutoff, algorithm reported as a risk score for each trisomy

- 0169U NUDT15 (nudix hydrolase 15) and TPMT (thiopurine S-methyltransferase) (eg, drug metabolism) gene analysis, common variants

- 0170U Neurology (autism spectrum disorder [ASD]), RNA, nextgeneration sequencing, saliva, algorithmic analysis, and results reported as predictive probability of ASD diagnosis

- 0171U Targeted genomic sequence analysis panel, acute myeloid leukemia, myelodysplastic syndrome, and myeloproliferative neoplasms, DNA analysis, 23 genes, interrogation for sequence variants, rearrangements and minimal residual disease, reported as presence/absence

- 0172U   Oncology (solid tumor as indicated by the label), somatic mutation analysis of BRCA1 (BRCA1, DNA repair associated), BRCA2 (BRCA2, DNA repair associated) and analysis of homologous recombination deficiency pathways, DNA, formalin-fixed paraffin-embedded tissue, algorithm quantifying tumor genomic instability score

- 0173U   Psychiatry (ie, depression, anxiety), genomic analysis panel, includes variant analysis of 14 genes

- 0174U   Oncology (solid tumor), mass spectrometric 30 protein targets, formalin-fixed paraffin-embedded tissue, prognostic and predictive algorithm reported as likely, unlikely, or uncertain benefit of 39 chemotherapy and targeted therapeutic oncology agents

- 0175U   Psychiatry (eg, depression, anxiety), genomic analysis panel, variant analysis of 15 genes

- 0176U   Cytolethal distending toxin B (CdtB) and vinculin IgG antibodies by immunoassay (ie, ELISA)

- 0177U   Oncology (breast cancer), DNA, PIK3CA (phosphatidylinositol-4,5-bisphosphate 3-kinase catalytic subunit alpha) gene analysis of 11 gene variants utilizing plasma, reported as PIK3CA gene mutation status

- 0178U   Peanut allergen-specific quantitative assessment of multiple epitopes using enzyme-linked immunosorbent assay (ELISA), blood, report of minimum eliciting exposure for a clinical reaction

- 0179U   Oncology (non-small cell lung cancer), cell-free DNA, targeted sequence analysis of 23 genes (single nucleotide variations, insertions and deletions, fusions without prior knowledge of partner/breakpoint, copy number variations), with report of significant mutation(s)

- 0180U   Red cell antigen (ABO blood group) genotyping (ABO), gene analysis Sanger/chain termination/conventional sequencing, ABO (ABO, alpha 1-3-N-acetylgalactosaminyltransferase and alpha 1-3-galactosyltransferase) gene, including subtyping, 7 exons

- 0181U   Red cell antigen (Colton blood group) genotyping (CO), gene analysis, AQP1 (aquaporin 1 [Colton blood group]) exon 1

- 0182U   Red cell antigen (Cromer blood group) genotyping (CROM), gene analysis, CD55 (CD55 molecule [Cromer blood group]) exons 1-10

- 0183U   Red cell antigen (Diego blood group) genotyping (DI), gene analysis, SLC4A1 (solute carrier family 4 member 1 [Diego blood group]) exon 19

- 0184U   Red cell antigen (Dombrock blood group) genotyping (DO), gene analysis, ART4 (ADP-ribosyltransferase 4 [Dombrock blood group]) exon 2

- 0185U   Red cell antigen (H blood group) genotyping (FUT1), gene analysis, FUT1 (fucosyltransferase 1 [H blood group]) exon 4

- 0186U   Red cell antigen (H blood group) genotyping (FUT2), gene analysis, FUT2 (fucosyltransferase 2) exon 2

- 0187U   Red cell antigen (Duffy blood group) genotyping (FY), gene analysis, ACKR1 (atypical chemokine receptor 1 [Duffy blood group]) exons 1-2

- 0188U   Red cell antigen (Gerbich blood group) genotyping (GE), gene analysis, GYPC (glycophorin C [Gerbich blood group]) exons 1-4

- 0189U   Red cell antigen (MNS blood group) genotyping (GYPA), gene analysis, GYPA (glycophorin A [MNS blood group]) introns 1, 5, exon 2

- 0190U   Red cell antigen (MNS blood group) genotyping (GYPB), gene analysis, GYPB (glycophorin B [MNS blood group]) introns 1, 5, pseudoexon 3

- 0191U   Red cell antigen (Indian blood group) genotyping (IN), gene analysis, CD44 (CD44 molecule [Indian blood group]) exons 2, 3, 6

- 0192U   Red cell antigen (Kidd blood group) genotyping (JK), gene analysis, SLC14A1 (solute carrier family 14 member 1 [Kidd blood group]) gene promoter, exon 9

- 0193U   Red cell antigen (JR blood group) genotyping (JR), gene analysis, ABCG2 (ATP binding cassette subfamily G member 2 [Junior blood group]) exons 2-26

- 0194U   Red cell antigen (Kell blood group) genotyping (KEL), gene analysis, KEL (Kell metallo-endopeptidase [Kell blood group]) exon 8

- 0195U   KLF1 (Kruppel-like factor 1), targeted sequencing (ie, exon 13)

- 0196U   Red cell antigen (Lutheran blood group) genotyping (LU), gene analysis, BCAM (basal cell adhesion molecule [Lutheran blood group]) exon 3

- 0197U   Red cell antigen (Landsteiner-Wiener blood group) genotyping (LW), gene analysis, ICAM4 (intercellular adhesion molecule 4 [Landsteiner-Wiener blood group]) exon 1

- 0198U   Red cell antigen (RH blood group) genotyping (RHD and RHCE), gene analysis Sanger/chain termination/ conventional sequencing, RHD (Rh blood group D antigen) exons 1-10 and RHCE (Rh blood group CcEe antigens) exon 5

- 0199U   Red cell antigen (Scianna blood group) genotyping (SC), gene analysis, ERMAP (erythroblast membrane associated protein [Scianna blood group]) exons 4, 12

- 0200U   Red cell antigen (Kx blood group) genotyping (XK), gene analysis, XK (X-linked Kx blood group) exons 1-3

- 0201U   Red cell antigen (Yt blood group) genotyping (YT), gene analysis, ACHE (acetylcholinesterase [Cartwright blood group]) exon 2

- **0202U** Infectious disease (bacterial or viral respiratory tract infection), pathogen-specific nucleic acid (DNA or RNA), 22 targets including severe acute respiratory syndrome coronavirus 2 (SARS-CoV-2), qualitative RT-PCR, nasopharyngeal swab, each pathogen reported as detected or not detected

- **0203U** Autoimmune (inflammatory bowel disease), mRNA, gene expression profiling by quantitative RT-PCR, 17 genes (15 target and 2 reference genes), whole blood, reported as a continuous risk score and classification of inflammatory bowel disease aggressiveness

- **0204U** Oncology (thyroid), mRNA, gene expression analysis of 593 genes (including BRAF, RAS, RET, PAX8, and NTRK) for sequence variants and rearrangements, utilizing fine needle aspirate, reported as detected or not detected

- **0205U** Ophthalmology (age-related macular degeneration), analysis of 3 gene variants (2 CFH gene, 1 ARMS2 gene), using PCR and MALDI-TOF, buccal swab, reported as positive or negative for neovascular age-related maculardegeneration risk associated with zinc supplements

- **0206U** Neurology (Alzheimer disease); cell aggregation using morphometric imaging and protein kinase C-epsilon (PKCe) concentration in response to amylospheroid treatment by ELISA, cultured skin fibroblasts, each reported as positive or negative for Alzheimer disease

- **+0207U** quantitative imaging of phosphorylated ERK1 and ERK2 in response to bradykinin treatment by in situ immunofluorescence, using cultured skin fibroblasts, reported as a probability index for Alzheimer disease (List separately in addition to code for primary procedure)

- **0208U** Oncology (medullary thyroid carcinoma), mRNA, gene expression analysis of 108 genes, utilizing fine needle aspirate, algorithm reported as positive or negative for medullary thyroid carcinoma

- **0209U** Cytogenomic constitutional (genome-wide) analysis, interrogation of genomic regions for copy number, structural changes and areas of homozygosity for chromosomal abnormalities

- **0210U** Syphilis test, non-treponemal antibody, immunoassay, quantitative (RPR)

- **0211U** Oncology (pan-tumor), DNA and RNA by next-generation sequencing, utilizing formalin-fixed paraffin-embedded tissue, interpretative report for single nucleotide variants, copy number alterations, tumor mutational burden, and microsatellite instability, with therapy association

- **0212U** Rare diseases (constitutional/heritable disorders), whole genome and mitochondrial DNA sequence analysis, including small sequence changes, deletions, duplications, short tandem repeat gene expansions, and variants in non-uniquely mappable regions, blood or saliva, identification and categorization of genetic variants, proband

- **0213U** Rare diseases (constitutional/heritable disorders), whole genome and mitochondrial DNA sequence analysis, including small sequence changes, deletions, duplications, short tandem repeat gene expansions, and variants in non-uniquely mappable regions, blood or saliva, identification and categorization of genetic variants, each comparator genome (eg, parent, sibling)

- **0214U** Rare diseases (constitutional/heritable disorders), whole exome and mitochondrial DNA sequence analysis, including small sequence changes, deletions, duplications, short tandem repeat gene expansions, and variants in non-uniquely mappable regions, blood or saliva, identification and categorization of genetic variants, proband

- **0215U** Rare diseases (constitutional/heritable disorders), whole exome and mitochondrial DNA sequence analysis, including small sequence changes, deletions, duplications, short tandem repeat gene expansions, and variants in non-uniquely mappable regions, blood or saliva, identification and categorization of genetic variants, each comparator exome (eg, parent, sibling)

- **0216U** Neurology (inherited ataxias), genomic DNA sequence analysis of 12 common genes including small sequence changes, deletions, duplications, short tandem repeat gene expansions, and variants in non-uniquely mappable regions, blood or saliva, identification and categorization of genetic variants

- **0217U** Neurology (inherited ataxias), genomic DNA sequence analysis of 51 genes including small sequence changes, deletions, duplications, short tandem repeat gene expansions, and variants in non-uniquely mappable regions, blood or saliva, identification and categorization of genetic variants

- **0218U** Neurology (muscular dystrophy), DMD gene sequence analysis, including small sequence changes, deletions, duplications, and variants in non-uniquely mappable regions, blood or saliva, identification and characterization of genetic variants

- **0219U** Infectious agent (human immunodeficiency virus), targeted viral next-generation sequence analysis (ie, protease [PR], reverse transcriptase [RT], integrase [INT]), algorithm reported as prediction of antiviral drug susceptibility

- **0220U** Oncology (breast cancer), image analysis with artificial intelligence assessment of 12 histologic and immunohistochemical features, reported as a recurrence score

- **0221U** Red cell antigen (ABO blood group) genotyping (ABO), gene analysis, next-generation sequencing, ABO (ABO, alpha 1-3-N-acetylgalactosaminyltransferase and alpha 1-3-galactosyltransferase) gene

- **0222U** Red cell antigen (RH blood group) genotyping (RHD and RHCE), gene analysis, next-generation sequencing, RH proximal promoter, exons 1-10, portions of introns 2-3

- **0223U** Infectious disease (bacterial or viral respiratory tract infection), pathogen-specific nucleic acid (DNA or RNA), 22 targets including severe acute respiratory syndrome coronavirus 2 (SARS-CoV-2), qualitative RT-PCR, nasopharyngeal swab, each pathogen reported as detected or not detected

- **0224U** Antibody, severe acute respiratory syndrome coronavirus 2 (SARS-CoV-2) (Coronarvirus disease [COVID-19]), inlcudes titer(s), when performed

● 0225U   Infectious disease (bacterial or viral respiratory tract infection) pathogen-specific DNA and RNA, 21 targets, including severe acute respiratory syndrome coronavirus 2 (SARS-CoV-2), amplified probe technique, including multiple reverse transcription for RNA targets, each analyte reported as detected or not detected

● 0226U   Surrogate viral neutralization test (sVNT), severe acute respiratory syndrome coronavirus 2 (SARS-CoV-2) (Coronavirus disease [COVID-19]), ELISA, plasma, serum

● 0240U   Infectious disease (viral respiratory tract infection), pathogen-specific RNA, 3 targets (severe acute respiratory syndrome coronavirus 2 [SARS-CoV-2], influenza A, influenza B), upper respiratory specimen, each pathogen reported as detected or not detected

● 0241U   Infectious disease (viral respiratory tract infection), pathogen-specific RNA, 4 targets (severe acute respiratory syndrome coronavirus 2 [SARS-CoV-2], influenza A, influenza B, respiratory syncytial virus [RSV]), upper respiratory specimen, each pathogen reported as detected or not detected

Medicine

● 90377   Rabies immune globulin, heat- and solvent/detergenttreated (RIg-HT S/D), human, for intramuscular and/or subcutaneous use

▲ 92227   Imaging of retina for detection or monitoring of disease; with remote clinical staff review and report, unilateral or bilateral

▲ 92228   with remote physician or other qualified health care professional interpretation and report, unilateral or bilateral

● 92229   point-of-care automated analysis and report, unilateral or bilateral

● 92517   Vestibular evoked myogenic potential (VEMP) testing, with interpretation and report; cervical (cVEMP)

● 92518   ocular (oVEMP)

● 92519   cervical (cVEMP) and ocular (oVEMP)

(92585   code deleted 2020 [2021 edition])

(92586   code deleted 2020 [2021 edition])

● 92650   Auditory evoked potentials; screening of auditory potential with broadband stimuli, automated analysis

● 92651   for hearing status determination, broadband stimuli, with interpretation and report

● 92652   for threshold estimation at multiple frequencies, with interpretation and report

● 92653   neurodiagnostic, with interpretation and report

(92992   code deleted 2020 [2021 edition])

(92993   code deleted 2020 [2021 edition])

● 93241   External electrocardiographic recording for more than 48 hours up to 7 days by continuous rhythm recording and storage; includes recording, scanning analysis with report, review and interpretation

● 93242   recording (includes connection and initial recording)

● 93243   scanning analysis with report

● 93244   review and interpretation

● 93245   External electrocardiographic recording for more than 7 days up to 15 days by continuous rhythm recording and storage; includes recording, scanning analysis with report, review and interpretation

● 93246   recording (includes connection and initial recording)

● 93247   scanning analysis with report

● 93248   review and interpretation

(94250   code deleted 2020 [2021 edition])

(94400   code deleted 2020 [2021 edition])

▲ 94617   Exercise test for bronchospasm, including pre- and post-spirometry, and pulse oximetry; with electrocardiographic recording(s)

● 94619   without electrocardiographic recording(s)

(94750   code deleted 2020 [2021 edition])

(94770   code deleted 2020 [2021 edition])

▲ 95070   Inhalation bronchial challenge testing (not including necessary to code for primary procedure) pulmonary function tests);, with histamine, methacholine, or similar compounds

(95071   code deleted 2020 [2021 edition])

Category II Codes

▲ 3170F   Baseline flow cytometry studies performed at time of diagnosis or prior to initiating treatment (HEM)1

Category III Codes

(0058T	code deleted 2020 [2021 edition])	
(0085T	code deleted 2020 [2021 edition])	
(0111T	code deleted 2020 [2021 edition])	
(0126T	code deleted 2020 [2021 edition])	
(0228T	code deleted 2020 [2021 edition])	
(0229T	code deleted 2020 [2021 edition])	
(0230T	code deleted 2020 [2021 edition])	
(0231T	code deleted 2020 [2021 edition])	
(0295T	code deleted 2020 [2021 edition])	
(0296T	code deleted 2020 [2021 edition])	
(0297T	code deleted 2020 [2021 edition])	
(0298T	code deleted 2020 [2021 edition])	
(0381T	code deleted 2020 [2021 edition])	
(0382T	code deleted 2020 [2021 edition])	
(0383T	code deleted 2020 [2021 edition])	
(0384T	code deleted 2020 [2021 edition])	
(0385T	code deleted 2020 [2021 edition])	
0386T	code deleted 2020 [2021 edition])	
(0396T	code deleted 2020 [2021 edition])	
(0400T	code deleted 2020 [2021 edition])	
(0401T	code deleted 2020 [2021 edition])	
(0405T	code deleted 2020 [2021 edition])	

● **0623T** Automated quantification and characterization of coronary atherosclerotic plaque to assess severity of coronary disease, using data from coronary computed tomographic angiography; data preparation and transmission, computerized analysis of data, with review of computerized analysis output to reconcile discordant data, interpretation and report

● **0624T** data preparation and transmission

● **0625T** computerized analysis of data from coronary computed tomographic angiography

● **0626T** Review of computerized analysis output to reconcile discordant data, interpretation and report

● **0620T** Endovascular venous arterialization, tibial or peroneal vein, with transcatheter placement of intravascular stent graft(s) and closure by any method, including percutaneous or open vascular access, ultrasound guidance for vascular access when performed, all catheterization(s) and intraprocedural roadmapping and imaging guidance necessary to complete the intervention, all associated radiological supervision and interpretation, when performed

▲ **0577T** Electrophysiological evaluation of implantable cardioverter- defibrillator system with substernal electrode (includes defibrillation threshold evaluation, induction of arrhythmia, evaluation of sensing for arrhythmia termination, and programming or reprogramming of sensing or therapeutic parameters)

● **0614T** Removal and replacement of substernal implantable defibrillator pulse generator

● **0594T** Osteotomy, humerus, with insertion of an externally controlled intramedullary lengthening device, including intraoperative imaging, initial and subsequent alignment assessments, computations of adjustment schedules, and management of the intramedullary lengthening device

(0595T code deleted 2020 [2021 edition])

● **0596T** Temporary female intraurethral valve-pump (ie, voiding prosthesis); initial insertion, including urethral measurement

● **0597T** replacement

● **0598T** Noncontact real-time fluorescence wound imaging, for bacterial presence, location, and load, per session; first anatomic site (eg, lower extremity)

● +**0599T** each additional anatomic site (eg, upper extremity) (List separately in addition to code for primary procedure)d

● **0600T** Ablation, irreversible electroporation; 1 or more tumors per organ, including imaging guidance, when performed, percutaneous

● **0601T** 1 or more tumors per organ, including fluoroscopic and ultrasound guidance, when performed, open

● **0602T** Glomerular filtration rate (GFR) measurement(s), transdermal, including sensor placement and administration of a single dose of fluorescent pyrazine agent

- 0603T   Glomerular filtration rate (GFR) monitoring, transdermal, including sensor placement and administration of more than one dose of fluorescent pyrazine agent, each 24 hours

- 0604T   Optical coherence tomography (OCT) of retina, remote, patient-initiated image capture and transmission to a remote surveillance center, unilateral or bilateral; initial device provision, set-up and patient education on use of equipment

- 0605T   remote surveillance center technical support, data analyses and reports, with a minimum of 8 daily recordings, each 30 days

- 0606T   review, interpretation and report by the prescribing physician or other qualified health care professional of remote surveillance center data analyses, each 30 days

- 0607T   Remote monitoring of an external continuous pulmonary fluid monitoring system, including measurement of radiofrequency-derived pulmonary fluid levels, heart rate, respiration rate, activity, posture, and cardiovascular rhythm (eg, ECG data), transmitted to a remote 24-hour attended surveillance center; set-up and patient education on use of equipment

- 0608T   analysis of data received and transmission of reports to the physician or other qualified health care professional

- 0609T   Magnetic resonance spectroscopy, determination and localization of discogenic pain (cervical, thoracic, or lumbar); acquisition of single voxel data, per disc, on biomarkers (ie, lactic acid, carbohydrate, alanine, laal, propionic acid, proteoglycan, and collagen) in at least 3 discs

- 0610T   transmission of biomarker data for software analysis

- 0611T   postprocessing for algorithmic analysis of biomarker data for determination of relative chemical differences between discs

- 0612T   interpretation and report

- 0613T   Percutaneous transcatheter implantation of interatrial septal shunt device, including right and left heart catheterization, intracardiac echocardiography, and imaging guidance by the proceduralist, when performed

- 0615T   Eye-movement analysis without spatial calibration, with interpretation and report

- 0616T   Insertion of iris prosthesis, including suture fixation and repair or removal of iris, when performed; without removal of crystalline lens or intraocular lens, without insertion of intraocular lens

- 0617T   with removal of crystalline lens and insertion of intraocular lens

- 0618T   with secondary intraocular lens placement or intraocular lens exchange

- 0619T   Cystourethroscopy with transurethral anterior prostate commissurotomy and drug delivery, including transrectal ultrasound and fluoroscopy, when performed

- 0621T   Trabeculostomy ab interno by laser;

- 0622T   with use of ophthalmic endoscope

- 0627T   Percutaneous injection of allogeneic cellular and/or tissue-based product, intervertebral disc, unilateral or bilateral injection, with fluoroscopic guidance, lumbar; first level

- +0628T   each additional level (List separately in addition to code for primary procedure)

- 0629T   Percutaneous injection of allogeneic cellular and/or tissue-based product, intervertebral disc, unilateral or bilateral injection, with CT guidance, lumbar; first level

- +0630T   each additional level (List separately in addition to code for primary procedure)

- 0631T   Transcutaneous visible light hyperspectral imaging measurement of oxyhemoglobin, deoxyhemoglobin, and tissue oxygenation, with interpretation and report, per extremity

- 0632T   Percutaneous transcatheter ultrasound ablation of nerves innervating the pulmonary arteries, including right heart catheterization, pulmonary artery angiography, and all imaging guidance

- 0633T   Computed tomography, breast, including 3D rendering, when performed, unilateral; without contrast material

- 0634T   with contrast material(s)

- 0635T   without contrast, followed by contrast material(s)

- 0636T   Computed tomography, breast, including 3D rendering, when performed, bilateral; without contrast material(s)

- 0637T   with contrast material(s)

- 0638T   without contrast, followed by contrast material(s)

- 0639T   Wireless skin sensor thermal anisotropy measurement(s) and assessment of flow in cerebrospinal fluid shunt, including ultrasound guidance, when performed

This page intentionally left blank

The CPT® coding system includes two-digit modifier codes which are used to report that a service or procedure has been "altered or modified by some specific circumstance" without altering or modifying the basic definition or CPT code.

The proper use of CPT modifiers can speed up claim processing and increase reimbursement, while the improper use of CPT modifiers may result in claim delays or claim denials. In addition, using certain CPT modifiers, for example -22, too frequently may trigger a claims audit.

CPT MODIFIERS

-22   Increased procedural services

When the work required to provide a service is substantially greater than typically required, it may be identified by adding modifier -22 to the usual procedure code. Documentation must support the substantial additional work and the reason for the additional work (ie, increased intensity, time, technical difficulty of procedure, severity of patient's condition, physical and mental effort required). **Note**: This modifier should not be appended to an E/M service.

-23   Unusual anesthesia

Occasionally, a procedure, which usually requires either no anesthesia or local anesthesia, because of unusual circumstances must be done under general anesthesia. This circumstance may be reported by adding the modifier -23 to the procedure code of the basic service.

-24   Unrelated evaluation and management service by the same physician or other qualified health care professional during a postoperative period

The physician or other qualified health care professional may need to indicate that an evaluation and management service was performed during a postoperative period for a reason(s) unrelated to the original procedure. This circumstance may be reported by adding the modifier -24 to the appropriate level of E/M service.

-25   Significant, separately identifiable evaluation and management service by the same physician or other qualified health care professional on the same day of the procedure or other service

It may be necessary to indicate that on the day a procedure or service identified by a CPT code was performed, the patient's condition required a significant, separately identified E/M service above and beyond the other service provided or beyond the usual preoperative and postoperative care associated with the procedure that was performed. A significant, separately identifiable E/M service is defined or substantiated by documentation that satisfies the relevant criteria for the respective E/M service to be reported (see Evaluation and Management Services Guidelines for instructions on determining level of E/M service). The E/M service may be prompted by the symptom or condition for which the procedure and/or service was provided. As such, different diagnoses are not required for reporting of the E/M service on the same date. This circumstance may be reported by adding modifier -25 to the appropriate level of E/M service. **Note**: This modifier is not used to report an E/M service that resulted in a decision to perform surgery. See modifier -57. For significant, separately identifiable non-E/M services, see modifier -59.

-26   Professional component

Certain procedures are a combination of a physician or other qualified health care professional component and a technical component. When the physician or other qualified health care professional component is reported separately, the service may be identified by adding the modifier -26 to the usual procedure number.

-27   Multiple outpatient hospital evaluation and management encounters on the same date

For hospital outpatient reporting purposes, utilization of hospital resources related to separate and distinct E/M encounters performed in multiple outpatient hospital settings on the same date may be reported by adding modifier -27 to each appropriate level outpatient and/or emergency department E/M code(s). This modifier provides a means of reporting circumstances involving evaluation and management services provided by physician(s) in more than one (multiple) outpatient hospital setting(s) (eg, hospital emergency department, clinic). **Note**: This modifier is not to be used for physician reporting of multiple E/M services performed by the same physician on the same date. For physician reporting of all outpatient evaluation and management services provided by the same physician on the same date and performed in multiple outpatient setting(s) (eg, hospital emergency department, clinic), see Evaluation and Management, Emergency Department, or Preventive Medicine Services codes.

-32   Mandated services

Services related to *mandated* consultation and/or related services (eg, third party payer, governmental, legislative or regulatory requirement) may be identified by adding the modifier -32 to the basic procedure.

-33   Preventive service

When the primary purpose of the service is the delivery of an evidence based service in accordance with a US Preventive Services Task Force A or B rating in effect and other preventive services identified in preventive services mandates (legislative or regulatory), the service may be identified by adding -33 to the procedure. For separately reported services specifically identified as preventive, the modifier should not be used.

-47   Anesthesia by surgeon

Regional or general anesthesia provided by the surgeon may be reported by adding the modifier -47 to the basic service. (This does not include local anesthesia.) **Note**: Modifier -47 would not be used as a modifier for the Anesthesia procedures.

-50   Bilateral procedure

Unless otherwise identified in the listings, bilateral procedures that are performed at the same session, should be identified by adding modifier 50 to the appropriate 5 digit code. Note: This modifier should not be appended to designated "add-on" codes

This modifier is reported when bilateral procedures requiring a separate incision are performed during the SAME operative session. Proper reporting of this modifier on the CMS1500 health insurance claim form requires the CPT procedure code to be listed two times: first with no modifier, and the second time with modifier -50.

This modifier may not be used if the definition of the basic procedure code includes the term "bilateral."

-51   Multiple procedures

When multiple procedures, other than E/M services, Physical Medicine and Rehabilitation services, or provision of supplies (eg, vaccines), are performed at the same session by the same individual, the primary procedure or service may be reported as listed. The additional procedure(s) or service(s) may be identified by appending modifier -51 to the additional procedure or service code(s). **Note**: This modifier should not be appended to designated "add-on" codes.

-52   Reduced services

Under certain circumstances a service or procedure is partially reduced or eliminated at the discretion of the physician or other qualified health care professional. Under these circumstances the service provided can be identified by its usual procedure number and the addition of the modifier -52, signifying that the service is reduced. This provides a means of reporting reduced services without disturbing the identification of the basic service. **Note**: For hospital outpatient reporting of a previously scheduled procedure/service that is partially reduced or cancelled as a result of extenuating circumstances or those that threaten the well-being of the patient prior to or after administration of anesthesia, see modifiers -73 and -74 (see modifiers approved for ASC hospital outpatient use).

The intended use of this modifier is to report the reduction of a service without affecting provider profiles maintained by health insurance companies.

Modifier -52 is another frequently misused modifier. Some medical practices mistakenly use modifier -52 to mean "reduced fee" and use it as a discounting method. Not only is this incorrect, the provider may seriously damage their provider profile with health insurance companies. The proper use for modifier -52 is to report that a service was not completed, or some part of a multiple-part service was not performed. A fee reduction may be in order as well; however that is not the primary purpose of the modifier.

-53   Discontinued procedure

Under certain circumstances, the physician or other qualified health care professional may elect to terminate a surgical or diagnostic procedure. Due to extenuating circumstances or those that threaten the well-being of the patient, it may be necessary to indicate that a surgical or diagnostic procedure was started but discontinued. This circumstance may be reported by adding modifier -53 to the code reported by the individual for the discontinued procedure. **Note**: This modifier is not used to report the elective cancellation of a procedure prior to the patient's anesthesia induction and/or surgical preparation in the operating suite. For outpatient hospital/ambulatory surgery center (ASC) reporting of a previously scheduled procedure/service that is partially reduced or cancelled as a result of extenuating circumstances or those that threaten the well-being of the patient prior to or after administration of anesthesia, see modifiers -73 and -74 (see modifiers approved for ASC hospital outpatient use).

-54   Surgical care only

When 1 physician or other qualified health care professional performs a surgical procedure and another provides preoperative and/or postoperative management, surgical services may be identified by adding modifier -54 to the usual procedure number.

-55   Postoperative management only

When 1 physician or other qualified health care professional performed the postoperative management and another performed the surgical procedure, the postoperative component may be identified by adding modifier -55 to the usual procedure number.

-56   Preoperative management only

When 1 physician or other qualified health care professional performed the preoperative care and evaluation and another performed the surgical procedure, the preoperative component may be identified by adding modifier -56 to the usual procedure number.

-57   Decision for surgery

An evaluation and management service that resulted in the initial decision to perform the surgery may be identified by adding the modifier -57 to the appropriate level of E/M service.

-58   Staged or related procedure or service by the same physician or other qualified health care professional during the postoperative period

It may be necessary to indicate that the performance of a procedure or service during the postoperative period was: (a) planned or anticipated (staged); (b) more extensive than the original procedure; or (c) for therapy following a surgical procedure. This circumstance may be reported by adding modifier -58 to the staged or related procedure. **Note**: For treatment of a problem that requires a return to the operating/procedure room (eg, unanticipated clinical condition), see modifier -78.

-59   Distinct Procedural Service

Under certain circumstances, it may be necessary to indicate that a procedure or service was distinct or independent from other non-E/M services performed on the same day. Modifier -59 is used to identify procedures/services, other than E/M services, that are not normally reported together, but are appropriate under the circumstances. Documentation must support a different session, different procedure or surgery, different site or organ system, separate incision/excision, separate lesion, or separate injury (or area of injury in extensive injuries) not ordinarily encountered or performed on the same day by the same individual. However, when another already established modifier is appropriate it should be used rather than modifier -59. Only if no more descriptive modifier is available, and the use of modifier -59 best explains the circumstances, should modifier -59 be used. **Note**: Modifier -59 should not be appended to an E/M service. To report a separate and distinct E/M service with a non-E/M service performed on the same date, see modifier -25.

-62   Two surgeons

When 2 surgeons work together as primary surgeons performing distinct part(s) of a procedure, each surgeon should report his/her distinct operative work by adding modifier -62 to the procedure code and any associated add-on code(s) for that procedure as long as both surgeons continue to work together as primary surgeons. Each surgeon should report the co-surgery once using the same procedure code. If additional procedure(s) (including add-on procedure(s) are performed during the same surgical session, separate code(s) may also be reported with modifier -62 added. **Note**: If a co-surgeon acts as an assistant in the performance of additional procedure(s), other than those reported with the modifier -62, during the same surgical session, those services may be reported using separate procedure code(s) with modifier -80 or modifier -82 added, as appropriate.

-63 Procedure performed on infants less than 4 kg

Procedures performed on neonates and infants up to a present body weight of 4 kg may involve significantly increased complexity and physician or other qualified health care professional work commonly associated with these patients. This circumstance may be reported by adding modifier 63 to the procedure number. Note: Unless otherwise designated, this modifier may only be appended to procedures/services listed in the 20100-69990 code series and 92920, 92928, 92953, 92960, 92986, 92987, 92990, 92997, 92998, 93312, 93313, 93314, 93315, 93316, 93317, 93318, 93452, 93505, 93530, 93531, 93532, 93533, 93561, 93562, 93563, 93564, 93568, 93580, 93582, 93590, 93591, 93592, 93615, 93616 from the Medicine/Cardiovascular section. Modifier 63 should not be appended to any CPT codes listed in the Evaluation and Management Services, Anesthesia, Radiology, Pathology/Laboratory, or Medicine sections (other than those identified above from the Medicine/Cardiovascular section).

-66 Surgical team

Under some circumstances, highly complex procedures (requiring the concomitant services of several physicians or other qualified health care professionals, often of different specialties, plus other highly skilled specially trained personnel, various types of complex equipment) are carried out under the "surgical team" concept. Such circumstances may be identified by each participating individual with the addition of modifier -66 to the basic procedure number used for reporting services.

-73 Discontinued out-patient procedure prior to anesthesia administration

Due to extenuating circumstances or those that threaten the well being of the patient, the physician may cancel a surgical or diagnostic procedure subsequent to the patient's surgical preparation (including sedation when provided, and being taken to the room where the procedure is to be performed), but prior to the administration of anesthesia (local, regional block(s) or general). Under these circumstances, the intended service that is prepared for but cancelled can be reported by its usual procedure number and the addition of the modifier -73.

Note: The elective cancellation of a service prior to the administration of anesthesia and/or surgical preparation of the patient should not be reported. For physician reporting of a discontinued procedure, see modifier -53.

-74 Discontinued out-patient procedure after anesthesia administration

Due to extenuating circumstances or those that threaten the well being of the patient, the physician may terminate a surgical or diagnostic procedure after the administration of anesthesia (local, regional block(s), general) or after the procedure was started (incision made, intubation started, scope inserted, etc.). Under these circumstances, the procedure started but terminated can be reported by its usual procedure number and the addition of the modifier -74. **Note**: The elective cancellation of a service prior to the administration of anesthesia and/or surgical preparation of the patient should not be reported. For physician reporting of a discontinued procedure, see modifier -53.

-76 Repeat procedure or service by same physician or other qualified health care professional

It may be necessary to indicate that a procedure or service was repeated by the same physician or other qualified health care professional subsequent to the original procedure or service. This circumstance may be reported by adding modifier -76 to the repeated procedure or service. **Note**: This modifier should not be appended to an E/M service.

-77 Repeat procedure by another physician or other qualified health care professional

It may be necessary to indicate that a basic procedure or service was repeated by another physician or other qualified health care professional subsequent to the original procedure or service. This circumstance may be reported by adding modifier -77 to the repeated procedure or service. **Note**: This modifier should not be appended to an E/M service.

-78 Unplanned return to the operating/procedure room by the same physician or other qualified health care professional following initial procedure for a related procedure during the postoperative period

It may be necessary to indicate that another procedure was performed during the postoperative period of the initial procedure (unplanned procedure following initial procedure). When this procedure is related to the first and requires the use of an operating/procedure room, it may be reported by adding modifier -78 to the related procedure. (For repeat procedures, see modifier -76.)

-79 Unrelated procedure or service by the same physician or other qualified health care professional during the postoperative period

The individual may need to indicate that the performance of a procedure or service during the postoperative period was unrelated to the original procedure. This circumstance may be reported by using modifier -79. (For repeat procedures on the same day, see '-76.')

-80 Assistant surgeon

Surgical assistant services may be identified by adding the modifier -80 to the usual procedure number(s).

-81 Minimum assistant surgeon

Minimum surgical assistant services are identified by adding the modifier -81 to the usual procedure number.

-82 Assistant surgeon (when qualified resident surgeon not available)

The unavailability of a qualified resident surgeon is a prerequisite for use of modifier -82 appended to the usual procedure code number(s).

-90 Reference (outside) laboratory

When laboratory procedures are performed by a party other than the treating or reporting physician or other qualified health care professional, the procedure may be identified by adding modifier -90 to the usual procedure number.

-91 Repeat clinical diagnostic laboratory test

In the course of treatment of the patient, it may be necessary to repeat the same laboratory test on the same day to obtain subsequent (multiple) test results. Under these circumstances, the laboratory test performed can be identified by its usual procedure number and the addition of modifier -91. **Note**: This modifier may not be used when tests are rerun to confirm initial results; due to testing problems with specimens or equipment; or for any other reason when a normal, one-time, reportable result is all that is required. This modifier may not be used when other code(s) describe a series of tests results (eg, glucose tolerance tests, evocative/suppression testing). This modifier may only be used for laboratory test(s) performed more than once on the same day on the same patient.

-92 Alternative Laboratory Platform Testing

When laboratory testing is being performed using a kit or transportable instrument that wholly or in part consists of a single use, disposable analytical chamber, the service may be identified by adding modifier 92 to the usual laboratory procedure code (HIV testing 86701-86703, and 87389). The test does not require permanent dedicated space, hence by its design may be hand carried or transported to the vicinity of the patient for immediate testing at that site, although location of the testing is not in itself determinative of the use of this modifier.

-95 Synchronous Telemedicine Service Rendered Via a Real-Time Interactive Audio and Video Telecommunications System

Synchronous telemedicine service is defined as a real-time interaction between a physician or other qualified health care professional and a patient who is located at a distant site from the physician or other qualified health care professional. The totality of the communication of information exchanged between the physician or other qualified health care professional and the patient during the course of the synchronous telemedicine service must be of an amount and nature that would be sufficient to meet the key components and/or requirements of the same service when rendered via a face-to-face interaction. Modifier 95 may only be appended to the services listed in Appendix P of CPT. Appendix P is the list of CPT codes for services that are typically performed face-to-face but may be rendered via a real-time (synchronous) interactive audio and video telecommunications system.

-96 Habilitative services

Habilitative Services: When a service or procedure that may be either habilitative or rehabilitative in nature is provided for habilitative purposes, the physician or other qualified health care professional may add modifier 96 to the service or procedure code to indicate that the service or procedure provided was a habilitative service. Habilitative services help an individual learn skills and functioning for daily living that the individual has not yet developed, and then keep and/or improve those learned skills. Habilitative services also help an individual keep, learn, or improve skills and functioning for daily living.

-97 **Rehabilitative services**

Rehabilitative Services: When a service or procedure that may be either habilitative or rehabilitative in nature is provided for rehabilitative purposes, the physician or other qualified health care professional may add modifier 97 to the service or procedure code to indicate that the service or procedure provided was a rehabilitative service. Rehabilitative services help an individual keep, get back, or improve skills and functioning for daily living that have been lost or impaired because the individual was sick, hurt, or disabled.

-99 **Multiple modifiers**

Under certain circumstances two or more modifiers may be necessary to completely delineate a service. In such situations modifier -99 should be added to the basic procedure, and other applicable modifiers may be listed as part of the description of the service.

ANESTHESIA PHYSICAL STATUS MODIFIERS

The Physical Status modifiers are consistent with the American Society of Anesthesiologists ranking of patient physical status, and distinguishing various levels of complexity of the anesthesia provided. All anesthesia services are reported by use of the anesthesia five-digit procedure code (00100-01999) with the appropriate physical status modifier appended. For example, 00100-P1

Under certain circumstances, when another established modifier(s) is appropriate, it should be used in addition to the physical status modifier. i.e., 00100-P4-53

P1   A normal healthy patient

P2   A patient with mild systemic disease

P3   A patient with severe systemic disease

P4   A patient with severe systemic disaease that is a constant threat to life

P5   A moribund patient who is not expected to survive without the operation

P6   A declared brain-dead patient whose organs are being removed for donor purposes

CATEGORY II MODIFIERS

The following performance measurement modifiers may be used with Category II codes to indicate that a service specified in the associated measure(s) was considered byt, due to either medical, patient, or system circumstance(s) documented in the medical record, the service was not provided. These modifiers serve as denominator exclusions from the performance measure. The user should note that not all listed measures provide for exclusions.

Category II modifiers should only be reported with Category II codes—they should not be reported with Category I or Category III codes. In addition, the modifiers in the Category II section should only be used where specified in the guidelines, reporting instructions, parenthetic notes, or code descriptor language listed in the Category II section (code listing and the Alphabetical Clinical Topics Listing).

1P   Performance Measure Exclusion Modifier due to Medical Reasons

Reasons include:

- Not indicated (absence of organ/limb, already received/performed, other)
- Contraindicated (patient allergic history, potential adverse drug interaction, other)
- Other medical reasons

2P   Performance Measure Exclusion Modifier due to Patient Reasons

Reasons include:

- Patient declinde
- Economic, social, or religious reasons

- Other patient reasons

3P   Performance Measure Exclusion Modifier due to System Reasons

Reasons include:

- Resources to perform the services not available
- Insurance coverage/payor-related limitations
- Other reason attributable to health care delivery system

Modifier 8P is intended to be used as a reporting modifier to allow the reporting of circumstances when an action described in a measure's numerator is not performed and the reason is not otherwise specified

8P   Performance measure reporting modifier—action not performed, reason not otherwise specified

LEVEL II (HCPCS/NATIONAL) MODIFIERS

HCPCS modifiers, defined and managed by The Centers for Medicare and Medicaid Services (CMS), are two digit modifier codes which may be either alpha (all letters) or alphanumeric (letters plus numbers). Some HCPCS modifiers may be used with CPT codes to modify procedures and services on health insurance claim forms filed for Medicare patients. See the most current edition of HCPCS for a complete list.

This page intentionally left blank

ANATOMICAL ILLUSTRATIONS

A fundamental knowledge and understanding of basic human anatomy and physiology is a prerequisite for accurate CPT© procedure coding. While a comprehensive treatment of anatomy and physiology is beyond the scope of this text, the large scale, full color anatomical illustrations on the following pages are designed to facilitate the procedure coding process for both beginning and experienced coders.

The illustrations provide an anatomical perspective of procedure coding by providing a side-by-side view of the major systems of the human body and a corresponding list of the most common CPT procedural categories used to report medical, surgical and diagnostic services performed on the illustrated system.

The CPT procedural categories listed on the left facing page of each anatomical illustration are code ranges only and should not be used for coding. These categories are provided as "pointers" to the appropriate section of CPT, where the definitive code may be found.

PLATE 1. SKIN AND SUBCUTANEOUS TISSUE - MALE

Skin, Subcutaneous and Accessory Structures

Introduction and Removal	10030-10036
Incision and Drainage	10040-10180
Debridement	11000-11047
Paring or Cutting	11055-11057
Biopsy	11102-11107
Removal of Skin Tags	11200-11201
Shaving of Lesions	11300-11313
Excision-Benign Lesions	11400-11471
Excision-Malignant Lesions	11600-11646

Nails	11719-11765

Pilondial Cyst	11770-11772

Repair (Closure)

Repair-Simple	12001-12021
Repair-Intermediate	12031-12057
Repair-Complex	13100-13160
Adjacent Tissue Transfer	14000-14350
Skin Replacement Surgery	15002-15278
Flaps (Skin and/or Deep Tissues)	15570-15777
Pressure Ulcers	15920-15999
Burns, Local Treatment	16000-16036

Destruction

Destruction, Benign or Premalignant Lesions	17000-17250
Destruction, Malignant Lesions	17260-17286
Mohs' Micrographic Surgery	17311-17315
Other Destruction Procedures	17340-17999

Laboratory Services

Skin Tests, Immunology	86485-86580
Skin Tests, Allergy	95004-95199

Visit and Medicine Services

E/M Services	99202-99499
Special Dermatological Procedures	96900-96999

Male Figure
(Anterior View)

Parietal region

Temporal region

Frontal region

Orbital region

Nasal region

Oral region

Mental region

Anterior neck region

Lateral neck region

Infraclavicular region

Deltoid region

Sternal region

Pectoral region

Axillary region

Brachial region

Hypochondriac region

Epigastric region

Cubital region

Umbilical region

Antebrachial region

Lateral abdominal region

Inguinal region

Pubic region

Femoral region

Knee region

Crural region

PLATE 2. SKIN AND SUBCUTANEOUS TISSUE - FEMALE

Skin, Subcutaneous and Accessory Structures

Introduction and Removal	10030-10036
Incision and Drainage	10040-10180
Debridement	11000-11047
Paring or Cutting	11055-11057
Biopsy	11102-11107
Removal of Skin Tags	11200-11201
Shaving of Lesions	11300-11313
Excision-Benign Lesions	11400-11471
Excision-Malignant Lesions	11600-11646

Nails
11719-11765

Pilondial Cyst
11770-11772

Repair (Closure)

Repair-Simple	12001-12021
Repair-Intermediate	12031-12057
Repair-Complex	13100-13160
Adjacent Tissue Transfer	14000-14350
Skin Replacement Surgery	15002-15278
Flaps (Skin and/or Deep Tissues)	15570-15777
Pressure Ulcers	15920-15999
Burns, Local Treatment	16000-16036

Destruction

Destruction, Benign or Premalignant Lesions	17000-17250
Destruction, Malignant Lesions	17260-17286
Mohs' Micrographic Surgery	17311-17315
Other Destruction Procedures	17340-17999

Laboratory Services

Skin Tests, Immunology	86485-86580
Skin Tests, Allergy	95004-95199

Visit and Medicine Services

E/M Services	99202-99499
Special Dermatological Procedures	96900-96999

Female Figure
(Anterior View)

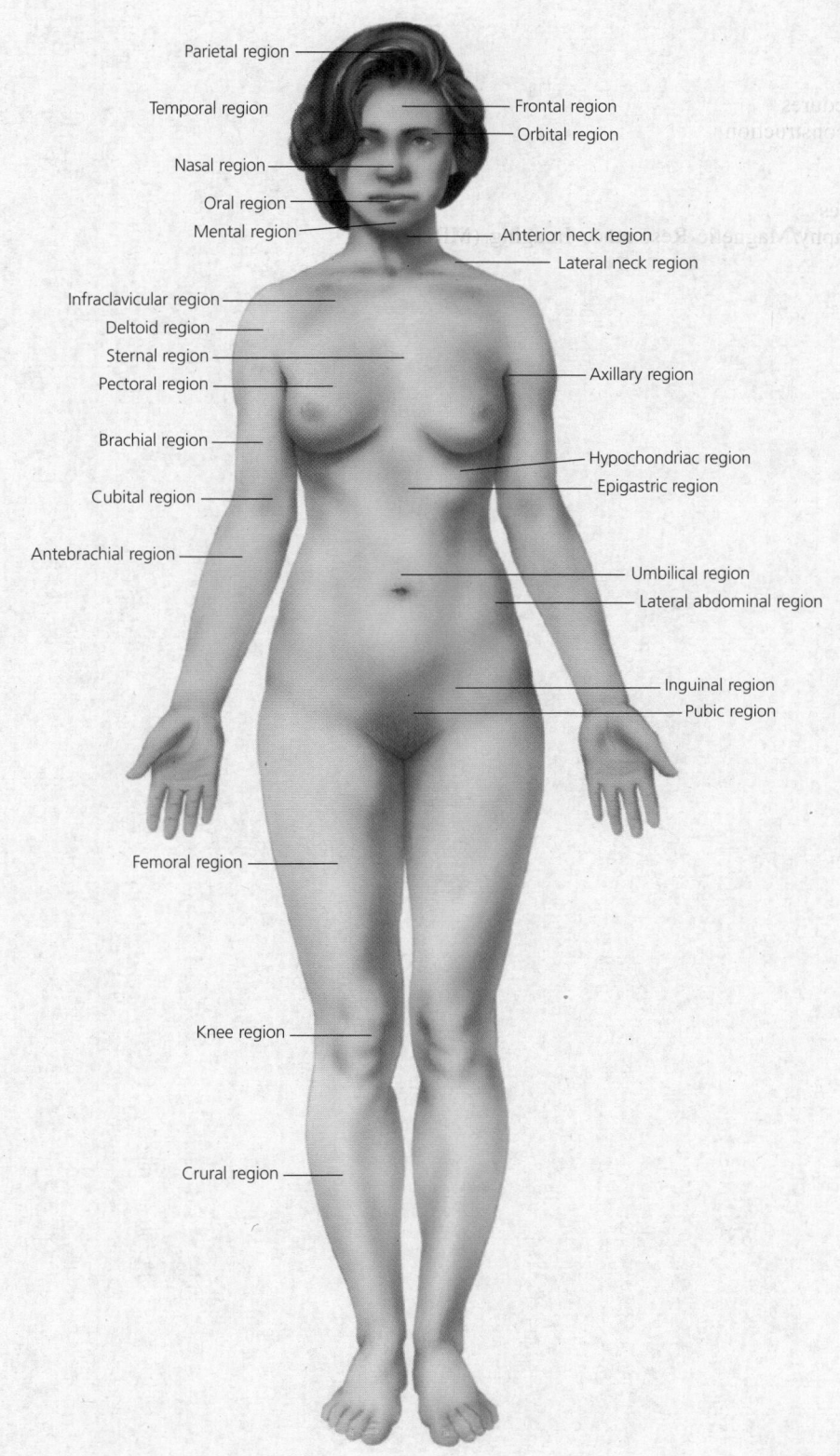

Parietal region

Temporal region

Frontal region

Orbital region

Nasal region

Oral region

Mental region

Anterior neck region

Lateral neck region

Infraclavicular region

Deltoid region

Sternal region

Pectoral region

Axillary region

Brachial region

Hypochondriac region

Cubital region

Epigastric region

Antebrachial region

Umbilical region

Lateral abdominal region

Inguinal region

Pubic region

Femoral region

Knee region

Crural region

PLATE 3. FEMALE BREAST

Breast

Incision	19000-19030
Excision	19081-19272
Introduction	19281-19298
Mastectomy Procedures	19300-19307
Repair and/or Reconstruction	19316-19396
Other Procedures	19499

Radiology Services

Breast Mammography/Magnetic Resonance Imaging (MRI)	77046-77067

E/M Services 99202-99499

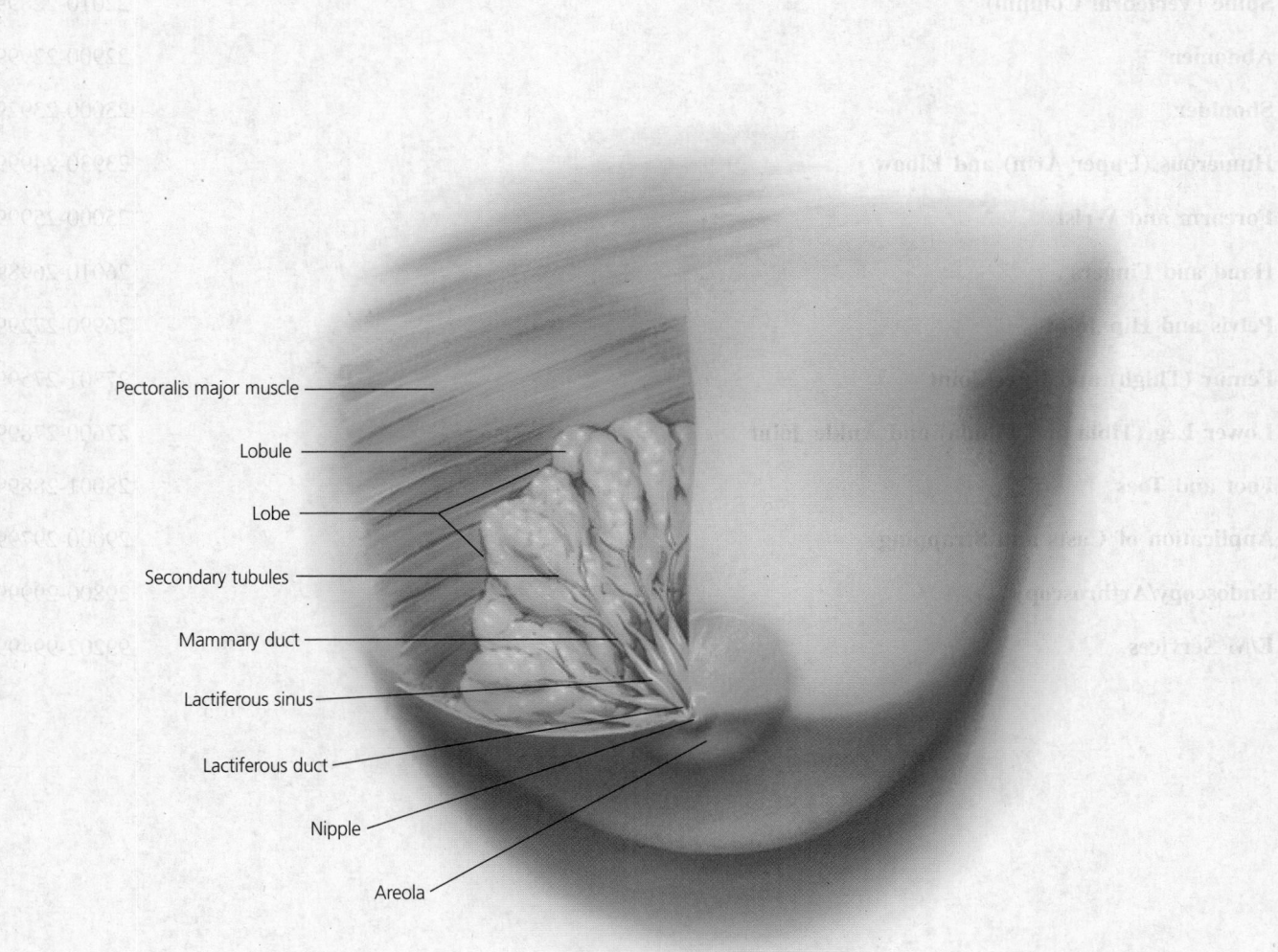

Pectoralis major muscle

Lobule

Lobe

Secondary tubules

Mammary duct

Lactiferous sinus

Lactiferous duct

Nipple

Areola

PLATE 4. MUSCULAR SYSTEM AND CONNECTIVE TISSUE - ANTERIOR VIEW

General	20100-20999
Head	21010-21499
Neck (Soft Tissues) and Thorax	21501-21899
Back and Flank	21920-21936
Spine (Vertebral Column)	22010-22899
Abdomen	22900-22999
Shoulder	23000-23929
Humerous (Upper Arm) and Elbow	23930-24999
Forearm and Wrist	25000-25999
Hand and Fingers	26010-26989
Pelvis and Hip Joint	26990-27299
Femur (Thigh) and Knee Joint	27301-27599
Lower Leg (Tibia and Fibula) and Ankle Joint	27600-27899
Foot and Toes	28001-28899
Application of Casts and Strapping	29000-29799
Endoscopy/Arthroscopy	29800-29999
E/M Services	99202-99499

Muscular System
(Anterior View)

Temporalis m.
Orbicularis oculi m.
Masseter m.
Sternocleidomastoid m.
Trapezius m.
Levator scapulae m.
Deltoid m.
Pectoralis major m.
Serratus anterior m.
Biceps m.
External abdominal oblique m.
Brachialis m.
Brachioradialis m.
Extensor carpi radialis longus m.
Palmaris longus m.
Flexor carpi radialis m.
Superficial inguinal ring
Tensor fasciae latae m.
Sartorius m.
Rectus femoris m.
Adductor longus m.
Vastus lateralis m.
Iliotibial tract
Vastus medialis m.
Lateral patellar retinaculum
Tibialis anterior m.
Gastrocnemius m.
Extensor digitorum longus m.
Peroneus longus m.
Soleus m.
Peroneus brevis m.
Extensor hallucis longus m.
Extensor hallucis brevis m.
Extensor digitorum brevis m.

Frontalis m.
Buccinator
Orbicularis oris m.
Depressor anguli oris m.
Pectoralis minor m.
Internal intercostal m.
Coracobrachialis m.
Brachialis m.
Rectus sheath
Rectus abdominis m.
Linea alba
Internal abdominal oblique m.
Transversus abdominis m.
Flexor digitorum superficialis m.
Flexor pollicis longus m.
Abductor digiti minimi m.
Abductor pollicis brevis m.
Flexor pollicis brevis m.
Iliopsoas m.
Pectineus m.
Adductor brevis m.
Gracilis m.
Adductor magnus m.
Vastus medialis m.
Vastus lateralis m.
Sartorius m.
Patella
Patellar ligament
Medial patellar retinaculum
Gastrocnemius m.
Soleus m.
Tibia
Flexor digitorum longus m.
Extensor hallucis brevis m.
Abductor hallucis m.

PLATE 5. MUSCULAR SYSTEM AND CONNECTIVE TISSUE - POSTERIOR VIEW

General	20100-20999
Head	21010-21499
Neck (Soft Tissues) and Thorax	21501-21899
Back and Flank	21920-21936
Spine (Vertebral Column)	22010-22899
Abdomen	22900-22999
Shoulder	23000-23929
Humerous (Upper Arm) and Elbow	23930-24999
Forearm and Wrist	25000-25999
Hand and Fingers	26010-26989
Pelvis and Hip Joint	26990-27299
Femur (Thigh) and Knee Joint	27301-27599
Lower Leg (Tibia and Fibula) and Ankle Joint	27600-27899
Foot and Toes	28001-28899
Application of Casts and Strapping	29000-29799
Endoscopy/Arthroscopy	29800-29999
E/M Services	99202-99499

Muscular System
(Posterior View)

Frontalis m.
Temporoparietalis m.
Zygomaticus major m.
Masseter m.
Risorius m.
Trapezius m.
Deltoid m.
Infraspinatus m.
Teres minor m.
Teres major m.
Triceps m.
Latissimus dorsi m.
Brachialis m.
Brachioradialis m.
Extensor carpi radialis longus m.
Flexor carpi ulnaris m.
Extensor digitorum m.
Extensor carpi radialis brevis m.
Extensor carpi ulnaris m.
Abductor pollicis longus m.
Extensor pollicis brevis m.
Gluteus medius m.
Gluteus maximus m.

Biceps femoris m.
Adductor magnus m.
Iliotibial tract
Vastus lateralis m.
Semimembranosus m.
Semitendinosus m.

Gastrocnemius m.
Peroneus longus m.

Soleus m.
Calcaneal t. (Achilles)

Galea aponeurotica
Occipitalis m.
Sternocleidomastoid m.
Splenius capitis m.
Splenius cervicis m.
Levator scapulae m.
Supraspinatus m.
Rhomboid minor m.
Rhomboid major m.
Spinalis thoracis m.
Iliocostalis thoracis m.
Longissimus thoracis m.
Serratus posterior inferior m.
Brachioradialis m.
Extensor carpi radialis longus m.
External abdominal oblique m.
Supinator m.
Gluteus medius m.
Extensor pollicis longus m.
Gluteus minimus m.
Piriformis m.
Superior gemellus m.
Obturator internus m.
Inferior gemellus m.
Quadratus femoris m.
Adductor magnus m.

Gracilis m.
Biceps femoris m.
Semimembranosus m.

Plantaris m.
Popliteus m.
Soleus m.

Flexor digitorum longus m.
Peroneus longus m.
Flexor hallucis longus m.
Peroneus brevis m.

PLATE 6. MUSCULAR SYSTEM - SHOULDER AND ELBOW

General
Wound exploration - Trauma	20100-20103
Excision	20150-20251
Introduction or Removal	20500-20697
Replantation	20802-20838
Grafts of Implants	20900-20938
Other	20950-20999

Shoulder
Incision	23000-23044
Excision	23065-23220
Introduction or Removal	23330-23350
Repair, Revision and/or Reconstruction	23395-23491
Fracture and/or Dislocation	23500-23680
Manipulation	23700
Arthrodesis	23800-23802
Amputation	23900-23921
Other/Unlisted Procedures	23929

Humerous (Upper Arm) and Elbow
Incision	23930-24006
Excision	24065-24155
Introduction or Removal	24160-24220
Repair, Revision and/or Reconstruction	24300-24498
Fracture and/or Dislocation	24500-24685
Arthrodesis	24800-24802
Amputation	24900-24940
Other/Unlisted Procedure	24999

Application of Casts/Strapping
Body and Upper Extremity Casts and Strapping	29000-29280
Removal or Repair	29700-29750
Other	29799

Endoscopy/Arthroscopy
29805-29838

Radiology Services
73000-73225

E/M Services
99202-99499

Shoulder and Elbow
(Anterior View)

Coracoclavicular ligament
Acromioclavicular ligament
Coracoacromial ligament
Supraspinatus tendon
Coracohumeral ligament
Transverse humeral ligament
Tendon of long head of biceps muscle
Subscapularis tendon
Articular capsule

Acromion   Clavicle

Coracoid process
Scapular notch
Subscapular fossa
Head of humerus
Lesser tubercle
Greater tubercle
Scapula
Nutrient foramen
Humerus
Deltoid tuberosity

Articular capsule
Radial collateral ligament
Annular ligament
Ulnar collateral ligament

Interosseous membrane
Radius
Ulna

Lateral epicondyle
Capitulum
Coronoid fossa
Medial epicondyle
Trochlea
Coronoid process
Head of radius
Ulnar tuberosity
Radial tuberosity

PLATE 7. MUSCULAR SYSTEM - HAND AND WRIST

General
Wound exploration - Trauma	20100-20103
Excision	20150-20251
Introduction or Removal	20500-20697
Replantation	20802-20838
Grafts of Implants	20900-20938
Other	20950-20999

Forearm and Wrist
Incision	25000-25040
Excision	25065-25240
Introduction or Removal	25246-25259
Repair, Revision and/or Reconstruction	25260-25492
Fracture and/or Dislocation	25500-25695
Arthrodesis	25800-25830
Amputation	25900-25931
Other/Unlisted Procedure	25999

Hand and Fingers
Incision	26010-26080
Excision	26100-26262
Introduction or Removal	26320
Repair, Revision, and/or Reconstruction	26340-26596
Fracture and/or Dislocation	26600-26785
Arthrodesis	26820-26863
Amputation	26910-26952
Other/Unlisted Procedure	26989

Application of Casts/Strapping   29000-29280

Endoscopy/Arthroscopy   29840-29848

Radiology Services   73000-73225

E/M Services   99202-99499

Abductor pollicis longus muscle

Extensor pollicis brevis muscle

Extensor digitorum tendons

Extensor pollicis brevis tendon

Extensor pollicis longus tendon

Extensor carpi radialis brevis tendon

Extensor carpi radialis longus tendon

1st dorsal interosseous muscle

Extensor digiti minimi muscle

Extensor carpi ulnaris muscle

Extensor retinaculum

Extensor digiti minimi tendons

Extensor digitorum tendons

2nd, 3rd, 4th dorsal interosseous muscles

Brachioradialis tendon

Flexor carpi radialis tendon

Flexor pollicis longus muscle

Abductor pollicis longus tendon

Opponens pollicis muscle

Abductor pollicis brevis muscle

Flexor pollicis brevis muscle

Flexor digitorum superficialis muscle & tendons

Flexor carpi ulnaris tendon

Palmaris longus tendon

Opponens digiti minimi muscle

Flexor digiti minimi brevis muscle

Abductor digiti minimi muscle

Flexor digitorum superficialis tendons

Palmar interosseous muscles

Fibrous digital sheath:
anular part
cruciform part

Adductor pollicis muscle

Lumbrical muscles

Flexor digitorum profundus tendon

PLATE 8. MUSCULOSKELETAL SYSTEM - HIP AND KNEE

General

Wound exploration - Trauma	20100-20103
Excision	20150-20251
Introduction or Removal	20500-20697
Replantation	20802-20838
Grafts of Implants	20900-20938
Other	20950-20999

Pelvis and Hip Joint

Incision	26990-27036
Excision	27040-27080
Introduction or Removal	27086-27096
Repair, Revision, and/or Reconstruction	27097-27187
Fracture and/or dislocation	27193-27269
Manipulation	27275
Arthrodesis	27280-27286
Amputation	27290-27295
Other/Unlisted Procedure	27299

Femur (Thigh Region) and Knee Joint

Incision	27301-27310
Excision	27323-27365
Introduction or Removal	27369-37372
Repair, Revision, and/or Reconstruction	27380-27499
Fracture and/or Dislocation	27500-27566
Manipulation	27570
Arthrodesis	27580
Amputation	27590-27598
Other/Unlisted Procedure	27599

Application of Casts/Strapping	29305-29584
Endoscopy/Arthroscopy	29850-29889
Radiology Services	73500-73725
E/M Services	99202-99499

Hip and Knee
(Anterior View)

Sacral promontory
Sacrum
Iliac crest
Ilium
Anterior superior iliac spine
Spine of ischium
Anterior inferior iliac spine
Head of femur
Greater trochanter
Obturator foramen
Pubis
Lesser trochanter

Anterior longitudinal ligament
Iliolumbar ligament
Anterior sacroiliac ligament
Coccyx
Sacrotuberous ligament
Sacrospinous ligament
Inguinal ligament
Iliofemoral ligament
Pubofemoral ligament
Obturator membrane
Pubic symphysis
Femur

Medial epicondyle
Lateral epicondyle
Patella
Lateral condyles
Head of fibula
Tibial tuberosity
Medial condyles

Tibia

Fibula

Quadriceps femoris tendon
Medial patellar retinaculum
Fibular collateral ligament
Tibial collateral ligament
Lateral patellar retinaculum
Patellar ligament

Interosseous
membrane

PLATE 9. MUSCULOSKELETAL SYSTEM - FOOT AND ANKLE

General

Wound exploration - Trauma	20100-20103
Excision	20150-20251
Introduction or Removal	20500-20697
Replantation	20802-20838
Grafts of Implants	20900-20938
Other	20950-20999

Leg (Tibia and Fibula) and Ankle Joint

Incision	27600-27612
Excision	27613-27647
Introduction or Removal	27648
Repair, Revision and/or Reconstruction	27650-27745
Fracture and/or Dislocation	27750-27848
Manipulation	27860
Arthrodesis	27870-27871
Amputation	27880-27889
Other Procedures	27892-27899

Foot and Toes

Incision	28001-28035
Excision	28043-28175
Introduction or Removal	28190-28193
Repair, Revision, and/or Reconstruction	28200-28360
Fracture and/or Dislocation	28400-28675
Arthrodesis	28705-28760
Amputation	28800-28825
Other/Unlisted Procedures	28890-28899

Application of Casts/Strapping	29305-29584
Endoscopy/Arthroscopy	29891-29999
Radiology Services	73500-73725
E/M Services	99202-99499

Soleus muscle

Tibia

Flexor digitorum longus muscle

Flexor hallucis tendon

Achilles tendon

Medial malleolus

Tibialis posterior tendon

Retinaculum

Tibialis posterior tendon

Tibialis anterior tendon

Extensor hallucis brevis muscle

Abductor hallucis muscle

Tibialis anterior muscle

Peroneus brevis muscle

Peroneus longus tendon

Extensor digitorum longus muscle

Tibia

Fibula

Extensor hallucis longus muscle

Lateral malleous

Retinaculum

Peroneus longus tendon

Extensor digitorum brevis muscle

Calcaneus

Peroneus brevis tendon

Peroneus tertius tendon

Opponens digiti minimi muscle

Dorsal interosseous muscles

Extensor hallucis longus tendon

Extensor hallucis brevis muscle

Extensor digitorum longus tendons

PLATE 10. SKELETAL SYSTEM - ANTERIOR VIEW

General	20100-20999
Head	21010-21499
Neck (Soft Tissues) and Thorax	21501-21899
Back and Flank	21920-21936
Spine (Vertebral Column)	22010-22899
Abdomen	22900-22999
Shoulder	23000-23929
Humerous (Upper Arm) and Elbow	23930-24999
Forearm and Wrist	25000-25999
Hand and Fingers	26010-26989
Pelvis and Hip Joint	26990-27299
Femur (Thigh) and Knee Joint	27301-27599
Lower Leg (Tibia and Fibula) and Ankle Joint	27600-27899
Foot and Toes	28001-28899
Application of Casts and Strapping	29000-29799
Endoscopy/Arthroscopy	29800-29999
Radiology Services	70010-73725
Bone/Joint Studies	77071-77086
E/M Services	99202-99499

Skeletal System
(Anterior View)

Frontal bone — Parietal bone
Temporal bone — Orbit
Nasal conchae — Zygomatic bone
Maxilla — Nasal septum
Manubrium of sternum — Mandible
Coracoid process — Hyoid bone
Acromion — Clavicle
Greater tubercle — Coracoclavicular ligament
Head of humerus — Supraspinatus tendon
Scapula — Subscapularis tendon
Humerus — Body of sternum
True ribs (1–7) — Xiphoid process
False ribs (8–12) — Costal cartilages
Medial epicondyle — Anterior longitudinal ligament
Lateral epicondyle — Ulnar collateral ligament
Radius — Radial collateral ligament
Ulna — Annular ligament
Sacrum — L3
Anterior superior iliac spine — Iliac crest
Head of femur — Anterior sacroiliac ligament
Greater trochanter — Interosseous membrane
Inguinal ligament
Coccyx
Iliofemoral ligament
Pubic symphysis
Metacarpals
Proximal phalanges
Middle phalanges
Distal phalanges
Femur

Key to Carpal Bones
A Scaphoid
B Trapezium
C Trapezoid
D Capitate
E Lunate
F Pisiform
G Triquetral
H Hamate

Medial epicondyle — Quadriceps femoris tendon
Lateral epicondyle — Tibial collateral ligament
Patella — Fibular collateral ligament
Head of fibula — Patellar ligament
Tibial tuberosity — Tibia
Fibula
Interosseous membrane

Key to Tarsal Bones
J Intermediate cuneiform
K Lateral cuneiform
L Cuboid
M Talus
N Navicular
O Calcaneus
P Medial cuneiform

Medial malleolus
Lateral malleolus

PLATE 11. SKELETAL SYSTEM - POSTERIOR VIEW

General	20100-20999
Head	21010-21499
Neck (Soft Tissues) and Thorax	21501-21899
Back and Flank	21920-21936
Spine (Vertebral Column)	22010-22899
Abdomen	22900-22999
Shoulder	23000-23929
Humerous (Upper Arm) and Elbow	23930-24999
Forearm and Wrist	25000-25999
Hand and Fingers	26010-26989
Pelvis and Hip Joint	26990-27299
Femur (Thigh) and Knee Joint	27301-27599
Lower Leg (Tibia and Fibula) and Ankle Joint	27600-27899
Foot and Toes	28001-28899
Application of Casts and Strapping	29000-29799
Endoscopy/Arthroscopy	29800-29999
Radiology Services	70010-73725
Bone/Joint Studies	77071-77086
E/M Services	99202-99499

Skeletal System
(Posterior View)

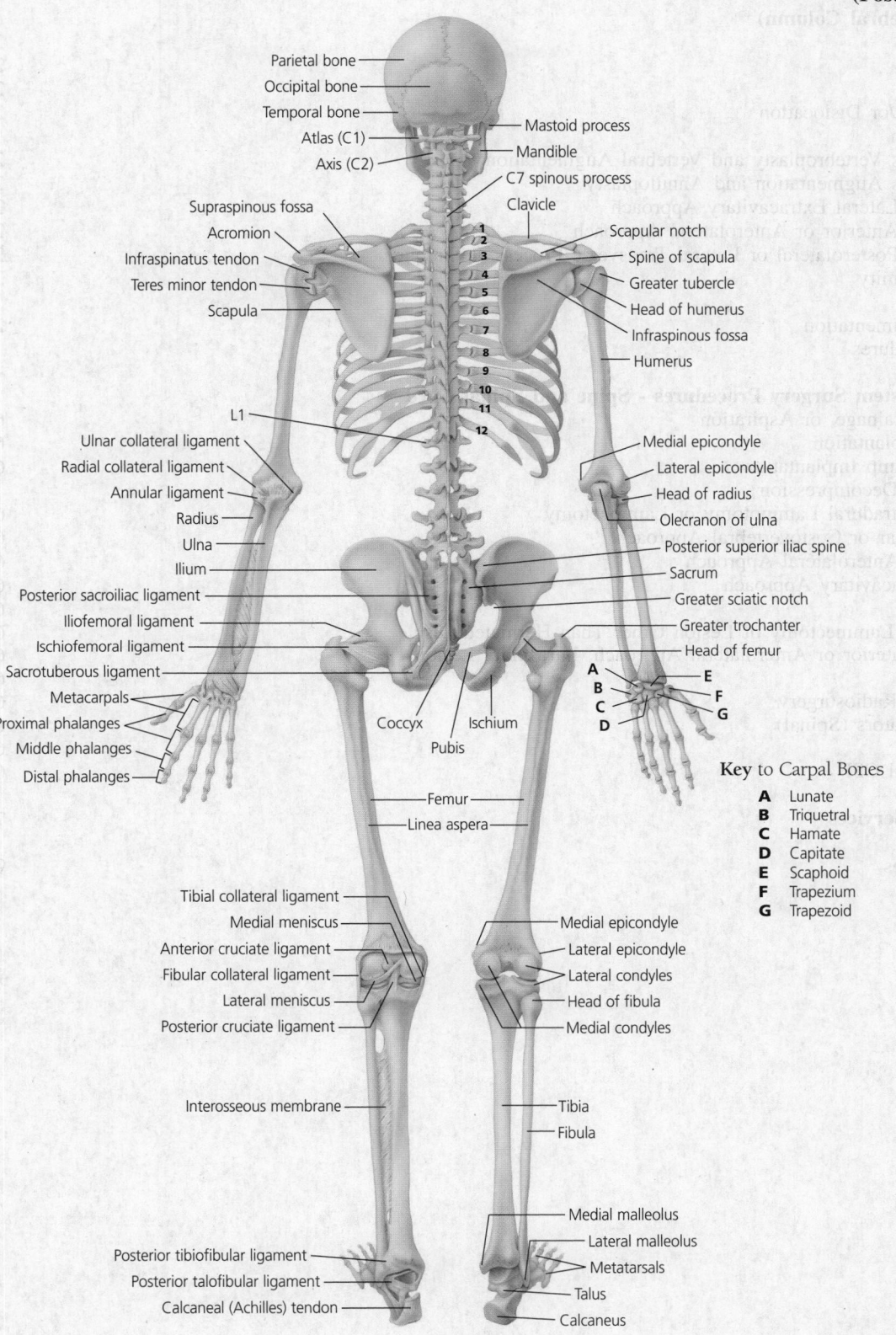

Parietal bone
Occipital bone
Temporal bone
Atlas (C1)
Axis (C2)
Mastoid process
Mandible
C7 spinous process
Clavicle
Supraspinous fossa
Acromion
Infraspinatus tendon
Teres minor tendon
Scapula
Scapular notch
Spine of scapula
Greater tubercle
Head of humerus
Infraspinous fossa
Humerus
L1
Ulnar collateral ligament
Radial collateral ligament
Annular ligament
Radius
Ulna
Ilium
Posterior sacroiliac ligament
Iliofemoral ligament
Ischiofemoral ligament
Sacrotuberous ligament
Metacarpals
Proximal phalanges
Middle phalanges
Distal phalanges
Medial epicondyle
Lateral epicondyle
Head of radius
Olecranon of ulna
Posterior superior iliac spine
Sacrum
Greater sciatic notch
Greater trochanter
Head of femur
Coccyx
Ischium
Pubis
Femur
Linea aspera
Tibial collateral ligament
Medial meniscus
Anterior cruciate ligament
Fibular collateral ligament
Lateral meniscus
Posterior cruciate ligament
Medial epicondyle
Lateral epicondyle
Lateral condyles
Head of fibula
Medial condyles
Interosseous membrane
Tibia
Fibula
Posterior tibiofibular ligament
Posterior talofibular ligament
Calcaneal (Achilles) tendon
Medial malleolus
Lateral malleolus
Metatarsals
Talus
Calcaneus

Key to Carpal Bones

A Lunate
B Triquetral
C Hamate
D Capitate
E Scaphoid
F Trapezium
G Trapezoid

PLATE 12. SKELETAL SYSTEM - VERTEBRAL COLUMN

Spine (Vertebral Column)

Incision	22010-22015
Excision	22100-22116
Osteotomy	22206-22226
Fracture and/or Dislocation	22310-22328
Manipulation	22505
Percutaneous Vertebroplasty and Vertebral Augmentation	22510-22515
Percutaneous Augmentation and Annuloplasty	22526-22527
Arthrodesis-Lateral Extracavitary Approach	22532-22534
Arthrodesis-Anterior or Anterolateral Approach	22548-22586
Arthrodesis-Posterolateral or Lateral Transverse Process Technique	22590-22634
Spine Deformity	22800-22819
Exploration	22830
Spinal Instrumentation	22840-22870
Other Procedures	22899

Nervous System Surgery Procedures - Spine and Spinal Cord

Injection, Drainage, or Aspiration	62263-62327
Catheter Implantation	62350-62355
Reservoir/Pump Implantation	62360-62370
Endoscopic Decompression	62380
Posterior Extradural Laminotomy or Laminectomy	63001-63051
Transpedicular or Costovertebral Approach	63055-63066
Anterior or Anterolateral Approach	63075-63091
Lateral Extracavitary Approach	63101-63103
Incision	63170-63200
Excision by Laminectomy of Lesion Other Than Herniated Disc	63250-63295
Excision, Anterior or Anterolateral Approach, Intraspinal Lesion	63300-63308
Stereotaxis	63600-63610
Stereotactic Radiosurgery	63620-63621
Neurostimulators (Spinal)	63650-63688
Repair	63700-63710
Shunt, Spinal CSF	63740-63746

Radiology Services	72020-72295

E/M Services	99202-99499

Vertebral Column
(Lateral View)

Atlas (C1)

Axis (C2)

Cervical
vertebrae
(C1–C7)

Cervical
curve

C7

T1

Intervertebral
discs

Thoracic
vertebrae
(T1–T12)

Thoracic
curve

Foveae for
ribs

T12

L1

Lumbar
vertebrae
(L1–L5)

Lumbar
curve

Intervertebral
foramina

L5

Sacrum

Pelvic
curve

Coccyx

PLATE 13. RESPIRATORY SYSTEM

Nose
Incision	30000-30020
Excision	30100-30160
Introduction	30200-30220
Removal of Foreign Body	30300-30320
Repair	30400-30630
Destruction	30801-30802
Other	30901-30999

Accessory Sinuses
Incision	31000-31090
Excision	31200-31230
Endoscopy	31231-31298
Other	31299

Larynx
Excision	31300-31420
Introduction	31500-31502
Endoscopy	31505-31579
Repair	31580-31592
Destruction	31595
Other	31599

Trachea and Bronchi
Incision	31600-31614
Endoscopy	31615-31654
Bronchial Thermoplasty	31660-31661
Introduction	31717-31730
Excision, Repair	31750-31830
Other	31899

Lungs and Pleura
Incision	32035-32225
Excision/Resection and Removal	32310-32540
Introduction and Removal	32550-32557
Destruction	32560-32562
Thoracoscopy	32601-32674
Stereotactic Radiation Therapy	32701
Repair	32800-32820
Lung Transplantation	32850-32856
Surgical Collapse Therapy; Thoracoplasty	32900-32960
Other Procedures	32994-32999

Radiology Services/Chest
	71010-71555

E/M Services
	99202-99499

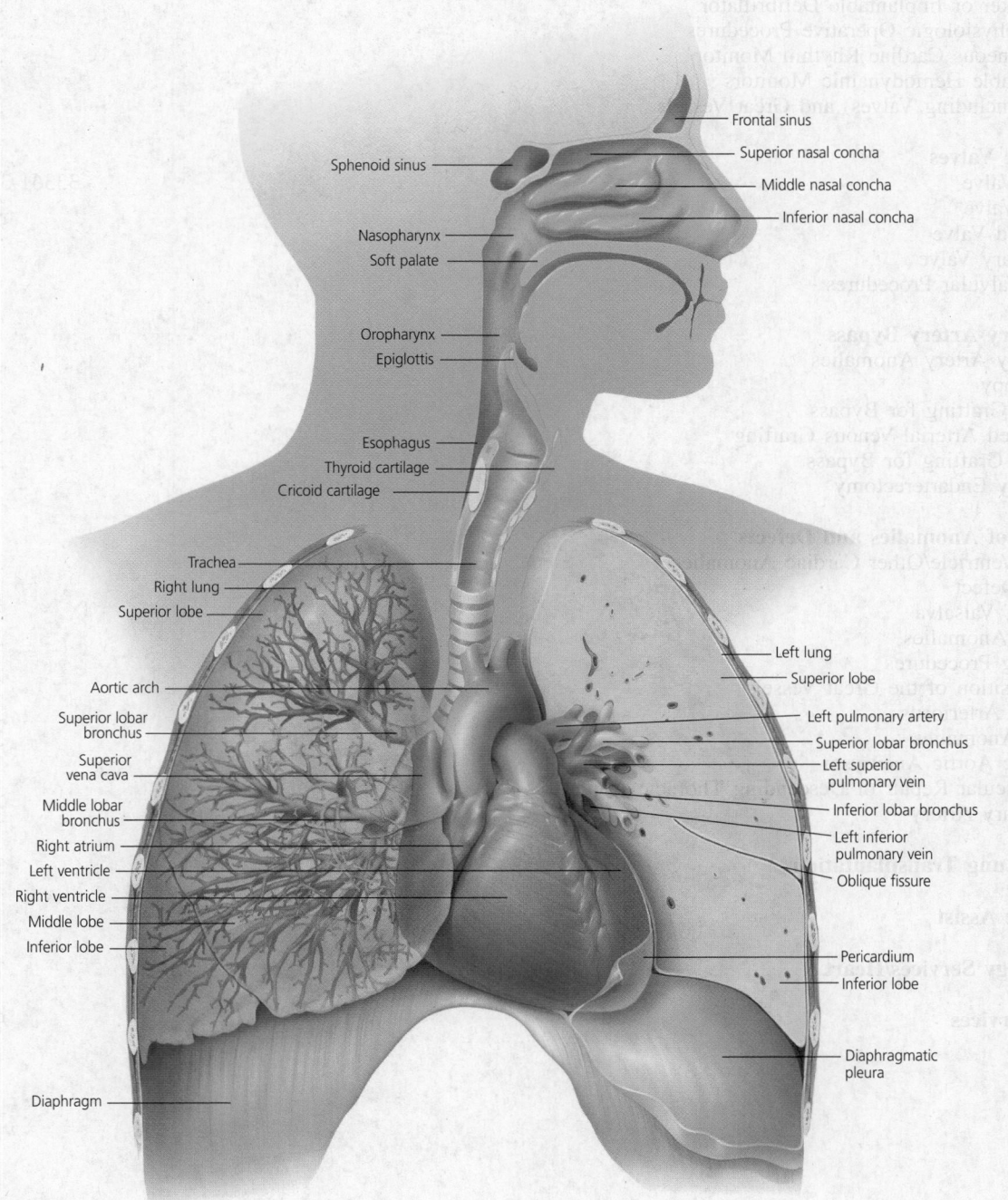

Frontal sinus

Sphenoid sinus

Superior nasal concha

Middle nasal concha

Inferior nasal concha

Nasopharynx

Soft palate

Oropharynx

Epiglottis

Esophagus

Thyroid cartilage

Cricoid cartilage

Trachea

Right lung

Superior lobe

Aortic arch

Superior lobar bronchus

Superior vena cava

Middle lobar bronchus

Right atrium

Left ventricle

Right ventricle

Middle lobe

Inferior lobe

Diaphragm

Left lung

Superior lobe

Left pulmonary artery

Superior lobar bronchus

Left superior pulmonary vein

Inferior lobar bronchus

Left inferior pulmonary vein

Oblique fissure

Pericardium

Inferior lobe

Diaphragmatic pleura

PLATE 14. HEART AND PERICARDIUM

General

Pericardium	33010-33050
Cardiac Tumor	33120-33130
Transmyocardial Revascularization	33140, 33141
Pacemaker or Implantable Defibrillator	33202-33275
Electrophysiologic Operative Procedures	33250-33266
Subcutaneous Cardiac Rhythm Monitor	33285-33286
Implantable Hemodynamic Monitors	33289
Heart (Including Valves) and Great Vessels	33300-33340

Cardiac Valves

Aortic Valve	33361-33417, 33440
Mitral Valve	33418-33430
Tricuspid Valve	33460-33468
Pulmonary Valve	33470-33478
Other Valvular Procedures	33496

Coronary Artery Bypass

Coronary Artery Anomalies	33500-33507
Endoscopy	33508
Venous Grafting for Bypass	33510-33516
Combined Arterial-Venous Grafting	33517-33530
Arterial Grafting for Bypass	33533-33548
Coronary Endarterectomy	33572

Repair of Anomalies and Defects

Single Ventricle/Other Cardiac Anomalies	33600-33622
Septal Defect	33641-33697
Sinus of Valsalva	33702-33722
Venous Anomalies	33724-33732
Shunting Procedures	33735-33768
Transposition of the Great Vessels	33770-33783
Truncus Arteriosus	33786-33788
Aortic Anomalies	33800-33853
Thoracic Aortic Aneurysm	33860-33877
Endovascular Repair of Descending Thoracic Aorta	33880-33891
Pulmonary Artery	33910-33926

Heart/Lung Transplantation	33927-33945
Cardiac Assist	33967-33993
Radiology Services/Heart	75557-75574
E/M Services	99202-99499

Heart
(External View)

Left common carotid artery

Brachiocephalic artery

Left subclavian artery

Aortic arch

Ligamentum arteriosum

Left pulmonary artery

Superior vena cava

Ascending aorta

Pulmonary trunk

Left auricle

Right coronary artery

Circumflex artery

Great cardiac vein

Right atrium

Right ventricle

Anterior descending (interventricular) artery

Anterior cardiac vein

Left ventricle

Right marginal artery

Small cardiac vein

Apex

Heart
(Internal View)

Superior vena cava

Right pulmonary artery branches

Aorta

Pulmonary trunk

Left pulmonary artery

Left pulmonary veins

Right pulmonary veins

Left atrium

Pulmonary semilunar valve

Aortic semilunar valve

Right atrium

Bicuspid (left AV) valve

Left ventricle

Tricuspid (right AV) valve

Papillary muscle

Interventricular septum

Chordae tendineae

Inferior vena cava

Myocardium

Right ventricle

Trabeculae carneae

63

PLATE 15. CIRCULATORY SYSTEM

Embolectomy/Thrombectomy
Arterial, With or Without Catheter   34001-34203
Venous, Direct or With Catheter   34401-34490

Venous Reconstruction   34501-34530

Repair
Endovascular Repair of Aneurysm   34701-34848
Direct Repair of Aneurysm   35001-35152
Repair Arteriovenous Fistula   35180-35190
Repair Blood Vessel Other Than for Fistula   35201-35286

Thromboendarterectomy   35301-35390

Angioscopy   35400

Bypass Graft   35500-35671

Composite Grafts   35681-35683

Transposition and Exploration/Revision
Arterial Transposition   35691-35697
Excision, Exploration, Repair, Revision   35700-35907

Vascular Injection Procedures
Intravenous   36000-36015
Intra-Arterial/Intra-Aortic   36100-36299
Venous   36400-36522
Central Venous Access   36555-36598
Arterial   36600-36660
Intraosseous   36680

Cannulization or Shunt and Other Procedures
Hemodialysis Access, Intervascular Cannulization, or Shunt Insertion   36800-36861
Dialysis Circuit   36901-36909
Portal Decompression Procedures   37140-37183
Transcatheter Procedures   37184-37218
Endovascular Revascularization   37220-37239, 37246-37249
Vascular Embolization and Occlusion   37241-37244
Intravascular Ultrasound Services   37252-37253
Endoscopy   37500-37501
Ligation and Other Procedures   37565-37799

Radiology Services   75600-75989

E/M Services   99202-99499

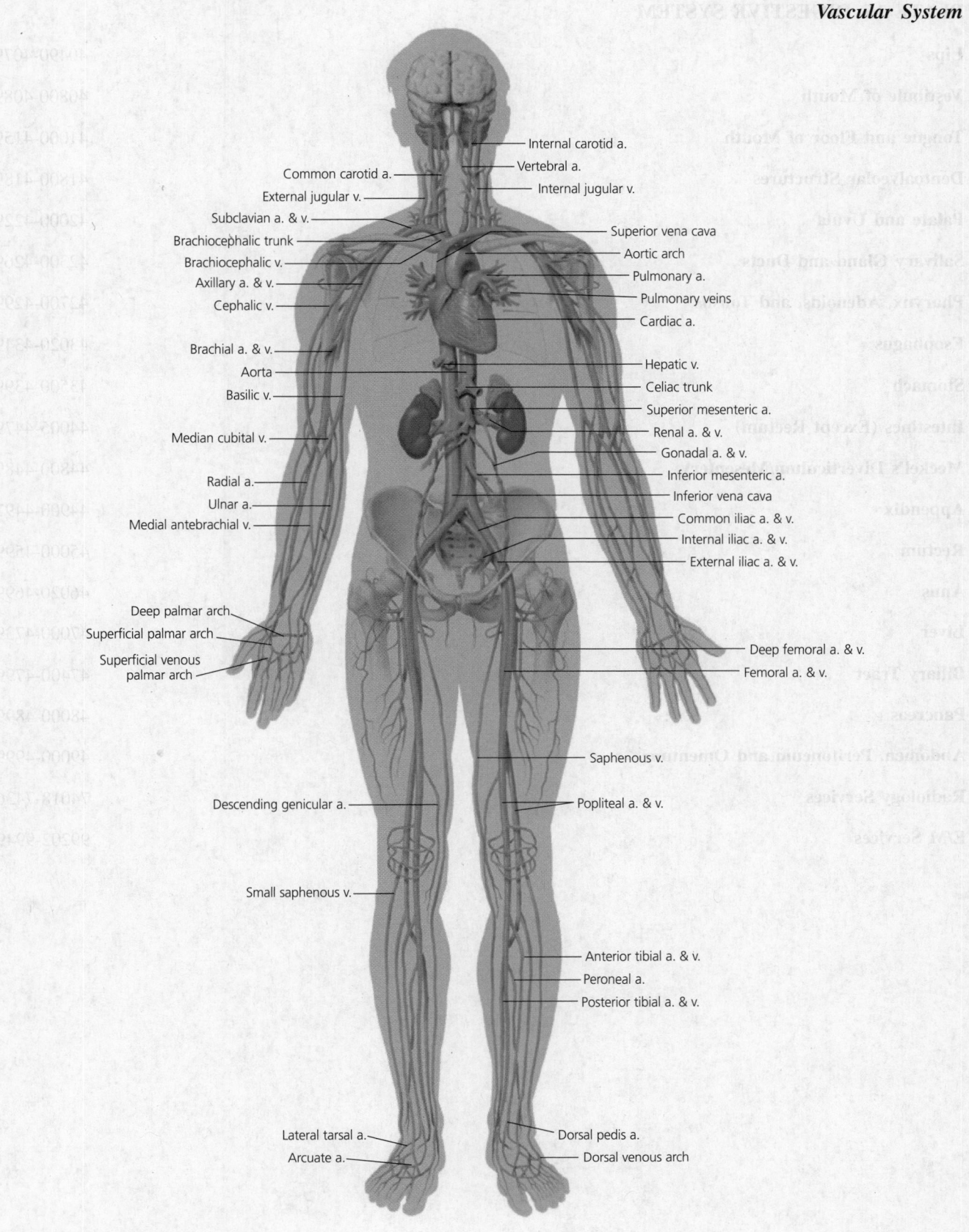

Internal carotid a.
Vertebral a.
Common carotid a.
External jugular v.
Internal jugular v.
Subclavian a. & v.
Brachiocephalic trunk
Brachiocephalic v.
Axillary a. & v.
Cephalic v.
Superior vena cava
Aortic arch
Pulmonary a.
Pulmonary veins
Cardiac a.
Brachial a. & v.
Aorta
Basilic v.
Median cubital v.
Hepatic v.
Celiac trunk
Superior mesenteric a.
Renal a. & v.
Gonadal a. & v.
Inferior mesenteric a.
Inferior vena cava
Common iliac a. & v.
Internal iliac a. & v.
External iliac a. & v.
Radial a.
Ulnar a.
Medial antebrachial v.
Deep palmar arch
Superficial palmar arch
Superficial venous palmar arch
Deep femoral a. & v.
Femoral a. & v.
Saphenous v.
Descending genicular a.
Popliteal a. & v.
Small saphenous v.
Anterior tibial a. & v.
Peroneal a.
Posterior tibial a. & v.
Lateral tarsal a.
Arcuate a.
Dorsal pedis a.
Dorsal venous arch

PLATE 16. DIGESTIVE SYSTEM

Lips	40490-40799
Vestibule of Mouth	40800-40899
Tongue and Floor of Mouth	41000-41599
Dentoalveolar Structures	41800-41899
Palate and Uvula	42000-42299
Salivary Gland and Ducts	42300-42699
Pharynx, Adenoids, and Tonsils	42700-42999
Esophagus	43020-43499
Stomach	43500-43999
Intestines (Except Rectum)	44005-44799
Meckel's Diverticulum/Mesentery	44800-44899
Appendix	44900-44979
Rectum	45000-45999
Anus	46020-46999
Liver	47000-47399
Biliary Tract	47400-47999
Pancreas	48000-48999
Abdomen, Peritoneum and Omentum	49000-49999
Radiology Services	74018-74363
E/M Services	99202-99499

Teeth

Tongue

Epiglottis

Pharynx

Larynx

Esophagus

Liver, left lobe

Stomach

Liver, right lobe

Rugae

Common hepatic duct

Aorta

Cystic duct

Portal vein

Common bile duct

Celiac trunk

Muscularis:
Oblique
Circular
Longitudinal

Pancreas

Superior mesenteric
vein & artery

Free tenia

Circular folds

Iliocecal valve

Semilunar fold

Cecum

Opening of appendix

Appendix

Levator ani muscle

External anal
sphincter muscles

PLATE 17. GENITOURINARY SYSTEM

Kidney
Incision	50010-50135
Excision	50200-50290
Renal Transplantation	50300-50380
Introduction	50382-50396, 50430-50437
Repair	50400-50540
Laparoscopy/Endoscopy	50541-50580
Other	50590-50593

Ureter
Incision	50600-50630
Excision	50650-50660
Introduction	50684-50690
Repair	50700-50940
Laparoscopy/Endoscopy	50945-50980

Bladder
Incision	51020-51080
Removal	51100-51102
Excision	51500-51597
Introduction	51600-51720
Urodynamics	51725-51798
Repair	51800-51980
Laparoscopy	51990-51999

Endoscopy—Cystoscopy—Urethroscopy—Cystourethroscopy   52000-52010

Transurethral Surgery
Urethra and Bladder	52204-52318
Ureter and Pelvis	52320-52356

Vesical Neck and Prostate   52400-52700

Urethra
Incision	53000-53085
Excision	53200-53275
Repair	53400-53520
Manipulation	53600-53665
Other Procedures	53850-53899

Radiology Services   74400-74485

E/M Services   99202-99499

Inferior vena cava

Adrenal gland

Kidney

Renal artery

Renal vein

Renal pelvis

Cortex

Medulla

Fibrous capsule

Major calyx

Minor calyx

Cortex

Renal pyramid

Renal column

Ureter

Abdominal aorta

Right common iliac vein

Right common iliac artery

Left common iliac artery

Left common iliac vein

Urinary bladder

Opening of ureter

Trigone

Urethra

PLATE 18. MALE REPRODUCTIVE SYSTEM

Penis
Incision	54000-54015
Destruction	54050-54065
Excision	54100-54164
Introduction	54200-54250
Repair	54300-54440
Manipulation	54450

Testis
Excision/Exploration	54500-54560
Repair	54600-54680
Laparoscopy	54690-54699

Epididymis
Incision/Excision	54700-54861
Repair	54900-54901

Tunica Vaginalis
Incision/Excision	55000-55041
Repair	55060

Scrotum
Incision/Excision	55100-55150
Repair	55175-55180

Vas Deferens
Incision/Excision	55200, 55250
Introduction	55300
Repair	55400
Suture	55450

Spermatic Cord
Excision	55500-55540
Laparoscopy	55550-55559

Seminal Vesicles
Incision	55600-55605
Excision	55650-55680

Prostate
Incision	55700-55725
Excision	55801-55865
Laparoscopy	55866
Other Procedures	55870-55899

E/M Services 99202-99499

Bladder

Trigone

Prostatic utricle

Prostatic urethra

Prostate

Bulbourethral gland

Membranous urethra

Bulb of penis

Crus of penis

Opening of bulbourethral gland

Corpus cavernosum

Deep artery of penis

Corpus spongiosum

Penile urethra

Corona

Glans penis

Prepuce

Urethral opening

Sigmoid colon

Peritoneum

Ampulla of ductus deferens

Urinary bladder

Seminal vesicle

Pubic symphysis

Ejaculatory duct

Prostate gland

Urogenital diaphragm

Corpus cavernosum

Corpus spongiosum

Urethra

Ductus deferens

Glans of penis

Testis

Epididymis

Rectum

Anus

PLATE 19. FEMALE REPRODUCTIVE SYSTEM

Vulva, Perineum and Introitus
Incision	56405-56442
Destruction	56501-56515
Excision	56605-56740
Repair	56800-56810
Endoscopy	56820, 56821

Vagina
Incision	57000-57023
Destruction	57061-57065
Excision	57100-57135
Introduction	57150-57180
Repair	57200-57335
Manipulation	57400-57415
Endoscopy/Laparoscopy	57420-57426

Cervix Uteri
Endoscopy	57452-57461
Excision	57500-57558
Repair	57700-57720
Manipulation	57800

Corpus Uteri
Excision	58100-58294
Introduction	58300-58356
Repair	58400-58540
Laparoscopy/Hysteroscopy	58541-58579, 58674

Oviduct
Incision	58600-58615
Laparoscopy	58660-58673, 58679
Excision	58700-58720
Repair	58740-58770

Ovary
Incision	58800-58825
Excision	58900-58960

In Vitro Fertilization   58970-58999

Radiology Services   74710-74775

E/M Services   99202-99499

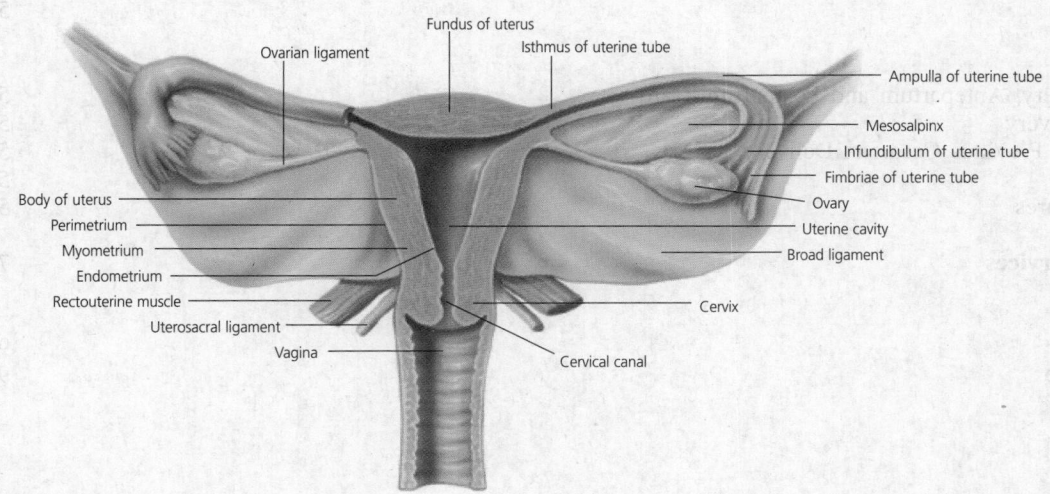

Fundus of uterus

Ovarian ligament

Isthmus of uterine tube

Ampulla of uterine tube

Mesosalpinx

Infundibulum of uterine tube

Fimbriae of uterine tube

Ovary

Uterine cavity

Broad ligament

Body of uterus

Perimetrium

Myometrium

Endometrium

Rectouterine muscle

Uterosacral ligament

Vagina

Cervix

Cervical canal

Sacrum

Sigmoid colon

Rectouterine pouch

Suspensory ligament of ovary

Uterine tube

Ovary

Round ligament of uterus

Uterus

Urinary bladder

Pubic symphysis

Urethra

Clitoris

Cervix

Rectum

Vagina

Anus

Labium minus

Labium majus

Vaginal opening

PLATE 20. PREGNANCY, CHILDBIRTH AND THE PUERPERIUM

Antepartum Services
Antepartum Services   59000-59076
Excision   59100-59160
Introduction   59200
Repair   59300-59350

Delivery
Vaginal Delivery, Antepartum and Postpartum Care   59400-59430
Cesarean Delivery   59510-59525
Delivery after Previous Cesarean Delivery   59610-59622
Abortion   59812-59857
Other Procedures   59866-59899

Radiology Services   74710-74775

E/M Services
E/M Services   99202-99499
Newborn Care   99460-99465

Vertebral column
Intervertebral disks
Spinous processes
Vertebral bodies
Spinal cord
Superior vena cava
Aorta
Pulmonary trunk
Lung
Heart
Right atrium
Inferior vena cava
Diaphragm
Right ventricle
Liver
Stomach
Transverse colon
Pancreas
Placenta
Uterus
Umbilical cord
Small intestine
Sacrum
Rectum
Cervix
Coccyx
Vagina
Bladder
Pubic symphysis
Urethra

PLATE 21. NERVOUS SYSTEM - BRAIN

Skull, Meninges, and Brain

Injection, Drainage, or Aspiration	61000-61070
Twist Drill, Burr Hole(s), or Trephine	61105-61253
Craniectomy or Craniotomy	61304-61576

Surgery of Skull Base Approach Procedures

Anterior Cranial Fossa	61580-61586
Middle Cranial Fossa	61590-61592
Posterior Cranial Fossa	61595-61598

Surgery of Skull Base Definitive Procedures

Base of Anterior Cranial Fossa	61600-61601
Base of Middle Cranial Fossa	61605-61613
Base of Posterior Cranial Fossa	61615-61616

Repair and/or Reconstruction of Surgical Defects of Skull Base	61618-61619
Endovascular Therapy	61623-61651
Surgery for Aneurysm, Arterio-Venous Malformation or Vascular Disease	61680-61711
Stereotaxis	61720-61791
Stereotactic Radiosurgery (Cranial)	61796-61800
Neurostimulators (Intra-Cranial)	61850-61888
Repair	62000-62148
Neuroendoscopy	62160-62165
Cerebrospinal Fluid (CSF) Shunt	62180-62258
Radiology Services	70010-70559
E/M Services	99202-99499

Brain
(Base View)

Cerebrum

Anterior communicating artery

Anterior cerebral artery

Middle cerebral artery

Posterior communicating artery

Posterior cerebral artery

Superior cerebellar artery

Basilar artery

Abducens nerve

Hypoglossal nerve (XII)

Accessory nerve (XI)

Vertebral artery

Anterior spinal artery

Spinal cord

Olfactory bulb

Olfactory tract (I)

Optic nerve (II)

Optic chiasm

Internal carotid artery

Pituitary gland

Oculomotor nerve (III)

Troclear nerve (IV)

Trigeminal nerve (V)

Pons

Abducens nerve (VI)

Facial nerve (VII)

Vestibulocochlear nerve (VIII)

Glossopharyngeal nerve (IX)

Vagus nerve (X)

Anterior inferior cerebellar artery

Medulla oblongata

Cerebellum

Posterior inferior cerebellar artery

PLATE 22. NERVOUS SYSTEM

Spine and Spinal Cord

Injection, Drainage or Aspiration	62263-62327
Catheter, Reservoir and Pump Implantation	62350-62370
Endoscopic Decompression of Neural Elements and/or Excision Herniated Intervertebral Disc	62380
Posterior Extradural Laminotomy or Laminectomy	63001-63051
Transpedicular or Costovertebral Approach for Posterolateral Extradural Exploration/Decompression	63055-63066
Anterior or Anterolateral Approach for Extradural Exploration/Decompression	63075-63091
Lateral Extracavitary Approach for Extradural Exploration/Decompression	63101-63103
Incision	63170-63200
Excision by Laminectomy of Lesion Other Than Herniated Disc	63250-63295
Excision, Anterior or Anterolateral Approach, Intraspinal Lesion	63300-63308
Stereotaxis	63600-63610
Sterotactic Radiosurgery (Spinal)	63620-63621
Neurostimulators (Spinal)	63650-63688
Repair	63700-63710
Shunt, Spinal CSF	63740-63746

Extracranial Nerves, Peripheral Nerves and Autonomic Nervous System

Introduction/Injection of Anesthetic Agent, Diagnostic or Therapeutic	64400-64530
Neurostimulators (Peripheral Nerve)	64553-64595
Destruction by Neurolytic Agent, Chemodenervation	64600-64681

Neuroplasty

	64702-64727

Transection or Avulsion

	64732-64772

Excision

Somatic Nerves	64774-64795
Sympathetic Nerves	64802-64823

Neurorrhaphy

Without Nerve Graft	64831-64876
With Nerve Graft	64885-64913
Other Procedures	64999

E/M Services

	99202-99499

Brain

Cerebrum

Brain stem

Cerebellum

Cervical plexus

Lateral cord

Spinal cord

Medial cord

Brachial plexus

Posterior cord

Phrenic nerve

Musculocutaneous nerve

Intercostal nerves

Ulnar nerve

Median nerve

Subcostal nerve

Radial nerve

Iliohypogastric nerve

Lumbar plexus

Ilioinguinal nerve

Genitofemoral nerve

Deep branch of radial nerve

Sacral plexus

Lateral femoral cutaneous nerve

Coccygeal plexus

Superficial branch of radial nerve

Femoral nerve

Obturator nerve

Pudendal nerve

Sciatic nerve

Muscular branches of femoral nerve

Saphenous nerve

Common peroneal nerve

Deep peroneal nerve

Superficial peroneal nerve

Tibial nerve

PLATE 23. EYE AND OCULAR ADNEXA

Eyeball
Removal of Eye	65091-65114
Secondary Implant(s) Procedures	65125-65175
Removal of Foreign Body	65205-65265
Repair of Laceration	65270-65290

Anterior Segment
Cornea Procedures	65400-65782
Anterior Chamber Procedures	65800-66030
Anterior Sclera Procedures	66130-66250
Iris, Ciliary Body Procedures	66500-66770
Lens Procedures	66820-66940
Intraocular Lens Procedures	66982-66986

Posterior Segment
Vitreous	67005-67043
Retina or Choroid Procedures	67101-67229
Posterior Sclera	67250-67255

Ocular Adnexa   67311-67399

Orbit   67400-67599

Eyelids
Incision/Excision	67700-67850
Tarsorrhaphy	67875-67882
Repair	67900-67924
Reconstruction	67930-67975

Conjunctiva
Incision and Drainage	68020-68040
Excision and/or Destruction	68100-68135
Injection	68200
Conjunctivoplasty	68320-68340

Lacrimal System
Incision/Excision	68400-68550
Repair	68700-68770
Probing and/or Related Procedures	68801-68850

E/M Services   99202-99499

Ophthalmological Services   92002-92287

Contact Lens, Prosthetics and Spectacles   92310-92499

Lateral rectus muscle

Conjunctiva

Canal of Schlemm

Zonular fibers

Iris

Lens

Cornea

Pupil

Aqueous humor

Anterior chamber

Posterior chamber

Ciliary body

Sclera

Ora serrata

Choroid

Medial rectus muscle

Vitreous body

Hyaloid canal

Macula lutea

Optic disc

Retinal vessels

Optic nerve

Nerve sheath

Retina

PLATE 24. AUDITORY SYSTEM

External Ear
Incision	69000-69090
Excision	69100-69155
Removal of Foreign Body	69200-69222
Repair	69300-69320
Other Procedures	69399

Middle Ear
Incision	69420-69450
Excision	69501-69554
Repair	69601-69676
Other Procedures	69700-69799

Inner Ear
Incision and/or Destruction	69801-69806
Excision	69905-69915
Introduction	69930
Other Procedures	69949

Temporal Bone, Middle Fossa Approach
69950-69979

Visit and Medicine Services
Vestibular Function Tests	92531-92548
Audiologic Function Tests	92550-92597
E/M Services	99202-99499

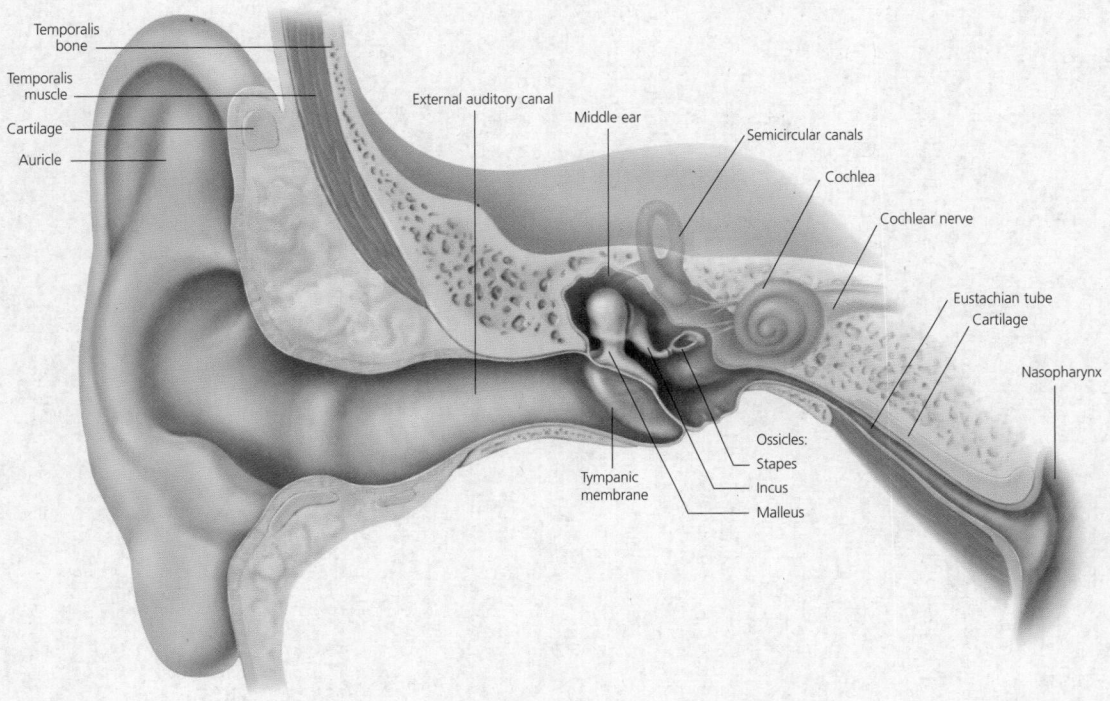

Temporalis bone

Temporalis muscle

Cartilage

Auricle

External auditory canal

Middle ear

Semicircular canals

Cochlea

Cochlear nerve

Eustachian tube

Cartilage

Nasopharynx

Ossicles:

Stapes

Incus

Malleus

Tympanic membrane

This page intentionally left blank.

EVALUATION & MANAGEMENT GUIDELINES

EVALUATION AND MANAGEMENT (E/M) SERVICES OVERVIEW

The first section of the CPT coding system is the evaluation and management (E/M) section, which includes procedure codes for visits and special care services. Within each subsection, the CPT codes are arranged first by patient category, then by the level of service.

The evaluation and management section of the CPT coding system includes codes for reporting visits, consultations, prolonged service, case management services, preventive medicine services, newborn care, and special services. The section is divided into categories such as office visits, hospital visits and consultations. Most of the categories are further divided into two or more subcategories.

The subcategories for evaluation and management services are further classified into levels of service that are identified by specific codes. The level of service classification is important because the physician work required to provide the service varies by the type of service, the place of service, and the patient's clinical status.

The basic format of the evaluation and management service codes and definitions is the same for most categories.

- *A unique five-digit CPT code number is listed*
- *The place and/or type of service is specified, for example "office consultation"*
- *The content of the service is defined, eg. "comprehensive history and comprehensive examination"*
- *The nature of the presenting problem(s) usually associated with a given level is described.*
- *The time typically required to provide the service is specified.*

EVALUATION AND MANAGEMENT SERVICES SUBSECTIONS

The Evaluation and Management section of the CPT book is divided into the following subsections:

Office or Other Outpatient Services	
New Patient	99202-99205
Established Patient	99211-99215
Hospital Observation Services	
Observation Care Discharge Services	99217
Initial Observation Care	99218-99220
Susbequent Observation Care	99224-99226
Hospital Inpatient Services	
Initial Hospital Care	99221-99223
Subsequent Hospital Care	99231-99233
Observation or Inpatient Care (including admission and discharge) Services	99234-99236
Hospital Discharge Services	99238-99239
Consultations	
Office or Other Outpatient Consultations	99241-99245
Inpatient Consultation	99251-99255
Emergency Department Services	99281-99288
Critical Care Services, Adult	99291-99292
Nursing Facility Services	
Initial Nursing Facility Care	99304-99306
Subsequent Nursing Facility Care	99307-99310
Nursing Facility Discharge Services	99315-99316
Other Nursing Facility Services	99318
Domiciliary, Rest Home, or Custodial Care Services	
New Patient	99324-99328
Established Patient	99334-99337
Domiciliary, Rest Home, or Home Care Plan Oversight	99339-99340

Home Services
    New Patient   99341-99345
    Established Patient   99347-99350
Prolonged Services
    With Direct Patient Contact   99354-99357
    Without Direct Patient Contact   99358-99359
    With Physician Supervision   99415, 99416
    Standby Services   99360
Case Management Services
    Medical Team Conferences   99366-99368
Care Plan Oversight Services   99374-99380
Preventive Medicine Services
    New Patient   99381-99387
    Established Patient   99391-99397
    Counseling Risk Factor Reduction and Behavior Change Intervention   99401-99429
Non Face-to-Face Physician Services
    Telephone Services   99441-99443
    Online Digital Evaluation and Management Services   99421-99423
    Interprofessional Telephone/Internet/Electronic Health Record Consultation   99446-99449, 99451, 99452
    Digitally Stored Data Services/Remote Physiologic Monitoring   99453-99454, 99091, 99473, 99474
    Remote Physiologic Monitoring Treatment Management Services   99457-99458
Special Evaluation and Management Services   99450-99456
Newborn Care Services   99460-99463
Delivery/Birthing Room Attendance and Resuscitation Services   99464-99465
Inpatient Neonatal Intensive Care Services and Pediatric and Neonatal Critical Care Services   99466-99486
Cognitive Assessment and Care Plan Services   99483
Care Management Services
    Chronic Care Management   99490-99491
    Complex Chronic Care Management   99487-99489
Psychiatric Collaborative Care Management Services   99492-99494
Transitional Care Management Services   99495-99496
Advance Care Planning   99497-99498
General Behavioral Health Integration Care Management   99484
Other Evaluation and Management Services   99499

All of these subsections have extensive notes that should be reviewed carefully prior to selecting codes for services located within the section.

E/M GUIDELINES OVERVIEW

The E/M guidelines have sections that are common to all E/M categories and sections that are category specific. Most of the categories and many of the subcategories of service have special guidelines or instructions unique to that category or subcategory. Where these are indicated, eg, "Inpatient Hospital Care," special instructions are presented before the listing of the specific E/M services codes. It is important to review the instructions for each category or subcategory. These guidelines are to be used by the reporting physician or other qualified health care professional to select the appropriate level of service. These guidelines do not establish documentation requirements or standards of care. The main purpose of documentation is to support care of the patient by current and future health care team(s).

There are two sets of guidelines: one for office or other outpatient services and another for the remaining E/M services. There are sections that are common to both (ie, Guidelines in Common). These guidelines are presented as Guidelines Common to all E/M Services, Guidelines for E/M Services (Hospital Observation, Hospital Inpatient, Consultations, Emergency Department, Nursing Facility, Domiciliary, Rest Home or Custodial Care, Home) and Guidelines for Office or Other Outpatient Services.

The main differences between the two sets of guidelines is that the office or other outpatient services use medical decision making (MDM) or time as the basis for selecting a code level, whereas the other E/M codes use history, examination, and MDM and only use time when counseling and/or coordination of care dominates the service. The definitions of time are different for different categories of services.

Summary of Guideline Differences		
Component(s) for Code Selection	Office or Other Outpatient Srevices	Other E/M Services (Hospital Observation, Hospital Inpatient, Consultations, Emergency Department, Nursing Facility, Domiciliary, Rest Home, or Custodial Care Home)
History and Examination	• As medically appropriate. • Not used in code selection	• Use key components (history, examination, MDM)
Medical Decision Making (MDM)	• May use MDM or total time on the date of the encounter.	• Use key components (history, examination, MDM)
Time	• May use MDM or total time on the date of the encounter.	• May use face-to-face or time at the bedside and on the patient's floor or unit when counseling and/or coordination of care dominates the service. • *Time is NOT a descriptive component for the emergency department levels of E/M services.*
MDM Elements	• Number and complexity of problems addresses at the encounter. • Amount and/or complexity of data to be reviewed and analyzed. • Rish of complications and/or morbidity or mortality of patient management.	• Number of diagnoses or management options. • Amount and/or complexity of data to be reviewed. • Risk of complications and/or morbidity or mortality.

CLASSIFICATION OF EVALUATION AND MANAGEMENT SERVICES

The E/M section is divided into broad categories such as office visits, hospital visits, and consultations. Most of the categories are further divided into two or more subcategories of E/M services. For example, there are two subcategories of office visits (new patient and established patient) and there are two subcategories of hospital visits (initial and subsequent). The subcategories of E/M services are further classified into levels of E/M services that are identified by specific codes.

The basic format of the levels of E/M services is the same for most categories. First, a unique code number is listed. Second, the place and/or type of service is specified, eg, office consultation. Third, the content of the service is defined. Fourth, time is specified. (A detailed discussion of time is provided following the Decision Tree for New vs Established Patients.)

DEFINITIONS OF COMMONLY USED TERMS

Certain key words and phrases are used throughout the E/M section. The following definitions are intended to reduce the potential for differing interpretations and to increase the consistency of reporting by physicians and other qualified health care professionals. The definitions in the E/M section are provided solely for the basis of code selection.

Some definitions are common to all categories of services and others are specific to one or more categories only.

GUIDELINES COMMON TO ALL E/M SERVICES

LEVELS OF E/M SERVICES

Within each category or subcategory of E/M service,there are three to five levels of E/M services available for reporting purposes. Levels of E/M services are not interchangeable among the different categories or subcategories of service. For example, the first level of E/M services in the subcategory of office visit, new patient, does not have the same definition as the first level of E/M services in the subcategory of office visit, established patient. Each level of E/M services may be used by all physicians or other qualified health care professionals.

NEW AND ESTABLISHED PATIENTS

Solely for the purposes of distinguishing between new and established patients, professional services are those face-to-face services rendered by physicians and other qualified health care professionals who may report evaluation and management services reported by a specific CPT code(s). A new patient is one who has not received any professional services from the physician/qualified health care professional or another physician/qualified health care professional of the exact same specialty and subspecialty who belongs to the same group practice, within the past three years.

Decision Tree for New vs Established Patients

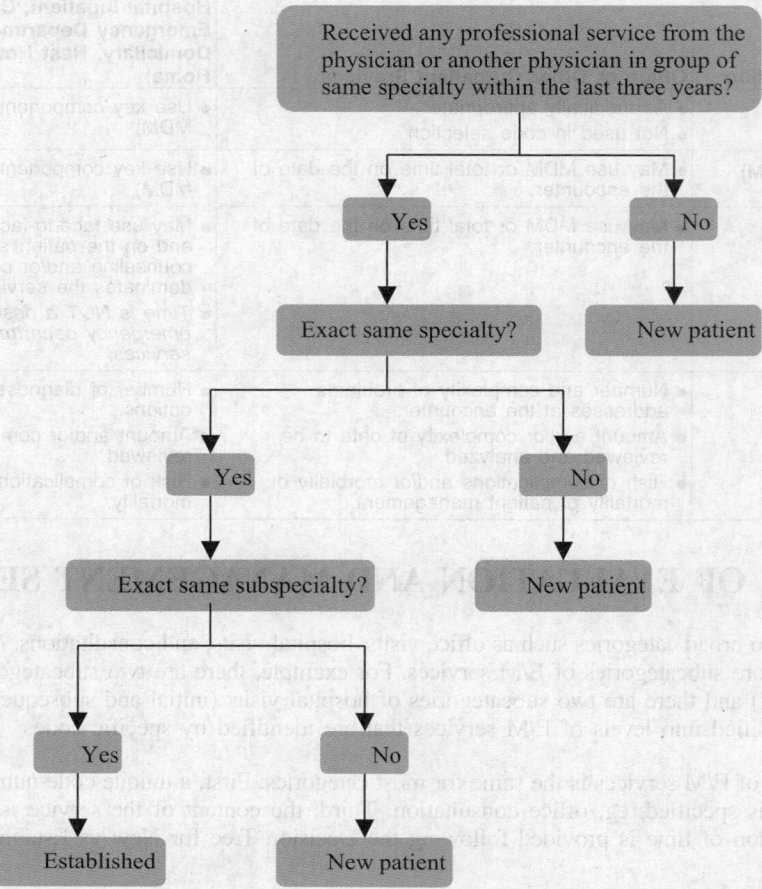

An established patient is one who has received professional services from the physician/qualified health care professional or another physician/qualified health care professional of the exact same specialty and subspecialty who belongs to the same group practice, within the past three years. See Decision Tree.

In the instance where a physician/qualified health care professional is on call for or covering for another physician/qualified health care professional, the patient's encounter will be classified as it would have been by the physician/qualified health care professional who is not available. When advanced practice nurses and physician assistants are working with physicians, they are considered as working in the exact same specialty and exact same subspecialties as the physician

No distinction is made between new and established patients in the emergency department. Evaluation and Management services in the emergency department category may be coded for any new or established patient who presents for treatment in the emergency department.

The decision tree above is provided to aid in determining whether to report the E/M service provided as a new or as an established patient encounter.

TIME

The inclusion of time in the definitions of levels of E/M services has been implicit in prior editions of the CPT codebook. The inclusion of time as an explicit factor beginning in CPT 1992 was done to assist in selecting the most appropriate level of E/M services. Beginning with CPT 2021, except for 99211, time alone may be used to select the appropriate code level for the office or other outpatient E/M services codes (99202, 99203, 99204, 99205, 99212, 99213, 99214, 99215). Different categories of services use time differently. It is important to review the instructions for each category.

Time is **not** a descriptive component for the emergency department levels of E/M services because emergency department services are typically provided on a variable intensity basis, often involving multiple encounters with several patients over an extended period of time. Therefore, it is often difficult to provide accurate estimates of the time spent face-to-face with the patient.

Time may be used to select a code level in office or other outpatient services whether or not counseling and/or coordination of care dominates the service. Time may only be used for selecting the level of the other E/M services when counseling and/or coordination of care dominates the service.

When time is used for reporting E/M services codes, the time defined in the service descriptors is used for selecting the appropriate level of services. The E/M services for which these guidelines apply require a face-to-face encounter with the physician or other qualified health care professional. For office or other outpatient services, if the physician's or other qualified health care professional's time is spent in the supervision of clinical staff who perform the face-to-face services of the encounter, use 99211.

A shared or split visit is defined as a visit in which a physician and other qualified health care professional(s) jointly provide the face-to-face and non-face-to-face work related to the visit. When time is being used to select the appropriate level of services for which time-based reporting of shared or split visits is allowed, the time personally spent by the physician and other qualified health care professional(s) assessing and managing the patient on the date of the encounter is summed to define total time. Only distinct time should be summed for shared or split visits (ie, when two or more individuals jointly meet with or discuss the patient, only the time of one individual should be counted).

When prolonged time occurs, the appropriate prolonged services code may be reported. The appropriate time should be documented in the medical record when it is used as the basis for code selection.

Face-to-face time (outpatient consultations [99241, 99242, 99243, 99244, 99245], domiciliary, rest home, or custodial services [99324, 99325, 99326, 99327, 99328, 99334, 99335, 99336, 99337], home services [99341, 99342, 99343, 99344, 99345, 99347, 99348, 99349, 99350], cognitive assessment and care plan services [99483]): For coding purposes, face-to-face time for these services is defined as only that time spent face-to-face with the patient and/or family. This includes the time spent performing such tasks as obtaining a history, examination, and counseling the patient.

Unit/floor time (hospital observation services [99218, 99219, 99220, 99224, 99225, 99226, 99234, 99235, 99236], hospital inpatient services [99221, 99222, 99223, 99231, 99232, 99233], inpatient consultations [99251, 99252, 99253, 99254, 99255], nursing facility services [99304, 99305, 99306, 99307, 99308, 99309, 99310, 99315, 99316, 99318]): For coding purposes, time for these services is defined as unit/floor time, which includes the time present on the patient's hospital unit and at the bedside rendering services for that patient. This includes the time to establish and/or review the patient's chart, examine the patient, write notes, and communicate with other professionals and the patient's family.

Total time on the date of the encounter (office or other outpatient services [99202, 99203, 99204, 99205, 99212, 99213, 99214, 99215]): For coding purposes, time for these services is the total time on the date of the encounter. It includes both the face-to-face and non-face-to-face time personally spent by the physician and/or other qualified health care professional(s) on the day of the encounter (includes time in activities that require the physician or other qualified health care professional and does not include time in activities normally performed by clinical staff).

Physician/other qualified health care professional time includes the following activities, when performed:

- preparing to see the patient (eg, review of tests)
- obtaining and/or reviewing separately obtained history
- performing a medically appropriate examination and/or evaluation
- counseling and educating the patient/family/caregiver
- ordering medications, tests, or procedures
- referring and communicating with other health care professionals (when not separately reported)
- documenting clinical information in the electronic or other health record
- independently interpreting results (not separately reported) and communicating results to the patient/ family/caregiver
- care coordination (not separately reported)

CONCURRENT CARE AND TRANSFER OF CARE

Concurrent care is the provision of similar services (eg, hospital visits) to the same patient by more than one physician or other qualified health care professional on the same day. When concurrent care is provided, no special reporting is required. Transfer of care is the process whereby a physician or other qualified health care professional who is providing management for some or all of a patient's problems relinquishes this responsibility to another physician or other qualified health care professional who explicitly agrees to accept this responsibility and who, from the initial encounter, is not providing consultative services. The physician or other qualified health care professional transferring care is then no longer providing care for these problems though he or she may continue providing care for other conditions when appropriate. Consultation codes should not be reported by the physician or other qualified health care professional who has agreed to accept transfer of care before an initial evaluation but are appropriate to report if the decision to accept transfer of care cannot be made until after the initial consultation evaluation, regardless of site of service.

COUNSELING

Counseling is a discussion with a patient and/or family concerning one or more of the following areas:

- Diagnostic results, impressions, and/or recommended diagnostic studies;

- Prognosis;

- Risks and benefits of management (treatment) options;

- Instructions for management (treatment) and/or follow-up;

- Importance of compliance with chosen management (treatment) options;

- Risk factor reduction; and

- Patient and family education. (Psychotherapy, see 90832-90834,90836-90840)

SERVICES REPORTED SEPARATELY

Any specifically identifiable procedure or service (ie, identified with a specific CPT code) performed on the date of E/M services may be reported separately. The actual performance and/or interpretation of diagnostic tests/studies during a patient encounter are not included in determining the levels of E/M services when reported separately. Physician performance of diagnostic tests/studies for which specific CPT codes are available may be reported separately, in addition to the appropriate E/M code. The physician's interpretation of the results of diagnostic tests/studies (ie, professional component) with preparation of a separate distinctly identifiable signed written report may also be reported separately, using the appropriate CPT code and, if required, with modifier 26 appended. If a test/study is independently interpreted in order to manage the patient as part of the E/M service, but is not separately reported, it is part of MDM.

The physician or other qualified health care professional may need to indicate that on the day a procedure or service identified by a CPT code was performed, the patient's condition required a significant separately identifiable E/M service. The E/M service may be caused or prompted by the symptoms or condition for which the procedure and/or service was provided. This circumstance may be reported by adding modifier 25 to the appropriate level of E/M service. As such, different diagnoses are not required for reporting of the procedure and the E/M services on the same date.

GUIDELINES FOR HOSPITAL OBSERVATION, HOSPITAL INPATIENT, CONSULTATIONS, EMERGENCY DEPARTMENT, NURSING FACILITY, DOMICILIARY, REST HOME OR CUSTODIAL CARE, AND HOME E/M SERVICES

LEVELS OF E/M SERVICES

The descriptors for the levels of evaluation and management services recognize seven components, six of which are used in defining the levels of evaluation and management services. These components are:

- History;

- Examination;

- Medical decision making;

- Counseling;

- Coordination of care;

- Nature of presenting problem; and

- TIme.

The first three of these components (history, examination, and medical decision making) are considered the **key** components in selecting a level of evaluation and management services. (See "Determine the Extent of History Obtained")

The next three components (counseling, coordination of care, and the nature of the presenting problem) are considered **contributory** factors in the majority of encounters. Although the first two of these contributory factors are important evaluation and management services, it is not required that these services be provided at every patient encounter.

Coordination of care with other physicians, other health care professionals, or agencies without a patient encounter on that day is coded using the case management codes.

The final component, time, is discussed in detail following the Decision Tree for New vs Established Patients.

CHIEF COMPLAINT

A chief complaint is a concise statement describing the symptom, problem, condition, diagnosis or other factor that is the reason for the encounter, usually stated in the patient's words.

HISTORY OF PRESENT ILLNESS

A chronological description of the development of the patient's present illness from the first sign and/or symptom to the present. This includes a description of location, quality, severity, timing, context, modifying factors and associated signs and symptoms significantly related to the presenting problem(s).

NATURE OF PRESENTING PROBLEM

A presenting problem is a disease, condition, illness, injury, symptom, sign, finding, complaint, or other reason for encounter, with or without a diagnosis being established at the time of the encounter. The evaluation and management codes recognize five types of presenting problems that are defined as follows:

Minimal: a problem that may not require the presence of the physician or other qualified health care professional, but service is provided under the physician's or other qualified health care professional's supervision.

Self-limited or minor: a problem that runs a definite and prescribed course, is transient in nature, and is not likely to permanently alter health status.

Low severity: a problem where the risk of morbidity without treatment is low; there is little to no risk of mortality without treatment; full recovery without functional impairment is expected.

Moderate severity: a problem where the risk of morbidity without treatment is moderate; there is moderate risk of mortality without treatment; uncertain prognosis OR increased probability of prolonged functional impairment.

High severity: a problem where the risk of morbidity without treatment is high to extreme; there is a moderate to high risk of mortality without treatment OR high probability of severe, prolonged functional impairment.

PAST HISTORY

A review of the patient's past experiences with illnesses, injuries, and treatments that includes significant information about:

- Prior major illnesses and injuries;
- Prior operations;
- Prior hospitalizations;
- Current medications;
- Allergies (eg, drug, food);
- Age appropriate immunization status;
- Age appropriate feeding/dietary status.

FAMILY HISTORY

A review of medical events in the patient's family that includes significant information about:

- The health status or cause of death of parents, siblings, and children;
- Specific diseases related to problems identified in the Chief Complaint or History of the Present Illness, and/or System Review;
- Diseases of family members which may be hereditary or place the patient at risk.

SOCIAL HISTORY

An age appropriate review of past and current activities that includes significant information about:

- Marital status and/or living arrangements;
- Current employment;
- Occupational history;
- Military history;
- Use of drugs, alcohol, and tobacco;
- Level of education;
- Sexual history;
- Other relevant social factors

SYSTEM REVIEW (REVIEW OF SYSTEMS)

An inventory of body systems obtained through a series of questions seeking to identify signs and/or symptoms that the patient may be experiencing or has experienced. For the purposes of the CPT codebook, the following elements of a system review have been identified:

- Constitutional symptoms (fever, weight loss, etc.)
- Eyes
- Ears, nose, mouth, throat
- Cardiovascular
- Respiratory
- Gastrointestinal
- Genitourinary
- Musculoskeletal
- Integumentary (skin and/or breast)
- Neurological
- Psychiatric
- Endocrine
- Hematologic/lymphatic
- Allergic/immunologic

The review of systems helps define the problem, clarify the differential diagnosis, identify needed testing, or serves as baseline data on other systems that might be affected by any possible management options.

INSTRUCTIONS FOR SELECTING A LEVEL OF E/M SERVICE FOR HOSPITAL OBSERVATION, HOSPITAL INPATIENT, CONSULTATIONS, EMERGENCY DEPARTMENT, NURSING FACILITY, DOMICILIARY, REST HOME, OR CUSTODIAL CARE, AND HOME E/M SERVICES

REVIEW THE LEVEL OF E/M SERVICE DESCRIPTORS AND EXAMPLES IN THE SELECTED CATEGORY OR SUBCATEGORY

The descriptors for the levels of evaluation and management services recognize seven components, six of which are used in defining the levels of evaluation and management services. These components are:

- History;
- Examination;
- Medical decision making;
- Counseling;
- Coordination of care;
- Nature of presenting problem; and
- Time.

The first three of these components (ie, history, examination, and medical decision making) should be considered the **key** components in selecting the level of E/M services. An exception to this rule is in the case of visits that consist predominantly of counseling or coordination of care.

The nature of the presenting problem and time are provided in some levels to assist the physician in determining the appropriate level of E/M service.

DETERMINE THE EXTENT OF HISTORY OBTAINED

The extent of the history is dependent upon clinical judgment and on the nature of presenting problems(s). The levels of evaluation and management services recognize four types of history that are defined as follows:

Problem focused: chief complaint; brief history of present illness or problem.

Expanded problem focused: chief complaint; brief history of present illness; problem pertinent system review.

Detailed: chief complaint; extended history of present illness; problem pertinent system review extended to include a review of a limited number of additional systems; **pertinent** past, family, and/or social history **directly related to the patient's problems**.

Comprehensive: chief complaint; extended history of present illness; review of systems which is directly related to the problem(s) identified in the history of the present illness plus a review of all additional body systems; **complete** past, family, and social history.

The comprehensive history obtained as part of the preventive medicine evaluation and management service is not problem-oriented and does not involve a chief complaint or present illness. It does, however, include a comprehensive system review and comprehensive or interval past, family, and social history as well as a comprehensive assessment/history of pertinent risk factors.

DETERMINE THE EXTENT OF EXAMINATION PERFORMED

The extent of the examination performed is dependent on clinical judgment and on the nature of the presenting problem(s). The levels of evaluation and management services recognize four types of examination that are defined as follows:

Problem focused: a limited examination of the affected body area or organ system.

Expanded problem focused: a limited examination of the affected body area or organ system and other symptomatic or related organ system(s).

Detailed: an extended examination of the affected body area(s) and other symptomatic or related organ system(s).

Comprehensive: a general multi-system examination or a complete examination of a single organ system. **Note**: the comprehensive examination performed as part of the preventive medicine evaluation and management service is multisystem, but its extent is based on age and risk factors identified.

For the purposes of these CPT definitions, the following body areas are recognized:

- Head, including the face
- Neck
- Chest, including breasts and axilla
- Abdomen
- Genitalia, groin, buttocks
- Back
- Each extremity

For the purposes of these CPT definitions, the following organ systems are recognized:

- Eyes
- Ears, nose, mouth, and throat
- Cardiovascular
- Respiratory
- Gastrointestinal
- Genitourinary
- Musculoskeletal
- Skin
- Neurologic
- Psychiatric
- Hematologic/lymphatic/immunologic

DETERMINE COMPLEXITY OF MEDICAL DECISION MAKING

Medical decision making refers to the complexity of establishing a diagnosis and/or selecting a management option as measured by:

- The number of possible diagnoses and/or the number of management options that must be considered;
- The amount and/or complexity of medical records, diagnostic tests, and/or other information that must be obtained, reviewed, and analyzed; and
- The risk of significant complications, morbidity, and/or mortality, as well as comorbidities, associated with the patient's presenting problems(s), the diagnostic procedure(s) and/or the possible management options.

Four types of medical decision making are recognized: straightforward; low complexity; moderate complexity; and high complexity. To qualify for a given type of decision making, two of the three elements in Table 1 must be met or exceeded.

Comorbidities/underlying diseases, in and of themselves, are not considered in selecting a level of evaluation and management services unless their presence significantly increases the complexity of the medical decision making.

Table 1: Complexity of Medical Decision Making

Number of diagnoses or management options	Amount and/or complexity of data to be reviewed	Risk of complications and/or morbidity or mortality	Type of decision making
Minimal	Minimal or none	Minimal	**Straightforward**
Limited	Limited	Low	**Low complexity**
Multiple	Moderate	Moderate	**Moderate complexity**
Extensive	Extensive	High	**High complexity**

SELECT THE APPROPRIATE LEVEL OF EVALUATION AND MANAGEMENT SERVICES BASED ON THE FOLLOWING

1. For the following categories/subcategories, **all of the key components**, (ie, history, examination, and medical decision making), must meet or exceed the stated requirements to qualify for a particular level of E/M service: initial observation care; initial hospital care; observation or inpatient hospital care (including admission and discharge services); office or other outpatient consultations; inpatient consultations;.emergency department services; initial nursing facility care; other nursing facility services; domiciliary care, new patient; and home services, new patient.

2. For the following categories/subcategories, **two of the three key components** (ie, history, examination, and medical decision making) must meet or exceed the stated requirements to qualify for a particular level of E/M services: subsequent observation care; subsequent hospital care; subsequent nursing facility care; domiciliary care, established patient; and home services, established patient.

3. When counseling and/or coordination of care dominates (more than 50%) the encounter with the patient and/or family (face-to-face time in the office or other outpatient setting or floor/unit time in the hospital or nursing facility), then **time** shall be considered the key or controlling factor to qualify for a particular level of E/M services. This includes time spent with parties who have assumed responsibility for the care of the patient or decision making whether or not they are family members (eg, foster parents, person acting in locum parentis, legal guardian). The extent of counseling and/or coordination of care must be documented in the medical record.

GUIDELINES FOR OFFICE OR OTHER OUTPATIENT E/M SERVICES

HISTORY AND/OR EXAMINATION

Office or other outpatient services include a medically appropriate history and/or physical examination, when performed. The nature and extent of the history and/or physical examination are determined by the treating physician or other qualified health care professional reporting the service. The care team may collect information and the patient or caregiver may supply information directly (eg, by electronic health record [EHR] portal or questionnaire) that is reviewed by the reporting physician or other qualified health care professional. The extent of history and physical examination is not an element in selection of the level of office or other outpatient codes.

NUMBER AND COMPLEXITY OF PROBLEMS ADDRESSED AT THE ENCOUNTER

One element used in selecting the level of office or other outpatient services is the number and complexity of the problems that are addressed at an encounter. Multiple new or established conditions may be addressed at the same time and may affect MDM. Symptoms may cluster around a specific diagnosis and each symptom is not necessarily a unique condition. Comorbidities/underlying diseases, in and of themselves, are not considered in selecting a level of E/M services unless they are addressed, and their presence increases the amount and/or complexity of data to be reviewed and analyzed or the risk of complications and/or morbidity or mortality of patient management. The final diagnosis for a condition does not, in and of itself, determine the complexity or risk, as extensive evaluation may be required to reach the conclusion that the signs or symptoms do not represent a highly morbid condition. Multiple problems of a lower severity may, in the aggregate, create higher risk due to interaction.

Definitions for the elements of MDM (see Table 3, Levels of Medical Decision Making) for other office or other outpatient services are:

Problem: A problem is a disease, condition, illness, injury, symptom, sign, finding, complaint, or other matter addressed at the encounter, with or without a diagnosis being established at the time of the encounter.

Problem addressed: A problem is addressed or managed when it is evaluated or treated at the encounter by the physician or other qualified health care professional reporting the service. This includes consideration of further testing or treatment that may not be elected by virtue of risk/benefit analysis or patient/parent/guardian/ surrogate choice. Notation in the patient's medical record that another professional is managing the problem without additional assessment or care coordination documented does not qualify as being addressed or managed by the physician or other qualified health care professional reporting the service. Referral without evaluation (by history, examination, or diagnostic study[ies]) or consideration of treatment does not qualify as being addressed or managed by the physician or other qualified health care professional reporting the service.

Minimal problem: A problem that may not require the presence of the physician or other qualified health care professional, but the service is provided under the physician's or other qualified health care professional's supervision (see 99211).

Self-limited or minor problem: A problem that runs a definite and prescribed course, is transient in nature, and is not likely to permanently alter health status.

Stable, chronic illness: A problem with an expected duration of at least one year or until the death of the patient. For the purpose of defining chronicity, conditions are treated as chronic whether or not stage or severity changes (eg, uncontrolled diabetes and controlled diabetes are a single chronic condition). "Stable" for the purposes of categorizing MDM is defined by the specific treatment goals for an individual patient. A patient who is not at his or her treatment goal is not stable, even if the condition has not changed and there is no short-term threat to life or function. For example, in a patient with persistently poorly controlled blood pressure for whom better control is a goal is not stable, even if the pressures are not changing and the patient is asymptomatic, the risk of morbidity without treatment is significant. Examples may include well-controlled hypertension, non-insulin-dependent diabetes, cataract, or benign prostatic hyperplasia.

Acute, uncomplicated illness or injury: A recent or new short-term problem with low risk of morbidity for which treatment is considered. There is little to no risk of mortality with treatment, and full recovery without functional impairment is expected. A problem that is normally self-limited or minor but is not resolving consistent with a definite and prescribed course is an acute, uncomplicated illness. Examples may include cystitis, allergic rhinitis, or a simple sprain.

Chronic illness with exacerbation, progression, or side effects of treatment: A chronic illness that is acutely worsening, poorly controlled, or progressing with an intent to control progression and requiring additional supportive care or requiring attention to treatment for side effects but that does not require consideration of hospital level of care.

Undiagnosed new problem with uncertain prognosis: A problem in the differential diagnosis that represents a condition likely to result in a high risk of morbidity without treatment. An example may be a lump in the breast.

Acute illness with systemic symptoms: An illness that causes systemic symptoms and has a high risk of morbidity without treatment. For systemic general symptoms, such as fever, body aches, or fatigue in a minor illness that may be treated to alleviate symptoms, shorten the course of illness, or to prevent complications, see the definitions for self-limited or minor problem or acute, uncomplicated illness or injury. Systemic symptoms may not be general but may be single system. Examples may include pyelonephritis, pneumonitis, or colitis.

Acute, complicated injury: An injury which requires treatment that includes evaluation of body systems that are not directly part of the injured organ, the injury is extensive, or the treatment options are multiple and/or associated with risk of morbidity. An example may be a head injury with brief loss of consciousness.

Chronic illness with severe exacerbation, progression, or side effects of treatment: The severe exacerbation or progression of a chronic illness or severe side effects of treatment that have significant risk of morbidity and may require hospital level of care.

Acute or chronic illness or injury that poses a threat to life or bodily function: An acute illness with systemic symptoms, an acute complicated injury, or a chronic illness or injury with exacerbation and/or progression or side effects of treatment, that poses a threat to life or bodily function in the near term without treatment. Examples may include acute myocardial infarction, pulmonary embolus, severe respiratory distress, progressive severe rheumatoid arthritis, psychiatric illness with potential threat to self or others, peritonitis, acute renal failure, or an abrupt change in neurologic status.

Test: Tests are imaging, laboratory, psychometric, or physiologic data. A clinical laboratory panel (eg, basic metabolic panel [80047]) is a single test. The differentiation between single or multiple unique tests is defined in accordance with the CPT code set.

External: External records, communications and/or test results are from an external physician, other qualified health care professional, facility, or health care organization.

External physician or other qualified health care professional: An external physician or other qualified health care professional who is not in the same group practice or is of a different specialty or subspecialty. This includes licensed professionals who are practicing independently. The individual may also be a facility or organizational provider such as from a hospital, nursing facility, or home health care agency.

Independent historian(s): An individual (eg, parent, guardian, surrogate, spouse, witness) who provides a history in addition to a history provided by the patient who is unable to provide a complete or reliable history (eg, due to developmental stage, dementia, or psychosis) or because a confirmatory history is judged to be necessary. In the case where there may be conflict or poor communication between multiple historians and more than one historian is needed, the independent historian requirement is met.

Independent interpretation: The interpretation of a test for which there is a CPT code and an interpretation or report is customary. This does not apply when the physician or other qualified health care professional is reporting the service or has previously reported the service for the patient. A form of interpretation should be documented but need not conform to the usual standards of a complete report for the test.

Appropriate source: For the purpose of the discussion of management data element (see Table 3, Levels of Medical Decision Making), an appropriate source includes professionals who are not health care professionals but may be involved in the management of the patient (eg, lawyer, parole officer, case manager, teacher). It does not include discussion with family or informal caregivers.

Risk: The probability and/or consequences of an event. The assessment of the level of risk is affected by the nature of the event under consideration. For example, a low probability of death may be high risk, whereas a high chance of a minor, self-limited adverse effect of treatment may be low risk. Definitions of risk are based upon the usual behavior and thought processes of a physician or other qualified health care professional in the same specialty. Trained clinicians apply common language usage meanings to terms such as high, medium, low, or minimal risk and do not require quantification for these definitions (though quantification may be provided when evidence-based medicine has established probabilities). For the purposes of MDM, level of risk is based upon consequences of the problem(s) addressed at the encounter when appropriately treated. Risk also includes MDM related to the need to initiate or forego further testing, treatment, and/or hospitalization.

Morbidity: A state of illness or functional impairment that is expected to be of substantial duration during which function is limited, quality of life is impaired, or there is organ damage that may not be transient despite treatment.

Social determinants of health: Economic and social conditions that influence the health of people and communities. Examples may include food or housing insecurity.

Drug therapy requiring intensive monitoring for toxicity: A drug that requires intensive monitoring is a therapeutic agent that has the potential to cause serious morbidity or death. The monitoring is performed for assessment of these adverse effects and not primarily for assessment of therapeutic efficacy. The monitoring should be that which is generally accepted practice for the agent but may be patient-specific in some cases. Intensive monitoring may be long-term or short-term. Long-term intensive monitoring is not performed less than quarterly. The monitoring may be performed with a laboratory test, a physiologic test, or imaging. Monitoring by history or examination does not qualify. The monitoring affects the level of MDM in an encounter in which it is considered in the management of the patient. Examples may include monitoring for cytopenia in the use of an antineoplastic agent between dose cycles or the short-term intensive monitoring of electrolytes and renal function in a patient who is undergoing diuresis. Examples of monitoring that do not qualify include monitoring glucose levels during insulin therapy, as the primary reason is the therapeutic effect (even if hypoglycemia is a concern); or annual electrolytes and renal function for a patient on a diuretic, as the frequency does not meet the threshold.

OTHER DEFINITIONS OF NATURE OF THE PRESENTING PROBLEM

In addition to the above five specific definitions found in the CPT coding system, there are other definitions found in the E.M Service codes used to report Subsequent Hospital Care and Follow-Up Inpatient Consultations. See Table 2 for these additional definitions.

Table 2: Other Definitions of Nature of Presenting Problems

Evaluation and Management Codes	Nature of Presenting Problem(s) Defined	Equivalent To
99231	Stable, recovering or improving	Self-limited or minor
99232	Inadequate response or minor complication	Low to moderate severity
99233	Significant complication or new problem	Moderate to high severity

INSTRUCTIONS FOR SELECTING A LEVEL OF OFFICE OR OTHER OUTPATIENT E/M SERVICES

Select the appropriate level of E/M services based on the following:

1.   The level of the MDM as defined for each service, or

2.   The total time for E/M services performed on the date of the encounter.

MEDICAL DECISION MAKING

MDM includes establishing diagnoses, assessing the status of a condition, and/or selecting a management option. MDM in the office or other outpatient services codes is defined by three elements:

- The number and complexity of problem(s) that are addressed during the encounter.

- The amount and/or complexity of data to be reviewed and analyzed. These data include medical records, tests, and/or other information that must be obtained, ordered, reviewed, and analyzed for the encounter. This includes information obtained from multiple sources or interprofessional communications that are not reported separately and interpretation of tests that are not reported separately. Ordering a test is included in the category of test result(s) and the review of the test result is part of the encounter and not a subsequent encounter. Data are divided into three categories:

  - Tests, documents, orders, or independent historian(s). (Each unique test, order, or document is counted to meet a threshold number.)

  - Independent interpretation of tests.

  - Discussion of management or test interpretation with external physician or other qualified health care professional or appropriate source.

- The risk of complications and/or morbidity or mortality of patient management decisions made at the visit, associated with the patient's problem(s), the diagnostic procedure(s), treatment(s). This includes the possible management options selected and those considered but not selected, after shared MDM with the patient and/or family. For example, a decision about hospitalization includes consideration of alternative levels of care.

  Examples may include a psychiatric patient with a sufficient degree of support in the outpatient setting or the decision to not hospitalize a patient with advanced dementia with an acute condition that would generally warrant inpatient care, but for whom the goal is palliative treatment.

Four types of MDM are recognized: straightforward, low, moderate, and high. The concept of the level of MDM does not apply to 99211.

Shared MDM involves eliciting patient and/or family preferences, patient and/or family education, and explaining risks and benefits of management options.

MDM may be impacted by role and management responsibility.

When the physician or other qualified health care professional is reporting a separate CPT code that includes interpretation and/or report, the interpretation and/or report should not count toward the MDM when selecting a level of office or other outpatient services.

When the physician or other qualified health care professional is reporting a separate service for discussion of management with a physician or another qualified health care professional, the discussion is not counted toward the MDM when selecting a level of office or other outpatient services.

The Levels of Medical Decision Making (MDM) table (Table 3) is a guide to assist in selecting the level of MDM for reporting an office or other outpatient E/M services code. The table includes the four levels of MDM (ie, straightforward, low, moderate, high) and the three elements of MDM (ie, number and complexity of problems addressed at the encounter, amount and/or complexity of data reviewed and analyzed, and risk of complications and/or morbidity or mortality of patient management). To qualify for a particular level of MDM, two of the three elements for that level of MDM must be met or exceeded. **See Table 3: Levels of Medical Decision Making (MDM).**

Table 3: Levels of Medical Decision Making (MDM)

Code	Level of MDM (Based on 2 out of 3 Elements of MDM)	Number and Complexity of Problems Addressed at the Encounter	Amount and/or Complexity of Data to be Reviewed and Analyzed *Each unique test, order or document contributes to the combination of 2 or combination of 3 in Category 1 below.*	Risk of Complications and/or Morbidity or Mortality of Patient Management
		Elements of Medical Decision Making		
99211	N/A	N/A	N/A	N/A
99202 99212	Straightforward	**Minimal** • 1 self-limited or minor problem	**Minimal or none**	**Minimal risk of morbidity from additional diagnostic testing or treatment**
99203 99213	Low	**Low** • 2 or more self-limited or minor problems; **or** • 1 stable chronic illness; **or** • 1 acute, uncomplicated illness or injury	**Limited** *(Must meet the requirements of at least 1 of the 2 categories)* **Category 1: Tests and documents** Any combination of 2 from the following: • Review of prior external note(s) from each unique source* • Review of the result(s) of each unite test* • Ordering of each unique test **or** **Category 2: Assessment requireing an independent historian(s)** *(For the categories of independent interpretation of tests and discussion of management or test interpretation, see moderate or high)*	**Low risk of morbidity from additional diagnostic testing or treatment**
99204 99214	Moderate	**Moderate** • 1 or more chronic illnesses with exacerbation, progression, or side effects of treatment; **or** • 2 or more stable, chronic illnesses; **or** • 1 undiagnosed new problem with uncertain prognosis; **or** • 1 acute illness with systemic symptoms; **or** • 1 acute complicated injury	**Moderate** *(Must meet the requirements of at least 1 out of 3 categories)* **Category 1: Tests, documents, or independent historian9s)** Any combination of 3 from the following: • Review of prior external note(s) from each unique source • Review of the result(s) of each unique test • Ordering of each unique test • Assessment requiring an independent historian(s) **or** **Category 2: Independent interpretation of tests** • Independent interpretation of a test performed by another physician/other qualified health care professional (not separately reported) **or** **Category 3: Discussion of management or test interpretation** • Discussion of management or test interpretation with external physician/ other qualified health care professional / appropriate source (not separately reported)	**Moderate risk of morbidity from additional diagnostic testing or treatment** *Examples only:* • Prescription drug management • Decision regarding minor surgery with identified patient or procedure risk factors • Decision regarding elective major surgery without identified patient or procedure risk factors • Diagnosis or treatment significantly limited by social determinants of health

continued

		Elements of Medical Decision Making		
Code	Level of MDM (Based on 2 out of 3 Elements of MDM)	Number and Complexity of Problems Addressed at the Encounter	Amount and/or Complexity of Data to be Reviewed and Analyzed *Each unique test, order or document contributes to the combination of 2 or combination of 3 in Category 1 below.	Risk of Complications and/or Morbidity or Mortality of Patient Management
99205 99215	High	**High** • 1 or more chronic illnesses with severe exacerbation, progression, or side effects of treatment; **or** • 1 acute or chronic illness or injury that poses a threat to life or bodily function	**Extensive** *(Must meet the requirements of at least 2 out of 3 categories)* **Category 1: Tests, documents, or independent historian(s)** Any combination of 3 from the following: • Review of prior external note(s) from each unique source* • Review of the result(s) of each unique test* • Ordering of each unique test* • Assessment requiring an independent historian(s) **or** **Category 2: Independent interpretation of tests** • Independent interpretation of a test performed by another physician/other qualified health care professional (not separately reported); **or** **Category 3: Discussion of management or test interpretation** • Discussion of management or test interpretation with external physician/other qualified health care professional/appropriate source (not separately reported)	**High risk of morbidity from additional diagnostic testing or treatment** *Examples only:* • Drug therapy requiring intensive monitoring for toxicity • Decision regarding elective major surgery with identified patient or procedure risk factors • Decision regarding elective major surgery • Decision regarding hospitalization • Decision not to resuscitate or to de-escalate care because of poor prognosis

TIME

For instructions on using time to select the level of office or other outpatient E/M services code, see the *Time* subsection in *Guidelines Common to All E/M Services*.

UNLISTED SERVICE

An E/M service may be provided that is not listed in this section of the CPT codebook. When reporting such a service, the appropriate "Unlisted" code may be used to indicate the service, identifying it by "Special Report" as discussed in the following paragraph. The "Unlisted Services" and accompanying codes for the evaluation and management section are as follows:

99429   Unlisted preventive medicine service
99499   Unlisted evaluation and management service

SPECIAL REPORT

An unlisted service or one that is unusual, variable, or new may require a special report demonstrating the medical appropriateness of the service. Pertinent information should include an adequate definition or description of the nature, extent, and need for the procedure; and the time, effort, and equipment necessary to provide the service. Additional items that may be included are complexity of symptoms, final diagnosis, pertinent physical findings, diagnostic and therapeutic procedures, concurrent problems, and follow-up care.

CLINICAL EXAMPLES

Clinical examples of the codes for E/M services are provided to assist in understanding the meaning of the descriptors and selecting the correct code. These are listed in Appendix C of the AMA's book. Each example was developed by the specialties shown. The same problem, when seen by different specialties, may involve different amounts of work. Therefore, the appropriate level of encounter should be reported using the descriptors rather than the examples.

DIAGNOSTIC TESTS OR STUDIES

The performance of diagnostic tests or studies for which specific CPT codes are available is not included in the levels of evaluation and management services. Any diagnostic tests or studies performed by the physician for which specific CPT codes are available should be coded separately, in addition to the appropriate evaluation and management service code.

EVALUATION AND MANAGEMENT SERVICES MODIFIERS

Evaluation and management services may be modified under certain circumstances. When applicable, the modifying circumstance should be identified by reporting the appropriate modifier code in addition to the basic service. Modifiers which may be used with evaluation and management service codes are:

-24 Unrelated evaluation and management service by the same physician during a postoperative period

-25 Significant, separately identifiable evaluation and management service by the same physician on the same day of the procedure or other service

-32 Mandated services

-52 Reduced services

-57 Decision for surgery

EVALUATION AND MANAGEMENT SERVICES DOCUMENTATION GUIDELINES

Documentation in the medical record of all services provided is critical for reimbursement and audit liability. If the provider reported a service or procedure on the health insurance claim form but did not document it, or document it completely, in the patient's medical records, from the point of view of Medicare or private health insurance company auditors, the service was not performed, can't be reported, and therefore will not be paid for.

Millions of dollars are reclaimed from physicians and other medical professionals annually by Medicare and other third party payers because the medical record documentation does not support the services and procedures reported. Providers can protect their medical practices from audit liability by following the most current documentation guidelines published by CMS.

The following documentation guidelines for evaluation and management services were developed jointly by the American Medical Association (AMA) and CMS. The stated goal of CMS in publishing these guidelines is to provide physicians and health insurance claims reviewers with advice about preparing or reviewing documentation for evaluation and management services.

In developing and testing the validity of these guidelines, special emphasis was placed on assuring that they:

- *are consistent with the clinical descriptors and definitions contained in CPT,*
- *would be widely accepted by clinicians and minimize any changes in record-keeping practices; and*
- *would be interpreted and applied uniformly by users across the country.*

WHAT IS DOCUMENTATION AND WHY IS IT IMPORTANT?

Medical record documentation is required to record pertinent facts, findings, and observations about an individual's health history including past and present illnesses, examinations, tests, treatments, and outcomes. The medical record chronologically documents the care of the patient and is an important element contributing to high quality care. The medical record facilitates:

- *the ability of the physician and other medical professionals to evaluate and plan the patient's immediate treatment, and to monitor his/her health care over time;*

- *communication and continuity of care among physicians and other medical professionals involved in the patient's care;*

- *accurate and timely claims review and payment;*

- *appropriate utilization review and quality of care evaluations; and*

- *collection of data that may be useful for research and education.*

An appropriately documented medical record can reduce many of the hassles associated with claims processing and may serve as a legal document to verify the care provided, if necessary.

WHAT DO THIRD PARTY PAYERS WANT AND WHY?

Because payers have a contractual obligation to enrollees, they may require reasonable documentation that services are consistent with the insurance coverage provided. They may request information to validate:

- *the site of service;*

- *the medical necessity and appropriateness of the diagnostic and/or therapeutic services provided; and/or*

- *that services provided have been accurately reported.*

GENERAL PRINCIPLES OF MEDICAL RECORD DOCUMENTATION

The principles of documentation listed below are applicable to all types of medical and surgical services in all settings. For evaluation and management (E/M) services, the nature and amount of physician work and documentation varies by type of service, place of service and the patient's status. The general principles listed below may be modified to account for these variable circumstances in providing evaluation and management services.

1. *The medical record should be complete and legible.*

2. *The documentation of each patient encounter should include:*
   - *the reason for the encounter as well as relevant history, physical examination findings and prior diagnostic test results;*
   - *an assessment, clinical impression or diagnosis;*
   - *a plan for care; and*
   - *the date and legible identity of the observer.*

3. *If not documented, the rationale for ordering diagnostic and other ancillary services should be easily inferred.*

4. *Past and present diagnoses should be accessible to the treating and/or consulting physician.*

5. *Appropriate health risk factors should be identified.*

6. *The patient's progress, response to and changes in treatment, and revision of diagnosis should be documented.*

7. *CPT and ICD-9-CM codes reported on the health insurance claim form or patient billing statement should be supported by the documentation in the medical record.*

DOCUMENTATION OF EVALUATION AND MANAGEMENT SERVICES

This section provides definitions and documentation guidelines for the three key components of evaluation and management services and for visits which consist predominately of counseling or coordination of care. The three key components—history, examination, and medical decision making—appear in the descriptors for office and other outpatient services, hospital observation services, hospital inpatient services, consultations, emergency department services, nursing facility services, domiciliary care services, and home services. Note that Documentation Guidelines are identified by the symbol •DG.

The E/M descriptors recognize seven components which are used in defining the levels of service. These components are:

- *History*
- *Examination*
- *Medical decision making*
- *Counseling*
- *Coordination of care*
- *Nature of presenting problem*
- *Time*

The first three (i.e., history, examination and medical decision making) are the key components in selecting the level of evaluation and management services. However, with visits that consist predominantly of counseling or coordination of care, time is the key or controlling factor to qualify for a particular level of evaluation and management service.

Because the level of evaluation and management service is dependent on two or three key components, performance and documentation of one component (e.g., examination) at the highest level does not necessarily mean that the encounter in its entirety qualifies for the highest level of evaluation and management service.

These documentation guidelines for evaluation and management services reflect the needs of the typical adult population. For certain groups of patients, the recorded information may vary slightly from that described here.

Specifically, the medical records of infants, children, adolescents and pregnant women may have additional or modified information recorded in each history and examination area.

As an example, newborn records may include under history of the present illness, the details of the mother's pregnancy and the infant's status at birth; social history focused on family structure; family history focused on congenital anomalies and hereditary disorders in the family. In addition, the content of a pediatric examination will vary with the age and development of the child. Although not specifically defined in these documentation guidelines, these patient group variations on history and examination are appropriate.

DOCUMENTATION OF HISTORY

The levels of evaluation and management services are based on four types of history (Problem Focused, Expanded Problem Focused, Detailed, and Comprehensive). Each type of history includes some or all of the following elements:

- *Chief complaint*
- *History of present illness*
- *Review of systems*
- *Past, family and/or social history*

The extent of history of present illness, review of systems and past, family and/or social history that is obtained and documented is dependent upon clinical judgement and the nature of the presenting problem(s).

Present History	Review of Systems	Past, Family or Social History	Type of History
Brief	N/A	N/A	*Problem Focused*
Brief	Problem Pertinent	N/A	*Expanded Problem Focused*
Extended	Extended	Pertinent	*Detailed*
Extended	Complete	Complete	*Comprehensive*

The above chart shows the progression of the elements required for each type of history. To qualify for a given type of history all three elements in the table must be met. (A chief complaint is indicated at all levels.)

●*DG:* *The chief complaint, review of systems and past, family and/or social history may be listed as separate elements of history, or they may be included in the description of the history of the present illness.*

●*DG:* *A review of systems and/or a past, family and/or social history obtained during an earlier encounter does not need to be re-recorded if there is evidence that the physician reviewed and updated the previous information. This may occur when a physician updates his or her own record or in an institutional setting or group practice where many physicians use a common record. The review and update may be documented by:*

- *describing any new review of systems and/or past, family and/or social history information or noting there has been no change in the information; and*

- *noting the date and location of the earlier review of systems and/or past, family and/or social history.*

●*DG:* *The review of systems and/or past, family and/or social history may be recorded by ancillary staff or on a form completed by the patient. To document that the physician reviewed the information, there must be a notation supplementing or confirming the information recorded by others.*

●*DG:* *If the physician is unable to obtain a history from the patient or other source, the record should describe the patient's condition or other circumstance which precludes obtaining a history.*

Definitions and specific documentation guidelines for each of the elements of history are listed below.

CHIEF COMPLAINT

The chief complaint is "a concise statement describing the symptom, problem, condition, diagnosis, or other factor that is the reason for the encounter, usually stated in the patient's words."

●*DG:* *The medical record should clearly reflect the chief complaint.*

HISTORY OF PRESENT ILLNESS

The history of present illness is "a chronological description of the development of the patient's present illness from the first sign and/or symptom to the present." It includes the following elements:

- *Location*
- *Quality*
- *Severity*
- *Duration*
- *Timing*
- *Context*
- *Modifying factors*
- *Associated signs and symptoms*

Brief *and* **extended** *history of present illnesses are distinguished by the amount of detail needed to accurately characterize the clinical problem(s). A* **brief** *history of present illness consists of one to three elements of the history of present illness.*

●*DG:* *The medical record should describe at least one to three elements of the present illness (history of present illness).*

An **extended** *history of present illness consists of at least four elements of the history of present illness or the status of at least three chronic or inactive conditions.*

●*DG:* *Medical record should describe at least four elements of the present illness (history of present illness), or the status of at least three chronic or inactive conditions.*

REVIEW OF SYSTEMS

A review of systems is "an inventory of body systems obtained through a series of questions seeking to identify signs and/or symptoms which the patient may be experiencing or has experienced." For purposes of review of systems, the following systems are recognized:

- Constitutional symptoms (e.g., fever, weight loss)
- Eyes
- Ears, Nose, Mouth, Throat
- Neck
- Cardiovascular
- Respiratory
- Gastrointestinal
- Genitourinary
- Musculoskeletal
- Integumentary (skin and/or breast)
- Neurological
- Psychiatric
- Endocrine
- Hematologic/Lymphatic
- Allergic/Immunologic

A **problem pertinent** review of systems inquires about the system directly related to the problem(s) identified in the history of present illness.

●**DG:** The patient's positive responses and pertinent negatives for the system related to the problem should be documented.

An **extended** review of systems inquires about the system directly related to the problem(s) identified in the history of present illness and a limited number of additional systems.

●**DG:** The patient's positive responses and pertinent negatives for two to nine systems should be documented.

A **complete** review of systems inquires about the system(s) directly related to the problem(s) identified in the history of present illness plus all additional body systems.

●**DG:** At least ten organ systems must be reviewed. Those systems with positive or pertinent negative responses must be individually documented. For the remaining systems, a notation indicating all other systems are negative is permissible. In the absence of such a notation, at least ten systems must be individually documented.

PAST, FAMILY AND/OR SOCIAL HISTORY

The past, family and/or social history consists of a review of the following areas:

- Past history: the patient's past experiences with illnesses, operations, injuries and treatments.
- Family history: a review of medical events in the patient's family, including diseases which may be hereditary or place the patient at risk.
- Social history: an age appropriate review of past and current activities.

For certain categories of evaluation and management services that include only an interval history, it is not necessary to record information about the past, family and/or social history. Those categories are subsequent hospital care, follow-up inpatient consultations and subsequent nursing facility care.

A **pertinent** past, family and/or social history is a review of the history area(s) directly related to the problem(s) identified in the history of present illness.

●**DG:** At least one specific item from any of the three history areas must be documented for a pertinent past, family and/or social history

A **complete** past, family and/or social history is of a review of two or all three of the past, family and/or social history areas, depending on the category of the evaluation and management service. A review of all three history areas is required for services that by their nature include a comprehensive assessment or reassessment of the patient. A review of two of the three history areas is sufficient for other services.

- **●DG:** At least one specific item from two of the three history areas must be documented for a complete past, family and/or social history for the following categories of evaluation and management services: office or other outpatient services, established patient; emergency department; domiciliary care, established patient; and home care, established patient.

- **●DG:** At least one specific item from each of the three history areas must be documented for a complete past, family and/or social history for the following categories of evaluation and management services: office or other outpatient services, new patient; hospital observation services; hospital inpatient services, initial care; consultations; comprehensive nursing facility assessments; domiciliary care, new patient; and home care, new patient.

DOCUMENTATION OF EXAMINATION

The levels of E/M services are based on four types of examination:

- Problem Focused — "a limited examination of the affected body area or organ system."
- Expanded Problem Focused — "a limited examination of the affected body area or organ system and any other symptomatic or related body organ system(s)."
- Detailed — "an extended examination of the affected body area(s) and other symptomatic or related organ system(s)."
- Comprehensive — "a general multi-system examination, or complete examination of a single organ system."

These types of examinations have been defined for general multi-system and the following single organ systems:

- Cardiovascular
- Ears, Nose, Mouth and Throat
- Eyes
- Genitourinary (Female)
- Genitourinary (Male)
- Hematologic/Lymphatic/Immunologic
- Musculoskeletal
- Neurological
- Psychiatric
- Respiratory
- Skin

A general multi-system examination or a single organ system examination may be performed by any physician regardless of specialty. The type (general multi-system or single organ system) and content of examination are selected by the examining physician and are based upon clinical judgement, the patient's history, and the nature of the presenting problem(s).

The content and documentation requirements for each type and level of examination are summarized below and described in detail in tables beginning on page 116. In the tables, organ systems and body areas recognized by CPT for purposes of describing examinations are shown in the left column. The content, or individual elements, of the examination pertaining to that body area or organ system are identified by bullets (●) in the right column.

Parenthetical examples, (e.g., ...), have been used for clarification and to provide guidance regarding documentation. Documentation for each element must satisfy any numeric requirements (such as "Measurement of any three of the following seven...") included in the description of the element. Elements with multiple components but with no specific numeric requirement (such as "Examination of liver and spleen") require documentation of at least one component. It is possible for a given examination to be expanded beyond what is defined here. When that occurs, findings related to the additional systems and/or areas should be documented.

- **●DG:** Specific abnormal and relevant negative findings of the examination of the affected or symptomatic body area(s) or organ system(s) should be documented. A notation of "abnormal" without elaboration is insufficient.

●*DG:* *Abnormal or unexpected findings of the examination of any asymptomatic body area(s) or organ system(s) should be described.*

●*DG:* *A brief statement or notation indicating "negative" or "normal" is sufficient to document normal findings related to unaffected area(s) or asymptomatic organ system(s).*

GENERAL MULTI-SYSTEM EXAMINATIONS

To qualify for a given level of multi-system examination, the following content and documentation requirements should be met:

● *Problem Focused Examination — should include performance and documentation of one to five elements identified by a bullet (●) in one or more organ system(s) or body area(s).*

● *Expanded Problem Focused Examination — should include performance and documentation of at least six elements identified by a bullet (●) in one or more organ system(s) or body area(s).*

● *Detailed Examination — should include at least six organ systems or body areas. For each system/area selected, performance and documentation of at least two elements identified by a bullet (●) is expected. Alternatively, a detailed examination may include performance and documentation of at least twelve elements identified by a bullet (●) in two or more organ systems or body areas.*

● *Comprehensive Examination — should include at least nine organ systems or body areas. For each system/area selected, all elements of the examination identified by a bullet (●) should be performed, unless specific directions limit the content of the examination. For each area/system, documentation of at least two elements identified by a bullet is expected.*

SINGLE ORGAN SYSTEM EXAMINATIONS

Variations among single organ system examinations in the organ systems and body areas identified in the left columns and in the elements of the examinations described in the right columns reflect differing emphases among specialties. To qualify for a given level of single organ system examination, the following content and documentation requirements should be met:

● *Problem Focused Examination — should include performance and documentation of one to five elements identified by a bullet (●), whether in a box with a shaded or unshaded border.*

● *Expanded Problem Focused Examination — should include performance and documentation of at least six elements identified by a bullet (●), whether in a box with a shaded or unshaded border.*

● *Detailed Examination — examinations other than the eye and psychiatric examinations should include performance and documentation of at least twelve elements identified by a bullet (●), whether in box with a shaded or unshaded border.*

Eye and psychiatric examinations should include the performance and documentation of at least nine elements identified by a bullet (●), whether in a box with a shaded or unshaded border.

● *Comprehensive Examination — should include performance of all elements identified by a bullet (●), whether in a shaded or unshaded box. Documentation of every element in each box with a shaded border and at least one element in each box with an unshaded border is expected.*

Documentation of every element in each box with a shaded border and at least one element in each box with an unshaded border is expected.

GENERAL MULTI-SYSTEM EXAMINATION

SYSTEM/BODY AREA	ELEMENTS OF EXAMINATION
Constitutional	• *Measurement of any three of the following seven vital signs: 1) sitting or standing blood pressure, 2) supine blood pressure, 3) pulse rate and regularity, 4) respiration, 5) temperature, 6) height, 7) weight (May be measured and recorded by ancillary staff)*
	• *General appearance of patient (e.g., development, nutrition, body habitus, deformities, attention to grooming)*
Eyes	• *Inspection of conjunctivae and lids*
	• *Examination of pupils and irises (e.g., reaction to light and accommodation, size and symmetry)*
	• *Ophthalmoscopic examination of optic discs (e.g., size, C/D ratio, appearance) and posterior segments (e.g., vessel changes, exudates, hemorrhages)*
Ears, Nose, Mouth, Throat	• *External inspection of ears and nose (e.g., overall and appearance, scars, lesions, masses)*
	• *Otoscopic examination of external auditory canals and tympanic membranes*
	• *Assessment of hearing (e.g., whispered voice, finger rub, tuning fork)*
	• *Inspection of nasal mucosa, septum and turbinates*
	• *Inspection of lips, teeth and gums*
	• *Examination of oropharynx: oral mucosa, salivary glands, hard and soft palates, tongue, tonsils and posterior pharynx*
Neck	• *Examination of neck (e.g., masses, overall appearance, symmetry, tracheal position, crepitus)*
	• *Examination of thyroid (e.g., enlargement, tenderness, mass)*
Respiratory	• *Assessment of respiratory effort (e.g., intercostal retractions, use of accessory muscles, diaphragmatic movement)*
	• *Percussion of chest (e.g., dullness, flatness, hyperresonance)*
	• *Palpation of chest (e.g., tactile fremitus)*
	• *Auscultation of lungs (e.g., breath sounds, adventitious sounds, rubs)*
Cardiovascular	• *Palpation of heart (e.g., location, size, thrills)*
	• *Auscultation of heart with notation of abnormal sounds and murmurs*
	Examination of:
	• *Carotid arteries (e.g., pulse amplitude, bruits)*
	• *Abdominal aorta (e.g., size, dbruits)*
	• *Femoral arteries (e.g., pulse amplitude, bruits)*
	• *Pedal pulses (e.g., pulse amplitude)*
	• *Extremities for edema and/or varicosities*
Chest (Breasts)	• *Inspection of breasts (e.g., symmetry, nipple discharge)*
	• *Palpation of breasts and axillae (e.g., masses or lumps, tenderness)*
Gastrointestinal (Abdomen)	• *Examination of abdomen with notation of presence of masses or tenderness*
	• *Examination of liver and spleen*

- Examination for presence or absence of hernia
- Examination (when indicated) of anus, perineum and rectum, including sphincter tone, presence of hemorrhoids, rectal masses
- Obtain stool sample for occult blood test when indicated

Genitourinary Male
- Examination of the scrotal contents (e.g., hydrocele, spermatocele, tenderness of cord, testicular mass)
- Examination of the penis
- Digital rectal examination of prostate gland (e.g., size, symmetry, nodularity, tenderness)

Genitourinary Female
- Pelvic examination (with or without specimen collection for smears and cultures), including:
- Examination of external genitalia (e.g., general appearance, hair distribution, lesions) and vagina (e.g., general appearance, estrogen effect, discharge, lesions, pelvic support, cystocele, rectocele)
- Examination of urethra (e.g., masses, tenderness, scarring)
- Examination of bladder (e.g., fullness, masses, tenderness)
- Cervix (e.g., general appearance, lesions, discharge)
- Uterus (e.g., size, contour, position, mobility, tenderness, consistency, descent or support)
- Adnexa/parametria (e.g., masses, tenderness, organomegaly, nodularity)

Lymphatic
Palpation of lymph nodes in two or more areas:
- Neck
- Axillae
- Groin
- Other

Musculoskeletal
- Examination of gait and station
- Inspection and/or palpation of digits and nails (eg clubbing, cyanosis, inflammatory conditions, petechiae, ischemia, infections, nodes)
- Examination of joints, bones and muscles of one or more of the following six areas: 1) head and neck; 2) spine, ribs and pelvis; 3) right upper extremity; 4) left upper extremity; 5) right lower extremity; and 6) left lower extremity. The examination of a given area includes:
- Inspection and/or palpation with notation of presence of any misalignment, asymmetry, crepitation, defects, tenderness, masses, effusions
- Assessment of range of motion with notation of any pain, crepitation or contracture
- Assessment of stability with notation of any dislocation (luxation), subluxation or laxity
- Assessment of muscle strength and tone (e.g., flaccid, cog wheel, spastic) with notation of any atrophy or abnormal movements

Skin
- Inspection of skin and subcutaneous tissue (e.g., rashes, lesions, ulcers)
- Palpation of skin and subcutaneous tissue (e.g., induration, subcutaneous nodules, tightening)

Neurologic
- Test cranial nerves with notation of any deficits
- Examination of deep tendon reflexes with notation of pathological reflexes (e.g., Babinski)
- Examination of sensation (e.g., by touch, pin, vibration, proprioception)

Psychiatric
- Description of patient's judgment and insight

Brief assessment of mental status including:

- *Orientation to time, place and person*
- *Recent and remote memory*
- *Mood and affect (e.g., depression, anxiety, agitation)*

CONTENT AND DOCUMENTATION REQUIREMENTS

Level of Exam	Perform and Document:
Problem Focused	One to five elements identified by a bullet.
Expanded Problem Focused	At least six elements identified by a bullet.
Detailed	At least two elements identified by a bullet from each of six areas/systems OR at least twelve elements identified by a bullet in two or more areas/systems.
Comprehensive	Perform all elements identified by a bullet in at least nine organ systems or body areas and document at least two elements identified by a bullet from each of nine areas/systems.

CARDIOVASCULAR EXAMINATION

SYSTEM/BODY AREA	ELEMENTS OF EXAMINATION
Constitutional	• Measurement of any three of the following seven vital signs: 1) sitting or standing blood pressure, 2) supine blood pressure, 3) pulse rate and regularity, 4) respiration, 5) temperature, 6) height, 7) weight (May be measured and recorded by ancillary staff)
	• General appearance of patient (e.g., development, nutrition, body habitus, deformities, attention to grooming)
Head and Face	
Eyes	• Inspection of conjunctivae and lids (e.g., xanthelasma)
Ears, Nose, Mouth and Throat	• Inspection of teeth, gums and palate
	• Inspection of oral mucosa with notation of presence of pallor or cyanosis
Neck	• Examination of jugular veins (e.g., distension; a, v or cannon a waves)
	• Examination of thyroid (e.g., enlargement, tenderness, mass)
Respiratory	• Assessment of respiratory effort (e.g., intercostal retractions, use of accessory muscles, diaphragmatic movement)
	• Auscultation of lungs (e.g., breath sounds, adventitious sounds, rubs)
Cardiovascular	• Palpation of heart (e.g., location, size and forcefulness of the point of maximal impact; thrills; lifts; palpable S3 or S4)
	• Auscultation of heart including sounds, abnormal sounds and murmurs
	• Measurement of blood pressure in two or more extremities when indicated (e.g., aortic dissection, coarctation)
	Examination of:
	• Carotid arteries (e.g., waveform, pulse amplitude, bruits, apical-carotid delay)
	• Abdominal aorta (e.g., size, bruits)
	• Femoral arteries (e.g., pulse amplitude, bruits)
	• Pedal pulses (e.g., pulse amplitude)
	• Extremities for peripheral edema and/or varicosities
Chest (Breasts)	
Gastrointestinal (Abdomen)	• Examination of abdomen with notation of presence (Abdomen) of masses or tenderness
	• Examination of liver and spleen
	• Obtain stool sample for occult blood from patients who are being considered for thrombolytic or anticoagulant therapy
Genitourinary	
Lymphatic	
Musculoskeletal	• Examination of the back with notation of kyphosis or scoliosis
	• Examination of gait with notation of ability to undergo exercise testing and/or participation in exercise programs

- *Assessment of muscle strength and tone (e.g., flaccid, cog wheel, spastic) with notation of any atrophy and abnormal movements*

Extremities	• *Inspection and palpation of digits and nails (e.g., clubbing, cyanosis, inflammation, petechiae, ischemia, infections, Osler's nodes)*
Skin	• *Inspection and/or palpation of skin and subcutaneous tissue (e.g., stasis dermatitis, ulcers, scars, xanthomas)*
Neurological/Psychiatric	*Brief assessment of mental status including:* • *Orientation to time, place and person* • *Mood and affect (e.g., depression, anxiety, agitation)*

CONTENT AND DOCUMENTATION REQUIREMENTS

Level of Exam	*Perform and Document:*
Problem Focused	*One to five elements identified by a bullet.*
Expanded Problem Focused	*At least six elements identified by a bullet.*
Detailed	*At least twelve elements identified by a bullet.*
Comprehensive	*Perform all elements identified by a bullet; document every element in each box with a shaded border and at least one element in each box with an unshaded border.*

EAR, NOSE AND THROAT EXAMINATION

SYSTEM/BODY AREA	ELEMENTS OF EXAMINATION
Constitutional	• Measurement of any three of the following seven vital signs: 1) sitting or standing blood pressure, 2) supine blood pressure, 3) pulse rate and regularity, 4) respiration, 5) temperature, 6) height, 7) weight (May be measured and recorded by ancillary staff) • General appearance of patient (e.g., development, nutrition, body habitus, deformities, attention to grooming) • Assessment of ability to communicate (e.g., use of sign language or other communication aids) and quality of voice
Head and Face	• Inspection of head and face (e.g., overall appearance, scars, lesions and masses) • Palpation and/or percussion of face with notation of presence or absence of sinus tenderness • Examination of salivary glands • Assessment of facial strength
Eyes	• Test ocular motility including primary gaze alignment
Ears, Nose, Mouth and Throat	• Otoscopic examination of external auditory canals and tympanic membranes including pneumo-otoscopy with notation of mobility of membranes • Assessment of hearing with tuning forks and clinical speech reception thresholds (e.g., whispered voice, finger rub) • External inspection of ears and nose (e.g., overall appearance, scars, lesions and masses) • Inspection of nasal mucosa, septum and turbinates • Inspection of lips, teeth and gums • Examination of oropharynx: oral mucosa, hard and soft palates, tongue, tonsils and posterior pharynx (e.g., asymmetry, lesions, hydration of mucosal surfaces) • Inspection of pharyngeal walls and pyriform sinuses (e.g., pooling of saliva, asymmetry, lesions) • Examination by mirror of larynx including the condition of the epiglottis, false vocal cords, true vocal cords and mobility of larynx (Use of mirror not required in children) • Examination by mirror of nasopharynx including appearance of the mucosa, adenoids, posterior choanae and eustachian tubes (Use of mirror not required in children)
Neck	• Examination of neck (e.g., masses, overall appearance, symmetry, tracheal position, crepitus) • Examination of thyroid (e.g., enlargement, tenderness, mass)
Respiratory	• Inspection of chest including symmetry, expansion and/or assessment of respiratory effort (e.g., intercostal retractions, use of accessory muscles, diaphragmatic movement) • Auscultation of lungs (e.g., breath sounds, adventitious sounds, rubs)
Cardiovascular	• Auscultation of heart with notation of abnormal sounds and murmurs • Examination of peripheral vascular system by observation (e.g., swelling, varicosities) and palpation (e.g., pulses, temperature, edema, tenderness)
Chest (Breasts)	
Gastrointestinal (Abdomen)	
Genitourinary	

Lymphatic	• *Palpation of lymph nodes in neck, axillae, groin and/or other location*
Musculoskeletal	
Extremities	
Skin	
Neurological/Psychiatric	• *Test cranial nerves with notation of any deficits*
	Brief assessment of mental status including:
	• *Orientation to time, place and person*
	• *Mood and affect (e.g., depression, anxiety, agitation)*

CONTENT AND DOCUMENTATION REQUIREMENTS

Level of Exam	*Perform and Document:*
Problem Focused	*One to five elements identified by a bullet.*
Expanded Problem Focused	*At least six elements identified by a bullet.*
Detailed	*At least twelve elements identified by a bullet.*
Comprehensive	*Perform all elements identified by a bullet; document every element in each box with a shaded border and at least one element in each box with an unshaded border.*

EYE EXAMINATION

SYSTEM/BODY AREA	ELEMENTS OF EXAMINATION
Constitutional	
Head and Face	
Eyes	• Test visual acuity (Does not include determination of refractive error) • Gross visual field testing by confrontation • Test ocular motility including primary gaze alignment • Inspection of bulbar and palpebral conjunctivae • Examination of ocular adnexae including lids (e.g., ptosis or lagophthalmos), lacrimal glands, lacrimal drainage, orbits and preauricular lymph nodes • Examination of pupils and irises including shape, direct and consensual reaction (afferent pupil), size (e.g., anisocoria) and morphology • Slit lamp examination of the corneas including epithelium, stroma, endothelium, and tear film • Slit lamp examination of the anterior chambers including depth, cells, and flare • Slit lamp examination of the lenses including clarity, anterior and posterior capsule, cortex, and nucleus • Measurement of intraocular pressures (except in children and patients with trauma or infectious disease) • Ophthalmoscopic examination through dilated pupils (unless contraindicated) of • Optic discs including size, C/D ratio, appearance (e.g., atrophy, cupping, tumor elevation) and nerve fiber layer • Posterior segments including retina and vessels (e.g., exudates and hemorrhages)
Ears, Nose, Mouth and Throat	
Neck	
Respiratory	
Cardiovascular	
Chest (Breasts)	
Gastrointestinal (Abdomen)	
Genitourinary	
Lymphatic	
Musculoskeletal	
Extremities	
Skin	
Neurological/Psychiatric	Brief assessment of mental status including: • Orientation to time, place and person

- *Mood and affect (e.g., depression, anxiety, agitation)*

CONTENT AND DOCUMENTATION REQUIREMENTS

Level of Exam	Perform and Document:
Problem Focused	One to five elements identified by a bullet.
Expanded Problem Focused	At least six elements identified by a bullet.
Detailed	At least nine elements identified by a bullet.
Comprehensive	Perform all elements identified by a bullet; document every element in each box with a shaded border and at least one element in each box with an unshaded border.

GENITOURINARY EXAMINATION

SYSTEM/BODY AREA	ELEMENTS OF EXAMINATION
Constitutional	• Measurement of any three of the following seven vital signs: 1) sitting or standing blood pressure, 2) supine blood pressure, 3) pulse rate and regularity, 4) respiration, 5) temperature, 6) height, 7) weight (May be measured and recorded by ancillary staff) • General appearance of patient (e.g., development, nutrition, body habitus, deformities, attention to grooming)
Head and Face	
Eyes	
Ears, Nose, Mouth and Throat	
Neck	• Examination of neck (e.g., masses, overall appearance, symmetry, tracheal position, crepitus) • Examination of thyroid (e.g., enlargement, tenderness, mass)
Respiratory	• Assessment of respiratory effort (e.g., intercostal retractions, use of accessory muscles, diaphragmatic movement) • Auscultation of lungs (e.g., breath sounds, adventitious sounds, rubs)
Cardiovascular	• Auscultation of heart with notation of abnormal sounds and murmurs • Examination of peripheral vascular system by observation (e.g., swelling, varicosities) and palpation (e.g., pulses, temperature, edema, tenderness)
Chest (Breasts)	[See genitourinary (female)]
Gastrointestinal (Abdomen)	• Examination of abdomen with notation of presence of masses or tenderness • Examination for presence or absence of hernia • Examination of liver and spleen • Obtain stool sample for occult blood test when indicated
Genitourinary (male)	• Inspection of anus and perineum Examination (with or without specimen collection for smears and cultures) of genitalia including: • Scrotum (e.g., lesions, cysts, rashes) • Epididymides (e.g., size, symmetry, masses) • Testes (e.g., size, symmetry, masses) • Urethral meatus (e.g., size, location, lesions, discharge) • Penis (e.g., lesions, presence or absence of foreskin, foreskin retractability, plaque, masses, scarring, deformities) Digital rectal examination including: • Prostate gland (e.g., size, symmetry, nodularity, tenderness) • Seminal vesicles (e.g., symmetry, tenderness, masses, enlargement) • Sphincter tone, presence of hemorrhoids, rectal masses
Genitourinary (female)	Includes at least seven of the following eleven elements identified by bullets:

- *Inspection and palpation of breasts (e.g., masses or lumps, tenderness, symmetry, nipple discharge)*
- *Digital rectal examination including sphincter tone, presence of hemorrhoids, rectal masses*

Pelvic examination (with or without specimen collection for smears and cultures) including:

- *External genitalia (e.g., general appearance, hair distribution, lesions)*
- *Urethral meatus (e.g., size, location, lesions, prolapse)*
- *Urethra (e.g., masses, tenderness, scarring)*
- *Bladder (e.g., fullness, masses, tenderness)*
- *Vagina (e.g., general appearance, estrogen effect, discharge, lesions, pelvic support, cystocele, rectocele)*
- *Cervix (e.g., general appearance, lesions, discharge)*
- *Uterus (e.g., size, contour, position, mobility, tenderness, consistency, descent or support)*
- *Adnexa/parametria (e.g., masses, tenderness, organomegaly, nodularity)*
- *Anus and perineum*

Lymphatic	• *Palpation of lymph nodes in neck, axillae, groin and/or other location*
Musculoskeletal	
Extremities	
Skin	• *Inspection and/or palpation of skin and subcutaneous tissue (e.g., rashes, lesions, ulcers)*
Neurological/Psychiatric	*Brief assessment of mental status including:*
	• *Orientation (e.g., time, place and person) and*
	• *Mood and affect (e.g., depression, anxiety, agitation)*

CONTENT AND DOCUMENTATION REQUIREMENTS

Level of Exam	Perform and Document:
Problem Focused	*One to five elements identified by a bullet.*
Expanded Problem Focused	*At least six elements identified by a bullet.*
Detailed	*At least twelve elements identified by a bullet.*
Comprehensive	*Perform all elements identified by a bullet; document every element in each box with a shaded border and at least one element in each box with an unshaded border.*

HEMATOLOGIC, LYMPHATIC, AND/OR IMMUNOLOGIC EXAMINATION

SYSTEM/BODY AREA	ELEMENTS OF EXAMINATION
Constitutional	• Measurement of any three of the following seven vital signs: 1) sitting or standing blood pressure, 2) supine blood pressure, 3) pulse rate and regularity, 4) respiration, 5) temperature, 6) height, 7) weight (May be measured and recorded by ancillary staff)
	• General appearance of patient (e.g., development, nutrition, body habitus, deformities, attention to grooming)
Head and Face	• Palpation and/or percussion of face with notation of presence or absence of sinus tenderness
Eyes	• Inspection of conjunctivae and lids
Ears, Nose, Mouth and Throat	• Otoscopic examination of external auditory canals and tympanic membranes
	• Inspection of nasal mucosa, septum and turbinates
	• Inspection of teeth and gums
	• Examination of oropharynx (e.g., oral mucosa, hard and soft palates, tongue, tonsils, posterior pharynx)
Neck	• Examination of neck (e.g., masses, overall appearance, symmetry, tracheal position, crepitus)
	• Examination of thyroid (e.g., enlargement, tenderness, mass)
Respiratory	• Assessment of respiratory effort (e.g., intercostal retractions, use of accessory muscles, diaphragmatic movement)
	• Auscultation of lungs (e.g., breath sounds, adventitious sounds, rubs)
Cardiovascular	• Auscultation of heart with notation of abnormal sounds and murmurs
	• Examination of peripheral vascular system by observation (e.g., swelling, varicosities) and palpation (e.g., pulses, temperature, edema, tenderness)
Chest (Breasts)	
Gastrointestinal (Abdomen)	• Examination of abdomen with notation of presence of masses or tenderness
	• Examination of liver and spleen
Genitourinary	
Lymphatic	• Palpation of lymph nodes in neck, axillae, groin, and/or other location
Musculoskeletal	
Extremities	• Inspection and palpation of digits and nails (e.g., clubbing, cyanosis, inflammation, petechiae, ischemia, infections, nodes)
Skin	• Inspection and/or palpation of skin and subcutaneous tissue (e.g., rashes, lesions, ulcers, ecchymoses, bruises)
Neurological/Psychiatric	Brief assessment of mental status including:
	• Orientation to time, place and person

● *Mood and affect (e.g., depression, anxiety, agitation)*

CONTENT AND DOCUMENTATION REQUIREMENTS

Level of Exam	*Perform and Document:*
Problem Focused	*One to five elements identified by a bullet.*
Expanded Problem Focused	*At least six elements identified by a bullet.*
Detailed	*At least twelve elements identified by a bullet.*
Comprehensive	*Perform all elements identified by a bullet; document every element in each box with a shaded border and at least one element in each box with an unshaded border.*

MUSCULOSKELETAL EXAMINATION

SYSTEM/BODY AREA	ELEMENTS OF EXAMINATION
Constitutional	• Measurement of any three of the following seven vital signs: 1) sitting or standing blood pressure, 2) supine blood pressure, 3) pulse rate and regularity, 4) respiration, 5) temperature, 6) height, 7) weight (May be measured and recorded by ancillary staff) • General appearance of patient (e.g., development, nutrition, body habitus, deformities, attention to grooming)
Head and Face	
Eyes	
Ears, Nose, Mouth and Throat	
Neck	
Respiratory	
Cardiovascular	• Examination of peripheral vascular system by observation (e.g., swelling, varicosities) and palpation (e.g., pulses, temperature, edema, tenderness)
Chest (Breasts)	
Gastrointestinal (Abdomen)	
Genitourinary	
Lymphatic	• Palpation of lymph nodes in neck, axillae, groin and/or other location
Musculoskeletal	• Examination of gait and station • Examination of joint(s), bone(s) and muscle(s)/tendon(s) of four of the following six areas: 1) head and neck; 2) spine, ribs and pelvis; 3) right upper extremity; 4) left upper extremity; 5) right lower extremity; and 6) left lower extremity. The examination of a given area includes: • Inspection, percussion and/or palpation with notation of any misalignment, asymmetry, crepitation, defects, tenderness, masses or effusions • Assessment of range of motion with notation of any pain (e.g., straight leg raising), crepitation or contracture • Assessment of stability with notation of any dislocation (luxation), subluxation or laxity • Assessment of muscle strength and tone (e.g., flaccid, cog wheel, spastic) with notation of any atrophy or abnormal movements NOTE: For the comprehensive level of examination, all four of the elements identified by a bullet must be performed and documented for each of four anatomic areas. For the three lower levels of examination, each element is counted separately for each body area. For example, assessing range of motion in two extremities constitutes two elements.
Extremities	[See musculoskeletal and skin]
Skin	• Inspection and/or palpation of skin and subcutaneous tissue (e.g., scars, rashes, lesions, cafe-au-lait spots, ulcers) in four of the following six areas: 1) head and neck; 2) trunk; 3) right upper extremity; 4) left upper extremity; 5) right lower extremity; and 6) left lower extremity.

NOTE: *For the comprehensive level, all four areas must be examined and documented. For the three lower levels, each body area is counted separately. For example, inspection and/or palpation of the skin and subcutaneous tissue of two extremities constitutes two elements.*

Neurological/Psychiatric	● *Test coordination (e.g., finger/nose, heel/knee/shin, rapid alternating movements in the upper and lower extremities, evaluation of fine motor coordination in young children)*
	● *Examination of deep tendon reflexes and/or nerve stretch test with notation of pathological reflexes (e.g., Babinski)*
	● *Examination of sensation (e.g., by touch, pin, vibration, proprioception)*
	Brief assessment of mental status including
	● *Orientation to time, place and person*
	● *Mood and affect (e.g., depression, anxiety, agitation)*

CONTENT AND DOCUMENTATION REQUIREMENTS

Level of Exam	*Perform and Document:*
Problem Focused	*One to five elements identified by a bullet.*
Expanded Problem Focused	*At least six elements identified by a bullet.*
Detailed	*At least twelve elements identified by a bullet.*
Comprehensive	*Perform all elements identified by a bullet; document every element in each box with a shaded border and at least one element in each box with an unshaded border.*

NEUROLOGICAL EXAMINATION

SYSTEM/BODY AREA	ELEMENTS OF EXAMINATION
Constitutional	• *Measurement of any three of the following seven vital signs: 1) sitting or standing blood pressure, 2) supine blood pressure, 3) pulse rate and regularity, 4) respiration, 5) temperature, 6) height, 7) weight (May be measured and recorded by ancillary staff)* • *General appearance of patient (e.g., development, nutrition, body habitus, deformities, attention to grooming)*
Head and Face	
Eyes	• *Ophthalmoscopic examination of optic discs (e.g., size, C/D ratio, appearance) and posterior segments (e.g., vessel changes, exudates, hemorrhages)*
Ears, Nose, Mouth and Throat	
Neck	
Respiratory	
Cardiovascular	• *Examination of carotid arteries (e.g., pulse amplitude, bruits)* • *Auscultation of heart with notation of abnormal sounds and murmurs* • *Examination of peripheral vascular system by observation (e.g., swelling, varicosities) and palpation (e.g., pulses, temperature, edema, tenderness)*
Chest (Breasts)	
Gastrointestinal (Abdomen)	
Genitourinary	
Lymphatic	
Musculoskeletal	• *Examination of gait and station* *Assessment of motor function including:* • *Muscle strength in upper and lower extremities* • *Muscle tone in upper and lower extremities (e.g., flaccid, cog wheel, spastic) with notation of any atrophy or abnormal movements (e.g., fasciculation, tardive dyskinesia)*
Extremities	*[See musculoskeletal]*
Skin	
Neurological/Psychiatric	*Evaluation of higher integrative functions including:* • *Orientation to time, place and person* • *Recent and remote memory* • *Attention span and concentration* • *Language (e.g., naming objects, repeating phrases, spontaneous speech)* • *Fund of knowledge (e.g., awareness of current events, past history, vocabulary)* *Test the following cranial nerves:*

- 2nd cranial nerve (e.g., visual acuity, visual fields, fundi)

- 3rd, 4th and 6th cranial nerves (e.g., pupils, eye movements)

- 5th cranial nerve (e.g., facial sensation, corneal reflexes)

- 7th cranial nerve (e.g., facial symmetry, strength)

- 8th cranial nerve (e.g., hearing with tuning fork, whispered voice and/or finger rub)

- 9th cranial nerve (e.g., spontaneous or reflex palate movement)

- 11th cranial nerve (e.g., shoulder shrug strength)

- 12th cranial nerve (e.g., tongue protrusion)

- Examination of sensation (e.g., by touch, pin, vibration, proprioception)

- Examination of deep tendon reflexes in upper and lower extremities with notation of pathological reflexes (e.g., Babinski)

- Test coordination (e.g., finger/nose, heel/knee/shin, rapid alternating movements in the upper and lower extremities, evaluation of fine motor coordination in young children)

CONTENT AND DOCUMENTATION REQUIREMENTS

Level of Exam	Perform and Document:
Problem Focused	One to five elements identified by a bullet.
Expanded Problem Focused	At least six elements identified by a bullet.
Detailed	At least twelve elements identified by a bullet.
Comprehensive	Perform all elements identified by a bullet; document every element in each box with a shaded border and at least one element in each box with an unshaded border.

PSYCHIATRIC EXAMINATION

SYSTEM/BODY AREA	ELEMENTS OF EXAMINATION
Constitutional	• Measurement of any three of the following seven vital signs: 1) sitting or standing blood pressure, 2) supine blood pressure, 3) pulse rate and regularity, 4) respiration, 5) temperature, 6) height, 7) weight (May be measured and recorded by ancillary staff) • General appearance of patient (e.g., development, nutrition, body habitus, deformities, attention to grooming)
Head and Face	
Eyes	
Ears, Nose, Mouth and Throat	
Neck	
Respiratory	
Cardiovascular	
Chest (Breasts)	
Gastrointestinal (Abdomen)	
Genitourinary	
Lymphatic	
Musculoskeletal	• Assessment of muscle strength and tone (e.g., flaccid, cog wheel, spastic) with notation of any atrophy and abnormal movements • Examination of gait and station
Extremities	
Skin	
Neurological	
Psychiatric	• Description of speech including: rate; volume; articulation; coherence; and spontaneity with notation of abnormalities (e.g., perseveration, paucity of language) • Description of thought processes including: rate of thoughts; content of thoughts (e.g., logical vs. illogical, tangential); abstract reasoning; and computation • Description of associations (e.g., loose, tangential, circumstantial, intact) • Description of abnormal or psychotic thoughts including: hallucinations; delusions; preoccupation with violence; homicidal or suicidal ideation; and obsessions • Description of the patient's judgment (e.g., concerning everyday activities and social situations) and insight (e.g., concerning psychiatric condition) Complete mental status examination including: • Orientation to time, place and person • Recent and remote memory • Attention span and concentration

● *Language (e.g., naming objects, repeating phrases)*

● *Fund of knowledge (e.g., awareness of current events, past history, vocabulary)*

● *Mood and affect (e.g., depression, anxiety, agitation, hypomania, lability)*

CONTENT AND DOCUMENTATION REQUIREMENTS

Level of Exam	*Perform and Document:*
Problem Focused	*One to five elements identified by a bullet.*
Expanded Problem Focused	*At least six elements identified by a bullet.*
Detailed	*At least nine elements identified by a bullet.*
Comprehensive	*Perform all elements identified by a bullet; document every element in each box with a shaded border and at least one element in each box with an unshaded border.*

RESPIRATORY EXAMINATION

SYSTEM/BODY AREA	ELEMENTS OF EXAMINATION
Constitutional	• *Measurement of any three of the following seven vital signs: 1) sitting or standing blood pressure, 2) supine blood pressure, 3) pulse rate and regularity, 4) respiration, 5) temperature, 6) height, 7) weight (May be measured and recorded by ancillary staff)*
	• *General appearance of patient (e.g., development, nutrition, body habitus, deformities, attention to grooming)*
Head and Face	
Eyes	
Ears, Nose, Mouth and Throat	• *Inspection of nasal mucosa, septum and turbinates*
	• *Inspection of teeth and gums*
	• *Examination of oropharynx (e.g., oral mucosa, hard and soft palates, tongue, tonsils and posterior pharynx)*
Neck	• *Examination of neck (e.g., masses, overall appearance, symmetry, tracheal position, crepitus)*
	• *Examination of thyroid (e.g., enlargement, tenderness, mass)*
	• *Examination of jugular veins (e.g., distension; a, v or cannon a waves)*
Respiratory	• *Inspection of chest with notation of symmetry and expansion*
	• *Assessment of respiratory effort (e.g., intercostal retractions, use of accessory muscles, diaphragmatic movement)*
	• *Percussion of chest (e.g., dullness, flatness, hyperresonance)*
	• *Palpation of chest (e.g., tactile fremitus)*
	• *Auscultation of lungs (e.g., breath sounds, adventitious sounds, rubs)*
Cardiovascular	• *Auscultation of heart including sounds, abnormal sounds and murmurs*
	• *Examination of peripheral vascular system by observation (e.g., swelling, varicosities) and palpation (e.g., pulses, temperature, edema, tenderness)*
Chest (Breasts)	
Gastrointestinal (Abdomen)	• *Examination of abdomen with notation of presence of masses or tenderness*
	• *Examination of liver and spleen*
Genitourinary	
Lymphatic	• *Palpation of lymph nodes in neck, axillae, groin and/or other location*
Musculoskeletal	• *Assessment of muscle strength and tone (e.g., flaccid, cog wheel, spastic) with notation of any atrophy and abnormal movements*
	• *Examination of gait and station*
Extremities	• *Inspection and palpation of digits and nails (e.g., clubbing, cyanosis, inflammation, petechiae, ischemia, infections, nodes)*

Skin	• *Inspection and/or palpation of skin and subcutaneous tissue (e.g., rashes, lesions, ulcers)*
Neurological/Psychiatric	*Brief assessment of mental status including:*
	• *Orientation to time, place and person*
	• *Mood and affect (e.g., depression, anxiety, agitation)*

CONTENT AND DOCUMENTATION REQUIREMENTS

Level of Exam	*Perform and Document:*
Problem Focused	*One to five elements identified by a bullet.*
Expanded Problem Focused	*At least six elements identified by a bullet.*
Detailed	*At least twelve elements identified by a bullet.*
Comprehensive	*Perform all elements identified by a bullet; document every element in each box with a shaded border and at least one element in each box with an unshaded border.*

SKIN EXAMINATION

SYSTEM/BODY AREA	ELEMENTS OF EXAMINATION
Constitutional	• *Measurement of any three of the following seven vital signs: 1) sitting or standing blood pressure, 2) supine blood pressure, 3) pulse rate and regularity, 4) respiration, 5) temperature, 6) height, 7) weight (May be measured and recorded by ancillary staff)* • *General appearance of patient (e.g., development, nutrition, body habitus, deformities, attention to grooming)*
Head and Face	
Eyes	• *Inspection of conjunctivae and lids*
Ears, Nose, Mouth and Throat	• *Inspection of lips, teeth and gums* • *Examination of oropharynx (e.g., oral mucosa, hard and soft palates, tongue, tonsils, posterior pharynx)*
Neck	• *Examination of thyroid (e.g., enlargement, tenderness, mass)*
Respiratory	
Cardiovascular	• *Examination of peripheral vascular system by observation (e.g., swelling, varicosities) and palpation (e.g., pulses, temperature, edema, tenderness)*
Chest (Breasts)	
Gastrointestinal (Abdomen)	• *Examination of liver and spleen* • *Examination of anus for condyloma and other lesions*
Genitourinary	
Lymphatic	• *Palpation of lymph nodes in neck, axillae, groin and/or other location*
Musculoskeletal	
Extremities	• *Inspection and palpation of digits and nails (e.g., clubbing, cyanosis, inflammation, petechiae, ischemia, infections, nodes)*
Skin	• *Palpation of scalp and inspection of hair of scalp, eyebrows, face, chest, pubic area (when indicated) and extremities* *Inspection and/or palpation of skin and subcutaneous tissue (e.g., rashes, lesions, ulcers, susceptibility to and presence of photo damage) in eight of the following ten areas:* • *Head, including the face and* • *Neck* • *Chest, including breasts and axillae* • *Abdomen* • *Genitalia, groin, buttocks* • *Back* • *Right upper extremity*

- *Left upper extremity*
- *Right lower extremity*
- *Left lower extremity*

NOTE: For the comprehensive level, the examination of at least eight anatomic areas must be performed and documented. For the three lower levels of examination, each body area is counted separately. For example, inspection and/or palpation of the skin and subcutaneous tissue of the right upper extremity and the left upper extremity constitutes two elements.

- *Inspection of eccrine and apocrine glands of skin and subcutaneous tissue with identification and location of any hyperhidrosis, chromhidroses or bromhidrosis*

Neurological/Psychiatric	*Brief assessment of mental status including:*
	• *Orientation to time, place and person*
	• *Mood and affect (e.g., depression, anxiety, agitation)*

CONTENT AND DOCUMENTATION REQUIREMENTS

Level of Exam	Perform and Document:
Problem Focused	*One to five elements identified by a bullet.*
Expanded Problem Focused	*At least six elements identified by a bullet.*
Detailed	*At least twelve elements identified by a bullet.*
Comprehensive	*Perform all elements identified by a bullet; document every element in each box with a shaded border and at least one element in each box with an unshaded border.*

DOCUMENTATION OF THE COMPLEXITY OF MEDICAL DECISION MAKING

The levels of evaluation and management services recognize four types of medical decision making (straight-forward, low complexity, moderate complexity and high complexity). Medical decision making refers to the complexity of establishing a diagnosis and/or selecting a management option as measured by:

- the number of possible diagnoses and/or the number of management options that must be considered;
- the amount and/or complexity of medical records, diagnostic tests, and/or other information that must be obtained, reviewed and analyzed; and
- the risk of significant complications, morbidity and/or mortality, as well as comorbidities, associated with the patient's presenting problem(s), the diagnostic procedure(s) and/or the possible management options.

The following chart illustrates the progression of the elements required for each level of medical decision making. To qualify for a given type of decision making, two of the three elements in the table must be either met or exceeded.

NUMBER OF DIAGNOSES OR MANAGEMENT OPTIONS

The number of possible diagnoses and/or the number of management options that must be considered is based on the number and types of problems addressed during the encounter, the complexity of establishing a diagnosis and the management decisions that are made by the physician.

Generally, decision making with respect to a diagnosed problem is easier than that for an identified but undiagnosed problem. The number and type of diagnostic tests employed may be an indicator of the number of possible diagnoses. Problems which are improving or resolving are less complex than those which are worsening or failing to change as expected. The need to seek advice from others is another indicator of complexity of diagnostic or management problems.

- **DG:** *For each encounter, an assessment, clinical impression, or diagnosis should be documented. It may be explicitly stated or implied in documented decisions regarding management plans and/or further evaluation.*

  - *For a presenting problem with an established diagnosis, the record should reflect whether the problem is: a) improved, well controlled, resolving or resolved; or, b) inadequately controlled, worsening, or failing to change as expected.*

  - *For a presenting problem without an established diagnosis, the assessment or clinical impression may be stated in the form of differential diagnoses or as a "possible", "probable", or "rule out" (R/O) diagnosis.*

Number of Diagnoses	Amount of Data to Review	Risk of Complication	Type of Decision Making
Minimal	Minimal or none	Minimal	Straightforward
Limited	Limited	Low	Low Complexity
Multiple	Moderate	Moderate	Moderate Complexity
Extensive	Extensive	High	High Complexity
Each of the elements of medical decision making is described in the text below			

- **DG:** *The initiation of, or changes in, treatment should be documented. Treatment includes a wide range of management options including patient instructions, nursing instructions, therapies, and medications.*

- **DG:** *If referrals are made, consultations requested or advice sought, the record should indicate to whom or where the referral or consultation is made or from whom the advice is requested.*

AMOUNT AND/OR COMPLEXITY OF DATA TO BE REVIEWED

The amount and complexity of data to be reviewed is based on the types of diagnostic testing ordered or reviewed. A decision to obtain and review old medical records and/or obtain history from sources other than the patient increases the amount and complexity of data to be reviewed.

Discussion of contradictory or unexpected test results with the physician who performed or interpreted the test is an indication of the complexity of data being reviewed. On occasion the physician who ordered a test may personally review the image, tracing or specimen to supplement information from the physician who prepared the test report or interpretation; this is another indication of the complexity of data being reviewed.

•**DG:** If a diagnostic service (test or procedure) is ordered, planned, scheduled, or performed at the time of the evaluation and management encounter, the type of service, e.g., lab or x-ray, should be documented.

•**DG:** The review of lab, radiology and/or other diagnostic tests should be documented. A simple notation such as "WBC elevated" or "chest x-ray unremarkable" is acceptable. Alternatively, the review may be documented by initialing and dating the report containing the test results.

•**DG:** A decision to obtain old records or decision to obtain additional history from the family, caretaker or other source to supplement that obtained from the patient should be documented.

•**DG:** Relevant findings from the review of old records, and/or the receipt of additional history from the family, caretaker or other source to supplement that obtained from the patient should be documented. If there is no relevant information beyond that already obtained, that fact should be documented. A notation of "Old records reviewed" or "additional history obtained from family" without elaboration is insufficient.

•**DG:** The results of discussion of laboratory, radiology or other diagnostic tests with the physician who performed or interpreted the study should be documented.

•**DG:** The direct visualization and independent interpretation of an image, tracing or specimen previously or subsequently interpreted by another physician should be documented.

RISK OF SIGNIFICANT COMPLICATIONS, MORBIDITY AND/OR MORTALITY

The risk of significant complications, morbidity, and/or mortality is based on the risks associated with the presenting problem(s), the diagnostic procedure(s), and the possible management options.

•**DG:** Comorbidities/underlying diseases or other factors that increase the complexity of medical decision making by increasing the risk of complications, morbidity, and/or mortality should be documented.

•**DG:** If a surgical or invasive diagnostic procedure is ordered, planned or scheduled at the time of the evaluation and management encounter, the type of procedure, e.g., laparoscopy, should be documented.

•**DG:** If a surgical or invasive diagnostic procedure is performed at the time of the evaluation and management encounter, the specific procedure should be documented.

•**DG:** The referral for or decision to perform a surgical or invasive diagnostic procedure on an urgent basis should be documented or implied.

The Table of Risk on the following page may be used to help determine whether the risk of significant complications, morbidity, and/or mortality is minimal, low, moderate, or high. Because the determination of risk is complex and not readily quantifiable, the table includes common clinical examples rather than absolute measures of risk. The assessment of risk of the presenting problem(s) is based on the risk related to the disease process anticipated between the present encounter and the next one. The assessment of risk of selecting diagnostic procedures and management options is based on the risk during and immediately following any procedures or treatment. The highest level of risk in any one category (presenting problem(s), diagnostic procedure(s), or management options) determines the overall risk.

DOCUMENTATION OF AN ENCOUNTER DOMINATED BY COUNSELING OR COORDINATION OF CARE

In the case where counseling and/or coordination of care dominates (more than 50%) of the physician/patient and/or family encounter (face-to-face time in the office or other or outpatient setting, floor/unit time in the hospital or nursing facility), time is considered the key or controlling factor to qualify for a particular level of evaluation and management services.

•**DG:** If the physician elects to report the level of service based on counseling and/or coordination of care, the total length of time of the encounter (face-to-face or floor time, as appropriate) should be documented and the record should describe the counseling and/or activities to coordinate care.

TABLE OF RISK

LEVEL OF RISK	PRESENTING PROBLEM(S)	DIAGNOSTIC PROCEDURES	MANAGEMENT OPTIONS
Minimal	• One self-limited or minor problem, (eg, cold, insect bite, tinea corporis)	• Laboratory tests requiring venipuncture • Chest x-rays • EKG/EEG • Urinalysis • Ultrasound, (eg, echocardiography) • KOH prep	• Rest • Gargles • Elastic bandages • Superficial dressings
Low	• Two or more self-limited or minor problems • One stable chronic illness, (eg, well controlled hypertension, non-insulin dependent diabetes, cataract, BPH) • Acute uncomplicated illness or injury, (eg, cystitis, allergic rhinitis, simple sprain)	• Physiologic tests not under stress, (eg, pulmonary function tests) • Non-cardiovascular imaging studies with contrast,(eg, barium enema) • Superficial needle biopsies • Clinical laboratory tests requiring arterial puncture • Skin biopsies	• Over-the-counter drugs • Minor surgery with no identified risk factors • Physical therapy • Occupational therapy • IV fluids without additives
Moderate	• One or more chronic illnesses with mild exacerbation, progression, or side effects of treatment • Two or more stable chronic illnesses • Undiagnosed new problem with uncertain prognosis, (eg, lump in breast) • Acute illness with systemic symptoms, (eg, pyelonephritis, pneumonitis, colitis) • Acute complicated injury, (eg, head injury with brief loss of consciousness)	• Physiologic tests under stress, (eg, cardiac stress test, fetal contraction stress test) • Diagnostic endoscopies with no identified risk factors • Deep needle or incisional biopsy • Cardiovascular imaging studies with contrast and no identified risk factors, (eg, arteriogram, cardiac catheterization) • Obtain fluid from body cavity, (eg, lumbar puncture, thoracentesis, culdocentesis)	• Minor surgery with identified risk factors • Elective major surgery (open, percutaneous or endoscopic) with no identified risk factors • Prescription drug management • Therapeutic nuclear medicine • IV fluids with additives • Closed treatment of fracture or dislocation without manipulation
High	• One or more chronic illnesses with severe exacerbation, progression, or side effects of treatment • Acute or chronic illnesses or injuries that pose a threat to life or bodily function, (eg, multiple trauma, acute MI, pulmonary embolus, severe respiratory distress, progressive severe rheumatoid arthritis, psychiatric illness with potential threat to self or others, peritonitis, acute renal failure) • An abrupt change in neurologic status, (eg, seizure, TIA, weakness, sensory loss)	• Cardiovascular imaging studies with contrast with identified risk factors • Cardiac electrophysiological tests • Diagnostic endoscopies with identified risk factors • Discography	• percutaneous or endoscopic) with identified risk factors • Emergency major surgery (open, percutaneous or endoscopic) • Parenteral controlled substances • Drug therapy requiring intensive monitoring for toxicity • Decision not to resuscitate or to de-escalate care because of poor prognosis

EVALUATION AND MANAGEMENT CODING VISUAL MATRIX

Many people are visually oriented, which means they perceive and learn better when presented with pictures, graphics, shapes, and colors. The following Evaluation and Management Coding Visual Matrix is designed to assist visually oriented readers to quickly grasp the sections and choices available.

The Evaluation and Management Coding Visual Matrix reinforces that each Evaluation and Management code is selected from a choice of 1) history, 2) examination 3) medical decision making and 4) presenting problem components. Some Evaluation and Management codes include a time unit; measured as either face-to-face time or bedside/floor or unit time.

Color Key — Significance

- Components required
- History & examination choices
- Medical decision-making choices
- Presenting problem (severity) choices

Office/Other Outpatient Services (New Patients)

Components required: Not applicable for this section	99202	99203	99204	99205
History & Exam				
Problem focused				
Expanded problem focused				
Detailed				
Comprehensive				
Medically appropriate	●	●	●	●
Medical Decision Making				
Straightforward	●			
Low level/complexity		●		
Moderate level/complexity			●	
High level/complexity				●
Presenting Problem (Severity)				
Not applicable to this section				
Typical Time: Face-to-Face	15-29	30-44	45-59	60-74

Office/Other Outpatient Services (Established Patients)

Components required: Not applicable	99211	99212	99213	99214	99215
History & Exam					
Problem focused					
Expanded problem focused					
Detailed					
Comprehensive					
Medically appropriate		●	●	●	●
Medical Decision Making					
Straightforward		●			
Low level/complexity			●		
Moderate level/complexity				●	
High level/complexity					●
Presenting Problem (Severity)					
Not applicable to this section					
Typical Time: Face-to-Face		10-19	20-29	30-39	40-54

Initial Observation Care (New/Established Patients)

Components required: 3 of 3	99218	99219	99220
History & Exam			
Detailed or comprehensive	●		
Comprehensive		●	●
Straightforward or low	●		
Moderate		●	
High			●
Presenting Problem (Severity)			
Low	●		
Moderate		●	
High			●
Typical Time: Bedside/Floor/Unit	30	50	70

Subsequent Observation Care (New/Established Patients)

Components required: 2 of 3	99224	99225	99226
History & Exam			
Problem focused	●		
Expanded problem focused		●	
Detailed			●
Medical Decision Making			
Straightforward or low	●		
Moderate		●	
High			●
Presenting Problem (Severity)			
Stable/recovering/improving	●		
Responding inadequately/minor complication		●	
Unstable/significant complication/new problem			●
Typical Time: Bedside/Floor/Unit	15	25	35

Initial Hospital Care (New/Established Patients)

Components required: 3 of 3	99221	99222	99223
History & Exam			
Detailed or comprehensive	●		
Comprehensive		●	●
Straightforward or low	●		
Moderate		●	
High			●
Presenting Problem (Severity)			
Low	●		
Moderate		●	
High			●
Typical Time: Bedside/Floor/Unit	30	50	70

Subsequent Hospital Care (New/Established Patients)

Components required: 2 of 3	99231	99232	99233
History & Exam			
Problem focused	●		
Expanded problem focused		●	
Detailed			●
Medical Decision Making			
Straightforward or low	●		
Moderate		●	
High			●
Presenting Problem (Severity)			
Stable/recovering/improving	●		
Responding inadequately/minor complication		●	
Unstable/significant complication/new problem			●
Typical Time: Bedside/Floor/Unit	15	25	35

Observation/Inpatient Care Services (New/Established Patients) (Including Admission and Discharge Services)

Components required: 3 of 3	99234	99235	99236
History & Exam			
Detailed or comprehensive	●		
Comprehensive		●	●
Straightforward or low	●		
Moderate		●	
High			●
Presenting Problem (Severity)			
Low	●		
Moderate		●	
High			●
Typical Time:	40	50	55

Office/Other Outpatient Consultations (New/Established Patients)

Components required: 3 of 3	99241	99242	99243	99244	99245
History & Exam					
Problem focused	●				
Expanded problem focused		●			
Detailed			●		
Comprehensive				●	●
Medical Decision Making					
Straightforward	●	●			
Low			●		
Moderate				●	
High					●
Presenting Problem (Severity)					
Self-limited or minor	●				
Low		●			
Moderate			●		
Moderate to high				●	●
Typical Time: Face-to-Face	15	30	40	60	80

Inpatient Consultations (New/Established Patients)

Components required: 3 of 3	99251	99252	99253	99254	99255
History & Exam					
Problem focused	●				
Expanded problem focused		●			
Detailed			●		
Comprehensive				●	●
Medical Decision Making					
Straightforward	●	●			
Low			●		
Moderate				●	
High					●
Presenting Problem (Severity)					
Self-limited or minor	●				
Low		●			
Moderate			●		
Moderate to high				●	●
Typical Time: Bedside/Floor/Unit	20	40	55	80	110

Emergency Department Services (New/Established Patients)

Components required: 3 of 3	99281	99282	99283	99284	99285
History & Exam					
Problem focused	●				
Expanded problem focused		●	●		
Detailed				●	
Comprehensive					●
Medical Decision Making					
Straightforward	●				
Low		●			
Moderate			●	●	
High					●
Presenting Problem (Severity)					
Self-limited or minor	●				
Low to moderate		●			
Moderate			●		
High				●	
High severity/immediate significant threat to life or physiological function					●
Typical Time: Not applicable					

Initial Nursing Facility Care (New/Established Patients)

Components required: 3 of 3	99304	99305	99306
History & Exam			
Detailed or comprehensive	●		
Comprehensive		●	●
Medical Decision Making			
Straightforward or low	●		
Moderate		●	
High			●
Presenting Problem (Severity)			
Low	●		
Moderate		●	
High			●
Typical Time: Bedside/Floor/Unit	25	35	45

Subsequent Nursing Facility Services

Components required: 2 of 3	99307	99308	99309	99310
History & Exam				
Problem focused	●			
Expanded problem focused		●		
Detailed			●	
Comprehensive				●
Medical Decision Making				
Straightforward	●			
Low		●		
Moderate			●	
High				●
Presenting Problem (Severity)				
Stable/recovering/improving	●			
Responding inadequately to therapy/minor complication		●		
Significant complication/significant new problem			●	
Unstable/significant new problem requiring immediate physician attention				●
Typical Time: Bedside/Floor/Unit	10	15	25	35

Domiciliary, Rest Home, Or Custodial Care Services (New Patient)

Components required: 3 of 3	99324	99325	99326	99327	99328
History & Exam					
Problem focused	●				
Expanded problem focused		●			
Detailed			●		
Comprehensive				●	●
Medical Decision Making					
Straightforward	●				
Low		●			
Moderate			●	●	
High					●
Presenting Problem (Severity)					
Low	●				
Moderate		●			
Moderate to high			●		
High				●	
Unstable/significant new problem requiring immediate attention					●
Typical Time: Face-to-Face	20	30	45	60	75

Domiciliary, Rest Home, or Custodial Care Services (Established Patient)

Components required: 2 of 3	99334	99335	99336	99337
History & Exam				
Problem focused	●			
Expanded problem focused		●		
Detailed			●	
Comprehensive				●
Medical Decision Making				
Straightforward	●			
Low		●		
Moderate			●	
Moderate to high				●
Presenting Problem (Severity)				
Self-limited or minor	●			
Low to moderate		●		
Moderate to high			●	
Moderate to high/unstable/significant new problem				●
Typical Time: Face-to-Face	15	25	40	60

Home Services (New Patients)

Components required: 3 of 3	99341	99342	99343	99344	99345
History & Exam					
Problem focused	●				
Expanded problem focused		●			
Detailed			●		
Comprehensive				●	●
Medical Decision Making					
Straightforward	●				
Low		●			
Moderate			●	●	
High					●
Presenting Problem (Severity)					
Low	●				
Moderate		●			
Moderate to high			●		
High				●	
Unstable/significant new problem					●
Typical Time: Face-to-Face	20	30	45	60	75

Home Services (Established Patient)

Components required: 2 of 3	99347	99348	99349	99350
History & Exam				
Problem focused	●			
Expanded problem focused		●		
Detailed			●	
Comprehensive				●
Medical Decision Making				
Straightforward	●			
Low		●		
Moderate			●	
Moderate to high				●
Presenting Problem (Severity)				
Self-limited or minor	●			
Low to moderate		●		
Moderate to high			●	
Moderate to high/unstable/significant new problem				●
Typical Time: Face-to-Face	15	25	40	60

This page intentionally left blank.

EVALUATION AND MANAGEMENT

OFFICE OR OTHER OUTPATIENT SERVICES

The key coding issues are the extent of history obtained, the extent of examination performed, and the complexity of medical decision making. Additional reporting issues include counseling and/or coordination of care, the nature of presenting problem(s), and the duration of face-to-face time spent with the patient and/or family.

CODING RULES

1. *A patient is considered an outpatient until admitted as an inpatient to a health care facility.*

2. *If outpatient evaluation and management services are provided in conjunction with, or result in, an inpatient admission, the service is reported using CPT codes for initial hospital care.*

3. *CPT codes in this section may also be used to report the services provided by a physician to a patient in an observation area of a hospital.*

4. *Laboratory tests, radiology services, and diagnostic or therapeutic procedures performed in conjunction with evaluation and management services are reported in addition to the basic evaluation and management service.*

5. *Supplies and materials provided by the physician over and above those usually included with the evaluation and management or other services rendered may be listed separately. List all drugs, trays, supplies and materials provided.*

The following codes are used to report evaluation and management services provided in the office or in an outpatient or other ambulatory facility. A patient is considered an outpatient until inpatient admission to a health care facility occurs.

To report services provided to a patient who is admitted to a hospital or nursing facility in the course of an encounter in the office or other ambulatory facility, see the notes for initial hospital inpatient care, or initial nursing facility care.

For services provided in the emergency department, see 99281-99288.

For observation care, see 99217-99226.

For observation or inpatient care services (including admission and discharge services), see 99234-99236.

NEW PATIENT

(**99201**   deleted 2020 [2021 Edition]. To report, use 99202)

▲★**99202**   Office or other outpatient visit for the evaluation and management of a new patient, which requires a medically appropriate history and/or examination and straightforward medical decision making. When using time for code selection, 15-29 minutes of total time is spent on the date of the encounter.

▲★**99203**   Office or other outpatient visit for the evaluation and management of a new patient, which requires a medically appropriate history and/or examination and low level of medical decision making.When using time for code selection, 30-44 minutes of total time is spent on the date of the encounter.

▲★**99204**   Office or other outpatient visit for the evaluation and management of a new patient, which requires a medically appropriate history and/or examination and moderate level of medical decision making. When using time for code selection, 45-59 minutes of total time is spent on the date of the encounter.

▲★**99205**   Office or other outpatient visit for the evaluation and management of a new patient, which requires a medically appropriate history and/or examination and high level of medical decision making. When using time for code selection, 60-74 minutes of total time is spent on the date of the encounter.

(For services 75 minutes or longer, use prolonged services code 99417)

ESTABLISHED PATIENT

▲ 99211   Office or other outpatient visit for the evaluation and management of an established patient, that may not require the presence of a physician or other qualified health care professional. Usually, the presenting problem(s) are minimal.

▲★99212   Office or other outpatient visit for the evaluation and management of an established patient, which requires amedically appropriate history and/or examination and straightforward medical decision making.

When using time for code selection, 10-19 minutes of total time is spent on the date of the encounter.

▲★99213   Office or other outpatient visit for the evaluation and management of an established patient, which requires a medically appropriate history and/or examination and low level of medical decision making.

When using time for code selection, 20-29 minutes of total time is spent on the date of the encounter.

▲★99214   Office or other outpatient visit for the evaluation and management of an established patient, which requires a medically appropriate history and/or examination and moderate level of medical decision making.

When using time for code selection, 30-39 minutes of total time is spent on the date of the encounter.

▲★99215   Office or other outpatient visit for the evaluation and management of an established patient, which requires a medically appropriate history and/or examination and high level of medical decision making.

When using time for code selection, 40-54 minutes of total time is spent on the date of the encounter.

(For services 55 minutes or longer, use prolonged services code 99417)

HOSPITAL OBSERVATION SERVICES

Occasionally a physician will watch or "observe" a patient in an area of an inpatient hospital designated as an "observation" area. This area is frequently located in or near the emergency room, and the observation typically after any acute care is rendered.

The purpose of the observation is to determine if the patient's condition requires inpatient hospitalization. Patients considered under observation status may be discharged from the observation area or admitted to the hospital as an inpatient.

All observation care services are "per day" and should be coded only once per date of service. CPT code 99217 is used to report all services provided on discharge from "observation status" if the discharge is on other than the initial date of "observation status."

The following codes are used to report evaluation and management services provided to patients designated/admitted as "observation status" in a hospital. It is not necessary that the patient be located in an observation area designated by the hospital.

If such an area does exist in a hospital (as a separate unit in the hospital, in the emergency department, etc.), these codes are to be utilized if the patient is placed in such an area.

For definitions of key components and commonly used terms, please see Evaluation and Management Services Guidelines.

OBSERVATION CARE DISCHARGE SERVICES

Observation care discharge of a patient from "observation status" includes final examination of the patient, discussion of the hospital stay, instructions for continuing care, and preparation of dishcarge records. For observation or inpatient hospital care including the admission and discharge of the patient on the same date, see codes 99234-99236 as appropriate.

99217   Observation care discharge day management (This code is to be utilized to report all services provided to a patient on discharge from outpatient hospital "observation status" if the discharge is on other than the initial date of "observation status." To report services to a patient designated as "observation status" or "inpatient status" and discharged on the same date, use codes for Observation or Inpatient Care Services [including Admission and Discharge Services, 99234-99236 as appropriate]).

INITIAL OBSERVATION CARE

NEW OR ESTABLISHED PATIENT

The following codes are used to report the encounter(s) by the supervising physician or other qualified health care professional with the patient when designated as outpatient hospital "observation status." This refers to the initiation of observation status, supervision of the care plan for observation, and performance of periodic reassessments. For observation encounters by other physicians, see office or other outpatient consultation codes (99241-99245) or subsequent observation care codes (99224-99226) as appropriate.

To report services provided to a patient who is admitted to the hospital after receiving hospital observation care services on the same date, see the notes for initial hospital inpatient care (later in this section). For observation care services on other than the initial or discharge date, see subsequent observation services codes (99224-99226). For a patient admitted to the hospital on a date subsequent to the date of observation status, the hospital admission would be reported with the appropriate initial hospital care code (99221-99223). For a patient admitted and discharged from observation or inpatient status on the same date, the services should be reported with codes 99234-99236 as appropriate. Do not report observation discharge (99217) in conjunction with a hospital admission (99221-99223).

When "observation status" is initiated in the course of an encounter in another site of service (eg, hospital emergency department, office, nursing facility) all evaluation and management services provided by the supervising physician or other qualified health care professional in conjunction with initiating "observation status" are considered part of the initial observation care when performed on the same date. The observation care level of service reported by the supervising physician or other qualified health care professional should include the services related to initiating "observation status" provided in the other sites of service as well as in the observation setting.

Evaluation and management services including new or established patient office or other outpatient services (99202-99215), emergency department services (99281-99285), nursing facility services (99304-99318), domiciliary, rest home, or custodial care services (99324-99337), home services (99341-99350), and preventive medicine services (99381-99429) on the same date related to the admission to "observation status" should not be reported separately.

These codes may not be utilized for post-operative recovery if the procedure is considered part of the surgical "package." These codes apply to all evaluation and management services that are provided on the same date of initiating "observation status."

99218 Initial observation care, per day, for the evaluation and management of a patient which requires these 3 key components:

- A detailed or comprehensive history;
- A detailed or comprehensive examination; and
- Medical decision making that is straightforward or of low complexity.

Counseling and/or coordination of care with other physicians, other qualified health care professionals, or agencies are provided consistent with the nature of the problem(s) and the patient's and/or family's needs.

Usually, the problem(s) requiring admission to outpatient hospital "observation status" are of low severity. Typically 30 minutes are spent at the bedside and on the patient's hospital floor or unit.

99219 Initial observation care, per day, for the evaluation and management of a patient, which requires these 3 key components:

- A comprehensive history;
- A comprehensive examination; and
- Medical decision making of moderate complexity.

Counseling and/or coordination of care with other physicians, other qualified health care professionals, or agencies are provided consistent with the nature of the problem(s) and the patient's and/or family's needs.

Usually, the problem(s) requiring admission to outpatient hospital "observation status" are of moderate severity. Typically 50 minutes are spent at the bedside and on the patient's hospital floor or unit.

99220 Initial observation care, per day, for the evaluation and management of a patient, which requires these 3 key components:

- A comprehensive history;
- A comprehensive examination; and

- Medical decision making of high complexity.

Counseling and/or coordination of care with other physicians, other qualified health care professionals, or agencies are provided consistent with the nature of the problem(s) and the patient's and/or family's needs.

Usually, the problem(s) requiring admission to outpatient hospital "observation status" are of high severity. Typically 70 minutes are spent at the bedside and on the patient's hospital floor or unit.

SUBSEQUENT OBSERVATION CARE

All levels of subsequent observation care include reviewing the medical record and reviewing the results of diagnostic studies and changes in the patient's status (ie., changes in history, physical condition, and response to management) since the last assessment.

99224 Subsequent observation care, per day, for the evaluation and management of a patient, which requires at least 2 of these 3 key components:

- problem focused interval history;
- problem focused examination;
- medical decision making that is straightforward or of low complexity.

Counseling and/or coordination of care with other physicians, other qualified health care professionals, or agencies are provided consistent with the nature of the problem(s) and the patient's and/or family's needs.

Usually, the patient is stable, recovering, or improving. Typically 15 minutes are spent at the bedside and on the patient's hospital floor or unit.

99225 Subsequent observation care, per day, for the evaluation and management of a patient, which requires at least 2 of these 3 key components:

- an expanded problem focused interval history;
- an expanded problem focused examination;
- medical decision making of moderate complexity

Counseling and/or coordination of care with other physicians, other qualified health care professionals, or agencies are provided consistent with the nature of the problem(s) and the patient's and/or family's needs.

Usually, the patient is responding inadequately to therapy or has developed a minor complication. Typically 25 are spent minutes at the bedside and on the patient's hospital floor or unit.

99226 Subsequent observation care, per day, for the evaluation and management of a patient, which requires at least 2 of these 3 key components:

- a detailed interval history;
- a detailed examination
- medical decision making of high complexity.

Counseling and/or coordination of care with other physicians, other qualified health care professionals, or agencies are provided consistent with the nature of the problem(s) and the patient's and/or family's needs.

Usually, the patient is unstable or has developed a significant complication or a significant new problem. Typically 35 minutes are spent at the bedside and on the patient's hospital floor or unit.

HOSPITAL INPATIENT SERVICES

Hospital inpatient services refer to hospital visits during the course of an inpatient hospital stay. The services may be provided by the patient's primary physician and/or other physicians in the event of multiple illnesses or injuries. Evaluation and management codes 99221-99239 are used to report services provided in the hospital. The key coding issues are the extent of history obtained, the extent of examination performed, and the complexity of medical decision making. Additional reporting issues include counseling and/or coordination of care, the nature of presenting problem(s), and the time spent at the bedside and on the patient's facility floor or unit.

CODING RULES

1. *CPT codes defined as Initial Hospital Care are used to report the first hospital inpatient encounter with the patient by the admitting physician.*

2. *The admitting physician should report all service related to the admission provided in all other locations.*

3. *For observation care or inpatient hospital care services provided to patients who are admitted and discharged on the same date, report with CPT codes 99234-99236 from the Observation or Inpatient Care services subsections.*

The following codes are used to report evaluation and management services provided to hospital inpatients. Hospital inpatient services include those services provided to patients in a "partial hospital" setting. These codes are to be used to report these partial hospitalization services. See also psychiatry notes in the full text of the CPT code set.

For definitions of key components and commonly used terms, please see Evaluation and Management Services Guidelines. For Hospital Observation Services, see 99218-99220, 99224-99226. For a patient admitted and discharged from observation or inpatient status on the same date, the services should be reported with codes 99234-99236 as appropriate.

INITIAL HOSPITAL CARE

NEW OR ESTABLISHED PATIENT

The following codes are used to report the first hospital inpatient encounter with the patient by the admitting physician.

For initial inpatient encounters by physicians other than the admitting physician, see initial inpatient consultation codes (99251-99255) or subsequent hospital care codes (99231-99233) as .appropriate.

For admission services for the neonate (28 days of age or younger) requiring intensive observation, frequent interventions, and other intensive care services, see 99477.

When the patient is admitted to the hospital as an inpatient in the course of an encounter in another site of service (eg, hospital emergency department, observation status in a hospital, office, nursing facility), all evaluation and mangement services provided by that physician in conjunction with that admission are considered part of the initial hospital care when performed on the same date as the admission. The inpatient care level of service reported by the admitting physician should include the services related to the admission he/she provided in the other sites of service as well as in the inpatient setting.

Evaluation and management services including new or established patient office or other outpatient services (99202-99215), emergency department services (99281-99285), nursing facility services (99304-99318), domiciliary, rest home, or custodial care services (99324-99337), home services (99341-99350), and preventive medicine services (99381-99397) on the same date related to the admission to "observation status" should not be reported separately. For a patient admitted and discharged from observation or inpatient status on the same date, the services should be reported with codes 99234-99236 as appropriate.

99221 Initial hospital care, per day, for the evaluation and management of a patient which requires these three key components:

- a detailed or comprehensive history;

- a detailed or comprehensive examination; and

- medical decision making that is straightforward or of low complexity.

Counseling and/or coordination of care with other physicians, other qualified health care professionals, or agencies are provided consistent with the nature of the problem(s) and the patient's and/or family's needs.

Usually, the problem(s) requiring admission are of low severity. Typically 30 minutes are spent at the bedside and on the patient's hospital floor or unit.

99222 Initial hospital care, per day, for the evaluation and management of a patient, which requires these three key components:

- a comprehensive history;
- a comprehensive examination; and
- medical decision making of moderate complexity.

Counseling and/or coordination of care with other physicians, other qualified health care professionals, or agencies are provided consistent with the nature of the problem(s) and the patient's and/or family's needs.

Usually, the problem(s) requiring admission are of moderate severity. Typically 50 minutes are spent at the bedside and on the patient's hospital floor or unit.

99223 Initial hospital care, per day, for the evaluation and management of a patient, which requires these three key components:

- a comprehensive history;
- a comprehensive examination; and
- medical decision making of high complexity.

Counseling and/or coordination of care with other physicians, other qualified health care professionals, or agencies are provided consistent with the nature of the problem(s) and the patient's and/or family's needs.

Usually, the problem(s) requiring admission are of high severity. Typically 70 minutes are spent at the bedside and on the patient's hospital floor or unit.

99224 This code is out of order. See page 144.

99225 This code is out of order. See page 144.

99226 This code is out of order. See page 144.

SUBSEQUENT HOSPITAL CARE

All levels of subsequent hospital care include reviewing the medical record and reviewing the results of diagnostic studies and changes in the patient's status (i.e., changes in history, physical condition and response to management) since the last assessment.

★ **99231** Subsequent hospital care, per day, for the evaluation and management of a patient, which requires at least two of these three key components:

- a problem focused interval history;
- a problem focused examination;
- medical decision making that is straightforward or of low complexity.

Counseling and/or coordination of care with other physicians, other qualified health care professionals, or agencies are provided consistent with the nature of the problem(s) and the patient's and/or family's needs.

Usually, the patient is stable, recovering or improving. Typically 15 minutes are spent at the bedside and on the patient's hospital floor or unit.

★ **99232** Subsequent hospital care, per day, for the evaluation and management of a patient, which requires at least two of these three key components:

- an expanded problem focused interval history;
- an expanded problem focused examination;
- medical decision making of moderate complexity.

Counseling and/or coordination of care with other physicians, other qualified health care professionals, or agencies are provided consistent with the nature of the problem(s) and the patient's and/or family's needs.

Usually, the patient is responding inadequately to therapy or has developed a minor complication. Typically 25 minutes are spent at the bedside and on the patient's hospital floor or unit.

★ **99233** Subsequent hospital care, per day, for the evaluation and management of a patient, which requires at least two of these three key components:

- a detailed interval history;
- a detailed examination;
- medical decision making of high complexity.

Counseling and/or coordination of care with other physicians, other qualified health care professionals, or agencies are provided consistent with the nature of the problem(s) and the patient's and/or family's needs.

Usually, the patient is unstable or has developed a significant complication or a significant new problem. Typically 35 minutes are spent at the bedside and on the patient's hospital floor or unit.

OBSERVATION OR INPATIENT CARE SERVICES (INCLUDING ADMISSION AND DISCHARGE SERVICES)

The following codes are used to report observation or inpatient hospital care services provided to patients admitted and discharged on the same date of sevice. When a patient is admitted to the hospital from observation status on the same date, only the initial hospital care code should be reported. The initial hospital care code reported by the admitting physician or other qualified health care professional should include the services related to the observation status services he/she provided on the same date of inpatient admission.

When "observation status" is initiated in the course of an encounter in another site of service (eg, hospital emergency department, office, nursing facility), all evaluation and management services provided by the supervising physician or other qualified health care professional in conjunction with initiating "observation status" are considered part of the initial observation care when performed on the same date. The observation care level of service should include the services related to initiating "observation status" provided in the other sites of services as well as in the observation setting when provided by the same individual.

For patients admitted to observation or inpatient care and discharged on a different date, see codes 99218-99220, 99224-99226, 99217, or 99221-99223, 99238, and 99239.

99234 Observation or inpatient hospital care, for the evaluation and management of a patient including admission and discharge on the same date which requires these three key components:

- a detailed or comprehensive history;
- a detailed or comprehensive examination; and
- medical decision making that is straightforward or of low complexity.

Counseling and/or coordination of care with other physicians, other qualified health care professionals, or agencies are provided consistent with the nature of the problem(s) and the patient's and/or family's needs.

Usually the presenting problem(s) requiring admission are of low severity. Typically 40 minutes are spent at the bedside and on the patient's hospital floor or unit.

99235 Observation or inpatient hospital care, for the evaluation and management of a patient including admission and discharge on the same date which requires these three key components:

- a comprehensive history;
- a comprehensive examination; and
- medical decision making of moderate complexity.

Counseling and/or coordination of care with other physicians, other qualified health care professionals, or agencies are provided consistent with the nature of the problem(s) and the patient's and/or family's needs.

Usually the presenting problem(s) requiring admission are of moderate severity. Typically, 50 minutes are spent at the bedside and on the patient's hospital floor or unit.

99236 Observation or inpatient hospital care, for the evaluation and management of a patient including admission and discharge on the same date which requires these three key components:

- a comprehensive history;
- a comprehensive examination; and
- medical decision making of high complexity.

Counseling and/or coordination of care with other physicians, other qualified health care professionals, or agencies are provided consistent with the nature of the problem(s) and the patient's and/or family's needs.

Usually the presenting problem(s) requiring admission are of high severity. Typically, 55 minutes are spent at the bedside and on the patient's floor or unit.

HOSPITAL DISCHARGE SERVICES

The hospital discharge day management codes are to be used to report the total duration of time spent by a physician for final hospital discharge of a patient. The codes include, as appropriate, final examination of the patient, discussion of the hospital stay, even if the time spent by the physician on that date is not continuous, instructions for continuing care to all relevant caregivers, and preparation of discharge records, prescriptions and referral forms. For a patient admitted and discharged from observation or inpatient status on the same date, the services should be reported with codes 99234-99236 as appropriate.

99238 Hospital discharge day management; 30 minutes or less

99239 more than 30 minutes

(These codes are to be utilized to report all services provided to a patient on the date of discharge, if other than the initial date of inpatient status. To report services to a patient who is admitted as an inpatient and discharged on the same date, see codes 99234-99236 for observation or inpatient hospital care including the admission and discharge of the patient on the same date. To report concurrent care services provided by a individual other than the physician or qualified health care professional performing the discharge day management service, use subsequent hospital care codes [99231-99233] on the day of discharge.)

(For Observation Care Discharge, use 99217)

(For observation or inpatient hospital care including the admission and discharge of the patient on the same date, see 99234-99236)

(For Nursing Facility Care Discharge, 99315, 99316)

(For discharge services provided to newborns admitted and discharged on the same date, use 99463)

CONSULTATIONS

A consultation is a type of evaluation and management service provided at the request of another physician or appropriate source to either recommend care for a specific condition or problem or to determine whether to accept responsibility for ongoing management of the patient's entire care or for the care of a specific condition or problem.

A physician consultant may initiate diagnostic and/or therapeutic services at the same or subsequent visit.

A "consultation" initiated by a patient and/or family, and not requested by a physician or other appropriate source (eg, physician assistant, nurse practitioner, doctor of chiropractic, physical therapist, occupational therapist, speech-language pathologist, psychologist, social worker, lawyer, or insurance company) is not reported using the consultation codes, but may be reported using the office visit, home service, or domiciliary/rest home care codes as appropriate.

The written or verbal request for consult may be made by a physician or other appropriate source and documented in the patient's medical record by either the consulting or requesting physician or appropriate source. The consultant's opinion and any services that were ordered or performed must also be documented in the patient's medical record and sommunicated by written report to the requesting physician or other appropriate source.

If a consultation is mandated (eg, by a third-party payer) modifier 32 should also be reported.

Any specifically identifiable procedure (ie, identified with a specific CPT code) performed on or subsequent to the date of the initial consultation should be reported separately.

If subsequent to the completion of a consultation the consultant assumes responsibility for management of a portion or all of the patient's condition(s), the appropriate Evaluation and Management services code for the site of service should be reported. In the hospital or nursing facility setting, the consulting consultant should use the appropriate inpatient consultation code for the initial encounter and then subsequent hospital or nursing facility care codes. In the office setting, the consultant should use the appropriate office or other outpatient consultation codes and then the established patient office or other outpatient services codes.

To report services provided to a patient who is admitted to a hospital or nursing facility in the course of an encounter in the office or other ambulatory facility, see the notes for Initial Hospital Inpatient Care or Initial Nursing Facility Care. For definitions of key components and commonly used terms, please see Evaluation and Management Services Guidelines.

CODING GUIDELINES

A consultation is the process of taking a history, performing a physical examination, and ordering and interpreting appropriate diagnostic tests for the purpose of rendering an expert opinion about a patient's illness and/or injury. E/M service codes 99241-99275 are used to report office, inpatient, and confirmatory consultation services provided to new or established patients. The key coding issues are the location of the service, the extent of history obtained, the extent of examination performed, and the complexity of medical decision making. Additional reporting issues include counseling and/or coordination of care, the nature of presenting problem(s), and the time, depending on location, spent either face to face with the patient and/or family or at the bedside and on the patient's facility floor or unit.

Coding Rules

1. *The request for a consultation from the attending physician or other appropriate source and the need for a consultation must be documented in the patient's medical record.*

2. *The consultant's opinion and any services that were ordered or performed must be documented in the patient's medical record and communicated to the requesting physician or source.*

3. *Consultations that are initiated by request from the patient and/or family may be reported using codes for confirmatory consultations or office services as appropriate.*

4. *If a confirmatory consultation is required by a third party, such as a Peer Review Organization (PRO), modifier -32 should be added to the basic service.*

5. *Any specifically identifiable procedure performed on or subsequent to the date of the initial consultation is reported separately.*

6. *If the consultant subsequently assumes responsibility for management of all or a portion of the patient's condition(s), then either hospital services or office services are used as appropriate.*

Consultation service codes may not be billed to Medicare for services rendered on or after January 1, 2010. Physicians must use visit/outpatient or inpatient hospital evaluation and management codes to bill Medicare for consultation services. Telehealth consultation may be reported using the appropriate HCPCS G-codes.

Medicare Cross-Walk from Consultation Codes to Outpatient/Hospital Codes

CMS published a cross-walk from consultation codes to outpatient/hospital codes for the purpose of establishing budget neutrality. According to CMS the cross-walks are not billing guidance and physicians should bill the E/M code appropriate for the service provided. For office based consultations, the selection of E/M visit codes is based on whether the patient is a new or established patient. For hospital consultations, the selection of appropriate E/M codes is based on the location of the consultation in either an acute care hospital or nursing home and the level of history, exam, and medical decision making.

Office Consultation Codes			Inpatient Consultation Codes		
Source	Destination	Mapping*	Source	Destination	Mapping*
99241	99202	50%	99251	99221	70%
	99211	50%		99304	30%
99242	99202	50%	99252	99221	35%
	99212	50%		99222	35%
99243	99203	50%		99304	15%
	99213	50%		99305	15%
99244	99204	50%	99253	99222	70%
	99214	50%		99305	30%
99245	99205	50%	99254	99222	35%
	99215	50%		99223	35%
				99305	15%
				99306	15%
			99255	99223	70%
				99306	30%

Separate Procedure   Unlisted Procedure   CCI Comp. Code   Non-specific Procedure   **149**

OFFICE OR OTHER OUTPATIENT CONSULTATIONS

NEW OR ESTABLISHED PATIENT

The following codes are used to report consultations provided in the office or in an outpatient or other ambulatory facility, including hospital observation services, home services, domiciliary, rest home or emergency department (see the preceding consultation definition above). Follow-up visits in the consultant's office or other outpatient facility that are initiated by the consultant or patient are reported using the appropriate codes for established patients, office visits (99211-99215), domiciliary, rest home (99334-99337), or home (99347-99350). If an additional request for an opinion or advice regarding the same or a new problem is received from another physician or other appropriate source and documented in the medical record, the office consultation codes may be used again. Services that constitute transfer of care (ie, are provided for the managment of the patient's entire care or for the care of a specific condition or problem) are reported with the appropriate new or established patient codes for office or other outpatient visits, domiciliary, rest home services, or home services.

★ **99241**   Office consultation for a new or established patient, which requires these three key components:

- • a problem focused history;
- • a problem focused examination; and
- • straightforward medical decision making.

Counseling and/or coordination of care with other physicians, other qualified health care professionals, or agencies are provided consistent with the nature of the problem(s) and the patient's and/or family's needs.

Usually, the presenting problem(s) are self limited or minor. Typically 15 minutes are spent face-to-face with the patient and/or family.

Medicare Cross-Walk:

Report 99202 instead of 99241 for new patients.
Report 99211 instead of 99241 for established patients.

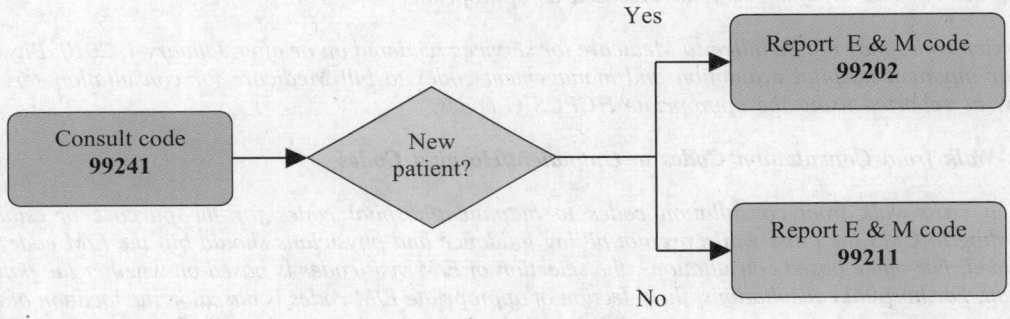

★ **99242**   Office consultation for a new or established patient, which requires these three key components:

- • an expanded problem focused history;
- • an expanded problem focused examination; and
- • straightforward medical decision making.

Counseling and/or coordination of care with other physicians, other qualified health care professionals, or agencies are provided consistent with the nature of the problem(s) and the patient's and/or family's needs.

Usually, the presenting problem(s) are of low severity. Typically 30 minutes are spent face-to-face with the patient and/or family.

Medicare Cross-Walk:

Report 99202 instead of 99242 for new patients.
Report 99212 instead of 99242 for established patients.

---

150   • New Code   ▲ Revised Code   + Add-On Code   ⊘ Modifier -51 Exempt   ★ Telemedicine

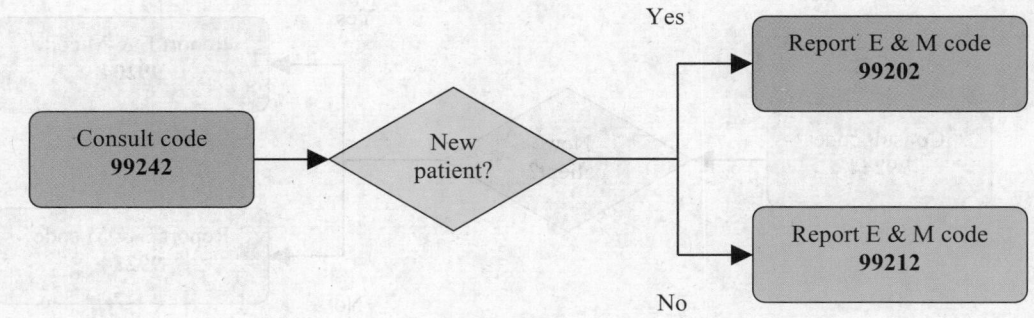

★ **99243**   Office consultation for a new or established patient, which requires these three key components:

- a detailed history;
- a detailed examination; and
- medical decision making of low complexity.

Counseling and/or coordination of care with other physicians, other qualified health care professionals, or agencies are provided consistent with the nature of the problem(s) and the patient's and/or family's needs.

Usually, the presenting problem(s) are of moderate severity. Typically 40 minutes are spent face-to-face with the patient and/or family.

Medicare Cross-Walk:

Report 99203 instead of 99243 for new patients.
Report 99213 instead of 99243 for established patients

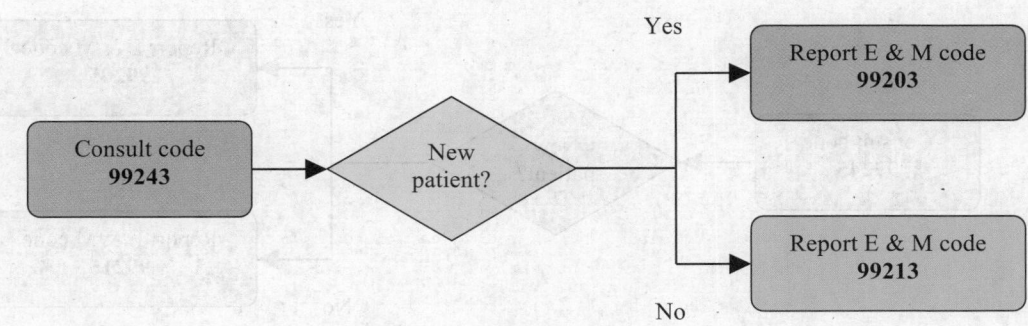

★ **99244**   Office consultation for a new or established patient, which requires these three key components:

- a comprehensive history;
- a comprehensive examination; and
- medical decision making of moderate complexity.

Counseling and/or coordination of care with other physicians, other qualified health care professionals, or agencies are provided consistent with the nature of the problem(s) and the patient's and/or family's needs.

Usually, the presenting problem(s) are of moderate to high severity. Typically 60 minutes are spent face-to-face with the patient and/or family.

Medicare Cross-Walk:

Report 99204 instead of 99244 for new patients.
Report 99214 instead of 99244 for established patients.

| Separate Procedure | Unlisted Procedure | CCI Comp. Code | Non-specific Procedure | **151** |

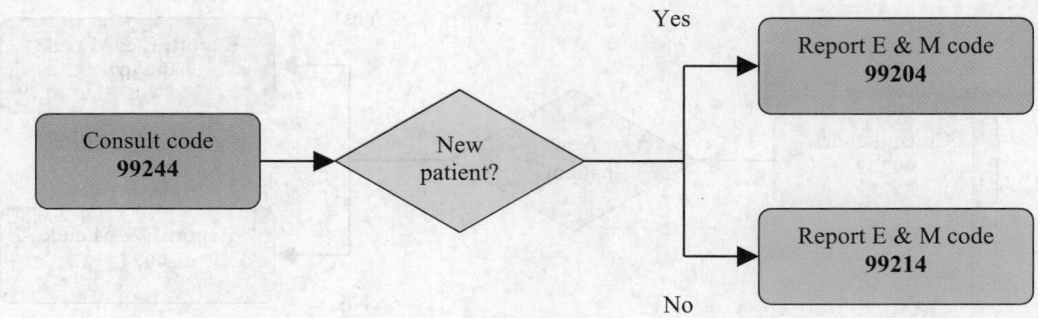

★ **99245** Office consultation for a new or established patient, which requires these three key components:

- a comprehensive history;
- a comprehensive examination; and
- medical decision making of high complexity.

Counseling and/or coordination of care with other physicians, other qualified health care professionals, or agencies are provided consistent with the nature of the problem(s) and the patient's and/or family's needs.

Usually, the presenting problem(s) are of moderate to high severity. Typically 80 minutes are spent face-to-face with the patient and/or family.

Medicare Cross-Walk:

Report 99205 instead of 99245 for new patients.
Report 99215 instead of 99245 for established patients.

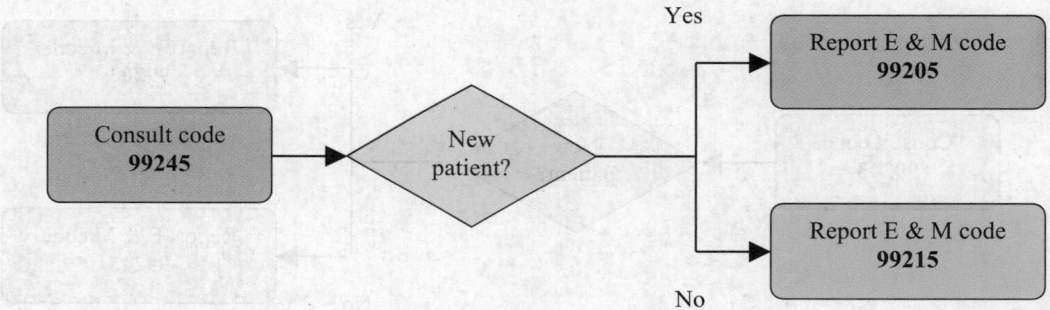

INPATIENT CONSULTATIONS

NEW OR ESTABLISHED PATIENT

The following codes are used to report physician or other qualified health care professional consultations provided to hospital inpatients, residents of nursing facilities, or patients in a partial hospital setting. Only one consultation should be reported by a consultant per admission. Subsequent services during the same admission are reported using Subsequent Hospital Care codes (99231-99233) or Subsequent Nursing Facility Care codes (99307-99310), including services to complete the initial consultation, monitor progress, revise recommendations, or address a new problem. Use subsequent hospital care codes (99231-99233) or subsequent nursing facility care codes (99307-99310) to report transfer of care services.

When an inpatient consultation is performed on a date that a patient is admitted to a hospital or nursing facility, all E/M services provided by the consultant related to the admission are reported with the inpatient consultation service code (99251-99255). If a patient is admitted after an oupatient consultation (office, emergency department, etc.), and the patient is not seen on the unit on the date of admission, only report the outpatient consultation code (99241-99245). If the patient is seen by the consultant on the unit on the date of admission, report all E/M services provided by the consultant related to the admission with either the inpatient consultation code (99251-99255) or with the initial inpatient admission service code (99221-99223). Do not report both an outpatient consultation (99241-99245) and inpatient consultation (99251-99255) for services related to the same inpatient stay.

When transfer of care services are provided on a date subsequent to the outpatient consultation, use the subsequent hospital care codes (99231-99233) or subsequent nursing facility care codes (99307-99310).

★ **99251**   Inpatient consultation for a new or established patient, which requires these three key components:

- a problem focused history;
- a problem focused examination; and
- straightforward medical decision making.

Counseling and/or coordination of care with other physicians, other qualified health care professionals, or agencies are provided consistent with the nature of the problem(s) and the patient's and/or family's needs.

Usually, the presenting problem(s) are self limited or minor. Typically 20 minutes are spent at the bedside and on the patient's hospital floor or unit.

Medicare Cross-Walk:

Report 99221 instead of 99251 for acute hospital consultations.
Report 99304 instead of 99251 for nursing home consultations.

★ **99252**   Inpatient consultation for a new or established patient, which requires these three key components:

- an expanded problem focused history;
- an expanded problem focused examination; and
- straightforward medical decision making.

Counseling and/or coordination of care with other physicians, other qualified health care professionals, or agencies are provided consistent with the nature of the problem(s) and the patient's and/or family's needs.

Usually, the presenting problem(s) are of low severity. Typically 40 minutes are spent at the bedside and on the patient's hospital floor or unit.

Medicare Cross-Walk:

Report 99221 or 99222 instead of 99252 for acute hospital consultations.
Report 99304 or 99305 instead of 99252 for nursing home consultations.

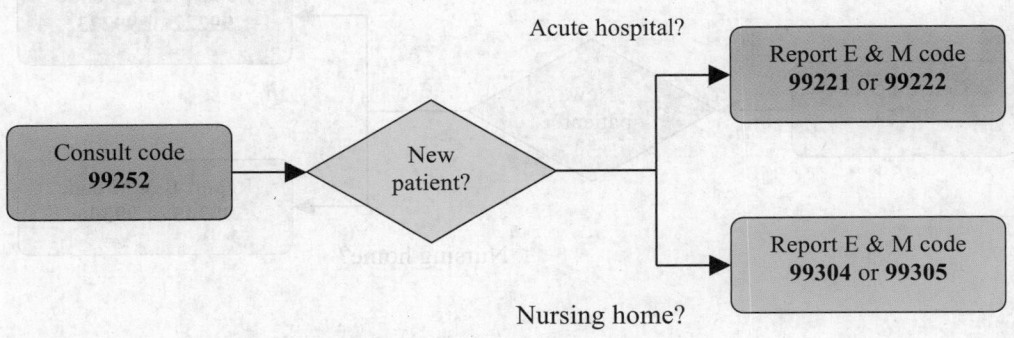

| | Separate Procedure | | Unlisted Procedure | | CCI Comp. Code | | Non-specific Procedure | **153** |

★ **99253** Inpatient consultation for a new or established patient, which requires these three key components:

- a detailed history;
- a detailed examination; and
- medical decision making of low complexity.

Counseling and/or coordination of care with other physicians, other qualified health care professionals, or agencies are provided consistent with the nature of the problem(s) and the patient's and/or family's needs.

Usually, the presenting problem(s) are of moderate severity. Typically 55 minutes are spent at the bedside and on the patient's hospital floor or unit.

Medicare Cross-Walk:

Report 99222 instead of 99253 for acute hospital consultations.
Report 99305 instead of 99253 for nursing home consultations

★ **99254** Inpatient consultation for a new or established patient, which requires three key components:

- a comprehensive history;
- a comprehensive examination; and
- medical decision making of moderate complexity.

Counseling and/or coordination of care with other physicians, other qualified health care professionals, or agencies are provided consistent with the nature of the problem(s) and the patient's and/or family's needs.

Usually, the presenting problem(s) are of moderate to high severity. Typically 80 minutes are spent at the bedside and on the patient's hospital floor or unit.

Medicare Cross-Walk:

Report 99222 or 99223 instead of 99254 for acute hospital consultations.
Report 99305 or 99306 instead of 99254 for nursing home consultations.

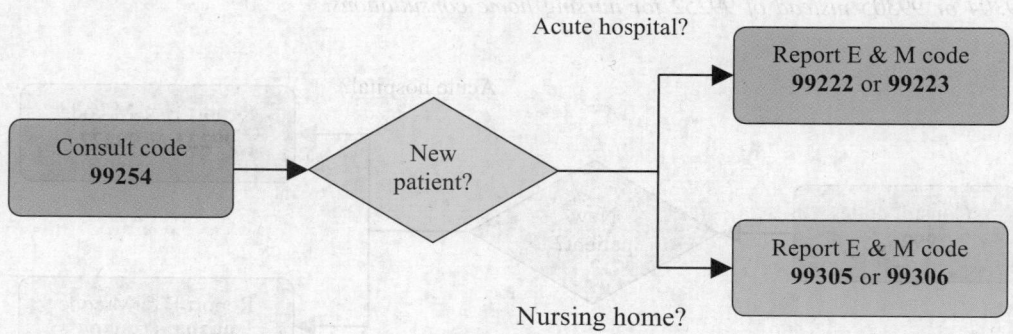

● New Code   ▲ Revised Code   ✛ Add-On Code   ⊘ Modifier -51 Exempt   ★ Telemedicine

★ **99255** Inpatient consultation for a new or established patient, which requires these three key components:

- a comprehensive history;
- a comprehensive examination; and
- medical decision making of high complexity.

Counseling and/or coordination of care with other physicians, other qualified health care professionals, or agencies are provided consistent with the nature of the problem(s) and the patient's and/or family's needs.

Usually, the presenting problem(s) are of moderate to high severity. Typically 110 minutes are spent at the bedside and on the patient's hospital floor or unit.

Medicare Cross-Walk:

Report 99223 instead of 99255 for acute hospital consultations.
Report 99306 instead of 99255 for nursing home consultations.

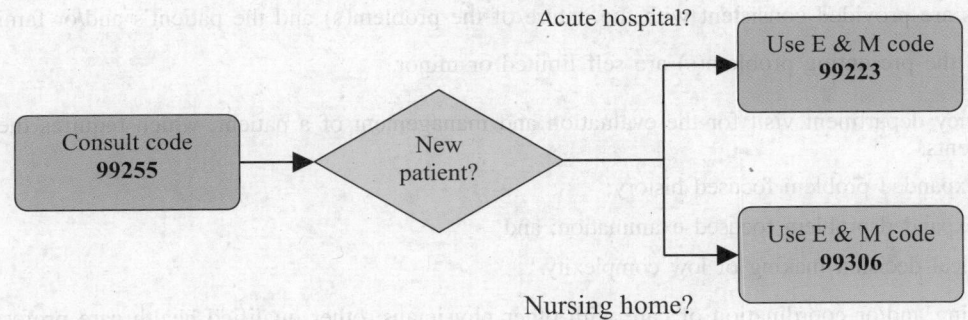

EMERGENCY DEPARTMENT SERVICES

Evaluation and management codes 99281-99288 are used to report services provided to new or established patients in the emergency department. The emergency department is defined as a facility for the treatment of patients with emergent conditions. The emergency department must be attached to a hospital and operate on a 24/7 basis.

The key coding issues for evaluation and management emergency services are the extent of history obtained, the extent of examination performed, and the complexity of medical decision making. Additional reporting issues include counseling and/or coordination of care, and the nature of presenting problem(s).

Time is not a descriptive component for evaluation and management services provided in the emergency department. These services are typically provided on a variable intensity basis, often involving multiple encounters with several patients over an extended period of time. Therefore, it is difficult for physicians to provide accurate estimates of the time spent face-to-face with the patient in the emergency department.

CODING RULES

1. *No distinction is made between new and established patients in the emergency department.*

2. *If the emergency department is used for observation or inpatient care services, report using codes from the Observation Care services subsection of the CPT coding system.*

3. *For critical care services provided in the emergency department, use the appropriate codes from the Critical Care subsection of the CPT coding system.*

EMERGENCY DEPARTMENT SERVICES

NEW OR ESTABLISHED PATIENT

The following codes are used to report evaluation and management services provided in the emergency department. No distinction is made between new and established patients in the emergency department.

An emergency department is defined as an organized hospital-based facility for the provision of unscheduled episodic services to patients who present for immediate medical attention. The facility must be available 24 hours a day.

For critical care services provided in the emergency department, see Critical Care notes and 99291, 99292.

For evaluation and management services provided to a patient in an observation area of a hospital, see 99217-99220.

For observation or inpatient care services (including admission and discharge services), see 99234-99236.

99281 Emergency department visit for the evaluation and management of a patient, which requires these three key components:

- a problem focused history;
- a problem focused examination; and
- straightforward medical decision making.

Counseling and/or coordination of care with other physicians, other qualified health care professionals, or agencies are provided consistent with the nature of the problem(s) and the patient's and/or family's needs.

Usually, the presenting problem(s) are self limited or minor.

99282 Emergency department visit for the evaluation and management of a patient, which requires these three key components:

- an expanded problem focused history;
- an expanded problem focused examination; and
- medical decision making of low complexity.

Counseling and/or coordination of care with other physicians, other qualified health care professionals, or agencies are provided consistent with the nature of the problem(s) and the patient's and/or family's needs.

Usually, the presenting problem(s) are of low to moderate severity.

99283 Emergency department visit for the evaluation and management of a patient, which requires these three key components:

- an expanded problem focused history;
- an expanded problem focused examination; and
- medical decision making of moderate complexity.

Counseling and/or coordination of care with other physicians, other qualified health care professionals, or agencies are provided consistent with the nature of the problem(s) and the patient's and/or family's needs.

Usually, the presenting problem(s) are of moderate severity.

99284 Emergency department visit for the evaluation and management of a patient, which requires these three key components:

- a detailed history;
- a detailed examination; and
- medical decision making of moderate complexity.

Counseling and/or coordination of care with other physicians, other qualified health care professionals, or agencies are provided consistent with the nature of the problem(s) and the patient's and/or family's needs.

Usually, the presenting problem(s) are of high severity, and require urgent evaluation by the physician or other qualified health care professional but do not pose an immediate significant threat to life or physiologic function.

99285 Emergency department visit for the evaluation and management of a patient, which requires these three key components within the constraints imposed by the urgency of the patient's clinical condition and/or mental status:

- a comprehensive history;

- a comprehensive examination; and
- medical decision making of high complexity.

Counseling and/or coordination of care with other physicians, other qualified health care professionals, or agencies are provided consistent with the nature of the problem(s) and the patient's and/or family's needs.

Usually, the presenting problem(s) are of high severity and pose an immediate significant threat to life or physiologic function.

OTHER EMERGENCY SERVICES

In directed emergency care, advanced life support, the physician or other qualified health care professional is located in a hospital emergency or critical care department, and is in two-way voice communication with ambulance or rescue personnel outside the hospital. Direction of the performance of necessary medical procedures includes but is not limited to: telemetry of cardiac rhythm; cardiac and/or pulmonary resuscitation; endotracheal or esophageal obturator airway intubation; administration of intravenous fluids and/or administration of intramuscular, intratracheal or subcutaneous drugs; and/or electrical conversion of arrhythmia.

99288   Physician or other qualified health care professional direction of emergency medical systems (EMS) emergency care, advanced life support

CRITICAL CARE SERVICES

Critical care is the direct delivery by a physician(s) or other qualified health care professional of medical care for a critically ill or critically injured patient. A critical illness or injury acutely impairs one or more vital organ systems such that there is a high probability of imminent or life threatening deterioration in the patient's condition. Critical care involves high complexity decision making to assess, manipulate, and support vital system function(s) to treat single or multiple vital organ system failure and/or to prevent further life threatening deterioration of the patient's condition. Examples of vital organ system failure include, but are not limited to: central nervous system failure, circulatory failure, shock, renal, hepatic, metabolic, and/or respiratory failure. Although critical care typically requires interpretation of multiple physiologic parameters and/or application of advanced technology(s), critical care may be provided in life threatening situations when these elements are not present. Critical care may be provided on multiple days, even if no changes are made in the treatment rendered to the patient, provided that the patient's condition continues to require the level of attention described above.

Providing medical care to a critically ill, injured, or post-operative patient qualifies as a critical care service only if both the illness or injury and the treatment being provided meet the above requirements. Critical care is usually, but not always, given in a critical care area, such as the coronary care unit, intensive care unit, pediatric intensive care unit, respiratory care unit, or the emergency care facility.

Inpatient critical care services provided to infants 29 days through 71 months of age are reported with pediatric critical care codes 99471-99476. The pediatric critical care codes are reported as long as the infant/young child qualifies for critical care services during the hospital stay through 71 months of age. Inpatient critical care services provided to neonates (28 days of age or younger) are reported with the neonatal critical care codes 99468 and 99469. The neonatal critical care codes are reported as long as the neonate qualifies for critical care services during the hospital stay through the 28th postnatal day. The reporting of the pediatric and neonatal critical care services is not based on time or the type of unit (eg, pediatric or neonatal critical care unit) and it is not dependent upon the type of physician or other qualified health care professional delivering the care. To report critical care services provided in the outpatient setting (eg, emergency department or office), for neonates and pediatric patients up through 71 months of age, see the critical care codes 99291, 99292. If the same individual provides critical care services for a neonatal or pediatric patient in both the outpatient and inpatient settings on the same day, report only the appropriate neonatal or pediatric critical care code 99468-99472 for all critical care services provided on that day. Also report 99291-99292 for neonatal or pediatric critical care services provided by the individual providing critical care at one facility but transferring the patient to another facility. Critical care services provided by a second individual of a different specialty not reporting a per day neonatal or pediatric critical care code can be reported with codes 99291-99292. For additional instructions reporting these services, see the Neonatal and Pediatric Critical Care section and codes 99468-99476.

Services for a patient who is not critically ill but happens to be in a critical care unit are reported using other appropriate E/M codes. Critical care and other E/M services may be provided to the same patient on the same date by the same physician.

Critical care and other E/M services may be provided to the same patient on the same date by the same individual.

For reporting by professionals, the following services are included in critical care when performed during the critical period by the physician(s) providing critical care: the interpretation of cardiac output measurements (93561, 93562), chest X-rays (71045,

71046), pulse oximetry (94760, 94761, 94762), blood gases, and collection and interpretation of physiologic data (eg., ECGs, blood pressures, hematologic data); gastric intubation (43752, 43753); temporary transcutaneous pacing (92953); ventilatory management (94002-94004, 94660, 94662); and vascular access procedures (36000, 36410, 36415, 36591, 36600). Any services performed that are not included in this listing should be reported separately. Facilities may report the above services separately.

Codes 99291, 99292 should be reported for the attendance during the transport of critically ill or critically injured patients older than 24 months of age to or from a facility or hospital. For transport services of critically ill or critically injured pediatric patients 24 months of age or younger, see 99466, 99467.

Codes 99291, 99292 are used to report the total duration of time spent in provision of critical care services to a critically ill or critically injured patient, even if the time spent providing care on that date is not continuous. For any given period of time spent providing critical care services, the individual must devote his or her full attention to the patient and, therefore, cannot provide services to any other patient during the same period of time.

Time spent with the individual patient should be recorded in the patient's record. The time that can be reported as critical care is the time spent engaged in work directly related to the individual patient's care whether that time was spent at the immediate bedside or elsewhere on the floor or unit. For example, time spent on the unit or at the nursing station on the floor reviewing test results or imaging studies, discussing the critically ill patient's care with other medical staff or documenting critical care services in the medical record would be reported as critical care, even though it does not occur at the bedside. Also, when the patient is unable to lacks capacity to participate in discussions, time spent on the floor or unit with family members or surrogate decision makers obtaining a medical history, reviewing the patient's condition or prognosis, or discussing treatment or limitation(s) of treatment may be reported as critical care, provided that the conversation bears directly on the management of the patient.

Time spent in activities that occur outside of the unit or off the floor (eg, telephone calls whether taken at home, in the office or elsewhere in the hospital) may not be reported as critical care since the individual is not immediately available to the patient. Time spent in activities that do not directly contribute to the treatment of the patient may not be reported as critical care, even if they are performed in the critical care unit (eg, participation in administration meetings or telephone calls to discuss other patients). Time spent performing separately reportable procedures or services should not be included in the time reported as critical care time.

Code 99291 is used to report the first 30-74 minutes of critical care on a given date. It should be used only once per date even if the time spent by the individual is not continuous on that date. Critical care of less than 30 minutes total duration on a given date should be reported with the appropriate E/M code.

Code 99292 is used to report additional block(s) of time, of up to 30 minutes each beyond the first 74 minutes. (See table)

CORRECT CODING CHART FOR CRITICAL CARE SERVICES

DURATION OF CRITICAL CARE	CODE(S) TO REPORT
less than 30 minutes	appropriate E/M codes
30-74 minutes	99291 once
75-104 minutes	99291 once and 99292 once
105-134 minutes	99291 once and 99292 twice
135-164 minutes	99291 once and 99292 three times
165-194 minutes	99291 once and 99292 four times
195 minutes or longer	99291 and 99292 as appropriate (see example above)

CODING RULES

1. *The critical care CPT codes are used to report the total duration of time spent by a physician providing constant attention to a critically ill patient.*

2. *Critical care code 99291 is used to report the first 30-74 minutes of critical care on a given day. It should be reported only once per day even if the time spent is not continuous on that day.*

3. *Critical care 99292 is used to report each additional 30 minutes beyond the first 74 minutes.*

4. *Other procedures which are not considered included in the critical care services, for example, suturing of lacerations, setting of fractures, reduction of joint dislocations, lumbar puncture, peritoneal lavage and bladder tap, are reported separately.*

CRITICAL CARE SERVICES

99291   Critical care, evaluation and management of the critically ill or critically injured patient; first 30-74 minutes

+ 99292   each additional 30 minutes (List separately in addition to code for primary service)

(Use 99292 in conjunction with 99291)

NURSING FACILITY SERVICES

The following codes are used to report evaluation and management services to patients in nursing facilities (formerly called skilled nursing facilities [SNFs], intermediate care facilities [ICFs], or long-term care facilities [LTCFs]).

These codes should also be used to report evaluation and management services provided to a patient in a psychiatric residential treatment center (a facility or a distinct part of a facility for psychiatric care, which provides a 24-hour therapeutically planned and professionally staffed group living and learning environment). If procedures such as medical psychotherapy are provided in addition to evaluation and management services, these should be reported in addition to the E/M services provided.

Nursing facilities that provide convalescent, rehabilitative, or long-term care are required to conduct comprehensive accurate, standardized, and reproducible assessments of each resident's functional capacity using a Resident Assessment Instrument (RAI). All RAIs include the Minimum Data Set (MDS), Resident Assessment Protocols (RAPs), and utilization guidelines. The MDS is the primary screening and assessment tool; the RAPs trigger the identification of potential problems and provide guidelines for follow-up assessments.

Physicians have a central role in assuring that all residents receive thorough assessments and that medical plans of care are instituted or revised to enhance or maintain the resident's physical and psychosocial functioning. This role includes providing input in the development of the MDS and a multi-disciplinary plan of care, as required by regulations pertaining to the care of nursing facility residents.

Two major subcategories of nursing facility services are recognized: Initial Nursing Facility Care, and Subsequent Nursing Facility Care. Both subcategories apply to new or established patients.

For definitions of key components and commonly used terms, please see Evaluation and Management Services Guidelines.

(For care plan oversight services provided to nursing facility residents, see 99379-99380)

CODING RULES

1. *If a patient is admitted to the nursing facility after receiving services in the physician's office or hospital emergency department, all evaluation and management services are considered inclusive in the initial nursing facility care.*

2. *With the exception of hospital discharge services, evaluation and management service on the same date provided in locations other than the nursing facility that are related to the admission should not be coded separately.*

3. *When reporting these CPT codes to Medicare include the HCPCS Level II modifier -SP or -MP, or HCPCS Level III modifier if specified by the local Medicare carrier.*

INITIAL NURSING FACILITY CARE

NEW OR ESTABLISHED PATIENT

When the patient is admitted to the nursing facility in the course of an encounter in another site of service (eg, hospital emergency department, office), all evaluation and management services provided by that physician in conjunction with that admission are considered part of the initial nursing facility care when performed on the same date as the admission or readmission. The nursing facility care level of service reported by the admitting physician should include the services related to the admission he/she provided in the other sites of service as well as in the nursing facility setting.

Hospital discharge or observation discharge services performed on the same date of nursing facility admission or readmission may be reported separately. For a patient discharged from inpatient status on the same date of nursing facility admission or readmission, the hospital discharge services should be reported with codes 99238, 99239 as appropriate. For a patient discharged from observation status on the same date of nursing facility admission or readmission, the observation care discharge services should be reported with code 99217. For a patient admitted and discharged from observation or inpatient status on the same date, see codes 99234-99236.

(For nursing facility care discharge, see 99315, 99316)

99304 Initial nursing facility care, per day, for the evaluation and management of a patient which requires these three key components:

- a detailed or comprehensive history;
- a detailed or comprehensive examination;
- and medical decision making that is straightforward or of low complexity.

Counseling and/or coordination of care with other physicians, other qualified health care professionals, or agencies are provided consistent with the nature of the problem(s) and the patient's and/or family's needs.

Usually, the problem(s) requiring admission are of low severity. Typically 25 minutes are spent at the bedside and on the patient's facility floor or unit.

99305 Initial nursing facility care, per day, for the evaluation and management of a patient which requires these three key components:

- a comprehensive history;
- a comprehensive examination;
- and medical decision making of moderate complexity.

Counseling and/or coordination of care with other physicians, other qualified health care professionals, or agencies are provided consistent with the nature of the problem(s) and the patient's and/or family's needs.

Usually, the problem(s) requiring admission are of moderate severity. Typically 35 minutes are spent at the bedside and on the patient's facility floor or unit.

99306 Initial nursing facility care, per day, for the evaluation and management of a patient, which requires these three key components:

- a comprehensive history;
- a comprehensive examination;
- and medical decision making of high complexity.

Counseling and/or coordination of care with other physicians, other qualified health care professionals, or agencies are provided consistent with the nature of the problem(s) and the patient's and/or family's needs.

Usually, the problem(s) requiring admission are of high severity. Typically 45 minutes are spent at the bedside and on the patient's facility floor or unit.

SUBSEQUENT NURSING FACILITY CARE

All levels of subsequent nursing facility care include reviewing the medical record and reviewing the results of diagnostic studies and changes in the patient's status (ie, changes in history, physical condition, and response to management) since the last assessment by the physician or other qualified health care professional.

★ **99307** Subsequent nursing facility care, per day, for the evaluation and management of a patient, which requires at least two of these three key components:

- a problem focused interval history;
- a problem focused examination;
- straightforward medical decision making.

Counseling and/or coordination of care with other physicians, other qualified health care professionals, or agencies are provided consistent with the nature of the problem(s) and the patient's and/or family's needs.

Usually, the patient is stable, recovering, or improving. Typically 10 minutes are spent at the bedside and on the patient's facility floor or unit.

★ **99308** Subsequent nursing facility care, per day, for the evaluation and management of a patient, which requires at least two of these three key components:

- an expanded problem focused interval history;
- an expanded problem focused examination;
- medical decision making of low complexity.

Counseling and/or coordination of care with other physicians, other qualified health care professionals, or agencies are provided consistent with the nature of the problem(s) and the patient's and/or family's needs.

Usually, the patient is responding inadequately to therapy or has developed a minor complication. Typically 15 minutes are spent at the bedside and on the patient's facility floor or unit.

★ **99309** Subsequent nursing facility care, per day, for the evaluation and management of a patient, which requires at least two of these three key components:

- a detailed interval history;
- a detailed examination;
- medical decision making of moderate complexity.

Counseling and/or coordination of care with other physicians, other qualified health care professionals, or agencies are provided consistent with the nature of the problem(s) and the patient's and/or family's needs.

Usually, the patient has developed a significant complication or a significant new problem. Typically 25 minutes are spent at the bedside and on the patient's facility floor or unit.

★ **99310** Subsequent nursing facility care, per day, for the evaluation and management of a patient, which requires at least two of these three key components:

- a comprehensive interval history;
- a comprehensive examination;
- medical decision making of high complexity.

Counseling and/or coordination of care with other physicians, other qualified health care professionals, or agencies are provided consistent with the nature of the problem(s) and the patient's and/or family's needs.

The patient may be unstable or may have developed a significant new problem requiring immediate physician attention. Typically 35 minutes are spent at the bedside and on the patient's facility floor or unit.

NURSING FACILITY DISCHARGE SERVICES

The nursing facility discharge day management codes are to be used to report the total duration of time spent by a physician or other qualified health care professional for the final nursing facility discharge of a patient. The codes include, as appropriate, final examination of the patient, discussion of the nursing facility stay, even if the time spent on that date is not continuous. Instructions are given for continuing care to all relevant caregivers, and preparation of discharge records, prescriptions and referral forms.

99315 Nursing facility discharge day management; 30 minutes or less

99316 more than 30 minutes

OTHER NURSING FACILITY SERVICES

99318 Evaluation and management of a patient involving an annual nursing facility assessment, which requires these three key components:

- a detailed interval history;
- a comprehensive examination;
- and medical decision making that is of low to moderate complexity.

Counseling and/or coordination of care with other physicians, other qualified health care professionals, or agencies are provided consistent with the nature of the problem(s) and the patient's and/or family's needs.

Usually, the patient is stable, recovering, or improving. Typically 30 minutes are spent at the bedside and on the patient's facility floor or unitr.

(Do not report 99318 on the same date of service as nursing facility services codes 99304-99316)

DOMICILIARY, REST HOME (eg, BOARDING HOME), OR CUSTODIAL CARE SERVICES

E/M service codes 99324-99340 are used to report services provided to a new or established patient in domiciliary, rest home or custodial care facility. The key coding issues are the extent of history obtained, the extent of examination performed, and the complexity of medical decision making. Additional reporting issues include counseling and/or coordination of care, and the nature of presenting problems.

When reporting these CPT codes to Medicare include HCPCS modifier -SP or -MP to indicate single or multiple patients seen during the visit. Consult the local Medicare intermediary before using these modifiers.

The following codes are used to report evaluation and management services in a facility which provides room, board and other personal assistance services, generally on a long-term basis. These codes include evaluation and management services provided in an assisted living facility, group home, custodial care, and intermediate care facilities.

The facility's services do not include a medical component.

For definitions of key components and commonly used terms, please see Evaluation and Management Services Guidelines.

(For care plan oversight services provided to a patient in a domiciliary facility under the care of a home health agency, see 99374, 99375, and for hospice agency, see 99377, 99378. For care plan oversight provided to a patient under hospice or home health agency care, see 99339, 99340)

NEW PATIENT

99324 Domiciliary or rest home visit for the evaluation and management of a new patient, which requires these three key components:

- a problem focused history;
- a problem focused examination; and
- straightforward medical decision making.

Counseling and/or coordination of care with other physicians, other qualified health care professionals, or agencies are provided consistent with the nature of the problem(s) and the patient's and/or family's needs.

Usually, the presenting problem(s) are of low severity. Typically 20 minutes are spent with the patient and/or family or caregiver.

99325 Domiciliary or rest home visit for the evaluation and management of a new patient, which requires these three key components:

- an expanded problem focused history;
- an expanded problem focused examination; and
- medical decision making of low complexity.

Counseling and/or coordination of care with other physicians, other qualified health care professionals, or agencies are provided consistent with the nature of the problem(s) and the patient's and/or family's needs.

Usually, the presenting problem(s) are of moderate severity. Typically 30 minutes are spent with the patient and/or family or caregiver.

99326 Domiciliary or rest home visit for the evaluation and management of a new patient, which requires these three key components:

- a detailed history;
- a detailed examination; and
- medical decision making of moderate complexity.

Counseling and/or coordination of care with other physicians, other qualified health care professionals, or agencies are provided consistent with the nature of the problem(s) and the patient's and/or family's needs.

Usually, the presenting problem(s) are of moderate to high severity. Typically 45 minutes are spent with the patient and/or family or caregiver.

99327 Domiciliary or rest home visit for the evaluation and management of a new patient, which requires these three key components:

- a comprehensive history;
- a comprehensive examination; and
- medical decision making of moderate complexity.

Counseling and/or coordination of care with other physicians, other qualified health care professionals, or agencies are provided consistent with the nature of the problem(s) and the patient's and/or family's needs.

Usually, the presenting problem(s) are of high severity. Typically 60 minutes are spent with the patient and/or family or caregiver.

99328 Domiciliary or rest home visit for the evaluation and management of a new patient, which requires these three key components:

- a comprehensive history;
- a comprehensive examination; and
- medical decision making of high complexity.

Counseling and/or coordination of care with other physicians, other qualified health care professionals, or agencies are provided consistent with the nature of the problem(s) and the patient's and/or family's needs.

Usually, the patient is unstable or has developed a significant new problem requiring immediate physician attention. Typically 75 minutes are spent with the patient and/or family or caregiver.

ESTABLISHED PATIENT

99334 Domiciliary or rest home visit for the evaluation and management of an established patient, which requires at least two of these three key components:

- a problem focused interval history;
- a problem focused examination;
- straightforward medical decision making.

Counseling and/or coordination of care with other physicians, other qualified health care professionals, or agencies are provided consistent with the nature of the problem(s) and the patient's and/or family's needs.

Usually, the presenting problem(s) are self-limited or minor. Typically 15 minutes are spent with the patient and/or family or caregiver.

99335 Domiciliary or rest home visit for the evaluation and management of an established patient, which requires at least two of these three key components:

- an expanded problem focused interval history;
- an expanded problem focused examination;
- medical decision making of low complexity.

Counseling and/or coordination of care with other physicians, other qualified health care professionals, or agencies are provided consistent with the nature of the problem(s) and the patient's and/or family's needs.

Usually, the presenting problem(s) are of low to moderate severity. Typically 25 minutes are spent with the patient and/or family or caregiver.

99336 Domiciliary or rest home visit for the evaluation and management of an established patient, which requires at least two of these three key components:

- a detailed interval history;

- a detailed examination;
- medical decision making of moderate complexity.

Counseling and/or coordination of care with other physicians, other qualified health care professionals, or agencies are provided consistent with the nature of the problem(s) and the patient's and/or family's needs.

Usually, the presenting problem(s) are of moderate to high severity. Typically 40 minutes are spent with the patient and/or family or caregiver.

99337 Domiciliary or rest home visit for the evaluation and management of an established patient, which requires at least two of these three key components:

- a comprehensive interval history;
- a comprehensive examination;
- and medical decision making of moderate to high complexity.

Counseling and/or coordination of care with other physicians, other qualified health care professionals, or agencies are provided consistent with the nature of the problem(s) and the patient's and/or family's needs.

Usually, the presenting problem(s) are of moderate to high severity. The patient may be unstable or may have developed a significant new problem requiring immediate physician attention. Typically 60 minutes are spent with the patient and/or family or caregiver.

DOMICILIARY, REST HOME (eg, ASSISTED LIVING FACILITY), OR HOME CARE PLAN OVERSIGHT SERVICES

(For instructions on the use of 99339, 99340, see introductory notes for 99374-99380)

(For care plan oversight services for patients under the care of a home health agency, hospice, or nursing facility, see 99374-99380)

(Do not report 99339, 99340 for time reported with 98966, 98967, 98968, 99421, 99422, 99423, 99441, 99442, 99443)

99339 Individual physician supervision of a patient (patient not present) in home, domiciliary or rest home (eg, assisted living facility) requiring complex and multidisciplinary care modalities involving regular physician development and/or revision of care plans, review of subsequent reports of patient status, review of related laboratory and other studies, communication (including telephone calls) for purposes of assessment or care decisions with health care professional(s), family member(s), surrogate decision maker(s) (eg, legal guardian) and/or key caregiver(s) involved in patient's care, integration of new information into the medical treatment plan and/or adjustment of medical therapy, within a calendar month; 15-29 minutes

99340   30 minutes or more

(Do not report 99339, 99340 for patients under the care of a home health agency, enrolled in a hospice program, or for nursing facility residents)

(Do not report 99339, 99340 during the same month with 99487-99489)

(Do not report 99339, 99340 when performed during the service time of codes 99495 or 99496)

HOME SERVICES

The following codes are used to report evaluation and management services provided in a home. Home may be defined as a private residence, temporary lodging, or short term accommodation (eg, hotel, campground, hostel, or cruise ship).

For definitions of key components and commonly used terms, please see Evaluation and Management Services Guidelines.

>(For care plan oversight services provided to a patient in the home under the care of a home health agency, see 99374-99375, and for hospice agency, see 99377, 99378. For care plan oversight provided to a patient under hospice or home health agency care, see 99339, 99340))

NEW PATIENT

99341 Home visit for the evaluation and management of a new patient, which requires these three key components:

- a problem focused history;
- a problem focused examination; and
- straightforward medical decision making.

Counseling and/or coordination of care with other physicians, other qualified health care professionals, or agencies are provided consistent with the nature of the problem(s) and the patient's and/or family's needs.

Usually, the presenting problem(s) are of low severity. Typically 20 minutes are spent face-to-face with the patient and/or family.

99342 Home visit for the evaluation and management of a new patient, which requires these three key components:

- an expanded problem focused history;
- an expanded problem focused examination; and
- medical decision making of low complexity.

Counseling and/or coordination of care with other physicians, other qualified health care professionals, or agencies are provided consistent with the nature of the problem(s) and the patient's and/or family's needs.

Usually, the presenting problem(s) are of moderate severity. Typically 30 minutes are spent face-to-face with the patient and/or family.

99343 Home visit for the evaluation and management of a new patient, which requires these three key components:

- a detailed history;
- a detailed examination; and
- medical decision making of moderate complexity.

Counseling and/or coordination of care with other physicians, other qualified health care professionals, or agencies are provided consistent with the nature of the problem(s) and the patient's and/or family's needs.

Usually, the presenting problem(s) are of moderate to high severity. Typically 45 minutes ar spent face-to-face with the patient and/or family.

99344 Home visit for the evaluation and management of a new patient, which requires these three components:

- a comprehensive history;
- a comprehensive examination; and
- medical decision making of moderate complexity.

Counseling and/or coordination of care with other physicians, other qualified health care professionals, or agencies are provided consistent with the nature of the problem(s) and the patient's and/or family's needs.

Usually, the presenting problem(s) are of high severity. Typically 60 minutes are spent face-to-face with the patient and/or family.

99345 Home visit for the evaluation and management of a new patient, which requires these three key components:

- a comprehensive history;
- a comprehensive examination; and
- medical decision making of high complexity.

Counseling and/or coordination of care with other physicians, other qualified health care professionals, or agencies are provided consistent with the nature of the problem(s) and the patient's and/or family's needs.

Usually, the patient is unstable or has developed a significant new problem requiring immediate physician attention. Typically 75 minutes are spent face-to-face with the patient and/or family.

ESTABLISHED PATIENT

99347 Home visit for the evaluation and management of an established patient, which requires at least two of these three key components:

- a problem focused interval history;
- a problem focused examination;
- straightforward medical decision making.

Counseling and/or coordination of care with other physicians, other qualified health care professionals, or agencies are provided consistent with the nature of the problem(s) and the patient's and/or family's needs.

Usually, the presenting problem(s) are self-limited or minor. Typically 15 minutes are spent face-to-face with the patient and/or family.

99348 Home visit for the evaluation and management of an established patient, which requires at least two of these three key components:

- an expanded problem focused interval history;
- an expanded problem focused examination;
- medical decision making of low complexity.

Counseling and/or coordination of care with other physicians, other qualified health care professionals, or agencies are provided consistent with the nature of the problem(s) and the patient's and/or family's needs.

Usually, the presenting problem(s) are of low to moderate severity. Typically 25 minutes are spent face-to-face with the patient and/or family.

99349 Home visit for the evaluation and management of an established patient, which requires at least two of these three key components:

- a detailed interval history;
- a detailed examination;
- medical decision making of moderate complexity.

Counseling and/or coordination of care with other physicians, other qualified health care professionals, or agencies are provided consistent with the nature of the problem(s) and the patient's and/or family's needs.

Usually, the presenting problem(s) are moderate to high severity. Typically 40 minutes are spent face-to-face with the patient and/or family.

99350 Home visit for the evaluation and management of an established patient, which requires at least two of these three key components:

- a comprehensive interval history;
- a comprehensive examination;
- medical decision making of moderate to high complexity.

Counseling and/or coordination of care with other physicians, other qualified health care professionals, or agencies are provided consistent with the nature of the problem(s) and the patient's and/or family's needs.

● New Code   ▲ Revised Code   + Add-On Code   ⊘ Modifier -51 Exempt   ★ Telemedicine

Usually, the presenting problem(s) are of moderate to high severity. The patient may be unstable or may have developed a significant new problem requiring immediate physician attention. Typically 60 minutes are spent face-to-face with the patient and/or family.

PROLONGED SERVICES

PROLONGED SERVICE WITH DIRECT PATIENT CONTACT (EXCEPT WITH OFFICE OR OTHER OUTPATIENT SERVICES)

Codes 99354-99357 are used when a physician or other qualified health care professional provides prolonged service(s) involving direct patient contact that is provided beyond the usual service in either the inpatient, observation or outpatient setting, except with office or other outpatient services (99202, 99203, 99204, 99205, 99212, 99213, 99214, 99215). Direct patient contact is face-to-face and includes additional non-face-to-face services on the patient's floor or unit in the hospital or nursing facility during the same session. This service is reported in addition to the primary procedure. Appropriate codes should be selected for supplies provided or other procedures performed in the care of the patient during this period.

Codes 99354-99355 are used to report the total duration of face-to-face time spent by a physician or other qualified health care professional on a given date providing prolonged service in the outpatient setting, even if the time spent by the physician or other qualified health care professional on that date is not continuous. Codes 99356-99357 are used to report the total duration of time spent by a physician or other qualified health care professional at the bedside and on the patient's floor or unit in the hospital or nursing facility on a given date providing prolonged service to a patient, even if the time spent by the physician or other qualified health care professional on that date is not continuous.

Time spent performing separately reported services other than the E/M or psychotherapy service is not counted toward the prolonged services time.

Code 99354 or 99356 is used to report the first hour of prolonged service on a given date, depending on the place of service.

Either code should be used only once per date, even if the time spent by the physician or other qualified health care professional is not continuous on that date. Prolonged service of less than 30 minutes total duration on a given date is not separately reported.

Code 99355 or 99357 is used to report each additional 30 minutes beyond the first hour, depending on the place of service. Either code may also be used to report the final 15-30 minutes of prolonged service on a given date. Prolonged service of less than 15 minutes beyond the first hour or less than 15 minutes beyond the final 30 minutes is not reported separately.

The use of the time based add-on codes requires that the primary evaluation and management service have a typical or specified time published in the CPT codebook.

For E/M services that require prolonged clinical staff time and may include face-to-face services by the physician or other qualified health care professional, use 99415, 99416. Do not report 99354, 99355 with 99415, 99416, 99417.

For prolonged total time in addition to office or other outpatient services (ie, 99205, 99215), use 99417.

The following table illustrates the correct reporting of prolonged physician or other qualified health care professional service with direct patient contact in the inpatient or observation setting beyond the usual service time.

The following table illustrates the correct reporting of prolonged physician or other qualified health care professional service with direct patient contact in the office setting beyond the usual service time.

TOTAL DURATION OF PROLONGED SERVICES	CODE(S)
less than 30 minutes	Not reported separately
30-74 minutes (30 minutes - 1 hr. 14 min.)	99356 once
75-104 minutes (1 hr. 15 min. - 1 hr. 44 min.)	99356 once and 99357 once
105 minutes or more (1 hr. 45 min. or more)	99356 once and 99357 twice or more for each additional 30 mins.

▲★+99354　　Prolonged service(s) in the outpatient setting requiring direct patient contact beyond the time of the usual service; first hour (List separately in addition to code for outpatient Evaluation and Management or psychotherapy service, except with office or other outpatient services [99202, 99203, 99204, 99205, 99212, 99213, 99214, 99215])

　　　　　　(Use 99354 in conjunction with 90837, 90847, 99241-99245, 99324-99337, 99341-99350, 99483)

(Do not report 99354 in conjunction with 99202, 99203, 99204, 99205, 99212, 99213, 99214, 99215, 99415, 99416, 99417)

▲★+99355 each additional 30 minutes (List separately in addition to code for prolonged service)

(Use 99355 in conjunction with 99354)

(Do not report 99355 in conjunction with 99202, 99203, 99204, 99205, 99212, 99213, 99214, 99215, 99415, 99416, 99417)

▲+99356 Prolonged service in the inpatient or observation setting, requiring unit/floor time beyond the usual service; first hour (List separately in addition to code for inpatient or observation Evaluation and Management service)

(Use 99356 in conjunction with codes 99218-99220, 99221-99223, 99224-99226, 99231-99233, 99234-99236, 99251-99255, 99304-99310)

+ 99357 each additional 30 minutes (List separately in addition to code for prolonged physician service)

(Use 99357 in conjunction with 99356)

PROLONGED SERVICE WITHOUT DIRECT PATIENT CONTACT

Codes 99358 and 99359 are used when a prolonged service is provided that is neither face-to-face time in the outpatient, inpatient, or observation setting, nor additional unit/floor time in the hospital or nursing facility setting. Codes 99358, 99359 may be used during the same session of an evaluation and management service, except office or other outpatient services (99202, 99203, 99204, 99205, 99212, 99213, 99214, 99215). For prolonged total time in addition to office or other outpatient services (ie, 99205, 99215) on the same date of service without direct patient contact, use 99417. Codes 99358, 99359 may also be used for prolonged services on a date other than the date of a face-to-face encounter.

This service is to be reported in relation to other physician or other qualified health care professional services, including evaluation and management services at any level. This prolonged service may be reported on a different date than the primary service to which it is related. For example, extensive record review may relate to a previous evaluation and management service performed at an earlier date. However, it must relate to a service or patient where (face-to-face) patient care has occurred or will occur and relate to ongoing patient management.

Codes 99358 and 99359 are used to report the total duration of non-face-to-face time spent by a physician or other qualified health care professional on a given date providing prolonged service, even if the time spent by the physician or other qualified health care professional on that date is not continuous. Code 99358 is used to report the first hour of prolonged service on a given date regardless of the place of service. It should be used only once per date.

Prolonged service of less than 30 minutes total duration on a given date is not separately reported.

Code 99359 is used to report each additional 30 minutes beyond the first hour. It may also be used to report the final 15 to 30 minutes of prolonged service on a given date.

Prolonged service of less than 15 minutes beyond the first hour or less than 15 minutes beyond the final 30 minutes is not reported separately.

Do not report 99358, 99359 for time without direct patient contact reported in other services such as care plan oversight services (99339, 99340, 99374-99380), chronic care management by a physician or other qualified health care professional (99491), home and outpatient INR monitoring (93792, 93793), medical team conferences (99366-99368), interprofessional telephone/Internet/electronic health record consultations (99446, 99447, 99448, 99449, 99451, 99452), or online digital evaluation and management services (99421, 99422, 99423).

99358 Prolonged evaluation and management service before and/or after direct patient care; first hour

+ 99359 each additional 30 minutes (List separately in addition to code for prolonged physician service)

(Use 99359 in conjunction with 99358)

(Do not report 99358, 99359 on the same date of service as 99202, 99203, 99204, 99205, 99212, 99213, 99214, 99215, 99417)

 ● New Code ▲ Revised Code + Add-On Code ⊘ Modifier -51 Exempt ★ Telemedicine

TOTAL DURATION OF PROLONGED SERVICES WITHOUT DIRECT FACE-TO-FACE CONTACT	CODE(S)
less than 30 minutes	Not reported separately
30-74 minutes	99358 once
75-104 minutes	99358 once and 99359 once
105 minutes or more	99358 once and 99359 twice or more for each additional 30 mins.

PROLONGED CLINICAL STAFF SERVICES WITH PHYSICIAN OR OTHER QUALIFIED HEALTH CARE PROFESSIONAL SUPERVISION

Codes 99415, 99416 are used when a prolonged evaluation and management (E/M) service is provided in the office or outpatient setting that involves prolonged clinical staff face-to-face time beyond the highest total time of the E/M service, as stated in the ranges of time in the code descriptions. The physician or qualified health care professional is present to provide direct supervision of the clinical staff. This service is reported in addition to the designated E/M services and any other services provided at the same session as E/M services.

Codes 99415, 99416 are used to report the total duration of face-to-face time spent by clinical staff on a given date providing prolonged service in the office or other outpatient setting, even if the time spent by the clinical staff on that date is not continuous. Time spent performing separately reported services other than the E/M service is not counted toward the prolonged services time.

Code 99415 is used to report the first hour of prolonged clinical staff service on a given date. Code 99415 should be used only once per date, even if the time spent by the clinical staff is not continuous on that date. Prolonged service of less than 30 minutes total duration on a given date is not separately reported because the clinical staff time involved is included in the E/M codes. The highest total time in the time ranges of the code descriptions is used in defining when prolonged services time begins. For example, prolonged clinical staff services for 99214 begin after 39 minutes, and 99415 is not reported until at least 69 minutes total face-to-face clinical staff time has been performed. When face-to-face time is noncontiguous, use only the face-to-face time provided to the patient by the clinical staff.

Code 99416 is used to report each additional 30 minutes of prolonged clinical staff service beyond the first hour. Code 99416 may also be used to report the final 15-30 minutes of prolonged service on that date. Prolonged service of less than 15 minutes beyond the first hour or less than 15 minutes beyond the final 30 minutes is not reported separately.

Codes 99415, 99416 may be reported for no more than two simultaneous patients. The use of the time-based add-on codes requires that the primary E/M service has a time published in the CPT code set.

For prolonged services by the physician or other qualified health care professional, see 99354, 99355, 99417. Do not report 99415, 99416 with 99354, 99355, 99417.

Facilities may not report 99415, 99416.

▲+**99415**   Prolonged clinical staff service (the service beyond the highest time in the range of total time of the service) during an evaluation and management service in the office or outpatient setting, direct patient contact with physician supervision; first hour (List separately in addition to code for outpatient Evaluation and Management service)

(Use 99415 in conjunction with 99202, 99203, 99204, 99205, 99212, 99213, 99214, 99215)

(Do not report 99415 in conjunction with 99354, 99355, 99417)

▲+**99416**   each additional 30 minutes (List separately in addition to code for prolonged service)

(Use 99416 in conjunction with 99415)

(Do not report 99416 in conjunction with 99354, 99355, 99417)

The Total Duration of Prolonged Services Table illustrates the correct reporting of prolonged services provided by clinical staff with physician supervision in the office setting beyond the initial 30 minutes of clinical staff time:

TOTAL DURATION OF PROLONGED SERVICES	CODE(s)
less than 30 minutes	Not reported separately
30-74 minutes (30 minutes - 1 hr. 14 min.)	99415 once
75-104 minutes (1 hr. 15 min. - 1 hr. 44 min.)	99415 once and 99416 once
105 minutes or more (1 hr. 45 min. or more)	99415 once and 99416 twice or more for each additional 30 mins

PROLONGED SERVICE WITH OR WITHOUT DIRECT PATIENT CONTACT ON THE DATE OF AN OFFICE OR OTHER OUTPATIENT SERVICE

Code 99417 is used to report prolonged total time (ie, combined time with and without direct patient contact) provided by the physician or other qualified health care professional on the date of office or other outpatient services (ie, 99205, 99215). Code 99417 is only used when the office or other outpatient service has been selected using time alone as the basis and only after the minimum time required to report the highest-level service (ie, 99205 or 99215) has been exceeded by 15 minutes. To report a unit of 99417, 15 minutes of additional time must have been attained. Do not report 99417 for any additional time increment of less than 15 minutes.

The listed time ranges for 99205 (ie, 60-74 minutes) and 99215 (ie, 40-54 minutes) represent the complete range of time for which each code may be reported. Therefore, when reporting 99417, the initial time unit of 15 minutes should be added once the minimum time in the primary E/M code has been surpassed by 15 minutes. For example, to report the initial unit of 99417 for a new patient encounter (99205), do not report 99417 until at least 15 minutes of time has been accumulated beyond 60 minutes (ie, 75 minutes) on the date of the encounter. For an established patient encounter (99215), do not report 99417 until at least 15 minutes of time has been accumulated beyond 40 minutes (ie, 55 minutes) on the date of the encounter.

Time spent performing separately reported services other than the E/M service is not counted toward the time to report 99205, 99215 and prolonged services time.

For prolonged services on a date other than the date of a face-to-face encounter, including office or other outpatient services (99202, 99203, 99204, 99205, 99212, 99213, 99214, 99215), see 99358, 99359. For E/M services that require prolonged clinical staff time and may include face-to-face services by the physician or other QHP, see 99415, 99416. Do not report 99417 in conjunction with 99354, 99355, 99358, 99359, 99415, 99416.

Prolonged services of less than 15 minutes total time is not reported on the date of office or other outpatient service when the highest level is reached (ie, 99205, 99215).

●★+99417   Prolonged office or other outpatient evaluation and management service(s) beyond the minimum required time of the primary procedure which has been selected using total time, requiring total time with or without direct patient contact beyond the usual service, on the date of the primary service, each 15 minutes of total time (List separately in addition to codes 99205, 99215 for office or other outpatient Evaluation and Management services)

(Use 99417 in conjunction with 99205, 99215)

(Do not report 99417 on the same date of service as 99354, 99355, 99358, 99359, 99415, 99416)

(Do not report 99417 for any time unit less than 15 minutes)

TOTAL DURATION OF NEW PATIENT OFFICE OR OTHER OUTPATIENT SERVICES (USE WITH 99205)	CODE(s)
less than 75 minutes	Not reported separately
75-89 minutes	99205 once and 99417 once
90-104 minutes	99205 once and 99417 twice
105 minutes or more	99205 once and 99417 three times or more for each additional 30 mins

TOTAL DURATION OF ESTABLISHED PATIENT OFFICE OR OTHER OUTPATIENT SERVICES (USE WITH 99215)	CODE(s)
less than 55 minutes	Not reported separately
55-69 minutes	99215 once and 99417 once
70-84 minutes	99215 once and 99417 twice
85 minutes or more	99215 once and 99417 three times or more for each additional 30 mins

STANDBY SERVICES

Code 99360 is used to report physician or other qualified health care professional standby services that are requested by another individual and that involve prolonged attendance without direct (face-to-face) patient contact. Care or services may not be provided to other patients during this period. This code is not used to report time spent proctoring another individual. It is also not used if the period of standby ends with the performance of a procedure subject to a surgical package by the individual who was on standby.

Code 99360 is used to report the total duration of time spent on a given date on standby. Standby service of less than 30 minutes total duration on a given date is not reported separately.

COMPARISON OF PROLONGED SERVICE CODES (99354, 99355, 99356, 99357, 99358, 99359, 99417) TABLE

CODE	PATIENT CONTACT	MINIMUM REPORTABLE PROLONGED SERVICE TIME (SINGLE DATE OF SERVICE)	USE IN CONJUNCTION WITH	*DO NOT REPORT WITH	OTHER PROLONGED SERVICE(S) REPORTABLE ON SAME DATE OF SERVICE
+99354	Face-to-Face Only	30 minutes (beyond listed typical time)	90837, 90847, 989241, 99245, 99324-99337, 99341,99350, 99483	99202-99205, 99212-99215, 99415, 99416, 99417	99358, 99359
+99355	Face-to-Face Only	Each additional 15 minutes (beyond 99354)	99354	99202-99205, 99212-99215, 99415, 99416, 99417	99358, 99359
+99356	Face-to-Face and Unit/Floor Time	30 minutes (beyond listed typcial time)	90837, 90847, 99218-99220, 99221-99223, 99224-99226, , 99231-99233, 99234-99236, 99251-99255, 99304-99310		99358, 99359
+99357	Face-to-Face and Unit/Floor Time	Each additional 15 minutes (beyond 99356)	99356		99358, 99359
99358	Non Face-to-Face Only	30 minutes	Must relate to a service where face-to-face care has or will occur. This is not an add-on code and is not used in conjunction with a base code	99202-99205, 99212-99215, 99417 On same date of service	99354, 99356
+99359	Non Face-to-Face Only	Each additional 15 minutes (beyond 99358)	99358	99202-99205, 99212-99215, 99417 On same date of service	99354, 99356
+99417	Face-to-Face and/or Non Face-to-Face	Reported with 99205, 75 minutes or more Reported with 99215, 55 minutes or more	99205, 99215	99354, 99355, 99358, 99359, 99415, 99416	N/A

*Do not count the time of any separately reported service as prolonged services time.
99533 is for prolonged services time beyond 99354 and may be reported in multiple units
99357 is for prolonged services time beyonn 99356 and may be reported in multiple units
99359 is for prolonged services time beyond 99358 and may be reported multiple times
99417 is for prolonged services time beyond 99205 or 99215 and may be reported in multiple units of at least 15 minutes.

Second and subsequent periods of standby beyond the first 30 minutes may be reported only if a full 30 minutes of standby was provided for each unit of service reported.

99360   Standby service, requiring prolonged attendance, each 30 minutes (eg, operative standby, standby for frozen section, for cesarean/high risk delivery, for monitoring EEG)

(For hospital mandated on call services, see 99026, 99027)

(99360 may be reported in addition to 99460, 99465 as appropriate)

(Do not report 99360 in conjunction with 99464)

CASE MANAGEMENT SERVICES

Case management is a process in which a physician or another qualified health care professional is responsible for direct care of a patient and, additionally, for coordinating, managing access to, initiating, and/or supervising other health care services needed by the patient. .

ANTICOAGULANT MANAGEMENT

(**99363**   deleted 2017 [2018 edition]. To report, see 93792, 93793.)

(**99364**   deleted 2017 [2018 edition]. To report, see 93792, 93793.)

MEDICAL TEAM CONFERENCES

Medical team conferences include face-to-face participation by a minimum of three qualified health care professionals from different specialties or disciplines (each of whom provide direct care to the patient), with or without the presence of the patient, family member(s), community agencies, surrogate decision maker(s) (eg., legal guardian), and/or caregiver(s). The participants are actively involved in the development, revision, coordination, and implementation of health care services needed by the patient. Reporting participants shall have performed face-to-face evaluations or treatments of the patient, independent of any team conference, within the previous 60 days.

Physicians or other qualified health care professionals who may report evaluation and management services should report their time spent in a team conference with the patient and/or family present using evaluation and management (E/M) codes (and time as the key controlling factor for code selection when counseling and/or coordination of care dominates the service). These introductory guidelines do not apply to services reported using E/M codes (see E/M services guidelines). However, the individual must be directly involved with the patient, providing face-to-face services outside of the conference visit with other physicians, other qualified health care professionals, or agencies.

Reporting participants shall document their participation in the team conference as well as their contributed information and subsequent treatment recommendations.

No more than one individual from the same specialty may report 99366-99368 at the same encounter.

Individuals should not report 99366-99368 when their participation in the medical team conference is part of a facility or organizational service contractually provided by the organizational or facility.

The team conference starts at the beginning of the review of an individual patient and ends at the conclusion of the review. Time related to record keeping and report generation is not reported. The reporting participant shall be present for all time reported. The time reported is not limited to the time that the participant is communicating to the other team members or patient and/or family. Time reported for medical team conferences may not be used in the determination of time for other services such as care plan oversight (99374-99380), home, domiciliary, or rest home care plan oversight (99339-99340), prolonged services (99354-99359), psychotherapy, or any E/M service. For team conferences where the patient is present for any part of the duration of the conference, nonphysician qualified health care professionals (eg, speech-language pathologists, physical therapists, occupational therapist, social workers, dieticians) report the team conference face-to-face code 99366.

MEDICAL TEAM CONFERENCE, DIRECT (FACE-TO-FACE) CONTACT WITH PATIENT AND/OR FAMILY

99366   Medical team conference with interdisciplinary team of health care professionals, face-to-face with patient and/or family, 30 minutes or more, participation by nonphysician qualified health care professional

(Team conference services of less than 30 minutes duration are not reported separately)

(For team conference services by a physician with patient and/or family present, see Evaluation and Management services)

(Do not report 99366 during the same month with 99439, 99487, 99489, 99490, 99491)

MEDICAL TEAM CONFERENCE, WITHOUT DIRECT (FACE-TO-FACE) CONTACT WITH PATIENT AND/OR FAMILY

99367   Medical team conference with interdisciplinary team of health care professionals, patient and/or family not present, 30 minutes or more; participation by physician

99368   participation by nonphysician qualified health care professional

(Team conference services of less than 30 minutes duration are not reported separately)

(Do not report 99367, 99368 during the same month with 99439, 99487, 99489, 99490, 99491)

CARE PLAN OVERSIGHT SERVICES

Care plan oversight services are reported separately from codes for office/ outpatient, hospital, home, nursing facility or domiciliary or non face-to-face services. The complexity and approximate time of the care plan oversight services provided within a 30-day period determine code selection. Only one individual may report services for a given period of time, to reflect the sole or predominant supervisory role with a particular patient. These codes should not be reported for supervision of patients in nursing facilities or under the care of home health agencies unless they require recurrent supervision of therapy.

The work involved in providing very low intensity or infrequent supervision services is included in the pre- and post-encounter work for home, office/outpatient and nursing facility or domiciliary visit codes.

CODING RULES

1.   *Evaluation and management services are not inclusive of care plan oversight services. Care plan oversight is coded separately.*

2.   *Care plan oversight services may be coded only by a single physician for each patient during a specific period of time.*

(For care plan oversight services of patients in the home, domiciliary, or rest home [eg, assisted living facility] see 99339, 99340, and for hospice agency, see 99377, 99378))

(Do not report 99374-99380 for time reported with 98966, 98967, 98968, 99421, 99422, 99423, 99441, 99442, 99443)

(Do not report 99374-99378 during the same month with 99487-99489)

(Do not report 99374-99380 when performed during the service time of codes 99495 or 99496)

99374   Supervision of a patient under care of home health agency (patient not present) in home, domiciliary or equivalent environment (eg, Alzheimer's facility) requiring complex and multidisciplinary care modalities involving regular development and/or revision of care plans by that individual, review of subsequent reports of patient status, review of related laboratory and other studies, communication (including telephone calls) for purposes of assessment or care decisions with health care professional(s), family member(s), surrogate decision maker(s) (eg., legal guardian) and/or key caregiver(s) involved in patient's care, integration of new information into the medical treatment plan and/or adjustment of medical therapy, within a calendar month; 15-29 minutes

99375   30 minutes or more

99377   Supervision of a hospice patient (patient not present) requiring complex and multidisciplinary care modalities involving regular development and/or revision of care plans by that individual, review of subsequent reports of patient status, review of related laboratory and other studies, communication (including telephone calls) for purposes of assessment or care decisions with health care professional(s), family member(s), surrogate decision maker(s) (eg, legal guardian) and/or key caregiver(s) involved in patient's care, integration of new information into the medical treatment plan and/or adjustment of medical therapy, within a calendar month; 15-29 minutes

---

Separate Procedure   Unlisted Procedure   CCI Comp. Code   Non-specific Procedure   **173**

99378   30 minutes or more

99379   Supervision of a nursing facility patient (patient not present) requiring complex and multidisciplinary care modalities involving regular development and/or revision of care plans by that individual, review of subsequent reports of patient status, review of related laboratory and other studies, communication (including telephone calls) for purposes of assessment or care decisions with health care professional(s), family member(s), surrogate decision maker(s) (eg, legal guardian) and/or key caregiver(s) involved in patient's care, integration of new information into the medical treatment plan and/or adjustment of medical therapy, within a calendar month; 15-29 minutes

99380   30 minutes or more

PREVENTIVE MEDICINE SERVICES

The following codes are used to report the preventive medicine evaluation and management of infants, children, adolescents, and adults.

The extent and focus of the services will largely depend on the age of the patient.

If an abnormality is encountered or a preexisting problem is addressed in the process of performing this preventive medicine evaluation and management service, and if the problem or abnormality is significant enough to require additional work to perform the key components of a problem-oriented evaluation and management service, then the appropriate office/ outpatient code 99202, 99203, 99204, 99205, 99211, 99212, 99213, 99214, 99215 should also be reported. Modifier 25 should be added to the office/outpatient code to indicate that a significant, separately identifiable evaluation and management service was provided on the same day as the preventive medicine service. The appropriate preventive medicine service is additionally reported.

An insignificant or trivial problem/abnormality that is encountered in the process of performing the preventive medicine evaluation and management service and which does not require additional work and the performance of the key components of a problem-oriented E/M service should not be reported.

The "comprehensive" nature of the preventive medicine services codes 99381-99397 reflects an age- and genderappropriate history/exam and is not synonymous with the "comprehensive" examination required in evaluation and management codes 99202-99350.

Codes 99381-99397 include counseling/anticipatory guidance/risk factor reduction interventions which are provided at the time of the initial or periodic comprehensive preventive medicine examination. (Refer to codes 99401, 99402, 99403, 99404, 99411, and 99412 for reporting those counseling/anticipatory guidance/risk factor reduction internventions that are provided at an encounter separate from the preventive medicine examination.)

(For behavior change intervention, see 99406, 99407, 99408, 99409)

Vaccine/toxoid products, immunization administrations, ancillary studies involving laboratory, radiology, other procedures, or screening tests (eg, vision, hearing, developmental) identified with a specific CPT code are reported separately. For immunization administration and vaccine risk/benefit counseling, see 90460, 90461, 90470-90474. For vaccine/toxoid products, see 90476-90749.

CODING RULES

1. *The selection of Preventive Medicine codes is mostly dependent upon the age of the patient.*

2. *Preventive medicine codes are coded only in the absence of illness. If illness, injury is discovered during provision of a preventive medicine service, office/outpatient evaluation and management codes are coded.*

3. *Immunizations and diagnostic studies involving laboratory or radiology, or other procedures are not included in the preventive medicine service and should be coded separately.*

NEW PATIENT

99381   Initial comprehensive preventive medicine evaluation and management of an individual including an age and gender appropriate history, examination, counseling/anticipatory guidance/risk factor reduction interventions, and the ordering of laboratory/diagnostic procedures, new patient; infant (age under 1 year)

99382	early childhood (age 1 through 4 years)	
99383	late childhood (age 5 through 11 years)	
99384	adolescent (age 12 through 17 years)	
99385	18-39 years	
99386	40-64 years	
99387	65 years and over	

ESTABLISHED PATIENT

99391 Periodic comprehensive preventive medicine reevaluation and management of an individual including an age and gender appropriate history, examination, counseling/anticipatory guidance/risk factor reduction interventions, and the ordering of laboratory/diagnostic procedures, established patient; infant (age under 1 year)

99392	early childhood (age 1 through 4 years)	
99393	late childhood (age 5 through 11 years)	
99394	adolescent (age 12 through 17 years)	
99395	18-39 years	
99396	40-64 years	
99397	65 years and over	

COUNSELING RISK FACTOR REDUCTION AND BEHAVIOR CHANGE INTERVENTION

NEW OR ESTABLISHED PATIENT

These codes are used to report services provided face-to-face by a physician or other qualified health care professional for the purpose of promoting health and preventing illness or injury. They are distinct from evaluation and management (E/M) services that may be reported separately with modifier 25 when performed. Risk factor reduction services are used for persons without a specific illness for which the counseling might otherwise be used as part of treatment.

Preventive medicine counseling and risk factor reduction interventions will vary with age and should address such issues as family problems, diet and exercise, substance use, sexual practices, injury prevention, dental health, and diagnostic and laboratory test results available at the time of the encounter.

Behavior change interventions are for persons who have a behavior that is often considered an illness itself, such as tobacco use and addiction, substance abuse/misuse, or obesity. Behavior change services may be reported when performed as part of the treatment of condition(s) related to or potentially exacerbated by the behavior or when performed to change the harmful behavior that has not yet resulted in illness. Any E/M services reported on the same day must be distinct and reported with modifier 25, and time spent providing these services may not be used as a basis for the E/M code selection. Behavior change services involve specific validated interventions of assessing readiness for change and barriers to change, advising a change in behavior, assisting by providing specific suggested actions and motivational counseling, and arranging for services and follow-up.

For counseling groups of patients with symptoms or established illness, use 99078.

Health behavior assessment and intervention services (96156, 96158, 96159, 96164, 96165, 96167, 96168, 96170, 96171) should not be reported on the same day as codes 99401-99412.

Preventive Medicine, Individual Counseling

99401 Preventive medicine counseling and/or risk factor reduction intervention(s) provided to an individual (separate procedure); approximately 15 minutes

---

99402	approximately 30 minutes
99403	approximately 45 minutes
99404	approximately 60 minutes

Behavior Change Interventions, Individual

★ 99406   Smoking and tobacco use cessation counseling visit; intermediate, greater than 3 minutes up to 10 minutes

★ 99407   intensive, greater than 10 minutes

(Do not report 99407 in conjunction with 99406)

★ 99408   Alcohol and/or substance (other than tobacco) abuse structured screening (eg, AUDIT, DAST), and brief intervention (SBI) services; 15 to 30 minutes

(Do not report services of less than 15 minutes with 99408)

★ 99409   greater than 30 minutes

(Do not report 99409 in conjunction with 99408)

(Do not report 99408, 99409 in conjunction with 96160, 96161)

(Use 99408, 99409 only for initial screening and brief intervention)

Preventive Medicine, Group Counseling

99411   Preventive medicine counseling and/or risk factor reduction intervention(s) provided to individuals in a group setting (separate procedure); approximately 30 minutes

99412   approximately 60 minutes

99415   Code out of order. See page 169

99416   Code out of order. See page 169

99417   Code out of order. See page 170

OTHER PREVENTIVE MEDICINE SERVICES

99421   Code out of order. See page 178

99422   Code out of order. See page 178

99423   Code out of order. See page 178

99429   Unlisted preventive medicine service

NON-FACE-TO-FACE SERVICES

TELEPHONE SERVICES

Telephone services are non-face-to-face evaluation and management (E/M) services provided to a patient using the telephone by a physician or other qualified health care professional, who may report evaluation and management services. These codes are used to report episodes of patient care initiated by an established patient or guardian of an established patient. If the telephone service ends with a decision to see the patient within 24 hours or next available urgent visit appointment, the code is not reported; rather the encounter is considered part of the preservice work of the subsequent E/M service, procedure, and visit. Likewise, if the telephone call refers to an E/M service performed and reported by that individual within the previous seven days (either requested or unsolicited patient follow-up) or within the postoperative period of the previously completed procedure, then the service(s) is considered part of that previous E/M service or procedure. (Do not report 99441-99443, if 99421, 99422, 99423 have been reported by the same provider in the previous seven days for the same problem.)

> (For telephone services provided by a qualified nonphysician health care professional who may not report evaluation and management services [eg, speech-language pathologists, physical therapists, occupational therapists, social workers, dieticians], see 98966-98968)

99439 This code is out of order. See page 191

99441 Telephone evaluation and management service by a physician or other qualified health care professional who may report evaluation and management services provided to an established patient, parent, or guardian not originating from a related E/M service provided within the previous 7 days nor leading to an E/M service or procedure within the next 24 hours or soonest available appointment; 5-10 minutes of medical discussion

99442 11-20 minutes of medical discussion

99443 21-30 minutes of medical discussion

> (Do not report 99441-99443 when using 99339-99340, 99374-99380 for the same call[s])

> (Do not report 99441-99443 for home and outpatient INR monitoring when reporting 93792, 93793)

> (Do not report 99441-99443 during the same month with 99487-99489)

> (Do not report 99441-99443 when performed during the service time of codes 99495 or 99496)

ONLINE DIGITAL EVALUATION AND MANAGEMENT SERVICES

Online digital evaluation and management (E/M) services (99421, 99422, 99423) are patient-initiated services with physicians or other qualified health care professionals (QHPs). Online digital E/M services require physician or other QHP's evaluation, assessment, and management of the patient. These services are not for the nonevaluative electronic communication of test results, scheduling of appointments, or other communication that does not include E/M. While the patient's problem may be new to the physician or other QHP, the patient is an established patient. Patients initiate these services through Health Insurance Portability and Accountability Act (HIPAA)-compliant secure platforms, such as electronic health record (EHR) portals, secure email, or other digital applications, which allow digital communication with the physician or other QHP.

Online digital E/M services are reported once for the physician's or other QHP's cumulative time devoted to the service during a seven-day period. The seven-day period begins with the physician's or other QHP's initial, personal review of the patient-generated inquiry. Physician's or other QHP's cumulative service time includes review of the initial inquiry, review of patient records or data pertinent to assessment of the patient's problem, personal physician or other QHP interaction with clinical staff focused on the patient's problem, development of management plans, including physician or other QHP generation of prescriptions or ordering of tests, and subsequent communication with the patient through online, telephone, email, or other digitally supported communication, which does not otherwise represent a separately reported E/M service. All professional decision making, assessment, and subsequent management by physicians or other QHPs in the same group practice contribute to the cumulative service time of the patient's online digital E/M service. Online digital E/M services require permanent documentation storage (electronic or hard copy) of the encounter.

If within seven days of the initiation of an online digital E/M service, a separately reported E/M visit occurs, then the physician or other QHP work devoted to the online digital E/M service is incorporated into the separately reported E/M visit (eg, additive of visit time for a timebased E/M visit or additive of decision-making complexity for a key component-based E/M visit). This includes E/M visits and procedures that are provided through synchronous telemedicine visits using interactive audio and video telecommunication equipment, which are reported with modifier 95 appended to the E/M service code. If the patient initiates an online digital inquiry for the same or a related problem within seven days of a previous E/M service, then the online digital visit is not reported. If the online digital inquiry is related to a surgical procedure and occurs during the postoperative period of a previously completed procedure, then the online digital E/M service is not reported separately. If the patient generates the initial online digital inquiry for a new problem within seven days of a previous E/M visit that addressed a different problem, then the online digital E/M service may be reported separately. If the patient presents a new, unrelated problem during the seven-day period of an online digital E/M service, then the physician's or other QHP's time spent on evaluation, assessment, and management of the additional problem is added to the cumulative service time of the online digital E/M service for that seven-day period.

> (For online digital E/M services provided by a qualified nonphysician health care professional who may not report the physician or other qualified health care professional E/M services [eg, speech-language

pathologists, physical therapists, occupational therapists, social workers, dietitians], see 98970, 98971, 98972)

99421   Online digital evaluation and management service, for an established patient, for up to 7 days, cumulative time during the 7 days; 5-10 minutes

99422   11-20 minutes

99423   21 or more minutes

(Report 99421, 99422, 99423 once per 7-day period)

(Clinical staff time is not calculated as part of cumulative time for 99421, 99422, 99423)

(Do not report online digital E/M services for cumulative service time less than 5 minutes)

(Do not count 99421, 99422, 99423 time otherwise reported with other services)

(Do not report 99421, 99422, 99423 on a day when the physician or other qualified health care professional reports E/M services [99202, 99203, 99204, 99205, 99212, 99213, 99214, 99215, 99241, 99242, 99243, 99244, 99245])

(Do not report 99421, 99422, 99423 when using 99091, 99339, 99340, 99374, 99375, 99377, 99378, 99379, 99380, 99487, 99489 for the same communication[s])

(Do not report 99421, 99422, 99423 for home and outpatient INR monitoring when reporting 93792, 93793)

(**99444**   deleted 2019 [2020 Edition]. To report, see 99421, 99422, 99423)

INTERPROFESSIONAL TELEPHONE/INTERNET CONSULTATIONS

The consultant should use codes 99446, 99447, 99448, 99449, 99451 to report interprofessional telephone/Internet/electronic health record consultations. An interprofessional telephone/Internet/electronic health record consultation is an assessment and management service in which a patient's treating (eg, attending or primary) physician or other qualified health care professional requests the opinion and/or treatment advice of a physician with specific specialty expertise (the consultant) to assist the treating physician or other qualified health care professional in the diagnosis and/or management of the patient's problem without patient face-to-face contact with the consultant.

The patient for whom the interprofessional telephone/Internet/electronic health record consultation is requested may be either a new patient to the consultant or an established patient with a new problem or an exacerbation of an existing problem. However, the consultant should not have seen the patient in a face-toface encounter within the last 14 days. When the telephone/Internet/electronic health record consultation leads to a transfer of care or other face-to-face service (eg, a surgery, a hospital visit, or a scheduled office evaluation of the patient) within the next 14 days or next available appointment date of the consultant, these codes are not reported.

Review of pertinent medical records, laboratory studies, imaging studies, medication profile, pathology specimens, etc is included in the telephone/Internet/electronic health record consultation service and should not be reported separately when reporting 99446, 99447, 99448, 99449, 99451. The majority of the service time reported (greater than 50%) must be devoted to the medical consultative verbal or Internet discussion. If greater than 50% of the time for the service is devoted to data review and/or analysis, 99446, 99447, 99448, 99449 should not be reported. However, the service time for 99451 is based on total review and interprofessional-communication time.

If more than one telephone/Internet/electronic health record contact(s) is required to complete the consultation request (eg, discussion of test results), the entirety of the service and the cumulative discussion and information review time should be reported with a single code. Codes 99446, 99447, 99448, 99449, 99451 should not be reported more than once within a seven-day interval.

The written or verbal request for telephone/Internet/electronic health record advice by the treating/requesting physician or other qualified health care professional should be documented in the patient's medical record, including the reason for the request. Codes 99446, 99447, 99448, 99449 conclude with a verbal opinion report and written report from the consultant to the treating/requesting physician or other qualified health care professional. Code 99451 concludes with only a written report.

Telephone/Internet/electronic health record consultations of less than five minutes should not be reported. Consultant communications with the patient and/or family may be reported using 98966, 98967, 98968, 99421, 99422, 99423, 99441, 99442, 99443, and the time related to these services is not used in reporting 99446, 99447, 99448, 99449. Do not report 99358, 99359 for any time within the service period, if reporting 99446, 99447, 99448, 99449, 99451.

When the sole purpose of the telephone/Internet/electronic health record communication is to arrange a transfer of care or other face-to-face service, these codes are not reported.

The treating/requesting physician or other qualified health care professional may report 99452 if spending 16-30 minutes in a service day preparing for the referral and/or communicating with the consultant. Do not report 99452 more than once in a 14-day period. The treating/requesting physician or other qualified health care professional may report the prolonged service codes 99354, 99355, 99356, 99357 for the time spent on the interprofessional telephone/Internet/electronic health record discussion with the consultant (eg, specialist) if the time exceeds 30 minutes beyond the typical time of the appropriate E/M service performed and the patient is present (on-site) and accessible to the treating/requesting physician or other qualified health care professional. If the interprofessional telephone/Internet/electronic health record assessment and management service occurs when the patient is not present and the time spent in a day exceeds 30 minutes, then the non-face-to-face prolonged service codes 99358, 99359 may be reported by the treating/requesting physician or other qualified health care professional.

> (For telephone services provided by a physician to a patient, see 99441, 99442, 99443)

> (For telephone services provided by a qualified health care professional to a patient, see 98966, 98967, 98968)

> (For online digital E/M services provided by a physician or other qualified health care professional to a patient, see 99421, 99422, 99423)

99446 Interprofessional telephone/Internet/electronic health record assessment and management service provided by a consultative physician, including a verbal and written report to the patient's treating/requesting physician or other qualified health care professional; 5-10 minutes of medical consultative discussion and review

99447 11-20 minutes of medical consultative discussion and review

99448 21-30 minutes of medical consultative discussion and review

99449 31 minutes or more of medical consultative discussion and review

99451 Interprofessional telephone/Internet/electronic health record assessment and management service provided by a consultative physician, including a written report to the patient's treating/requesting physician or other qualified health care professional, 5 minutes or more of medical consultative time

99452 Interprofessional telephone/Internet/electronic health record referral service(s) provided by a treating/requesting physician or other qualified health care professional, 30 minutes

DIGITALLY STORED DATA SERVICES/REMOTE PHYSIOLOGIC MONITORING

Codes 99453 and 99454 are used to report remote physiologic monitoring services (eg, weight, blood pressure, pulse oximetry) during a 30-day period. To report 99453, 99454, the device used must be a medical device as defined by the FDA, and the service must be ordered by a physician or other qualified health care professional. Code 99453 may be used to report the setup and patient education on use of the device(s). Code 99454 may be used to report supply of the device for daily recording or programmed alert transmissions. Codes 99453, 99454 are not reported if monitoring is less than 16 days. Do not report 99453, 99454 when these services are included in other codes for the duration of time of the physiologic monitoring service (eg, 95250 for continuous glucose monitoring requires a minimum of 72 hours of monitoring).

Code 99091 should be reported no more than once in a 30-day period to include the physician or other qualified health care professional time involved with data accession, review and interpretation, modification of care plan as necessary (including communication to patient and/or caregiver), and associated documentation.

If the services described by 99091 or 99474 are provided on the same day the patient presents for an evaluation and management (E/M) service to the same provider, these services should be considered part of the E/M service and not reported separately.

Do not report 99091 for time in the same calendar month when used to meet the criteria for care plan oversight services (99374, 99375, 99377, 99378, 99379, 99380), home, domiciliary, or rest home care plan oversight services (99339, 99340), remote

---

physiologic monitoring services (99457), or personally performed chronic care management (99491). Do not report 99091 if other more specific codes exist (eg, 93227, 93272 for cardiographic services; 95250 for continuous glucose monitoring). Do not report 99091 for transfer adn interpretation of data from hospital or clinical laboratory computers.

Code 99453 is reported for each episode of care. For coding remote monitoring of physiologic parameters, an episode of care is defined as beginning when the remote monitoring physiologic service is initiated, and ends with attainment of targeted treatment goals.

99453 Remote monitoring of physiologic parameter(s) (eg, weight, blood pressure, pulse oximetry, respiratory flow rate), initial; set-up and patient education on use of equipment

(Do not report 99453 more than once per episode of care)

(Do not report 99453 for monitoring of less than 16 days)

99454 device(s) supply with daily recording(s) or programmed alert(s) transmission, each 30 days

(For physiologic monitoring treatment management services, use 99457)

(Do not report 99454 for monitoring of less than 16 days)

(Do not report 99453, 99454 in conjunction with codes for more specific physiologic parameters [eg, 93296, 94760])

(For self-measured blood pressure monitoring, see 99473, 99474)

99091 Collection and interpretation of physiologic data (eg, ECG, blood pressure, glucose monitoring) digitally stored and/or transmitted by the patient and/or caregiver to the physician or other qualified health care professional, qualified by education, training, licensure/regulation (when applicable) requiring a minimum of 30 minutes of time, each 30 days

(Do not report 99091 in conjunction with 99457)

(Do not report 99091 for time in a calendar month when used to meet the criteria for 99339, 99340, 99374, 99375, 99377, 99378, 99379, 99380, 99457, 99491)

99473 Self-measured blood pressure using a device validated for clinical accuracy; patient education/training and device calibration

(Do not report 99473 more than once per device)

(For ambulatory blood pressure monitoring, see 93784, 93786, 93788, 93790)

99474 separate self-measurements of two readings one minute apart, twice daily over a 30-day period (minimum of 12 readings), collection of data reported by the patient and/or caregiver to the physician or other qualified health care professional, with report of average systolic and diastolic pressures and subsequent communication of a treatment plan to the patient

(Do not report 99473, 99474 in the same calendar month as 93784, 93786, 93788, 93790, 99091, 99439, 99453, 99454, 99457, 99487, 99489, 99490, 99491)

(Do not report 99474 more than once per calendar month)

REMOTE PHYSIOLOGIC MONITORING TREATMENT MANAGEMENT SERVICES

Remote physiologic monitoring treatment management services are provided when clinical staff/physician/other qualified health care professional use the results of remote physiological monitoring to manage a patient under a specific treatment plan. To report remote physiological monitoring, the device used must be a medical device as defined by the FDA, and the service must be ordered by a physician or other qualified health care professional. Do not use 99457, 99458 for time that can be reported using more specific monitoring services (eg, for the patient that requires reevaluation of medication regimen and/or changes in treatment). Codes 99457, 99458 may be reported during the same service period as chronic care management services (99439, 99487, 99489, 99490, 99491), transitional care management services (99495, 99496), and behavioral health integration services (99484, 99492, 99493, 99494); however, time spent performing these services should remain separate and no time should be counted toward the required time for both services in a single month. Codes 99457, 99458 require a live, interactive communication with the patient/caregiver. For the first completed 20 minutes of clinical staff/physician/other qualified health care professional time in a calendar month report 99457, and report 99458 for each additional completed 20 minutes. Do not report

99457, 99458 for services of less than 20 minutes. Report 99457 one time regardless of the number of physiologic monitoring modalities performed in a given calendar month.

Do not count any time on a day when the physician or other qualified health care professional reports an E/M service (office or other outpatient services 99202, 99203, 99204, 99205, 99211, 99212, 99213, 99214, 99215, domiciliary, rest home services 99324, 99325, 99326, 99327, 99328, 99334, 99335, 99336, 99337, home services 99341, 99342, 99343, 99344, 99345, 99347, 99348, 99349, 99350, inpatient services 99221, 99222, 99223, 99231, 99232, 99233, 99251, 99252, 99253, 99254, 99255). Do not count any time related to other reported services (eg, 93290, 93793, 99291, 99292).

99457 Remote physiologic monitoring treatment management services, clinical staff/physician/other qualified health care professional time in a calendar month requiring interactive communication with the patient/caregiver during the month; first 20 minutes

(Report 99457 once each 30 days, regardless of the number of parameters monitored)

(Do not report 99457 for services of less than 20 minutes)

(Do not report 99457 in conjunction with 93264, 99091)

(Do not report 99457 in the same month as 99473, 99474)

+ 99458 each additional 20 minutes (List separately in addition to code for primary procedure)

(Use 99458 in conjunction with 99457)

(Do not report 99458 for services of less than 20 minutes)

SPECIAL EVALUATION AND MANAGEMENT SERVICES

The following codes are used to report evaluations performed to establish baseline information prior to life or disability insurance certificates being issued. This service is performed in the office or other setting, and applies to both new and established patients When using these codes, no active management of the problem(s) is undertaken during the encounter..

If other evaluation and management services and/or procedures are performed on the same date, the appropriate E/M or procedure code(s) should be reported in addition to these codes.

BASIC LIFE AND/OR DISABILITY EVALUATION SERVICES

99450 Basic life and/or disability examination that includes:
- measurement of height, weight and blood pressure;
- completion of a medical history following a life insurance pro forma;
- collection of blood sample and/or urinalysis complying with "chain of custody" protocols; and
- completion of necessary documentation/certificates.

99451 This code is out of order. See page 179

99452 This code is out of order. See page 179

99453 This code is out of order. See page 180

99454 This code is out of order. See page 180

WORK RELATED OR MEDICAL DISABILITY EVALUATION SERVICES

99455 Work related or medical disability examination by the treating physician that includes:
- completion of a medical history commensurate with the patient's condition;
- performance of an examination commensurate with the patient's condition;
- formulation of a diagnosis, assessment of capabilities and stability, and calculation of impairment;
- development of future medical treatment plan; and

- completion of necessary documentation/certificates and report.

99456 Work related or medical disability examination by other than the treating physician that includes:
- completion of a medical history commensurate with the patient's condition;
- performance of an examination commensurate with the patient's condition;
- formulation of a diagnosis, assessment of capabilities and stability, and calculation of impairment;
- development of future medical treatment plan; and
- completion of necessary documentation/certificates and report.

(Do not report 99455, 99456 in conjunction with 99080 for the completion of Workman's Compensation forms)

99457 This code is out of order. See page 181

99458 This code is out of order. See page 181

NEWBORN CARE SERVICES

The following codes are used to report the services provided to newborns (birth through the first 28 days) in several different settings. Use of the normal newborn codes is limited to the initial care of the newborn in the first days after birth prior to home discharge.

Evaluation and Management (E/M) services for the newborn include maternal and/or fetal and newborn history, newborn physical examination(s), ordering of diagnostic tests and treatments, meetings with the family, and documentation in the medical record.

When delivery room attendance services (99464) or delivery room resuscitation services (99465) are required, report these in addition to normal newborn services E/M codes.

For E/M services provided to newborns who are other than normal, see codes for hospital inpatient services (99221-99233) and neonatal intensive and critical care services (99466-99469, 99477-99480). When normal newborn services are provided by the same individual on the same date that the newborn later becomes ill and receives additional intensive or critical care services, report the appropriate E/M code with modifier 25 for these services in addition to the normal newborn code..

Procedures (eg, 54150, newborn circumcision) are not included with the normal newborn codes, and when performed, should be reported in addition to the newborn services.

When newborns are seen in follow-up after the date of discharge in the office or outpatient setting, see 99202-99215, 99381, 99391 as appropriate.

99460 Initial hospital or birthing center care, per day, for evaluation and management of normal newborn infant

99461 Initial care, per day, for evaluation and management of normal newborn infant seen in other than hospital or birthing center

99462 Subsequent hospital care, per day, for evaluation and management of normal newborn

99463 Initial hospital or birthing center care, per day, for evaluation and management of normal newborn infant admitted and discharged on the same date

(For newborn Hospital discharge services provided on a date subsequent to the admission date, see 99238, 99239)

DELIVERY/BIRTHING ROOM ATTENDANCE AND RESUSCITATION SERVICES

99464 Attendance at delivery (when requested by the delivering physician or other qualified health care professional) and initial stabilization of newborn

(99464 may be reported in conjunction with 99460, 99468, 99477)

(Do not report 99464 in conjunction with 99465)

99465 Delivery/birthing room resuscitation, provision of positive pressure ventilation and/or chest compressions in the presence of acute inadequate ventilation and/or cardiac output

(99465 may be reported in conjunction with 99460, 99468, 99477)

(Do not report 99465 in conjunction with 99464)

(Procedures that are performed as a necessary part of the resuscitation [eg, intubation, vascular lines] are reported separately in addition to 99465. In order to report these procedures, they must be performed as a necessary component of the resuscitation and not as a convenience before admission to the neonatal intensive care unit)

INPATIENT NEONATAL INTENSIVE CARE SERVICES AND PEDIATRIC AND NEONATAL CRITICAL CARE SERVICES

PEDIATRIC CRITICAL CARE PATIENT TRANSPORT

Codes 99466, 99467 are used to report the physical attendance and direct face-to-face care by a physician during the interfacility transport of a critically ill or critically injured pediatric patient 24 months of age or younger. Codes 99485, 99486 are used to report the control physician's non-face-to-face supervision of interfacility transport of a critically ill or critically injured pediatric patient 24 months of age or younger. These codes are not reported together for the same patient by the same physician. For the purpose of reporting 99466 and 99467, face-to-face care begins when the physician assumes primary responsibility of the pediatric patient at the referring facility, and ends when the receiving facility accepts responsibility for the pediatric patient's care. Only the time the physician spends in direct face-to-face contact with the patient during the transport should be reported. Pediatric patient transport services involving less than 30 minutes of face-to-face physician care should not be reported using 99466, 99467. Procedure(s) or services(s) performed by other members of the transporting team may not be reported by the supervising physician.

Codes 99485, 99486 may be used to report control physician's non-face-to-face supervision of interfacility pediatric critical care transport, which includes all twoway communication between the control physician and the specialized transport team prior to transport, at the referring facility and during transport of the patient back to the receiving facility. The "control" physician is the physician directing transport services. These codes do not include pretransport communication between the control physician and the referring facility before or following patient transport. These codes may only be reported for patients 24 months of age or younger who are critically ill or critically injured. The control physician provides treatment advice to a specialized transport team who are present and delivering the hands-on patient care. The control physician does not report any services provided by the specialized transport team. The control physician's non-face-to-face time begins with the first contact by the control physician with the specialized transport team and ends when the patient's care is handed over to the receiving facility team. Refer to 99466 and 99467 for face-to-face transport care of the critically ill/injured patient. Time spent with the individual patient's transport team and reviewing data submissions should be recorded. Code 99485 is used to report the first 16-45 minutes of direction on a given date and should only be used once even if time spent by the physician is discontinuous. Do not report services of 15 minutes or less or any time when another physician is reporting 99466, 99467. Do not report 99485 or 99486 in conjunction with 99466, 99467 when performed by the same physician.

For the definition of the critically injured pediatric patient, see the Neonatal and Pediatric Critical Care Services section.

The non-face-to-face direction of emergency care to a patient's transporting staff by a physician located in a hospital or other facility by two-way communication is not considered direct face-to-face care and should not be reported with 99466, 99467. Physician-directed non-face-to-face emergency care through outside voice communication to transporting staff personnel is reported with 99288 or 99485, 99486 based upon the age and clinical condition of the patient.

Emergency department services (99281-99285), initial hospital care (99221-99223), critical care (99291, 99292), initial date neonatal intensive (99477) or critical care (99468) may only be reported after the patient has been admitted to the emergency department, the inpatient floor, or the critical care unit of the receiving facility. If inpatient critical care services are reported in the referring facility prior to transfer to the receiving hospital, use the critical care codes (99291, 99292).

The following services are included when performed during the pediatric patient transport by the physician providing critical care and may not be reported separately: routine monitoring evaluations (eg, heart rate, respiratory rate, blood pressure, and pulse oximetry), the interpretation of cardiac output measurements (93562), chest X rays (71045, 71046), pulse oximetry (94760, 94761, 94762), blood gases and information data stored in computers (eg, ECGs, blood pressures, hematologic data), gastric intubation (43752, 43753), temporary transcutaneous pacing (92953), ventilatory management (94002, 94003, 94660, 94662), and vascular access procedures (36000, 36400, 36405, 36406, 36415, 36591, 36600). Any services performed which are not listed above should be reported separately.

| | Separate Procedure | | Unlisted Procedure | | CCI Comp. Code | | Non-specific Procedure | **183** |

CPT codes and descriptions only ©2020 American Medical Association. All rights reserved.

Services provided by the specialized transport team during non-face-to-face transport supervision are not reported by the control physician.

Code 99466 is used to report the first 30 to 74 minutes of direct face-to-face time with the transport pediatric patient and should be reported only once on a given date. Code 99467 is used to report each additional 30 minutes provided on a given date. Face-to-face services of less than 30 minutes should not be reported with these codes.

Code 99485 is used to report the first 30 minutes of non-face-to-face supervision of an interfacility transport of a critically ill or critically injured pediatric patient and should be reported only once per date of service. sOnly the communication time spent by the supervising physician with the specialty transport team members during an interfacility transport should be reported. Code 99486 is used to report each additional 30 minutes beyond the initial 30 minutes. Non-face-to-face interfacility transport of 15 minutes or less is not reported.

(For total body and selective head cooling of neonates, use 99184)

99466   Critical care face-to-face services, during an interfacility transport of critically ill or critically injured pediatric patient, 24 months of age or less; first 30-74 minutes of hands-on care during transport

+ 99467   each additional 30 minutes (list separately in addition to code for primary service)

(Use 99467 in conjunction with 99466)

(Critical care of less than 30 minutes total duration should be reported with the appropriate E/M code)

99485   Supervision by a control physician of interfacility transport care of the critically ill or critically injured pediatric patient, 24 month of age or younger, includes two-way communication with transport team before transport, at the referring facility and during the transport, including data interpretation and report, first 30 minutes.

+ 99486   each additional 30 minutes (List separately in addition to code for primary procedure)

(Use 99486 in conjunction with 99485)

(For physician direction of emergency medical systems supervision for a pediatric patient older than 24 months of age, or at any age if not critically ill or injured, use 99288)

(Do not report 99485, 99486 with any other services reported by the control physician for the same period)

(Do not report 99485, 99486 in conjunction with 99466, 99467 when performed by the same physician)

INPATIENT NEONATAL AND PEDIATRIC CRITICAL CARE

The same definitions for critical care services apply to the adult, child and neonate.

Codes 99468, 99469 may be used to report the services of directing the inpatient care of a critically ill neonate or infant 28 days of age or younger. They represent care starting with the date of admission (99468) for critical care services and all subsequent day(s) (99469) that the neonate remains in critical care. These codes may be reported only by a single individual and only once per calendar day, per patient. Initial inpatient neonatal critical care (99468) may only be reported once per hospital admission. If readmitted for neonatal critical care services during the same hospital stay, then report the subsequent inpatient neonatal critical care code (99469) for the first day of readmission to critical care, and 99469 for each day of critical care following readmission.

The initial inpatient neonatal critical care code (99468) can be used in addition to 99464 or 99465 as appropriate, when the physician or other qualified health care professional is present for the delivery (99464) or resuscitation (99465) is required. Other procedures performed as a necessary part of the resuscitation (eg, endotracheal intubation [31500]) may also be reported separately, when performed as part of the pre-admission delivery room care. In order to report these procedures separately, they must be performed as a necessary component of the resuscitation and not simply as a convenience before admission to the neonatal intensive care unit.

Codes 99471-99476 may be used to report the services of directing the inpatient care of a critically ill infant or young child from 29 days of postnatal age through 5 years of age. They represent care starting with the date of admission (99471, 99475) for pediatric critical care services and all subsequent day(s) (99472, 99476) that the infant or child remains in critical condition. These codes may only be reported by a single individual and only once per calendar day, per patient. Services for the critically ill or critically injured child 6 years of age or older would be reported with the time-based critical care codes (99291, 99292). Initial inpatient critical care (99471, 99475) may only be reported once per hospital admission. If readmitted to the pediatric critical care unit during the same hospital stay, then report the subsequent inpatient pediatric critical care code 99472 or 99476 for the first day of readmission to critical care and 99472 or 99476 for each day of critical care following readmission.

The pediatric and neonatal critical care codes include those procedures listed for the critical care codes (99291, 99292). In addition, the following procedures are also included (and are not separately reported by professionals, but may be reported by facilities) in the pediatric and neonatal critical care service codes (99468-99472, 99475, 99476), and the intensive care services codes (99477- 99480):

Any services performed that are not included in these listings may be reported separately. For initiation of selective head or total body hypothermia in the critically ill neonate, report 99184. Facilities may report the included services separately.

Invasive or non-invasive electronic monitoring of vital signs

Vascular access procedures

> Peripheral vessel catheterization (36000)
> Other arterial catheters (36140, 36620)
> Umbilical venous catheters (36510)
> Central vessel catheterization (36555)
> Vascular access procedures (36400, 36405, 36406)
> Vascular punctures (36420, 36600)
> Umbilical arterial catheters (36660)

Airway and ventilation management

> Endotracheal intubation (31500)
> Ventilatory management (94002-94004)
> Bedside pulmonary function testing (94375)
> Surfactant administration (94610)
> Continuous positive airway pressure (CPAP) (94660)

Monitoring or interpretation of blood gases or oxygen saturation (94760-94762)

Car Seat Evaluation (94780-94781)

Transfusion of blood components (36430, 36440)

Oral or nasogastric tube placement (43752)

Suprapubic bladder aspiration (51100)

Bladder catheterization (51701, 51702)

Lumbar puncture (62270)

Any services performed which are not listed above may be reported separately.

When a neonate or infant is not critically ill but requires intensive observation, frequent interventions, and other intensive care services, the Continuing Intensive Care Services codes (99477-99480) should be used to report these services.

To report critical care services provided in the outpatient setting (eg., emergency department or office) for neonates and pediatric patients of any age, see the Critical Care codes 99291, 99292. If the same individual provides critical care services for a neonatal or pediatric patient less than 6 years of age in both the outpatient and inpatient settings on the same day, report only the appropriate Neonatal or Pediatric Critical Care codes 99468-99476 for all critical care services provided on that day. Critical care services provided by a second individual of a different specialty not reporting a per-day neonatal or pediatric critical care code can be reported with 99291, 99292.

When critical care services are provided to neonates or pediatric patients less than 6 years of age at two separate institutions by an individual from a different group on the same date of service, the individual from the referring institution should report their critical care services with the critical care codes (99291, 99292) and the receiving institution should report the appropriate initial day of care code 99468, 99471, 99475 for the same date of service.

Critical care services to a pediatric patient six years of age or older are reported with the critical care codes 99291, 99292.

| | Separate Procedure | | Unlisted Procedure | | CCI Comp. Code | | Non-specific Procedure | **185** |

When the critically ill neonate or pediatric patient improves and is transferred to a lower level of care to another individual in another group within the same facility, the transferring individual does not report a per day critical care service. subsequent hospital care (99231-99233) or time-based critical care services (99291-99292) is reported, as appropriate based upon the condition of the neonate or child. The receiving individual reports subsequent intensive care (99478- 99480) or subsequent hospital care (99231-99233) services, as appropriate based upon the condition of the neonate or child.

When the neonate or infant becomes critically ill on a day when initial or subsequent intensive care services (99477-99480), hospital services (99221-99233), or normal newborn services (99460, 99461, 99462) have been performed by one individual and is transferred to a critical care level of care provided by a different individual in a different group, the transferring individual reports either the time-based critical care services performed (99291, 99292) for the time spent providing critical care to the patient, the intensive care service (99477-99480), hospital care services (99221-99233), or normal newborn service ((99460, 99461, 99462) performed, but only one service. The receiving individual reports initial or subsequent inpatient neonatal or pediatric critical care (99468-99476), as appropriate based upon the patient's age and whether this is the first or subsequent admission to the critical care unit for the hospital stay.

When a newborn becomes critically ill on the same day they have already received normal newborn care (99460, 99461, 99462), and the same individual or group assumes critical care, report initial critical care service (99468) with modifier 25 in addition to the normal newborn code.

When a neonate, infant, or child requires initial critical care services on the same day the patient already has received hospital care or intensive care services by the same individual or group, only the initial critical care service code (99468, 99471, 99475) is reported.

Time-based critical care services (99291, 99292) are not reportable by the same individual or different individual of the same specialty and same group, when neonatal or pediatric critical care services (9468-99476) may be reported for the same patient on the same day. Tim-based critical care services (99291, 99292) may be reported by an individual of a different specialty from either the same or different group on the same day that neonatal or pediatric critical care services are reported. Critical care interfacility transport face-to-face (99466, 99467) or supervisory (99485, 99486) services may be reported by the same or different individual of the same specialty and same group, when neonatal or pediatric critical care services (99468-99476) are reported for the same patient on the same day.

99468   Initial inpatient neonatal critical care, per day, for the evaluation and management of a critically ill neonate, 28 days of age or younger

99469   Subsequent inpatient neonatal critical care, per day, for the evaluation and management of a critically ill neonate, 28 days of age or younger

99471   Initial inpatient pediatric critical care, per day, for the evaluation and management of a critically ill infant or young child, 29 days through 24 months of age

99472   Subsequent inpatient pediatric critical care, per day, for the evaluation and management of a critically ill infant or young child, 29 days through 24 months of age

99473   This code is out of order. See page 180

99474   This code is out of order. See page 180

99475   Initial inpatient pediatric critical care, per day, for the evaluation and management of a critically ill infant or young child, 2 through 5 years of age

99476   Subsequent inpatient pediatric critical care, per day, for the evaluation and management of a critically ill infant or young child, 2 through 5 years of age

INITIAL AND CONTINUING INTENSIVE CARE SERVICES

Code 99477 represents the initial day of inpatient care for the child who is not critically ill but requires intensive observation, frequent interventions, and other intensive care services. Codes 99478-99480 are used to report the subsequent day services of directing the continuing intensive care of the low birth weight (LBW 1500-2500 grams) present body weight infant, very low birth weight (VLBW less than 1500 grams) present body weight infant, or normal (2501-5000 grams) present body weight newborn who does not meet the definition of critically ill but continues to require intensive observation, frequent interventions, and other intensive care services. These services are for infants and neonates who are not critically ill but continue to require intensive cardiac and respiratory monitoring, continuous and/or frequent vital sign monitoring, heat maintenance, enteral and/or parenteral nutritional adjustments, laboratory and oxygen monitoring, and constant observation by the health care team under direct supervision of the physician or other qualified health care professional. Codes 99477-99480 may be reported by a single individual and only once per day, per patient in a given facility. If readmitted to the intensive care unit during the same hospital stay, report 99478-99480 for the first day of intensive care and for each successive day that the child requires intensive care services.

These codes include the same procedures that are outlined in the Neonatal and Pediatric Critical Care Services section and these services should not be separately reported.

The initial day neonatal intensive care code (99477) can be used in addition to 99464 or 99465 as appropriate, when the physician or other qualified health care professional is present for the delivery (99464) or resuscitation (99465) is required. In this situation, report 99477 with modifier 25. Other procedures performed as a necessary part of the resuscitation (eg, endotracheal intubation [31500]) are also reported separately when performed as part of the pre-admission delivery room care. In order to report these procedures separately, they must be performed as a necessary component of the resuscitation and not simply as a convenience before admission to the neonatal intensive care unit.

The same procedures are included as bundled services with the neonatal intensive care codes as those listed for the neonatal (99468, 99469) and pediatric (99471-99476) critical care codes.

When the neonate or infant improves after the initial day and no longer requires intensive care services and is transferred to a lower level of care, the transferring individual does not report a per day intensive care service. Subsequent hospital care (99231-99233) or subsequent normal newborn care (99460, 99462) is reported as appropriate based upon the condition of the neonate or infant. If the transfer to a lower level of care occurs on the same day as initial intensive care services were provided by the transferring individual, 99477 may be reported.

When the neonate or infant is transferred after the initial day within the same facility to the care of another individual in a different group, both individuals report subsequent hospital care (99231-99233) services. The receiving individual reports subsequent hospital care (99231-99233) or subsequent normal newborn care (99462).

When the neonate or infant becomes critically ill on a day when initial or subsequent intensive care services (99477-99480) have been reported by one individual and is transferred to a critical care level of care provided by a different individual from a different group, the transferring individual reports either the time-based critical care services performed (99291-99292) for the time spent providing critical care to the patient, or the initial or subsequent intensive care (99477-99480) services, but not both. The receiving individual reports initial or subsequent inpatient neonatal or pediatric critical care (99468-99476) based upon the patient's age and whether this is the first or subsequent admission to critical care for the same hospital stay.

When the neonate or infant becomes critically ill on a day when initial or subsequent intensive care services (99477-99480) have been performed by the same individual or group, report only initial or subsequent inpatient neonatal or pediatric critical care (99468-99476) based upon the patient's age and whether this is the first or subsequent admission to critical care for the same hospital stay.

For the subsequent care of the sick neonate younger than 28 days of age, but more than 5000 grams who does not require intensive or critical care services, use 99231-99233.

99477 Initial hospital care, per day, for the evaluation and management of the neonate, 28 days of age or less, who requires intensive observation, frequent interventions, and other intensive care services

(For the initiation of inpatient care of the normal newborn, report 99460)

(For the initiation of care of the critically ill neonate, use 99468)

(For initiation of inpatient hospital care of the ill neonate not requiring intensive observation, frequent interventions, and other intensive care services, see 99221-99223)

99478 Subsequent intensive care, per day, for the evaluation and management of the recovering very low birth weight infant (present body weight less than 1500 grams)

99479 Subsequent intensive care, per day, for the evaluation and management of the recovering low birth weight infant (present body weight of 1500-2500 grams)

99480 Subsequent intensive care, per day, for the evaluation and management of the recovering infant (present body weight of 2501-5000 grams)

| Separate Procedure | Unlisted Procedure | CCI Comp. Code | Non-specific Procedure | **187** |

COGNITIVE ASSESSMENT AND CARE PLAN SERVICES

Cognitive assessment and care plan services are provided when a comprehensive evaluation of a new or existing patient, who exhibits signs and/or symptoms of cognitive impairment, is required to establish or confirm a diagnosis, etiology and severity for the condition. This service includes a thorough evaluation of medical and psychosocial factors, potentially contributing to increased morbidity. Do not report cognitive assessment and care plan services if any of the required elements are not performed or are deemed unnecessary for the patient's condition. For these services, see the appropriate evaluation and management code. A single physician or other qualified health care professional should not report 99483 more than once every 180 days.

Services for cognitive assessment and care plan include a cognition-relevant history, as well as an assessment of factors that could be contributing to cognitive impairment, including, but not limited to, psychoactive medication, chronic pain syndromes, infection, depression and other brain disease (eg, tumor, stroke, normal pressure hydrocephalus). Medical decision making includes current and likely progression of the disease, assessing the need for referral for rehabilitative, social, legal, financial, or community-based services, meal, transportation, and other personal assistance services.

99483   Assessment of and care planning for a patient with cognitive impairment, requiring an independent historian, in the office or other outpatient, home or domiciliary or rest home, with all of the following required elements:

- Cognition-focused evaluation including a pertinent history and examination;

- Medical decision making of moderate or high complexity;

- Functional assessment (eg, basic and instrumental activities of daily living), including decision-making capacity;

- Use of standardized instruments for staging of dementia (eg, functional assessment staging test [FAST], clinical dementia rating [CDR]);

- Medication reconciliation and review for high-risk medications;

- Evaluation for neuropsychiatric and behavioral symptoms, including depression, including use of standardized screening instrument(s);

- Evaluation of safety (eg, home), including motor vehicle operation;

- Identification of caregiver(s), caregiver knowledge, caregiver needs, social supports, and the willingness of caregiver to take on caregiving tasks;

- Development, updating or revision, or review of an Advance Care Plan;

- Creation of a written care plan, including initial plans to address any neuropsychiatric symptoms, neurocognitive symptoms, functional limitations, and referral to community resources as needed (eg, rehabilitation services, adult day programs, support groups) shared with the patient and/or caregiver with initial education and support.

Typically, 50 minutes are spent face-to-face with the patient and/or family or caregiver.

(Do not report 99483 in conjunction with E/M services [99202, 99203, 99204, 99205, 99211, 99212, 99213, 99214, 99215, 99241, 99242, 99243, 99244, 99245, 99324, 99325, 99326, 99327, 99328, 99334, 99335, 99336, 99337, 99341, 99342, 99343, 99344, 99345, 99347, 99348, 99349, 99350, 99366, 99367, 99368, 99497, 99498]; psychiatric diagnostic procedures [90785, 90791, 90792]; brief emotional/behavioral assessment [96127]; psychological or neuropsychological test administration [96146]; health risk assessment administration [96160, 96161]; medication therapy management services [99605, 99606, 99607])

99484   This code is out of order. See page 197

99485   This code is out of order. See page 183

99486   This code is out of order. See page 183

CARE MANAGEMENT SERVICES

Care management services are management and support services provided by clinical staff, under the direction of a physician or other qualified health care professional, or may be provided personally by a physician or other qualified health care professional to a patient residing at home or in a domiciliary, rest home, or assisted living facility. Services include establishing, implementing, revising, or monitoring the care plan, coordinating the care of other professionals and agencies, and educating the patient or caregiver about the patient's condition, care plan, and prognosis. The physician or other qualified health care professional provides or oversees the management and/or coordination of services, as needed, for all medical conditions, psychosocial needs, and activities of daily living.

A comprehensive plan of care for health problems is based on a physical, mental, cognitive, social, functional, and environmental evaluation. It is intended to provide a simple and concise overview of the patient, and be a useful resource for patients, caregivers, health care professionals, and others, as necessary.

A typical plan of care is not limited to, but may include:

- Problem list
- Expected outcome and prognosis
- Measurable treatment goals
- Cognitive assessment
- Functional assessment
- Symptom management
- Planned interventions
- Medical management
- Environmental evaluation
- Caregiver assessment
- Interaction and coordination with outside resources and other health care professionals and others, as necessary
- Summary of advance directives

The above elements are intended to be a guide for creating a meaningful plan of care rather than a strict set of requirements, so should be addressed only as appropriate for the individual.

The plan of care should include specific and achievable goals for each condition and be relevant to the patient's well-being and lifestyle. When possible, the treatment goals should also be measurable and time bound. The plan should be updated periodically based on status or goal changes. The entire care plan should be reviewed at least annually.

An electronic and/or printed plan of care must be documented and shared with the patient and/or caregiver.

Codes 99487, 99489, 99490, 99491 are reported only once per calendar month and 99439 is reported no more than twice per calendar month. Codes 99439, 99487, 99489, 99490, 99491 may only be reported by the single physician or other qualified health care professional who assumes the care management role with a particular patient for the calendar month.

For 99439, 99487, 99489, 99490 the face-to-face and non-face-to-face time spent by the clinical staff in communicating with the patient and/or family, caregivers, other professionals, and agencies; creating, revising, documenting, and implementing the care plan; or teaching self-management is used in determining the care management clinical staff time for the month. Only the time of the clinical staff of the reporting professional is counted. Only count the time of one clinical staff member when two or more clinical staff members are meeting about the patient. For 99491, only count the time personally spent by the physician or other qualified health care professional. Do not count any of the clinical staff time spent on the day of an initiating visit (the creation of the care plan, initial explanation to the patient and/or caregiver, and obtaining consent).

Care management activities performed by clinical staff, or personally by the physician or other qualified health care professional, typically include:

- communication and engagement with patient, family members, guardian or caretaker, surrogate decision makers, and/or other professionals regarding aspects of care;
- communication with home health agencies and other community services utilized by the patient;
- collection of health outcomes data and registry documentation;
- patient and/or family/caregiver education to support self management, independent living, and activities of daily living;
- assessment and support for treatment regimen adherence and medication management;

- identification of available community and health resources;

- facilitating access to care and services needed by the patient and/or family;

- management of care transitions not reported as part of transitional care management (99495, 99496);

- ongoing review of patient's status, including review of laboratory and other studies not reported as part of an E/M service, noted above;

- development, communication, and maintenance of a comprehensive care plan.

The care management office/practice must have the following capabilities:

- provide 24/7 access to physicians or other qualified health care professionals or clinical staff including providing patients/caregivers with a means to make contact with health care professionals in the practice to address urgent needs regardless of the time of day or day of week;

- provide continuity of care with a designated member of the care team with whom the patient is able to schedule successive routine appointments;

- provide timely access and management for follow-up after an emergency department visit or facility discharge;

- utilize an electronic health record system so that care providers have timely access to clinical information;

- use a standardized methodology to identify patients who require care management services;

- have an internal care management process/function whereby a patient identified as meeting the requirements for these services starts receiving them in a timely manner; use a form and format in the medical record that is standardized within the practice;

- be able to engage and educate patients and caregivers as well as coordinate care among all service professionals, as appropriate for each patient;

- reporting physician or other qualified health care professional oversees activities of the care team;

- all care team members providing services are clinically integrated.

Each minute of service time is counted toward only one service. Do not count any time and activities used to meet criteria for another reported service. However, time of clinical staff and time of a physician or other qualified health care professional are distinct when each provides a distinct, separately reportable service to the same patient during the same period of time (eg, calendar month). A list of services not reported in the same calendar month as 99439, 99487, 99489, 99490 is provided in the parenthetical instructions following 99439, 99489. See the parenthetical instruction below 99491 for a list of services not separately reported in the same calendar month that 99491 is reported. Do not report 99439, 99487, 99489, 99490 when reporting 99491 for the same calendar month. If the care management services are performed within the postoperative period of a reported surgery, the same individual may not report 99439, 99487, 99489, 99490, 99491. For service time used for reporting 99439, 99487, 99489, 99490, 99491, do not also include service time used to report 99421, 99422, 99423.

Care management may be reported in any calendar month during which the clinical staff time or physician or other qualified health care professional personal time requirements are met.

When behavioral or psychiatric collaborative care management services are also provided, 99484, 99492, 99493, 99494 may be reported in addition.

CHRONIC CARE MANAGEMENT SERVICES

Chronic care management services are provided when medical and/or psychosocial needs of the patient require establishing, implementing, revising, or monitoring the care plan. Patients who receive chronic care management services have two or more chronic continuous or episodic health conditions that are expected to last at least 12 months, or until the death of the patient, and that place the patient at significant risk of death, acute exacerbation/decompensation, or functional decline. Code 99490 is reported when, during the calendar month, at least 20 minutes of clinical staff time is spent in care management activities. Code 99439 is reported in conjunction with 99490 for each additional 20 minutes of clinical staff time spent in care management activities during the calendar month up to a maximum of 60 minutes total time (ie, 99439 may only be reported twice per calendar month). Code 99491 is reported when 30 minutes of physician or other qualified health care professional personal time is spent in care management activities. Do not report 99439, 99490 in the same calendar month as 99491. If reporting 99491, do not count any physician or other qualified health care professional time on the date of a face-to-face E/M encounter towards the time used in reporting 99491.

▲ **99490**   Chronic care management services with the following required elements:

- multiple (two or more) chronic conditions expected to last at least 12 months, or until the death of the patient,
- chronic conditions place the patient at significant risk of death, acute exacerbation/decompensation, or functional decline,
- comprehensive care plan established, implemented, revised, or monitored;

first 20 minutes of clinical staff time directed by a physician or other qualified health care professional, per calendar month.

●+**99439**   each additional 20 minutes of clinical staff time directed by a physician or other qualified health care professional, per calendar month (List separately in addition to code for primary procedure)

(Use 99439 in conjunction with 99490)

(Chronic care management services of less than 20 minutes duration, in a calendar month, are not reported separately)

(Chronic care management services of 60 minutes or more and requiring moderate or high complexity medical decision making may be reported using 99487, 99489)

(Do not report 99439 more than twice per calendar month)

(Do not report 99439, 99490 in the same calendar month with 90951-90970, 99339, 99340, 99374, 99375, 99377, 99378, 99379, 99380, 99487, 99489, 99491, 99605, 99606, 99607)

(Do not report 99439, 99490 for service time reported with 93792, 93793, 98960, 98961, 98962, 98966, 98967, 98968, 98970, 98971, 98972, 99071, 99078, 99080, 99091, 99358, 99359, 99366, 99367, 99368, 99421, 99422, 99423, 99441, 99442, 99443, 99605, 99606, 99607)

TOTAL DURATION OF STAFF CARE MANAGEMENT SERVICES	CHRONIC CARE MANAGEMENT
less than 20 minutes	Not reported separately
20 to 39 minutes	99490 once
40 to 59 minutes	99490 once and 99439 once
60 minutes or more (1 hour or more)	99490 once and 99439 twice (also see 99487)

99491   Chronic care management services, provided personally by a physician or other qualified health care professional, at least 30 minutes of physician or other qualified health care professional time, per calendar month, with the following required elements:

- multiple (two or more) chronic conditions expected to last at least 12 months, or until the death of the patient;
- chronic conditions place the patient at significant risk of death, acute exacerbation/decompensation, or functional decline;
- comprehensive care plan established, implemented, revised, or monitored.

(Do not report 99491 in the same calendar month with 90951-90970, 99339, 99340, 99374, 99375, 99377, 99378, 99379, 99380, 99439, 99487, 99489, 99490, 99605, 99606, 99607)

(Do not report 99491 for service time reported with 93792, 93793, 98960, 98961, 98962, 98966, 98967, 98968, 99071, 99078, 99080, 99091, 99358, 99359, 99366, 99367, 99368, 99421, 99422, 99423, 99441, 99442, 99443)

(Do not report 99491 when performed during the service time of 99495, 99496, if reporting 99495, 99496)

COMPLEX CHRONIC CARE MANAGEMENT SERVICES

Complex chronic care management services are provided during a calendar month that includes criteria for chronic care management services including establishing, revising, implementing, or monitoring the care plan; medical, functional, and/or psychosocial problems requiring medical decision making of moderate or high complexity; and clinical staff care management services for at least 60 minutes, under the direction of a physician or other qualified health care professional. Medical decision making as defined in the Evaluation and Management (E/M) guidelines is determined by the problems addressed by the reporting individual during the month.

Patients who require complex chronic care management services may be identified by practice-specific or other published algorithms that recognize multiple illnesses, multiple medication use, inability to perform activities of daily living, requirement for caregiver, and/or repeat admissions or emergency department visits. Typical adult patients who receive complex chronic care management services are treaeted with three or more prescription medications and may be receiving other types of therapeutic interventions (eg., physical therapy, occupational therapy). Typical pediatric patients receive three or more therapeutic interventions (eg., medications, nutritional support, respiratory therapy). All patients have two or more chronic continuous or episodic health conditions that are expected to last at least 12 months, or until the death of the patient, and that place the patient at significant risk of death, acute exaggeration/decompensation, or functional decline. Typical patients have complex diseases and morbidities and, as a result, demonstrate one or more of the following:

- need for the coordination of a number of specialties and services;

- inability to perform activities of daily living and/or cognitive impairment resulting in poor adherence to the treatment plan without substantial assistance from caregiver;

- psychiatric and other medical comorbidities (eg., dementia and chronic obstructive pulmonary disease or substance abuse and diabetes) that complicate their care; and/or

- social support requirements or difficulty with access to care.

Total Duration of Staff Care Management Services	Complex Chronic Care Management
Less than 60minutes	Not reported separately
60 to 89 minutes (1 hr. - 1 hr. 29 min.)	99487
90 to 119 minutes (1 hr. 30 min. - 1 hr. 59 min.)	99487 AND 99489 x 1
120 minutes or more (2 hours or more)	99487 AND 99489 x 2 AND 99489 for each additional 30 minutes

▲ **99487**   Complex chronic care management services, with the following required elements:

- multiple (two or more) chronic conditions expected to last at least 12 months, or until the death of the patient,

- chronic conditions place the patient at significant risk of death, acute exacerbation/decompensation, or functional decline,

- comprehensive care plan established, implemented, revised, or monitored

- moderate or high complexity medical decision making;

first 60 minutes of clinical staff time directed by a physician or other qualified health care professional, per calendar month.

(Complex chronic care management services of less than 60 minutes duration, in a calendar month, are not reported separately)

▲ **+99489**   each additional 30 minutes of clinical staff time directed by a physician or other qualified health care professional, per calendar month (List separately in addition to code for primary procedure)

(Report 99489 in conjunction with 99487)

(Do not report 99489 for care management services of less than 30 minutes additional to the first 60 minutes of complex chronic care management services during a calendar month)

(Do not report 99487, 99489 during the same calendar month with 90951-90970, 99339, 99340, 99374, 99375, 99377, 99378, 99379, 99380, 99439, 99490, 99491, 99605, 99606, 99607)

(Do not report 99487, 99489 for service time reported with 93792, 93793, 98960, 98961, 98962, 98966, 98967, 98968, 98969, 98970, 98971, 98972, 99071, 99078, 99080, 99091, 99358, 99359, 99366, 99367, 99368, 99421, 99422, 99423, 99441, 99442, 99443, 99605, 99606, 99607)

99490   This code is out of order. See page 191

99491   This code is out of order. See page 191

PSYCHIATRIC COLLABORATIVE CARE MANAGEMENT SERVICES

Psychiatric collaborative care services are provided under the direction of a treating physician or other qualified health care professional (see definitions below) during a calendar month. These services are reported by the treating physician or other qualified health care professional and include the services of the treating physician or other qualified health care professional, the behavioral health care manager (see definition below), and the psychiatric consultant (see definition below), who has contracted directly with the treating physician or other qualified health care professional, to provide consultation. Patients directed to the behavioral health care manager typically have behavioral health signs and/or symptoms or a newly diagnosed behavioral health condition, may need help in engaging in treatment, have not responded to standard care delivered in a nonpsychiatric setting, or require further assessment and engagement, prior to consideration of referral to a psychiatric care setting.

These services are provided when a patient requires a behavioral health care assessment; establishing, implementing, revising, or monitoring a care plan; and provision of brief interventions.

The following definitions apply to this section:

Definitions

Episode of care patients are treated for an episode of care, which is defined as beginning when the patient is directed by the treating physician or other qualified health care professional to the behavioral health care manager and ending with:

- the attainment of targeted treatment goals, which typically results in the discontinuation of care management services and continuation of usual followup with the treating physician or other qualified healthcare professional; or

- failure to attain targeted treatment goals culminating in referral to a psychiatric care provider for ongoing treatment of the behavioral health condition; or

- lack of continued engagement with no psychiatric collaborative care management services provided over a consecutive six month calendar period (break in episode)

A new episode of care starts after a break in episode of six calendar months or more.

Health care professionals refers to the treating physician or other qualified health care professional who directs the behavioral health care manager and continues to oversee the patient's care, including prescribing medications, providing treatments for medical conditions, and making referrals to specialty care when needed. Evaluation and management (E/M) and other services may be reported separately by the same physician or other qualified health care professional during the same calendar month.

Behavioral health care manager refers to clinical staff with a masters-/doctoral-level education or specialized training in behavioral health who provides care management services as well as an assessment of needs, including the administration of validated rating scales, the development of a care plan, provision of brief interventions, ongoing collaboration with the treating physician or other qualified health care professional, maintenance of a registry, all in consultation with a psychiatric consultant. Services are provided both face-toface and non-face-to-face and psychiatric consultation is provided minimally on a weekly basis, typically non-face-to-face.

The behavioral health care manager providing other services in the same calendar month, such as psychiatric evaluation (90791, 90792), psychotherapy (90832, 90833, 90834, 90836, 90837, 90838), psychotherapy for crisis (90839, 90840), family psychotherapy (90846, 90847), multiple family group psychotherapy (90849), group psychotherapy (90853), smoking and tobacco use cessation counseling (99406, 99407), and alcohol and/or substance abuse structured screening and brief intervention services (99408, 99409), may report these services separately. Activities for services reported separately are not included in the time applied to 99492, 99493, 99494.

Psychiatric consultant refers to a medical professional, who is trained in psychiatry or behavioral health, and qualified to prescribe the full range of medications. The psychiatric consultant advises and makes recommendations, as needed, for psychiatric and other medical care, including psychiatric and other medical differential diagnosis, treatment strategies regarding appropriate therapies, medication management, medical management of complications associated with treatment of psychiatric disorders, and referral for specialty services, which are typically communicated to the treating physician or other qualified health care professional through the behavioral health care manager.

| | Separate Procedure | | Unlisted Procedure | | CCI Comp. Code | | Non-specific Procedure | **193** |

Type of Service	Total Duration of Collaborative Care Management Over Calendar Month	Code(s)
Initial - 70 minutes	Less than 36 minutes	Not reported separately
	36-85 minutes (36 minutes - 1 hr. 25 minutes)	99492
Initial plus each additional increment up to 30 minutes	86-116 minutes (1 hr. 26 minutes - 1 hr. 56 minutes)	99492 once AND 99494 once
Subsequent - 60 minutes	Less than 31 minutes	Not reported separately
	31-75 minutes (31 minutes - 1 hr. 15 minustes)	99493
Subsequent plus each additional increment up to 30 minutes	76-105 minutes (1 hr. 16 minutes - 1 hr. 45 minutes)	99493 once AND 99494 once

The psychiatric consultant typically does not see the patient or prescribe medications, except in rare circumstances. The psychiatric consultant may provide services in the calendar month described by other codes, such as evaluation and management (E/M) services and psychiatric evaluation (90791, 90792). These services may be reported separately by the psychiatric consultant. Activities for services reported separately are not included in the services reported using 99492, 99493, 99494.

Do not report 99492 and 99493 in the same calendar month.

99492 Initial psychiatric collaborative care management, first 70 minutes in the first calendar month of behavioral health care manager activities, in consultation with a psychiatric consultant, and directed by the treating physician or other qualified health care professional, with the following required elements:

- outreach to and engagement in treatment of a patient directed by the treating physician or other qualified health care professional;

- initial assessment of the patient, including administration of validated rating scales, with the development of an individualized treatment plan;

- review by the psychiatric consultant with modifications of the plan if recommended;

- entering patient in a registry and tracking patient follow-up and progress using the registry, with appropriate documentation, and participation in weekly caseload consultation with the psychiatric consultant; and

- provision of brief interventions using evidence-based techniques such as behavioral activation, motivational interviewing, and other focused treatment strategies.

99493 Subsequent psychiatric collaborative care management, first 60 minutes in a subsequent month of behavioral health care manager activities, in consultation with a psychiatric consultant, and directed by the treating physician or other qualified health care professional, with the following required elements:

- tracking patient follow-up and progress using the registry, with appropriate documentation;

- participation in weekly caseload consultation with the psychiatric consultant;

- ongoing collaboration with and coordination of the patient's mental health care with the treating physician or other qualified health care professional and any other treating mental health providers;

- additional review of progress and recommendations for changes in treatment, as indicated, including medications, based on recommendations provided by the psychiatric consultant;

- provision of brief interventions using evidence-based techniques such as behavioral activation, motivational interviewing, and other focused treatment strategies;

- monitoring of patient outcomes using validated rating scales; and

- relapse prevention planning with patients as they achieve remission of symptoms and/or other treatment goals and are prepared for discharge from active treatment.

+99494 Initial or subsequent psychiatric collaborative care management, each additional 30 minutes in a calendar month of behavioral health care manager activities, in consultation with a psychiatric consultant, and directed by the treating physician or other qualified health care professional (List separately in addition to code for primary procedure)

(Use 99494 in conjunction with 99492, 99493)

● New Code ▲ Revised Code + Add-On Code ⊘ Modifier -51 Exempt ★ Telemedicine

TRANSITIONAL CARE MANAGEMENT SERVICES

Codes 99495 and 99496 are used to report transitional care management services (TCM). These services are for a new or established patient whose medical and/or physchosocial problems require moderate or high complexity medical decision making during transitions in care from an inpatient hospital setting (including acute hospital, rehabilitation hospital, long-tem acute care hospital), partial hospital, observation status in a hospital, or skilled nursing facility/nursing facility, to the patient's community setting (home, domiciliary, rest home or assisted living). TCM commences upon the date of discharge and continues for the next 29 days.

TCM is comprised of one face-to-face visit within the specified time frames, in combination with non-face-to-face services that may be performed by the physician or other qualified health care professional and/or licensed clinical staff under his/her direction.

Non-face-to-face services provided by clinical staff, under the direction of the physician or other qualified health care professional, may include:

- communication (with patient, family members, guardian or caretaker, surrogate decision makers, and/or other professionals) regarding aspects of care;

- communication with home health agencies and other community services utilized by the patient;

- patient and/or family/caretaker education to support self-management, independent living, and activities of daily living;

- assessment and support for treatment regimen adherence and medication management;

- identification of available community and health resources;

- facilitating access to care and services needed by the patient and/or family.

Non-face-to-face services provided by the physician or other qualified health care professional may include:

- obtaining and reviewing the discharge information (eg, discharge summary, as available, or continuity of care documents);

- reviewing need for or follow-up on pending diagnostic tests and treatments;

- interaction with other qualified health care professionals who will assume or reassume care of the patient's system-specific problems;

- education of patient, family, guardian, and/or caregiver;

- establishment or reestablishment of referrals and arranging for needed community resources;

- assistance in scheduling any required follow-up with community providers and services.

TCM requires a face-to-face visit, initial patient contact, and medication reconciliation within specified time frames. The first face-to-face visit is part of the TCM service and not reported separately. Additional E/M services provided on subsequent dates after the first face-to-face visit may be reported separately. TCM requires an interactive contact with the patient or caregiver, as appropriate, within two business days of discharge. The contact may be direct (face-to-face), by telephone, or by electronic means. Medication reconciliation and management must occur no later than the date of the face-to-face visit.

These services address any needed coordination of care performed by multiple disciplines and community service agencies. The reporting individual provides or oversees the management and/or coordination of services, as needed, for all medical conditions, psychosocial needs, and activities of daily living support by providing first contact and continuous access.

Medical decision making and the date of the first face-to-face visit are used to select and report the appropriate TCM code. For 99496, the face-to-face visit must occur within 7 calendar days of the date of discharge, and medical decision making must be of high complexity. For 99495, the face-to-face visit must occur within 14 calendar days of the date of discharge, and medical decision making must be of at least moderate complexity.

Type of Medical Decision Making	Face-to-face visit within 7 days	Face-to-face visit within 8 to 14 days
Moderate complexity	99495	99495
High complexity	99496	99495

Medical decision making is defined by the E/M Services Guidelines. The medical decision making over the service period reported is used to define the medical decision making of TCM. Documentation includes the timing of the initial post-discharge communication with the patient or caregivers, date of the face-to-face visit, and the complexity of the medical decision making.

Only one individual may report these services and only once per patient within 30 days of discharge. Another TCM may not be reported by the same individual or group for any subsequent discharge(s) within the 30 days. The same individual may report hospital or observation discharge services and TCM. However, the discharge service may not constitute the required face-to-face visit. The same individual should not report TCM services provided in the postoperative period of a service that the individual reported.

A physician or other qualified health care professional who reports codes 99495, 99496 may not report care plan oversight services (99339, 99340, 99374-99380), prolonged services without direct patient contact (99358, 99359), home and outpatient INR monitoring (93792, 93793), medical team conferences (99366-99368), education and training (98960-98962, 99071, 99078), telephone services (98966-98968, 99441-99443), end stage renal disease services (90951-90970), preparation of special reports (99080), analysis of data (99091), complex chronic care coordination services (99487-99489), medication therapy management services (99605-99607), during the time period covered by the transitional care management services codes. When reporting 99495, 99496, do not report 99421, 99422, 99423 during the same time period.

★ **99495** Transitional care management services with the following required elements:

- Communication (direct contact, telephone, electronic) with the patient and/or caregiver within 2 business days of discharge
- Medical decision making of at least moderate complexity during the service period
- Face-to-face visit withing 14 calendar days of discharge

★ **99496** Transitional care management services with the following required elements:

- Communication (direct contact, telephone, electronic) with the patient and/or caregiver within 2 business days of discharge
- Medical decision making of high complexity during the service period
- Face-to-face visit within 7 calendar days of discharge

(Do not report 99495, 99496 in conjunction with 93792, 93793)

(Do not report 90951-90970, 98960-98962, 98966, 98967, 98968, 99071, 99078, 99080, 99091, 99339, 99340, 99358, 99359, 99366-99368, 99374-99380, 99441, 99442, 99443, 99487-99489, 99605-99607, when performed during the service time of code 99495 or 99496)

ADVANCE CARE PLANNING

Codes 99497, 99498 are used to report the face-to-face service between a physician or other qualified health care professional and a patient, family member, or surrogate in counseling and discussing advance directives, with or without completing relevant legal forms. An advance directive is a document appointing an agent and/or recording the wishes of a patient pertaining to his/her medical treatment at a future time should he/she lack decisional capacity at that time. Examples of written advanced directives include, but are not limited to, Health Care Proxy, Durable Power of Attorney for Health Care, Living Will, and Medical Orders for Life Sustaining Treatment (MOLST).

When using codes 99497, 99498, no active management of the problems is undertaken during the time period reported.

Codes 99497, 99498 may be reported separately if these services are performed on the same day as another Evaluation and Management service (99202-99215, 99217, 99218, 99219, 99220, 99221, 99222, 99223, 99224, 99225, 99226, 99231, 99232, 99233, 99234, 99235, 99236, 99238, 99239, 99241, 99242, 99243, 99244, 99245, 99251, 99252, 99253, 99254, 99255, 99281, 99282, 99283, 99284, 99285, 99304, 99305, 99306, 99307, 99308, 99309, 99310, 99315, 99316, 99318, 99324, 99325, 99326, 99327, 99328, 99334, 99335, 99336, 99337, 99341, 99342, 99343, 99344, 99345, 99347, 99348, 99349, 99350, 99381-99397, 99495, 99496).

99497 Advance care planning including the explanation and discussion of advance directives such a standard forms (with completion of such forms, when performed), by the physician or other qualified health care professional; first 30 minutes, face-to-face with the patient, family members, and/or surrogate.

+ **99498** each additional 30 minutes (List separately in addition to code for primary procedure)

(Use 99498 in conjunction with 99497)

(Do not report 99497 and 99498 on the same date of service as 99291, 99292, 99468, 99469, 99471, 99472, 99475, 99476, 99477, 99478, 99479, 99480, 99483.)

GENERAL BEHAVIORAL HEALTH INTEGRATION CARE MANAGEMENT

General behavioral health integration care management services (99484) are reported by the supervising physician or other qualified health care professional. The services are performed by clinical staff for a patient with a behavioral health (including substance use) condition that requires care management services (face-to-face or non-face-to-face) of 20 or more minutes in a calendar month. A treatment plan as well as the specified elements of the service description is required. The assessment and treatment plan is not required to be comprehensive and the office/practice is not required to have all the functions of chronic care management (99439, 99487, 99489, 99490). Code 99484 may be used in any outpatient setting, as long as the reporting professional has an ongoing relationship with the patient and clinical staff and as long as the clinical staff is available for face-to-face services with the patient.

The reporting professional must be able to perform the evaluation and management (E/M) services of an initiating visit. General behavioral integration care management (99484) and chronic care management services may be reported by the same professional in the same month, as long as distinct care management services are performed. Behavioral health integration care management (99484) and psychiatric collaborative care management (99492, 99493, 99494) may not be reported by the same professional in the same month. Behavioral health care integration clinical staff are not required to have qualifications that would permit them to separately report services (eg, psychotherapy), but, if qualified and they perform such services, they may report such services separately, as long as the time of the service is not used in reporting 99484.

99484   Care management services for behavioral health conditions, at least 20 minutes of clinical staff time, directed by a physician or other qualified health care professional, per calendar month, with the following required elements:

- initial assessment or follow-up monitoring, including the use of applicable validated rating scales;
- behavioral health care planning in relation to behavioral/psychiatric health problems, including revision for patients who are not progressing or whose status changes;
- facilitating and coordinating treatment such as psychotherapy, pharmacotherapy, counseling and/or psychiatric consultation; and
- continuity of care with a designated member of the care team.

(Do not report 99484 in conjunction with 99492, 99493, 99494 in the same calendar month)

(E/M services, including care management services [99439, 99487, 99489, 99490, 99495, 99496], and psychiatric services [90785-90899] may be reported separately by the same physician or other qualified health care professional on the same day or during the same calendar month, but time and activities used to meet criteria for another reported service do not count toward meeting criteria for 99484)

OTHER EVALUATION AND MANAGEMENT SERVICES

99499   Unlisted evaluation and management service

Separate Procedure   Unlisted Procedure   CCI Comp. Code   Non-specific Procedure   **197**

This page intentionally left blank.

ANESTHESIA OVERVIEW

Services involving administration of anesthesia are reported by the use of the anesthesia five-digit procedure code (00100-01999) plus modifier codes (defined under "Anesthesia Modifiers" later in these Guidelines).

The reporting of anesthesia services is appropriate by or under the responsible supervision of a physician. These services may include but are not limited to general, regional, supplementation of local anesthesia, or other supportive services in order to afford the patient the anesthesia care deemed optimal by the anesthesiologist during any procedure. These services include the usual preoperative and postoperative visits, the anesthesia care during the procedure, the administration of fluids and/or blood and the usual monitoring services (eg, ECG, temperature, blood pressure, oximetry, capnography, and mass spectrometry). Unusual forms of monitoring (eg, intra-arterial, central venous, and Swan-Ganz) are not included.

Items used by all physicians in reporting their services are presented in the Introduction. Some of the commonalities are repeated in this section for the convenience of those physicians referring to this section on Anesthesia. Other definitions and items unique to anesthesia are also listed.

To report moderate (conscious) sedation provided by a physician also performing the service for which conscious sedation is being provided, see codes 99151, 99152, 99153.

When a second physician other than the health care professional performing the diagnostic or therapeutic services provides moderate (conscious) sedation in the facility setting (eg, hospital, outpatient hospital/ambulatory surgery center, skilled nursing facility), the second physician reports the associated moderate sedation procedure/service 99155, 99156, 99157; when these services are performed by the second physician in the nonfacility setting (eg, physician office, freestanding imaging center), codes 99155, 99156, 99157 would not be reported. Moderate sedation does not include minimal sedation (anxiolysis), deep sedation, or monitored anesthesia care (00100-01999).

To report regional or general anesthesia provided by a physician also performing the services for which the anesthesia is being provided, see modifier 47 in Appendix A.

KEY POINTS ABOUT ANESTHESIA CODING

1. *Time recording for anesthesia services starts with patient preparation for anesthesia induction and ends when the anesthesiologist or anesthetist has completed his/her services and transfers responsibility for postoperative supervision.*

2. *Consultations and/or other evaluation and management services which are not included in the administration or supervising the administration of anesthesia, regardless of location provided, are reporting using CPT codes from the evaluation and management section of the CPT book.*

3. *Any supplies and/or materials provided by the anesthesiologist or anesthetist which are not considered to be included in the standard service may be coded separately.*

4. *Multiple procedures provided on the same date of service should be coded separately.*

5. *Any service which may be considered rare, unusual, variable or not defined should be supported with a special report which clearly defines the need for the unusual service. These services are generally coded with an unlisted CPT code or by adding modifier -22 to the CPT code which defines the procedure.*

TIME REPORTING

Time for anesthesia services and procedures should be reported based on customs in the local area of practice. Anesthesia time begins when the anesthesiologist or anesthetist begins to prepare the patient for the induction of anesthesia in the operating room (or equivalent area) and ends when the anesthesiologist is no longer in personal attendance of the patient, i.e. when the patient is placed under postoperative supervision and care.

ANESTHESIA SERVICES

Non-anesthesia services rendered in the office, home, or hospital; consultation; and other medical services are listed in the Evaluation and Management Services section (99202- 99499 series). "Special Services, Procedures, and Reports" (99000-99082 series) are listed in the Medicine section.

SUPPLIES AND MATERIALS

Supplies and materials provided (eg, sterile trays, drugs) over and above those usually included with the office visit or anesthesia services rendered may be listed separately. Drugs, tray supplies, and materials provided should be listed and identified with 99070 or the appropriate supply code. For Medicare claims, HCPCS Level II codes should be used to report supplies and materials.

SEPARATE OR MULTIPLE PROCEDURES

When multiple surgical procedures are performed during a single anesthetic administration, the anesthesia code representing the most complex procedure is reported. The anesthesia time reported is the combined total for all surgical procedures.

UNLISTED SERVICE OR PROCEDURE

An anesthesia service or procedure may be provided that is not listed in the CPT codebook. When reporting such service(s), the appropriate "Unlisted Procedure" code should be used to indicate the service, identifying it by "Special Report" as discussed below. The "Unlisted Procedures" and accompanying code for Anesthesia is as follows:

01999   Unlisted anesthesia procedure(s)

SPECIAL REPORT

A service that is rarely provided, unusual, variable, or new may require a special report. Pertinent information should include an adequate definition or description of the nature, extent, and need for the procedure and the time, effort, and equipment necessary to provide the service.

ANESTHESIA SERVICE MODIFIERS

All anesthesia services are reported by use of the anesthesia five-digit procedure code (00100-01999) plus the addition of a physical status modifier. The use of other optional modifiers may be appropriate.

PHYSICAL STATUS MODIFIERS

-P1   A normal healthy patient.

-P2   A patient with a mild systemic disease.

-P3   A patient with severe systemic disease.

-P4   A patient with severe systemic disease that is a constant threat to life.

-P5   A moribund patient who is not expected to survive without the operation.

-P6   A declared brain-dead patient whose organs are being removed for donor purposes.

These six levels are consistent with the American Society of Anesthesiologists (ASA) ranking of patient physical status. Physical status is included in the CPT codebook to distinguish among various levels of complexity of the anesthesia service provided. Example: 00100-P1

OTHER ANESTHESIA SERVICE MODIFIERS

Under certain circumstances, medical services and procedures may need to be further modified. Other CPT coding system modifiers commonly used with ANESTHESIA services include:

-22   Unusual services

-23   Anesthesia

-32   Mandated services

-51   Multiple procedures

QUALIFYING CIRCUMSTANCES FOR ANESTHESIA

More than one qualifying circumstance may be selected. Many anesthesia services are provided under particularly difficult circumstances, depending on factors such as extraordinary condition of patient, notable operative conditions, and/or unusual risk factors. This section includes a list of important qualifying circumstances that significantly affect the character of the anesthesia service provided. These procedures would not be reported alone but would be reported as additional procedure numbers qualifying an anesthesia procedure or service.

In the case of difficult and/or extraordinary circumstances such as extreme youth or age, extraordinary condition of the patient, and/or unusual risk factors it may be appropriate to report one or more of the following qualifying circumstances in addition to the anesthesia services.

+ 99100   Anesthesia for patient of extreme age, younger than 1 year and older than 70 (List separately in addition to code for primary anesthesia procedure)

(For procedure performed on infants younger than 1 year of age at time of surgery, see 00326, 00561, 00834, 00836)

+ 99116   Anesthesia complicated by utilization of total body hypothermia (List separately in addition to code for primary anesthesia procedure)

+ 99135   Anesthesia complicated by utilization of controlled hypotension (List separately in addition to code for primary anesthesia procedure)

+ 99140   Anesthesia complicated by emergency conditions (specify) (List separately in addition to code for primary anesthesia procedure)

(An emergency is defined as existing when delay in treatment of the patient would lead to a significant increase in the threat to life or body part)

| | Separate Procedure | | Unlisted Procedure | | CCI Comp. Code | | Non-specific Procedure | **201** |

This page intentionally left blank.

● New Code ▲ Revised Code ➕ Add-On Code ⊘ Modifier -51 Exempt ★ Telemedicine

ANESTHESIA CODES

HEAD

00100 Anesthesia for procedures on salivary glands, including biopsy

00102 Anesthesia for procedures on plastic repair of cleft lip

00103 Anesthesia for reconstructive procedures of eyelid (eg, blepharoplasty, ptosis surgery)

00104 Anesthesia for electroconvulsive therapy

00120 Anesthesia for procedures on external, middle, and inner ear including biopsy; not otherwise specified

00124   otoscopy

00126   tympanotomy

00140 Anesthesia for procedures on eye; not otherwise specified

00142   lens surgery

00144   corneal transplant

00145   vitreoretinal surgery

00147   iridectomy

00148   ophthalmoscopy

00160 Anesthesia for procedures on nose and accessory sinuses; not otherwise specified

00162   radical surgery

00164   biopsy, soft tissue

00170 Anesthesia for intraoral procedures, including biopsy; not otherwise specified

00172   repair of cleft palate

00174   excision of retropharyngeal tumor

00176   radical surgery

00190 Anesthesia for procedures on facial bones or skull; not otherwise specified

00192   radical surgery (including prognathism)

00210 Anesthesia for intracranial procedures; not otherwise specified

00211   craniotomy or craniectomy for evacuation of hematoma

00212   subdural taps

00214   burr holes, including ventriculography

00215   cranioplasty or elevation of depressed skull fracture, extradural (simple or compound)

| Separate Procedure | Unlisted Procedure | CCI Comp. Code | Non-specific Procedure | **203** |

00216	vascular procedures
00218	procedures in sitting position
00220	cerebrospinal fluid shunting procedures
00222	electrocoagulation of intracranial nerve

NECK

00300	Anesthesia for all procedures on the integumentary system, muscles and nerves of head, neck, and posterior trunk, not otherwise specified
00320	Anesthesia for all procedures on esophagus, thyroid, larynx, trachea and lymphatic system of neck; not otherwise specified, age 1 year or older
00322	needle biopsy of thyroid

(For procedures on cervical spine and cord, see 00600, 00604, 00670)

| 00326 | Anesthesia for all procedures on the larynx and trachea in children less than 1 year of age |

(Do not report 00326 in conjunction with code 99100)

| 00350 | Anesthesia for procedures on major vessels of neck; not otherwise specified |
| 00352 | simple ligation |

(For arteriography, use 01916)

THORAX (CHEST WALL AND SHOULDER GIRDLE)

00400	Anesthesia for procedures on the integumentary system on the extremities, anterior trunk and perineum; not otherwise specified
00402	reconstructive procedures on breast (eg, reduction or augmentation mammoplasty, muscle flaps)
00404	radical or modified radical procedures on breast
00406	radical or modified radical procedures on breast with internal mammary node dissection
00410	electrical conversion of arrhythmias
00450	Anesthesia for procedures on clavicle and scapula; not otherwise specified
00454	biopsy of clavicle
00470	Anesthesia for partial rib resection; not otherwise specified
00472	thoracoplasty (any type)
00474	radical procedures (eg, pectus excavatum)

INTRATHORACIC

| 00500 | Anesthesia for all procedures on esophagus |
| 00520 | Anesthesia for closed chest procedures; (including bronchoscopy) not otherwise specified |

● New Code ▲ Revised Code + Add-On Code ⊘ Modifier -51 Exempt ★ Telemedicine

00522   needle biopsy of pleura

00524   pneumocentesis

00528   mediastinoscopy and diagnostic thoracoscopy not utilizing 1 lung ventilation

(For tracheobronchial reconstruction, use 00539)

00529   mediastinoscopy and diagnostic thoracoscopy utilizing 1 lung ventilation

00530   Anesthesia for permanent transvenous pacemaker insertion

00532   Anesthesia for access to central venous circulation

00534   Anesthesia for transvenous insertion or replacement of pacing cardioverter/defibrillator

(For transthoracic approach, use 00560)

00537   Anesthesia for cardiac electrophysiologic procedures including radiofrequency ablation

00539   Anesthesia for tracheobronchial reconstruction

00540   Anesthesia for thoracotomy procedures involving lungs, pleura, diaphragm, and mediastinum (including surgical thoracoscopy); not otherwise specified

00541   utilizing 1 lung ventilation

(For thoracic spine and cord anesthesia procedures via an anterior transthoracic approach, see 00625-00626)

00542   decortication

00546   pulmonary resection with thoracoplasty

00548   intrathoracic procedures on the trachea and bronchi

00550   Anesthesia for sternal debridement

00560   Anesthesia for procedures on heart, pericardial sac, and great vessels of chest; without pump oxygenator

00561   with pump oxygenator, younger than one year of age

(Do not report 00561 in conjunction with 99100, 99116, and 99135)

00562   with pump oxygenator, age 1 year or older, for all non-coronary bypass procedures (eg. valve procedures) or for re-operation for coronary bypass more than 1 month after original operation)

00563   with pump oxygenator with hypothermic circulatory arrest

00566   Anesthesia for direct coronary artery bypass grafting; without pump oxygenator

00567   with pump oxygenator

00580   Anesthesia for heart transplant or heart/lung transplant

SPINE AND SPINAL CORD

00600   Anesthesia for procedures on cervical spine and cord; not otherwise specified

(For percutaneous image-guided spine and spinal cord anesthesia procedures, see 01935, 01936)

Separate Procedure   Unlisted Procedure   CCI Comp. Code   Non-specific Procedure   **205**

00604	procedures with patient in the sitting position
00620	Anesthesia for procedures on thoracic spine and cord; not otherwise specified
00625	Anesthesia for procedures on the thoracic spine and cord, via an anterior transthoracic approach; not utilizing 1 lung ventilation
00626	utilizing 1 lung ventilation

(For anesthesia for thoractomy procedures other than spinal, see 00540-00541)

00630	Anesthesia for procedures in lumbar region; not otherwise specified
00632	lumbar sympathectomy
00635	diagnostic or therapeutic lumbar puncture
00640	Anesthesia for manipulation of the spine or for closed procedures on the cervical, thoracic or lumbar spine
00670	Anesthesia for extensive spine and spinal cord procedures (eg, spinal instrumentation or vascular procedures)

UPPER ABDOMEN

00700	Anesthesia for procedures on upper anterior abdominal wall; not otherwise specified
00702	percutaneous liver biopsy
00730	Anesthesia for procedures on upper posterior abdominal wall
00731	Anesthesia for upper gastrointestinal endoscopic procedures, endoscope introduced proximal to duodenum; not otherwise specified
00732	endoscopic retrograde cholangiopancreatography (ERCP)

(For combined upper and lower gastrointestinal endoscopic procedures, use 00813)

(00740	deleted 2017 [2018 edition]. To report, see 00731, 00732.)
00750	Anesthesia for hernia repairs in upper abdomen; not otherwise specified
00752	lumbar and ventral (incisional) hernias and/or wound dehiscence
00754	omphalocele
00756	transabdominal repair of diaphragmatic hernia
00770	Anesthesia for all procedures on major abdominal blood vessels
00790	Anesthesia for intraperitoneal procedures in upper abdomen including laparoscopy; not otherwise specified
00792	partial hepatectomy or management of liver hemorrhage (excluding liver biopsy)
00794	pancreatectomy, partial or total (eg, Whipple procedure)
00796	liver transplant (recipient)

(For harvesting of liver, use 01990)

| 00797 | gastric restrictive procedure for morbid obesity |

● New Code ▲ Revised Code + Add-On Code ⊘ Modifier -51 Exempt ★ Telemedicine

LOWER ABDOMEN

00800   Anesthesia for procedures on lower anterior abdominal wall; not otherwise specified

00802   panniculectomy

(**00810**   deleted 2017 [2018 edition]. To report, see 00811, 00812, 00813.)

00811   Anesthesia for lower intestinal endoscopic procedures, endoscope introduced distal to duodenum; not otherwise specified

00812   screening colonoscopy

(Report 00812 to describe anesthesia for any screening colonoscopy regardless of ultimate findings)

00813   Anesthesia for combined upper and lower gastrointestinal endoscopic procedures, endoscope introduced both proximal to and distal to the duodenum

00820   Anesthesia for procedures on lower posterior abdominal wall

00830   Anesthesia for hernia repairs in lower abdomen; not otherwise specified

00832   ventral and incisional hernias

(For hernia repairs in the infant 1 year of age or younger, see 00834, 00836)

00834   Anesthesia for hernia repairs in the lower abdomen not otherwise specified, under 1 year of age

(Do not report 00834 in conjunction with code 99100)

00836   Anesthesia for hernia repairs in the lower abdomen not otherwise specified, infants less than 37 weeks gestational age at birth and less than 50 weeks gestational age at time of surgery

(Do not report 00836 in conjunction with code 99100)

00840   Anesthesia for intraperitoneal procedures in lower abdomen including laparoscopy; not otherwise specified

00842   amniocentesis

00844   abdominoperineal resection

00846   radical hysterectomy

00848   pelvic exenteration

00851   tubal ligation/transection

00860   Anesthesia for extraperitoneal procedures in lower abdomen, including urinary tract; not otherwise specified

00862   renal procedures, including upper 1/3 of ureter, or donor nephrectomy

00864   total cystectomy

00865   radical prostatectomy (suprapubic, retropubic)

00866   adrenalectomy

00868   renal transplant (recipient)

(For donor nephrectomy, use 00862)

Separate Procedure   Unlisted Procedure   CCI Comp. Code   Non-specific Procedure   **207**

(For harvesting kidney from brain-dead patient, use 01990)

00870	cystolithotomy
00872	Anesthesia for lithotripsy, extracorporeal shock wave; with water bath
00873	without water bath
00880	Anesthesia for procedures on major lower abdominal vessels; not otherwise specified
00882	inferior vena cava ligation

PERINEUM

(For perineal procedures on the integumentary system, muscles and nerves, see 00300, 00400)

00902	Anesthesia for; anorectal procedure
00904	radical perineal procedure
00906	vulvectomy
00908	perineal prostatectomy
00910	Anesthesia for transurethral procedures (including urethrocystoscopy); not otherwise specified
00912	transurethral resection of bladder tumor(s)
00914	transurethral resection of prostate
00916	post-transurethral resection bleeding
00918	with fragmentation, manipulation and/or removal of ureteral calculus
00920	Anesthesia for procedures on male genitalia (including open urethral procedures); not otherwise specified
00921	vasectomy, unilateral or bilateral
00922	seminal vesicles
00924	undescended testis, unilateral or bilateral
00926	radical orchiectomy, inguinal
00928	radical orchiectomy, abdominal
00930	orchiopexy, unilateral or bilateral
00932	complete amputation of penis
00934	radical amputation of penis with bilateral inguinal lymphadenectomy
00936	radical amputation of penis with bilateral inguinal and iliac lymphadenectomy
00938	insertion of penile prosthesis (perineal approach)
00940	Anesthesia for vaginal procedures (including biopsy of labia, vagina, cervix or endometrium); not otherwise specified

---

● New Code ▲ Revised Code + Add-On Code ⊘ Modifier -51 Exempt ★ Telemedicine

00942   colpotomy, vaginectomy, colporrhaphy and open urethral procedures

00944   vaginal hysterectomy

00948   cervical cerclage

00950   culdoscopy

00952   hysteroscopy and/or hysterosalpingography

PELVIS (EXCEPT HIP)

01112   Anesthesia for bone marrow aspiration and/or biopsy, anterior or posterior iliac crest

01120   Anesthesia for procedures on bony pelvis

01130   Anesthesia for body cast application or revision

01140   Anesthesia for interpelviabdominal (hindquarter) amputation

01150   Anesthesia for radical procedures for tumor of pelvis, except hindquarter amputation

01160   Anesthesia for closed procedures involving symphysis pubis or sacroiliac joint

01170   Anesthesia for open procedures involving symphysis pubis or sacroiliac joint

01173   Anesthesia for open repair of fracture disruption of pelvis or column fracture involving acetabulum

(**01180**   deleted 2017 [2018 edition])

(**01190**   deleted 2017 [2018 edition])

UPPER LEG (EXCEPT KNEE)

01200   Anesthesia for all closed procedures involving hip joint

01202   Anesthesia for arthroscopic procedures of hip joint

01210   Anesthesia for open procedures involving hip joint; not otherwise specified

01212   hip disarticulation

01214   total hip arthroplasty

01215   revision of total hip arthroplasty

01220   Anesthesia for all closed procedures involving upper 2/3 of femur

01230   Anesthesia for open procedures involving upper 2/3 of femur; not otherwise specified

01232   amputation

01234   radical resection

01250   Anesthesia for all procedures on nerves, muscles, tendons, fascia, and bursae of upper leg

01260   Anesthesia for all procedures involving veins of upper leg, including exploration

01270	Anesthesia for procedures involving arteries of upper leg, including bypass graft; not otherwise specified
01272	femoral artery ligation
01274	femoral artery embolectomy

KNEE AND POPLITEAL AREA

01320	Anesthesia for all procedures on nerves, muscles, tendons, fascia, and bursae of knee and/or popliteal area
01340	Anesthesia for all closed procedures on lower 1/3 of femur
01360	Anesthesia for all open procedures on lower 1/3 of femur
01380	Anesthesia for all closed procedures on knee joint
01382	Anesthesia for diagnostic arthroscopic procedures of knee joint
01390	Anesthesia for all closed procedures on upper ends of tibia, fibula, and/or patella
01392	Anesthesia for all open procedures on upper ends of tibia, fibula, and/or patella
01400	Anesthesia for open or surgical arthroscopic procedures on knee joint; not otherwise specified
01402	total knee arthroplasty
01404	disarticulation at knee
01420	Anesthesia for all cast applications, removal, or repair involving knee joint
01430	Anesthesia for procedures on veins of knee and popliteal area; not otherwise specified
01432	arteriovenous fistula
01440	Anesthesia for procedures on arteries of knee and popliteal area; not otherwise specified
01442	popliteal thromboendarterectomy, with or without patch graft
01444	popliteal excision and graft or repair for occlusion or aneurysm

LOWER LEG (BELOW KNEE, INCLUDES ANKLE AND FOOT)

01462	Anesthesia for all closed procedures on lower leg, ankle, and foot
01464	Anesthesia for arthroscopic procedures of ankle and/or foot
01470	Anesthesia for procedures on nerves, muscles, tendons, and fascia of lower leg, ankle, and foot; not otherwise specified
01472	repair of ruptured Achilles tendon, with or without graft
01474	gastrocnemius recession (eg, Strayer procedure)
01480	Anesthesia for open procedures on bones of lower leg, ankle, and foot; not otherwise specified
01482	radical resection (including below knee amputation)
01484	osteotomy or osteoplasty of tibia and/or fibula

● New Code ▲ Revised Code ✛ Add-On Code ⊘ Modifier -51 Exempt ★ Telemedicine

01486   total ankle replacement

01490   Anesthesia for lower leg cast application, removal, or repair

01500   Anesthesia for procedures on arteries of lower leg, including bypass graft; not otherwise specified

01502   embolectomy, direct or with catheter

01520   Anesthesia for procedures on veins of lower leg; not otherwise specified

01522   venous thrombectomy, direct or with catheter

SHOULDER AND AXILLA

Includes humeral head and neck, sternoclavicular joint, acromioclavicular joint, and shoulder joint

01610   Anesthesia for all procedures on nerves, muscles, tendons, fascia, and bursae of shoulder and axilla

01620   Anesthesia for all closed procedures on humeral head and neck, sternoclavicular joint, acromioclavicular joint, and shoulder joint

01622   Anesthesia for diagnostic arthroscopic procedures of shoulder joint

01630   Anesthesia for open or surgical arthroscopic procedures on humeral head and neck, sternoclavicular joint, acromioclavicular joint, and shoulder joint; not otherwise specified

01634   shoulder disarticulation

01636   interthoracoscapular (forequarter) amputation

01638   total shoulder replacement

01650   Anesthesia for procedures on arteries of shoulder and axilla; not otherwise specified

01652   axillary-brachial aneurysm

01654   bypass graft

01656   axillary-femoral bypass graft

01670   Anesthesia for all procedures on veins of shoulder and axilla

01680   Anesthesia for shoulder cast application, removal or repair; not otherwise specified

(01682   deleted 2017 [2018 edition])

UPPER ARM AND ELBOW

01710   Anesthesia for procedures on nerves, muscles, tendons, fascia, and bursae of upper arm and elbow; not otherwise specified

01712   tenotomy, elbow to shoulder, open

01714   tenoplasty, elbow to shoulder

01716   tenodesis; rupture of long tendon of biceps

01730   Anesthesia for all closed procedures on humerus and elbow

---

Separate Procedure   Unlisted Procedure   CCI Comp. Code   Non-specific Procedure   **211**

01732   Anesthesia for diagnostic arthroscopic procedures of elbow joint

01740   Anesthesia for open or surgical arthroscopic procedures of the elbow; not otherwise specified

01742   osteotomy of humerus

01744   repair of nonunion or malunion of humerus

01756   radical procedures

01758   excision of cyst or tumor of humerus

01760   total elbow replacement

01770   Anesthesia for procedures on arteries of upper arm and elbow; not otherwise specified

01772   embolectomy

01780   Anesthesia for procedures on veins of upper arm and elbow; not otherwise specified

01782   phleborrhaphy

FOREARM, WRIST, AND HAND

01810   Anesthesia for all procedures on nerves, muscles, tendons, fascia, and bursae of forearm, wrist, and hand

01820   Anesthesia for all closed procedures on radius, ulna, wrist, or hand bones

01829   Anesthesia for diagnostic arthroscopic procedures on the wrist

01830   Anesthesia for open or surgical arthroscopic/endoscopic procedures on distal radius, distal ulna, wrist, or hand joints; not otherwise specified

01832   total wrist replacement

01840   Anesthesia for procedures on arteries of forearm, wrist, and hand; not otherwise specified

01842   embolectomy

01844   Anesthesia for vascular shunt, or shunt revision, any type (eg, dialysis)

01850   Anesthesia for procedures on veins of forearm, wrist, and hand; not otherwise specified

01852   phleborrhaphy

01860   Anesthesia for forearm, wrist, or hand cast application, removal, or repair

RADIOLOGICAL PROCEDURES

01916   Anesthesia for diagnostic arteriography/venography

(Do not report 01916 in conjunction with therapeutic codes 01924-01926, 01930-01933)

01920   Anesthesia for cardiac catheterization including coronary angiography and ventriculography (not to include Swan-Ganz catheter)

01922   Anesthesia for non-invasive imaging or radiation therapy

---

   ● New Code   ▲ Revised Code   + Add-On Code   ⊘ Modifier -51 Exempt   ★ Telemedicine

01924 Anesthesia for therapeutic interventional radiologic procedures involving the arterial system; not otherwise specified

01925 carotid or coronary

01926 intracranial, intracardiac, or aortic

01930 Anesthesia for therapeutic interventional radiologic procedures involving the venous/lymphatic system (not to include access to the central circulation); not otherwise specified

01931 intrahepatic or portal circulation (eg, transvenous intrahepatic portosystemic shunt(s) (TIPS))

01932 intrathoracic or jugular

01933 intracranial

01935 Anesthesia for percutaneous image guided procedures on the spine and spinal cord; diagnostic

01936 therapeutic

BURN EXCISIONS OR DEBRIDEMENT

01951 Anesthesia for second and third degree burn excision or debridement with or without skin grafting, any site, for total body surface area (TBSA) treated during anesthesia and surgery; less than four percent total body surface area

01952 between four and nine percent of total body surface area

+ **01953** each additional nine percent total body surface area or part thereof (List separately in addition to code for primary procedure)

(Use 01953 in conjunction with code 01952)

OBSTETRIC

01958 Anesthesia for external cephalic version procedure

01960 Anesthesia for vaginal delivery only

01961 Anesthesia for cesarean delivery only

01962 Anesthesia for urgent hysterectomy following delivery

01963 Anesthesia for cesarean hysterectomy without any labor analgesia/anesthesia care

01965 Anesthesia for incomplete or missed abortion procedures

01966 Anesthesia for induced abortion procedures

01967 Neuraxial labor analgesia/anesthesia for planned vaginal delivery (this includes any repeat subarachnoid needle placement and drug injection and/or any necessary replacement of an epidural catheter during labor)

+ **01968** Anesthesia for cesarean delivery following neuraxial labor analgesia/anesthesia (List separately in addition to code for primary procedure performed)

(Use 01968 in conjunction with code 01967)

+ **01969** Anesthesia for cesarean hysterectomy following neuraxial labor analgesia/anesthesia (List separately in addition to code for primary procedure performed)

| Separate Procedure | Unlisted Procedure | CCI Comp. Code | Non-specific Procedure | **213** |

(Use 01969 in conjunction with code 01967)

OTHER PROCEDURES

01990   Physiological support for harvesting of organ(s) from brain-dead patient

01991   Anesthesia for diagnostic or therapeutic nerve blocks and injections (when block or injection is performed by a different physician or other qualified health care professional); other than the prone position

01992   prone position

(Do not report code 01991 or 01992 in conjunction with 99151, 99152, 99153, 99155, 99156, 99157)

(When regional intravenous administration of local anesthetic agent or other medication in the upper or lower extremity is used as the anesthetic for a surgical procedure, report the appropriate anesthesia code. To report a Bier block for pain management, use 64999.)

(For intra-arterial or intravenous therapy for pain management, see 96373, 96374.)

01996   Daily hospital management of epidural or subarachnoid continuous drug administration

(Report code 01996 for daily hospital management of continuous epidural or subarachnoid drug administration performed after insertion of an epidural or subarachnoid catheter placed primarily for anesthesia administration during an operative session, but retained for post-operative pain management)

01999   Unlisted anesthesia procedure(s)

● New Code   ▲ Revised Code   ＋ Add-On Code   ⊘ Modifier -51 Exempt   ★ Telemedicine

SURGERY SECTION OVERVIEW

The third section of the CPT coding system is the surgery section, and it includes surgical procedure codes for all body areas. Within each subsection, the CPT codes are arranged by anatomical site.

It is essential to understand the organization of the CPT surgery section in order to locate the correct procedure code. Understanding other or alternative terms which may apply to a procedure, injury, illness or condition may also make the location of the appropriate procedure easier and faster.

All procedures listed in the surgery section of the CPT book include local, metacarpal/digital block or topical anesthesia if used, the surgical procedure, and normal uncomplicated follow-up care. For diagnostic surgical procedures, follow-up care includes only the care related to recovery from the diagnostic procedure. For therapeutic surgical procedures, follow-up care includes only the care which would usually be included in the surgical service. Any complications resulting in additional services are not considered to be included and should be coded separately.

KEY POINTS ABOUT SURGERY SERVICES

- Evaluation and management services provided by surgeons in the office, home or hospital, plus consultations and other medical services are coded using evaluation and management service codes.

- Any supplies and/or materials provided by the surgeon which are not considered to be included in the standard service may be coded separately.

GLOBAL SURGICAL PACKAGE

Third-party payers differ in their definition of a surgical or global surgical package concept. Medicare defines the global surgical package as follows:

- The surgeon's initial evaluation or consultation will be paid separately.

- There is a one day preoperative period covered under the global surgical package.

- Included in the package are all intraoperative services that are considered to be usual and necessary. Separate billing of these services would be considered unbundling.

- Any treatment of complications by the surgeon not requiring a return to the operating room is included in the package.

- The surgical package contains a standard 90-day postoperative period which includes all visits to the physician during that time unless the visit is for a totally different reason than that for the surgery.

- In cases of organ transplant, immunosuppressive therapy is not included in the global package.

- Minor surgical procedures are those with a 0 or 10-day postoperative period, and are excluded from the surgical package definition.

SPECIAL REPORT

Surgical procedures which are rarely provided, unusual or vary significantly from the standard definition may require a special report. When preparing reports to accompany health insurance claim forms the provider should include a description of the nature, extent, and need for the procedure, and the time, effort, and equipment necessary to provides the service. Try to keep these reports as brief and simple as possible. Additional items which may be needed are:

- complexity of symptoms
- final diagnosis
- pertinent physical findings
- diagnostic and therapeutic procedures
- concurrent problems
- follow-up care

MULTIPLE SURGICAL PROCEDURES

It is common for several surgical procedures to be performed at the same operative session. When multiple procedures are performed on the same day or at the same session, the "major" procedure or service is listed first followed by secondary, additional, or "lessor" procedures or services. CPT modifier -51 is added to all procedures following the first one.

Reporting multiple procedures incorrectly may have a serious impact on reimbursement from health insurance payers. An inexperienced health insurance biller may simply list the procedures on the health insurance claim form in the order dictated or described in the operative report.

There are two critical decisions related to reporting multiple surgical procedures correctly; namely: 1) The order in which the procedures are listed on the health insurance claim form, and 2) whether or not to list the additional procedures with full or reduced fees.

ORDER OF LISTING MULTIPLE PROCEDURES

The first procedure to be listed when reporting services under the multiple procedure rule is the procedure with the highest fee. Additional procedures should be listed in descending order by fee. Modifier -51 should be added to each additional procedure.

All third party payers will reduce the allowance for the additional procedures, typically by 50 percent for the second procedure, and 50 to 75 percent for the third and subsequent procedures. Listing the procedures in descending order by fee minimizes the possibility of an incorrect reduction.

BILLING FULL VERSUS REDUCED FEES

The full fee should be listed for each procedure coded on the health insurance claim form as part of multiple surgical procedures. Third party payers will automatically reduce the allowances for the additional procedures by a specific formula. Listing all multiple procedures with full fees in descending fee order (the procedure with the highest fee first, the procedure with the next highest fee second, et cetera) will result in the maximum total allowable reimbursement for the provider or the insured.

After the maximum benefit has been paid by the health insurance company, the balance remaining, less any patient co-insurance or deductible requirements, should be written off. Note that billing practices vary in different areas of the country. Providers should continue to use the method that is customary or required by third party payers in the provider's practice location.

SEPARATE PROCEDURE

Some surgical procedures are considered to be an integral part of a more extensive surgical procedure. In this circumstance, the integral procedure is not coded. When the integral procedure is performed independently and is unrelated to other services, it should be listed as a "separate procedure."

SUPPLIES AND MATERIALS

Supplies and materials provided (eg, sterile trays, drugs) over and above those usually included with the office visit or anesthesia services rendered may be listed separately. Drugs, tray supplies, and materials provided should be listed and identified with 99070 or the appropriate supply code. For Medicare claims, HCPCS Level II codes should be used to report supplies and materials.

UNLISTED SERVICE OR PROCEDURE

A surgical service or procedure may be provided that is not listed in the current edition of the CPT codebook. When reporting such a service, the appropriate "Unlisted Procedure" code may be used to indicate the service, identifying it by "Special Report" as discussed below. The following list of "Unlisted Procedures" may be reported for Surgery Services:

15999	Unlisted procedure, excision pressure ulcer
17999	Unlisted procedure, skin, mucous membrane and subcutaneous tissue
19499	Unlisted procedure, breast
20999	Unlisted procedure, musculoskeletal system, general
21089	Unlisted maxillofacial prosthetic procedure
21299	Unlisted craniofacial and maxillofacial procedure
21499	Unlisted musculoskeletal procedure, head
21899	Unlisted procedure, neck or thorax
22899	Unlisted procedure, spine

22999	Unlisted procedure, abdomen, musculoskeletal system
23929	Unlisted procedure, shoulder
24999	Unlisted procedure, humerus or elbow
25999	Unlisted procedure, forearm or wrist
26989	Unlisted procedure, hands or fingers
27299	Unlisted procedure, pelvis or hip joint
27599	Unlisted procedure, femur or knee
27899	Unlisted procedure, leg or ankle
28899	Unlisted procedure, foot or toes
29799	Unlisted procedure, casting or strapping
29999	Unlisted procedure, arthroscopy
30999	Unlisted procedure, nose
31299	Unlisted procedure, accessory sinuses
31599	Unlisted procedure, larynx
31899	Unlisted procedure, trachea, bronchi
32999	Unlisted procedure, lungs and pleura
33999	Unlisted procedure, cardiac surgery
36299	Unlisted procedure, vascular injection
37501	Unlisted vascular endoscopy procedure
37799	Unlisted procedure, vascular surgery
38129	Unlisted laparoscopy procedure, spleen
38589	Unlisted laparoscopy procedure, lymphatic system
38999	Unlisted procedure, hemic or lymphatic system
39499	Unlisted procedure, mediastinum
39599	Unlisted procedure, diaphragm
40799	Unlisted procedure, lips
40899	Unlisted procedure, vestibule of mouth
41599	Unlisted procedure, tongue, floor of mouth
41899	Unlisted procedure, dentoalveolar structures
42299	Unlisted procedure, palate, uvula
42699	Unlisted procedure, salivary glands or ducts
42999	Unlisted procedure, pharynx, adenoids, or tonsils
43289	Unlisted laparoscopy procedure, esophagus
43499	Unlisted procedure, esophagus
43659	Unlisted laparoscopy procedure, stomach
43999	Unlisted procedure, stomach
44238	Unlisted laparoscopy procedure, intestine (except rectum)
44799	Unlisted procedure, small intestine
44899	Unlisted procedure, Meckel's diverticulum and the mesentery
44979	Unlisted laparoscopy procedure, appendix
45399	Unlisted procedure, colon
45499	Unlisted laparoscopy procedure, rectum
45999	Unlisted procedure, rectum
46999	Unlisted procedure, anus
47379	Unlisted laparoscopic procedure, liver
47399	Unlisted procedure, liver
47579	Unlisted laparoscopy procedure, biliary tract
47999	Unlisted procedure, biliary tract
48999	Unlisted procedure, pancreas
49329	Unlisted laparoscopy procedure, abdomen, peritoneum and omentum
49659	Unlisted laparoscopy procedure, hernioplasty, herniorrhaphy, herniotomy
49999	Unlisted procedure, abdomen, peritoneum and omentum
50549	Unlisted laparoscopy procedure, renal
50949	Unlisted laparoscopy procedure, ureter
51999	Unlisted laparoscopy procedure, bladder
53899	Unlisted procedure, urinary system
54699	Unlisted laparoscopy procedure, testis
55559	Unlisted laparoscopy procedure, spermatic cord
55899	Unlisted procedure, male genital system
58578	Unlisted laparoscopy procedure, uterus

58579	Unlisted hysteroscopy procedure, uterus
58679	Unlisted laparoscopy procedure, oviduct, ovary
58999	Unlisted procedure, female genital system (nonobstetrical)
59897	Unlisted fetal invasive procedure, including ultrasound guidance, when performed
59898	Unlisted laparoscopy procedure, maternity care and delivery
59899	Unlisted procedure, maternity care and delivery
60659	Unlisted laparoscopy procedure, endocrine system
60699	Unlisted procedure, endocrine system
64999	Unlisted procedure, nervous system
66999	Unlisted procedure, anterior segment of eye
67299	Unlisted procedure, posterior segment
67399	Unlisted procedure, extraocular muscle
67599	Unlisted procedure, orbit
67999	Unlisted procedure, eyelids
68399	Unlisted procedure, conjunctiva
68899	Unlisted procedure, lacrimal system
69399	Unlisted procedure, external ear
69799	Unlisted procedure, middle ear
69949	Unlisted procedure, inner ear
69979	Unlisted procedure, temporal bone, middle fossa approach

SURGERY SUBSECTIONS

The SURGERY section of the CPT coding system is divided into 19 subsections:

General	10004-10021
Integumentary System	10030-19499
Musculoskeletal System	20100-29999
Respiratory System	30000-32999
Cardiovascular System	33010-37799
Hemic and Lymphatic Systems	38100-38999
Mediastinum and Diaphragm	39000-39599
Digestive System	40490-49999
Urinary System	50010-53899
Male Genital System	54000-55899
Reproductive System Procedures	55920
Intersex Surgery	55970-55980
Female Genital System	56405-58999
Maternity Care and Delivery	59000-59899
Endocrine System	60000-60699
Nervous System	61000-64999
Eye and Ocular Adnexa	65091-68899
Auditory System	69000-69979
Operating Microscope	69990

Each sub-section of the SURGERY section of the CPT coding system is divided into organs then into procedures involving anatomic sites. Each anatomic site is further separated into surgical processes such as incision, excision, repair, removal, amputation, etc.

IMAGING GUIDANCE

When imaging guidance or imaging supervision and interpretation is included in a surgical procedure, guidelines for image documentation and report, included in the guidelines for Radiology (including Nuclear Medicine and Diagnostic Ultrasound) will apply. Imaging guidance should not be reported for use of a nonimaging-guided tracking or localizing system (eg, radar signals, electromagnetic signals). Imaging guidance should only be reported when an imaging modality (eg, radiography, fluoroscopy, ultrasonography, magnetic resonance imaging, computed tomography, or nuclear medicine) is used and is appropriately documented.

SURGERY SECTION MODIFIERS

Due to various circumstances, surgical procedures may be considered to be modified in comparison to the full or complete procedure. Modified procedures are identified by reporting a two-digit modifier to the CPT procedure code(s). The following CPT modifiers may be coded with surgical procedures:

-22	Unusual Procedural Services
-26	Professional Component
-32	Mandated Services
-47	Anesthesia by Surgeon
-50	Bilateral Procedure
-51	Multiple Procedures
-52	Reduced Services
-54	Surgical Care Only
-55	Postoperative Management Only
-56	Preoperative Management Only
-57	Decision for Surgery
-58	Staged or Related Procedure or Service by the Same Physician During the Postoperative Period
-62	Two Surgeons
-66	Surgical Team
-76	Repeat Procedure by Same Physician
-77	Repeat Procedure by Another Physician
-78	Return to the Operating Room for a Related Procedure During the Postoperative Period
-79	Unrelated Procedure or Service by the Same Physician During the Postoperative Period
-80	Assistant Surgeon
-81	Minimum Assistant Surgeon
-82	Assistant Surgeon (when qualified resident surgeon not available)
-90	Reference (Outside) Laboratory
-99	Multiple modifiers

ADD-ON CODES

Some of the listed procedures are commonly carried out in addition to the primary procedure performed. These additional or supplemental procedures are designated as add-on codes with the : symbol and they are listed in Appendix D of the CPT codebook. Add-on codes in CPT 2020 can be readily identified by specific descriptor nomenclature that includes phrases such as "each additional" or "(List separately in addition to primary procedure)."

The add-on code concept in CPT 2020 applies only to addon procedures or services performed by the same physician. Add-on codes describe additional intra-service work associated with the primary procedure, eg, additional digit(s), lesion(s), neurorrhaphy(s), vertebral segment(s), tendon(s), joint(s).

	Separate Procedure	Unlisted Procedure	CCI Comp. Code	Non-specific Procedure	**219**

Add-on codes are always performed in addition to the primary service or procedure and must never be reported as a stand-alone code. When the add-on procedure can be reported bilaterally and is performed bilaterally, the appropriate add-on code is reported twice, unless the code descriptor, guidelines, or parenthetical instructions for that particular add-on code instructs otherwise. Do not report modifier 50, Bilateral procedures, in conjunction with add-on codes. All add-on codes in the CPT code set are exempt from the multiple procedure concept. See the definitions of modifier 50 and 51 in Appendix A.

Many surgical procedures are performed secondary to primary surgical procedures. These procedures are classified as "additional" or "supplemental" procedures and are designated as "add-on" codes in the CPT coding system. "Add-on" CPT codes are identified in the CPT code book by a black plus sign "+" placed to the left of the code number.

Many of the CPT "Add-on" codes are further identified by phrases included within the descriptions of the definition of the CPT code or include the phrase "(List separately in addition to primary procedure)" following the definition. Examples of CPT codes identified as "add-on" codes include:

+ 11008   Removal of prosthetic material or mesh, abdominal wall for infection (eg, for chronic or recurrent mesh infection or necrotizing soft tissue infection) (list separately in addition to code for primary procedure)

+ 19295   Image guided placement, metallic localization clip, percutaneous, during breast biopsy/aspiration (List separately in addition to code for primary procedure)

MEDICAL AND SURGICAL SUPPLIES

HCPCS Level II codes for medical and surgical supplies, A4000-A4999, may be used to report supplies and materials provided to Medicare patients if the supplies and materials are not considered to be included with or part of the basic service(s) or procedure(s).

SURGERY CODES

GENERAL

FINE NEEDLE ASPIRATION (FNA) BIOPSY

A fine needle aspiration (FNA) biopsy is performed when material is aspirated with a fine needle and the cells are examined cytologically. A core needle biopsy is typically performed with a larger bore needle to obtain a core sample of tissue for histopathologic evaluation. FNA biopsy procedures are performed with or without imaging guidance. Imaging guidance codes (eg, 76942, 77002, 77012, 77021) may not be reported separately with 10004, 10005, 10006, 10007, 10008, 10009, 10010, 10011, 10012, 10021. Codes 10004, 10005, 10006, 10007, 10008, 10009, 10010, 10011, 10012, 10021 are reported once per lesion sampled in a single session.

When more than one FNA biopsy is performed on separate lesions at the same session, same day, same imaging modality, use the appropriate imaging modality add-on code for the second and subsequent lesion(s). When more than one FNA biopsy is performed on separate lesions, same session, same day, using different imaging modalities, report the corresponding primary code with modifier 59 for each additional imaging modality and corresponding add-on codes for subsequent lesions sampled. This instruction applies regardless of whether the lesions are ipsilateral or contralateral to each other, and/or whether they are in the same or different organs/structures. When FNA biopsy and core needle biopsy both are performed on the same lesion, same session, same day using the same type of imaging guidance, do not separately report the imaging guidance for the core needle biopsy. When FNA biopsy is performed on one lesion and core needle biopsy is performed on a separate lesion, same session, same day using the same type of imaging guidance, both the core needle biopsy and the imaging guidance for the core needle biopsy may be reported separately with modifier 59. When FNA biopsy is performed on one lesion and core needle biopsy is performed on a separate lesion, same session, same day using different types of imaging guidance, both the core needle biopsy and the imaging guidance for the core needle biopsy may be reported with modifier 59.

10004   Code is out of order. See page 221

10005   Code is out of order. See page 221

10006   Code is out of order. See page 222

10007   Code is out of order. See page 222

10008   Code is out of order. See page 222

10009   Code is out of order. See page 222

10010   Code is out of order. See page 222

10011   Code is out of order. See page 222

10012   Code is out of order. See page 222

10021   Fine needle aspiration biopsy, without imaging guidance; first lesion

(10022   deleted 2018 [2019 Edition]. To report, see 10005, 10006, 10007, 10008, 10009, 10010, 10011, 10012)

+ 10004   each additional lesion (List separately in addition to code for primary procedure)

     (Use 10004 in conjunction with 10021)

     (Do not report 10004, 10021 in conjunction with 10005, 10006, 10007, 10008, 10009, 10010, 10011, 10012 for the same lesion)

     (For evaluation of fine needle aspirate, see 88172, 88173, 88177)

10005   Fine needle aspiration biopsy, including ultrasound guidance; first lesion

+ 10006   each additional lesion (List separately in addition to code for primary procedure)

(Use 10006 in conjunction with 10005)

(Do not report 10005, 10006 in conjunction with 76942)

(For evaluation of fine needle aspirate, see 88172, 88173, 88177)

10007   Fine needle aspiration biopsy, including fluoroscopic guidance; first lesion

+ 10008   each additional lesion (List separately in addition to code for primary procedure)

(Use 10008 in conjunction with 10007)

(Do not report 10007, 10008 in conjunction with 77002)

(For evaluation of fine needle aspirate, see 88172, 88173, 88177)

10009   Fine needle aspiration biopsy, including CT guidance; first lesion

+ 10010   each additional lesion (List separately in addition to code for primary procedure)

(Use 10010 in conjunction with 10009)

(Do not report 10009, 10010 in conjunction with 77012)

(For evaluation of fine needle aspirate, see 88172, 88173, 88177)

10011   Fine needle aspiration biopsy, including MR guidance; first lesion

+ 10012   each additional lesion (List separately in addition to code for primary procedure)

(Use 10012 in conjunction with 10011)

(Do not report 10011, 10012 in conjunction with 77021)

(For evaluation of fine needle aspirate, see 88172, 88173, 88177)

(For percutaneous needle biopsy other than fine needle aspiration, see 19081-19086 for breast, 20206 for muscle, 32400 for pleura, 32408 for lung or mediastinum, 42400 for salivary gland, 47000 for liver, 48102 for pancreas, 49180 for abdominal or retroperitoneal mass, 50200 for kidney, 54500 for testis, 54800 for epididymis, 60100 for thyroid, 62267 for nucleus pulposus, intervertebral disc, or paravertebral tissue, 62269 for spinal cord)

(For percutaneous image-guided fluid collection drainage by catheter of soft tissue [eg, extremity, abdominal wall, neck], use 10030)

INTEGUMENTARY SYSTEM

SKIN, SUBCUTANEOUS AND ACCESSORY STRUCTURES

INTRODUCTION AND REMOVAL

10030 Image-guided fluid collection drainage by catheter (eg, abscess, hematoma, seroma, lymphocele, cyst), soft tissue (eg, extremity, abdominal wall, neck), percutaneous

(Report 10030 for each individual collection drained with a separate catheter)

(Do not report 10030 in conjunction with 75989, 76942, 77002, 77003, 77012, 77021)

(For image-guided fluid collection drainage, percutaneous or transvaginal/transrectal of visceral, peritoneal, or retroperitoneal collections, see 49405-49407)

Soft tissue marker placement with imaging guidance is reported with 10035 and 10036. If a more specific site descriptor than soft tissue is applicable (eg, breast), use the site-specific codes for marker placement at that site. Report 10035 and 10036 only once per target, regardless of how many markers (eg, clips, wires, pellets, radioactive seeds) are used to mark that target.

10035 Placement of soft tissue localization device(s) (eg, clip, metallic pellet, wire/needle, radioactive seeds), percutaneous, including imaging guidance; first lesion.

+ 10036 each additional lesion (List separately in addition to code for primary procedure)

(Use 10036 in conjunction with 10035)

(Do not report 10035, 10036 in conjunction with 76942, 77002, 77012, 77021)

(To report a second procedure on the same side or contralateral side, use 10036)

INCISION AND DRAINAGE

(For excision, see 11400, et seq)

10040 Acne surgery (eg, marsupialization, opening or removal of multiple milia, comedones, cysts, pustules)

10060 Incision and drainage of abscess (eg, carbuncle, suppurative hidradenitis, cutaneous or subcutaneous abscess, cyst, furuncle, or paronychia); simple or single

10061 complicated or multiple

10080 Incision and drainage of pilonidal cyst; simple

10081 complicated

(For excision of pilonidal cyst, see 11770-11772)

10120 Incision and removal of foreign body, subcutaneous tissues; simple

10121 complicated

(To report wound exploration due to penetrating trauma without laparotomy or thoracotomy, see 20100-20103, as appropriate)

(To report debridement associated with open fracture(s) and/or dislocation(s), use 11010-11012, as appropriate)

10140 Incision and drainage of hematoma, seroma or fluid collection

(If imaging guidance is performed, see 76942, 77012, 77021)

10160 Puncture aspiration of abscess, hematoma, bulla, or cyst

(If imaging guidance is performed, see 76942, 77002, 77012, 77021)

10180   Incision and drainage, complex, postoperative wound infection

(For secondary closure of surgical wound, see 12020, 12021, 13160)

DEBRIDEMENT

Wound debridements (11042-11047) are reported by depth of tissue that is removed and by surface area of the wound. These services may be reported for injuries, infections, wounds and chronic ulcers. When performing debridement of a single wound, report depth using the deepest level of tissue removed. In multiple wounds, sum the surface area of those wounds that are at the same depth, but do not combine sums from different depths. For example: When bone is debrided from a 4 sq cm heel ulcer and from a 10 sq cm ischial ulcer, report the work with a single code, 11044. When subcutaneous tissue is debrided from a 16 sq cm dehisced abdominal wound and a 10 sq cm thigh wound, report the work with 11042 for the first 20 sq cm and 11045 for the second 6 sq cm. If all four wounds were debrided on the same day, use modifier 59 with 11042 or 11044 as appropriate.

(For dermabrasions, see 15780-15783)

(For nail debridement, see 11720-11721)

(For burn(s), see 16000-16035)

(For pressure ulcers, see 15920-15999)

11000   Debridement of extensive eczematous or infected skin; up to 10% of body surface

(For abdominal wall or genitalia debridement for necrotizing soft tissue infection, see 11004-11006)

+ **11001**   each additional 10% of the body surface, or part thereof (List separately in addition to code for primary procedure)

(Use 11001 in conjunction with code 11000)

11004   Debridement of skin, subcutaneous tissue, muscle and fascia for necrotizing soft tissue infection; external genitalia and perineum

11005   abdominal wall, with or without fascial closure

11006   external genitalia, perineum and abdominal wall, with or without fascial closure

(If orchiectomy is performed, use 54520)

(If testicular transplantation is performed, use 54680)

+ **11008**   Removal of prosthetic material or mesh, abdominal wall for infection (eg, for chronic or recurrent mesh infection or necrotizing soft tissue infection) (list separately in addition to code for primary procedure)

(Use 11008 in conjunction with 10180, 11004-11006)

(Report skin grafts or flaps separately when performed for closure at the same session as 11004-11008)

(When insertion of mesh is used for closure, use 49568)

11010   Debridement including removal of foreign material at the site of an open fracture and/or an open dislocation (eg, excisional debridement); skin and subcutaneous tissues

11011   skin, subcutaneous tissue, muscle fascia, and muscle

11012   skin, subcutaneous tissue, muscle fascia, muscle, and bone

(For debridement of skin, ie, epidermis and/or dermis only, see 97597, 97598)

(For active wound care management, see 97597, 97598)

(For debridement of burn wounds, see 16020-16030)

11042   Debridement, subcutaneous tissue (includes epidermis and dermis, if performed); first 20 sq cm or less

(For debridement of skin [ie., epidermis and/or dermis only], see 97597, 97598)

+ 11045   each additional 20 sq cm or part thereof (list separately in addition to code for primary procedure)

(Use 11045 in conjunction with 11042)

11043   Debridement, muscle and/or fascia (includes epidermis, dermis, and subcutaneous tissue, if performed); first 20 sq cm or less

+ 11046   each additional 20 sq cm, or part thereof (list separately in addition to code for primary procedure)

(Use 11046 in conjunction with 11043)

11044   Debridement, bone (includes epidermis, dermis, subcutaneous tissue, muscle and/or fascia, if performed); first 20 sq cm or less

11045   This code is out of order. See page 225

11046   This code is out of order. See page 225

+ 11047   each additional 20 sq cm, or part thereof (list separately in addition to code for primray procedure

(Do not report 11042-11047 in conjunction with 97597-97602 for the same wound)

(Use 11047 in conjunction with 11044)

PARING OR CUTTING

(To report destruction, see 17000-17004)

11055   Paring or cutting of benign hyperkeratotic lesion (eg, corn or callus); single lesion

11056   two to four lesions

11057   more than four lesions

BIOPSY

The use of a biopsy procedure code (eg, 11102, 11103, 11104, 11105, 11106, 11107) indicates that the procedure to obtain tissue solely for diagnostic histopathologic examination was performed independently, or was unrelated or distinct from other procedures/services provided at that time. Biopsies performed on different lesions or different sites on the same date of service may be reported separately, as they are not considered components of other procedures.

During certain surgical procedures in the integumentary system, such as excision, destruction, or shave removals, the removed tissue is often submitted for pathologic examination. The obtaining of tissue for pathology during the course of these procedures is a routine component of such procedures. This obtaining of tissue is not considered a separate biopsy procedure and is not separately reported

Partial-thickness biopsies are those that sample a portion of the thickness of skin or mucous membrane and do not penetrate below the dermis or lamina propria. Fullthickness biopsies penetrate into tissue deep to the dermis or lamina propria, into the subcutaneous or submucosal space.

Sampling of stratum corneum only, by any modality (eg, skin scraping, tape stripping) does not constitute a skin biopsy procedure and is not separately reportable.

An appropriate biopsy technique is selected based on optimal tissue-sampling considerations for the type of neoplastic, inflammatory, or other lesion requiring a tissue diagnosis. Biopsy of the skin is reported under three distinct techniques:

Tangential biopsy (eg, shave, scoop, saucerize, curette) is performed with a sharp blade, such as a flexible biopsy blade, obliquely oriented scalpel or curette to remove a sample of epidermal tissue with or without portions of underlying dermis. The intent of a tangential biopsy (11102, 11103) is to obtain a tissue sample from a lesion for the purpose of diagnostic pathologic examination. Biopsy of lesions by tangential technique (11102, 11103) is not considered an excision. Tangential biopsy technique may be represented by a superficial sample and does not involve the full thickness of the dermis, which could result in portions of the lesion remaining in the deeper layers of the dermis.

For therapeutic removal of epidermal or dermal lesion(s) using shave technique, see 11300-11313.

An indication for a shave removal (11300-11313) procedure may include a symptomatic lesion that rubs on waistband or bra, or any other reason why an elevated lesion is being completely removed with the shave technique, suggesting a therapeutic intent. It is the responsibility of the physician or qualified health care professional performing the procedure to clearly indicate the purpose of the procedure.

Punch biopsy requires a punch tool to remove a fullthickness cylindrical sample of skin. The intent of a punch biopsy (11104, 11105) is to obtain a cylindrical tissue sample of a cutaneous lesion for the purpose of diagnostic pathologic examination. Simple closure of the defect is included in the service. Manipulation of the biopsy defect to improve wound approximation is included in simple closure.

Incisional biopsy requires the use of a sharp blade (not a punch tool) to remove a full-thickness sample of tissue via a vertical incision or wedge, penetrating deep to the dermis, into the subcutaneous space. The intent of an incisional biopsy (11106, 11107) is to obtain a fullthickness tissue sample of a skin lesion for the purpose of diagnostic pathologic examination. This type of biopsy may sample subcutaneous fat, such as those performed for the evaluation of panniculitis. Although closure is usually performed on incisional biopsies, simple closure is not separately reported.

(For complete lesion excision with margins, see 11400-11646)

When multiple biopsy techniques are performed during the same encounter, only one primary lesion biopsy code (11102, 11104, 11106) is reported. Additional biopsy codes should be selected based on the following convention:

If multiple biopsies of the same type are performed, the primary code for that biopsy should be used along with the corresponding add-on code(s).

If an incisional biopsy is performed, report 11106 in combination with a tangential (11103), punch (11105), or incisional biopsy (11107) for the additional biopsy procedures.

If a punch biopsy is performed, report 11104 in combination with a tangential (11103), or punch (11105), for the additional biopsy procedures.

If multiple tangential biopsies are performed, report tangential biopsy (11102) in combination with 11103 for the additional tangential biopsy procedures.

When two or more biopsies of the same technique (ie, tangential, punch, or incisional) are performed on separate/additional lesions, use the appropriate add-on code (11103, 11105, 11107) to specify each additional biopsy. When two or three different biopsy techniques (ie, tangential, punch, or incisional) are performed to sample separate/additional lesions, select the appropriate biopsy code (11102, 11104, 11106) plus an additional add-on code (11103, 11105, 11107) for each additional biopsy performed.

The following table provides an illustration of the appropriate use of these codes for multiple biopsies:

Procedures Performed	CPT Code(s) Reported
2 tangential biopsies	11102 once, 11103 once
3 punch biopsies	11104 once, 11105 twice
2 incisional biopsies	11106 once, 11107 once
1 incisional biopsy, 1 tangential biopsy and 1 punch biopsy	11106 once, 11103 once, 11105 once
1 punch biopsy adn 2 tangential biopsies	11104 once, 11103 twice

    (For biopsy of nail unit, use 11755)

    (For biopsy, intranasal, use 30100)

    (For biopsy of lip, use 40490)

    (For biopsy of vestibule of mouth, use 40808)

    (For biopsy of tongue, anterior two-thirds, use 41100)

    (For biopsy of floor of mouth, use 41108)

(For biopsy of penis, use 54100)

(For biopsy of vulva or perineum, see 56605, 56606)

(For biopsy of eyelid skin including lid margin, use 67810)

(For biopsy of conjunctiva, use 68100)

(For biopsy of ear, use 69100)

(**11100**   deleted 2018 [2019 Edition]. To report, see 11102, 11104, 11106)

(**11101**   deleted 2018 [2019 Edition]. To report, see 11103, 11105, 11107)

11102   Tangential biopsy of skin (eg, shave, scoop, saucerize, curette); single lesion

+ **11103**   each separate/additional lesion (List separately in addition to code for primary procedure)

(Report 11103 in conjunction with 11102, 11104, 11106, when different biopsy techniques are performed to sample separate/additional lesions for each type of biopsy technique used)

11104   Punch biopsy of skin (including simple closure, when performed); single lesion

+ **11105**   each separate/additional lesion (List separately in addition to code for primary procedure)

(Report 11105 in conjunction with 11104, 11106, when different biopsy techniques are performed to sample separate/additional lesions for each type of biopsy technique used)

11106   Incisional biopsy of skin (eg, wedge) (including simple closure, when performed); single lesion

+ **11107**   each separate/additional lesion (List separately in addition to code for primary procedure)

(Report 11107 in conjunction with 11106)

REMOVAL OF SKIN TAGS

Removal by scissoring or any sharp method, ligature strangulation, electrosurgical destruction or combination of treatment modalities, including chemical destruction or electrocauterization of wound, with or without local anesthesia.

11200   Removal of skin tags, multiple fibrocutaneous tags, any area; up to and including 15 lesions

+ **11201**   each additional 10 lesions, or part thereof (List separately in addition to code for primary procedure)

(Use 11201 in conjunction with code 11200)

SHAVING OF EPIDERMAL OR DERMAL LESIONS

Many of the procedure codes listed in the integumentary system subsection of the CPT manual are designated in centimeters or square centimeters. Many physicians document sizes using inches or millimeters. Make sure to verify, and convert if necessary, measurements before assigning a code.

To be able to code lesion removal appropriately, the site, size in centimeters, method of removal and morphology must be documented in the medical record. Always code morphology from the pathology report.

Excision of lesion codes are determined by the diameter of the actual lesion, not the specimen sent to pathology. However, the size of the specimen can be used when the size of the lesion cannot be located in the operative report or elsewhere in the medical record.

When more than one dimension of a lesion is provided in the documentation, select the code based on the largest size. For example, if the dimensions indicated are 3 cm x 2 cm x 1.5 cm, the lesion should be coded as 3 cm. Excision of benign and malignant lesions includes anesthesia and simple repair of the defect site.

Shaving is the sharp removal by transverse incision or horizontal slicing to remove epidermal and dermal lesions without a full-thickness dermal excision. This includes local anesthesia, chemical or electrcauterization ofthe wound. The wound does not require suture closure.

11300 Shaving of epidermal or dermal lesion, single lesion, trunk, arms or legs; lesion diameter 0.5 cm or less

11301 lesion diameter 0.6 to 1.0 cm

11302 lesion diameter 1.1 to 2.0 cm

11303 lesion diameter over 2.0 cm

11305 Shaving of epidermal or dermal lesion, single lesion, scalp, neck, hands, feet, genitalia; lesion diameter 0.5 cm or less

11306 lesion diameter 0.6 to 1.0 cm

11307 lesion diameter 1.1 to 2.0 cm

11308 lesion diameter over 2.0 cm

11310 Shaving of epidermal or dermal lesion, single lesion, face, ears, eyelids, nose, lips, mucous membrane; lesion diameter 0.5 cm or less

11311 lesion diameter 0.6 to 1.0 cm

11312 lesion diameter 1.1 to 2.0 cm

11313 lesion diameter over 2.0 cm

EXCISION OF BENIGN LESIONS

Excision (including simple closure) of benign lesions of skin (eg., neoplasm, cicatricial, fibrous, inflammatory, congenital, cystic lesions) includes local anesthesia. See appropriate size and area below. For shave removal, see 11300 et seq., and for electrosurgical and other methods, see 17000 et seq..

Excision is defined as full-thickness (through the dermis) removal of a lesion, inlcuding margins, and includes simple (non-layered) closure when performed. Report separately each benign lesion excised. Code selection is determined by measuring the greatest clinical diameter of the apparent lesion plus that margin required for complete excision (lesion diameter plus the most narrow margins required equals the excised diameter). The margins refer to the most narrow margin required to adequately excise the lesion, based on the individual judgment. The measurement of lesion plus margin is made prior to excision. The excised diameter is the same whether the surgical defect is repaired in a linear fashion, or reconstructed (eg, with a skin graft).

The closure of defects created by incision, excision, or trauma may require intermediate or complex closure. Repair by intermediate or complex closure should be reported separately. For excision of benign lesions requiring more than simple closure, i.e., requiring intermediate or complex closure, report 11400-11446 in addition to appropriate intermediate (12031-12057) or complex closure (13100-13153) codes. For reconstructive closure, see 15002-15261, 15570-15770. For excision performed in conjunction with adjacent tissue transfer, report only the adjacent tissue transfer code (14000-14302). Excision of lesion (11400-11446) is not separately reportable with adjacent tissue transfer.

> (For destruction [eg, laser surgery, electrosurgery, cryosurgery, chemosurgery, surgical curette] of benign lesions other than skin tags or cutaneous vascular proliferative lesions, see 17110, 17111; premalignant lesions, see 17000, 17003, 17004; cutaneous vascular proliferative lesions, see 17106, 17107, 17108; malignant lesions, see 17260-17286)

> (For excision of cicatricial lesion[s] [eg, full thickness excision, through the dermis], see 11400-11446)

> (For incisional removal of burn scar, see 16035, 16036)

> (For fractional ablative laser fenestration for functional improvement of traumatic or burn scars, see 0479T, 0480T)

11400 Excision, benign lesion including margins, except skin tag (unless listed elsewhere), trunk, arms or legs; excised diameter 0.5 cm or less

11401 excised diameter 0.6 to 1.0 cm

● New Code ▲ Revised Code ✛ Add-On Code ⊘ Modifier -51 Exempt ★ Telemedicine

11402	excised diameter 1.1 to 2.0 cm
11403	excised diameter 2.1 to 3.0 cm
11404	excised diameter 3.1 to 4.0 cm
11406	excised diameter over 4.0 cm

(For unusual or complicated excision, add modifier -22)

11420	Excision, benign lesion including margins, except skin tag (unless listed elsewhere), scalp, neck, hands, feet, genitalia; excised diameter 0.5 cm or less
11421	excised diameter 0.6 to 1.0 cm
11422	excised diameter 1.1 to 2.0 cm
11423	excised diameter 2.1 to 3.0 cm
11424	excised diameter 3.1 to 4.0 cm
11426	excised diameter over 4.0 cm

(For unusual or complicated excision, add modifier -22)

11440	Excision, other benign lesion including margins (unless listed elsewhere), face, ears, eyelids, nose, lips, mucous membrane; excised diameter 0.5 cm or less
11441	excised diameter 0.6 to 1.0 cm
11442	excised diameter 1.1 to 2.0 cm
11443	excised diameter 2.1 to 3.0 cm
11444	excised diameter 3.1 to 4.0 cm
11446	excised diameter over 4.0 cm

(For unusual or complicated excision, add modifier -22)

(For eyelids involving more than skin, see also 67800 et seq.)

11450	Excision of skin and subcutaneous tissue for hidradenitis, axillary; with simple or intermediate repair
11451	with complex repair
11462	Excision of skin and subcutaneous tissue for hidradenitis, inguinal; with simple or intermediate repair
11463	with complex repair
11470	Excision of skin and subcutaneous tissue for hidradenitis, perianal, perineal, or umbilical; with simple or intermediate repair
11471	with complex repair

(When skin graft or flap is used for closure, use appropriate procedure code in addition)

(For bilateral procedure, add modifier -50)

EXCISION OF MALIGNANT LESIONS

Excision (including simple closure) of malignant lesions of skin (eg., basal cell carcinoma, squamous cell carcinoma, melanoma) includes local anesthesia. (See appropriate size and body area below.) For destruction of malignant lesions of skin, see destruction codes 17260-17286.

The closure of defects created by incision, excision, or trauma may require intermediate or complex closure. Repair by intermediate or complex closure should be reported separately. For excision of malignant lesions requiring more than simple closure, i.e., requiring intermediate or complex closure, report 11600-11646 in addition to appropriate intermediate (12031-12057) or complex closure (13100-13153) codes. For reconstructive closure, see 15002-15261, 15570-15770. For excision performed in conjunction with adjacent tissue transfer, report only the adjacent tissue transfer code (14000-14302). Excision of lesion (11600-11646) is not separately reportable with adjacent tissue transfer.

When frozen section pathology shows the margins of excision were not adequate, an additional excision may be necessary for complete tumor removal. Use only one code to report the additional excision and re-excision(s) based on the final widest excised diameter required for complete tumor removal at the same operative session. To report a re-excised procedure performed to widen margins at a subsequent operative session, see codes 11600-11646, as appropriate. Append modifier 58 if the re-excision procedure is performed during the postoperative period of the primary excision procedure.

11600	Excision, malignant lesion including margins, trunk, arms, or legs; excised diameter 0.5 cm or less
11601	excised diameter 0.6 to 1.0 cm
11602	excised diameter 1.1 to 2.0 cm
11603	excised diameter 2.1 to 3.0 cm
11604	excised diameter 3.1 to 4.0 cm
11606	excised diameter over 4.0 cm
11620	Excision, malignant lesion including margins, scalp, neck, hands, feet, genitalia; excised diameter 0.5 cm or less
11621	excised diameter 0.6 to 1.0 cm
11622	excised diameter 1.1 to 2.0 cm
11623	excised diameter 2.1 to 3.0 cm
11624	excised diameter 3.1 to 4.0 cm
11626	excised diameter over 4.0 cm
11640	Excision, malignant lesion including margins, face, ears, eyelids, nose, lips; excised diameter 0.5 cm or less
11641	excised diameter 0.6 to 1.0 cm
11642	excised diameter 1.1 to 2.0 cm
11643	excised diameter 2.1 to 3.0 cm
11644	excised diameter 3.1 to 4.0 cm
11646	excised diameter over 4.0 cm

(For eyelids involving more than skin, see also 67800 et seq)

NAILS

(For drainage of paronychia or onychia, see 10060, 10061)

11719   Trimming of nondystrophic nails, any number

11720   Debridement of nail(s) by any method(s); 1 to 5

11721   6 or more

11730   Avulsion of nail plate, partial or complete, simple; single

+ **11732**   each additional nail plate (List separately in addition to code for primary procedure)

(Use 11732 in conjunction with code 11730)

11740   Evacuation of subungual hematoma

11750   Excision of nail and nail matrix, partial or complete, (eg, ingrown or deformed nail) for permanent removal;

(**11752**   deleted 2016 [2017 edition]. See 26236, 28124, 28160)

(For pinch graft, use 15050)

11755   Biopsy of nail unit (eg, plate, bed, matrix, hyponychium, proximal and lateral nail folds) (separate procedure)

11760   Repair of nail bed

11762   Reconstruction of nail bed with graft

11765   Wedge excision of skin of nail fold (eg, for ingrown toenail)

PILONIDAL CYST

11770   Excision of pilonidal cyst or sinus; simple

11771   extensive

11772   complicated

(For incision of pilonidal cyst, see 10080, 10081)

INTRODUCTION

11900   Injection, intralesional; up to and including seven lesions

11901   more than seven lesions

(11900, 11901 are not to be used for preoperative local anesthetic injection)

(For veins, see 36470, 36471)

(For intralesional chemotherapy administration, see 96405, 96406)

11920   Tattooing, intradermal introduction of insoluble opaque pigments to correct color defects of skin, including micropigmentation; 6.0 sq cm or less

11921   6.1 to 20.0 sq cm

+ **11922**   each additional 20.0 sq cm or part thereof (List separately in addition to code for primary procedure)

Separate Procedure   Unlisted Procedure   CCI Comp. Code   Non-specific Procedure   **231**

(Use 11922 in conjunction with code 11921)

11950 Subcutaneous injection of filling material (eg, collagen); 1 cc or less

11951   1.1 to 5.0 cc

11952   5.1 to 10.0 cc

11954   over 10.0 cc

11960 Insertion of tissue expander(s) for other than breast, including subsequent expansion

(Do not report 11960 in conjunction with 11971, 13160, 29848, 64702-64726)

(For insertion of tissue expander in breast reconstruction, use 19357)

▲ **11970** Replacement of tissue expander with permanent implant

▲ **11971** Removal of tissue expander without insertion of implant

(Do not report 11971 in conjunction with 11960, 11970)

(For removal of breast-tissue expander and replacement with breast implant, use 11970)

11976 Removal, implantable contraceptive capsules

11980 Subcutaneous hormone pellet implantation (implantation of estradiol and/or testosterone pellets beneath the skin)

11981 Insertion, non-biodegradable drug delivery implant

(For manual preparation and insertion of deep [eg, subfascial], intramedullary, or intra-articular drug-delivery device, see 20700, 20702, 20704)

(Do not report 11981 in conjunction with 20700, 20702, 20704)

11982 Removal, non-biodegradable drug delivery implant

(For removal of deep [eg, subfascial], intramedullary, or intra-articular drug-delivery device, see 20701, 20703, 20705)

(Do not report 11982 in conjunction with 20701, 20703, 20705)

11983 Removal with reinsertion, non-biodegradable drug delivery implant

REPAIR (CLOSURE)

To be able to code wound repair appropriately, the site, length of wound in centimeters and type of repair must be documented in the medical record. Review the definitions of simple, intermediate and complex repair in the current CPT coding system.

Use the codes in this section to designate wound closure utilizing sutures, staples, or tissue adhesives (eg., 2-cyanoacrylate), either singly or in combination with each other, or in combination with adhesive strips. Wound closure utilizing adhesive strips as the sole repair material should be coded using the appropriate E/M code.

Definitions

Simple repair is used when the wound is superficial, eg., involving primarily epidermis or dermis, or subcutaneous tissues without significant involvement of deeper structures, and requires simple one layer closure. This includes local anesthesia and chemical or electrocauterization of wounds not closed.

Intermediate repair includes the repair of wounds that, in addition to the above, require layered closure of one or more of the deeper layers of subcutaneous tissue and superficial (non-muscle) fascia, in addition to the skin (epidermal and dermal) closure. It includes limited undermining (defined as a distance less than the maximum width of the defect, measured perpendicular to the closure line, along at least one entire edge of the defect). Single-layer closure of heavily contaminated wounds that have required extensive cleaning or removal of particulate matter also constitutes intermediate repair.

Complex repair includes the repair of wounds that, in addition to the requirements for intermediate repair, require at least one of the following: exposure of bone, cartilage, tendon, or named neurovascular structure; debridement of wound edges (eg, traumatic lacerations or avulsions); extensive undermining (defined as a distance greater than or equal to the maximum width of the defect, measured perpendicular to the closure line along at least one entire edge of the defect); involvement of free margins of helical rim, vermilion border, or nostril rim; placement of retention sutures. Necessary preparation includes creation of a limited defect for repairs or the debridement of complicated lacerations or avulsions. Complex repair does not include excision of benign (11400-11446) or malignant (11600-11646) lesions, excisional preparation of a wound bed (15002-15005) or debridement of an open fracture or open dislocation.

Instuctions for listing services at time of wound repair:

1. The repaired wound(s) should be measured and recorded in centimeters, whether curved, angular or stellate.

2. When multiple wounds are repaired, add together the lengths of those in the same classification (see above) and from all anatomic sites that are grouped together into the same code descriptor. For example, add together the lengths of intermediate repairs to the trunk and extremities Do not add lengths of repairs from different groupings of anatomic sites (eg, face and extremities). Also, do not add together lengths of different classifications (eg, intermediate and complex repairs).

When more than one classification of wounds is repaired, list the more complicated as the primary procedure and the less complicated as the secondary procedure, using modifier 59.

3. Decontamination and/or debridement: Debridement is considered a separate procedure only when gross contamination requires prolonged cleansing, when appreciable amounts of devitalized or contaminated tissue are removed, or when debridement is carried out separately without immediate primary closure.

> (For extensive debridement of soft tissue and/or bone, not associated with open fracture(s) and/or dislocation(s) resulting from penetrating and/or blunt trauma, see 11042-11047.)

> (For extensive debridement of subcutaneous tissue, muscle fascia, muscle, and/or bone associated with open fracture(s) and/or dislocation(s), see 11010-11012.)

4. Involvement of nerves, blood vessels and tendons: Report under appropriate system (Nervous, Cardiovascular, Musculoskeletal) for repair of these structures. The repair of these associated wounds is included in the primary procedure unless it qualifies as a complex repair, in which case modifier 59 applies.

Simple ligation of vessels in an open wound is considered as part of any wound closure.

Simple "exploration" of nerves, blood vessels, or tendons exposed in an open wound is also considered part of the essential treatment of the wound and is not a separate procedure unless appreciable dissection is required. If the wound requires enlargement, extension of dissection (to determine penetration), debridement, removal of foreign body(s), ligation or coagulation of minor subcutaneous and/or muscular blood vessel(s) of the subcutaneous tissue, muscle fascia, and/or muscle, not requiring thoracotomy or laparotomy, use codes 20100-20103, as appropriate.

REPAIR — SIMPLE

Sum of lengths of repairs for each group of anatomic sites.

12001	Simple repair of superficial wounds of scalp, neck, axillae, external genitalia, trunk and/or extremities (including hands and feet); 2.5 cm or less
12002	2.6 cm to 7.5 cm
12004	7.6 cm to 12.5 cm
12005	12.6 cm to 20.0 cm
12006	20.1 cm to 30.0 cm
12007	over 30.0 cm

12011	Simple repair of superficial wounds of face, ears, eyelids, nose, lips and/or mucous membranes; 2.5 cm or less
12013	2.6 cm to 5.0 cm
12014	5.1 cm to 7.5 cm
12015	7.6 cm to 12.5 cm
12016	12.6 cm to 20.0 cm
12017	20.1 cm to 30.0 cm
12018	over 30.0 cm
12020	Treatment of superficial wound dehiscence; simple closure
12021	with packing

(For extensive or complicated secondary wound closure, use 13160)

REPAIR — INTERMEDIATE

Sum of lengths of repairs for each group of anatomic sites.

12031	Repair, intermediate of wounds of scalp, axillae, trunk and/or extremities (excluding hands and feet); 2.5 cm or less
12032	2.6 cm to 7.5 cm
12034	7.6 cm to 12.5 cm
12035	12.6 cm to 20.0 cm
12036	20.1 cm to 30.0 cm
12037	over 30.0 cm
12041	Repair, intermediate wounds of neck, hands, feet and/or external genitalia; 2.5 cm or less
12042	2.6 cm to 7.5 cm
12044	7.6 cm to 12.5 cm
12045	12.6 cm to 20.0 cm
12046	20.1 cm to 30.0 cm
12047	over 30.0 cm
12051	Repair, intermediate wounds of face, ears, eyelids, nose, lips and/or mucous membranes; 2.5 cm or less
12052	2.6 cm to 5.0 cm
12053	5.1 cm to 7.5 cm
12054	7.6 cm to 12.5 cm
12055	12.6 cm to 20.0 cm

● New Code   ▲ Revised Code   + Add-On Code   ⊘ Modifier -51 Exempt   ★ Telemedicine

| 12056 | 20.1 cm to 30.0 cm |
| 12057 | over 30.0 cm |

REPAIR — COMPLEX

Reconstructive procedures, complicated wound closure. Sum of lengths of repairs for each group of anatomic sites.

(For full thickness repair of lip or eyelid, see respective anatomical subsections)

| 13100 | Repair, complex, trunk; 1.1 cm to 2.5 cm |

(For 1.0 cm or less, see simple or intermediate repairs)

| 13101 | 2.6 cm to 7.5 cm |
| + 13102 | each additional 5 cm or less (List separately in addition to code for primary procedure) |

(Use 13102 in conjunction with code 13101)

| 13120 | Repair, complex, scalp, arms, and/or legs; 1.1 cm to 2.5 cm |

(For 1.0 cm or less, see simple or intermediate repairs)

| 13121 | 2.6 cm to 7.5 cm |
| + 13122 | each additional 5 cm or less (List separately in addition to code for primary procedure) |

(Use 13122 in conjunction with 13121)

| 13131 | Repair, complex, forehead, cheeks, chin, mouth, neck, axillae, genitalia, hands and/or feet; 1.1 cm to 2.5 cm |

(For 1.0 cm or less, see simple or intermediate repairs)

| 13132 | 2.6 cm to 7.5 cm |
| + 13133 | each additional 5 cm or less (List separately in addition to code for primary procedure) |

(Use 13133 in conjunction with 13132)

(For 1.0 cm or less, see simple or intermediate repairs)

13151	Repair, complex, eyelids, nose, ears and/or lips; 1.1 cm to 2.5 cm
13152	2.6 cm to 7.5 cm
+ 13153	each additional 5 cm or less (List separately in addition to code for primary procedure)

(Use 13153 in conjunction with 13152)

| 13160 | Secondary closure of surgical wound or dehiscence, extensive or complicated |

(Do not report 13160 in conjunction with 11960)

(For packing or simple secondary wound closure, see 12020, 12021)

ADJACENT TISSUE TRANSFER OR REARRANGEMENT

For full-thickness repair of lip or eyelid, see respective anatomical subsections.

Codes 14000-14302 are used for excision (including lesion) and/or repair by adjacent tissue transfer or rearrangement (eg., Z-plasty, W-plasty, V-Y plasty, rotation flap, random island flap, advancement flap). When applied in repairing lacerations, the procedures listed must be performed by the surgeon to accomplish the repair. They do not apply to direct closure or rearrangement of traumatic wounds incidentally resulting in these configurations. Undermining alone of adjacent tissues to achieve closure, without additional incisions, does not constitute adjacent tissue transfer. See complex repair codes 13100-13160. The excision of a benign lesion (11400-11446) or a malignant lesion (11600-11646) is not separately reportable with codes 14000-14302.

Skin graft necessary to close secondary defect is considered an additional procedure. For purposes of code selection, the term "defect" includes the primary and secondary defects. The primary defect resulting from the excision and the secondary defect resulting from flap design to perform the reconstruction are measured together to determine the code.

14000   Adjacent tissue transfer or rearrangement, trunk; defect 10 sq cm or less

14001   defect 10.1 sq cm to 30.0 sq cm

14020   Adjacent tissue transfer or rearrangement, scalp, arms and/or legs; defect 10 sq cm or less

14021   defect 10.1 sq cm to 30.0 sq cm

14040   Adjacent tissue transfer or rearrangement, forehead, cheeks, chin, mouth, neck, axillae, genitalia, hands and/or feet; defect 10 sq cm or less

14041   defect 10.1 sq cm to 30.0 sq cm

14060   Adjacent tissue transfer or rearrangement, eyelids, nose, ears and/or lips; defect 10 sq cm or less

14061   defect 10.1 sq cm to 30.0 sq cm

(For eyelid, full thickness, see 67961 et seq)

14301   Adjacent tissue transfer or rearrangement, any area; defect 30.1 sq cm to 60.0 sq cm

+ **14302**   each additional 30.0 sq cm, or part thereof (List separately in addition to code for primary procedure)

(Use 14302 in conjunction with 14301)

14350   Filleted finger or toe flap, including preparation of recipient site

SKIN REPLACEMENT SURGERY

Skin replacement surgery consists of surgical preparation and topical placement of an autograft (including tissue cultured autograft) or skin substitute graft (ie, homograft, allograft, xenograft). The graft is anchored using the individual's choice of fixation. When services are performed in the office, routine dressing supplies are not reported separately.

The following definition should be applied to those codes that reference "100 sq cm or 1% of body area of infants and children" when determining the involvement of body size: The measurement of 100 sq cm is applicable to adults and children 10 years of age and older; and percentages of body surface area apply to infants and children younger than 10 years of age. The measurements apply to the size of the recipient area.

Procedures involving wrist and/or ankle are reported with codes that include arm or leg in the descriptor.

When a primary procedure requires a skin substitute or skin autograft for definitive skin closure (eg, orbitectomy, radical mastectomy, or deep tumor removal) use 15100-15278 in conjunction with primary procedure.

For biological implant for soft tissue reinforcement, use 15777 in conjunction with primary procedure.

The supply of skin substitute graft(s) should be reported separately in conjunction with 15271-15278.

Definitions

Surgical preparation codes 15002-15005 for skin replacement surgery describe the initial services related to preparing a clean and viable wound surface for placement of an autograft, flap, skin substitute graft or for negatie pressure wound therapy. In come cases, closure may be possible using adjacent tissue transfer (14000-14061) or complex repair (13100-13153). In add cases, appreciable nonviable tissue is removed to treat a burn, traumatic wound or a necrotizing infection. The clean wound bed may also be created by incisional release of a scar contracture resulting in a surface defect from separation of tissues. The intent is to heal the wound by primary intention, or by the use of negative pressure wound therapy. Patient conditions may require the

---

closure or application of graft, flap, or skin substitute to be delayed, but in all cases the intent is to include these treatments or negative pressure wound therapy to heal the wound. Do not report 15002-15005 for removal of nonviable tissue/debris in a chronic wound (eg, venous or diabetic) when the wound is left to heal by secondary intention. See active wound management codes (97597, 97598) and debridement codes (11042-11047) for this service. For necrotizing soft tissue infections in specific anatomic locations, see 11004-11008.

Select the appropriate code from 15002-15005 based upon location and size of the resultant defect. For multiple wounds, sum the surface area of all wounds from all anatomic sites that are grouped together into the same code descriptor. For example, sum the surface area of all wounds on the trunk and arms. Do not sum wounds from different groupings of anatomic sites (eg, face and arms). Use 15002 or 15004, as appropriate, for excisions and incisional releases resulting in wounds up to and including 100 sq cm of surface area. Use 15003 or 15005 for each additional 100 sq cm or part thereof.

Autografts/tissue cultured autografts include the harvest and or application of an autologous skin graft. Repair of donor site requiring skin graft or local flaps is reported separately. Removal of current graft and/or simple cleansing of the wound is included, when performed. Do not report 97602. Debridement is considered a separate procedure only when gross contamination requires prolonged cleansing, when appreciable amounts of devialized or contaminated tissue ar removed, or when debridement is carried out separately without immediate primary closure.

Selecte the appropriate code from 15040-15261 based upon type of autograft and location and size of the defect. The measurements apply to the size of the recipient area. For multiple wounds, sum teh surface area of all wounds from all anatomic sites that are grouped together into the same code descriptor.

Skin substitute grafts include non-autologous human skin (dermal or epidermal, cellular and acellular) grafts (eg, homograft, allograft), non-human skin substitute grafts (ie, xenograft), and biological products that form a sheet scaffolding for skin growth. These codes are not to be reported for application of non-graft wound dressings (eg, gel, powder, ointment, foam, liquid) or injected skin substitutes. Application of non-graft wound dressings is not separately reportable. Removal of current graft and/or simple cleansing of the wound is included, when performed. Do not report 97602. Debridement is considered a separate procedure only when gross contamination requires prolonged cleansing, when appreciable amounts of devitalized or contaminated tissue are removed, or when debridement is carried out separately without immediate primary closure.

Select the appropriate code from 15271-15278 based upon location and size of the defect. For multiple wounds, sum the surface area of all wounds from all anatomic sites that are grouped together into the same code descriptor. For example, sum the surface area of all wounds on the trunk and arms. Do not sum wounds from different groupings of anatomic sites (eg, face and arms). The supply of skin substitute graft(s) should be reported separately in conjunction with 15271, 15272, 15273, 15274, 15275, 15276, 15277, 15278. For biologic implant for soft tissue reinforcement, use 15777 in conjunction with code for primary procedure.

Surgical Preparation

15002 Surgical preparation or creation of recipient site by excision of open wounds, burn eschar, or scar (including subcutaneous tissues), or incisional release of scar contracture, trunk, arms, legs; first 100 sq cm or 1% of body area of infants and children

(For linear scar revision, see 13100-13153)

+ **15003** each additional 100 sq cm, or part thereof, or each additional 1% of body area of infants and children (List separately in addition to code for primary procedure)

(Use 15003 in conjunction with 15002)

15004 Surgical preparation or creation of recipient site by excision of open wounds, burn eschar, or scar (including subcutaneous tissues), or incisional release of scar contracture, face, scalp, eyelids, mouth, neck, ears, orbits, genitalia, hands, feet and/or multiple digits; 1500405 first 100 sq cm or 1% of body area of infants and children

+ **15005** each additional 100 sq cm or part thereof, or each additional 1% of body area of infants and children (List separately in addition to code for primary procedure)

(Use 15005 in conjunction with 15004)

Autografts/Tissue Cultured Autograft

15040 Harvest of skin for tissue cultured skin autograft, 100 sq cm or less

15050 Pinch graft, single or multiple, to cover small ulcer, tip of digit, or other minimal open area (except on face), up to defect size 2 cm diameter

15100 Split-thickness autograft, trunk, arms, legs; first 100 sq cm or less, or one percent of body area of infants and children (except 15050)

+ **15101** each additional 100 sq cm, or each additional one percent of body area of infants and children, or part thereof (List separately in addition to code for primary procedure)

(Use 15101 in conjunction with code 15100)

15110 Epidermal autograft, trunk, arms, legs; first 100 sq cm or less, or one percent of body area of infants and children

+ **15111** each additional 100 sq cm, or each additional one percent of body area of infants and children, or part thereof (List separately in addition to code for primary procedure)

(Use 15111 in conjunction with 15110)

15115 Epidermal autograft, face, scalp, eyelids, mouth, neck, ears, orbits, genitalia, hands, feet, and/or multiple digits; first 100 sq cm or less, or one percent of body area of infants and children

+ **15116** each additional 100 sq cm, or each additional one percent of body area of infants and children, or part thereof (List separately in addition to code for primary procedure)

(Use 15116 in conjunction with 15115)

15120 Split-thickness autograft, face, scalp, eyelids, mouth, neck, ears, orbits, genitalia, hands, feet, and/or multiple digits; first 100 sq cm or less, or one percent of body area of infants and children (except 15050)

+ **15121** each additional 100 sq cm, or each additional one percent of body area of infants and children, or part thereof (List separately in addition to code for primary procedure)

(Use 15121 in conjunction with code 15120)

(For eyelids, see also 67961-67975)

15130 Dermal autograft, trunk, arms, legs; first 100 sq cm or less, or one percent of body area of infants and children

+ **15131** each additional 100 sq cm, or each additional one percent of body area of infants and children, or part thereof (List separately in addition to code for primary procedure)

(Use 15131 in conjunction with 15130)

15135 Dermal autograft, face, scalp, eyelids, mouth, neck, ears, orbits, genitalia, hands, feet, and/or multiple digits; first 100 sq cm or less, or one percent of body area of infants and children

+ **15136** each additional 100 sq cm, or each additional one percent of body area of infants and children, or part thereof (List separately in addition to code for primary procedure)

(Use 15136 in conjunction with 15135)

15150 Tissue cultured skin autograft, trunk, arms, legs; first 25 sq cm or less

+ **15151** additional 1 sq cm to 75 sq cm (List separately in addition to code for primary procedure)

(Do not report 15151 more than once per session)

(Use 15151 in conjunction with 15150)

+ **15152** each additional 100 sq cm, or each additional 1% of body area of infants and children, or part thereof (List separately in addition to code for primary procedure)

(Use 15152 in conjunction with 15151)

● New Code   ▲ Revised Code   ✛ Add-On Code   ⊘ Modifier -51 Exempt   ★ Telemedicine

15155   Tissue cultured skin autograft, face, scalp, eyelids, mouth, neck, ears, orbits, genitalia, hands, feet, and/or multiple digits; first 25 sq cm or less

+ **15156**   additional 1 sq cm to 75 sq cm (List separately in addition to code for primary procedure)

     (Do not report 15156 more than once per session)

     (Use 15156 in conjunction with 15155)

+ **15157**   each additional 100 sq cm, or each additional 1% of body area of infants and children, or part thereof (List separately in addition to code for primary procedure)

     (Use 15157 in conjunction with 15156)

15200   Full thickness graft, free, including direct closure of donor site, trunk; 20 sq cm or less

+ **15201**   each additional 20 sq cm or part thereof (List separately in addition to code for primary procedure)

     (Use 15201 in conjunction with 15200)

15220   Full thickness graft, free, including direct closure of donor site, scalp, arms, and/or legs; 20 sq cm or less

+ **15221**   each additional 20 sq cm or part thereof (List separately in addition to code for primary procedure)

     (Use 15221 in conjunction with 15220)

15240   Full thickness graft, free, including direct closure of donor site, forehead, cheeks, chin, mouth, neck, axillae, genitalia, hands, and/or feet; 20 sq cm or less

     (For finger tip graft, use 15050)

     (For repair of syndactyly, fingers, see 26560-26562)

+ **15241**   each additional 20 sq cm or part thereof (List separately in addition to code for primary procedure)

     (Use 15241 in conjunction with code 15240)

15260   Full thickness graft, free, including direct closure of donor site, nose, ears, eyelids, and/or lips; 20 sq cm or less

+ **15261**   each additional 20 sq cm or part thereof (List separately in addition to code for primary procedure)

     (Use 15261 in conjunction with code 15260)

     (For eyelids, see also 67961-67975)

     (Repair of donor site requiring skin graft or local flaps is considered a separate procedure)

Skin Substitute Grafts

The supply of skin substitute graft(s) should be reported separately in conjunction with 15271-15278. For biologic implant for soft tissue reinforcement, use 15777 in conjunction with code for primary procedure.

15271   Application of skin substitute graft to trunk, arms, legs, total wound surface area up to 100 sq cm; first 25 sq cm or less wound surface area

+ **15272**   each additional 25 sq cm wound surface area, or part thereof (List separately in addition to code for primary procedure)

     (Use 15272 in conjunction with 15271)

     (For total wound surface area greater than or equal to 100 sq cm, see 15273, 15274)

     (Do not report 15271, 15272 in conjunction with 15273, 15274)

15273 Application of skin substitute graft to trunk, arms, legs, total wound surface area greater than or equal to 100 sq cm; first 100 sq cm wound surface area, or 1% of body area of infants and children

+ 15274 each additional 100 sq cm wound surface area, or part thereof, or each additional 1% of body area of infants and children, or part thereof (List separately in addition to code for primary procedure)

(Use 15274 in conjunction with 15273)

(For total wound surface area up to 100 sq cm, see 15271, 15272)

15275 Application of skin substitute graft to face, scalp, eyelids, mouth, neck, ears, orbits, genitalia, hands, feet, and/or multiple digits, total wound surface area up to 100 sq cm; first 25 sq cm or less wound surface area

+ 15276 each additional 25 sq cm wound surface area, or part thereof (List separately in addition to code for primary procedure)

(Use 15276 in conjunction with 15275)

(For total wound surface area greater than or equal to 100 sq cm, see 15277, 15278)

(Do not report 15275, 15276 in conjunction with 15277, 15278)

15277 Application of skin substitute graft to face, scalp, eyelids, mouth, neck, ears, orbits, genitalia, hands, feet, and/or multiple digits, total wound surface area greater than or equal to 100 sq cm; first 100 sq cm wound surface area, or 1% of body area of infants and children

+ 15278 each additional 100 sq cm wound surface area, or part thereof, or each additional 1% of body area of infants and children, or part thereof (List separately in addition to code for primary procedure)

(Use 15278 in conjunction with 15277)

(For total wound surface area up to 100 sq cm, see 15275, 15276)

(Do not report 15271-15278 in conjunction with 97602)

FLAPS (SKIN AND/OR DEEP TISSUES)

The regions listed refer to the recipient area (not the donor site) when a flap is being attached in a transfer or to a final site.

The regions listed refer to a donor site when a tube is formed for later transfer or when a "delay" of flap occurs prior to the transfer. Codes 15733-15738 are described by donor site of the muscle, myocutaneous, or fasciocutaneous flap.

Codes 15570-15738 do not include extensive immobilization (eg., large plaster casts and other immobilizing devices are considered additional separate procedures).

A repair of a donor site requiring a skin graft or local flaps is considered an additional separate procedure.

(For microvascular flaps, see 15756-15758)

(For flaps without inclusion of a vascular pedicle, see 15570-15576)

(For adjacent tissue transfer flaps, see 14000-14302)

15570 Formation of direct or tubed pedicle, with or without transfer; trunk

15572 scalp, arms, or legs

15574 forehead, cheeks, chin, mouth, neck, axillae, genitalia, hands or feet

15576 eyelids, nose, ears, lips, or intraoral

15600 Delay of flap or sectioning of flap (division and inset); at trunk

15610 at scalp, arms, or legs

15620   at forehead, cheeks, chin, neck, axillae, genitalia, hands, or feet

15630   at eyelids, nose, ears, or lips

15650   Transfer, intermediate, of any pedicle flap (eg, abdomen to wrist, Walking tube), any location

(For eyelids, nose, ears, or lips, see also anatomical area)

(For revision, defatting or rearranging of transferred pedicle flap or skin graft, see 13100-14302)

15730   Midface flap (ie, zygomaticofacial flap) with preservation of vascular pedicle(s)

15731   Forehead flap with preservation of vascular pedicle (eg, axial pattern flap, paramedian forehead flap)

(For muscle, myocutaneous, or fasciocutaneous flap of the head or neck, use 15733)

(**15732**   deleted 2017 [2018 edition]. To report myocutaneous or fasciocutaneous flap, use 15733.)

15733   Muscle, myocutaneous, or fasciocutaneous flap; head and neck with named vascular pedicle (ie, buccinators, genioglossus, temporalis, masseter, sternocleidomastoid, levator scapulae)

(For forehead flap with preservation of vascular pedicle, use 15731)

(For anterior pericranial flap on named vascular pedicle, for repair of extracranial defect, use 15731)

(For repair of head and neck defects using non-axial pattern advancement flaps [including lesion] and/or repair by adjacent tissue transfer or rearrangement [eg, Z-plasty, W-plasty, V-Y plasty, rotation flap, random island flap, advancement flap], see 14040, 14041, 14060, 14061, 14301, 14302)

15734   trunk

15736   upper extremity

15738   lower extremity

OTHER FLAPS AND GRAFTS

Code 15740 describes a cutaneous flap, transposed into a nearby but not immediately adjacent defect, with a pedicle that incorporates an anatomically named axial vessel into its design. The flap is typically transferred through a tunnel underneath the skin and sutured into its new position. The donor site is closed directly.

Neurovascular pedicle procedures are reported with 15750. This code includes not only skin but also a functional motor or sensory nerve(s). The flap serves to reinnervate a damaged portion of the body dependent on touch or movement (eg, thumb).

Repair of donor site requiring skin graft or local flaps should be reported as an additional procedure.

For random island flaps, V-Y subcutaneous flaps, advancement flaps, and other flaps from adjacent areas without clearly defined anatomically named axial vessels, see 14000-14302.

Code 15769 may be used to report autologous soft tissue grafts, such as fat, dermis, fascia, or other soft tissues, which are harvested from the patient using an excisional technique. The autologous soft tissue grafts are then placed into a defect during the same operation. Autologous grafts that are already defined in the CPT code set, including skin, bone, nerve, tendon, fascia lata or vessels, should be reported with the specific codes for each tissue type. For harvesting, preparation or injection(s) of platelet-rich plasma, use 0232T.

Codes 15771, 15772, 15773, 15774 may be used to report autologous fat grafting when the adipose cells are harvested via a liposuction technique, prepared with minimal manipulation, and then injected via cannula in multiple small aliquots to the defect. The regions listed refer to the recipient area (not the donor site). Volumes are based on total injectate. For multiple sites of injection, sum the total volume of injectate to anatomic sites that are grouped together into the same code descriptor. Do not report 11950, 11951, 11952, 11954 in conjunction with 15771, 15772, 15773, 15774, for the same anatomic site.

15740   Flap; island pedicle requiring identification and dissection of an anatomically named axial vessel

15750   neurovascular pedicle

15756   Free muscle or myocutaneous flap with microvascular anastomosis

(Do not report code 69990 in addition to code 15756)

15757   Free skin flap with microvascular anastomosis

(Do not report code 69990 in addition to code 15757)

15758   Free fascial flap with microvascular anastomosis

(Do not report code 69990 in addition to code 15758)

15760   Graft; composite (eg, full thickness of external ear or nasal ala), including primary closure, donor area

15769   This code is out of order. See page 242

15770   derma-fat-fascia

15769   Grafting of autologous soft tissue, other, harvested by direct excision (eg, fat, dermis, fascia)

(For injection[s] of platelet-rich plasma, use 0232T)

15771   Grafting of autologous fat harvested by liposuction technique to trunk, breasts, scalp, arms, and/or legs; 50 cc or less injectate

(Report 15771 only once per session)

+ **15772**   each additional 50 cc injectate, or part thereof (List separately in addition to code for primary procedure)

(Use 15772 in conjunction with 15771)

15773   Grafting of autologous fat harvested by liposuction technique to face, eyelids, mouth, neck, ears, orbits, genitalia, hands, and/or feet; 25 cc or less injectate

(Report 15773 only once per session)

+ **15774**   each additional 25 cc injectate, or part thereof (List separately in addition to code for primary procedure)

(Use 15774 in conjunction with 15773)

(Do not report 15769, 15771, 15772, 15773, 15774 in conjunction with 15876, 15877, 15878, 15879, 0232T, 0481T, 0489T, 0490T)

(For injection[s], autologous white blood cell concentrate [autologous protein solution], any site, including image guidance, harvesting and preparation, when performed, use 0481T)

15775   Punch graft for hair transplant; 1 to 15 punch grafts

15776   more than 15 punch grafts

(For strip transplant, use 15220)

+ **15777**   Implantation of biologic implant (eg, acellular dermal matrix) for soft tissue reinforcement (ie, breast, trunk) (List separately in addition to code for primary procedure)

(For implantation of biologic implants for soft tissue reinforcement in tissues other than breast and trunk, use 17999)

(For bilateral breast procedure, report 15777 twice. Do not report modifier 50 in conjunction with 15777)

(For implantation of mesh or other prosthesis for open incisional or ventral hernia repair, use 49568 in conjunction with 49560-49566)

(For insertion of mesh or other prosthesis for closure of a necrotizing soft tissue infectino wound, use 49568 in conjunction with 11004-11006)

(For topical application of skin substitute graft to a wound surface, see 15271-15278)

(For repair of anorectal fistula with plug (eg, porcine small intestine submucosa [SIS]), use 46707)

(For insertion of mesh or other prosthesis for repair of pelvic floor defect, use 57267)

(For implantation of non-biologic or synthetic implant for fascial reinforcement of the abdominal wall, use 0437T)

(The supply of biologic implant should be reported separately in conjunction with 15777)

OTHER PROCEDURES

15780   Dermabrasion; total face (eg, for acne scarring, fine wrinkling, rhytids, general keratosis)

15781   segmental, face

15782   regional, other than face

15783   superficial, any site, (eg, tattoo removal)

15786   Abrasion; single lesion (eg, keratosis, scar)

+ **15787**   each additional 4 lesions or less (List separately in addition to code for primary procedure)

(Use 15787 in conjunction with code 15786)

15788   Chemical peel, facial; epidermal

15789   dermal

15792   Chemical peel, nonfacial; epidermal

15793   dermal

15819   Cervicoplasty

15820   Blepharoplasty, lower eyelid;

15821   with extensive herniated fat pad

15822   Blepharoplasty, upper eyelid;

15823   with excessive skin weighting down lid

(For bilateral blepharoplasty, add modifier -50)

15824   Rhytidectomy; forehead

(For repair of brow ptosis, use 67900)

15825   neck with platysmal tightening (platysmal flap, P-flap)

15826   glabellar frown lines

15828   cheek, chin, and neck

15829   superficial musculoaponeurotic system (SMAS) flap

(For bilateral rhytidectomy, add modifier -50)

15830   Excision, excessive skin and subcutaneous tissue (includes lipectomy); abdomen, infraumbilical panniculectomy

(Do not report 15830 in conjunction with 12031-12037, 13100-13102, 14000, 14001, 14302 for the same wound)

15832   thigh

15833   leg

15834   hip

15835   buttock

15836   arm

15837   forearm or hand

15838   submental fat pad

15839   other area

(For bilateral procedure, add modifier -50)

15840   Graft for facial nerve paralysis; free fascia graft (including obtaining fascia)

(For bilateral procedure, add modifier -50)

15841   free muscle graft (including obtaining graft)

15842   free muscle flap by microsurgical technique

(Do not report code 69990 in addition to code 15842)

15845   regional muscle transfer

(For intravenous fluorescein examination of blood flow in graft or flap, use 15860)

(For nerve transfers, decompression, or repair, see 64831-64876, 64905, 64907, 69720, 69725, 69740, 69745, 69955)

+ **15847**   Excision, excessive skin and subcutaneous tissue (includes lipectomy), abdomen (eg, abdominoplasty) (includes umbilical transposition and fascial plication) (List separately in addition to code for primary procedure)

(Use 15847 in conjunction with 15830)

(For abdominal wall hernia repair, see 49491-49587)

(To report other abdominoplasty, use 17999)

15850   Removal of sutures under anesthesia (other than local), same surgeon

15851   Removal of sutures under anesthesia (other than local), other surgeon

15852   Dressing change (for other than burns) under anesthesia (other than local)

15860   Intravenous injection of agent (eg, fluorescein) to test vascular flow in flap or graft

---

● New Code   ▲ Revised Code   + Add-On Code   ⊘ Modifier -51 Exempt   ★ Telemedicine

15876 Suction assisted lipectomy; head and neck

15877 trunk

15878 upper extremity

15879 lower extremity

(Do not report 15876, 15877, 15878, 15879 in conjunction with 15771, 15772, 15773, 15774, 0489T, 0490T)

(For harvesting of adipose tissue for autologous adiposederived regenerative cell therapy, use 0489T)

(For autologous fat grafting harvested by liposuction technique, see 15771, 15772, 15773, 15774)

PRESSURE ULCERS (DECUBITUS ULCERS)

15920 Excision, coccygeal pressure ulcer, with coccygectomy; with primary suture

15922 with flap closure

15931 Excision, sacral pressure ulcer, with primary suture;

15933 with ostectomy

15934 Excision, sacral pressure ulcer, with skin flap closure;

15935 with ostectomy

15936 Excision, sacral pressure ulcer, in preparation for muscle or myocutaneous flap or skin graft closure;

15937 with ostectomy

(For repair of defect using muscle or myocutaneous flap, use code(s) 15734 and/or 15738 in addition to 15936, 15937. For repair of defect using split skin graft, use codes 15100 and/or 15101 in addition to 15936, 15937)

15940 Excision, ischial pressure ulcer, with primary suture;

15941 with ostectomy (ischiectomy)

15944 Excision, ischial pressure ulcer, with skin flap closure;

15945 with ostectomy

15946 Excision, ischial pressure ulcer, with ostectomy, in preparation for muscle or myocutaneous flap or skin graft closure

(For repair of defect using muscle or myocutaneous flap, use code(s) 15734 and/or 15738 in addition to 15946. For repair of defect using split skin graft, use codes 15100 and/or 15101 in addition to 15946)

15950 Excision, trochanteric pressure ulcer, with primary suture;

15951 with ostectomy

15952 Excision, trochanteric pressure ulcer, with skin flap closure;

15953 with ostectomy

15956 Excision, trochanteric pressure ulcer, in preparation for muscle or myocutaneous flap or skin graft closure;

Separate Procedure   Unlisted Procedure   CCI Comp. Code   Non-specific Procedure   **245**

15958   with ostectomy

(For repair of defect using muscle or myocutaneous flap, use code(s) 15734 and/or 15738 in addition to 15956, 15958. For repair of defect using split skin graft, use codes 15100 and/or 15101 in addition to 15956, 15958)

15999   Unlisted procedure, excision pressure ulcer

(For free skin graft to close ulcer or donor site, see 15002 et seq)

BURNS, LOCAL TREATMENT

Procedures 16000-16036 refer to local treatment of burned surface only. Codes 16020-16030 include the application of materials (eg, dressings) not described in 15100-15278.

List percentage of body surface involved and depth of burn.

For necessary related medical services (eg., hospital visits, detention) in management of burned patients, see appropriate services in E/M and Medicine sections.

For the application of skin grafts or skin substitutes, see 15100-15777.

(For fractional ablative laser fenestration for functional improvement of traumatic or burn scars, see 0479T, 0480T)

16000   Initial treatment, first degree burn, when no more than local treatment is required

16020   Dressings and/or debridement of partial-thickness burns, initial or subsequent; small (less than 5% total body surface area)

16025   medium (eg, whole face or whole extremity, or 5% to 10% total body surface area)

16030   large (eg, more than 1 extremity, or greater than 10% total body surface area)

16035   Escharotomy; initial incision

+ **16036**   each additional incision (List separately in addition to code for primary procedure)

(Use 16036 in conjunction with code 16035)

(For debridement, curettement of burn wound, see 16020-16030)

DESTRUCTION

Destruction means the ablation of benign, premalignant or malignant tissues by any method, with or without curetement, including local anesthesia, and not usually requiring closure.

Any method includes electrosurgery, cryosurgery, laser and chemical treatment. Lesions include condylomata, papillomata, molluscum contagiosum, herpetic lesions, warts (ie, common, plantar, flat), milia or other benign premalignant (eg., actinic keratoses), or malignant lesions.

(For destruction of lesion(s) in specific anatomic sites, see 40820, 46900-46917, 46924, 54050-54057, 54065, 56501, 56515, 57061, 57065, 67850, 68135)

(For laser treatment for inflammatory skin disease, see 96920-96922)

(For paring or cutting of benign hyperkeratotic lesions (eg, corns or calluses), see 11055-11057)

(For sharp removal or electrosurgical destruction of skin tags and fibrocutaneous tags, see 11200, 11201)

(For cryotherapy of acne, use 17340)

(For initiation or follow-up care of topical chemotherapy (eg, 5-FU or similar agents), see appropriate office visits)

(For shaving of epidermal or dermal lesions, see 11300-11313)

● New Code   ▲ Revised Code   + Add-On Code   ⊘ Modifier -51 Exempt   ★ Telemedicine

(For excision of cicatricial lesion[s] [eg, full thickness excision, through the dermis], see 11400-11446)

(For incisional removal of burn scar, see 16035, 16036)

(For fractional ablative laser fenestration for functional improvement of traumatic or burn scars, see 0479T, 0480T)

DESTRUCTION, BENIGN OR PREMALIGNANT LESIONS

17000   Destruction (eg, laser surgery, electrosurgery, cryosurgery, chemosurgery, surgical curettement), premalignant lesions (eg, actinic keratoses); first lesion

+ 17003   second through 14 lesions, each (List separately in addition to code for first lesion)

(Use 17003 in conjunction with 17000)

(For destruction of common or plantar warts, see 17110-17111)

17004   Destruction (eg, laser surgery, electrosurgery, cryosurgery, chemosurgery, surgical curettement), premalignant lesions (eg, actinic keratoses), 15 or more lesions

(Do not report 17004 in conjunction with codes 17000-17003)

17106   Destruction of cutaneous vascular proliferative lesions (eg, laser technique); less than 10 sq cm

17107   10.0 to 50.0 sq cm

17108   over 50.0 sq cm

17110   Destruction (eg, laser surgery, electrosurgery, cryosurgery, chemosurgery, surgical curettement), of benign lesions other than skin tags or cutaneous vascular proliferative lesions; up to 14 lesions

17111   15 or more lesions

(For destruction of extensive cutaneous neurofibroma over 50-100 lesions, see 0419T, 0420T)

17250   Chemical cauterization of granulation tissue (ie, proud flesh)

(Do not report 17250 with removal or excision codes for the same lesion)

(Do not report 17250 when chemical cauterization is used to achieve wound hemostasis)

(Do not report 17250 in conjunction with 97597, 97598, 97602 for the same lesion)

DESTRUCTION, MALIGNANT LESIONS, ANY METHOD

17260   Destruction, malignant lesion (eg, laser surgery, electrosurgery, cryosurgery, chemosurgery, surgical curettement), trunk, arms or legs; lesion diameter 0.5 cm or less

17261   lesion diameter 0.6 to 1.0 cm

17262   lesion diameter 1.1 to 2.0 cm

17263   lesion diameter 2.1 to 3.0 cm

17264   lesion diameter 3.1 to 4.0 cm

17266   lesion diameter over 4.0 cm

17270   Destruction, malignant lesion (eg, laser surgery, electrosurgery, cryosurgery, chemosurgery, surgical curettement), scalp, neck, hands, feet, genitalia; lesion diameter 0.5 cm or less

17271   lesion diameter 0.6 to 1.0 cm

17272	lesion diameter 1.1 to 2.0 cm
17273	lesion diameter 2.1 to 3.0 cm
17274	lesion diameter 3.1 to 4.0 cm
17276	lesion diameter over 4.0 cm
17280	Destruction, malignant lesion, (eg, laser surgery, electrosurgery, cryosurgery, chemosurgery, surgical curettement), face, ears, eyelids, nose, lips, mucous membrane; lesion diameter 0.5 cm or less
17281	lesion diameter 0.6 to 1.0 cm
17282	lesion diameter 1.1 to 2.0 cm
17283	lesion diameter 2.1 to 3.0 cm
17284	lesion diameter 3.1 to 4.0 cm
17286	lesion diameter over 4.0 cm

MOHS MICROGRAPHIC SURGERY

Mohs micrographic surgery is a technique for the removal of complex or ill-defined skin cancer with histologic examination of 100% of the surgical margins. It involves removing a skin cancer one layer at a time and examining these layers under a microscope immediately after they are removed. This procedure allows for a close examination of each layer of skin to detect cancer cells. It also allows a minimal amount of tissue to be removed while ensuring complete removal of all the cancer cells. A local anesthetic is injected into the skin before the surgery. The physician begins to remove the skin cancer and a small amount of healthy tissue, one layer of skin at a time. Each tissue layer is prepared and examined under the microscope for cancer cells. Surgery is complete when no more cancer cells are detected.

If repair is performed, use separate repair, flap, or graft codes. If a biopsy of a suspected skin cancer is performed on the same day as Mohs surgery because there was no prior pathology confirmation of a diagnosis, then report a diagnostic skin biopsy (11102, 11104, 11106) and frozen section pathology (88331) with modifier 59 to distinguish from the subsequent definitive surgical procedure of Mohs surgery.

(If additional special pathology procedures, stains or immunostains are required, see 88311-88314, 88342)

(Do not report 88314 in conjunction with 17311-17315 for routine frozen section stain (eg., hematoxylin and eosin, toluidine blue) performed during Mohs surgery. When a nonroutine histochemical stain on frozen tissue is utilized, report 88314 with modifier -59)

(Do not report 88302-88309 on the same specimen as part of the Mohs surgery)

17311	Mohs micrographic technique, including removal of all gross tumor, surgical excision of tissue specimens, mapping, color coding of specimens, microscopic examination of specimens by the surgeon, and histopathologic preparation including routine stain(s) (eg, hematoxylin and eosin, toluidine blue), head, neck, hands, feet, genitalia, or any location with surgery directly involving muscle, cartilage, bone, tendon, major nerves, or vessels; first stage, up to 5 tissue blocks
+ 17312	each additional stage after the first stage, up to 5 tissue blocks (List separately in addition to code for primary procedure)

(Use 17312 in conjunction with 17311)

17313	Mohs micrographic technique, including removal of all gross tumor, surgical excision of tissue specimens, mapping, color coding of specimens, microscopic examination of specimens by the surgeon, and histopathologic preparation including routine stain(s) (eg, hematoxylin and eosin, toluidine blue), of the trunk, arms, or legs; first stage, up to 5 tissue blocks
+ 17314	each additional stage after the first stage, up to 5 tissue blocks (List separately in addition to code for primary procedure)

● New Code   ▲ Revised Code   + Add-On Code   ⊘ Modifier -51 Exempt   ★ Telemedicine

(Use 17314 in conjunction with 17313)

+ 17315   Mohs micrographic technique, including removal of all gross tumor, surgical excision of tissue specimens, mapping, color coding of specimens, microscopic examination of specimens by the surgeon, and histopathologic preparation including routine stain(s) (eg, hematoxylin and eosin, toluidine blue), each additional block after the first 5 tissue blocks, any stage (List separately in addition to code for primary procedure)

(Use 17315 in conjunction with 17311-17314)

OTHER PROCEDURES

17340   Cryotherapy (CO_2 slush, liquid N_2) for acne

17360   Chemical exfoliation for acne (eg, acne paste, acid)

17380   Electrolysis epilation, each 1/2 hour

(For actinotherapy, use 96900)

17999   Unlisted procedure, skin, mucous membrane and subcutaneous tissue

BREAST

Fine needle aspiration biopsies, core biopsies, open incisional or excisional biopsies, and related procedures performed to procure tissue from a lesion for which an established diagnosis exists are not to be reported separately at the time of a lesion excision unless performed on a different lesion or on the contralateral breast. However, if a diagnosis is not established, and the decision to perform the excision or mastectomy is dependent on the results of the biopsy, then the biopsy is separately reported. Modifier -58 may be used appropriately to indicate that the biopsy and the excision or mastectomy are staged or planned procedures.

Because excision of lesions occurs in the course of performing a mastectomy, breast excisions are not separately reported from a mastectomy unless performed to establish the malignant diagnosis before proceeding to the mastectomy. Specifically CPT codes 19110-19126 (breast excision) are in general included in all mastectomy CPT codes 19140-19240 of the same side. However, if the excision is performed to obtain tissue to determine pathologic diagnosis of malignancy prior to proceeding to a mastectomy, the excision is separately reportable with the mastectomy. Modifier -58 should be utilized in this situation.

Use of other integumentary codes for incision and closure are included in the codes describing various breast excision or mastectomy codes. Because of the frequent need to excise lymph node or muscle tissue in conjunction with mastectomies, these procedures have been included in the CPT coding for mastectomy. It would be inappropriate to separately report ipsilateral lymph node excision in conjunction with the appropriate mastectomy codes. However, sentinel lymph node biopsy is separately reported when performed prior to a localized excision of breast or a mastectomy with or without lymphadenectomy.

Open biopsy or excision of sentinel lymph node(s) should be reported as follows: axillary (CPT codes 38500 or 38525), deep cervical (CPT code 38510), internal mammary (CPT code 38530). (CPT code 38740 (axillary lymphadenectomy; superficial) should not be reported for a sentinel lymph node biopsy. Sentinel lymph node biopsy of superficial axillary lymph node(s) is correctly reported as CPT code 38500 (biopsy or excision of lymph node(s), superficial) which includes the removal of one or more discretely identified superficial lymph nodes. By contrast a superficial axillary lymphadenectomy (CPT code 38740) requires removal of all superficial axillary adipose tissue with all lymph nodes in this adipose tissue.)

In the circumstance where a breast lesion is identified and it is determined to be medically necessary to biopsy or excise the contralateral lymph nodes, use of the biopsy or lymph node dissection codes (using the appropriate anatomic modifier, -LT or -RT for left or right) would be acceptable. Additionally, breast reconstruction codes that include the insertion of a prosthetic implant are not to be reported with CPT codes that describe the insertion of a breast prosthesis only.

The CPT coding for breast procedures generally refers to unilateral procedures; when performed bilaterally, modifier -50 would be appropriate. This is identified parenthetically, where appropriate, in the CPT narrative.

INCISION

19000   Puncture aspiration of cyst of breast;

+ 19001   each additional cyst (List separately in addition to code for primary procedure)

| Separate Procedure | Unlisted Procedure | CCI Comp. Code | Non-specific Procedure | **249** |

(Use 19001 in conjunction with code 19000)

(If imaging guidance is performed, see 76942, 77021)

19020   Mastotomy with exploration or drainage of abscess, deep

19030   Injection procedure only for mammary ductogram or galactogram

(For radiological supervision and interpretation, see 77053, 77054)

Breast biopsy procedures may be performed via a percutaneous or open approach and with or without imaging guidance.

Percutaneous image-guided breast biopsies, including the placement of breast localization device(s), when performed, are reported with 19081, 19082, 19083, 19084, 19085, 19086. Imaging codes 76098, 76942, 77002, 77021 may not be separately reported for the same lesion. When more than one percutaneous breast biopsy with or without localization device placement is performed using the same imaging modality, use an addon code whether the additional service(s) is on the same or contralateral breast. If additional percutaneous biopsies with or without localization device placements are performed using different imaging modalities, report another primary code for each additional biopsy with or without localization device placement performed using a different image guidance modality.

To report bilateral image-guided breast biopsies, report 19081, 19083, 19085 for the initial biopsy. The contralateral and each additional breast image-guided biopsy are then reported with 19082, 19084, 19086.

Percutaneous breast biopsies without imaging guidance are reported with 19100.

Open incisional breast biopsy (19101) does not include imaging guidance. However, if an open incisional biopsy is performed after image-guided placement of a localization device, the appropriate image-guided localization device placement code (19281, 19282, 19283, 19284, 19285, 19286, 19287, 19288) may also be reported.

Percutaneous cryosurgical ablation of a fibroadenoma (19105) includes ultrasound guidance and, therefore, 76940, 76942 may not be separately reported. Code 19105 may only be reported once per cryoprobe insertion site, even if several adjacent lesions are ablated.

Open excision of a breast lesion (eg, lesions of breast duct[s], cyst[s], benign or malignant tumor[s]), without specific attention to adequate surgical margins, with or without the preoperative placement of radiological markers are reported with 19110, 19112, 19120, 19125, 19126. If an open excision of a breast lesion is performed after image-guided placement of a localization device, the appropriate image-guided localization device placement code (19281, 19282, 19283, 19284, 19285, 19286, 19287, 19288) may also be reported.

To report bilateral procedures for 19100, 19101, 19105, 19110, 19112, 19120, report modifier 50 with the procedure code.

19081   Biopsy, breast, with placement of breast localization device(s) (eg, clip, metallic pellet), when performed, and imaging of the biopsy specimen, when performed, percutaneous; first lesion, including stereotactic guidance

+ 19082   each additional lesion, including stereotactic guidance (List separately in addition to code for primary procedure)

(Use 19082 in conjunction with 19081)

19083   Biopsy, breast, with placement of breast localization device(s) (eg, clip, metallic pellet), when performed, and imaging of the biopsy specimen, when performed, percutaneous; first lesion, including ultrasound guidance

+ 19084   each additional lesion, including ultrasound guidance (List separately in addition to code for primary procedure)

(Use 19084 in conjunction with 19083)

19085   Biopsy, breast, with placement of breast localization device(s) (eg, clip, metallic pellet), when performed, and imaging of the biopsy specimen, when performed, percutaneous; first lesion, including magnetic resonance guidance

+ 19086   each additional lesion, including magnetic resonance guidance (List separately in addition to code for primary procedure)

     (Use 19086 in conjunction with 19085)

     (Do not report 19081-19086 in conjunction with 19281-19288, 76098, 76942, 77002, 77021 for same lesion)

19100   Biopsy of breast; percutaneous, needle core, not using imaging guidance (separate procedure)

     (For fine needle aspiration biopsy, see 10004, 10005, 10006, 10007, 10008, 10009, 10010, 10011, 10012, 10021)

19101   open, incisional

     (For placement of percutaneous localization clip with imaging guidance, see 19281-19288)

19105   Ablation, cryosurgical, of fibroadenoma, including ultrasound guidance, each fibroadenoma

     (Do not report 19105 in conjunction with 76940, 76942)

     (For cryoablation of malignant breast tumor[s], use 0581T)

     (For adjacent lesions treated with one cryoprobe insertion, report once)

19110   Nipple exploration, with or without excision of a solitary lactiferous duct or a papilloma lactiferous duct

19112   Excision of lactiferous duct fistula

19120   Excision of cyst, fibroadenoma, or other benign or malignant tumor, aberrant breast tissue, duct lesion, nipple or areolar lesion (except 19300), open, male or female, 1 or more lesions

19125   Excision of breast lesion identified by preoperative placement of radiological marker, open; single lesion

+ 19126   each additional lesion separately identified by a preoperative radiological marker (List separately in addition to code for primary procedure)

     (Use 19126 in conjunction with code 19125)

     (Intraoperative placement of clip[s] is not separately reported)

(19260   deleted 2019 [2020 Edition]. To report, use 21601)

(19271   deleted 2019 [2020 Edition]. To report, use 21602)

(19272   deleted 2019 [2020 Edition]. To report, use 21603)

INTRODUCTION

Percutaneous image-guided placement of breast localization device(s) without image-guided breast biopsy(ies) is reported with 19281, 19282, 19283, 19284, 19285, 19286, 19287, 19288. When more than one localization device placement without image-guided biopsy is performed using the same imaging modality, report an add-on code whether the additional service(s) is on the same or contralateral breast. If additional localization device placements without image-guided biopsy(ies) are performed using different imaging modalities, report another primary code for each additional localization device placement without imageguided biopsy performed using a different image guidance modality.

To report bilateral image-guided placement of localization devices report 19281, 19283, 19285, or 19287 for the initial lesion localized. The contra-lateral and each additional breast image-guided localization device placement is reported with code 19282, 19284, 19286 or 19288.

When an open breast biopsy or open excision of a breast lesion is performed after image-guided percutaneous placement of a localization device, the appropriate image-guided localization device placement code (19281, 19282, 19283, 19284, 19285, 19286, 19287, 19288) may also be reported.

Code 19294 is used to report the preparation of the tumor cavity with placement of an intraoperative radiation therapy applicator concurrent with partial mastectomy (19301, 19302).

Codes 19296, 19297, 19298 describe placement of radiotherapy catheters (afterloading expandable or afterloading brachytherapy) into the breast for interstitial radioelement application either concurrent or on a separate date from a partial mastectomy procedure. Imaging guidance is included and may not be separately reported.

19281 Placement of breast localization device(s) (eg, clip, metallic pellet, wire/needle, radioactive seeds), percutaneous; first lesion, including mammographic guidance

+ **19282** each additional lesion, including mammographic guidance (List separately in addition to code for primary procedure)

(Use 19282 in conjunction with 19281)

19283 Placement of breast localization device(s) (eg, clip, metallic pellet, wire/needle, radioactive seeds), percutaneous; first lesion, including stereotactic guidance

+ **19284** each additional lesion, including stereotactic guidance (List separately in addition to code for primary procedure)

(Use 19284 in conjunction with 19283)

19285 Placement of breast localization device(s) (eg, clip, metallic pellet, wire/needle, radioactive seeds), percutaneous; first lesion including ultrasound guidance

+ **19286** each additional lesion, including ultrasound guidance (List separately in addition to code for primary procedure)

(Use 19286 in conjunction with 19285)

19287 Placement of breast localization device(s) (eg, clip, metallic pellet, wire/needle, radioactive seeds), percutaneous; first lesion, including magnetic resonance guidance

+ **19288** each additional lesion, including magnetic resonance guidance (List separately in addition to code for primary procedure)

(Use 19288 in conjunction with 19287)

(Do not report 19281-19288 in conjunction with 19081-19086, 76942, 77002, 77021 for same lesion)

(For surgical specimen radiography, use 76098)

(To report image-guided placement of breast localization devices during image-guided biopsy, see 19081-19086. To report image-guided placement of breast localization devices without image-guided biopsy, see 19281-19288)

+ **19294** Preparation of tumor cavity, with placement of a radiation therapy applicator for intraoperative radiation therapy (IORT) concurrent with partial mastectomy (List separately in addition to code for primary procedure)

(Use 19294 in conjunction with 19301, 19302)

19296 Placement of radiotherapy afterloading expandable catheter (single or multichannel) into the breast for interstitial radioelement application following partial mastectomy, includes imaging guidance; on date separate from partial mastectomy

+ **19297** concurrent with partial mastectomy (List separately in addition to code for primary procedure)

(Use 19297 in conjunction with 19160 or 19162)

19298 Placement of radiotherapy after loading brachytherapy catheters (multiple tube and button type) into the breast for interstitial radioelement application following (at the time of or subsequent to) partial mastectomy, includes imaging guidance

---

● New Code   ▲ Revised Code   + Add-On Code   ⊘ Modifier -51 Exempt   ★ Telemedicine

MASTECTOMY PROCEDURES

Mastectomy procedures (with the exception of gynecomastia [19300]) are performed either for treatment or prevention of breast cancer.

Code 19301 describes a partial mastectomy where only a portion of the ipsilateral breast tissue is removed (eg, lumpectomy, tylectomy, quadrantectomy, segmentectomy). When a complete axillary lymphadenectomy is performed in addition to a partial mastectomy, report 19302. When breast tissue is removed for breast-size reduction and not for treatment or prevention of breast cancer, report 19318 (reduction mammaplasty).

Code 19303 describes total removal of ipsilateral breast tissue with or without removal of skin and/or nipples (eg, nipple-sparing), for treatment or prevention of breast cancer. Code 19303 does not include excision of pectoral muscle(s) and/or axillary and internal mammary lymph nodes. When a total mastectomy is performed for gynecomastia, report 19300.

Codes 19305, 19306, 19307 describe radical procedures that include total removal of the ipsilateral breast tissue, including the nipple for treatment of breast cancer and excision of pectoral muscle(s) and/or axillary lymph nodes and/or internal mammary lymph nodes.

To report bilateral procedures for 19300, 19301, 19302, 19303, 19305, 19306, 19307, report modifier 50 with the procedure code.

19300   Mastectomy for gynecomastia

(For breast tissue removed for breast-size reduction for other than gynecomastia, use 19318)

19301   Mastectomy, partial (eg, lumpectomy, tylectomy, quadrantectomy, segmentectomy);

19302   with axillary lymphadenectomy

(For placement of radiotherapy afterloading balloon/brachytherapy catheters, see 19296-19298)

(Intraoperative placement of clip[s] is not separately reported)

(For the preparation of tumor cavity with placement of an intraoperative radiation therapy applicator concurrent with partial mastectomy, use 19294)

(For radiofrequency spectroscopy, real time, intraoperative margin assessment, at the time of partial mastectomy, with report, use 0546T)

19303   Mastectomy, simple, complete

(Intraoperative placement of clip[s] is not separately reported)

(For immediate or delayed insertion of implant, see 19340, 19342)

(For gynecomastia, use 19300)

(19304   deleted 2019 [2020 Edition])

(For breast tissue removed for breast-size reduction for gynecomastia, use 19300)

(For breast tissue removed for breast-size reduction for other than gynecomastia, use 19318)

19305   Mastectomy, radical, including pectoral muscles, axillary lymph nodes

(Intraoperative placement of clip[s] is not separately reported)

(For immediate or delayed insertion of implant, see 19340, 19342)

19306   Mastectomy, radical, including pectoral muscles, axillary and internal mammary lymph nodes (Urban type operation)

(Intraoperative placement of clip[s] is not separately reported)

(For immediate or delayed insertion of implant, see 19340, 19342)

19307 Mastectomy, modified radical, including axillary lymph nodes, with or without pectoralis minor muscle, but excluding pectoralis major muscle

(Intraoperative placement of clip[s] is not separately reported)

(For immediate or delayed insertion of implant, see 19340, 19342)

REPAIR AND/OR RECONSTRUCTION

Breast reconstruction is performed to repair defects due to congenital anomaly or loss of breast tissue after a surgical excision. The goal of breast reconstruction is to correct the anatomic defect and to restore form and breast symmetry. A breast can be reconstructed using a single technique or a combination of techniques, and each technique can stand alone. In addition, both breasts may be reconstructed at the same time, but may use different techniques or a combination of techniques. In many instances breast reconstruction requires more than one planned procedure or may require revisions.

The native breast may be altered using different techniques. The breast and breast mound can be lifted with a mastopexy (19316), reduced in volume with a breast reduction (19318), or augmented with a breast implant (19325).

Post-mastectomy breast reconstruction may be performed using a variety of techniques. An implant-based reconstruction involves placement of a device filled with fluid (eg, saline, silicone gel) to provide volume to the breast. In immediate reconstruction, an implant is primarily placed at the time of a mastectomy (19340). In delayed reconstruction, an implant is placed at any date separate from the mastectomy (19342). This includes placement of any new implant or replacement of an existing implant within the mastectomy defect or reconstructed breast. The removal of an intact breast implant for replacement is included in 19342.

A breast implant cannot always be placed due to the lack of an adequate skin envelope. Code 19357 describes insertion of a tissue expander, which is a device that is surgically implanted to create an adequately sized pocket for subsequent insertion of a permanent implant. A tissue expander is an inflatable device placed beneath the skin and chest muscle, into which saline is injected over a period of weeks in the office to create the implant pocket. The tissue expander is eventually removed and may be replaced with a permanent breast implant (11970). Placement of either a breast implant (19340, 19342) or tissue expander (19357) may be reported separately when performed with flap reconstruction (19361, 19364, 19367, 19368, 19369).

Code 11970 describes the removal of a tissue expander with concurrent insertion of a permanent breast implant. Code 11970 includes removal of the expander, minor revisions to the breast capsule and placement of the new breast implant. Code 19370 may be reported in addition to 11970 if more extensive capsular revision is performed. Code 11971 describes the removal of a tissue expander without the replacement of an expander or implant.

Autologous breast reconstruction involves harvesting a flap of skin, subcutaneous fat and/or muscle from one area of the body and relocating the tissue to the anterior chest to create a new breast mound. Flap reconstruction may be performed at the time of mastectomy or in a delayed fashion depending on patient preference and other oncologic treatments.

Code 19361 describes breast reconstruction with a flap composed of the latissimus dorsi muscle including some of the overlying skin and subcutaneous fat to reconstruct the breast mound. This flap is left on its vascular pedicle and tunneled beneath the armpit skin to the anterior chest to rebuild the breast. The blood supply to the flap is left attached to its origin in the axilla. To give the breast mound additional volume, a tissue expander or permanent breast implant may be placed beneath the latissimus flap. Placement of either a breast implant (19340, 19342) or tissue expander (19357) may be reported separately.

Code 19364 describes a microsurgical free tissue transfer of skin and subcutaneous fat and/or muscle for breast reconstruction. This code includes the flap harvest, microsurgical anastomosis of one artery and two veins with use of an operating microscope, flap inset as a breast mound, and donor-site closure. Typical free flaps include free transverse rectus abdominis myocutaneous (f TRAM), deep inferior epigastric perforator (DIEP), superficial inferior epigastric artery (SIEA), or gluteal artery perforator (GAP) flaps.

Code 19367 describes a single-pedicled transverse rectus abdominis myocutaneous (TRAM) flap, in which skin, subcutaneous fat, and a large portion of the rectus abdominis muscle from the lower abdomen is moved beneath the upper abdominal wall skin up to the chest to rebuild the breast. The blood supply to the flap is left attached to its origin in the abdomen.

Code 19368 describes "supercharging" of a singlepedicled TRAM flap. This is typically performed to increase blood flow in TRAM flaps with marginal circulation to ensure flap survival. In addition to the standard unipedicle TRAM procedure, the inferior epigastric artery and/or veins are also anastomosed to recipient vessels in the chest using microsurgical techniques.

Code 19369 describes a bipedicled TRAM flap in which skin, subcutaneous fat, and both rectus muscles are harvested for the reconstruction of a single breast. The dual-blood supply to the flap is left attached to its origins in the abdomen.

Secondary and ancillary breast-reconstruction procedures include nipple reconstruction (19350), implant adjustments through revisions to the breast capsule (19370), or removal of the entire breast capsule via a complete capsulectomy (19371) to achieve correct breast tissue positioning. In addition, procedures may be performed on the contralateral breast to create symmetry (19316, 19318, 19325). Removal of an intact breast implant without replacement is reported with 19328. Removal of a ruptured breast implant, including the implant contents, is reported with 19330. A complete capsulectomy (19371) includes removal of the breast implant and all intracapsular contents.

Code 19380 describes a revision of a reconstructed breast, including significant excision of tissue re-advancement or re-inset of flaps. For autologous reconstruction, 19380 includes revisions of the flap position on the chest wall, removal of portions of the flap (via direct excision or liposuction), re-shaping of the flap, or scar revisions. However, if a limited procedure is performed with a defined code (eg, scar revision) then the more specific code should be used. The placement of a new implant (19342) or autologous fat grafting for increased volume (15771, 15772) may be separately reportable. For implant-based reconstruction, 19380 includes revisions to the skin and capsule when performed together. The exchange for a new or different size/shape/type of implant (19342) or autologous fat grafting for increased volume/contour irregularities (15771, 15772) may be reported separately. Nipple reconstruction is reported with 19350 and includes local flaps (14000, 14001), areolar skin grafting (15100, 15200, 15201), and subsequent tattooing (11920, 11921, 11922).

Code 19396 describes the formation of a moulage cast ofa patient's chest defect. The mold is used to fabricate aspecific, custom-made implant that fits the patient'sdefect.

(To report bilateral procedures, report modifier -50 with the procedure code)

(For biologic implant for soft tissue reinforcement, use 15777 in conjunction with primary procedure)

19316 Mastopexy

▲ **19318** Breast reduction

(**19324** deleted 2020 [2021 edition]. To report breast augmentation with fat grafting, see 15771, 15772)

▲ **19325** Breast augmentation with implant

(For fat grafting performed in conjunction with 19325, see 15771, 15772)

▲ **19328** Removal of intact breast implant

(Do not report 19328 for removal of tissue expander)

(Do not report 19328 in conjunction with 19370)

(For removal of tissue expander with placement of breast implant, use 11970)

(For removal of tissue expander without replacement, use 11971)

▲ **19330** Removal of ruptured breast implant, including implant contents (eg, saline, silicone gel)

(Do not report 19330 for removal of ruptured tissue expander)

(For removal of ruptured tissue expander with placement of breast implant, use 11970)

(For removal of ruptured tissue expander without replacement, use 11971)

(For placement of new breast implant during same operative session, use 19342)

▲ **19340** Insertion of breast implant on same day of mastectomy (ie, immediate)

▲ **19342** Insertion or replacement of breast implant on separate day from mastectomy

(Do not report 19342 in conjunction with 19328 for removal of implant in same breast)

(For removal of tissue expander and replacement with breast implant, use 11970)

(For supply of implant, use 99070)

Separate Procedure   Unlisted Procedure   CCI Comp. Code   Non-specific Procedure   **255**

19350   Nipple/areola reconstruction

(Do not report 19350 in conjunction with 11920, 11921, 11922, 14000, 14001, 15100, 15200, 15201)

19355   Correction of inverted nipples

▲ **19357**   Tissue expander placement in breast reconstruction, including subsequent expansion(s)

▲ **19361**   Breast reconstruction; with latissimus dorsi flap

(For insertion of breast implant with latissimus dorsi flap on same day of mastectomy, use 19340)

(For insertion of breast implant with latissimus dorsi flap on day separate from mastectomy, use 19342)

(For insertion of tissue expander with latissimus dorsi flap, use 19357)

▲ **19364**   with free flap (eg, fTRAM, DIEP, SIEA, GAP flap)

(Do not report code 69990 in addition to code 19364)

(**19366**   deleted 2020 [2021 edition]).

▲ **19367**   with single-pedicled transverse rectus abdominis myocutaneous (TRAM) flap

▲ **19368**   with single-pedicled transverse rectus abdominis myocutaneous (TRAM) flap, requiring separate microvascular anastomosis (supercharging)

(Do not report code 69990 in addition to code 19368)

▲ **19369**   with bipedicled transverse rectus abdominis myocutaneous (TRAM) flap

(19361, 19364, 19367, 19368, 19369 include harvesting of the flap, closure of the donor site, insetting and shaping the flap)

▲ **19370**   Revision of peri-implant capsule, breast, including capsulotomy, capsulorrhaphy, and/or partial capsulectomy

(Do not report 19370 in conjunction with 19328 for removal and replacement of same implant to access capsule)

(For removal and replacement with new implant, use 19342)

▲ **19371**   Peri-implant capsulectomy, breast, complete, including removal of all intracapsular contents

(Do not report 19371 in conjunction with 19328, 19330)

(Do not report 19371 in conjunction with 19370 in same breast)

(For removal and replacement with new implant, use 19342)

▲ **19380**   Revision of reconstructed breast (eg, significant removal of tissue, re-advancement and/or re-inset of flaps in autologous reconstruction or significant capsular revision combined with soft tissue excision in implant-based reconstruction)

(Do not report 19380 in conjunction with 12031, 12032, 12034, 12035, 12036, 12037, 13100, 13101, 13102, 15877, 19316, 19318, 19370, for the same breast)

19396   Preparation of moulage for custom breast implant

OTHER PROCEDURES

19499   Unlisted procedure, breast

   ● New Code   ▲ Revised Code   + Add-On Code   ⊘ Modifier -51 Exempt   ★ Telemedicine

MUSCULOSKELETAL SYSTEM

Musculoskeletal procedure codes include the application and removal of the initial cast or traction device. Use codes in range 29000 to 29999 to report subsequent cast or traction-device applications. Review the instructional notes under the "Application of Casts and Strapping" to identify other uses for these codes.

The procedures and services listed in this section of the CPT coding system include the application and removal of the first cast or traction device only. Subsequent replacement of the cast and/or traction device may be coded using the cast and strapping procedure CPT codes appearing at the end of the section.

MISCELLANEOUS CODING RULES

Most bone, cartilage and fascia graft procedures include obtaining of the graft by the operating surgeon. When a surgical associate obtains the graft for the operating surgeon, the additional service should be coded and coded separately using CPT codes from the 20900-20926 range. In addition, a surgical modifier for assistant surgeon or co-surgeon should be included when reporting the associates services.

CPT codes 20100-20103 relate to treatment of wounds resulting from penetrating trauma (e.g., gunshot, stab wound). Use these codes for wound explorations only if the procedure does not require a thoracotomy or laparotomy and/or repairs to major structure(s) or major blood vessels.

The term "complicated" appears in some narratives in the musculoskeletal subsection. This term implies that an infection occurred, treatment was delayed, or the surgery took longer than usual to perform. Send supporting documentation when the codes containing this descriptor are assigned.

An intermediate repair associated with a musculoskeletal surgery is an integral portion of the surgery and should not be coded separately.

Code the injection codes according to the location of the joint injected or aspirated. Example: small joint = fingers, toes; intermediate joint = wrist, elbow; and major joint = shoulder, hip, or knee.

When removing a foreign body or performing soft tissue biopsy, determine the site and whether or not the foreign body/biopsy is superficial or deep.

FRACTURES

Remember to differentiate between the type of fracture and the type of treatment when coding fractures. Review the meanings of open and closed treatment of fractures. Dislocations must also be coded with emphasis on whether the treatment is open or closed.

When coding the re-reduction of a fracture and/or dislocation performed by the primary physician, add modifier -76 to the procedure code. If the re-reduction were performed by another physician, then modifier -77 would be added to the procedure code.

DEFINITIONS

In orthopedic medicine, fractures are classified as closed or open (compound) and simple or multi-fragmentary (formerly comminuted).

Closed treatment

Closed fractures are those in which the skin is intact, i.e. not surgically open. A closed reduction re-aligns a bone by manipulation without surgery. Sometimes it is not possible for the physician to get the bones in the right position with a closed reduction. If this happens, traction can be put on the bones to gently pull them into position. Traction is usually used for a short period of time and before other forms of treatment are used.

Open treatment

Open (compound) fractures involve wounds that communicate with the fracture and may expose bone to contamination. Open injuries carry an elevated risk of infection; they require antibiotic treatment and usually urgent surgical treatment (debridement). This involves removal of all dirt, contamination, and dead tissue. An open reduction and internal fixation of the bone requires an orthopedic surgeon. The surgery requires cutting open the skin of the area over the fracture so bone fragments can be put back

MUSC-SKEL 20000

into place and the bone fixated or held in place. The bone fragments are held in place with special screws or by attaching metal plates to the bone. Pins that go through the bone or rods that go inside the length of the bone are used to keep the bone in place.

Percutaneous skeletal fixation

Percutaneous skeletal fixation defines fracture treatment which is neither open or closed. Prior to fixation a closed reduction may be performed if necessary for alignment of the broken bones. Pins or screws are then put through the skin and bone above and below the fracture, usually under x-ray guidance. The pins or screws are connected to metal bars on the outside of the skin to form a frame around the fracture. This frame keeps the bone pieces in place.

Simple fractures

Simple fractures are fractures that occur along one line, splitting the bone into two pieces, while multi-fragmentary fractures involve the bone splitting into multiple pieces. A simple, closed fracture is much easier to treat and has a much better prognosis than an open, contaminated fracture. Other considerations in fracture care are displacement (fracture gap) and angulation. If angulation or displacement is large, reduction (manipulation) of the bone may be required and, in adults, frequently requires surgical care. These injuries may take longer to heal than injuries without displacement or angulation

Additional coding rules

- *Codes for obtaining autogenous bone grafts, cartilage, tendon, fascia lata grafts or other tissues through separate incisions are to be used only when the graft is not already listed as part of the basic procedure.*

- *Re-reduction of a fracture and/or dislocation performed in the primary physician may be identified by the addition of modifier -76 to the usual procedure.*

- *Codes for external fixation are to be used only when external fixation is not already listed as part of the basic procedure.*

GENERAL

INCISION

(**20005**   deleted 2018 [2019 Edition])

(For incision and drainage of subfascial soft tissue abscess, see appropriate incision and drainage for specific anatomic sites)

WOUND EXPLORATION—TRAUMA (EG, PENETRATING GUNSHOT, STAB WOUND)

20100-20103 relate to wound(s) resulting from penetrating trauma. These codes describe surgical exploration and enlargement of the wound, extension of dissection (to determine penetration), debridement, removal of foreign body(s), ligation or coagulation of minor subcutaneous and/or muscular blood vessel(s), of the subcutaneous tissue, muscle fascia, and/or muscle, not requiring thoracotomy or laparotomy. If a repair is done to major structure(s) or major blood vessel(s) requiring thoracotomy or laparotomy, then those specific code(s) would supersede the use of codes 20100-20103. To report simple, intermediate, or complex repair of wound(s) that do not require enlargement of the wound, extension of dissection, etc., as stated above, use specific Repair code(s) in the Integumentary System section.

20100   Exploration of penetrating wound (separate procedure); neck

20101   chest

20102   abdomen/flank/back

20103   extremity

EXCISION

20150   Excision of epiphyseal bar, with or without autogenous soft tissue graft obtained through same fascial incision

20200   Biopsy, muscle; superficial

20205   deep

● New Code   ▲ Revised Code   ✚ Add-On Code   ⊘ Modifier -51 Exempt   ★ Telemedicine

20206   Biopsy, muscle, percutaneous needle

(If imaging guidance is performed, see 76942, 77002, 77012, 77021)

(For fine needle aspiration biopsy, see 10004, 10005, 10006, 10007, 10008, 10009, 10010, 10011, 10012, 10021)

(For evaluation of fine needle aspirate, see 88172-88173)

(For excision of muscle tumor, deep, see specific anatomic section)

20220   Biopsy, bone, trocar, or needle; superficial (eg, ilium, sternum, spinous process, ribs)

20225   deep (eg, vertebral body, femur)

(Do not report 20225 in conjunction with 22510, 22511, 22512, 22513, 22514, 22515, 0200T, 0201T, when performed at the same level)

(For bone marrow biopsy[ies] and/or aspiration[s], see 38220, 38221, 38222)

(For radiologic supervision and interpretation, see 77002, 77012, 77021)

20240   Biopsy, bone, open; superficial (eg, sternum, spinous process, rib, patella, olecranon process, calcaneus, tarsal, metatarsal, carpal, metacarpal, phalanx)

20245   deep (eg, humeral shaft, ischium, femoral shaft)

20250   Biopsy, vertebral body, open; thoracic

20251   lumbar or cervical

(For sequestrectomy, osteomyelitis or drainage of bone abscess, see anatomical area)

INTRODUCTION OR REMOVAL

(For injection procedure for arthrography, see anatomical area)

(For injection of autologous adipose-derived regenerative cells, see 0489T, 0490T)

20500   Injection of sinus tract; therapeutic (separate procedure)

20501   diagnostic (sinogram)

(For radiological supervision and interpretation, use 76080)

(For contrast injection[s] and radiological assessment of gastrostomy, duodenostomy, jejunostomy, gastrojejunostomy, or cecostomy [or other colonic] tube including fluoroscopic imaging guidance, use 49465)

20520   Removal of foreign body in muscle or tendon sheath; simple

20525   deep or complicated

20526   Injection, therapeutic (eg, local anesthetic, corticosteroid), carpal tunnel

20527   Injection, enzyme (eg, collagenase), palmar fascial cord (ie, Dupuytren's contracture)

(For manipulation of palmar fascial cord (ie, Dupuytren's cord) post enzyme injection (eg, collagenase), use 26341)

20550   Injection(s); single tendon sheath, or ligament, aponeurosis (eg, plantar "fascia")

(For injection of Morton's neuroma, see 64455, 64632)

20551   single tendon origin/insertion

(Do not report 20550, 20551 in conjunction with 0232T, 0481T)

(For harvesting, preparation, and injection[s] of platelet-rich plasma, use 0232T)

20552 Injection(s); single or multiple trigger point(s), 1 or 2 muscle(s)

20553 single or multiple trigger point(s), 3 or more muscle(s)

(Do not report 20552, 20553 in conjunction with 20560, 20561 for the same muscle[s])

(If imaging guidance is performed, see 76942, 77002, 77021)

20560 Needle insertion(s) without injection(s); 1 or 2 muscle(s)

20561 3 or more muscles

20555 Placement of needles or catheters into muscle and/or soft tissue for subsequent interstitial radioelement application (at the time of or subsequent to the procedure)

(For placement of devices into the breast for interstitial radioelement application, see 19296-19298)

(For placement of needles, catheters, or devices into muscle or soft tissue of the head and neck, for interstitial radioelement application, use 41019)

(For placement of needles or catheters for interstitial radioelement application into prostate, use 55875)

(For placement of needles or catheters into the pelvic organs or genitalia [except prostate] for interstitial radioelement application, use 55920)

(For interstitial radioelement application, see 77770, 77771, 77772, 77778)

(For imaging guidance, see 76942, 77002, 77012, 77021)

20560 This code is out of order. See page 260

20561 This code is out of order. See page 260

20600 Arthrocentesis, aspiration and/or injection, small joint or bursa (eg, fingers, toes); without ultrasound guidance

20604 with ultrasound guidance, with permanent recording and reporting

(Do not report 20600, 20604 in conjunction with 76942, 0489T, 0490T)

(If fluoroscopic, CT, or MRI guidance is performed, see 77002, 77012, 77021)

20605 Arthrocentesis, aspiration and/or injection, intermediate joint or bursa (eg, temporomandibular, acromioclavicular, wrist, elbow or ankle, olecranon bursa); without ultrasound guidance

20606 with ultrasound guidance, with permanent recording and reporting

(Do not report 20605, 20606 in conjunction with 76942)

(If fluoroscopic, CT, or MRI guidance is performed, see 77002, 77012, 77021)

20610 Arthrocentesis, aspiration and/or injection, major joint or bursa (eg, shoulder, hip, knee, subacromial bursa); without ultrasound guidance

20611 with ultrasound guidance, with permanent recording and reporting

(Do not report 20610, 20611 in conjunction with 27369, 76942)

(If fluoroscopic, CT, or MRI guidance is performed, see 77002, 77012, 77021)

20612 Aspiration and/or injection of ganglion cyst(s) any location

---

● New Code ▲ Revised Code + Add-On Code ⊘ Modifier -51 Exempt ★ Telemedicine

(To report multiple ganglion cyst aspirations/injections, use 20612 and append modifier -59)

20615   Aspiration and injection for treatment of bone cyst

20650   Insertion of wire or pin with application of skeletal traction, including removal (separate procedure)

20660   Application of cranial tongs, caliper, or stereotactic frame, including removal (separate procedure)

20661   Application of halo, including removal; cranial

20662   pelvic

20663   femoral

20664   Application of halo, including removal, cranial, 6 or more pins placed, for thin skull osteology (eg, pediatric patients, hydrocephalus, osteogenesis imperfecta)

20665   Removal of tongs or halo applied by another individual

20670   Removal of implant; superficial, (eg, buried wire, pin or rod) (separate procedure)

20680   deep (eg, buried wire, pin, screw, metal band, nail,rod or plate)

(For removal of sinus tarsi implant, use 0510T)

(For removal and reinsertion of sinus tarsi implant, use 0511T)

20690   Application of a uniplane (pins or wires in 1 plane), unilateral, external fixation system

20692   Application of a multiplane (pins or wires in more than 1 plane), unilateral, external fixation system (eg, Ilizarov, Monticelli type)

20693   Adjustment or revision of external fixation system requiring anesthesia (eg, new pin[s] or wire[s] and/or new ring[s] or bar[s])

20694   Removal, under anesthesia, of external fixation system

20696   Application of multiplane (pins or wires in more than 1 plane), unilateral, external fixation with stereotactic computer-assisted adjustment (eg, spatial frame), including imaging; initial and subsequent alignment(s), assessment(s), and computation(s) of adjustment schedule(s)

(Do not report 20696 in conjunction with 20692, 20697)

⊘ **20697**   exchange (ie, removal and replacement) of strut, each)

(Do not report 20697 in conjunction with 20692, 20696)

Manual preparation involves the mixing and preparation of antibiotics or other therapeutic agent(s) with a carrier substance by the physician or other qualified health care professional during the surgical procedure and then shaping the mixture into a drugdelivery device(s) (eg, beads, nails, spacers) for placement in the deep (eg, subfascial) intramedullary or intraarticular space(s). Codes 20700, 20702, 20704 are addon codes for the manual preparation and insertion of the drug-delivery device during the associated primary surgical procedure listed with each add-on code. Codes 20701, 20703, 20705 are add-on codes for the removal of drug-delivery device(s) during the associated primary surgical procedures listed in the parenthetical codes associated with each add-on code. Insertion of a prefabricated drug device(s) may not be reported with 20700, 20702, 20704. Report 20680, if removal of drugdelivery device(s) is performed alone. Report 20700, 20701, 20702, 20703, 20704, 20705 once per anatomic location.

+ **20700**   Manual preparation and insertion of drug-delivery device(s), deep (eg, subfascial) (List separately in addition to code for primary procedure)

(Use 20700 in conjunction with 11010, 11011, 11012, 11043, 11044, 11046, 11047, 20240, 20245, 20250, 20251, 21010, 21025, 21026, 21501, 21502, 21510, 21627, 21630, 22010, 22015, 23030, 23031, 23035,

23040, 23044, 23170, 23172, 23174, 23180, 23182, 23184, 23334, 23335, 23930, 23931, 23935, 24000, 24134, 24136, 24138, 24140, 24147, 24160, 25031, 25035, 25040, 25145, 25150, 25151, 26070, 26230, 26235, 26236, 26990, 26991, 26992, 27030, 27070, 27071, 27090, 27301, 27303, 27310, 27360, 27603, 27604, 27610, 27640, 27641, 28001, 28002, 28003, 28020, 28120, 28122)

(Do not report 20700 in conjunction with 11981)

+ **20701** Removal of drug-delivery device(s), deep (eg, subfascial)

(List separately in addition to code for primary procedure)

(Use 20701 in conjunction with 11010, 11011, 11012, 11043, 11044, 11046, 11047, 20240, 20245, 20250, 20251, 21010, 21025, 21026, 21501, 21502, 21510, 21627, 21630, 22010, 22015, 23030, 23031, 23035, 23040, 23044, 23170, 23172, 23174, 23180, 23182, 23184, 23334, 23335, 23930, 23931, 23935, 24000, 24134, 24136, 24138, 24140, 24147, 24160, 25031, 25035, 25040, 25145, 25150, 25151, 26070, 26230, 26235, 26236, 26990, 26991, 26992, 27030, 27070, 27071, 27090, 27301, 27303, 27310, 27360, 27603, 27604, 27610, 27640, 27641, 28001, 28002, 28003, 28020, 28120, 28122)

(Do not report 20701 in conjunction with 11982)

+ **20702** Manual preparation and insertion of drug-delivery device(s), intramedullary (List separately in addition to code for primary procedure

(Use 20702 in conjunction with 20680, 20690, 20692, 20694, 20802, 20805, 20838, 21510, 23035, 23170, 23180, 23184, 23515, 23615, 23935, 24134, 24138, 24140, 24147, 24430, 24516, 25035, 25145, 25150, 25151, 25400, 25515, 25525, 25526, 25545, 25574, 25575, 27245, 27259, 27360, 27470, 27506, 27640, 27720)

(Do not report 20702 in conjunction with 11981)

+ **20703** Removal of drug-delivery device(s), intramedullary (List separately in addition to code for primary procedure)

(Use 20703 in conjunction with 20690, 20692, 20694, 20802, 20805, 20838, 21510, 23035, 23170, 23180, 23184, 23515, 23615, 23935, 24134, 24138, 24140, 24147, 24430, 24516, 25035, 25145, 25150, 25151, 25400, 25515, 25525, 25526, 25545, 25574, 25575, 27245, 27259, 27360, 27470, 27506, 27640, 27720)

(Do not report 20703 in conjunction with 11982)

+ **20704** Manual preparation and insertion of drug-delivery device(s), intra-articular (List separately in addition to code for primary procedure)

(Use 20704 in conjunction with 22864, 22865, 23040, 23044, 23334, 24000, 24160, 25040, 25250, 25251, 26070, 26075, 26080, 26990, 27030, 27090, 27301, 27310, 27603, 27610, 28020)

(Do not report 20704 in conjunction with 11981, 27091, 27488)

+ **20705** Removal of drug-delivery device(s), intra-articular (List separately in addition to code for primary procedure)

(Use 20705 in conjunction with 22864, 22865, 23040, 23044, 23334, 24000, 24160, 25040, 25250, 25251, 26070, 26075, 26080, 26990, 27030, 27090, 27301, 27310, 27603, 27610, 28020)

(Do not report 20705 in conjunction with 11982, 23335, 27091, 27125, 27130, 27134, 27137, 27138, 27236, 27438, 27446, 27486, 27487, 27488)

REPLANTATION

20802 Replantation, arm (includes surgical neck of humerus through elbow joint), complete amputation

(To report replantation of incomplete arm amputation, see specific code(s) for repair of bone(s), ligament(s), tendon(s), nerve(s), or blood vessel(s) with modifier -52)

20805 Replantation, forearm (includes radius and ulna to radial carpal joint), complete amputation

(To report replantation of incomplete forearm amputation, see specific code(s) for repair of bone(s), ligament(s), tendon(s), nerve(s), or blood vessel(s) with modifier -52)

● New Code   ▲ Revised Code   + Add-On Code   ⊘ Modifier -51 Exempt   ★ Telemedicine

20808 Replantation, hand (includes hand through metacarpophalangeal joints), complete amputation

(To report replantation of incomplete hand amputation, see specific code(s) for repair of bone(s), ligament(s), tendon(s), nerve(s), or blood vessel(s) with modifier -52)

20816 Replantation, digit, excluding thumb (includes metacarpophalangeal joint to insertion of flexor sublimis tendon), complete amputation

(To report replantation of incomplete digit amputation excluding thumb, see specific code(s) for repair of bone(s), ligament(s), tendon(s), nerve(s), or blood vessel(s) with modifier -52)

20822 Replantation, digit, excluding thumb (includes distal tip to sublimis tendon insertion), complete amputation

(To report replantation of incomplete digit amputation excluding thumb, see specific code(s) for repair of bone(s), ligament(s), tendon(s), nerve(s), or blood vessel(s) with modifier -52)

20824 Replantation, thumb (includes carpometacarpal joint to MP joint), complete amputation

(To report replantation of incomplete thumb amputation, see specific code(s) for repair of bone(s), ligament(s), tendon(s), nerve(s), or blood vessel(s) with modifier -52)

20827 Replantation, thumb (includes distal tip to MP joint), complete amputation

(To report replantation of incomplete thumb amputation, see specific code(s) for repair of bone(s), ligament(s), tendon(s), nerve(s), or blood vessel(s) with modifier -52)

(To report replantation of complete leg amputation see specific code(s) for repair of bone(s), ligament(s), tendon(s), nerve(s), or blood vessel(s) with modifier -52)

(To report replantation of incomplete leg amputation, see specific code(s) for repair of bone(s), ligament(s), tendon(s), nerve(s), or blood vessel(s) with modifier -52)

20838 Replantation, foot, complete amputation

(To report replantation of incomplete foot amputation, see specific code(s) for repair of bone(s), ligament(s), tendon(s), nerve(s), or blood vessel(s) with modifier -52)

GRAFTS (OR IMPLANTS)

Codes for obtaining autogenous bone, cartilage, tendon, fascia lata grafts, bone marrow, or other tissues through separate skin/fascial incisions should be reported separately, unless the code descriptor references the harvesting of the graft or implant (eg, includes obtaining graft). Autologous grafts that are already defined in the CPT code set, including skin, bone, nerve, tendon, fascia lata, or vessels, should be reported with the more specific codes for each tissue type. Code 15769 may be used for other autologous soft tissue grafts harvested by direct excision. See 15771, 15772, 15773, 15774 for autologous fat grafting harvested by liposuction technique.

Do not append modifier 62 to bone graft codes 20900-20938.

(For spinal surgery bone graft(s) see codes 20930-20938)

20900 Bone graft, any donor area; minor or small (eg, dowel or button)

20902 major or large

20910 Cartilage graft; costochondral

20912 nasal septum

(For ear cartilage, use 21235)

20920 Fascia lata graft; by stripper

20922 by incision and area exposure, complex or sheet

20924 Tendon graft, from a distance (eg, palmaris, toe extensor, plantaris)

(**20926** deleted 2019 [2020 Edition])

(To report autologous soft tissue grafts harvested by direct excision, use 15769)

(To report autologous fat grafting harvested by liposuction technique, see 15771, 15772, 15773, 15774)

+ **20930** Allograft, morselized, or placement of osteopromotive material, for spine surgery only (List separately in addition to code for primary procedure)

(Use 20930 in conjunction with 22319, 22532, 22533, 22548-22558, 22590-22612, 22630, 22633, 22634, 22800-22812)

+ **20931** Allograft, structural, for spine surgery only (List separately in addition to code for primary procedure)

(Use 20931 in conjunction with 22319, 22532-22533, 22548-22558, 22590-22612, 22630, 22633, 22634, 22800-22812)

+ **20932** Allograft, includes templating, cutting, placement and internal fixation, when performed; osteoarticular, including articular surface and contiguous bone (List separately in addition to code for primary procedure)

(Do not report 20932 in conjunction with 20933, 20934, 23200, 24152, 27078, 27090, 27091, 27448, 27646, 27647, 27648)

+ **20933** hemicortical intercalary, partial (ie, hemicylindrical) (List separately in addition to code for primary procedure)

(Do not report 20933 in conjunction with 20932, 20934, 23200, 24152, 27078, 27090, 27091, 27448, 27646, 27647, 27648)

+ **20934** intercalary, complete (ie, cylindrical) (List separately in addition to code for primary procedure)

(Do not report 20934 in conjunction with 20932, 20933, 20955, 20956, 20957, 20962, 23146, 23156, 23200, 24116, 24126, 24152, 25126, 25136, 27078, 27090, 27091, 27130, 27132, 27134, 27138, 27236, 27244, 27356, 27448, 27638, 27646, 27647, 27648, 28103, 28107)

(Insertion of joint prosthesis may be separately reported)

(Use 20932, 20933, 20934 in conjunction with 23210, 23220, 24150, 25170, 27075, 27076, 27077, 27365, 27645, 27704)

+ **20936** Autograft for spine surgery only (includes harvesting the graft); local (eg, ribs, spinous process, or laminar fragments) obtained from same incision (List separately in addition to code for primary procedure)

(Use 20936 in conjunction with 22319, 22532, 22533, 22548-22558, 22590-22612, 22630, 22633, 22634, 22800-22812)

+ **20937** morselized (through separate skin or fascial incision) (List separately in addition to code for primary procedure)

(Use 20937 in conjunction with 22319, 22532, 22533, 22548-22558, 22590-22612, 22630, 22633, 22634, 22800-22812)

+ **20938** structural, bicortical or tricortical (through separate skin or fascial incision) (List separately in addition to code for primary procedure)

(Use 20938 in conjunction with 22319, 22532, 22533, 22548-22558, 22590-22612, 22630, 22633, 22634, 22800-22812)

(For aspiration of bone marrow for bone grafting, spine surgery only, use 20939)

+ **20939** Bone marrow aspiration for bone grafting, spine surgery only, through separate skin or fascial incision (List separately in addition to code for primary procedure)

● New Code ▲ Revised Code + Add-On Code ⊘ Modifier -51 Exempt ★ Telemedicine

(Use 20939 in conjunction with 22319, 22532, 22533, 22534, 22548, 22551, 22552, 22554, 22556, 22558, 22590, 22595, 22600, 22610, 22612, 22630, 22633, 22634, 22800, 22802, 22804, 22808, 22810, 22812)

(For bilateral procedure, report 20939 twice. Do not report modifier 50 in conjunction with 20939)

(For aspiration of bone marrow for the purpose of bone grafting, other than spine surgery and other therapeutic musculoskeletal applications, use 20999)

(For bone marrow aspiration[s] for platelet-rich stem cell injection, use 0232T)

(For diagnostic bone marrow aspiration[s], see 38220, 38222)

OTHER PROCEDURES

20950 Monitoring of interstitial fluid pressure (includes insertion of device,eg, wick catheter technique, needle manometer technique) in detection of muscle compartment syndrome

20955 Bone graft with microvascular anastomosis; fibula

20956   iliac crest

20957   metatarsal

20962   other than fibula, iliac crest, or metatarsal

(Do not report code 69990 in addition to codes 20955-20962)

20969 Free osteocutaneous flap with microvascular anastomosis; other than iliac crest, metatarsal, or great toe

20970   iliac crest

20972   metatarsal

20973   great toe with web space

(Do not report code 69990 in addition to codes 20969-20973)

(For great toe, wrap-around procedure, use 26551)

⊘ **20974** Electrical stimulation to aid bone healing; noninvasive (nonoperative)

⊘ **20975**   invasive (operative)

20979 Low intensity ultrasound stimulation to aid bone healing, noninvasive (nonoperative)

20982 Ablation therapy for reduction or eradication of 1 or more bone tumors (eg, metastasis) including adjacent soft tissue when involved by tumor extension, percutaneous, including imaging guidance when performed; radiofrequency

20983   cryoablation

(Do not report 20982, 20983 in conjunction with 76940, 77002, 77013, 77022)

+ **20985** Computer-assisted surgical navigational procedure for musculoskeletal procedures - image-less (List separately in addition to code for primary procedure)

(Do not report 20985 in conjunction with 61781-61783)

(For computer-assisted navigational procedures with image guidance based on pre-operative and intraoperatively obtained images, see 0054T, 0055T)

20999 Unlisted procedure, musculoskeletal system, general

HEAD

Skull, facial bones, and temporomandibular joint.

INCISION

(For incision and drainage procedures, cutaneous/subcutaneous, see 10060, 10061)

(For removal of embedded foreign body from dentoalveolar structure, see 41805, 41806)

21010   Arthrotomy, temporomandibular joint

(To report bilateral procedures, report 21010 with modifier -50)

EXCISION

21011   Excision, tumor, soft tissue of face or scalp, subcutaneous; less than 2 cm

21012   2 cm or greater

(For excision of benign lesions of cutaneous origin [eg, sebaceous cyst], see 11420-11426)

21013   Excision, tumor, soft tissue of face and scalp, subfascial (eg, subgaleal, intramuscular); less than 2 cm

21014   2 cm or greater

21015   Radical resection of tumor (eg, sarcoma), soft tissue of face or scalp; less than 2 cm

(To report excision of skull tumor for osteomyelitis, use 61501)

21016   2 cm or greater

(For radical resection of tumor[s] of cutaneous origin [eg, melanoma], see 11620-11646)

21025   Excision of bone (eg, for osteomyelitis or bone abscess); mandible

21026   facial bone(s)

21029   Removal by contouring of benign tumor of facial bone (eg, fibrous dysplasia)

21030   Excision of benign tumor or cyst of maxilla or zygoma by enucleation and curettage

21031   Excision of torus mandibularis

21032   Excision of maxillary torus palatinus

21034   Excision of malignant tumor of maxilla or zygoma

21040   Excision of benign tumor or cyst of mandible, by enucleation and/or curettage

(For enucleation and/or curettage of benign cysts or tumors of mandible not requiring osteotomy, use 21040)

(For excision of benign tumor or cyst of mandible requiring osteotomy, see 21046-21047)

21044   Excision of malignant tumor of mandible;

21045   radical resection

(For bone graft, use 21215)

21046   Excision of benign tumor or cyst of mandible; requiring intra-oral osteotomy (eg, locally aggressive or destructive lesion(s))

● New Code   ▲ Revised Code   + Add-On Code   ⊘ Modifier -51 Exempt   ★ Telemedicine

21047   requiring extra-oral osteotomy and partial mandibulectomy (eg, locally aggressive or destructive lesion(s))

21048 Excision of benign tumor or cyst of maxilla; requiring intra-oral osteotomy (eg, locally aggressive or destructive lesion(s))

21049   requiring extra-oral osteotomy and partial maxillectomy (eg, locally aggressive or destructive lesion(s))

21050 Condylectomy, temporomandibular joint (separate procedure)

(For bilateral procedures, report 21050 with modifier -50)

21060 Meniscectomy, partial or complete, temporomandibular joint (separate procedure)

(For bilateral procedures, report 21060 with modifier -50)

21070 Coronoidectomy (separate procedure)

(For bilateral procedures, report 21070 with modifier -50)

MANIPULATION

21073 Manipulation of temporomandibular joint(s) (TMJ), therapeutic, requiring an anesthesia service (ie, general or monitored anesthesia care)

(For TMJ manipulation without an anesthesia service [ie, general or monitored anesthesia care], see 97140, 98925-98929, 98943)

(For closed treatment of temporomandibular dislocation, see 21480, 21485)

HEAD PROSTHESIS

Codes 21076-21089 describe professional services for the rehabilitation of patients with oral, facial, or other anatomical deficiencies by means of prostheses, such as an artificial eye, ear, or nose or intraoral obturator to close a cleft. Codes 21076-21089 should only be used when the physician or other qualified health care professional actually designs and prepares the prosthesis (ie., not prepared by an outside laboratory).

(For application or removal of caliper or tongs, see 20660, 20665)

21076 Impression and custom preparation; surgical obturator prosthesis

21077   orbital prosthesis

21079   interim obturator prosthesis

21080   definitive obturator prosthesis

21081   mandibular resection prosthesis

21082   palatal augmentation prosthesis

21083   palatal lift prosthesis

21084   speech aid prosthesis

21085   oral surgical splint

21086   auricular prosthesis

21087   nasal prosthesis

21088   facial prosthesis

Other Procedures

21089   Unlisted maxillofacial prosthetic procedure

INTRODUCTION OR REMOVAL

21100   Application of halo type appliance for maxillofacial fixation, includes removal (separate procedure)

21110   Application of interdental fixation device for conditions other than fracture or dislocation, includes removal

(For removal of interdental fixation by another individual, see 20670-20680)

21116   Injection procedure for temporomandibular joint arthrography

(For radiological supervision and interpretation, use 70332. Do not report 77002 in addition to 70332)

REPAIR, REVISION AND/OR RECONSTRUCTION

(For cranioplasty, see 21179, 21180 and 62120, 62140-62147)

21120   Genioplasty; augmentation (autograft, allograft, prosthetic material)

21121   sliding osteotomy, single piece

21122   sliding osteotomies, 2 or more osteotomies (eg, wedge excision or bone wedge reversal for asymmetrical chin)

21123   sliding, augmentation with interpositional bone grafts (includes obtaining autografts)

21125   Augmentation, mandibular body or angle; prosthetic material

21127   with bone graft, onlay or interpositional (includes obtaining autograft)

21137   Reduction forehead; contouring only

21138   contouring and application of prosthetic material or bone graft (includes obtaining autograft)

21139   contouring and setback of anterior frontal sinus wall

21141   Reconstruction midface, LeFort I; single piece, segment movement in any direction (eg, for Long Face Syndrome), without bone graft

21142   2 pieces, segment movement in any direction, without bone graft

21143   3 or more pieces, segment movement in any direction, without bone graft

21145   single piece, segment movement in any direction, requiring bone grafts (includes obtaining autografts)

21146   2 pieces, segment movement in any direction, requiring bone grafts (includes obtaining autografts) (eg, ungrafted unilateral alveolar cleft)

21147   3 or more pieces, segment movement in any direction, requiring bone grafts (includes obtaining autografts) (eg, ungrafted bilateral alveolar cleft or multiple osteotomies)

21150   Reconstruction midface, LeFort II; anterior intrusion (eg, Treacher-Collins Syndrome)

21151   any direction, requiring bone grafts (includes obtaining autografts)

21154   Reconstruction midface, LeFort III (extracranial), any type, requiring bone grafts (includes obtaining autografts); without LeFort I

● New Code   ▲ Revised Code   ✛ Add-On Code   ⊘ Modifier -51 Exempt   ★ Telemedicine

21155 with LeFort I

21159 Reconstruction midface, LeFort III (extra and intracranial) with forehead advancement (eg, mono bloc), requiring bone grafts (includes obtaining autografts); without LeFort I

21160 with LeFort I

21172 Reconstruction superior-lateral orbital rim and lower forehead, advancement or alteration, with or without grafts (includes obtaining autografts)

 (For frontal or parietal craniotomy performed for craniosynostosis, use 61556)

21175 Reconstruction, bifrontal, superior-lateral orbital rims and lower forehead, advancement or alteration (eg, plagiocephaly, trigonocephaly, brachycephaly), with or without grafts (includes obtaining autografts)

 (For bifrontal craniotomy performed for craniosynostosis, use 61557)

21179 Reconstruction, entire or majority of forehead and/or supraorbital rims; with grafts (allograft or prosthetic material)

21180 with autograft (includes obtaining grafts)

 (For extensive craniectomy for multiple suture craniosynostosis, use only 61558 or 61559)

21181 Reconstruction by contouring of benign tumor of cranial bones (eg, fibrous dysplasia), extracranial

21182 Reconstruction of orbital walls, rims, forehead, nasoethmoid complex following intra- and extracranial excision of benign tumor of cranial bone (eg, fibrous dysplasia), with multiple autografts (includes obtaining grafts); total area of bone grafting less than 40 sq cm

21183 total area of bone grafting greater than 40 sq cm but less than 80 sq cm

21184 total area of bone grafting greater than 80 sq cm

 (For excision of benign tumor of cranial bones, see 61563, 61564)

21188 Reconstruction midface, osteotomies (other than LeFort type) and bone grafts (includes obtaining autografts)

21193 Reconstruction of mandibular rami, horizontal, vertical, C, or L osteotomy; without bone graft

21194 with bone graft (includes obtaining graft)

21195 Reconstruction of mandibular rami and/or body, sagittal split; without internal rigid fixation

21196 with internal rigid fixation

21198 Osteotomy, mandible, segmental;

21199 with genioglossus advancement

 (To report total osteotomy of the maxilla, see 21141-21160)

21206 Osteotomy, maxilla, segmental (eg, Wassmund or Schuchard)

21208 Osteoplasty, facial bones; augmentation (autograft, allograft, or prosthetic implant)

21209 reduction

21210 Graft, bone; nasal, maxillary or malar areas (includes obtaining graft)

 (For cleft palate repair, see 42200-42225)

21215   mandible (includes obtaining graft)

21230   Graft; rib cartilage, autogenous, to face, chin, nose or ear (includes obtaining graft)

21235   ear cartilage, autogenous, to nose or ear (includes obtaining graft)

          (To report graft augmentation of facial bones, use 21208)

21240   Arthroplasty, temporomandibular joint, with or without autograft (includes obtaining graft)

21242   Arthroplasty, temporomandibular joint, with allograft

21243   Arthroplasty, temporomandibular joint, with prosthetic joint replacement

21244   Reconstruction of mandible, extraoral, with transosteal bone plate (eg, mandibular staple bone plate)

21245   Reconstruction of mandible or maxilla, subperiosteal implant; partial

21246   complete

21247   Reconstruction of mandibular condyle with bone and cartilage autografts (includes obtaining grafts) (eg, for hemifacial microsomia)

21248   Reconstruction of mandible or maxilla, endosteal implant (eg, blade, cylinder); partial

21249   complete

          (To report midface reconstruction, see 21141-21160)

21255   Reconstruction of zygomatic arch and glenoid fossa with bone and cartilage (includes obtaining autografts)

21256   Reconstruction of orbit with osteotomies (extracranial) and with bone grafts (includes obtaining autografts) (eg, micro-ophthalmia)

21260   Periorbital osteotomies for orbital hypertelorism, with bone grafts; extracranial approach

21261   combined intra- and extracranial approach

21263   with forehead advancement

21267   Orbital repositioning, periorbital osteotomies, unilateral, with bone grafts; extracranial approach

21268   combined intra- and extracranial approach

21270   Malar augmentation, prosthetic material

          (For malar augmentation with bone graft, use 21210)

21275   Secondary revision of orbitocraniofacial reconstruction

21280   Medial canthopexy (separate procedure)

          (For medial canthoplasty, use 67950)

21282   Lateral canthopexy

21295   Reduction of masseter muscle and bone (eg, for treatment of benign masseteric hypertrophy); extraoral approach

21296   intraoral approach

● New Code   ▲ Revised Code   + Add-On Code   ⊘ Modifier -51 Exempt   ★ Telemedicine

OTHER PROCEDURES

21299 Unlisted craniofacial and maxillofacial procedure

FRACTURE AND/OR DISLOCATION

(For operative repair of skull fracture, see 62000-62010)

(To report closed treatment of skull fracture, use the appropriate Evaluation and Management code)

21310 Closed treatment of nasal bone fracture without manipulation

21315 Closed treatment of nasal bone fracture; without stabilization

21320   with stabilization

21325 Open treatment of nasal fracture; uncomplicated

21330   complicated, with internal and/or external skeletal fixation

21335   with concomitant open treatment of fractured septum

21336 Open treatment of nasal septal fracture, with or without stabilization

21337 Closed treatment of nasal septal fracture, with or without stabilization

21338 Open treatment of nasoethmoid fracture; without external fixation

21339   with external fixation

21340 Percutaneous treatment of nasoethmoid complex fracture, with splint, wire or headcap fixation, including repair of canthal ligaments and/or the nasolacrimal apparatus

21343 Open treatment of depressed frontal sinus fracture

21344 Open treatment of complicated (eg, comminuted or involving posterior wall) frontal sinus fracture, via coronal or multiple approaches

21345 Closed treatment of nasomaxillary complex fracture (LeFort II type), with interdental wire fixation or fixation of denture or splint

21346 Open treatment of nasomaxillary complex fracture (LeFort II type); with wiring and/or local fixation

21347   requiring multiple open approaches

21348   with bone grafting (includes obtaining graft)

21355 Percutaneous treatment of fracture of malar area, including zygomatic arch and malar tripod, with manipulation

21356 Open treatment of depressed zygomatic arch fracture (eg, Gillies approach)

21360 Open treatment of depressed malar fracture, including zygomatic arch and malar tripod

21365 Open treatment of complicated (eg, comminuted or involving cranial nerve foramina) fracture(s) of malar area, including zygomatic arch and malar tripod; with internal fixation and multiple surgical approaches

21366   with bone grafting (includes obtaining graft)

21385 Open treatment of orbital floor blowout fracture; transantral approach (Caldwell-Luc type operation)

Separate Procedure   Unlisted Procedure   CCI Comp. Code   Non-specific Procedure   **271**

21386 periorbital approach

21387 combined approach

21390 periorbital approach, with alloplastic or other implant

21395 periorbital approach with bone graft (includes obtaining graft)

21400 Closed treatment of fracture of orbit, except blowout; without manipulation

21401 with manipulation

21406 Open treatment of fracture of orbit, except blowout; without implant

21407 with implant

21408 with bone grafting (includes obtaining graft)

21421 Closed treatment of palatal or maxillary fracture (LeFort I type), with interdental wire fixation or fixation of denture or splint

21422 Open treatment of palatal or maxillary fracture (LeFort I type);

21423 complicated (comminuted or involving cranial nerve foramina), multiple approaches

21431 Closed treatment of craniofacial separation (LeFort III type) using interdental wire fixation of denture or splint

21432 Open treatment of craniofacial separation (LeFort III type); with wiring and/or internal fixation

21433 complicated (eg, comminuted or involving cranial nerve foramina), multiple surgical approaches

21435 complicated, utilizing internal and/or external fixation techniques (eg, head cap, halo device, and/or intermaxillary fixation)

(For removal of internal or external fixation device, use 20670)

21436 complicated, multiple surgical approaches, internal fixation, with bone grafting (includes obtaining graft)

21440 Closed treatment of mandibular or maxillary alveolar ridge fracture (separate procedure)

21445 Open treatment of mandibular or maxillary alveolar ridge fracture (separate procedure)

21450 Closed treatment of mandibular fracture; without manipulation

21451 with manipulation

21452 Percutaneous treatment of mandibular fracture, with external fixation

21453 Closed treatment of mandibular fracture with interdental fixation

21454 Open treatment of mandibular fracture with external fixation

21461 Open treatment of mandibular fracture; without interdental fixation

21462 with interdental fixation

21465 Open treatment of mandibular condylar fracture

21470   Open treatment of complicated mandibular fracture by multiple surgical approaches including internal fixation, interdental fixation, and/or wiring of dentures or splints

21480   Closed treatment of temporomandibular dislocation; initial or subsequent

21485   complicated (eg, recurrent requiring intermaxillary fixation or splinting), initial or subsequent

21490   Open treatment of temporomandibular dislocation

(For interdental wire fixation, use 21497)

(To report treatment of closed fracture of larynx, use the applicable Evaluation and Management codes)

21497   Interdental wiring, for condition other than fracture

OTHER PROCEDURES

21499   Unlisted musculoskeletal procedure, head

(For unlisted craniofacial or maxillofacial procedure, use 21299)

NECK (SOFT TISSUES) AND THORAX

(For cervical spine and back, see 21920 et seq)

(For injection of fracture site or trigger point, use 20550)

INCISION

(For incision and drainage of abscess or hematoma, superficial, see 10060, 10140)

21501   Incision and drainage, deep abscess or hematoma, soft tissues of neck or thorax;

(For posterior spine subfascial incision and drainage, see 22010-22015)

21502   with partial rib ostectomy

21510   Incision, deep, with opening of bone cortex (eg, for osteomyelitis or bone abscess), thorax

EXCISION

(For bone biopsy, see 20220-20251)

21550   Biopsy, soft tissue of neck or thorax

(For needle biopsy of soft tissue, use 20206)

21552   This code is out of order. See page 273

21554   This code is out of order. See page 273

21555   Excision, tumor, soft tissue of neck or anterior thorax, subcutaneous; less than 3 cm

21552   3 cm or greater

(For excision of benign lesions of cutaneous origin [eg, sebaceous cyst], see 11420-11426)

21556   Excision, tumor, soft tissue of neck or anterior thorax, subfascial (eg, intramuscular); less than 5 cm

21554   5 cm or greater

21557   Radical resection of tumor (eg, sarcoma), soft tissue of neck or anterior thorax; less than 5 cm

---

21558   5 cm or greater

(For radical resection of tumor[s] of cutaneous origin [eg, melanoma], see 11600-11620)

21600   Excision of rib, partial

(For radical resection of chest wall and rib cage for tumor, use 21601)

(For radical debridement of chest wall and rib cage for injury, see 11044, 11047)

21601   Excision of chest wall tumor including rib(s)

21602   Excision of chest wall tumor involving rib(s), with plastic reconstruction; without mediastinal lymphadenectomy

21603   with mediastinal lymphadenectomy

(Do not report 21601, 21602, 21603 in conjunction with 32100, 32503, 32504, 32551, 32554, 32555)

21610   Costotransversectomy (separate procedure)

21615   Excision first and/or cervical rib;

21616   with sympathectomy

21620   Ostectomy of sternum, partial

21627   Sternal debridement

(For debridement and closure, use 21750)

21630   Radical resection of sternum;

21632   with mediastinal lymphadenectomy

REPAIR, REVISION, AND/OR RECONSTRUCTION

(For superficial wound, see Integumentary System section under Repair, Simple)

21685   Hyoid myotomy and suspension

21700   Division of scalenus anticus; without resection of cervical rib

21705   with resection of cervical rib

21720   Division of sternocleidomastoid for torticollis, open operation; without cast application

(For transection of spinal accessory and cervical nerves, see 63191, 64722)

21725   with cast application

21740   Reconstructive repair of pectus excavatum or carinatum; open

21742   minimally invasive approach (Nuss procedure), without thoracoscopy

21743   minimally invasive approach (Nuss procedure), with thoracoscopy

21750   Closure of median sternotomy separation with or without debridement (separate procedure)

FRACTURE AND/OR DISLOCATION

(To report closed treatment of an uncomplicated rib fracture, use the Evaluation and Management codes)

21811	Open treatment of rib fracture(s) with internal fixation, includes thoracoscopic visualization when performed, unilateral; 1-3 ribs

(For bilateral procedure, report 21811 with modifier 50)

21812	4-6 ribs

(For bilateral procedure, report 21812 with modifier 50)

21813	7 or more ribs

(For bilateral procedure, report 21812 with modifier 50)

21820	Closed treatment of sternum fracture

21825	Open treatment of sternum fracture with or without skeletal fixation

(For sternoclavicular dislocation, see 23520-23532)

OTHER PROCEDURES

21899	Unlisted procedure, neck or thorax

BACK AND FLANK

EXCISION

21920	Biopsy, soft tissue of back or flank; superficial

21925	deep

(For needle biopsy of soft tissue, use 20206)

21930	Excision, tumor, soft tissue of back or flank, subcutaneous; less than 3 cm

21931	3 cm or greater

(For excision of benign lesions of cutaneous origin [eg, sebaceous cyst], see 11400-11406)

21932	Excision, tumor, soft tissue of back or flank, subfascial (eg, intramuscular); less than 5 cm

21933	5 cm or greater

21935	Radical resection of tumor (eg, sarcoma), soft tissue of back or flank; less than 5 cm

21936	5 cm or greater

(For radical resection of tumor[s] of cutaneous origin [eg, melanoma], see 11600-11606)

SPINE (VERTEBRAL COLUMN)

Cervical, thoracic and lumbar spine.

Within the spine section, bone grafting procedures are reported separately and in addition to arthrodesis. For bone grafts in other Musculoskeletal sections, see specific code(s) descriptor(s) and/or accompanying guidelines.

To report bone grafts performed after arthrodesis, see 20930-20938. Do not append modifier 62 to bone graft codes 20900-20938.

For example, posterior arthrodesis of L5-S1 for degenerative disc disease utilizing morselized autogenous iliac bone graft harvested through a separate fascial incision. Report as 22612 and 20937.

Within the spine section, instrumentation is reported separately and in addition to arthrodesis. To report instrumentation procedures performed with definitive vertebral procedure(s), see 22840-22855, 22859. Instrumentation procedure codes 22840-22848, 22853, 22854, 22859 are reported in addition to the definitive procedure(s). Modifier 62 may not be appended to the definitive or add-on spinal instrumentation procedure code(s) 22840-22848, 22850, 22852, 22853, 22854, 22859.

For example, posterior arthrodesis of L4-S1 utilizing morselized autogenous iliac bone graft harvested through separate fascial incision, and pedicle screw fixation. Report as 22612, 22614, 22842 and 20937.

When arthrodesis is performed in addition to another procedure, the arthrodesis should be reported in addition to the original procedure with modifier 51 (multiple procedures). Examples are after osteotomy, fracture care, vertebral corpectomy, and laminectomy. Bone grafts and instrumentation are never performed without arthrodesis.

For example, treatment of a burst fracture of L2 by corpectomy followed by arthrodesis of L1-L3, utilizing anterior instrumentation L1-L3 and structural allograft. Report as 63090, 22558-51, 22585, 22845, and 20931.

When two surgeons work together as primary surgeons performing distinct part(s) of a single reportable procedure, each surgeon should report his/her distince operative work by appending modifier 62 to the single definitive procedure code. If additional procedure(s) (including add-on procedure[s]) are performed during the same surgical session, separate code(s) may be reported by each co-surgeon, with modifier 62 appended.

For example, a 42-year-old male with a history of posttraumatic degenerative disc disease at L3-4 and L4-5 (internal disc disruption) underwent surgical repair. Surgeon A performed an anterior exposure of the spine with mobilization of the great vessels. Surgeon B performed anterior (minimal) discectomy and fusion at L3-4 and L4-5 using anterior interbody technique. Surgeon A report: 22558 append modifier 62, 22585 append modifier 62. Surgeon B report: 22558 append modifier 62, 22585 append modifier 62, 20931.

(Do not append modifier -62 to bone graft code 20931)

(For injection procedure for myelography, use 62284)

(For injection procedure for discography, see 62290, 62291)

(For injection procedure, chemonucleolysis, single or multiple leveles, use 62292)

(For injection procedure for facet joints, see 64490-64495, 64633--22-64636)

(For needle or trocar biopsy, see 20220-20225)

INCISION

22010   Incision and drainage, open, of deep abscess (subfascial), posterior spine; cervical, thoracic, or cervicothoracic

22015   lumbar, sacral, or lumbosacral

(Do not report 22015 in conjunction with 22010)

(Do not report 22015 in conjunction with instrumentation removal, 10180, 22850, 22852)

(For incision and drainage of abscess or hematoma, superficial, see 10060, 10140)

EXCISION

For the following codes, when two surgeons work together as primary surgeons performing distinct part(s) of partial vertebral body excision, each surgeon should report his/her distinct operative work by appending modifier 62 to the procedure code. In this situation, modifier 62 may be appended to the procedure code(s) 22100-22102, 22110-22114 and, as appropriate, to the associated additional vertebral segment add-on code(s) 22103, 22116 as long as both surgeons continue to work together as primary surgeons.

(For bone biopsy, see 20220-20251)

(To report soft tissue biopsy of back or flank, see 21920-21925)

(For needle biopsy of soft tissue, use 20206)

(To report excision of soft tissue tumor of back or flank, use 21930)

22100   Partial excision of posterior vertebral component (eg, spinous process, lamina or facet) for intrinsic bony lesion, single vertebral segment; cervical

22101   thoracic

22102   lumbar

      (For insertion of posterior spinous process distraction devices, see 22867, 22868, 22869, 22870)

+ 22103   each additional segment (List separately in addition to code for primary procedure)

      (Use 22103 in conjunction with codes 22100, 22101, 22102)

22110   Partial excision of vertebral body, for intrinsic bony lesion, without decompression of spinal cord or nerve root(s), single vertebral segment; cervical

22112   thoracic

22114   lumbar

+ 22116   each additional vertebral segment (List separately in addition to code for primary procedure)

      (Use 22116 in conjunction with codes 22110, 22112, 22114)

      (For complete or near complete resection of vertebral body, see vertebral corpectomy, 63081-63091)

      (For spinal reconstruction with bone graft (autograft, allograft) and/or methacrylate of cervical vertebral body, use 63081 and 22554 and 20931 or 20938)

      (For spinal reconstruction with bone graft (autograft, allograft) and/or methacrylate of thoracic vertebral body, use 63085 or 63087 and 22556 and 20931 or 20938)

      (For spinal reconstruction with bone graft (autograft, allograft) and/or methacrylate of lumbar vertebral body, use 63087 or 63090 and 22558 and 20931 or 20938)

      (For spinal reconstruction following vertebral body resection, use 63082 or 63086 or 63088 or 63091, and 22585)

      (For harvest of bone autograft for vertebral reconstruction, see 20931 or 20938)

      (For cervical spinal reconstruction with prosthetic replacement of resected vertebral bodies, see codes 63081 and 22554 and 20931 or 20938 and 22853, 22854, 22859)

      (For thoracic spinal reconstruction with prosthetic replacement of resected vertebral bodies, see codes 63085 or 63087 and 22556 and 20931 or 20938 and 22853, 22854, 22859)

      (For lumbar spinal reconstruction with prosthetic replacement of resected vertebral bodies, see codes 63087 or 63090 and 22558 and 20931 or 20938 and 22853, 22854, 22859)

      (For osteotomy of spine, see 22210-22226)

OSTEOTOMY

To report arthrodesis, see codes 22590-22632. (Report in addition to code[s] for the definitive procedure with modifier -51.)

To report instrumentation procedures, see 22840- 22855, 22859. (Report in addition to code[s] for the definitive procedure[s].) Do not append modifier 62 to spinal instrumentation codes 22840-22848, 22850, 22852, 22853, 22854, 22859.

To report bone graft procedures, see 20930-20938. (Report in addition to code[s] for the definitive procedure[s].) Do not append modifier -62 to bone graft codes 20900-20938.

For the following codes, when two surgeons work together as primary surgeons performing distinct part(s) of an anterior spine osteotomy, each surgeon should report his/her distinct operative work by appending modifier 62 to the procedure code. In this situation, modifier 62 may be appended to the procedure code(s) 22210-22214, 22220-22224 and, as appropriate, to associated additional segment add-on code(s) 22216, 22226 as long as both surgeons continue to work together as primary surgeons.

Spinal osteotomy procedures are reported when a portion(s) of the vertebral segment(s) is cut and removed in preparation for re-aligning the spine as part of a spinal deformity correction. For excision of an intrinsic lesion of the vertebra without deformity correction, see 22100-22116. For decompression of the spinal cord and/or nerve roots, see 63001-63308.

The three columns are defined as anterior (anterior two-thirds of the vertebral body), middle (posterior third of the vertebral body and pedicle), and posterior (articular facets, lamina, and spinous process).

22206 Osteotomy of spine, posterior or posterolateral approach, 3 columns, 1 vertebral segment (eg, pedicle/vertebral body subtraction); thoracic

(Do not report 22206 in conjunction with 22207)

22207 lumbar

(Do not report 22207 in conjunction with 22206)

+ **22208** each additional vertebral segment (List separately in addition to code for primary procedure)

(Use 22208 in conjunction with 22206, 22207)

(Do not report 22206, 22207, 22208 in conjunction with 22210-22226, 22830, 63001-63048, 63055-63066, 63075-63091, 63101-63103, when performed at the same level)

22210 Osteotomy of spine, posterior or posterolateral approach, 1 vertebral segment; cervical

22212 thoracic

22214 lumbar

+ **22216** each additional vertebral segment (List separately in addition to primary procedure)

(Use 22216 in conjunction with codes 22210, 22212, 22214)

22220 Osteotomy of spine, including diskectomy, anterior approach, single vertebral segment; cervical

22222 thoracic

22224 lumbar

+ **22226** each additional vertebral segment (List separately in addition to code for primary procedure)

(Use 22226 in conjunction with codes 22220, 22222, 22224)

(For vertebral corpectomy, see 63081-63091)

FRACTURE AND/OR DISLOCATION

To report arthrodesis, see codes 22590-22632. (Report in addition to code[s] for the definitive procedure with modifier -51.)

To report instrumentation procedures, see 22840- 22855, 22859. (Report in addition to code[s] for the definitive procedure[s].) Do not append modifier 62 to spinal instrumentation codes 22840-22848, 22850, 22852, 22853, 22854, 22859.

To report bone graft procedures, see 20930-20938. (Report in addition to code[s] for the definitive procedure[s].) Do not append modifier -62 to bone graft codes 20900-20938.

For the following codes, when two surgeons work together as primary surgeons performing distinct part(s) of open fracture and/or dislocation procedure(s), each surgeon should report his/her distinct operative work by appending modifier 62 to the procedure code. In this situation, modifier 62 may be appended to the procedure code(s) 22318-22327 and, as appropriate, the associated additional fracture vertebrae or dislocated segment add-on code 22328 as long as both surgeons continue to work together as primary surgeons.

(**22305** deleted 2016 [2017 edition]. To report, see the appropriate evaluation and management codes)

22310 Closed treatment of vertebral body fracture(s), without manipulation, requiring and including casting or bracing

(Do not report 22310 in conjunction with 22510, 22511, 22512, 22513, 22514, 22515, when performed at the same level)

22315 Closed treatment of vertebral fracture(s) and/or dislocation(s) requiring casting or bracing, with and including casting and/or bracing, by manipulation or traction

(Do not report 22315 in conjunction with 22510, 22511, 22512, 22513, 22514, 22515, when performed at the same level)

(For spinal subluxation, use 97140)

22318 Open treatment and/or reduction of odontoid fracture(s) and or dislocation(s) (including os odontoideum), anterior approach, including placement of internal fixation; without grafting

22319 with grafting

22325 Open treatment and/or reduction of vertebral fracture(s) and/or dislocation(s), posterior approach, 1 fractured vertebrae or dislocated segment; lumbar

(Do not report 22325 in conjunction with 22511, 22512, 22514, 22515, when performed at the same level)

22326 cervical

(Do not report 22326 in conjunction with 22510, 22512, when performed at the same level)

22327 thoracic

(Do not report 22327 in conjunction with 22510, 22512, 22513, 22515, when performed at the same level)

+ 22328 each additional fractured vertebrae or dislocated segment (List separately in addition to code for primary procedure)

(Use 22328 in conjunction with codes 22325, 22326, 22327)

(For treatment of vertebral fracture by the anterior approach, see corpectomy 63081-63091, and appropriate arthrodesis, bone graft and instrument codes)

(For decompression of spine following fracture, see 63001-63091; for arthrodesis of spine following fracture, see 22548-22632)

MANIPULATION

(For spinal manipulation without anesthesia, use 97140)

22505 Manipulation of spine requiring anesthesia, any region

PERCUTANEOUS VERTEBROPLASTY AND VERTEBRAL AUGMENTATION

Codes 22510, 22511, 22512, 22513, 22514, 22515 describe procedures for percutaneous vertebral augmentation that include vertebroplasty of the cervical, thoracic, lumbar, and sacral spine and vertebral augmentation of the thoracic and lumbar spine.

For the purposes of reporting 22510, 22511, 22512, 22513, 22514, 22515, "vertebroplasty" is the process of injecting a material (cement) into the vertebral body to reinforce the structure of the body using image guidance. "Vertebral augmentation" is the process of cavity creation followed by the injection of a material (cement) under image guidance. For 0200T and 0201T, "sacral augmentation (sacroplasty)" refers to the creation of a cavity within a sacral vertebral body followed by injection of a material to fill that cavity.

The procedure codes are inclusive of bone biopsy, when performed, and imaging guidance necessary to perform the procedure. Use one primary procedure code and an add-on code for additional levels. When treating the sacrum, sacral procedures are reported only once per encounter.

22510 Percutaneous vertebroplasty (bone biopsy included when performed), 1 vertebral body, unilateral or bilateral injection, inclusive of all imaging guidance; cervicothoracic

22511 lumbosacral

+ 22512 each additional cervicothoracic or lumbosacral vertebral body (List separately in addition to code for primary procedure)

(Use 22512 in conjunction with 22510, 22511)

(Do not report 22510, 22511, 22512 in conjunction with 20225, 22310, 22315, 22325, 22327, when performed at the same level as 22510, 22511, 22512)

22513 Percutaneous vertebral augmentation, including cavity creation (fracture reduction and bone biopsy included when performed) using mechanical device (eg, kyphoplasty), 1 vertebral body, unilateral or bilateral cannulation, inclusive of all imaging guidance; thoracic

22514 lumbar

+ 22515 each additional thoracic or lumbar vertebral body (list separately in addition to code for primary procedure)

(Use 22515 in conjunction with 22513, 22514)

(Do not report 22513, 22514, 22515 in conjunction with 20225, 22310, 22315, 22325, 22327, when performed at the same level as 22513, 22514, 22515)

PERCUTANEOUS AUGMENTATION AND ANNULOPLASTY

22526 Percutaneous intradiscal electrothermal annuloplasty, unilateral or bilateral including fluoroscopic guidance; single level

+ 22527 1 or more additional levels (List separately in addition to code for primary procedure)

(Use 22527 in conjunction with 22526)

(Do not report codes 22526, 22527 in conjunction with 77002, 77003)

(For percutaneous intradiscal annuloplasty using method other than electrothermal, use 22899)

ARTHRODESIS

Arthrodesis may be performed in the absence of other procedures and therefore when it is combined with another definitive procedure (eg., osteotomy, fracture care, vertebral corpectomy, or laminectomy), modifier 51 is appropriate. However, arthrodesis codes 22585, 22614, and 22632 are considered add-on procedure codes and should not be used with modifier 51.

To report instrumentation procedures, see 22840- 22855, 22859. (Codes 22840-22848, 22853, 22854, 22859 are reported in conjunction with code[s] for the definitive procedure[s]. When instrumentation reinsertion or removal is reported in conjunction with other definitive procedures, including arthrodesis, decompression, and exploration of fusion, append modifier 51 to 22849, 22850, 22852, and 22855.) To report exploration of fusion, use 22830. (When exploration is reported in conjunction with other definitive procedures, including arthrodesis and decompression, append modifier 51 to 22830.) Do not append modifier 62 to spinal instrumentation codes 22840-22848, 22850, 22852, 22853, 22854, 22859.

To report bone graft procedures, see 20930-20938. (Report in addition to code[s] for the definitive procedure[s].) Do not append modifier -62 to bone graft codes 20900-20938.

Lateral Extracavitary Approach Technique

22532 Arthrodesis, lateral extracavitary technique, including minimal diskectomy to prepare interspace (other than for decompression); thoracic

22533 lumbar

+ 22534 thoracic or lumbar, each additional vertebral segment (List separately in addition to code for primary procedure)

● New Code ▲ Revised Code **+** Add-On Code ⊘ Modifier -51 Exempt ★ Telemedicine

(Use 22534 in conjunction with 22532 and 22533)

Anterior or Anterolateral Approach Technique

Procedure codes 22554-22558 are for SINGLE interspace; for additional interspaces, use 22585. A vertebral interspace is the non-bony compartment between two adjacent vertebral bodies, which contains the intervertebral disc, and includes the nucleus pulposus, annulus fibrosus, and two cartilagenous endplates.

For the following codes, when two surgeons work together as primary surgeons performing distinct part(s) of an anterior interbody arthrodesis, each surgeon should report his/her distinct operative work by appending modifier 62 to the procedure code. In this situation, modifier 62 may be appended to the procedure code(s) 22548-22558 and, as appropriate, to the associated additional interspace add-on code 22585 as long as both surgeons continue to work together as primary surgeons.

22548 Arthrodesis, anterior transoral or extraoral technique, clivus-C1-C2 (atlas-axis), with or without excision of odontoid process

(For intervertebral disc excision by laminotomy or laminectomy, see 63020-63042)

22551 Arthrodesis, anterior interbody, including disc space preparation, discectomy, osteophytectomy and decompression of spinal cord and/or nerve roots, cervical below C2;

+ **22552**   each additional interspace (list separately in addition to code for separate procedure)

(Use 22552 in conjunction with 22551)

22554 Arthrodesis, anterior interbody technique, including minimal diskectomy to prepare interspace (other than for decompression); cervical below C2

(Do not report 22554 in conjunction with 63075, even if performed by a separate individual. To report anterior cervical discectomy and interbody fusion at the same level during the same session, use 22551)

22556   thoracic

22558   lumbar

(For arthrodesis using pre-sacral interbody technique, use 22586)

+ **22585**   each additional interspace (List separately in addition to code for primary procedure)

(Use 22585 in conjunction with codes 22554, 22556, 22558)

(Do not report 22585 in conjunction with 63075 even if performed by a separate individual. To report anterior cervical discectomy and interbody fusion at the same level during the same session, use 22552)

22586 Arthrodesis, pre-sacral interbody technique, including disc space preparation, discectomy, with posterior instrumentation, wiht image guidance, includes bone graft when performed, L5-S1 interspace

(Do not report 22586 in conjunction with 20930-20938, 22840, 22848, 72275, 77002, 77003, 77011, 77012)

Posterior, Posterolateral or Lateral Transverse Process Technique

To report instrumentation procedures, see 22840- 22855, 22859. (Report in addition to code[s] for the definitive procedure[s].) Do not append modifier 62 to spinal instrumentation codes 22840-22848, 22850, 22852, 22853, 22854, 22859

To report bone graft procedures, see 20930-20938. (Report in addition to code[s] for the definitive procedure[s].) Do not append modifier -62 to bone graft codes 20900-20938.

A vertebral segment describes the basic constituent part into which the spine may be divided. It represents a single complete vertebral bone with its associated articular processes and laminae. A vertebral interspace is the non-bony compartment between two adjacent vertebral bodies which contains the intervertebral disc, and includes the nucleus pulposus, annulus fibrosus, and two cartilagenous endplates.

22590 Arthrodesis, posterior technique, craniocervical (occiput-C2)

22595   Arthrodesis, posterior technique, atlas-axis (C1-C2)

22600   Arthrodesis, posterior or posterolateral technique, single level; cervical below C2 segment

22610   thoracic (with lateral transverse technique, when performed)

22612   lumbar (with lateral transverse technique, when performed)

     (Do not report 22612 in conjunction with 22630 for the same interspace and segment, use 22633)

+ 22614   each additional vertebral segment (List separately in addition to code for primary procedure)

     (Use 22614 in conjunction with 22600, 22610, 22612, 22630 or 22633 when performed at a different level. When performing a posterior or posterolateral technique for fusion/arthrodesis at an additional level, use 22614. When performing a posterior interbody fusion arthrodesis at an additional level, use 22632. When performing a combined posterior or posterolateral technique with posterior interbody arthrodesis at an additional level, use 22634)

     (For facet joint fusion, see 0219T-0222T)

     (For placement of a posterior intrafacet implant, see 0219T-0222T)

22630   Arthrodesis, posterior interbody technique, including laminectomy and/or diskectomy to prepare interspace (other than for decompression), single interspace; lumbar

     (Do not report 22630 in conjunction with 22612 for the same interspace and segment, use 22633)

+ 22632   each additional interspace (List separately in addition to code for primary procedure)

     (Use 22632 in conjunction with 22612, 22630, or 22633 when performed at a different level. When peforming a posterior interbody fusion arthrodesis at an additional level, use 22632. When performing a posterior or posterolateral technique for fusion/arthrodesis at an additional level, use 22614. When performing a combined posterior or posterolateral technique with posterior interbody arthrodesis at an additional level, use 22634)

22633   Arthrodesis, combined posterior or posterolateral technique with posterior interbody technique including laminectomy and/or discectomy sufficient to prepare interspace (other than for decompression), single interspace and segment; lumbar

     (Do not report with 22612 or 22630 at the same level)

+ 22634   each additional interspace and segment (List separately in addition to code for primary procedure)

     (Use 22634 in conjunction with 22633)

Spine Deformity (eg, Scoliosis, Kyphosis)

To report instrumentation procedures, see 22840- 22855, 22859. (Report in addition to code[s] for the definitive procedure[s].) Do not append modifier 62 to spinal instrumentation codes 22840-22848, 22850, 22852, 22853, 22854, 22859.

To report bone graft procedures, see 20930-20938. (Report in addition to code[s] for the definitive procedure[s].) Do not append modifier -62 to bone graft codes 20900-20938.

A vertebral segment describes the basic constituent part into which the spine may be divided. It represents a single complete vertebral bone with its associated articular processes and laminae.

For the following codes, when two surgeons work together as primary surgeons performing distinct part(s) of an arthrodesis for spinal deformity, each surgeon should report his/her distinct operative work by appending modifier 62 to the procedure code. In this situation, modifier 62 may be appended to procedure code(s) 22800-22819 as long as both surgeons continue to work together as primary surgeons.

22800   Arthrodesis, posterior, for spinal deformity, with or without cast; up to 6 vertebral segments

22802   7 to 12 vertebral segments

22804   13 or more vertebral segments

22808   Arthrodesis, anterior, for spinal deformity, with or without cast; 2 to 3 vertebral segments

22810   4 to 7 vertebral segments

22812   8 or more vertebral segments

22818   Kyphectomy, circumferential exposure of spine and resection of vertebral segment(s) (including body and posterior elements); single or 2 segments

22819   3 or more segments

(To report arthrodesis, see 22800-22804 and add modifier -51)

EXPLORATION

To report instrumentation procedures, see 22840- 22855, 22859. (Codes 22840-22848, 22853, 22854, 22859 are reported in conjunction with code[s] for the definitive procedure[s]. When instrumentation reinsertion or removal is reported in conjunction with other definitive procedures, including arthrodesis, decompression, and exploration of fusion, append modifier 51 to 22849, 22850, 22852, and 22855.) Code 22849 should not be reported with 22850, 22852, and 22855 at the same spinal levels. To report exploration of fusion, see 22830. (When exploration is reported in conjunction with other definitive procedures, including arthrodesis and decompression, append modifier 51 to 22830.)

(To report bone graft procedures, see 20930-20938)

22830   Exploration of spinal fusion

SPINAL INSTRUMENTATION

Segmental instrumentation is defined as fixation at each end of the construct and at least one additional interposed bony attachment.

Non-segmental instrumentation is defined as fixation at each end of the construct and may span several vertebral segments without attachment to the intervening segments.

Insertion of spinal instrumentation is reported separately and in addition to arthrodesis. Instrumentation procedure codes 22840-22848, 22853, 22854, 22859 are reported in addition to the definitive procedure(s). Do not append modifier 62 to spinal instrumentation codes 22840-22848, 22850, 22852, 22853, 22854, 22859.

To report bone graft procedures, see 20930-20938. (Report in addition to code[s] for definitive procedure[s].) Do not append modifier -62 to bone graft codes 20900-20938.

A vertebral segment describes the basic constituent part into which the spine may be divided. It represents a single complete vertebral bone with its associated articular processes and laminae. A vertebral interspace is the non-bony compartment between two adjacent vertebral bodies, which contains the intervertebral disc, and includes the nucleus pulposus, annulus fibrosus, and two cartilaginous endplates.

Codes 22849, 22850, 22852, and 22855 are subject to modifier 51 if reported with other definitive procedure(s), including arthrodesis, decompression, and exploration of fusion. Code 22849 should not be reported in conjincyion with 22850, 22852, and 22855 at the same spinal levels. Only the appropriate insertion code (22840-22848) should be reported when previously placed spinal instrumentation is being removed or revised during the same session where new instrumentation is inserted at levels including all or part of the previously instrumented segments. Do not report the reinsertion (22849) or removal (22850, 22852, 22855) procedures in addition to the insertion of the new instrumentation (22840-22848).

+ **22840**   Posterior non-segmental instrumentation (eg, Harrington rod technique, pedicle fixation across 1 interspace, atlantoaxial transarticular screw fixation, sublaminar wiring at C1, facet screw fixation) (List separately in addition to code for primary procedure)

(Use 22840 in conjunction with 22100-22102, 22110- 22114, 22206, 22207, 22210-22214, 22220-22224, 22310- 22327, 22532, 22533, 22548-22558, 22590-22612, 22630, 22633, 22634, 22800-22812, 63001-63030, 63040-63042, 63045-63047, 63050-63056, 63064, 63075, 63077, 63081, 63085, 63087, 63090, 63101, 63102, 63170-63290, 63300-63307)

+ 22841   Internal spinal fixation by wiring of spinous processes (List separately in addition to code for primary procedure)

> Use 22841 in conjunction with 22100-22102, 22110- 22114, 22206, 22207, 22210-22214, 22220-22224, 22310-22327, 22532, 22533, 22548-22558, 22590-22612, 22630, 22633, 22634, 22800-22812, 63001-63030, 63040-63042, 63045-63047, 63050-63056, 63064, 63075, 63077, 63081, 63085, 63087, 63090, 63101, 63102, 63170-63290, 63300-63307)

+ 22842   Posterior segmental instrumentation (eg, pedicle fixation, dual rods with multiple hooks and sublaminar wires); 3 to 6 vertebral segments (List separately in addition to code for primary procedure)

> (Use 22842 in conjunction with 22100-22102, 22110- 22114, 22206, 22207, 22210-22214, 22220-22224, 22310-22327, 22532, 22533, 22548-22558, 22590-22612, 22630, 22633, 22634, 22800-22812, 63001-63030, 63040-63042, 63045-63047, 63050-63056, 63064, 63075, 63077, 63081, 63085, 63087, 63090, 63101, 63102, 63170-63290, 63300-63307)

+ 22843   7 to 12 vertebral segments (List separately in addition to code for primary procedure)

> (Use 22843 in conjunction with 22100-22102, 22110-22114, 22206, 22207, 22210-22214, 22220-22224, 22310-22327, 22532, 22533, 22548-22558, 22590-22612, 22630, 22633, 22634, 22800-22812, 63001-63030, 63040-63042, 63045-63047, 63050-63056, 63064, 63075, 63077, 63081, 63085, 63087, 63090, 63101, 63102, 63170-63290, 63300-63307)

+ 22844   13 or more vertebral segments (List separately in addition to code for primary procedure)

> (Use 22844 in conjunction with 22100-22102, 22110-22114, 22206, 22207, 22210-22214, 22220-22224, 22310-22327, 22532, 22533, 22548-22558, 22590-22612, 22630, 22633, 22634, 22800-22812, 63001-63030, 63040-63042, 63045-63047, 63050-63056, 63064, 63075, 63077, 63081, 63085, 63087, 63090, 63101, 63102, 63170-63290, 63300-63307)

+ 22845   Anterior instrumentation; 2 to 3 vertebral segments (List separately in addition to code for primary procedure)

> (Use 22845 in conjunction with 22100-22102, 22110-22114, 22206, 22207, 22210-22214, 22220-22224, 22310-22327, 22532, 22533, 22548-22558, 22590-22612, 22630, 22633, 22634, 22800-22812, 63001-63030, 63040-63042, 63045-63047, 63050-63056, 63064, 63075, 63077, 63081, 63085, 63087, 63090, 63101, 63102, 63170-63290, 63300-63307)

+ 22846   4 to 7 vertebral segments (List separately in addition to code for primary procedure)

> (Use 22846 in conjunction with 22100-22102, 22110-22114, 22206, 22207, 22210-22214, 22220-22224, 22310-22327, 22532, 22533, 22548-22558, 22590-22612, 22630, 22633, 22634, 22800-22812, 63001-63030, 63040-63042, 63045-63047, 63050-63056, 63064, 63075, 63077, 63081, 63085, 63087, 63090, 63101, 63102, 63170-63290, 63300-63307)

+ 22847   8 or more vertebral segments (List separately in addition to code for primary procedure)

> (Use 22847 in conjunction with 22100-22102, 22110-22114, 22206, 22207, 22210-22214, 22220-22224, 22310-22327, 22532, 22533, 22548-22558, 22590-22612, 22630, 22633, 22634, 22800-22812, 63001-63030, 63040-63042, 63045-63047, 63050-63056, 63064, 63075, 63077, 63081, 63085, 63087, 63090, 63101, 63102, 63170-63290, 63300-63307)

+ 22848   Pelvic fixation (attachment of caudal end of instrumentation to pelvic bony structures) other than sacrum (List separately in addition to code for primary procedure)

> (Use 22848 in conjunction with 22100-22102, 22110-22114, 22206, 22207, 22210-22214, 22220-22224, 22310-22327, 22532, 22533, 22548-22558, 22590-22612, 22630, 22633, 22634, 22800-22812, 63001-63030, 63040-63042, 63045-63047, 63050-63056, 63064, 63075, 63077, 63081, 63085, 63087, 63090, 63101, 63102, 63170-63290, 63300-63307)

22849   Reinsertion of spinal fixation device

22850   Removal of posterior nonsegmental instrumentation (eg, Harrington rod)

22852   Removal of posterior segmental instrumentation

+ 22853 Insertion of interbody biomechanical device(s) (eg, synthetic cage, mesh) with integral anterior instrumentation for device anchoring (eg, screws, flanges), when performed, to intervertebral disc space in conjunction with interbody arthrodesis, each interspace (List separately in addition to code for primary procedure)

(Use 22853 in conjunction with 22100-22102, 22110-22114, 22206, 22207, 22210-22214, 22220-22224, 22310-22327, 22532, 22533, 22548-22558, 22590-22612, 22630, 22633, 22634, 22800-22812, 63001-63030, 63040-63042, 63045-63047, 63050-63056, 63064, 63075, 63077, 63081, 63085, 63087, 63090, 63101, 63102, 63170-63290, 63300-63307)

(Report 22853 for each treated intervertebral disc space)

+ 22854 Insertion of intervertebral biomechanical device(s) (eg, synthetic cage, mesh) with integral anterior instrumentation for device anchoring (eg, screws, flanges), when performed, to vertebral corpectomy(ies) (vertebral body resection, partial or complete) defect, in conjunction with interbody arthrodesis, each contiguous defect (List separately in addition to code for primary procedure)

(Use 22854 in conjunction with 22100-22102, 22110-22114, 22206, 22207, 22210-22214, 22220-22224, 22310-22327, 22532, 22533, 22548-22558, 22590-22612, 22630, 22633, 22634, 22800-22812, 63001-63030, 63040-63042, 63045-63047, 63050-63056, 63064, 63075, 63077, 63081, 63085, 63087, 63090, 63101, 63102, 63170-63290, 63300-63307)

+ 22859 Insertion of intervertebral biomechanical device(s) (eg, synthetic cage, mesh, methylmethacrylate) to intervertebral disc space or vertebral body defect without interbody arthrodesis, each contiguous defect (List separately in addition to code for primary procedure)

(Use 22859 in conjunction with 22100-22102, 22110- 22114, 22206, 22207, 22210-22214, 22220-22224, 22310-22327, 22532, 22533, 22548-22558, 22590-22612, 22630, 22633, 22634, 22800-22812, 63001-63030, 63040-63042, 63045-63047, 63050-63056, 63064, 63075, 63077, 63081, 63085, 63087, 63090, 63101, 63102, 63170-63290, 63300-63307)

(22853, 22854, 22859 may be reported more than once for noncontiguous defects)

(For application of an intervertebral bone device/graft, see 20930, 20931, 20936, 20937, 20938)

22855 Removal of anterior instrumentation

22856 Total disc arthroplasty (artificial disc), anterior approach, including discectomy with end plate preparation (includes osteophytectomy for nerve root or spinal cord decompression and microdissection); single interspace, cervical

(Do not report 22856 in conjunction with 22554, 22845, 22853, 22854, 22859, 63075, when performed at the same level)

(Do not report 22856 in conjunction with 69990)

(For additional interspace cervical total disc arthroplasty, use 22858)

+ 22858 second level, cervical (List separately in addition to code for primary procedure)

(Use 22858 in conjunction with 22856)

22857 Total disc arthroplasty (artificial disc), anterior approach, including discectomy to prepare interspace (other than for decompression), single interspace, lumbar

(Do not report 22857 in conjunction with 22558, 22845, 22853, 22854, 22859, 49010 when performed at the same level)

(For additional interspace, use Category III code 0163T)

22858 This code is out of order. See page 285

22859 This code is out of order. See page 285

22861 Revision including replacement of total disc arthroplasty (artificial disc), anterior approach, single interspace; cervical

---

(Do not report 22861 in conjunction with 22845, 22853, 22854, 22859, 22864, 63075 when performed at the same level)

(Do not report 22861 in conjunction with 69990)

(For additional interspace revision of cervical total disc arthroplasty, use 0098T)

22862   lumbar

(Do not report 22862 in conjunction with 22558, 22845, 22853, 22854, 22859, 22865, 49010 when performed at the same level)

(For additional interspace, use Category III code 0165T)

22864   Removal of total disc arthroplasty (artificial disc), anterior approach single interspace; cervical

(Do not report 22864 in conjunction with 22861, 69990)

(For additional interspace removal of cervical total disc arthroplasty, use 0095T)

22865   lumbar

(Do not report 22865 in conjunction with 49010)

(For additional interspace, use Category III code 0164T)

(22856-22865 include fluoroscopy when performed)

(For decompression, see 63001-63048)

22867   Insertion of interlaminar/interspinous process stabilization/distraction device, without fusion, including image guidance when performed, with open decompression, lumbar; single level

+ 22868   second level (List separately in addition to code for primary procedure)

(Use 22868 in conjunction with 22867)

(Do not report 22867, 22868 in conjunction with 22532, 22533, 22534, 22558, 22612, 22614, 22630, 22632, 22633, 22634, 22800, 22802, 22804, 22840, 22841, 22842, 22869, 22870, 63005, 63012, 63017, 63030, 63035, 63042, 63044, 63047, 63048, 77003 for the same level)

(For insertion of interlaminar/interspinous process stabilization/distraction device, without open decompression or fusion, see 22869, 22870)

22869   Insertion of interlaminar/interspinous process stabilization/distraction device, without open decompression or fusion, including image guidance when performed, lumbar; single level

+ 22870   second level (List separately in addition to code for primary procedure)

(Use 22870 in conjunction with 22869)

(Do not report 22869, 22870 in conjunction with 22532, 22533, 22534, 22558, 22612, 22614, 22630, 22632, 22633, 22634, 22800, 22802, 22804, 22840, 22841, 22842, 63005, 63012, 63017, 63030, 63035, 63042, 63044, 63047, 63048, 77003)

OTHER PROCEDURES

22899   Unlisted procedure, spine

ABDOMEN

EXCISION

22900   Excision, tumor, soft tissue of abdominal wall, subfascial (eg, intramuscular); less than 5 cm

22901   5 cm or greater

● New Code   ▲ Revised Code   + Add-On Code   ⊘ Modifier -51 Exempt   ★ Telemedicine

22902 Excision, tumor, soft tissue of abdominal wall, subcutaneous; less than 3 cm

22903   3 cm or greater

(For excision of benign lesions of cutaneous origin [eg, sebaceous cyst], see 11400-11406)

22904 Radical resection of tumor (eg, sarcoma), soft tissue of abdominal wall; less than 5 cm

22905   5 cm or greater

(For radical resection of tumor[s] of cutaneous origin [eg, melanoma], see 11600-11606)

OTHER PROCEDURES

22999 Unlisted procedure, abdomen, musculoskeletal system

SHOULDER

INCISION

23000 Removal of subdeltoid calcareous deposits, open

(For arthroscopic removal of bursal deposits, use 29999)

23020 Capsular contracture release (eg, Sever type procedure)

(For incision and drainage procedures, superficial, see 10040-10160)

23030 Incision and drainage, shoulder area; deep abscess or hematoma

23031   infected bursa

23035 Incision, bone cortex (eg, osteomyelitis or bone abscess), shoulder area

23040 Arthrotomy, glenohumeral joint, including exploration, drainage, or removal of foreign body

23044 Arthrotomy, acromioclavicular, sternoclavicular joint, including exploration, drainage, or removal of foreign body

EXCISION

23065 Biopsy, soft tissue of shoulder area; superficial

23066   deep

(For needle biopsy of soft tissue, use 20206)

23071 This code is out of order. See page 287

23073 This code is out of order. See page 287

23075 Excision, tumor, soft tissue of shoulder area, subcutaneous; less than 3 cm

23071   3 cm or greater

(For excision of benign lesions of cutaneous origin [eg, sebaceous cyst], see 11400-11406)

23076 Excision, tumor, soft tissue of shoulder area, subfascial (eg, intramuscular); less than 5 cm

23073   5 cm or greater

23077 Radical resection of tumor (eg, sarcoma), soft tissue of shoulder area; less than 5 cm

---

23078   5 cm or greater

(For radical resection of tumor[s] of cutaneous origin [eg, melanoma], see 11600-11606)

23100   Arthrotomy, glenohumeral joint, including biopsy

23101   Arthrotomy, acromioclavicular joint or sternoclavicular joint, including biopsy and/or excision of torn cartilage

23105   Arthrotomy; glenohumeral joint, with synovectomy, with or without biopsy

23106   sternoclavicular joint, with synovectomy, with or without biopsy

23107   Arthrotomy, glenohumeral joint, with joint exploration, with or without removal of loose or foreign body

23120   Claviculectomy; partial

(For arthroscopic procedure, use 29824)

23125   total

23130   Acromioplasty or acromionectomy, partial, with or without coracoacromial ligament release

23140   Excision or curettage of bone cyst or benign tumor of clavicle or scapula;

23145   with autograft (includes obtaining graft)

23146   with allograft

23150   Excision or curettage of bone cyst or benign tumor of proximal humerus;

23155   with autograft (includes obtaining graft)

23156   with allograft

23170   Sequestrectomy (eg, for osteomyelitis or bone abscess), clavicle

23172   Sequestrectomy (eg, for osteomyelitis or bone abscess), scapula

23174   Sequestrectomy (eg, for osteomyelitis or bone abscess), humeral head to surgical neck

23180   Partial excision (craterization, saucerization, or diaphysectomy) bone (eg, osteomyelitis), clavicle

23182   Partial excision (craterization, saucerization, or diaphysectomy) bone (eg, osteomyelitis), scapula

23184   Partial excision (craterization, saucerization, or diaphysectomy) bone (eg, osteomyelitis), proximal humerus

23190   Ostectomy of scapula, partial (eg, superior medial angle)

23195   Resection, humeral head

(For replacement with implant, use 23470)

23200   Radical resection of tumor; clavicle

23210   scapula

23220   Radical resection of tumor, proximal humerus

● New Code   ▲ Revised Code   ＋ Add-On Code   ⊘ Modifier -51 Exempt   ★ Telemedicine

INTRODUCTION OR REMOVAL

(For arthrocentesis or needling of bursa, use 20610)

(For K-wire or pin insertion or removal, see 20650, 20670, 20680)

23330 Removal of foreign body, shoulder; subcutaneous

(To report removal of foreign body, see 23330, 23333)

23333 deep (subfascial or intramuscular)

23334 Removal of prosthesis, includes debridement and synovectomy when performed; humeral or glenoid component

23335 humeral and glenoid components (eg, total shoulder)

(Do not report 23334, 23335 in conjunction with 23473, 23474 if a prosthesis [ie, humeral and/or glenoid component(s)] is being removed and replaced in the same shoulder during the same surgical session)

(To report removal of hardware, other than humeral and/or glenoid prosthesis, use 20680)

23350 Injection procedure for shoulder arthrography or enhanced CT/MRI shoulder arthrography

(For radiographic arthrography, radiological supervision and interpretation, use 73040. Fluoroscopy [77002] is inclusive of radiographic arthrography)

(When fluoroscopic guided injection is performed for enhanced CT arthrography, use 23350, 77002 and 73201 or 73202)

(When fluoroscopic guided injection is performed for enhanced MR arthrography, use codes 23350, 77002, and 73222 or 73223)

(For enhanced CT or enhanced MRI arthrography, use 77002 and either 73201, 73202, 73222 or 73223)

(To report biopsy of the shoulder and joint, see 29805-29826)

REPAIR, REVISION AND/OR RECONSTRUCTION

23395 Muscle transfer, any type, shoulder or upper arm; single

23397 multiple

23400 Scapulopexy (eg, Sprengels deformity or for paralysis)

23405 Tenotomy, shoulder area; single tendon

23406 multiple tendons through same incision

23410 Repair of ruptured musculotendinous cuff (eg, rotator cuff) open; acute

23412 chronic

(For arthroscopic procedure, use 29827)

23415 Coracoacromial ligament release, with or without acromioplasty

(For arthroscopic procedure, use 29826)

23420 Reconstruction of complete shoulder (rotator) cuff avulsion, chronic (includes acromioplasty)

23430 Tenodesis of long tendon of biceps

(For arthroscopic biceps tenodesis, use 29828)

Separate Procedure   Unlisted Procedure   CCI Comp. Code   Non-specific Procedure   **289**

23440 Resection or transplantation of long tendon of biceps

23450 Capsulorrhaphy, anterior; Putti-Platt procedure or Magnuson type operation

(To report arthroscopic thermal capsulorrhaphy, use 29999)

23455 with labral repair (eg, Bankart procedure)

(For arthroscopic procedure, use 29806)

23460 Capsulorrhaphy, anterior, any type; with bone block

23462 with coracoid process transfer

(To report open thermal capsulorrhaphy, use 23929)

23465 Capsulorrhaphy, glenohumeral joint, posterior, with or without bone block

(For sternoclavicular and acromioclavicular reconstruction, see 23530, 23550)

23466 Capsulorrhaphy, glenohumeral joint, any type multi-directional instability

23470 Arthroplasty, glenohumeral joint; hemiarthroplasty

23472 total shoulder (glenoid and proximal humeral replacement (eg, total shoulder))

(For removal of total shoulder implants, see 23334, 23335)

(For osteotomy, proximal humerus, use 24400)

23473 Revision of total shoulder arthroplasty, including allograft when performed; humeral **or** glenoid component

23474 humeral **and** glenoid component

(Do not report 23473, 23474 in conjunction with 23334, 23335 if a prosthesis [ie, humeral and/or glenoid component(s)] is being removed and replaced in the same shoulder during the same surgical session)

23480 Osteotomy, clavicle, with or without internal fixation;

23485 with bone graft for nonunion or malunion (includes obtaining graft and/or necessary fixation)

23490 Prophylactic treatment (nailing, pinning, plating or wiring) with or without methylmethacrylate; clavicle

23491 proximal humerus

FRACTURE AND/OR DISLOCATION

23500 Closed treatment of clavicular fracture; without manipulation

23505 with manipulation

23515 Open treatment of clavicular fracture, includes internal fixation, when performed

23520 Closed treatment of sternoclavicular dislocation; without manipulation

23525 with manipulation

23530 Open treatment of sternoclavicular dislocation, acute or chronic;

23532 with fascial graft (includes obtaining graft)

23540 Closed treatment of acromioclavicular dislocation; without manipulation

● New Code   ▲ Revised Code   ✛ Add-On Code   ⃠ Modifier -51 Exempt   ★ Telemedicine

23545 with manipulation

23550 Open treatment of acromioclavicular dislocation, acute or chronic;

23552 with fascial graft (includes obtaining graft)

23570 Closed treatment of scapular fracture; without manipulation

23575 with manipulation, with or without skeletal traction (with or without shoulder joint involvement)

23585 Open treatment of scapular fracture (body, glenoid or acromion) includes internal fixation when performed

23600 Closed treatment of proximal humeral (surgical or anatomical neck) fracture; without manipulation

23605 with manipulation, with or without skeletal traction

23615 Open treatment of proximal humeral (surgical or anatomical neck) fracture, includes internal fixation, when performed includes repair of tuberosity(-ies) when performed;

23616 with proximal humeral prosthetic replacement

23620 Closed treatment of greater humeral tuberosity fracture; without manipulation

23625 with manipulation

23630 Open treatment of greater humeral tuberosity fracture, includes internal fixation, when performed

23650 Closed treatment of shoulder dislocation, with manipulation; without anesthesia

23655 requiring anesthesia

23660 Open treatment of acute shoulder dislocation

(Repairs for recurrent dislocations, see 23450-23466)

23665 Closed treatment of shoulder dislocation, with fracture of greater humeral tuberosity, with manipulation

23670 Open treatment of shoulder dislocation, with fracture of greater humeral tuberosity, includes internal fixation, when performed

23675 Closed treatment of shoulder dislocation, with surgical or anatomical neck fracture, with manipulation

23680 Open treatment of shoulder dislocation, with surgical or anatomical neck fracture, includes internal fixation, when performed

MANIPULATION

23700 Manipulation under anesthesia, shoulder joint, including application of fixation apparatus (dislocation excluded)

ARTHRODESIS

23800 Arthrodesis, glenohumeral joint;

23802 with autogenous graft (includes obtaining graft)

AMPUTATION

23900 Interthoracoscapular amputation (forequarter)

Separate Procedure   Unlisted Procedure   CCI Comp. Code   Non-specific Procedure   **291**

23920	Disarticulation of shoulder;
23921	secondary closure or scar revision

OTHER PROCEDURES

23929	Unlisted procedure, shoulder

HUMERUS (UPPER ARM) AND ELBOW

The elbow area includes the head and neck of the radius and olecranon process.

INCISION

(For incision and drainage procedures, superficial, see 10040-10160)

23930	Incision and drainage, upper arm or elbow area; deep abscess or hematoma
23931	bursa
23935	Incision, deep, with opening of bone cortex (eg, for osteomyelitis or bone abscess), humerus or elbow
24000	Arthrotomy, elbow, including exploration, drainage, or removal of foreign body
24006	Arthrotomy of the elbow, with capsular excision for capsular release (separate procedure)

EXCISION

24065	Biopsy, soft tissue of upper arm or elbow area; superficial
24066	deep (subfascial or intramuscular)

(For needle biopsy of soft tissue, use 20206)

24071	This code is out of order. See page 292
24073	This code is out of order. See page 292
24075	Excision, tumor, soft tissue of upper arm or elbow area, subcutaneous; less than 3 cm
24071	3 cm or greater

(For excision of benign lesions of cutaneous origin [eg, sebaceous cyst], see 11400-11406)

24076	Excision, tumor, soft tissue of upper arm or elbow area, subfascial (eg, intramuscular); less than 5 cm
24073	5 cm or greater
24077	Radical resection of tumor (eg, sarcoma), soft tissue of upper arm or elbow area; less than 5 cm
24079	5 cm or greater

(For radical resection of tumor[s] of cutaneous origin [eg, melanoma], see 11600-11606)

24100	Arthrotomy, elbow; with synovial biopsy only
24101	with joint exploration, with or without biopsy, with or without removal of loose or foreign body
24102	with synovectomy
24105	Excision, olecranon bursa

● New Code   ▲ Revised Code   ✛ Add-On Code   ⊘ Modifier -51 Exempt   ★ Telemedicine

24110 Excision or curettage of bone cyst or benign tumor, humerus;

24115   with autograft (includes obtaining graft)

24116   with allograft

24120 Excision or curettage of bone cyst or benign tumor of head or neck of radius or olecranon process;

24125   with autograft (includes obtaining graft)

24126   with allograft

24130 Excision, radial head

(For replacement with implant, use 24366)

24134 Sequestrectomy (eg, for osteomyelitis or bone abscess), shaft or distal humerus

24136 Sequestrectomy (eg, for osteomyelitis or bone abscess), radial head or neck

24138 Sequestrectomy (eg, for osteomyelitis or bone abscess), olecranon process

24140 Partial excision (craterization, saucerization, or diaphysectomy) bone (eg, osteomyelitis), humerus

24145 Partial excision (craterization, saucerization, or diaphysectomy) bone (eg, osteomyelitis), radial head or neck

24147 Partial excision (craterization, saucerization, or diaphysectomy) bone (eg, osteomyelitis), olecranon process

24149 Radical resection of capsule, soft tissue, and heterotopic bone, elbow, with contracture release (separate procedure)

(For capsular and soft tissue release only, use 24006)

24150 Radical resection of tumor, shaft or distal humerus

24152 Radical resection of tumor, radial head or neck

24155 Resection of elbow joint (arthrectomy)

INTRODUCTION OR REMOVAL

(For K-wire or pin insertion or removal, see 20650, 20670, 20680)

(For arthrocentesis or needling of bursa or joint, use 20605)

24160 Removal of prosthesis, includes debridement and synovectomy when performed; humeral and ulnar components

(To report removal of foreign body, elbow, see 24200, 24201)

(To report removal of hardware from the distal humerus or proximal ulna, other than humeral and ulnar prosthesis, use 20680)

(Do not report 24160 in conjunction with 24370 or 24371 if a prosthesis [ie, humeral and/or ulnar component(s)] is being removed and replaced in the same elbow during the same surgical session)

24164   radial head

(To report removal of foreign body, elbow, see 24200, 24201)

(To report removal of hardware from proximal radius, other than radial head prosthesis, use 20680)

| Separate Procedure | Unlisted Procedure | CCI Comp. Code | Non-specific Procedure | **293** |

24200 Removal of foreign body, upper arm or elbow area; subcutaneous

24201 deep (subfascial or intramuscular)

24220 Injection procedure for elbow arthrography

(For radiological supervision and interpretation, use 73085. Do not report 77002 in addition to 73085)

(For injection of tennis elbow, use 20550)

REPAIR, REVISION, AND/OR RECONSTRUCTION

24300 Manipulation, elbow, under anesthesia

(For application of external fixation, see 20690 or 20692)

24301 Muscle or tendon transfer, any type, upper arm or elbow, single (excluding 24320-24331)

24305 Tendon lengthening, upper arm or elbow, each tendon

24310 Tenotomy, open, elbow to shoulder, each tendon

24320 Tenoplasty, with muscle transfer, with or without free graft, elbow to shoulder, single (Seddon-Brookes type procedure)

24330 Flexor-plasty, elbow (eg, Steindler type advancement);

24331 with extensor advancement

24332 Tenolysis, triceps

24340 Tenodesis of biceps tendon at elbow (separate procedure)

24341 Repair, tendon or muscle, upper arm or elbow, each tendon or muscle, primary or secondary (excludes rotator cuff)

24342 Reinsertion of ruptured biceps or triceps tendon, distal, with or without tendon graft

24343 Repair lateral collateral ligament, elbow, with local tissue

24344 Reconstruction lateral collateral ligament, elbow, with tendon graft (includes harvesting of graft)

24345 Repair medial collateral ligament, elbow, with local tissue

24346 Reconstruction medial collateral ligament, elbow, with tendon graft (includes harvesting of graft)

24357 Tenotomy, elbow, lateral or medial (eg, epicondylitis, tennis elbow, golfer's elbow); percutaneous

24358 debridement, soft tissue and/or bone, open

24359 debridement, soft tissue and/or bone, open with tendon repair or reattachment

(Do not report 24357-24359 in conjunction with 29837, 29838)

24360 Arthroplasty, elbow; with membrane (eg, fascial)

24361 with distal humeral prosthetic replacement

24362 with implant and fascia lata ligament reconstruction

24363 with distal humerus and proximal ulnar prosthetic replacement (eg, total elbow)

---

294 ● New Code ▲ Revised Code + Add-On Code ⊘ Modifier -51 Exempt ★ Telemedicine

(For revision of total elbow implant, see 24370, 24371)

24365 Arthroplasty, radial head;

24366   with implant

24370 Revision of total elbow arthroplasty, including allograft when performed; humeral **or** ulnar component

24371   humeral **and** ulnar component

(Do not report 24370, 24371 in conjunction with 24160 if a prosthesis [ie, humeral and/or ulnar component(s)] is being removed and replaced in the same elbow)

24400 Osteotomy, humerus, with or without internal fixation

24410 Multiple osteotomies with realignment on intramedullary rod, humeral shaft (Sofield type procedure)

24420 Osteoplasty, humerus (eg, shortening or lengthening) (excluding 64876)

24430 Repair of nonunion or malunion, humerus; without graft (eg, compression technique)

24435   with iliac or other autograft (includes obtaining graft)

(For proximal radius and/or ulna, see 25400-25420)

24470 Hemiepiphyseal arrest (eg, cubitus varus or valgus, distal humerus)

24495 Decompression fasciotomy, forearm, with brachial artery exploration

24498 Prophylactic treatment (nailing, pinning, plating or wiring), with or without methylmethacrylate, humeral shaft

FRACTURE AND/OR DISLOCATION

24500 Closed treatment of humeral shaft fracture; without manipulation

24505   with manipulation, with or without skeletal traction

24515 Open treatment of humeral shaft fracture with plate/screws, with or without cerclage

24516 Treatment of humeral shaft fracture, with insertion of intramedullary implant, with or without cerclage and/or locking screws

24530 Closed treatment of supracondylar or transcondylar humeral fracture, with or without intercondylar extension; without manipulation

24535   with manipulation, with or without skin or skeletal traction

24538 Percutaneous skeletal fixation of supracondylar or transcondylar humeral fracture, with or without intercondylar extension

24545 Open treatment of humeral supracondylar or transcondylar fracture, includes internal fixation, when performed; without intercondylar extension

24546   with intercondylar extension

24560 Closed treatment of humeral epicondylar fracture, medial or lateral; without manipulation

24565   with manipulation

24566 Percutaneous skeletal fixation of humeral epicondylar fracture, medial or lateral, with manipulation

24575 Open treatment of humeral epicondylar fracture, medial or lateral, includes internal fixation, when performed

24576 Closed treatment of humeral condylar fracture, medial or lateral; without manipulation

24577   with manipulation

24579 Open treatment of humeral condylar fracture, medial or lateral, includes internal fixation, when performed

(To report closed treatment of fractures without manipulation, see 24530, 24560, 24576, 24650, 24670)

(To report closed treatment of fractures with manipulation, see 24535, 24565, 24577, 24675)

24582 Percutaneous skeletal fixation of humeral condylar fracture, medial or lateral, with manipulation

24586 Open treatment of periarticular fracture and/or dislocation of the elbow (fracture distal humerus and proximal ulna and/or proximal radius);

24587   with implant arthroplasty

(See also 24361)

24600 Treatment of closed elbow dislocation; without anesthesia

24605   requiring anesthesia

24615 Open treatment of acute or chronic elbow dislocation

24620 Closed treatment of Monteggia type of fracture dislocation at elbow (fracture proximal end of ulna with dislocation of radial head), with manipulation

24635 Open treatment of Monteggia type of fracture dislocation at elbow (fracture proximal end of ulna with dislocation of radial head), includes internal fixation, when performed

24640 Closed treatment of radial head subluxation in child, nursemaid elbow, with manipulation

24650 Closed treatment of radial head or neck fracture; without manipulation

24655   with manipulation

24665 Open treatment of radial head or neck fracture, includes internal fixation or radial head excision, when performed;

24666   with radial head prosthetic replacement

24670 Closed treatment of ulnar fracture, proximal end (eg, olecranon or coronoid process[es]); without manipulation

24675   with manipulation

24685 Open treatment of ulnar fracture proximal end (eg, olecranon or coronoid process[es]), includes internal fixation, when performed

(Do not report 24685 in conjunction with 24100-24102)

ARTHRODESIS

24800 Arthrodesis, elbow joint; local

● New Code   ▲ Revised Code   + Add-On Code   ⊘ Modifier -51 Exempt   ★ Telemedicine

24802	with autogenous graft (includes obtaining graft)

AMPUTATION

24900	Amputation, arm through humerus; with primary closure
24920	open, circular (guillotine)
24925	secondary closure or scar revision
24930	re-amputation
24931	with implant
24935	Stump elongation, upper extremity
24940	Cineplasty, upper extremity, complete procedure

OTHER PROCEDURES

24999	Unlisted procedure, humerus or elbow

FOREARM AND WRIST

Radius, ulna, carpal bones, and joints.

INCISION

25000	Incision, extensor tendon sheath, wrist (eg, deQuervains disease)
	(For decompression median nerve or for carpal tunnel syndrome, use 64721)
25001	Incision, flexor tendon sheath, wrist (eg, flexor carpi radialis)
25020	Decompression fasciotomy, forearm and/or wrist, flexor OR extensor compartment; without debridement of nonviable muscle and/or nerve
25023	with debridement of nonviable muscle and/or nerve
	(For decompression fasciotomy with brachial artery exploration, use 24495)
	(For incision and drainage procedures, superficial, see 10040-10160)
	(For debridement, see also 11000-11044)
25024	Decompression fasciotomy, forearm and/or wrist, flexor AND extensor compartment; without debridement of nonviable muscle and/or nerve
25025	with debridement of nonviable muscle and/or nerve
25028	Incision and drainage, forearm and/or wrist; deep abscess or hematoma
25031	bursa
25035	Incision, deep, bone cortex, forearm and/or wrist (eg, osteomyelitis or bone abscess)
25040	Arthrotomy, radiocarpal or midcarpal joint, with exploration, drainage, or removal of foreign body

EXCISION

25065	Biopsy, soft tissue of forearm and/or wrist; superficial

---

25066   deep (subfascial or intramuscular)

(For needle biopsy of soft tissue, use 20206)

25071   This code is out of order. See page 3298

25073   This code is out of order. See page 298

25075   Excision, tumor, soft tissue of forearm and/or wrist area, subcutaneous; less than 3 cm

25071   3 cm or greater

(For excision of benign lesions of cutaneous origin [eg, sebaceous cyst], see 11400-11406)

25076   Excision, tumor, soft tissue of forearm and/or wrist area, subfascial (eg, intramuscular); less than 3 cm

25073   3 cm or greater

25077   Radical resection of tumor (eg, sarcoma), soft tissue of forearm and/or wrist area; less than 3 cm

25078   3 cm or greater

(For radical resection of tumor[s] of cutaneous origin [eg, melanoma], see 11600-11606)

25085   Capsulotomy, wrist (eg, contracture)

25100   Arthrotomy, wrist joint; with biopsy

25101   with joint exploration, with or without biopsy, with or without removal of loose or foreign body

25105   with synovectomy

25107   Arthrotomy, distal radioulnar joint including repair of triangular cartilage, complex

25109   Excision of tendon, forearm and/or wrist, flexor or extensor, each

25110   Excision, lesion of tendon sheath, forearm and/or wrist

25111   Excision of ganglion, wrist (dorsal or volar); primary

25112   recurrent

(For hand or finger, use 26160)

25115   Radical excision of bursa, synovia of wrist, or forearm tendon sheaths (eg, tenosynovitis, fungus, Tbc, or other granulomas, rheumatoid arthritis); flexors

25116   extensors, with or without transposition of dorsal retinaculum

(For finger synovectomies, use 26145)

25118   Synovectomy, extensor tendon sheath, wrist, single compartment;

25119   with resection of distal ulna

25120   Excision or curettage of bone cyst or benign tumor of radius or ulna (excluding head or neck of radius and olecranon process);

(For head or neck of radius or olecranon process, see 24120-24126)

25125   with autograft (includes obtaining graft)

● New Code   ▲ Revised Code   + Add-On Code   ⊘ Modifier -51 Exempt   ★ Telemedicine

25126	with allograft
25130	Excision or curettage of bone cyst or benign tumor of carpal bones;
25135	with autograft (includes obtaining graft)
25136	with allograft
25145	Sequestrectomy (eg, for osteomyelitis or bone abscess), forearm and/or wrist
25150	Partial excision (craterization, saucerization, or diaphysectomy) of bone (eg, for osteomyelitis); ulna
25151	radius

(For head or neck of radius or olecranon process, see 24145, 24147)

25170	Radical resection of tumor, radius or ulna
25210	Carpectomy; 1 bone

(For carpectomy with implant, see 25441-25445)

25215	all bones of proximal row
25230	Radial styloidectomy (separate procedure)
25240	Excision distal ulna partial or complete (eg, Darrach type or matched resection)

(For implant replacement, distal ulna, use 25442)

(For obtaining fascia for interposition, see 20920, 20922)

INTRODUCTION OR REMOVAL

(For K-wire, pin or rod insertion or removal, see 20650, 20670, 20680)

25246	Injection procedure for wrist arthrography

(For radiological supervision and interpretation, use 73115. Do not report 77002 in addition to 73115)

(For foreign body removal, superficial use 20520)

25248	Exploration with removal of deep foreign body, forearm or wrist
25250	Removal of wrist prosthesis; (separate procedure)
25251	complicated, including total wrist
25259	Manipulation, wrist, under anesthesia

(For application of external fixation, see 20690 or 20692)

REPAIR, REVISION, AND/OR RECONSTRUCTION

25260	Repair, tendon or muscle, flexor, forearm and/or wrist; primary, single, each tendon or muscle
25263	secondary, single, each tendon or muscle
25265	secondary, with free graft (includes obtaining graft), each tendon or muscle
25270	Repair, tendon or muscle, extensor, forearm and/or wrist; primary, single, each tendon or muscle

Separate Procedure	Unlisted Procedure	CCI Comp. Code	Non-specific Procedure	**299**

25272   secondary, single, each tendon or muscle

25274   secondary, with free graft (includes obtaining graft), each tendon or muscle

25275   Repair, tendon sheath, extensor, forearm and/or wrist, with free graft (includes obtaining graft) (eg, for extensor carpi ulnaris subluxation)

25280   Lengthening or shortening of flexor or extensor tendon, forearm and/or wrist, single, each tendon

25290   Tenotomy, open, flexor or extensor tendon, forearm and/or wrist, single, each tendon

25295   Tenolysis, flexor or extensor tendon, forearm and/or wrist, single, each tendon

25300   Tenodesis at wrist; flexors of fingers

25301   extensors of fingers

25310   Tendon transplantation or transfer, flexor or extensor, forearm and/or wrist, single; each tendon

25312   with tendon graft(s) (includes obtaining graft), each tendon

25315   Flexor origin slide (eg, for cerebral palsy, Volkmann contracture), forearm and/or wrist;

25316   with tendon(s) transfer

25320   Capsulorrhaphy or reconstruction, wrist, open (eg, capsulodesis, ligament repair, tendon transfer or graft) (includes synovectomy, capsulotomy and open reduction) for carpal instability

25332   Arthroplasty, wrist, with or without interposition, with or without external or internal fixation

        (For obtaining fascia for interposition, see 20920, 20922)

        (For prosthetic replacement arthroplasty, see 25441-25446)

25335   Centralization of wrist on ulna (eg, radial club hand)

25337   Reconstruction for stabilization of unstable distal ulna or distal radioulnar joint, secondary by soft tissue stabilization (eg, tendon transfer, tendon graft or weave, or tenodesis) with or without open reduction of distal radioulnar joint

        (For harvesting of fascia lata graft, see 20920, 20922)

25350   Osteotomy, radius; distal third

25355   middle or proximal third

25360   Osteotomy; ulna

25365   radius AND ulna

25370   Multiple osteotomies, with realignment on intramedullary rod (Sofield type procedure); radius OR ulna

25375   radius AND ulna

25390   Osteoplasty, radius OR ulna; shortening

25391   lengthening with autograft

25392   Osteoplasty, radius AND ulna; shortening (excluding 64876)

25393	lengthening with autograft
25394	Osteoplasty, carpal bone, shortening
25400	Repair of nonunion or malunion, radius OR ulna; without graft (eg, compression technique)
25405	with autograft (includes obtaining graft)
25415	Repair of nonunion or malunion, radius AND ulna; without graft (eg, compression technique)
25420	with autograft (includes obtaining graft)
25425	Repair of defect with autograft; radius OR ulna
25426	radius AND ulna
25430	Insertion of vascular pedicle into carpal bone (eg, Hori procedure)
25431	Repair of nonunion of carpal bone (excluding carpal scaphoid (navicular) (includes obtaining graft and necessary fixation), each bone
25440	Repair of nonunion, scaphoid carpal (navicular) bone, with or without radial styloidectomy (includes obtaining graft and necessary fixation)
25441	Arthroplasty with prosthetic replacement; distal radius
25442	distal ulna
25443	scaphoid carpal (navicular)
25444	lunate
25445	trapezium
25446	distal radius and partial or entire carpus (total wrist)
25447	Arthroplasty, interposition, intercarpal or carpometacarpal joints
	(For wrist arthroplasty, use 25332)
25449	Revision of arthroplasty, including removal of implant, wrist joint
25450	Epiphyseal arrest by epiphysiodesis or stapling; distal radius OR ulna
25455	distal radius AND ulna
25490	Prophylactic treatment (nailing, pinning, plating or wiring) with or without methylmethacrylate; radius
25491	ulna
25492	radius AND ulna

FRACTURE AND/OR DISLOCATION

(For application of external fixation in addition to internal fixation, use 20690 and the appropriate internal fixation code)

25500	Closed treatment of radial shaft fracture; without manipulation
25505	with manipulation

25515   Open treatment of radial shaft fracture, includes internal fixation, when performed

25520   Closed treatment of radial shaft fracture and closed treatment of dislocation of distal radioulnar joint (Galeazzi fracture/dislocation)

25525   Open treatment of radial shaft fracture, includes internal fixation, when performed, and closed treatment of distal radioulnar joint dislocation (Galeazzi fracture/dislocation), includes percutaneous skeletal fixation, when performed

25526   Open treatment of radial shaft fracture, includes internal fixation, when performed, and open treatment, of distal radioulnar joint dislocation (Galeazzi fracture/dislocation), includes internal fixation, when performed, includes repair of triangular fibrocartilage complex

25530   Closed treatment of ulnar shaft fracture; without manipulation

25535   with manipulation

25545   Open treatment of ulnar shaft fracture, includes internal fixation, when performed

25560   Closed treatment of radial and ulnar shaft fractures; without manipulation

25565   with manipulation

25574   Open treatment of radial AND ulnar shaft fractures, with internal fixation, when performed; of radius OR ulna

25575   of radius AND ulna

25600   Closed treatment of distal radial fracture (eg, Colles or Smith type) or epiphyseal separation, includes closed treatment of fracture of ulnar styloid, when performed; without manipulation

25605   with manipulation

     (Do not report 25600, 25605 in conjunction with 25650)

25606   Percutaneous skeletal fixation of distal radial fracture or epiphyseal separation

     (Do not report 25606 in conjunction with 25650)

     (For percutaneous treatment of ulnar styloid fracture, use 25651)

     (For open treatment of ulnar styloid fracture, use 25652)

25607   Open treatment of distal radial extra-articular fracture or epiphyseal separation, with internal fixation

     (Do not report 25607 in conjunction with 25650)

     (For percutaneous treatment of ulnar styloid fracture, use 25651)

     (For open treatment of ulnar styloid fracture, use 25652)

25608   Open treatment of distal radial intra-articular fracture or epiphyseal separation; with internal fixation of 2 fragments

     (Do not report 25608 in conjunction with 25609)

25609   with internal fixation of 3 or more fragments

     (Do not report 25608, 25609 in conjunction with 25650)

     (For percutaneous treatment of ulnar styloid fracture, use 25651)

     (For open treatment of ulnar styloid fracture, use 25652)

25622 Closed treatment of carpal scaphoid (navicular) fracture; without manipulation

25624   with manipulation

25628 Open treatment of carpal scaphoid (navicular) fracture, includes internal fixation, when performed

25630 Closed treatment of carpal bone fracture (excluding carpal scaphoid [navicular]); without manipulation, each bone

25635   with manipulation, each bone

25645 Open treatment of carpal bone fracture (other than carpal scaphoid [navicular]), each bone

25650 Closed treatment of ulnar styloid fracture

(Do not report 25650 in conjunction with 25600, 25605, 25607-25609)

25651 Percutaneous skeletal fixation of ulnar styloid fracture

25652 Open treatment of ulnar styloid fracture

25660 Closed treatment of radiocarpal or intercarpal dislocation, 1 or more bones, with manipulation

25670 Open treatment of radiocarpal or intercarpal dislocation, 1 or more bones

25671 Percutaneous skeletal fixation of distal radioulnar dislocation

25675 Closed treatment of distal radioulnar dislocation with manipulation

25676 Open treatment of distal radioulnar dislocation, acute or chronic

25680 Closed treatment of trans-scaphoperilunar type of fracture dislocation, with manipulation

25685 Open treatment of trans-scaphoperilunar type of fracture dislocation

25690 Closed treatment of lunate dislocation, with manipulation

25695 Open treatment of lunate dislocation

ARTHRODESIS

25800 Arthrodesis, wrist; complete, without bone graft (includes radiocarpal and/or intercarpal and/or carpometacarpal joints)

25805   with sliding graft

25810   with iliac or other autograft (includes obtaining graft)

25820 Arthrodesis, wrist; limited, without bone graft (eg, intercarpal or radiocarpal)

25825   with autograft (includes obtaining graft)

25830 Arthrodesis, distal radioulnar joint with segmental resection of ulna, with or without bone graft (eg, Sauve-Kapandji procedure)

AMPUTATION

25900 Amputation, forearm, through radius and ulna;

25905   open, circular (guillotine)

25907	secondary closure or scar revision
25909	re-amputation
25915	Krukenberg procedure
25920	Disarticulation through wrist;
25922	secondary closure or scar revision
25924	re-amputation
25927	Transmetacarpal amputation;
25929	secondary closure or scar revision
25931	re-amputation

OTHER PROCEDURES

25999	Unlisted procedure, forearm or wrist

HAND AND FINGERS

INCISION

26010	Drainage of finger abscess; simple
26011	complicated (eg, felon)
26020	Drainage of tendon sheath, digit and/or palm, each
26025	Drainage of palmar bursa; single, bursa
26030	multiple bursa
26034	Incision, bone cortex, hand or finger (eg, osteomyelitis or bone abscess)
26035	Decompression fingers and/or hand, injection injury (eg, grease gun)
26037	Decompressive fasciotomy, hand (excludes 26035)
	(For injection injury, use 26035)
26040	Fasciotomy, palmar (eg, Dupuytren's contracture); percutaneous
26045	open, partial
	(For palmar fasciotomy by enzyme injection (eg, collagenase), see 20527, 26341)
	(For fasciectomy, see 26121-26125)
26055	Tendon sheath incision (eg, for trigger finger)
26060	Tenotomy, percutaneous, single, each digit
26070	Arthrotomy, with exploration, drainage, or removal of loose or foreign body; carpometacarpal joint
26075	metacarpophalangeal joint, each

26080   interphalangeal joint, each

EXCISION

26100   Arthrotomy with biopsy; carpometacarpal joint, each

26105   metacarpophalangeal joint, each

26110   interphalangeal joint, each

26111   This code is out of order. See page 305

26113   This code is out of order. See page 305

26115   Excision, tumor or vascular malformation, soft tissue of hand or finger, subcutaneous; less than 1.5 cm

26111   1.5 cm or greater

          (For excision of benign lesions of cutaneous origin [eg, sebaceous cyst], see 11420-11426)

26116   Excision, tumor or vascular malformation, soft tissue of hand or finger, subfascial (eg, intramuscular); less than 1.5 cm

26113   1.5 cm or greater

26117   Radical resection of tumor (eg, sarcoma), soft tissue of hand or finger; less than 3 cm

26118   3 cm or greater

          (For radical resection of tumor[s] of cutaneous origin [eg, melanoma], see 11620-11626)

26121   Fasciectomy, palm only, with or without Z-plasty, other local tissue rearrangement, or skin grafting (includes obtaining graft)

26123   Fasciectomy, partial palmar with release of single digit including proximal interphalangeal joint, with or without Z-plasty, other local tissue rearrangement, or skin grafting (includes obtaining graft);

+ **26125**   each additional digit (List separately in addition to code for primary procedure)

          (Use 26125 in conjunction with code 26123)

          (For palmar fasciotomy by enzyme injection (eg, collagenase), see 20527, 26341)

          (For fasciotomy, see 26040, 26045)

26130   Synovectomy, carpometacarpal joint

26135   Synovectomy, metacarpophalangeal joint including intrinsic release and extensor hood reconstruction, each digit

26140   Synovectomy, proximal interphalangeal joint, including extensor reconstruction, each interphalangeal joint

26145   Synovectomy, tendon sheath, radical (tenosynovectomy), flexor tendon, palm and/or finger, each tendon

          (For tendon sheath synovectomies at wrist, see 25115, 25116)

26160   Excision of lesion of tendon sheath or joint capsule (eg, cyst, mucous cyst, or ganglion), hand or finger

          (For wrist ganglion, see 25111, 25112)

          (For trigger digit, use 26055)

26170   Excision of tendon, palm, flexor or extensor, single, each tendon

---

(Do not report 26170 in conjunction with 26390, 26415)

26180 Excision of tendon, finger, flexor or extensor, each tendon

(Do not report 26180 in conjunction with 26390, 26415)

26185 Sesamoidectomy, thumb or finger (separate procedure)

26200 Excision or curettage of bone cyst or benign tumor of metacarpal;

26205   with autograft (includes obtaining graft)

26210 Excision or curettage of bone cyst or benign tumor of proximal, middle, or distal phalanx of finger;

26215   with autograft (includes obtaining graft)

26230 Partial excision (craterization, saucerization, or diaphysectomy) bone (eg, osteomyelitis); metacarpal

26235   proximal or middle phalanx of finger

26236   distal phalanx of finger

26250 Radical resection of tumor, metacarpal

26260 Radical resection of tumor, proximal or middle phalanx of finger

26262 Radical resection of tumor, distal phalanx of finger

INTRODUCTION OR REMOVAL

26320 Removal of implant from finger or hand

(For removal of foreign body in hand or finger, see 20520, 20525)

REPAIR, REVISION, AND/OR RECONSTRUCTION

26340 Manipulation, finger joint, under anesthesia, each joint

(For application of external fixation, see 20690 or 20692)

26341 Manipulation, palmar fascial cord (ie, Dupuytren's cord), post enzyme injection (eg, collagenase), single cord

(For enzyme injection (eg, collagenase), palmar fascial cord (eg., Dupuytren's contracture), use 20527)

(Report custom orthotic fabrication/application separately)

26350 Repair or advancement, flexor tendon, not in zone 2 digital flexor tendon sheath (eg, no man's land); primary or secondary without free graft, each tendon

26352   secondary with free graft (includes obtaining graft), each tendon

26356 Repair or advancement, flexor tendon, in zone 2 digital flexor tendon sheath (eg, no man's land); primary, without free graft, each tendon

26357   secondary, without free graft, each tendon

26358   secondary with free graft (includes obtaining graft), each tendon

26370 Repair or advancement of profundus tendon, with intact superficialis tendon; primary, each tendon

26372   secondary with free graft (includes obtaining graft), each tendon

26373	secondary without free graft, each tendon
26390	Excision flexor tendon, with implantation of synthetic rod for delayed tendon graft, hand or finger, each rod
26392	Removal of synthetic rod and insertion of flexor tendon graft, hand or finger (includes obtaining graft), each rod
26410	Repair, extensor tendon, hand, primary or secondary; without free graft, each tendon
26412	with free graft (includes obtaining graft), each tendon
26415	Excision of extensor tendon, with implantation of synthetic rod for delayed tendon graft, hand or finger, each rod
26416	Removal of synthetic rod and insertion of extensor tendon graft (includes obtaining graft), hand or finger, each rod
26418	Repair, extensor tendon, finger, primary or secondary; without free graft, each tendon
26420	with free graft (includes obtaining graft) each tendon
26426	Repair of extensor tendon, central slip, secondary (eg, boutonniere deformity); using local tissue(s), including lateral band(s), each finger
26428	with free graft (includes obtaining graft), each finger
26432	Closed treatment of distal extensor tendon insertion, with or without percutaneous pinning (eg, mallet finger)
26433	Repair of extensor tendon, distal insertion, primary or secondary; without graft (eg, mallet finger)
26434	with free graft (includes obtaining graft)
	(For tenovaginotomy for trigger finger, use 26055)
26437	Realignment of extensor tendon, hand, each tendon
26440	Tenolysis, flexor tendon; palm OR finger, each tendon
26442	palm AND finger, each tendon
26445	Tenolysis, extensor tendon, hand or finger; each tendon
26449	Tenolysis, complex, extensor tendon, finger, including forearm, each tendon
26450	Tenotomy, flexor, palm, open, each tendon
26455	Tenotomy, flexor, finger, open, each tendon
26460	Tenotomy, extensor, hand or finger, open, each tendon
26471	Tenodesis; of proximal interphalangeal joint, each joint
26474	of distal joint, each joint
26476	Lengthening of tendon, extensor, hand or finger, each tendon
26477	Shortening of tendon, extensor, hand or finger, each tendon

26478 Lengthening of tendon, flexor, hand or finger, each tendon

26479 Shortening of tendon, flexor, hand or finger, each tendon

26480 Transfer or transplant of tendon, carpometacarpal area or dorsum of hand; without free graft, each tendon

26483 with free tendon graft (includes obtaining graft), each tendon

26485 Transfer or transplant of tendon, palmar; without free tendon graft, each tendon

26489 with free tendon graft (includes obtaining graft), each tendon

26490 Opponensplasty; superficialis tendon transfer type, each tendon

26492 tendon transfer with graft (includes obtaining graft), each tendon

26494 hypothenar muscle transfer

26496 other methods

(For thumb fusion in opposition, use 26820)

26497 Transfer of tendon to restore intrinsic function; ring and small finger

26498 all 4 fingers

26499 Correction claw finger, other methods

26500 Reconstruction of tendon pulley, each tendon; with local tissues (separate procedure)

26502 with tendon or fascial graft (includes obtaining graft) (separate procedure)

26508 Release of thenar muscle(s) (eg, thumb contracture)

26510 Cross intrinsic transfer, each tendon

26516 Capsulodesis, metacarpophalangeal joint; single digit

26517 2 digits

26518 3 or 4 digits

26520 Capsulectomy or capsulotomy; metacarpophalangeal joint, each joint

26525 interphalangeal joint, each joint

26530 Arthroplasty, metacarpophalangeal joint; each joint

(To report carpometacarpal joint arthroplasty, use 25447)

26531 with prosthetic implant, each joint

26535 Arthroplasty, interphalangeal joint; each joint

26536 with prosthetic implant, each joint

26540 Repair of collateral ligament, metacarpophalangeal or interphalangeal joint

---

● New Code ▲ Revised Code ✚ Add-On Code ⊘ Modifier -51 Exempt ★ Telemedicine

26541 Reconstruction, collateral ligament, metacarpophalangeal joint, single; with tendon or fascial graft (includes obtaining graft)

26542   with local tissue (eg, adductor advancement)

26545 Reconstruction, collateral ligament, interphalangeal joint, single, including graft, each joint

26546 Repair non-union, metacarpal or phalanx, (includes obtaining bone graft with or without external or internal fixation)

26548 Repair and reconstruction, finger, volar plate, interphalangeal joint

26550 Pollicization of a digit

26551 Transfer, toe-to-hand with microvascular anastomosis; great toe wrap-around with bone graft

    (For great toe with web space, use 20973)

26553   other than great toe, single

26554   other than great toe, double

    (Do not report code 69990 in addition to codes 26551-26554)

26555 Transfer, finger to another position without microvascular anastomosis

26556 Transfer, free toe joint, with microvascular anastomosis

    (Do not report code 69990 in addition to code 26556)

    (To report great toe-to-hand transfer, use 20973)

26560 Repair of syndactyly (web finger) each web space; with skin flaps

26561   with skin flaps and grafts

26562   complex (eg, involving bone, nails)

26565 Osteotomy; metacarpal, each

26567   phalanx of finger, each

26568 Osteoplasty, lengthening, metacarpal or phalanx

26580 Repair cleft hand

26587 Reconstruction of polydactylous digit, soft tissue and bone

    (For excision of polydactylous digit, soft tissue only, use 11200)

26590 Repair macrodactylia, each digit

26591 Repair, intrinsic muscles of hand, each muscle

26593 Release, intrinsic muscles of hand, each muscle

26596 Excision of constricting ring of finger, with multiple Z-plasties

    (To report release of scar contracture or graft repairs, see 11042, 14040-14041, or 15120, 15240)

Separate Procedure   Unlisted Procedure   CCI Comp. Code   Non-specific Procedure   **309**

FRACTURE AND/OR DISLOCATION

26600   Closed treatment of metacarpal fracture, single; without manipulation, each bone

26605   with manipulation, each bone

26607   Closed treatment of metacarpal fracture, with manipulation, with external fixation, each bone

26608   Percutaneous skeletal fixation of metacarpal fracture, each bone

26615   Open treatment of metacarpal fracture, single, includes internal fixation, when performed, each bone

26641   Closed treatment of carpometacarpal dislocation, thumb, with manipulation

26645   Closed treatment of carpometacarpal fracture dislocation, thumb (Bennett fracture), with manipulation

26650   Percutaneous skeletal fixation of carpometacarpal fracture dislocation, thumb (Bennett fracture), with manipulation

26665   Open treatment of carpometacarpal fracture dislocation, thumb (Bennett fracture), includes internal fixation, when performed

26670   Closed treatment of carpometacarpal dislocation, other than thumb, with manipulation, each joint; without anesthesia

26675   requiring anesthesia

26676   Percutaneous skeletal fixation of carpometacarpal dislocation, other than thumb, with manipulation, each joint

26685   Open treatment of carpometacarpal dislocation, other than thumb; includes internal fixation, when performed, each joint

26686   complex, multiple or delayed reduction

26700   Closed treatment of metacarpophalangeal dislocation, single, with manipulation; without anesthesia

26705   requiring anesthesia

26706   Percutaneous skeletal fixation of metacarpophalangeal dislocation, single, with manipulation

26715   Open treatment of metacarpophalangeal dislocation, single, includes internal fixation, when performed

26720   Closed treatment of phalangeal shaft fracture, proximal or middle phalanx, finger or thumb; without manipulation, each

26725   with manipulation, with or without skin or skeletal traction, each

26727   Percutaneous skeletal fixation of unstable phalangeal shaft fracture, proximal or middle phalanx, finger or thumb, with manipulation, each

26735   Open treatment of phalangeal shaft fracture, proximal or middle phalanx, finger or thumb, includes internal fixation, when performed, each

26740   Closed treatment of articular fracture, involving metacarpophalangeal or interphalangeal joint; without manipulation, each

26742   with manipulation, each

● New Code   ▲ Revised Code   ✚ Add-On Code   ⊘ Modifier -51 Exempt   ★ Telemedicine

26746	Open treatment of articular fracture, involving metacarpophalangeal or interphalangeal joint, includes internal fixation, when performed, each
26750	Closed treatment of distal phalangeal fracture, finger or thumb; without manipulation, each
26755	with manipulation, each
26756	Percutaneous skeletal fixation of distal phalangeal fracture, finger or thumb, each
26765	Open treatment of distal phalangeal fracture, finger or thumb, includes internal fixation, when performed, each
26770	Closed treatment of interphalangeal joint dislocation, single, with manipulation; without anesthesia
26775	requiring anesthesia
26776	Percutaneous skeletal fixation of interphalangeal joint dislocation, single, with manipulation
26785	Open treatment of interphalangeal joint dislocation, includes internal fixation, when performed, single

ARTHRODESIS

26820	Fusion in opposition, thumb, with autogenous graft (includes obtaining graft)
26841	Arthrodesis, carpometacarpal joint, thumb, with or without internal fixation;
26842	with autograft (includes obtaining graft)
26843	Arthrodesis, carpometacarpal joint, digit, other than thumb, each;
26844	with autograft (includes obtaining graft)
26850	Arthrodesis, metacarpophalangeal joint, with or without internal fixation;
26852	with autograft (includes obtaining graft)
26860	Arthrodesis, interphalangeal joint, with or without internal fixation;
+ 26861	each additional interphalangeal joint (List separately in addition to code for primary procedure)
	(Use 26861 in conjunction with code 26860)
26862	with autograft (includes obtaining graft)
+ 26863	with autograft (includes obtaining graft), each additional joint (List separately in addition to code for primary procedure)
	(Use 26863 in conjunction with code 26862)

AMPUTATION

	(For hand through metacarpal bones, use 25927)
26910	Amputation, metacarpal, with finger or thumb (ray amputation), single, with or without interosseous transfer
	(For repositioning see 26550, 26555)
26951	Amputation, finger or thumb, primary or secondary, any joint or phalanx, single, including neurectomies; with direct closure

---

26952   with local advancement flaps (V-Y, hood)

(For repair of soft tissue defect requiring split or full thickness graft or other pedicle flaps, see 15050-15758)

OTHER PROCEDURES

26989   Unlisted procedure, hands or fingers

PELVIS AND HIP JOINT

Including head and neck of femur.

INCISION

(For incision and drainage procedures, superficial, see 10040-10160)

26990   Incision and drainage, pelvis or hip joint area; deep abscess or hematoma

26991   infected bursa

26992   Incision, bone cortex, pelvis and/or hip joint (eg, osteomyelitis or bone abscess)

27000   Tenotomy, adductor of hip, percutaneous (separate procedure)

27001   Tenotomy, adductor of hip, open

(To report bilateral procedures, report 27001 with modifier -50)

27003   Tenotomy, adductor, subcutaneous, open, with obturator neurectomy

(To report bilateral procedures, report 27003 with modifier -50)

27005   Tenotomy, hip flexor(s), open (separate procedure)

27006   Tenotomy, abductors and/or extensor(s) of hip, open (separate procedure)

27025   Fasciotomy, hip or thigh, any type

(To report bilateral procedures, report 27025 with modifier -50)

27027   Decompression fasciotomy(ies), pelvic (buttock) compartment(s) (eg, gluteus medius-minimus, gluteus maximus, iliopsoas, and/or tensor fascia lata muscle), unilateral

(To report bilateral procedure, report 27027 with modifier 50)

27030   Arthrotomy, hip, with drainage (eg, infection)

27033   Arthrotomy, hip, including exploration or removal of loose or foreign body

27035   Denervation, hip joint, intrapelvic or extrapelvic intra-articular branches of sciatic, femoral, or obturator nerves

(For obturator neurectomy, see 64763, 64766)

27036   Capsulectomy or capsulotomy, hip, with or without excision of heterotopic bone, with release of hip flexor muscles (ie, gluteus medius, gluteus minimus, tensor fascia latae, rectus femoris, sartorius, iliopsoas)

EXCISION

27040   Biopsy, soft tissue of pelvis and hip area; superficial

27041   deep, subfascial or intramuscular

● New Code   ▲ Revised Code   + Add-On Code   ⊘ Modifier -51 Exempt   ★ Telemedicine

(For needle biopsy of soft tissue, use 20206)

27043　This code is out of order. See page 313

27045　This code is out of order. See page 313

27047　Excision, tumor, soft tissue of pelvis and hip area, subcutaneous; less than 3 cm

27043　　　3 cm or greater

(For excision of benign lesions of cutaneous origin [eg, sebaceous cyst], see 11400-11406)

27048　Excision, tumor, soft tissue of pelvis and hip area, subfascial (eg, intramuscular); less than 5 cm

27045　　　5 cm or greater

27049　Radical resection of tumor (eg, sarcoma), soft tissue of pelvis and hip area; less than 5 cm

27059　　　5 cm or greater

(For radical resection of tumor[s] of cutaneous origin [eg, melanoma], see 11600-11606)

27050　Arthrotomy, with biopsy; sacroiliac joint

27052　　　hip joint

27054　Arthrotomy with synovectomy, hip joint

27057　Decompression fasciotomy(ies), pelvic (buttock) compartment(s) (eg, gluteus medius-minimus, gluteus maximus, iliopsoas, and/or tensor fascia lata muscle) with debridement of nonviable muscle, unilateral

(To report bilateral procedure, report 27057 with modifier 50)

27059　This code is out of order. See page 313

27060　Excision; ischial bursa

27062　　　trochanteric bursa or calcification

(For arthrocentesis or needling of bursa, use 20610)

27065　Excision of bone cyst or benign tumor, wing of ilium, symphysis pubis, or greater trochanter of femur; superficial, includes autograft when performed

27066　　　deep (subfascial), includes autograft when performed

27067　　　with autograft requiring separate incision

27070　Partial excision, wing of ilium, symphysis pubis, or greater trochanter of femur, (craterization, saucerization) (eg, osteomyelitis or bone abscess); superficial

27071　　　deep (subfascial or intramuscular)

27075　Radical resection of tumor; wing of ilium, one pubic or ischial ramus or symphysis pubis

27076　　　ilium, including acetabulum, both pubic rami, or ischium and acetabulum

27077　　　innominate bone, total

27078　　　ischial tuberosity and greater trochanter of femur

27080 Coccygectomy, primary

(For pressure (decubitus) ulcer, see 15920, 15922 and 15931-15958)

INTRODUCTION OR REMOVAL

27086 Removal of foreign body, pelvis or hip; subcutaneous tissue

27087   deep (subfascial or intramuscular)

27090 Removal of hip prosthesis; (separate procedure)

27091   complicated, including total hip prosthesis, methylmethacrylate with or without insertion of spacer

27093 Injection procedure for hip arthrography; without anesthesia

(For radiological supervision and interpretation, use 73525. Do not report 77002 in conjunction with 73525)

27095   with anesthesia

(For radiological supervision and interpretation, use 73525. Do not report 77002 in conjunction with 73525)

27096 Injection procedure for sacroiliac joint, anesthetic/steroid, with image guidance (fluoroscopy or CT) including arthrography when performed

(27096 is to be used only with CT or fluoroscopic imaging confirmation of intra-articular needle positioning)

(If CT or fluoroscopic imaging is not performed, use 20552)

(Code 27096 is a unilateral procedure. For bilateral procedure, use modifier -50)

REPAIR, REVISION, AND/OR RECONSTRUCTION

27097 Release or recession, hamstring, proximal

27098 Transfer, adductor to ischium

27100 Transfer external oblique muscle to greater trochanter including fascial or tendon extension (graft)

27105 Transfer paraspinal muscle to hip (includes fascial or tendon extension graft)

27110 Transfer iliopsoas; to greater trochanter of femur

27111   to femoral neck

27120 Acetabuloplasty; (eg, Whitman, Colonna, Haygroves, or cup type)

27122   resection, femoral head (eg, Girdlestone procedure)

27125 Hemiarthroplasty, hip, partial (eg, femoral stem prosthesis, bipolar arthroplasty)

(For prosthetic replacement following fracture of the hip, use 27236)

27130 Arthroplasty, acetabular and proximal femoral prosthetic replacement (total hip arthroplasty), with or without autograft or allograft

27132 Conversion of previous hip surgery to total hip arthroplasty, with or without autograft or allograft

27134 Revision of total hip arthroplasty; both components, with or without autograft or allograft

27137	acetabular component only, with or without autograft or allograft
27138	femoral component only, with or without allograft
27140	Osteotomy and transfer of greater trochanter of femur (separate procedure)
27146	Osteotomy, iliac, acetabular or innominate bone;
27147	with open reduction of hip
27151	with femoral osteotomy
27156	with femoral osteotomy and with open reduction of hip
27158	Osteotomy, pelvis, bilateral (eg, congenital malformation)
27161	Osteotomy, femoral neck (separate procedure)
27165	Osteotomy, intertrochanteric or subtrochanteric including internal or external fixation and/or cast
27170	Bone graft, femoral head, neck, intertrochanteric or subtrochanteric area (includes obtaining bone graft)
27175	Treatment of slipped femoral epiphysis; by traction, without reduction
27176	by single or multiple pinning, in situ
27177	Open treatment of slipped femoral epiphysis; single or multiple pinning or bone graft (includes obtaining graft)
27178	closed manipulation with single or multiple pinning
27179	osteoplasty of femoral neck (Heyman type procedure)
27181	osteotomy and internal fixation
27185	Epiphyseal arrest by epiphysiodesis or stapling, greater trochanter of femur
27187	Prophylactic treatment (nailing, pinning, plating or wiring) with or without methylmethacrylate, femoral neck and proximal femur

FRACTURE AND/OR DISLOCATION

27197	Closed treatment of posterior pelvic ring fracture(s), dislocation(s), diastasis or subluxation of the ilium, sacroiliac joint, and/or sacrum, with or without anterior pelvic ring fracture(s) and/or dislocation(s) of the pubic symphysis and/or superior/inferior rami, unilateral or bilateral; without manipulation
27198	with manipulation, requiring more than local anesthesia (ie, general anesthesia, moderate sedation, spinal/epidural)
	(To report closed treatment of only anterior pelvic ring fracture(s) and/or dislocation(s) of the pubic symphysis and/or superior/inferior rami, unilateral or bilateral, use the appropriate evaluation and management services codes)
27200	Closed treatment of coccygeal fracture
27202	Open treatment of coccygeal fracture
27215	Open treatment of iliac spine(s), tuberosity avulsion, or iliac wing fracture(s), unilateral for pelvic bone fracture patterns that do not disrupt the pelvic ring, includes internal fixation, when performed

---

| Separate Procedure | Unlisted Procedure | CCI Comp. Code | Non-specific Procedure | **315** |

(To report bilateral procedure, report 27215 with modifier 50)

27216 Percutaneous skeletal fixation of posterior pelvic bone fracture and/or dislocation, for fracture patterns that disrupt the pelvic ring, unilateral (includes ipsilateral ilium, sacroiliac joint and/or sacrum)

(To report bilateral procedure, report 27216 with modifier 50)

(For percutaneous/minimally invasive arthrodesis of the sacroiliac joint without fracture and/or dislocation, use 27279)

27217 Open treatment of anterior pelvic bone fracture and/or dislocation for fracture patterns that disrupt the pelvic ring, unilateral, includes internal fixation, when performed (includes pubic symphysis and/or ipsilateral superior/inferior rami)

(To report bilateral procedure, report 27217 with modifier 50)

27218 Open treatment of posterior pelvic bone fracture and/or dislocation for fracture patterns that disrupt the pelvic ring, unilateral, includes internal fixation, when performed (includes ipsilateral ilium, sacroiliac joint and/or sacrum)

(To report bilateral procedure, report 27218 with modifier 50)

(For percutaneous/minimally invasive arthrodesis of the sacroiliac joint without fracture and/or dislocation, use 27279)

27220 Closed treatment of acetabulum (hip socket) fracture(s); without manipulation

27222 with manipulation, with or without skeletal traction

27226 Open treatment of posterior or anterior acetabular wall fracture, with internal fixation

27227 Open treatment of acetabular fracture(s) involving anterior or posterior (one) column, or a fracture running transversely across the acetabulum, with internal fixation

27228 Open treatment of acetabular fracture(s) involving anterior and posterior (two) columns, includes T-fracture and both column fracture with complete articular detachment, or single column or transverse fracture with associated acetabular wall fracture, with internal fixation

27230 Closed treatment of femoral fracture, proximal end, neck; without manipulation

27232 with manipulation, with or without skeletal traction

27235 Percutaneous skeletal fixation of femoral fracture, proximal end, neck

27236 Open treatment of femoral fracture, proximal end, neck, internal fixation or prosthetic replacement

27238 Closed treatment of intertrochanteric, pertrochanteric, or subtrochanteric femoral fracture; without manipulation

27240 with manipulation, with or without skin or skeletal traction

27244 Treatment of intertrochanteric, pertrochanteric or subtrochanteric femoral fracture; with plate/screw type implant, with or without cerclage

27245 with intramedullary implant, with or without interlocking screws and/or cerclage

27246 Closed treatment of greater trochanteric fracture, without manipulation

27248 Open treatment of greater trochanteric fracture, includes internal fixation, when performed

27250 Closed treatment of hip dislocation, traumatic; without anesthesia

● New Code ▲ Revised Code + Add-On Code ⊘ Modifier -51 Exempt ★ Telemedicine

27252   requiring anesthesia

27253   Open treatment of hip dislocation, traumatic, without internal fixation

27254   Open treatment of hip dislocation, traumatic, with acetabular wall and femoral head fracture, with or without internal or external fixation

(For treatment of acetabular fracture with fixation, see 27226, 27227)

27256   Treatment of spontaneous hip dislocation (developmental, including congenital or pathological), by abduction, splint or traction; without anesthesia, without manipulation

27257   with manipulation, requiring anesthesia

27258   Open treatment of spontaneous hip dislocation (developmental, including congenital or pathological), replacement of femoral head in acetabulum (including tenotomy, etc);

27259   with femoral shaft shortening

27265   Closed treatment of post hip arthroplasty dislocation; without anesthesia

27266   requiring regional or general anesthesia

27267   Closed treatment of femoral fracture, proximal end, head; without manipulation

27268   with manipulation

27269   Open treatment of femoral fracture, proximal end, head, includes internal fixation, when performed

(Do not report 27269 in conjunction with 27033, 27253)

MANIPULATION

27275   Manipulation, hip joint, requiring general anesthesia

ARTHRODESIS

27279   Arthrodesis, sacroiliac joint, percutaneous or minimally invasive (indirect visualization), with image guidance, includes obtaining bone graft when performed, and placement of transfixing device

(For bilateral procedure, report 27279 with modifier 50)

27280   Arthrodesis, open, sacroiliac joint, including obtaining bone graft, including instrumentation, when performed

(To report bilateral procedures, report 27280 with modifier -50)

(For percutaneous/minimally invasive arthrodesis of the sacroiliac joint without fracture and/or disloation,, use 27279)

27282   Arthrodesis, symphysis pubis (including obtaining graft)

27284   Arthrodesis, hip joint (including obtaining graft);

27286   with subtrochanteric osteotomy

AMPUTATION

27290   Interpelviabdominal amputation (hindquarter amputation)

27295   Disarticulation of hip

Separate Procedure   Unlisted Procedure   CCI Comp. Code   Non-specific Procedure   **317**

OTHER PROCEDURES

27299   Unlisted procedure, pelvis or hip joint

FEMUR (THIGH REGION) AND KNEE JOINT

Including tibial plateaus.

INCISION

(For incision and drainage of abscess or hematoma, superficial, see 10040-10160)

27301   Incision and drainage, deep abscess, bursa, or hematoma, thigh or knee region

27303   Incision, deep, with opening of bone cortex, femur or knee (eg, osteomyelitis or bone abscess)

27305   Fasciotomy, iliotibial (tenotomy), open

(For combined Ober-Yount fasciotomy, use 27025)

27306   Tenotomy, percutaneous, adductor or hamstring; single tendon (separate procedure)

27307   multiple tendons

27310   Arthrotomy, knee, with exploration, drainage, or removal of foreign body(eg, infection)

EXCISION

27323   Biopsy, soft tissue of thigh or knee area; superficial

27324   deep (subfascial or intramuscular)

(For needle biopsy of soft tissue, use 20206)

27325   Neurectomy, hamstring muscle

27326   Neurectomy, popliteal (gastrocnemius)

27327   Excision, tumor, soft tissue of thigh or knee area, subcutaneous; less than 3 cm

27337   3 cm or greater

(For excision of benign lesions of cutaneous origin [eg, sebaceous cyst], see 11400-11406))

27328   Excision, tumor, soft tissue of thigh or knee area, subfascial (eg, intramuscular); less than 5 cm

27339   5 cm or greater

27329   This code is out of order. See page 318

27330   Arthrotomy, knee; with synovial biopsy only

27331   including joint exploration, biopsy, or removal of loose or foreign bodies

27332   Arthrotomy, with excision of semilunar cartilage (meniscectomy) knee; medial OR lateral

27333   medial AND lateral

27334   Arthrotomy, with synovectomy, knee; anterior OR posterior

27335   anterior AND posterior including popliteal area

● New Code   ▲ Revised Code   ✚ Add-On Code   ⊘ Modifier -51 Exempt   ★ Telemedicine

27337	This code is out of order. See page 318	
27339	This code is out of order. See page 318	
27340	Excision, prepatellar bursa	
27345	Excision of synovial cyst of popliteal space (eg, Baker's cyst)	
27347	Excision of lesion of meniscus or capsule (eg, cyst, ganglion), knee	
27350	Patellectomy or hemipatellectomy	
27355	Excision or curettage of bone cyst or benign tumor of femur;	
27356	with allograft	
27357	with autograft (includes obtaining graft)	
+ 27358	with internal fixation (List in addition to code for primary procedure)	

(Use 27358 in conjunction with codes 27355, 27356 or 27357)

27360	Partial excision (craterization, saucerization, or diaphysectomy) bone, femur, proximal tibia and/or fibula (eg, osteomyelitis or bone abscess)
27329	Radical resection of tumor (eg, sarcoma), soft tissue of thigh or knee area; less than 5 cm
27364	5 cm or greater

(For radical resection of tumor[s] of cutaneous origin [eg, melanoma], see 11600-11606)

27365	Radical resection of tumor, femur or knee

(For radical resection of tumor, soft tissue of thigh or knee area, use 27329, 27364)

INTRODUCTION OR REMOVAL

27369	Injection procedure for contrast knee arthrography or contrast enhanced CT/MRI knee arthrography

(Use 27369 in conjunction with 73580, 73701, 73702, 73722, 73723)

(Do not report 27369 in conjunction with 20610, 20611, 29871)

(For arthrocentesis of the knee or injection of any material other than contrast for subsequent arthrography, see 20610, 20611)

(When fluoroscopic guided injection is performed for enhanced CT arthrography, use 27369, 77002, and 73701 or 73702)

(When fluoroscopic guided injection is performed for enhanced MR arthrography, use 27369, 77002, and 73722 or 73723)

(For arthroscopic lavage and drainage of the knee, use 29871)

(For radiographic arthrography, radiological supervision and interpretation, use 73580)

(27370	deleted 2018 [2019 Edition])

(For arthrocentesis of the knee or injection of any material other than contrast for subsequent arthrography, see 20610, 20611)

(For injection procedure for contrast knee arthrography or contrast enhanced CT/MRI knee arthrography, use 27369)

Separate Procedure   Unlisted Procedure   CCI Comp. Code   Non-specific Procedure   **319**

27372 Removal of foreign body, deep, thigh region or knee area

(For removal of knee prosthesis including "total knee," use 27488)

(For surgical arthroscopic knee procedures, see 29870-29887)

REPAIR, REVISION, AND/OR RECONSTRUCTION

27380 Suture of infrapatellar tendon; primary

27381 secondary reconstruction, including fascial or tendon graft

27385 Suture of quadriceps or hamstring muscle rupture; primary

27386 secondary reconstruction, including fascial or tendon graft

27390 Tenotomy, open, hamstring, knee to hip; single tendon

27391 multiple tendons, 1 leg

27392 multiple tendons, bilateral

27393 Lengthening of hamstring tendon; single tendon

27394 multiple tendons, 1 leg

27395 multiple tendons, bilateral

27396 Transplant or transfer (with muscle redirection or rerouting), thigh (eg., extensor to flexor); single tendon

27397 multiple tendons

27400 Transfer, tendon or muscle, hamstrings to femur (eg, Egger's type procedure)

27403 Arthrotomy with meniscus repair, knee

(For arthroscopic repair, use 29882)

27405 Repair, primary, torn ligament and/or capsule, knee; collateral

27407 cruciate

(For cruciate ligament reconstruction, use 27427)

27409 collateral and cruciate ligaments

(For ligament reconstruction, see 27427-27429)

27412 Autologous chondrocyte implantation, knee

(Do not report 27412 in conjunction with 15769, 15771, 15772, 15773, 15774, 27331, 27570)

(For harvesting of chondrocytes, use 29870)

27415 Osteochondral allograft, knee, open

(For arthroscopic implant of osteochondral allograft, use 29867)

(Do not report 27415 in conjunction with 27416)

27416 Osteochondral autograf(s), knee, open (eg, mosaicplasty) (includes harvesting of autograft[s])

● New Code   ▲ Revised Code   ＋ Add-On Code   ⊘ Modifier -51 Exempt   ★ Telemedicine

(Do not report 27416 in conjunction with 27415, 29870, 29871, 29875, 29884 when performed at the same session and/or 29874, 29877, 29879, 29885-29887 when performed in the same compartment)

(For arthroscopic osteochondral autograft of knee, use 29866)

27418   Anterior tibial tubercleplasty (eg, Maquet type procedure)

27420   Reconstruction of dislocating patella; (eg, Hauser type procedure)

27422   with extensor realignment and/or muscle advancement or release (eg, Campbell, Goldwaite type procedure)

27424   with patellectomy

27425   Lateral retinacular release open

(For arthroscopic lateral release, use 29873)

27427   Ligamentous reconstruction (augmentation), knee; extra-articular

27428   intra-articular (open)

27429   intra-articular (open) and extra-articular

(For primary repair of ligament(s) performed in addition to reconstruction, report 27405, 27407 or 27409 in addition to code 27427, 27428 or 27429)

27430   Quadricepsplasty (eg, Bennett or Thompson type)

27435   Capsulotomy, posterior capsular release; knee

27437   Arthroplasty, patella; without prosthesis

27438   with prosthesis

27440   Arthroplasty, knee, tibial plateau;

27441   with debridement and partial synovectomy

27442   Arthroplasty, femoral condyles or tibial plateau(s), knee;

27443   with debridement and partial synovectomy

27445   Arthroplasty, knee, hinge prosthesis (eg, Walldius type)

27446   Arthroplasty, knee, condyle and plateau; medial OR lateral compartment

27447   medial AND lateral compartments with or without patella resurfacing (total knee arthroplasty)

(For revision of total knee arthroplasty, use 27487)

(For removal of total knee prosthesis, use 27488)

27448   Osteotomy, femur, shaft or supracondylar; without fixation

(To report bilateral procedures, report 27448 with modifier -50)

27450   with fixation

(To report bilateral procedures, report 27450 with modifier -50)

27454   Osteotomy, multiple, with realignment on intramedullary rod, femoral shaft (eg, Sofield type procedure)

Separate Procedure   Unlisted Procedure   CCI Comp. Code   Non-specific Procedure   **321**

27455 Osteotomy, proximal tibia, including fibular excision or osteotomy (includes correction of genu varus [bowleg] or genu valgus [knock-knee]); before epiphyseal closure

(To report bilateral procedures, report 27455 with modifier -50)

27457 after epiphyseal closure

(To report bilateral procedures, report 27457 with modifier -50)

27465 Osteoplasty, femur; shortening (excluding 64876)

27466 lengthening

27468 combined, lengthening and shortening with femoral segment transfer

27470 Repair, nonunion or malunion, femur, distal to head and neck; without graft (eg, compression technique)

27472 with iliac or other autogenous bone graft (includes obtaining graft)

27475 Arrest, epiphyseal, any method (eg, epiphysiodesis); distal femur

27477 tibia and fibula, proximal

27479 combined distal femur, proximal tibia and fibula

27485 Arrest, hemiepiphyseal, distal femur or proximal tibia or fibula (eg, genu varus or valgus)

27486 Revision of total knee arthroplasty, with or without allograft; 1 component

27487 femoral and entire tibial component

27488 Removal of prosthesis, including total knee prosthesis, methylmethacrylate with or without insertion of spacer, knee

27495 Prophylactic treatment (nailing, pinning, plating or wiring) with or without methylmethacrylate, femur

27496 Decompression fasciotomy, thigh and/or knee, 1 compartment (flexor or extensor or adductor);

27497 with debridement of nonviable muscle and/or nerve

27498 Decompression fasciotomy, thigh and/or knee, multiple compartments;

27499 with debridement of nonviable muscle and/or nerve

FRACTURE AND/OR DISLOCATION

(For arthroscopic treatment of intercondylar spine(s) and tuberosity fracture(s) of the knee, see 29850, 29851)

(For arthroscopic treatment of tibial fracture, see 29855, 29856)

27500 Closed treatment of femoral shaft fracture, without manipulation

27501 Closed treatment of supracondylar or transcondylar femoral fracture with or without intercondylar extension, without manipulation

27502 Closed treatment of femoral shaft fracture, with manipulation, with or without skin or skeletal traction

27503 Closed treatment of supracondylar or transcondylar femoral fracture with or without intercondylar extension, with manipulation, with or without skin or skeletal traction

27506 Open treatment of femoral shaft fracture, with or without external fixation, with insertion of intramedullary implant, with or without cerclage and/or locking screws

27507 Open treatment of femoral shaft fracture with plate/screws, with or without cerclage

27508 Closed treatment of femoral fracture, distal end, medial or lateral condyle, without manipulation

27509 Percutaneous skeletal fixation of femoral fracture, distal end, medial or lateral condyle, or supracondylar or transcondylar, with or without intercondylar extension, or distal femoral epiphyseal separation

27510 Closed treatment of femoral fracture, distal end, medial or lateral condyle, with manipulation

27511 Open treatment of femoral supracondylar or transcondylar fracture without intercondylar extension, includes internal fixation, when performed

27513 Open treatment of femoral supracondylar or transcondylar fracture with intercondylar extension, includes internal fixation, when performed

27514 Open treatment of femoral fracture, distal end, medial or lateral condyle, includes internal fixation, when performed

27516 Closed treatment of distal femoral epiphyseal separation; without manipulation

27517 with manipulation, with or without skin or skeletal traction

27519 Open treatment of distal femoral epiphyseal separation, includes internal fixation, when performed

27520 Closed treatment of patellar fracture, without manipulation

27524 Open treatment of patellar fracture, with internal fixation and/or partial or complete patellectomy and soft tissue repair

27530 Closed treatment of tibial fracture, proximal (plateau); without manipulation

27532 with or without manipulation, with skeletal traction

(For arthroscopic treatment, see 29855, 29856)

27535 Open treatment of tibial fracture, proximal (plateau); unicondylar, includes internal fixation, when performed

27536 bicondylar, with or without internal fixation

(For arthroscopic treatment, see 29855, 29856)

27538 Closed treatment of intercondylar spine(s) and/or tuberosity fracture(s) of knee, with or without manipulation

(For arthroscopic treatment, see 29850, 29851)

27540 Open treatment of intercondylar spine(s) and/or tuberosity fracture(s) of the knee, includes internal fixation, when performed

27550 Closed treatment of knee dislocation; without anesthesia

27552 requiring anesthesia

27556 Open treatment of knee dislocation, includes internal fixation, when performed; without primary ligamentous repair or augmentation/reconstruction

27557 with primary ligamentous repair

27558   with primary ligamentous repair, with augmentation/ reconstruction

27560   Closed treatment of patellar dislocation; without anesthesia

(For recurrent dislocation, see 27420-27424)

27562   requiring anesthesia

27566   Open treatment of patellar dislocation, with or without partial or total patellectomy

MANIPULATION

27570   Manipulation of knee joint under general anesthesia (includes application of traction or other fixation devices)

ARTHRODESIS

27580   Arthrodesis, knee, any technique

AMPUTATION

27590   Amputation, thigh, through femur, any level;

27591   immediate fitting technique including first cast

27592   open, circular (guillotine)

27594   secondary closure or scar revision

27596   re-amputation

27598   Disarticulation at knee

OTHER PROCEDURES

27599   Unlisted procedure, femur or knee

LEG (TIBIA AND FIBULA) AND ANKLE JOINT

INCISION

27600   Decompression fasciotomy, leg; anterior and/or lateral compartments only

27601   posterior compartment(s) only

27602   anterior and/or lateral, and posterior compartment(s)

(For incision and drainage procedures, superficial, see 10040-10160)

(For decompression fasciotomy with debridement, see 27892-27894)

27603   Incision and drainage, leg or ankle; deep abscess or hematoma

27604   infected bursa

27605   Tenotomy, percutaneous, Achilles tendon (separate procedure); local anesthesia

27606   general anesthesia

27607   Incision (eg, osteomyelitis or bone abscess), leg or ankle

27610 Arthrotomy, ankle, including exploration, drainage, or removal of foreign body

27612 Arthrotomy, posterior capsular release, ankle, with or without Achilles tendon lengthening

(See also 27685)

EXCISION

27613 Biopsy, soft tissue of leg or ankle area; superficial

27614 deep (subfascial or intramuscular)

(For needle biopsy of soft tissue, use 20206)

27615 Radical resection of tumor (eg, sarcoma), soft tissue of leg or ankle area; less than 5 cm

27616 5 cm or greater

(For radical resection of tumor[s] of cutaneous origin [eg, melanoma], see 11600-11606)

27618 Excision, tumor, soft tissue of leg or ankle area, subcutaneous; less than 3 cm

27632 3 cm or greater

(For excision of benign lesions of cutaneous origin [eg, sebaceous cyst], see 11400-11406)

27619 Excision, tumor, soft tissue of leg or ankle area, subfascial (eg, intramuscular); less than 5 cm

27634 5 cm or greater

27620 Arthrotomy, ankle, with joint exploration, with or without biopsy, with or without removal of loose or foreign body

27625 Arthrotomy, with synovectomy, ankle;

27626 including tenosynovectomy

27630 Excision of lesion of tendon sheath or capsule (eg, cyst or ganglion), leg and/or ankle

27632 This code is out of order. See page 325

27634 This code is out of order. See page 325

27635 Excision or curettage of bone cyst or benign tumor, tibia or fibula;

27637 with autograft (includes obtaining graft)

27638 with allograft

27640 Partial excision (craterization, saucerization, or diaphysectomy) bone (eg, osteomyelitis); tibia

(For exostosis excision, use 27635)

27641 fibula

(For exostosis excision, use 27635)

27645 Radical resection of tumor; tibia

27646 fibula

27647	talus or calcaneus

INTRODUCTION OR REMOVAL

27648	Injection procedure for ankle arthrography

(For radiological supervision and interpretation use 73615. Do not report 77002 in addition to 73615)

(For ankle arthroscopy, see 29894-29898)

REPAIR, REVISION, AND/OR RECONSTRUCTION

27650	Repair, primary, open or percutaneous, ruptured Achilles tendon;
27652	with graft (includes obtaining graft)
27654	Repair, secondary, Achilles tendon, with or without graft
27656	Repair, fascial defect of leg
27658	Repair, flexor tendon, leg; primary, without graft, each tendon
27659	secondary, with or without graft, each tendon
27664	Repair, extensor tendon, leg; primary, without graft, each tendon
27665	secondary, with or without graft, each tendon
27675	Repair, dislocating peroneal tendons; without fibular osteotomy
27676	with fibular osteotomy
27680	Tenolysis, flexor or extensor tendon, leg and/or ankle; single, each tendon
27681	multiple tendons (through separate incision(s))
27685	Lengthening or shortening of tendon, leg or ankle; single tendon (separate procedure)
27686	multiple tendons (through same incision), each
27687	Gastrocnemius recession (eg, Strayer procedure)

(Toe extensors are considered as a group to be single tendon when transplanted into midfoot)

27690	Transfer or transplant of single tendon (with muscle redirection or rerouting); superficial (eg, anterior tibial extensors into midfoot)
27691	deep (eg, anterior tibial or posterior tibial through interosseous space, flexor digitorum longus, flexor hallucis longus, or peroneal tendon to midfoot or hind foot)
+ 27692	each additional tendon (List separately in addition to code for primary procedure)

(Use 27692 in conjunction with codes 27690, 27691)

27695	Repair, primary, disrupted ligament, ankle; collateral
27696	both collateral ligaments
27698	Repair, secondary disrupted ligament, ankle, collateral (eg, Watson-Jones procedure)
27700	Arthroplasty, ankle;

● New Code   ▲ Revised Code   + Add-On Code   ⊘ Modifier -51 Exempt   ★ Telemedicine

27702	with implant (total ankle)
27703	revision, total ankle
27704	Removal of ankle implant
27705	Osteotomy; tibia
27707	fibula
27709	tibia and fibula
27712	multiple, with realignment on intramedullary rod (eg, Sofield type procedure)

(For osteotomy to correct genu varus (bowleg) or genu valgus (knock-knee), see 27455-27457)

27715	Osteoplasty, tibia and fibula, lengthening or shortening
27720	Repair of nonunion or malunion, tibia; without graft, (eg, compression technique)
27722	with sliding graft
27724	with iliac or other autograft (includes obtaining graft)
27725	by synostosis, with fibula, any method
27726	Repair of fibula nonunion and/or malunion with internal fixation

(Do not reprt 27726 in conjunction with 27707)

27727	Repair of congenital pseudarthrosis, tibia
27730	Arrest, epiphyseal (epiphysiodesis), open; distal tibia
27732	distal fibula
27734	distal tibia and fibula
27740	Arrest, epiphyseal (epiphysiodesis), any method, combined, proximal and distal tibia and fibula;
27742	and distal femur

(For epiphyseal arrest of proximal tibia and fibula, use 27477)

| 27745 | Prophylactic treatment (nailing, pinning, plating or wiring) with or without methylmethacrylate, tibia |

FRACTURE AND/OR DISLOCATION

27750	Closed treatment of tibial shaft fracture (with or without fibular fracture); without manipulation
27752	with manipulation, with or without skeletal traction
27756	Percutaneous skeletal fixation of tibial shaft fracture (with or without fibular fracture) (eg, pins or screws)
27758	Open treatment of tibial shaft fracture, (with or without fibular fracture) with plate/screws, with or without cerclage
27759	Treatment of tibial shaft fracture (with or without fibular fracture) by intramedullary implant, with or without interlocking screws and/or cerclage

27760 Closed treatment of medial malleolus fracture; without manipulation

27762 with manipulation, with or without skin or skeletal traction

27766 Open treatment of medial malleolus fracture, includes internal fixation, when performed

27767 Closed treatment of posterior malleolus fracture; without manipulation

27768 with manipulation

27769 Open treatment of posterior malleolus fracture, includes internal fixation, when performed

(Do not report 27767-27769 in conjunction with 27808-27823)

27780 Closed treatment of proximal fibula or shaft fracture; without manipulation

27781 with manipulation

27784 Open treatment of proximal fibula or shaft fracture, includes internal fixation, when performed

27786 Closed treatment of distal fibular fracture (lateral malleolus); without manipulation

27788 with manipulation

27792 Open treatment of distal fibular fracture (lateral malleolus), includes internal fixation, when performed

(For treatment of tibia and fibula shaft fractures, see 27750-27759)

27808 Closed treatment of bimalleolar ankle fracture, (eg, lateral and medial malleoli, or lateral and posterior malleoli or medial and posterior malleoli); without manipulation

27810 with manipulation

27814 Open treatment of bimalleolar ankle fracture (eg, lateral and medial malleoli, or lateral and posterior malleoli, or medial and posterior malleoli), includes internal fixation, when performed

27816 Closed treatment of trimalleolar ankle fracture; without manipulation

27818 with manipulation

27822 Open treatment of trimalleolar ankle fracture, includes internal fixation, when performed, medial and/or lateral malleolus; without fixation of posterior lip

27823 with fixation of posterior lip

27824 Closed treatment of fracture of weight bearing articular portion of distal tibia (eg, pilon or tibial plafond), with or without anesthesia; without manipulation

27825 with skeletal traction and/or requiring manipulation

27826 Open treatment of fracture of weight bearing articular surface/portion of distal tibia (eg, pilon or tibial plafond), with internal fixation, when performed; of fibula only

27827 of tibia only

27828 of both tibia and fibula

27829 Open treatment of distal tibiofibular joint (syndesmosis) disruption, includes internal fixation, when performed

27830 Closed treatment of proximal tibiofibular joint dislocation; without anesthesia

27831   requiring anesthesia

27832 Open treatment of proximal tibiofibular joint dislocation, includes internal fixation, when performed, or with excision of proximal fibula

27840 Closed treatment of ankle dislocation; without anesthesia

27842   requiring anesthesia, with or without percutaneous skeletal fixation

27846 Open treatment of ankle dislocation, with or without percutaneous skeletal fixation; without repair or internal fixation

27848   with repair or internal or external fixation

(For surgical diagnostic arthroscopic procedures, see 29894-29898)

MANIPULATION

27860 Manipulation of ankle under general anesthesia (includes application of traction or other fixation apparatus)

ARTHRODESIS

27870 Arthrodesis, ankle, open

(For arthroscopic ankle arthrodesis, use 29899)

27871 Arthrodesis, tibiofibular joint, proximal or distal

AMPUTATION

27880 Amputation, leg, through tibia and fibula;

27881   with immediate fitting technique including application of first cast

27882   open, circular (guillotine)

27884   secondary closure or scar revision

27886   re-amputation

27888 Amputation, ankle, through malleoli of tibia and fibula (eg, Syme, Pirogoff type procedures), with plastic closure and resection of nerves

27889 Ankle disarticulation

OTHER PROCEDURES

27892 Decompression fasciotomy, leg; anterior and/or lateral compartments only, with debridement of nonviable muscle and/or nerve

(For decompression fasciotomy of the leg without debridement, use 27600)

27893   posterior compartment(s) only, with debridement of nonviable muscle and/or nerve

(For decompession fasciotomy of the leg without debridement, use 27601)

27894   anterior and/or lateral, and posterior compartment(s), with debridement of nonviable muscle and/or nerve

(For decompression fasciotomy of the leg without debridement, use 27602)

27899 Unlisted procedure, leg or ankle

FOOT AND TOES

INCISION

(For incision and drainage procedures, superficial, see 10040-10160)

28001 Incision and drainage, bursa, foot

28002 Incision and drainage below fascia, with or without tendon sheath involvement, foot; single bursal space

28003 multiple areas

28005 Incision, bone cortex (eg, osteomyelitis or bone abscess), foot

28008 Fasciotomy, foot and/or toe

(See also 28060, 28062, 28250)

28010 Tenotomy, percutaneous, toe; single tendon

28011 multiple tendons

(For open tenotomy, see 28230-28234)

28020 Arthrotomy, including exploration, drainage, or removal of loose or foreign body; intertarsal or tarsometatarsal joint

28022 metatarsophalangeal joint

28024 interphalangeal joint

28035 Release, tarsal tunnel (posterior tibial nerve decompression)

(For other nerve entrapments, see 64704, 64722)

EXCISION

28039 This code is out of order. See page 330

28041 This code is out of order. See page 330

28043 Excision, tumor, soft tissue of foot or toe, subcutaneous; less than 1.5 cm

28039 1.5 cm or greater

(For excision of benign lesions of cutaneous origin [eg, sebaceous cyst], see 11420-11426)

28045 Excision, tumor, soft tissue of foot or toe, subfascial (eg, intramuscular); less than 1.5 cm

28041 1.5 cm or greater

28046 Radical resection of tumor (eg, sarcoma), soft tissue of foot or toe; less than 3 cm

28047 3 cm or greater

(For radical resection of tumor[s] of cutaneous origin [eg, melanoma], see 11620-11626)

28050 Arthrotomy with biopsy; intertarsal or tarsometatarsal joint

28052 metatarsophalangeal joint

● New Code ▲ Revised Code ✚ Add-On Code ⊘ Modifier -51 Exempt ★ Telemedicine

28054	interphalangeal joint
28055	Neurectomy, intrinsic musculature of foot
28060	Fasciectomy, plantar fascia; partial (separate procedure)
28062	radical (separate procedure)

(For plantar fasciotomy, see 28008, 28250)

28070	Synovectomy; intertarsal or tarsometatarsal joint, each
28072	metatarsophalangeal joint, each
28080	Excision, interdigital (Morton) neuroma, single, each
28086	Synovectomy, tendon sheath, foot; flexor
28088	extensor
28090	Excision of lesion, tendon, tendon sheath, or capsule (including synovectomy) (eg, cyst or ganglion); foot
28092	toe(s), each
28100	Excision or curettage of bone cyst or benign tumor, talus or calcaneus;
28102	with iliac or other autograft (includes obtaining graft)
28103	with allograft
28104	Excision or curettage of bone cyst or benign tumor, tarsal or metatarsal, except talus or calcaneus;
28106	with iliac or other autograft (includes obtaining graft)
28107	with allograft
28108	Excision or curettage of bone cyst or benign tumor, phalanges of foot

(For partial excision of bossing or exostosis for phalanx in the foot, use 28124)

28110	Ostectomy, partial excision, fifth metatarsal head (bunionette) (separate procedure)
28111	Ostectomy, complete excision; first metatarsal head
28112	other metatarsal head (second, third or fourth)
28113	fifth metatarsal head
28114	all metatarsal heads, with partial proximal phalangectomy, excluding first metatarsal (eg, Clayton type procedure)
28116	Ostectomy, excision of tarsal coalition
28118	Ostectomy, calcaneus;
28119	for spur, with or without plantar fascial release
28120	Partial excision (craterization, saucerization, sequestrectomy, or diaphysectomy) bone (eg, osteomyelitis or bossing); talus or calcaneus

Separate Procedure	Unlisted Procedure	CCI Comp. Code	Non-specific Procedure	**331**

| 28122 | tarsal or metatarsal bone, except talus or calcaneus |

(For partial excision of talus or calcaneus, use 28120)

(For cheilectomy for hallux rigidus, use 28289)

28124	phalanx of toe
28126	Resection, partial or complete, phalangeal base, each toe
28130	Talectomy (astragalectomy)

(For calcanectomy, use 28118)

28140	Metatarsectomy
28150	Phalangectomy, toe, each toe
28153	Resection, condyle(s), distal end of phalanx, each toe
28160	Hemiphalangectomy or interphalangeal joint excision, toe, proximal end of phalanx, each
28171	Radical resection of tumor; tarsal (except talus or calcaneus)
28173	metatarsal
28175	phalanx of toe

(For talus or calcaneus, use 27647)

INTRODUCTION OR REMOVAL

28190	Removal of foreign body, foot; subcutaneous
28192	deep
28193	complicated

REPAIR, REVISION, AND/OR RECONSTRUCTION

28200	Repair, tendon, flexor, foot; primary or secondary, without free graft, each tendon
28202	secondary with free graft, each tendon (includes obtaining graft)
28208	Repair, tendon, extensor, foot; primary or secondary, each tendon
28210	secondary with free graft, each tendon (includes obtaining graft)
28220	Tenolysis, flexor, foot; single tendon
28222	multiple tendons
28225	Tenolysis, extensor, foot; single tendon
28226	multiple tendons
28230	Tenotomy, open, tendon flexor; foot, single or multiple tendon(s) (separate procedure)
28232	toe, single tendon (separate procedure)
28234	Tenotomy, open, extensor, foot or toe, each tendon

● New Code ▲ Revised Code + Add-On Code ⊘ Modifier -51 Exempt ★ Telemedicine

(For tendon transfer to midfoot or hindfoot, see 27690, 27691)

28238 Reconstruction (advancement), posterior tibial tendon with excision of accessory tarsal navicular bone (eg, Kidner type procedure)

(For subcutaneous tenotomy, see 28010, 28011)

(For transfer or transplant of tendon with muscle redirection or rerouting, see 27690-27692)

(For extensor hallucis longus transfer with great toe IP fusion (Jones procedure), use 28760)

28240 Tenotomy, lengthening, or release, abductor hallucis muscle

28250 Division of plantar fascia and muscle (eg, Steindler stripping) (separate procedure)

28260 Capsulotomy, midfoot; medial release only (separate procedure)

28261   with tendon lengthening

28262   extensive, including posterior talotibial capsulotomy and tendon(s) lengthening (eg, resistant clubfoot deformity)

28264 Capsulotomy, midtarsal (eg, Heyman type procedure)

28270 Capsulotomy; metatarsophalangeal joint, with or without tenorrhaphy, each joint (separate procedure)

28272   interphalangeal joint, each joint (separate procedure)

28280 Syndactylization, toes (eg, webbing or Kelikian type procedure)

28285 Correction, hammertoe (eg, interphalangeal fusion, partial or total phalangectomy)

28286 Correction, cock-up fifth toe, with plastic skin closure (eg, Ruiz-Mora type procedure)

28288 Ostectomy, partial, exostectomy or condylectomy, metatarsal head, each metatarsal head

28289 Hallux rigidus correction with cheilectomy, debridement and capsular release of the first metatarsophalangeal joint; without implant

28291   with implant

28292 Correction, hallux valgus (bunionectomy), with sesamoidectomy, when performed; with resection of proximal phalanx base, when performed, any method

28295 This code is out of order. See page 333

28296   with distal metatarsal osteotomy, any method

28295   with proximal metatarsal osteotomy, any method

28297   with first metatarsal and medial cuneiform joint arthrodesis; any method

28298   with proximal phalanx osteotomy, any method

28299   with double osteotomy, any method

28300 Osteotomy; calcaneus (eg, Dwyer or Chambers type procedure), with or without internal fixation

28302   talus

Separate Procedure   Unlisted Procedure   CCI Comp. Code   Non-specific Procedure   **333**

28304 Osteotomy, tarsal bones, other than calcaneus or talus;

28305   with autograft (includes obtaining graft) (eg, Fowler type)

28306 Osteotomy, with or without lengthening, shortening or angular correction, metatarsal; first metatarsal

28307   first metatarsal with autograft (other than first toe)

28308   other than first metatarsal, each

28309   multiple (eg, Swanson type cavus foot procedure)

28310 Osteotomy, shortening, angular or rotational correction; proximal phalanx, first toe (separate procedure)

28312   other phalanges, any toe

28313 Reconstruction, angular deformity of toe, soft tissue procedures only (eg, overlapping second toe, fifth toe, curly toes)

28315 Sesamoidectomy, first toe (separate procedure)

28320 Repair, nonunion or malunion; tarsal bones

28322   metatarsal, with or without bone graft (includes obtaining graft)

28340 Reconstruction, toe, macrodactyly; soft tissue resection

28341   requiring bone resection

28344 Reconstruction, toe(s); polydactyly

28345   syndactyly, with or without skin graft(s), each web

28360 Reconstruction, cleft foot

FRACTURE AND/OR DISLOCATION

28400 Closed treatment of calcaneal fracture; without manipulation

28405   with manipulation

28406 Percutaneous skeletal fixation of calcaneal fracture, with manipulation

28415 Open treatment of calcaneal fracture, includes internal fixation, when performed;

28420   with primary iliac or other autogenous bone graft (includes obtaining graft)

28430 Closed treatment of talus fracture; without manipulation

28435   with manipulation

28436 Percutaneous skeletal fixation of talus fracture, with manipulation

28445 Open treatment of talus fracture, includes internal fixation, when performed

28446 Open osteochondral autograft, talus (includes obtaining graft[s])

(Do not report 28446 in conjunction with 27705, 27707)

(For arthroscopic osteochondral talus graft, use 29892)

● New Code   ▲ Revised Code   ✛ Add-On Code   ⊘ Modifier -51 Exempt   ★ Telemedicine

(For open osteochondral allograft or repairs with industrial grafts, use 28899)

28450 Treatment of tarsal bone fracture (except talus and calcaneus); without manipulation, each

28455 with manipulation, each

28456 Percutaneous skeletal fixation of tarsal bone fracture (except talus and calcaneus), with manipulation, each

28465 Open treatment of tarsal bone fracture (except talus and calcaneus), includes internal fixation, when performed, each

28470 Closed treatment of metatarsal fracture; without manipulation, each

28475 with manipulation, each

28476 Percutaneous skeletal fixation of metatarsal fracture, with manipulation, each

28485 Open treatment of metatarsal fracture, includes internal fixation, when performed, each

28490 Closed treatment of fracture great toe, phalanx or phalanges; without manipulation

28495 with manipulation

28496 Percutaneous skeletal fixation of fracture great toe, phalanx or phalanges, with manipulation

28505 Open treatment of fracture great toe, phalanx or phalanges, includes internal fixation, when performed

28510 Closed treatment of fracture, phalanx or phalanges, other than great toe; without manipulation, each

28515 with manipulation, each

28525 Open treatment of fracture, phalanx or phalanges, other than great toe, includes internal fixation, when performed, each

28530 Closed treatment of sesamoid fracture

28531 Open treatment of sesamoid fracture, with or without internal fixation

28540 Closed treatment of tarsal bone dislocation, other than talotarsal; without anesthesia

28545 requiring anesthesia

28546 Percutaneous skeletal fixation of tarsal bone dislocation, other than talotarsal, with manipulation

28555 Open treatment of tarsal bone dislocation, includes internal fixation, when performed

28570 Closed treatment of talotarsal joint dislocation; without anesthesia

28575 requiring anesthesia

28576 Percutaneous skeletal fixation of talotarsal joint dislocation, with manipulation

28585 Open treatment of talotarsal joint dislocation, includes internal fixation, when performed

28600 Closed treatment of tarsometatarsal joint dislocation; without anesthesia

28605 requiring anesthesia

28606 Percutaneous skeletal fixation of tarsometatarsal joint dislocation, with manipulation

---

28615 Open treatment of tarsometatarsal joint dislocation, includes internal fixation, when performed

28630 Closed treatment of metatarsophalangeal joint dislocation; without anesthesia

28635   requiring anesthesia

28636 Percutaneous skeletal fixation of metatarsophalangeal joint dislocation, with manipulation

28645 Open treatment of metatarsophalangeal joint dislocation, includes internal fixation, when performed

28660 Closed treatment of interphalangeal joint dislocation; without anesthesia

28665   requiring anesthesia

28666 Percutaneous skeletal fixation of interphalangeal joint dislocation, with manipulation

28675 Open treatment of interphalangeal joint dislocation, includes internal fixation, when performed

ARTHRODESIS

28705 Arthrodesis; pantalar

28715   triple

28725   subtalar

28730 Arthrodesis, midtarsal or tarsometatarsal, multiple or transverse;

28735   with osteotomy (eg, flatfoot correction)

28737 Arthrodesis, with tendon lengthening and advancement, midtarsal, tarsal navicular-cuneiform (eg, Miller type procedure)

28740 Arthrodesis, midtarsal or tarsometatarsal, single joint

28750 Arthrodesis, great toe; metatarsophalangeal joint

28755   interphalangeal joint

28760 Arthrodesis, with extensor hallucis longus transfer to first metatarsal neck, great toe, interphalangeal joint (eg, Jones type procedure)

        (For hammertoe operation or interphalangeal fusion, use 28285)

AMPUTATION

28800 Amputation, foot; midtarsal (eg, Chopart type procedure)

28805   transmetatarsal

28810 Amputation, metatarsal, with toe, single

28820 Amputation, toe; metatarsophalangeal joint

28825   interphalangeal joint

        (For amputation of tuft of distal phalanx, use 11752)

OTHER PROCEDURES

28890   Extracorporeal shock wave, high energy, performed by a physician or other qualified health care professional, requiring anesthesia other than local, including ultrasound guidance, involving the plantar fascia

(For extracorporeal shock wave therapy involving musculoskeletal system not otherwise specified, see 0101T, 0102T)

(For extracorporeal shock wave therapy involving integumentary system not otherwise specified, see 0512T, 0513T)

(Do not report 28890 in conjunction with 0512T, 0513T, when treating the same area)

28899   Unlisted procedure, foot or toes

APPLICATION OF CASTS AND STRAPPING

CPT codes in this section are used only when the cast application or strapping is a replacement procedure performed during or after the period of follow-up care. An additional evaluation and management service code, dependent on location, is reportable only if significant identifiable other services are provided at the time of the cast application or strapping.

For coding cast or strap application in situations not involving surgery, for example, casting of a sprained ankle or knee, use the appropriate level of evaluation and management services code plus code 99070 or equivalent HCPCS Level II code to report casting materials.

The listed procedures apply when the cast application or strapping is a replacement procedure used during or aftre the period of follow-up care, or when the cast application or strapping is an initial service performed without a restorative treatment or procedure(s) to stabilize or protect a fracture, injury, or dislocation and/or to afford comfort to a patient. Restorative treatment or procedure(s) rendered by another individual following the application of the initial cast/splint/strap may be reported with a treatment of fracture and/or dislocation code.

An individual who applies the initial cast, strap, or splint and also assumes all of the subsequent fracture, dislocation, or injury care cannot use the application of casts and strapping codes as an initial service, since the first cast/splint or strap application is included in the treatment of fracture and/or dislocation codes. (See notes under Musculoskeletal System.) A temporary cast/splint/strap is not considered to be part of the preoperative care, and the use of the modifier 56 is not applicable. Additional evaluation and management services are reportable only if significant identifiable further services are provided at the time of the cast application or strapping.

If a cast application or strapping is provided as an initial service (eg, casting of a sprained ankle or knee) in which no other procedure or treatment (eg, surgical repair, reduction of a fracture, or joint dislocation) is performed or is expected to be performed by an individual rendering the initial care only, use the casting, strapping, and/or supply code (99070) in addition to an evaluation and management code as appropriate.

Listed procedures include removal of cast or strapping.

(For orthotics management and training, see 97760, 97761, 97763)

BODY AND UPPER EXTREMITY

Casts

29000   Application of halo type body cast (see 20661-20663 for insertion)

29010   Application of Risser jacket, localizer, body; only

29015   including head

29035   Application of body cast, shoulder to hips;

29040   including head, Minerva type

29044   including 1 thigh

29046	including both thighs
29049	Application, cast; figure-of-eight
29055	shoulder spica
29058	plaster Velpeau
29065	shoulder to hand (long arm)
29075	elbow to finger (short arm)
29085	hand and lower forearm (gauntlet)
29086	finger (eg, contracture)

Splints

29105	Application of long arm splint (shoulder to hand)
29125	Application of short arm splint (forearm to hand); static
29126	dynamic
29130	Application of finger splint; static
29131	dynamic

Strapping - Any Age

29200	Strapping; thorax
	(To report low back strapping, use 29799)
29240	shoulder (eg, Velpeau)
29260	elbow or wrist
29280	hand or finger

LOWER EXTREMITY

Casts

29305	Application of hip spica cast; 1 leg
29325	1 and one-half spica or both legs
	(For hip spica (body) cast, including thighs only, use 29046)
29345	Application of long leg cast (thigh to toes);
29355	walker or ambulatory type
29358	Application of long leg cast brace
29365	Application of cylinder cast (thigh to ankle)
29405	Application of short leg cast (below knee to toes);

● New Code ▲ Revised Code ＋ Add-On Code ⊘ Modifier -51 Exempt ★ Telemedicine

29425		walking or ambulatory type
29435		Application of patellar tendon bearing (PTB) cast
29440		Adding walker to previously applied cast
29445		Application of rigid total contact leg cast
29450		Application of clubfoot cast with molding or manipulation, long or short leg

(To report bilateral procedures, use 29450 with modifier -50)

Splints

29505	Application of long leg splint (thigh to ankle or toes)
29515	Application of short leg splint (calf to foot)

Strapping - Any Age

29520	Strapping; hip
29530	knee
29540	ankle and/or foot

(Do not report 29540 in conjunction with 29580, 29581, for the same extremity)

29550	toes
29580	Unna boot

(Do not report 29580 in conjunction with 29540, 29581, for the same extremity)

29581	Application of multi-layer compression system; leg (below knee), including ankle and foot

(Do not report 29581 in conjunction with 29540, 29580, for the same extremity)b

(Do not report 29520, 29530, 29540, 29550, 29580, 29581 in conjunction with 36465, 36466, 36468, 36470, 36471, 36473, 36474, 36475, 36476, 36478, 36479, 36482, 36483, for the same extremity)

(**29582**	deleted 2017 [2018 edition].)
(**29583**	deleted 2017 [2018 edition].)
29584	upper arm, forearm, hand and fingers

(Do not report 29584 in conjunction with 36465, 36466, 36468, 36470, 36471, 36473, 36474, 36475, 36476, 36478, 36479, 36482, 36483, for the same extremity)

REMOVAL OR REPAIR

29700		Removal or bivalving; gauntlet, boot or body cast
29705		full arm or full leg cast
29710		shoulder or hip spica, Minerva, or Risser jacket, etc.
29720		Repair of spica, body cast or jacket
29730		Windowing of cast

29740   Wedging of cast (except clubfoot casts)

29750   Wedging of clubfoot cast

    (To report bilateral procedures, use 29750 with modifier -50)

OTHER PROCEDURES

29799   Unlisted procedure, casting or strapping

ENDOSCOPY/ARTHROSCOPY

Surgical endoscopy/arthroscopy always includes a diagnostic endoscopy/ arthroscopy and is therefore never reported in addition to the surgical procedure. However, there are several arthroscopy procedures defined as separate procedures, indicating that the codes may be reported if the diagnostic arthroscopy is the only procedure performed.

Surgical endoscopy/arthroscopy always includes a diagnostic endoscropy/arthroscopy.

When arthroscopy is performed in conjunction with arthrotomy, add modifier 51.

Arthroscopic removal of loose body(ies) or foreign body(ies) (ie, 29819, 29834, 29861, 29874, 29894, 29904) may be reported only when the loose body(ies) or foreign body(ies) is equal to or larger than the diameter of the arthroscopic cannula(s) used for the specific procedure, and can only be removed through a cannula larger than that used for the specific procedure or through a separate incision or through a portal that has been enlarged to allow removal of the loose or foreign body(ies).

29800   Arthroscopy, temporomandibular joint, diagnostic, with or without synovial biopsy (separate procedure)

29804   Arthroscopy, temporomandibular joint, surgical

    (For open procedure, use 21010)

29805   Arthroscopy, shoulder, diagnostic, with or without synovial biopsy (separate procedure)

    (For open procedure, see 23065-23066, 23100-23101)

29806   Arthroscopy, shoulder, surgical; capsulorrhaphy

    (For open procedure, see 23450-23466)

    (To report thermal capsulorrhaphy, use 29999)

29807   repair of slap lesion

29819   with removal of loose body or foreign body

    (For open procedure, see 23040-23044, 23107)

29820   synovectomy, partial

    (For open procedure, see 23105)

29821   synovectomy, complete

    (For open procedure, see 23105)

▲ **29822**   debridement, limited, 1 or 2 discrete structures (eg, humeral bone, humeral articular cartilage, glenoid bone, glenoid articular cartilage, biceps tendon, biceps anchor complex, labrum, articular capsule, articular side of the rotator cuff, bursal side of the rotator cuff, subacromial bursa, foreign body[ies])

    (For open procedure, see specific open shoulder procedure performed)

▲ **29823**   debridement, extensive, 3 or more discrete structures (eg, humeral bone, humeral articular cartilage, glenoid bone, glenoid articular cartilage, biceps tendon, biceps anchor complex, labrum, articular

---

capsule, articular side of the rotator cuff, bursal side of the rotator cuff, subacromial bursa, foreign body[ies])

(For open procedure, see specific open shoulder procedure performed)

29824 distal claviculectomy including distal articular surface (Mumford procedure)

(For open procedure, use 23120)

29825 with lysis and resection of adhesions, with or without manipulation

(For open procedure, see specific open shoulder procedure performed)

+ 29826 decompression of subacromial space with partial acromioplasty, with coracoacromial ligament (ie, arch) release, when performed (List separately in addition to code for primary procedure

(For open procedure, use 23130 or 23415)

(Use 29826 in conjunction with 29806-29825, 29827, 29828)

29827 with rotator cuff repair

(For open or mini-open rotator cuff repair, use 23412)

(When arthroscopic distal clavicle resection is performed at the same setting, use 29824 and append modifier '-51')

29828 biceps tenodesis

(Do not report 29828 in conjunction with 29805, 29820, 29822)

(For open biceps tenodesis, use 23430)

29830 Arthroscopy, elbow, diagnostic, with or without synovial biopsy (separate procedure)

29834 Arthroscopy, elbow, surgical; with removal of loose body or foreign body

29835 synovectomy, partial

29836 synovectomy, complete

29837 debridement, limited

29838 debridement, extensive

29840 Arthroscopy, wrist, diagnostic, with or without synovial biopsy (separate procedure)

29843 Arthroscopy, wrist, surgical; for infection, lavage and drainage

29844 synovectomy, partial

29845 synovectomy, complete

29846 excision and/or repair of triangular fibrocartilage and/or joint debridement

29847 internal fixation for fracture or instability

29848 Endoscopy, wrist, surgical, with release of transverse carpal ligament

(Do not report 29848 in conjunction with 11960)

(For open procedure, use 64721)

| Separate Procedure | Unlisted Procedure | CCI Comp. Code | Non-specific Procedure | **341** |

29850 Arthroscopically aided treatment of intercondylar spine(s) and/or tuberosity fracture(s) of the knee, with or without manipulation; without internal or external fixation (includes arthroscopy)

29851 with internal or external fixation (includes arthroscopy)

(For bone graft, use 20900, 20902)

29855 Arthroscopically aided treatment of tibial fracture, proximal (plateau); nicondylar, includes internal fixation, when performed (includes arthroscopy)

29856 bicondylar, includes internal fixation, when performed (includes arthroscopy)

(For bone graft, use 20900, 20902)

29860 Arthroscopy, hip, diagnostic with or without synovial biopsy (separate procedure)

29861 Arthroscopy, hip, surgical; with removal of loose body or foreign body

29862 with debridement/shaving of articular cartilage (chondroplasty), abrasion arthroplasty, and/or resection of labrum

29863 with synovectomy

29914 with femoroplasty (ie, treatment of cam lesion)

29915 with acetabuloplasty (ie, treatment of pincer lesion)

(Do not report 29914, 29915 in conjunction with 29862, 29863)

29916 with labral repair

(Do not report 29916 in conjunction with 29915, 29862, 29863)

29866 Arthroscopy, knee, surgical; osteochondral autograft(s) (eg, mosaicplasty) (includes harvesting of the autograft[s])

(Do not report 29866 in conjunction with 29870, 29871, 29875, 29884 when performed at the same session and/or 29874, 29877, 29879, 29885-29887 when performed in the same compartment)

(For open osteochondral autograft of knee, use 27416)

29867 osteochondral allograft (eg, mosaicplasty)

(Do not report 29867 in conjunction with 27570, 29870, 29871, 29875, 29884 when performed at the same session and/or 29874, 29877, 29879, 29885-29887 when performed in the same compartment)

(Do not report 29867 in conjunction with 27415)

29868 meniscal transplantation (includes arthrotomy for meniscal insertion), medial or lateral

(Do not report 29868 in conjunction with 29870, 29871, 29875, 29880, 29883, 29884 when performed at the same session or 29874, 29877, 29881, 29882 when performed in the same compartment)

29870 Arthroscopy, knee, diagnostic, with or without synovial biopsy (separate procedure)

(For open autologous chondrocyte implantation of the knee, use 27412)

29871 Arthroscopy, knee, surgical; for infection, lavage and drainage

(Do not report 29871 in conjunction with 27369)

(For implantation of osteochondral graft for treatment of articular surface defect, see 27412, 27415, 29866, 29867)

● New Code ▲ Revised Code ✛ Add-On Code ⊘ Modifier -51 Exempt ★ Telemedicine

29873	with lateral release	

(For open lateral release, use 27425)

29874   for removal of loose body or foreign body (eg, osteochondritis dissecans fragmentation, chondral fragmentation)

29875   synovectomy, limited (eg, plica or shelf resection) (separate procedure)

29876   synovectomy, major, 2 or more compartments (eg, medial or lateral)

29877   debridement/shaving of articular cartilage (chondroplasty)

(When performed with arthroscopic meniscectomy, see 29880 or 29881)

29879   abrasion arthroplasty (includes chondroplasty where necessary) or multiple drilling or microfracture

29880   with meniscectomy (medial AND lateral, including any meniscal shaving) including debridement/shaving of articular cartilage (chondroplasty), same or separate compartment(s), when performed

29881   with meniscectomy (medial OR lateral, including any meniscal shaving) including debridement/shaving of articular cartilage (chondroplasty), same or separate compartment(s), when performed

29882   with meniscus repair (medial OR lateral)

29883   with meniscus repair (medial AND lateral)

(For meniscal transplantation, medial or lateral, knee, use 29868)

29884   with lysis of adhesions, with or without manipulation (separate procedure)

29885   drilling for osteochondritis dissecans with bone grafting, with or without internal fixation (including debridement of base of lesion)

29886   drilling for intact osteochondritis dissecans lesion

29887   drilling for intact osteochondritis dissecans lesion with internal fixation

29888   Arthroscopically aided anterior cruciate ligament repair/augmentation or reconstruction

29889   Arthroscopically aided posterior cruciate ligament repair/augmentation or reconstruction

(Procedures 29888 and 29889 should not be used with reconstruction procedures 27427-27429)

29891   Arthroscopy, ankle, surgical, excision of osteochondral defect of talus and/or tibia, including drilling of the defect

29892   Arthroscopically aided repair of large osteochondritis dissecans lesion, talar dome fracture, or tibial plafond fracture, with or without internal fixation (includes arthroscopy)

29893   Endoscopic plantar fasciotomy

29894   Arthroscopy, ankle (tibiotalar and fibulotalar joints), surgical; with removal of loose body or foreign body

29895   synovectomy, partial

29897   debridement, limited

29898   debridement, extensive

| ██ Separate Procedure | ░░ Unlisted Procedure | ▓▓ CCI Comp. Code | ▒▒ Non-specific Procedure | **343** |

29899   with ankle arthrodesis

(For open ankle arthrodesis, use 27870)

29900   Arthroscopy, metacarpophalangeal joint, diagnostic, includes synovial biopsy

(Do not report 29900 with 29901, 29902)

29901   Arthroscopy, metacarpophalangeal joint, surgical; with debridement

29902   with reduction of displaced ulnar collateral ligament (eg, Stener lesion)

29904   Arthroscropy, subtalar joint, surgical; with removal of loose body or foreign body

29905   with synovectomy

29906   with debridement

29907   with subtalar arthrodesis

29914   This code is out of order. See page 342

29915   This code is out of order. See page 342

29916   This code is out of order. See page 342

29999   Unlisted procedure, arthroscopy

● New Code   ▲ Revised Code   ✛ Add-On Code   ⊘ Modifier -51 Exempt   ★ Telemedicine

RESPIRATORY SYSTEM

CPT codes from this section of the CPT coding system are used to report invasive and surgical procedures performed on the nose, sinuses, larynx, trachea and bronchi, and the lungs and pleura.

MISCELLANEOUS CODING RULES

Functional Endoscopic Sinus Surgery (FESS) codes are coded based on the procedures described in the operative report or on the nasal sinus endoscopy report. Each FESS code represents a unilateral procedure. To express that a procedure was performed bilaterally requires the application of the modifier -50, bilateral procedure.

Indirect laryngoscopy involves the visualization of the larynx using a warm laryngeal mirror positioned at the back of the throat. Direct laryngoscopy involves the visualization using a rigid or fiberoptic endoscope. Operative direct laryngoscopy involves an endoscopic examination under general anesthesia.

To code nasal hemorrhages appropriately, documentation needs to substantiate whether the hemorrhage is anterior or posterior and how the hemorrhage is controlled. Control of anterior nasal hemorrhage typically involves the insertion of gauze packing, or anterior packing or performance of cauterization. Control of posterior nasal hemorrhage most likely requires the insertion of nasal stents, tampons, balloon catheters, or posterior packing.

NOSE

INCISION

30000 Drainage abscess or hematoma, nasal, internal approach

(For external approach, see 10060, 10140)

30020 Drainage abscess or hematoma, nasal septum

(For lateral rhinotomy, see specific application (eg, 30118, 30320))

EXCISION

30100 Biopsy, intranasal

(For biopsy skin of nose, see 11102, 11103, 11104, 11105, 11106, 11107)

30110 Excision, nasal polyp(s), simple

(30110 would normally be completed in an office setting)

(To report bilateral procedure, use 30110 with modifier -50)

30115 Excision, nasal polyp(s), extensive

(30115 would normally require the facilities available in a hospital setting)

(To report bilateral procedure, use 30115 with modifier -50)

30117 Excision or destruction (eg, laser), intranasal lesion; internal approach

30118 external approach (lateral rhinotomy)

30120 Excision or surgical planing of skin of nose for rhinophyma

30124 Excision dermoid cyst, nose; simple, skin, subcutaneous

30125 complex, under bone or cartilage

30130 Excision inferior turbinate, partial or complete, any method

---

Separate Procedure   Unlisted Procedure   CCI Comp. Code   Non-specific Procedure   **345**

(For excision of superior or middle turbinate, use 30999)

30140   Submucous resection inferior turbinate, partial or complete, any method

(Do not report 30130 or 30140 in conjunction with 30801, 30802, 30930)

(For submucous resection of superior or middle turbinate, use 30999)

(For endoscopic resection of concha bullosa of middle turbinate, use 31240)

(For submucous resection of nasal septum, use 30520)

30150   Rhinectomy; partial

30160   total

(For closure and/or reconstruction, primary or delayed, see Integumentary System, 13151-13160, 14060-14302, 15120, 15121, 15260, 15261, 15760, 20900-20912)

INTRODUCTION

30200   Injection into turbinate(s), therapeutic

30210   Displacement therapy (Proetz type)

30220   Insertion, nasal septal prosthesis (button)

REMOVAL OF FOREIGN BODY

30300   Removal foreign body, intranasal; office type procedure

30310   requiring general anesthesia

30320   by lateral rhinotomy

REPAIR

(For obtaining tissues for graft, see 15769, 20900, 20902, 20910, 20912, 20920, 20922, 20924, 21210)

(For correction of nasal defects using fat harvested via liposuction technique, see 15773, 15774)

30400   Rhinoplasty, primary; lateral and alar cartilages and/or elevation of nasal tip

(For columellar reconstruction, see 13151 et seq)

30410   complete, external parts including bony pyramid, lateral and alar cartilages, and/or elevation of nasal tip

30420   including major septal repair

30430   Rhinoplasty, secondary; minor revision (small amount of nasal tip work)

30435   intermediate revision (bony work with osteotomies)

30450   major revision (nasal tip work and osteotomies)

30460   Rhinoplasty for nasal deformity secondary to congenital cleft lip and/or palate, including columellar lengthening; tip only

30462   tip, septum, osteotomies

30465   Repair of nasal vestibular stenosis (eg, spreader grafting, lateral nasal wall reconstruction)

● New Code   ▲ Revised Code   ✛ Add-On Code   ⃠ Modifier -51 Exempt   ★ Telemedicine

(30465 excludes obtaining graft. For graft procedure, see 15769, 20900, 20902, 20910, 20912, 20920, 20922, 20924, 21210, 21235)

(30465 is used to report a bilateral procedure. For unilateral procedure, use modifier -52)

(Do not report 30465 in conjunction with 30468, when performed on the ipsilateral side)

(For repair of nasal vestibular lateral wall collapse with subcutaneous/submucosal lateral wall implant[s], use 30468)

● **30468** Repair of nasal valve collapse with subcutaneous/submucosal lateral wall implant(s)

(30468 is used to report a bilateral procedure. For unilateral procedure, use modifier 52)

(Do not report 30468 in conjunction with 30465, when performed on the ipsilateral side)

(For repair of nasal vestibular stenosis [eg, spreader grafting, lateral nasal wall reconstruction], use 30465)

(For repair of nasal vestibular stenosis or collapse without cartilage graft, lateral wall reconstruction, or subcutaneous/submucosal implant [eg, radiofrequency remodeling, lateral wall suspension, or stenting without graft or subcutaneous/submucosal implant], use 30999)

30520 Septoplasty or submucous resection, with or without cartilage scoring, contouring or replacement with graft

(For submucous resection of turbinates, use 30140)

30540 Repair choanal atresia; intranasal

30545   transpalatine

(Do not report modifier '-63' in conjunction with 30540, 30545)

30560 Lysis intranasal synechia

30580 Repair fistula; oromaxillary (combine with 31030 if antrotomy is included)

30600   oronasal

30620 Septal or other intranasal dermatoplasty (does not include obtaining graft)

30630 Repair nasal septal perforations

DESTRUCTION

30801 Ablation, soft tissue of inferior turbinates, unilateral or bilateral, any method (eg, electrocautery, radiofrequency ablation, or tissue volume reduction); superficial

(For ablation of superior or middle turbinates, use 30999)

30802   intramural (ie, submucosal)

(Do not report 30801 in conjunction with 30802)

(Do not report 30801, 30802, 30930 in conjunction with 30130 or 30140)

(For cautery performed for control of nasal hemorrhage, see 30901-30906)

OTHER PROCEDURES

30901 Control nasal hemorrhage, anterior, simple (limited cautery and/or packing) any method

(To report bilateral procedure, use 30901 with modifier -50)

30903 Control nasal hemorrhage, anterior, complex (extensive cautery and/or packing) any method

(To report bilateral procedure, use 30903 with modifier -50)

Separate Procedure   Unlisted Procedure   CCI Comp. Code   Non-specific Procedure   **347**

30905 Control nasal hemorrhage, posterior, with posterior nasal packs and/or cautery, any method; initial

30906   subsequent

30915 Ligation arteries; ethmoidal

30920   internal maxillary artery, transantral

(For ligation external carotid artery, use 37600)

30930 Fracture nasal inferior turbinate(s), therapeutic

(Do not report 30801, 30802, 30930 in conjunction with 30130 or 30140)

(For fracture of superior or middle turbinate(s), use 30999)

30999 Unlisted procedure, nose

ACCESSORY SINUSES

INCISION

31000 Lavage by cannulation; maxillary sinus (antrum puncture or natural ostium)

(To report bilateral procedure, use 31000 with modifier -50)

31002   sphenoid sinus

31020 Sinusotomy, maxillary (antrotomy); intranasal

(To report bilateral procedure, use 31020 with modifier -50)

31030   radical (Caldwell-Luc) without removal of antrochoanal polyps

(To report bilateral procedure, use 31030 with modifier -50)

31032   radical (Caldwell-Luc) with removal of antrochoanal polyps

(To report bilateral procedure, use 31032 with modifier -50)

31040 Pterygomaxillary fossa surgery, any approach

(For transantral ligation of internal maxillary artery, use 30920)

31050 Sinusotomy, sphenoid, with or without biopsy;

31051   with mucosal stripping or removal of polyp(s)

31070 Sinusotomy frontal; external, simple (trephine operation)

(For frontal intranasal sinusotomy, use 31276)

31075   transorbital, unilateral (for mucocele or osteoma, Lynch type)

31080   obliterative without osteoplastic flap, brow incision (includes ablation)

31081   obliterative, without osteoplastic flap, coronal incision (includes ablation)

31084   obliterative, with osteoplastic flap, brow incision

31085   obliterative, with osteoplastic flap, coronal incision

● New Code   ▲ Revised Code   ✛ Add-On Code   ⊘ Modifier -51 Exempt   ★ Telemedicine

31086   nonobliterative, with osteoplastic flap, brow incision

31087   nonobliterative, with osteoplastic flap, coronal incision

31090   Sinusotomy, unilateral, 3 or more paranasal sinuses (frontal, maxillary, ethmoid, sphenoid)

EXCISION

31200   Ethmoidectomy; intranasal, anterior

31201   intranasal, total

31205   extranasal, total

31225   Maxillectomy; without orbital exenteration

31230   with orbital exenteration (en bloc)

(For orbital exenteration only, see 65110 et seq)

(For skin graft, see 15120 et seq)

ENDOSCOPY

A surgical sinus endoscopy includes a sinusotomy (when appropriate) and diagnostic endoscopy.

Codes 31295-31298 describe dilation of sinus ostia by displacement of tissue, any method, and include fluoroscopy if performed.

Stereotactic computer-assisted navigation may be used to facilitate the performance of endoscopic sinus surgery, and may be reported with 61782.

Codes 31233-31298 are used to report unilateral procedures unless otherwise specified.

Codes 31231-31235 for diagnostic evaluation refer to employing a nasal/sinus endoscope to inspect the interior of the nasal cavity and the middle and superior meatus, the turbinates, and the spheno-ethmoid recess. Any time a diagnostic evaluation is performed all these areas would be inspected and a separate code is not reported for each area. To report these services when all of the elements are not fully examined (eg, judged not clinically pertinent), or because the clinical situation precludes such exam (eg, technically unable, altered anatomy), append modifier 52 if repeat examination is not planned, or modifier 53 if repeat examination is planned.

31231   Nasal endoscopy, diagnostic, unilateral or bilateral (separate procedure)

31233   Nasal/sinus endoscopy, diagnostic; with maxillary sinusoscopy (via inferior meatus or canine fossa puncture)

(Do not report 31233 in conjunction with 31256, 31267, 31295, when performed on the ipsilateral side)

31235   Nasal/sinus endoscopy, diagnostic; with sphenoid sinusoscopy (via puncture of sphenoidal face or cannulation of ostium)

(Do not report 31235 in conjunction with 31257, 31259, 31287, 31288, 31297, 31298, when performed on the ipsilateral side)

(To report endoscopic placement of a drug-eluting implant in the ethmoid sinus without any other nasal/sinus endoscopic surgical service, use 31299. To report endoscopic placement of a drug-eluting implant in the ethmoid sinus in conjunction with biopsy, polypectomy, or debridement, use 31237)

31237   Nasal/sinus endoscopy, surgical; with biopsy, polypectomy or debridement (separate procedure)

(Do not report 31237 in conjunction with 31238, 31253, 31254, 31255, 31256, 31257, 31259, 31267, 31276, 31287, 31288, 31290, 31291, 31292, 31293, 31294, when performed on the ipsilateral side)

31238   with control of nasal hemorrhage

(Do not report 31238 in conjunction with 31237, 31241, when performed on the ipsilateral side)

31239   with dacryocystorhinostomy

31240   with concha bullosa resection

31241   with ligation of sphenopalatine artery

(Do not report 31241 in conjunction with 31238, when performed on the ipsilateral side)

31253   This code is out of order. See page 350

31254   Nasal/sinus endoscopy, surgical with ethmoidectomy; partial (anterior)

(Do not report 31254 in conjunction with 31237, 31253, 31255, 31257, 31259, 31290, 31291, 31292, 31293, 31294, when performed on the ipsilateral side)

31255   total (anterior andposterior)

(Do not report 31255 in conjunction with 31237, 31253, 31254, 31257, 31259, 31276, 31287, 31288, 31290, 31291, 31292, 31293, 31294, when performed on the ipsilateral side)

31253   total (anterior and posterior), including frontal sinus exploration, with removal of tissue from frontal sinus, when performed

(Do not report 31253 in conjunction with 31237, 31254, 31255, 31276, 31290, 31291, 31292, 31293, 31294, 31296, 31298, when performed on the ipsilateral side)

31257   total (anterior and posterior), including sphenoidotomy

(Do not report 31257 in conjunction with 31235, 31237, 31254, 31255, 31259, 31287, 31288, 31290, 31291, 31292, 31293, 31294, 31297, 31298, when performed on the ipsilateral side)

31259   total (anterior and posterior), including sphenoidotomy, with removal of tissue from the sphenoid sinus

(Do not report 31259 in conjunction with 31235, 31237, 31254, 31255, 31257, 31287, 31288, 31290, 31291, 31292, 31293, 31294, 31297, 31298, when performed on the ipsilateral side)

31256   Nasal/sinus endoscopy, surgical, with maxillary antrostomy;

(Do not report 31256 in conjunction with 31233, 31237, 31267, 31295, when performed on the ipsilateral side)

31257   This code is out of order. See page 350

31259   This code is out of order. See page 350

31267   with removal of tissue from maxillary sinus

(Do not report 31267 in conjunction with 31233, 31237, 31256, 31295, when performed on the ipsilateral side)

31276   Nasal/sinus endoscopy, surgical, with frontal sinus exploration, including removal of tissue from frontal sinus, when performed

(Do not report 31276 in conjunction with 31237, 31253, 31255, 31296, 31298, when performed on the ipsilateral side)

31287   Nasal/sinus endoscopy, surgical, with sphenoidotomy;

(Do not report 31287 in conjunction with 31235, 31237, 31255, 31257, 31259, 31288, 31291, 31294, 31297, 31298, when performed on the ipsilateral side)

31288   with removal of tissue from the sphenoid sinus

(Do not report 31288 in conjunction with 31235, 31237, 31255, 31257, 31259, 31287, 31291, 31294, 31297, 31298, when performed on the ipsilateral side)

31290 Nasal/sinus endoscopy, surgical, with repair of cerebrospinal fluid leak; ethmoid region

(Do not report 31290 in conjunction with 31237, 31253, 31254, 31255, 31257, 31259, when performed on the ipsilateral side)

31291 sphenoid region

(Do not report 31291 in conjunction with 31237, 31253, 31254, 31255, 31257, 31259, 31287, 31288, when performed on the ipsilateral side)

31292 Nasal/sinus endoscopy, surgical, with orbital decompression; medial or inferior wall

(Do not report 31292 in conjunction with 31237, 31253, 31254, 31255, 31257, 31259, 31293, 31296, when performed on the ipsilateral side)

31293 medial and inferior wall

(Do not report 31293 in conjunction with 31237, 31253, 31254, 31255, 31257, 31259, 31292, when performed on the ipsilateral side)

31294 Nasal/sinus endoscopy, surgical, with optic nerve decompression

(Do not report 31294 in conjunction with 31237, 31253, 31254, 31255, 31257, 31259, 31287, 31288, when performed on the ipsilateral side)

31295 Nasal/sinus endoscopy, surgical, with dilation (eg, balloon dilation); maxillary sinus ostium, transnasal or via canine fossa

(Do not report 31295 in conjunction with 31233, 31256, 31267, when performed on the ipsilateral side)

31296 frontal sinua ostium

(Do not report 31296 in conjunction with 31253, 31276, 31297, 31298, when performed on the ipsilateral side)

31297 sphenoid sinus ostium

(Do not report 31297 in conjunction with 31235, 31257, 31259, 31287, 31288, 31296, 31298, when performed on the ipsilateral side)

31298 frontal and sphenoid sinus ostia

(Do not report 31298 in conjunction with 31235, 31253, 31257, 31259, 31276, 31287, 31288, 31296, 31297, when performed on the ipsilateral side)

OTHER PROCEDURES

(For hypophysectomy, transantral or transeptal approach, use 61548)

(For transcranial hypophysectomy, use 61546)

31299 Unlisted procedure, accessory sinuses

LARYNX

EXCISION

31300 Laryngotomy (thyrotomy, laryngofissure); with removal of tumor or laryngocele, cordectomy

(**31320** deleted 2017 [2018 edition].)

31360 Laryngectomy; total, without radical neck dissection

Separate Procedure   Unlisted Procedure   CCI Comp. Code   Non-specific Procedure   **351**

31365	total, with radical neck dissection
31367	subtotal supraglottic, without radical neck dissection
31368	subtotal supraglottic, with radical neck dissection
31370	Partial laryngectomy (hemilaryngectomy); horizontal
31375	laterovertical
31380	anterovertical
31382	antero-latero-vertical
31390	Pharyngolaryngectomy, with radical neck dissection; without reconstruction
31395	with reconstruction
31400	Arytenoidectomy or arytenoidopexy, external approach

(For endoscopic arytenoidecomy, use 31560)

| 31420 | Epiglottidectomy |

INTRODUCTION

31500	Intubation, endotracheal, emergency procedure
31502	Tracheotomy tube change prior to establishment of fistula tract

ENDOSCOPY

For endoscopic procedures, report appropriate endoscopy of each anatomic site examined. Laryngoscopy includes examination of the tongue base, larynx, and hypopharynx. The anatomic structures examined with this procedure include both midline (single anatomic sites) and paired structures. Midline, single anatomic sites include tongue base, vallecula, epiglottis, subglottis, and posterior pharyngeal wall. Paired structures include true vocal cords, arytenoids, false vocal cords, ventricles, pyriform sinuses, and aryepiglottic folds. For the purposes of reporting therapeutic interventions, all paired structures contained within one side of the larynx/ pharynx are considered unilateral. If using operating microscope, telescope, or both, use the applicable code only once per operative session.

31505	Laryngoscopy, indirect; diagnostic (separate procedure)
31510	with biopsy
31511	with removal of foreign body
31512	with removal of lesion
31513	with vocal cord injection
31515	Laryngoscopy direct, with or without tracheoscopy; for aspiration
31520	diagnostic, newborn

(Do not report modifier -63 in conjunction with 31520)

31525	diagnostic, except newborn
31526	diagnostic, with operating microscope or telescope

(Do not report 31526 in conjunction with 69990)

● New Code   ▲ Revised Code   ✛ Add-On Code   ⊘ Modifier -51 Exempt   ★ Telemedicine

31527   with insertion of obturator

31528   with dilation, initial

31529   with dilation, subsequent

31530   Laryngoscopy, direct, operative, with foreign body removal;

31531   with operating microscope or telescope

(Do not report code 69990 in addition to code 31531)

31535   Laryngoscopy, direct, operative, with biopsy;

31536   with operating microscope or telescope

(Do not report code 69990 in addition to code 31536)

31540   Laryngoscopy, direct, operative, with excision of tumor and/or stripping of vocal cords or epiglottis;

31541   with operating microscope or telescope

(Do not report code 69990 in addition to code 31541)

31545   Laryngoscopy, direct, operative, with operating microscope or telescope, with submucosal removal of non-neoplastic lesion(s) of vocal cord; reconstruction with local tissue flap(s)

31546   reconstruction with graft(s) (includes obtaining autograft)

(Do not report 31546 in conjunction with 15769, 15771, 15772, 15773, 15774 for graft harvest)

(For reconstruction of vocal cord with allograft, use 31599)

(Do not report 31545 or 31546 in conjunction with 31540, 31541, 69990)

31551   This code is out of order. See page 354

31552   This code is out of order. See page 354

31553   This code is out of order. See page 354

31554   This code is out of order. See page 355

31560   Laryngoscopy, direct, operative, with arytenoidectomy;

31561   with operating microscope or telescope

(Do not report code 69990 in addition to code 31561)

31570   Laryngoscopy, direct, with injection into vocal cord(s), therapeutic;

31571   with operating microscope or telescope

(Do not report 31571 in conjunction with 69990)

31572   This code is out of order. See page 354

31573   This code is out of order. See page 354

31574   This code is out of order. See page 354

31575   Laryngoscopy, flexible; diagnostic

(Do not report 31575 in conjunction with 31231, unless performed for a separate condition using a separate endoscope)

(Do not report 31575 in conjunction with 31572, 31573, 31574, 31576, 31577, 31578, 43197, 43198, 92511, 92612, 92614, 92616)

31576   with biopsy(ies)

(Do not report 31576 in conjunction with 31572, 31578)

31577   with removal of foreign body(s)

31578   with removal of lesion(s), non-laser

31572   with ablation or destruction of lesion(s) with laser, unilateral

(Do not report 31572 in conjunction with 31576, 31578)

(To report flexible endoscopic evaluation of swallowing, see 92612-92613)

(To report flexible endoscopic evaluation with sensory testing, see 92614-92615)

(To report flexible endoscopic evaluation of swallowing with sensory testing, see 92616-92617)

(For flexible laryngoscopy as part of flexible endoscopic evaluation of swallowing and/or laryngeal sensory testing by cine or video recording, see 92612-92617)

31573   with therapeutic injection(s) (eg, chemodenervation agent or corticosteroid, injected percutaneous, transoral, or via endoscope channel), unilateral

31574   with injection(s) for augmentation (eg, percutaneous, transoral), unilateral

31579 Laryngoscopy, flexible or rigid telescopic, with stroboscopy

REPAIR

31580 Laryngoplasty; for laryngeal web, with indwelling keel or stent insertion

(Do not report 31580 in conjunction with 31551, 31552, 31553, 31554)

(To report tracheostomy, see 31600, 31601, 31603, 31605, 31610)

(To report removal of the keel or stent, use 31599)

31551   for laryngeal stenosis, with graft, without indwelling stent placement, younger than 12 years of age

(Do not report graft separately if harvested through the laryngoplasty incision [eg, thyroid cartilage graft])

(Do not report 31551 in conjunction with 31552, 31553, 31554, 31580)

(To report tracheostomy, see 31600, 31601, 31603, 31605, 31610)

31552   for laryngeal stenosis, with graft, without indwelling stent placement, age 12 years or older

(Do not report graft separately if harvested through the laryngoplasty incision [eg, thyroid cartilage graft])

(Do not report 31552 in conjunction with 31551, 31553, 31554, 31580)

(To report tracheostomy, see 31600, 31601, 31603, 31605, 31610)

31553   for laryngeal stenosis, with graft, with indwelling stent placement, younger than 12 years of age

(Do not report graft separately if harvested through the laryngoplasty incision [eg, thyroid cartilage graft])

(Do not report 31553 in conjunction with 31551, 31552, 31554, 31580)

(To report tracheostomy, see 31600, 31601, 31603, 31605, 31610)

● New Code   ▲ Revised Code   ＋ Add-On Code   ⊘ Modifier -51 Exempt   ★ Telemedicine

(To report removal of the stent, use 31599)

31554   for laryngeal stenosis, with graft, with indwelling stent placement, age 12 years or older

(Do not report graft separately if harvested through the laryngoplasty incision [eg, thyroid cartilage graft])

(Do not report 31554 in conjunction with 31551, 31552, 31553, 31580)

(To report tracheostomy, see 31600, 31601, 31603, 31605, 31610)

(To report removal of the stent, use 31599)

31584   with open reduction and fixation of (eg, plating) of fracture, includes tracheostomy, if performed

(Do not report graft separately if harvested through the laryngoplasty incision [eg, thyroid cartilage graft])

31587 Laryngoplasty, cricoid split, without graft placement

(To report tracheostomy, see 31600, 31601, 31603, 31605, 31610)

31590 Laryngeal reinnervation by neuromuscular pedicle

31591 Laryngoplasty, medialization, unilateral

31592 Cricotracheal resection

(Do not report graft separately if harvested through cricotracheal resection incision [eg, trachealis muscle])

(Do not report local advancement and rotational flaps separately if performed through the same incision)

(To report tracheostomy, see 31600, 31601, 31603, 31605, 31610)

(To report excision of tracheal stenosis and anastomosis, see 31780, 31781

DESTRUCTION

(**31595** deleted 2018 [2019 Edition])

OTHER PROCEDURES

31599 Unlisted procedure, larynx

TRACHEA AND BRONCHI

INCISION

31600 Tracheostomy, planned (separate procedure);

31601   under 2 years

31603 Tracheostomy, emergency procedure; transtracheal

31605   cricothyroid membrane

31610 Tracheostomy, fenestration procedure with skin flaps

(For endotracheal intubation, use 31500)

(For tracheal aspiration under direct vision, use 31515)

31611 Construction of tracheoesophageal fistula and subsequent insertion of an alaryngeal speech prosthesis (eg, voice button, Blom-Singer prosthesis)

31612 Tracheal puncture, percutaneous with transtracheal aspiration and/or injection

31613 Tracheostoma revision; simple, without flap rotation

31614   complex, with flap rotation

ENDOSCOPY

For endoscopy procedures, code appropriate endoscopy of each anatomic site examined. Surgical bronchoscopy always includes diagnostic bronchoscopy when performed by the same physician. Codes 31622-31651, 31660, 31661 include fluoroscopic guidance, when performed.

Codes 31652 and 31653 are complete services used for sampling (eg, aspiration/biopsy) lymph node(s) or adjacent structure(s) utilizing endobronchial ultrasound (EBUS) and are reported separately. Code 31654 is an add-on code and should be reported for identifying one or more peripheral lesion(s) with transendoscopic ultrasound.

31615 Tracheobronchoscopy through established tracheostomy incision

(For tracheoscopy, see laryngoscopy codes 31515-31574)

(For bronchoscopy with endobronchial ultrasound [EBUS] guided transtracheal/transbronchial sampling of mediastinal and/or hilar lymph node stations or structures, see 31652, 31653. For transendoscopic ultrasound during bronchoscopic diagnostic or therapeutic intervention[s] for peripheral lesions[s], use 31654)

31622 Bronchoscopy, rigid or flexible, including fluoroscopic guidance, when performed; diagnostic, with cell washing, when performed (separate procedure)

31623   with brushing or protected brushings

31624   with bronchial alveolar lavage

31625   with bronchial or endobronchial biopsy(s), single or multiple sites

31626   with placement of fiducial markers, single or multiple

(Report supply of device separately)

+ **31627**   with computer-assisted, image-guided navigation (List separately in addition to code for primary procedure[s])

(31627 includes 3D reconstruction. Do not report 31627 in conjunction with 76376, 76377)

(Use 31627 in conjunction with 31615, 31622-31626, 31628-31631, 31635, 31636, 31638-31643)

31628   with transbronchial lung biopsy(s), single lobe

(31628 should be reported only once regardless of how many transbronchial lung biopsies are performed in a lobe)

(To report transbronchial lung biopsies performed on additional lobe, use 31632)

31629   with transbronchial needle aspiration biopsy(s), trachea, main stem and/or lobar bronchus(i)

(31629 should be reported only once for upper airway biopsies regardless of how many transbronchial needle aspiration biopsies are performed in the upper airway or in a lobe)

(To report transbronchial needle aspiration biopsies performed on additional lobe(s), use 31633)

31630   with tracheal/bronchial dilation or closed reduction of fracture

31631   with placement of tracheal stent(s) (includes tracheal/ bronchial dilation as required)

(For placement of bronchial stent, see 31636, 31637)

(For revision of tracheal/bronchial stent, use 31638)

● New Code   ▲ Revised Code   + Add-On Code   ⊘ Modifier -51 Exempt   ★ Telemedicine

+ 31632   with transbronchial lung biopsy(s), each additional lobe (List separately in addition to code for primary procedure)

(Use 31632 in conjunction with 31628)

(31632 should be reported only once regardless of how many transbronchial lung biopsies are performed in a lobe)

+ 31633   with transbronchial needle aspiration biopsy(s), each additional lobe (List separately in addition to code for primary procedure)

(Use 31633 in conjunction with 31629)

(31633 should be reported only once regardless of how many transbronchial needle aspiration biopsies are performed in the trachea or the additional lobe)

31634   with balloon occlusion, with assessment of air leak, with administration of occlusive substance (eg, fibrin glue), if performed

(Do not report 31534 in conjunction with 31647, 31651 at the same session)

31635   with removal of foreign body

(For removal of implanted bronchial valves, see 31648-31649)

31636   with placement of bronchial stent(s) (includes tracheal/bronchial dilation as required), initial bronchus

+ 31637   each additional major bronchus stented (List separately in addition to code for primary procedure)

(Use 31637 in conjunction with 31636)

31638   with revision of tracheal or bronchial stent inserted at previous session (includes tracheal/bronchial dilation as required)

31640   with excision of tumor

31641   with destruction of tumor or relief of stenosis by any method other than excision (eg, laser therapy, cryotherapy)

(For bronchoscopic photodynamic therapy, report 31641 in addition to 96570, 96571 as appropriate)

31643   with placement of catheter(s) for intracavitary radioelement application

(For intracavitary radioelement application, see 77761-77763, 77770, 77771, 77772)

31645   with therapeutic aspiration of tracheobronchial tree, initial

31646   with therapeutic aspiration of tracheobronchial tree, subsequent, same hospital stay

(For catheter aspiration of tracheobronchial tree with fiberscope at bedside, use 31725)

31647   with balloon occlusion, when performed, assessment of air leak, airway sizing, and insertion of bronchial valve(s), initial lobe

+ 31651   with balloon occlusion, when performed, assessment of air leak, airway sizing, and insertion of bronchial valve(s), each additional lobe (List separately in addition to code for primary procedure[s])

(Use 31651 in conjunction with 31647)

31648   with removal of bronchial valve(s), initial lobe

(For removal and insertion of a bronchial valve at the same session, see 31647, 31648, and 31651)

+ 31649   with removal of bronchial valve(s), each additional lobe (List separately in addition to code for primary procedure)

Separate Procedure   Unlisted Procedure   CCI Comp. Code   Non-specific Procedure   **357**

(Use 31649 in conjunction with 31648)

31651   Code out of order. See page 357

31652   with endobronchial ultrasound (EBUS) guided transtracheal and/or transbronchial sampling (eg, aspiration[s]/ biopsy[ies]), one or two mediastinal and/or hilar lymph node stations or structures

31653   with endobronchial ultrasound (EBUS) guided transtracheal and/or transbronchial sampling (eg, aspiration[s]/ biopsy[ies]), 3 or more mediastinal and/or hilar lymph node stations or structures

+ 31654   with transendoscopic endobronchial ultrasound (EBUS) during bronchoscopic diagnostic or therapeutic intervention(s) for peripheral lesion(s) (List separately in addition to code for primary procedure[s])

(Use 31654 in conjunction with 31622, 31623, 31624, 31625, 31626, 31628, 31629, 31640, 31643, 31645, 31646)

(For EBUS to access mediastinal or hilar lymph node station[s] or adjacent structure[s], see 31652, 31653)

(Report 31652, 31653, 31654 only once per session)

BRONCHIAL THERMOPLASTY

31660   Bronchoscopy, rigid or flexible, including fluoroscopic guidance, when performed; with bronchial thermoplasty, 1 lobe

31661   with bronchial thermoplasty, 2 or more lobes

INTRODUCTION

(For endotracheal intubation, use 31500)

(For tracheal aspiration under direct vision, see 31515)

31717   Catheterization with bronchial brush biopsy

31720   Catheter aspiration (separate procedure); nasotracheal

31725   tracheobronchial with fiberscope, bedside

31730   Transtracheal (percutaneous) introduction of needle wire dilator/stent or indwelling tube for oxygen therapy

EXCISION, REPAIR

31750   Tracheoplasty; cervical

31755   tracheopharyngeal fistulization, each stage

31760   intrathoracic

31766   Carinal reconstruction

31770   Bronchoplasty; graft repair

31775   excision stenosis and anastomosis

(For lobectomy and bronchoplasty, use 32501)

31780   Excision tracheal stenosis and anastomosis; cervical

31781   cervicothoracic

31785   Excision of tracheal tumor or carcinoma; cervical

● New Code   ▲ Revised Code   + Add-On Code   ⊘ Modifier -51 Exempt   ★ Telemedicine

31786	thoracic
31800	Suture of tracheal wound or injury; cervical
31805	intrathoracic
31820	Surgical closure tracheostomy or fistula; without plastic repair
31825	with plastic repair

(For repair tracheoesophageal fistula, see 43305, 43312)

31830	Revision of tracheostomy scar

OTHER PROCEDURES

31899	Unlisted procedure, trachea, bronchi

LUNGS AND PLEURA

Pleural cavity or lung biopsy procedures may be accomplished using a percutaneous, thorascopic (Video-Assisted Thoracoscopic Surgery [VATS]), or thoracotomy approach. They involve the removal of differing amounts of tissue for diagnosis. A biopsy may be performed using different techniques such as incision or wedge. Lung resection procedures include diagnostic and therapeutic procedures, including the removal of blebs, bullae, cysts, and benign or malignant tumors or lesions. These procedures may involve the removal of small portions of the lung or even an entire lung. Additionally, lung resection procedures may require the removal of adjacent structures. Both diagnostic lung biopsies and therapeutic lung resections can be performed utilizing a wedge technique. However, a diagnostic biopsy of a lung nodule using a wedge technique requires only that a tissue sample be obtained without particular attention to resection margins. A therapeutic wedge resection requires attention to margins and complete resection even when the wedge resection is ultimately followed by a more extensive resection. In the case of a wedge resection where intraoperative pathology consultation determines that a more extensive resection is required in the same anatomic location, it becomes classified as a diagnostic wedge resection (32507, 32668). When no more extensive resection is required, the same procedure is a therapeutic wedge resection (32505, 32666).

Pleural or lung biopsies or diagnostic wedge resections should be reported using codes 32096, 32097, 32098, 32400, 32408, 32507, 32607, 32608, 32609 or 32668. The open or thorasoscopic (VATS) therapeutic resection of lung mass or nodules via a wedge resection is reported using codes 32505, 32506, 32666 and 32667. More extensive anatomic lung resection procedures, which can be performed with either thoracotomy or thoracoscopic (VATS) approaches, include: segmentectomy, lobectomy, bilobectomy, and pneumonectomy.

When diagnostic biopsy(ies) of the lung are performed, regardless of the approach (ie, open or thoracoscopic [VATS]), or technique (eg, incisional resection, cautery resection, or stapled wedge), and the specimen is sent for intraoperative pathology consultation, and during that same operative session the surgeon uses these results to determine the extent of the necessary surgical resection that includes the anatomical location biopsied, only the most extensive procedure performed (eg, segmentectomy, lobectomy, thoracoscopic [VATS] lobectomy) should be reported.

The therapeutic wedge resection codes (32505, 32506, 32666, or 32667) should not be reported in addition to the more extensive lung procedure (eg, lobectomy) unless the therapeutic wedge resection was performed on a different lobe or on the contralateral lung, whether or not an intraoperative pathology consultation is used to determine the extent of lung resection. When a diagnostic wedge resection is followed by a more extensive procedure in the same anatomical location, report add-on codes 32507 or 32668 with the more extensive procedure(s). When a therapeutic wedge resection (32505, 32506, 32666 or 32667) is performed in a different lobe than the more extensive lung resection (eg, lobectomy), report the therapeutic wedge resection with modifier 59.

INCISION

32035	Thoracostomy; with rib resection for empyema
32036	with open flap drainage for empyema

(To report wound exploration due to penetrating trauma without thoracotomy, use 20101)

32096	Thoracotomy, with diagnostic biopsy(ies) of lung infiltrate(s) (eg, wedge, incisional), unilateral

(Do not report 32096 more than once per lung)

(Do not report 32096 in conjunction with 32440, 32442, 32445, 32488)

32097 Thoracotomy, with diagnostic biopsy(ies) of lung nodule(s) or mass(es) (eg, wedge, incisional), unilateral

(Do not report 32097 more than once per lung)

(Do not report 32097 in conjunction with 32440, 32442, 32445, 32488)

32098 Thoracotomy, with biopsy(ies) of pleura

(For repair of macroscopic hernia, see 13305-13312)

32100 Thoracotomy; with exploration

(Do not report 32100 in conjunction with 21601, 21602, 21603, 32503, 32504, 33955, 33956, 33957, 33963, 33964)

32110   with control of traumatic hemorrhage and/or repair of lung tear

32120   for postoperative complications

32124   with open intrapleural pneumonolysis

32140   with cyst(s) removal, includes pleural procedure when performed

32141   with resection-plication of bullae, includes any pleural procedure when performed

(For lung volume reduction, use 32491)

32150   with removal of intrapleural foreign body or fibrin deposit

32151   with removal of intrapulmonary foreign body

32160   with cardiac massage

(For segmental or other resections of lung, see 32480-32504)

32200 Pneumonostomy; with open drainage of abscess or cyst

(For percutaneous image-guided drainage of abscess or cyst of lungs or mediastinum by catheter placement, use 49405)

32215 Pleural scarification for repeat pneumothorax

32220 Decortication, pulmonary (separate procedure); total

32225   partial

EXCISION/RESECTION

32310 Pleurectomy, parietal (separate procedure)

32320 Decortication and parietal pleurectomy

32400 Biopsy, pleura; percutaneous needle

(If imaging guidance is performed, see 76942, 77002, 77012, 77021)

(For fine needle aspiration biopsy, see 10004, 10005, 10006, 10007, 10008, 10009, 10010, 10011, 10012, 10021)

● New Code   ▲ Revised Code   + Add-On Code   ⊘ Modifier -51 Exempt   ★ Telemedicine

A core needle biopsy is typically performed with a needle that is designed to obtain a core sample of tissue for histopathologic evaluation. A fine needle aspiration (FNA) biopsy is performed when material is aspirated with a fine needle and the cells are examined cytologically.

A core needle biopsy of the lung or mediastinum is most commonly performed with imaging guidance (ie, ultrasound, fluoroscopy, CT, MRI). Imaging guidance codes (ie, 76942, 77002, 77012, 77021) may not be reported separately with 32408. Code 32408 is reported once per lesion sampled in a single session.

Code 32408 includes all imaging guidance regardless of the number of imaging modalities used on the same lesion during the same session.

When more than one core needle biopsy of the lung or mediastinum with imaging guidance is performed on separate lesions at the same session on the same day, use 32408 once for each lesion with modifier 59 for the second and each additional core needle lung or mediastinal biopsy.

When a core needle biopsy of the lung or mediastinum with imaging guidance is performed at the same session as a core biopsy of a site other than the lung or mediastinum (eg, liver), both the core needle biopsy for the other site (eg, 47000) and the imaging guidance for that additional core needle biopsy may be reported separately with modifier 59.

When FNA biopsy and core needle biopsy of the lung or mediastinum are performed on the same lesion at the same session on the same day using the same type of imaging guidance, modifier 52 should be used with either the FNA biopsy code or the core lung or mediastinal biopsy code.

When FNA biopsy and core needle biopsy of the lung or mediastinum are performed on the same lesion at the same session on the same day using different types of imaging guidance, both image-guided biopsy codes may be reported separately and one of them should be appended with modifier 59.

When FNA biopsy is performed on one lesion and core needle biopsy of the lung or mediastinum is performed on a separate lesion at the same session on the same day using the same type of imaging guidance, both the modality-specific image-guided FNA biopsy code and 32408 may be reported separately and one of the codes should be appended with modifier 59.

When FNA biopsy is performed on one lesion and core needle biopsy of the lung or mediastinum is performed on a separate lesion at the same session on the same day using different types of imaging guidance, both the modality-specific image-guided FNA biopsy code and 32408 may be reported separately and one of the codes should be appended with modifier 59

(**32405** deleted 2020 [2021 edition]. To report percutaneous core needle biopsy of lung or mediastinum, use 32408)

● **32408** Core needle biopsy, lung or mediastinum, percutaneous, including imaging guidance, when performed

(Do not report 32408 in conjunction with 76942, 77002, 77012, 77021)

(For open biopsy of lung, see 32096, 32097. For open biopsy of mediastinum, see 39000 or 39010. For thoracoscopic [VATS] biopsy of lung, pleura, pericardium or mediastinal space structure, see 32604, 32606, 32607, 32608, 32609)

(For fine needle aspiration biopsy, see 10004, 10005, 10006, 10007, 10008, 10009, 10010, 10011, 10012, 10021)

REMOVAL

32440 Removal of lung, pneumonectomy;

32442 with resection of segment of trachea followed by broncho-tracheal anastomosis (sleeve pneumonectomy)

32445 extrapleural

(For extrapleural pneumonectomy, with empyemectomy, use 32445 and 32540)

(If lung resection is performed with chest wall tumor resection, report the appropriate chest wall tumor resection code [21601, 21602, 21603], in addition to lung resection code [32440-32445])

32480 Removal of lung, other than pneumonectomy; single lobe (lobectomy)

32482   2 lobes (bilobectomy)

32484   single segment (segmentectomy)

(For removal of lung with bronchoplasty, use 32501)

32486   with circumferential resection of segment of bronchus followed by broncho-bronchial anastomosis (sleeve lobectomy)

32488   with all remaining lung following previous removal of a portion of lung (completion pneumonectomy)

(For lobectomy or segmentectomy, with concomitant decortication, use 32320 and the appropriate removal of lung code)

32491   with resection-plication of emphysematous lung(s) (bullous or non-bullous) for lung volume reduction, sternal split or transthoracic approach, includes any pleural procedure, when performed

(If lung resection is performed with chest wall tumor resection, report the appropriate chest wall tumor resection code [21601, 21602, 21603] in addition to lung resection code [32480, 32482, 32484, 32486, 32488, 32505, 32506, 32507])

+ 32501   Resection and repair of portion of bronchus (bronchoplasty) when performed at time of lobectomy or segmentectomy (List separately in addition to code for primary procedure)

(Use 32501 in conjunction with codes 32480, 32482, 32484)

(32501 is to be used when a portion of the bronchus to preserved lung is removed and requires plastic closure to preserve function of that preserved lung. It is not to be used for closure for the proximal end of a resected bronchus.)

32503   Resection of apical lung tumor (eg, Pancoast tumor), including chest wall resection, rib(s) resection(s), neurovascular dissection, when performed; without chest wall reconstruction(s)

32504   with chest wall reconstruction

(Do not report 32503, 32504 in conjunction with 21601, 21602, 21603, 32100, 32551, 32554, 32555)

32505   Thoracotomy; with therapeutic wedge resection (eg, mass, nodule), initial

(Do not report 32505 in conjunction with 32440, 32442, 32445, 32488)

+ 32506   with therapeutic wedge resection (eg, mass or nodule), each additional resection, ipsilateral (List separately in addition to code for primary procedure)

(Report 32506 only in conjunction with 32505)

(If lung resection is performed with chest wall tumor resection, report the appropriate chest wall tumor resection code [21601, 21602, 21603], in addition to lung resection code [32480, 32482, 32484, 32486, 32488, 32505, 32506, 32507])

+ 32507   with diagnostic wedge resection followed by anatomic lung resection (List separately in addition to code for primary procedure)

(Report 32507 in conjunction with 32440, 32442, 32445, 32480, 32482, 32484, 32486, 32488, 32503, 32504)

32540   Extrapleural enucleation of empyema (empyemectomy)

(For extrapleural enucleation of empyema (empyemectomy) with lobectomy, use 32540 and the appropriate removal of lung code)

INTRODUCTION AND REMOVAL

32550   Insertion of indwelling tunneled pleural catheter with cuff

● New Code   ▲ Revised Code   + Add-On Code   ⊘ Modifier -51 Exempt   ★ Telemedicine

(Do not report 32550 in conjunction with 32554, 32555, 32556, 32557 when performed on the same side of the chest)

(If imaging guidance is performed, use 75989)

32551 Tube thoracostomy, includes connection to drainage system (eg, water seal), when performed, open (separate procedure)

(Do not report 32551 in conjunction with 33020, 33025, if pleural drain/chest tube is placed on the ipsilateral side)

32552 Removal of indwelling tunneled pleural catheter with cuff

32553 Placement of interstitial device(s) for radiation therapy guidance (eg, fiducial markers, dosimeter), percutaneous, intra thoracic, single or multiple

(Report supply of device separately)

(For imaging guidance, see 76942, 77002, 77012, 77021)

(For percutaneous placement of interstitial device[s] for intra-abdominal, intrapelvic, and/or retroperitoneal radiation therapy guidance, use 49411)

32554 Thoraqcentesis, needle or catheter, aspiration of the pleural space; without imaging guidance

32555   with imaging guidance

32556 Pleural drainage, percutaneous, with insertion of indwelling catheter; without imaging guidance

32557   with imaging guidance

(For insertion of indwelling tunneled pleural catheter with cuff, use 32550)

(For open procedure, use 32551)

(Do not report 32554-32557 in conjunction with 32550, 32551 when performed on the same side of the chest)

(Do not report 32554-32557 in conjunction with 75989, 76942, 77002, 77012, 77021)

DESTRUCTION

The instillation of a fibrinolytic agent may be performed multiple times per day over the course of several days. Code 32561 should be reported only once on the initial day treatment. Code 32562 should be reported only once on each subsequent day of treatment.

32560 Instillation, via chest tube/catheter, agent for pleurodesis (eg, talc for recurrent or persistent pneumothorax)

(For chest tube insertion, use 32551)

32561 Instillation(s), via chest tube/catheter, agent for fibrinolysis (eg, fibrinolytic agent for break up of multiloculated effusion); initial day

(For chest tube insertion, use 32551)

32562   subsequent day

(For chest tube insertion, use 32551)

THORACOSCOPY (VIDEO-ASSISTED THORACIC SURGERY [VATS])

Surgical thoracoscopy (video-assisted thoracic surgery [VATS]) always includes diagnostic thoracoscopy.

32601 Thoracoscopy, diagnostic (separate procedure); lungs, pericardial sac, mediastinal or pleural space, without biopsy

---

| | Separate Procedure | | Unlisted Procedure | | CCI Comp. Code | | Non-specific Procedure | **363** |

32604   pericardial sac, with biopsy

(For open pericardial biopsy, use 39010)

32606   mediastinal space, with biopsy

32607   Thoracoscopy; with diagnostic biopsy(ies) of lung infiltrate(s) (eg, wedge, incisional), unilateral

(Do not report 32607 more than once per lung)

(Do not report 32607 in conjunction with 32440, 32442, 32445, 32488, 32671)

32608   with diagnostic biopsy(ies) of lung nodule(s) or mass(es) (eg, wedge, incisional), unilateral

(Do not report 32608 more than once per lung)

(Do not report 32608 in conjunction with 32440, 32442, 32445, 32488, 32671)

32609   with biopsy(ies) of pleura

32650   Thoracoscopy, surgical; with pleurodesis (eg, mechanical or chemical)

32651   with partial pulmonary decortication

32652   with total pulmonary decortication, including intrapleural pneumonolysis

32653   with removal of intrapleural foreign body or fibrin deposit

32654   with control of traumatic hemorrhage

32655   with resection-plication of bullae, including any pleural procedure when performed

(For thoracoscopic [VATS] lung volume reduction surgery, use 32672)

32656   with parietal pleurectomy

32658   with removal of clot or foreign body from pericardial sac

32659   with creation of pericardial window or partial resection of pericardial sac for drainage

32661   with excision of pericardial cyst, tumor, or mass

32662   with excision of mediastinal cyst, tumor, or mass

32663   with lobectomy (single lobe)

(For thoracoscopic [VATS] segmentectomy, use 32669)

32664   with thoracic sympathectomy

32665   with esophagomyotomy (Heller type)

(For exploratory thoracoscopy, and exploratory throacoscopy with biopsy, see 32601-32609)

32666   with therapeutic wedge resection (eg, mass, nodule), initial unilateral

(To report bilateral procedure, report 32666 with modifier 50)

(Do not report 32666 in conjunction with 32440, 32442, 32445, 32488, 32671)

+ **32667**   with therapeutic wedge resection (eg, mass or nodule), each additional resection, ipsilateral (List separately in addition to code for primary procedure)

● New Code   ▲ Revised Code   + Add-On Code   ⊘ Modifier -51 Exempt   ★ Telemedicine

(Report 32667 only in conjunction with 32666)

(Do not report 32667 in conjunction with 32440, 32442, 32445, 32488, 32671)

+ 32668   with diagnostic wedge resection followed by anatomic lung resection (List separately in addition to code for primary procedure)

(Report 32668 in conjunction with 32440, 32442, 32445, 32480, 32482, 32484, 32486, 32488, 32503, 32504, 32663, 32669, 32670, 32671)

32669   with removal of a single lung segment (segmentectomy)

32670   with removal of two lobes (bilobectomy)

32671   with removal of lung (pneumonectomy)

32672   with resection-plication for emphysematous lung (bullous or non-bullous) for lung volume reduction (LVRS), unilateral includes any pleural procedure, when performed

32673   with resection of thymus, unilateral or bilateral

(For open thymectomy, see 60520, 60521, 60522)

(For open excision mediastinal cyst, see 39200. For open excision mediastinal tumor, use 39220)

(For exploratory thoracoscopy, and exploratory thoracoscopy with biopsy, see 32601-32609)

+ 32674   with mediastinal and regional lymphadenectomy (List separately in addition to code for primary procedure)

(On the right, mediastinal lymph nodes include the paratracheal, subcarinal, paraesophageal, and inferior pulmonary ligament)

(On the left, mediastinal lymph nodes include the aortopulmonary window, subcarinal, paraesophageal, and inferior pulmonary ligament)

(Report 32674 in conjunction with 21601, 31760, 31766, 31786, 32096-32200, 32220-32320, 32440-32491, 32503-32505, 32601-32663, 32666, 32669-32673, 32815, 33025, 33030, 33050-33130, 39200-39220, 39560, 39561, 43101, 43112, 43117, 43118, 43122, 43123, 43287, 43288, 43351, 60270, 60505)

(To report mediastinal and regional lymphadenectomy via thoracotomy, use 38746)

STEREOTACTIC RADIATION THERAPY

Thoracic stereotactic body radiation therapy (SRS/SBRT) is a distinct procedure which may involve collaboration between a surgeon and radiation oncologist. The surgeon identifies and delineates the target for therapy. The radiation oncologist reports the appropriate code(s) for clinical treatment planning, physics and dosimetry, treatment delivery and management from the Radiation Oncology section (see 77295, 77331, 77370, 77373, 77435). The same physician should not report target delineation services with radiation treatment management codes (77427-77499).

Target delineation involves specific determination of tumor borders to identify tumor volume and relationship with adjacent structures (eg, chest wall, intraparenchymal vasculature and atelectatic lung) and previously placed fiducial markers, when present. Target delineation also includes availability to identify and validate the thoracic target prior to treatment delivery when a difucial-less tracking system is utilized.

Do not report target delineation more than once per entire course of treatment when the treatment requires greater than one session.

32701   Thoracic target(s) delineation for stereotactic body radiation therapy (SRS/SBRT), (photon or particle beam), entire course of treatment

((Do not report 32701 in conjunction with 77261-77799)

(For placement of fiducial markers, see 31626, 32553)

REPAIR

32800 Repair lung hernia through chest wall

32810 Closure of chest wall following open flap drainage for empyema (Clagett type procedure)

32815 Open closure of major bronchial fistula

32820 Major reconstruction, chest wall (posttraumatic)

LUNG TRANSPLANTATION

Lung allotransplantation involves three distinct components of physician work:

1) **Cadaver donor pneumonectomy(s)**, which include(s) harvesting the allograft and cold preservation of the allograft (perfusing with cold preservation solution and cold maintenance) (use 32850).

2) **Backbench work:**

Preparation of a cadaver donor single lung allograft prior to transplantation, including dissection of the allograft from surrounding soft tissues to prepare the pulmonary venous/atrial cuff, pulmonary artery, and bronchus unilaterally (use 32855).

Preparation of a cadaver donor double lung allograft prior to transplantation, including dissection of the allograft from surrounding soft tissues to prepare the pulmonary venous/atrial cuff, pulmonary artery, and bronchus bilaterally (use 32856).

3) **Recipient lung allotransplantation**, which includes transplantation of a single or double lung allograft and care of the recipient (see 32851-32854).

(For ex-vivo assessment of marginal donor lung transplant, see 0494T, 0495T, 0496T)

32850 Donor pneumonectomy (including cold preservation), from cadaver donor

32851 Lung transplant, single; without cardiopulmonary bypass

32852 with cardiopulmonary bypass

32853 Lung transplant, double (bilateral sequential or en bloc); without cardiopulmonary bypass

32854 with cardiopulmonary bypass

32855 Backbench standard preparation of cadaver donor lung allograft prior to transplantation, including dissection of allograft from surrounding soft tissues to prepare pulmonary venous/atrial cuff, pulmonary artery, and bronchus; unilateral

32856 bilateral

(For repair or resection procedures on the donor lung, see 32491, 32505, 32506, 32507, 35216, 35276)

SURGICAL COLLAPSE THERAPY; THORACOPLASTY

(See also 32503, 32504)

32900 Resection of ribs, extrapleural, all stages

32905 Thoracoplasty, Schede type or extrapleural (all stages);

32906 with closure of bronchopleural fistula

(For open closure of major bronchial fistula, use 32815)

(For resection of first rib for thoracic outlet compression, see 21615, 21616)

32940 Pneumonolysis, extraperiosteal, including filling or packing procedures

---

● New Code   ▲ Revised Code   + Add-On Code   ⊘ Modifier -51 Exempt   ★ Telemedicine

32960   Pneumothorax, therapeutic, intrapleural injection of air

OTHER PROCEDURES

32994   This code is out of order. See page 367

32997   Total lung lavage (unilateral)

(For bronchoscopic bronchial alveolar lavage, use 31624)

32998   Ablation therapy for reduction or eradication of 1 or more pulmonary tumor(s) including pleura or chest wall when involved by tumor extension, percutaneous, including imaging guidance when performed, unilateral; radiofrequency

32994   cryoablation

(For bilateral procedure, report 32994, 32998 with modifier 50)

32999   Unlisted procedure, lungs and pleura

This page intentionally left blank

CARDIOVASCULAR SYSTEM

CPT codes from this section of the CPT coding system are used to report invasive and surgical procedures performed on the heart and pericardium, including pacemakers or defibrillators; cardiac valves; coronary arteries; aorta; and arteries and veins.

For coding services such as monitoring, operation of pump and other non-surgical services performed during cardiovascular surgery, see the Special Services CPT codes 99150, 99151, 99160-99162 or CPT codes 99291-99292 and 99190-99192 from the evaluation and management section of the CPT coding system.

MISCELLANEOUS CODING RULES

A pacemaker system includes a pulse generator containing electronics, a battery, and one or more electrodes (leads) inserted one of several ways. Pulse generators may be placed in a subcutaneous "pocket" created in either a subclavicular or intra-abdominal site. Electrodes may be inserted through a vein (transvenous) or on the surface of the heart (epicardial). A single chamber system includes a pulse generator, one electrode inserted into either the atrium or ventricle. A dual chamber system includes a pulse generator, one electrode inserted in the atrium, and one electrode inserted in the ventricle.

Assign two CPT codes when a pacemaker or cardioverter-defibrillator "battery"/pulse generator is replaced. One code should describe the removal of the old pulse generator and the other should describe the insertion of the new pulse generator.

Cardiac catheterization codes are classified in the Medicine Section of the CPT coding system. Insertion of a dilator into a vein prior to the placement of a catheter should not be separately coded.

Selective vascular catheterization should be coded to include introduction and all lesser order selective catheterization used in the approach (eg., the description for a selective right middle cerebral artery catheterization includes the introduction and placement catheterization of the right common and internal carotid arteries).

Additional second and/or third order arterial catheterizations within the same family of arteries supplied by a single first order artery should be expressed by 36218 or 36248. Additional first order or higher catheterizations in vascular families supplied by a first order vessel different from a previously selected and coded family should be separately coded using the conventions described above.

> (For monitoring, operation of pump and other nonsurgical services, see 99190-99192, 99291, 99292, 99354-99360)

> (For other medical or laboratory related services, see appropriate section)

> (For radiological supervision and interpretation, see 75600-75970)

HEART AND PERICARDIUM

PERICARDIUM

In order to report pericardial drainage with insertion of indwelling catheter (33017, 33018, 33019), the catheter needs to remain in place when the procedure is completed. Codes 33017, 33018, 33019 should not be reported when a catheter is placed to aspirate fluid and then removed at the conclusion of the procedure. Congenital cardiac anomaly for reporting percutaneous pericardial drainage with insertion of indwelling catheter is defined as abnormal situs (heterotaxy, dextrocardia, mesocardia), single ventricle anomaly/physiology, or any patient in the first 90-day postoperative period after repair of a congenital cardiac anomaly.

> (For thoracoscopic [VATS] pericardial procedures, see 32601, 32604, 32658, 32659, 32661)

(**33010** deleted 2019 [2020 Edition]. To report, see 33016, 33017, 33018, 33019)

(**33011** deleted 2019 [2020 Edition]. To report, see 33016, 33017, 33018, 33019)

(**33015** deleted 2019 [2020 Edition]. To report, see 33017, 33018, 33019)

33016 Pericardiocentesis, including imaging guidance, when performed

> (Do not report 33016 in conjunction with 76942, 77002, 77012, 77021)

| Separate Procedure | Unlisted Procedure | CCI Comp. Code | Non-specific Procedure | **369** |

33017 Pericardial drainage with insertion of indwelling catheter, percutaneous, including fluoroscopy and/or ultrasound guidance, when performed; 6 years and older without congenital cardiac anomaly

33018   birth through 5 years of age or any age with congenital cardiac anomaly

    (Do not report 33017, 33018 in conjunction with 75989, 76942, 77002, 77012, 77021)

    (Do not report 33016, 33017, 33018 in conjunction with 93303-93325 when echocardiography is performed solely for the purpose of pericardiocentesis guidance)

    (For CT-guided pericardial drainage, use 33019)

33019 Pericardial drainage with insertion of indwelling catheter, percutaneous, including CT guidance

    (Do not report 33019 in conjunction with 75989, 76942, 77002, 77012, 77021)

33020 Pericardiotomy for removal of clot or foreign body (primary procedure)

33025 Creation of pericardial window or partial resection for drainage

    (Do not report 33020, 33025 in conjunction with 32551, if pleural drain/chest tube is placed on the ipsilateral side)

    (For thoracoscopic [VATS] pericardial window, use 32659)

33030 Pericardiectomy, subtotal or complete; without cardiopulmonary bypass

33031   with cardiopulmonary bypass

33050 Resection of pericardial cyst or tumor electrode(s); atrial

    (For open pericardial biopsy, use 39010)

    (For thoracoscopic [VATS] resection of pericardial cyst, tumor or mass, use 32661)

CARDIAC TUMOR

33120 Excision of intracardiac tumor, resection with cardiopulmonary bypass

33130 Resection of external cardiac tumor

TRANSMYOCARDIAL REVASCULARIZATION

33140 Transmyocardial laser revascularization, by thoracotomy (separate procedure)

+ **33141**   performed at the time of other open cardiac procedure(s) (List separately in addition to code for primary procedure)

    (Use 33141 in conjunction with codes 33390, 33391, 33404-33496, 33510-33536, 33542)

PACEMAKER OR IMPLANTABLE DEFIBRILLATOR

A pacemaker system with lead(s) includes a pulse generator containing electronics, battery, and one or more leads. A lead consists of one or more electrodes as well as conductor wires, insulation, and a fixation mechanism. Pulse generators are placed in a subcutaneous "pocket" created in either a subclavicular site or just above the abdominal muscles just below the rib cage. Leads may be inserted through a vein (transvenous) or they may be placed on the surface of the heart (epicardial). The epicardial location of leads requires a thoracotomy for insertion.

A single chamber pacemaker system with lead includes a pulse generator and one electrode inserted in either the atrium or ventricle. A dual chamber pacemaker system with two leads includes a pulse generator and one lead inserted in the right atrium and one lead inserted in the right ventricle. In certain circumstances, an additional lead may be required to achieve pacing of the left ventricle (bi-ventricular pacing). In this event, transvenous (cardiac vein) placement of the lead should be separately reported using code 33224 or 33225. Epicardial placement of the lead should be separately reported using 33202-33203.

A leadless cardiac pacemaker system includes a pulse generator with built-in battery and electrode for implantation in a cardiac chamber via a transcatheter approach. For implantation of a leadless pacemaker system, use 33274. Insertion, replacement, or removal of a leadless pacemaker system includes insertion of a catheter into the right ventricle.

Right heart catheterization (93451, 93453, 93456, 93457, 93460, 93461, 93530, 93531, 93532, 93533) may not be reported in conjunction with leadless pacemaker insertion and removal codes 33274, 33275 unless complete right heart catheterization is performed for an indication distinct from the leadless pacemaker procedure.

Like a pacemaker system, an implantable defibrillator system includes a pulse generator and electrodes. Three general categories of implantable defibrillators exist: transvenous implantable pacing cardioverter-defibrillator (ICD), subcutaneous implantable defibrillator (S-ICD), and substernal implantable cardioverter-defibrillator. Implantable pacing cardioverter-defibrillator devices use a combination of antitachycardia pacing, low-energy cardioversion or defibrillating shocks to treat ventricular tachycardia or ventricular fibrillation. The subcutaneous implantable defibrillator uses a single subcutaneous electrode to treat ventricular tachyarrhythmias. The substernal implantable cardioverter-defibrillator uses at least one substernal electrode to perform defibrillation, cardioversion, and antitachycardia pacing. Subcutaneous implantable defibrillators differ from transvenous implantable pacing cardioverter-defibrillators in that subcutaneous defibrillators do not provide antitachycardia pacing or chronic pacing. Substernal implantable defibrillators differ from both subcutaneous and transvenous implantable pacing cardioverter-defibrillators in that they provide antitachycardia pacing, but not chronic pacing.

Implantable defibrillator pulse generators may be implanted in a subcutaneous infraclavicular, axillary, or abdominal pocket. Removal of an implantable defibrillator pulse generator requires opening of the existing subcutaneous pocket and disconnection of the pulse generator from its electrode(s). A thoracotomy (or laparotomy in the case of abdominally placed pulse generators).

The electrodes (leads) of an implantable defibrillator system may be positioned within the atrial and/or ventricular chambers of the heart via the venous system (transvenously), or placed on the surface of the heart (epicardial), or positioned under the skin overlying the heart (subcutaneous). Electrode positioning on the epicardial surface of the heart requires a thoracotomy or thoracoscopic placement of the leads. Epicardial placement of electrode(s) may be separately reported using 33202, 33203. The electrode (lead) of a subcutaneous implantable defibrillator system is tunneled under the skin to the left parasternal margin. Subcutaneous placement of electrode may be reported using 33270 or 33271. The electrode (lead) of a substernal implantable defibrillator system is tunneled subcutaneously and placed into the substernal anterior mediastinum without entering the pericardial cavity and may be reported using 0571T, 0572T. In certain circumstances, an additional electrode may be required to achieve pacing of the left ventricle (bi-ventricular pacing). In this event, transvenous (cardiac vein) placement of the electrode may be separately reported using 33224 or 33225.

Removal of a transvenous electrode(s) may first be attempted by transvenous extraction (33234, 33235, or 33244). However, if transvenous extraction is unsuccessful, a thoracotomy may be required to remove the electrodes (33238 or 33243). Use 33212, 33213, 33221, 33230, 33231, 33240 as appropriate, in addition to the thoracotomy or endoscopic epicardial lead placement codes (33202 or 33203) to report the insertion of the generator if done by the same physician during the same session. Removal of a subcutaneous implantable defibrillator electrode may be separately reported using 33272. For removal of a leadless pacemaker system without replacement, use 33275. For removal and replacement of a leadless pacemaker system during the same session, use 33274.

When the "battery" of a pacemaker system with lead(s) or implantable defibrillator is changed, it is actually the pulse generator that is changed. Removal of only the pacemaker or implantable defibrillator pulse generator is reported with 33233 or 33241. If only a pulse generator is inserted or replaced without any right atrial and/or right ventricular lead(s) inserted or replaced, report the appropriate code for only pulse generator insertion or replacement based on the number of final existing lead(s) (33227, 33228, 33229 and 33262, 33263, 33264). Do not report removal of a pulse generator (33233 or 33241) separately for this service. Insertion of a new pulse generator, when existing lead(s) are already in place and when no prior pulse generator is removed, is reported with 33212, 33213, 33221, 33230, 33231, 33240. When a pulse generator insertion involves the insertion or replacement of one or more right atrial and/or right ventricular lead(s) or subcutaneous lead(s), use system codes 33206, 33207, 33208 for pacemaker, 33249 for implantable pacing cardioverter-defibrillator, or 33270 for subcutaneous implantable defibrillator. When reporting the system insertion or replacement codes, removal of a pulse generator (33233 or 33241) may be reported separately, when performed. In addition, extraction of leads 33234, 33235 or 33244 for transvenous or 33272 for subcutaneous may be reported separately, when performed. An exception involves a pacemaker upgrade from single to dual system that includes removal of pulse generator, replacement of new pulse generator, and insertion of new lead, reported with 33214.

Revision of a skin pocket is included in 33206-33249, 33262, 33263, 33264, 33270, 33271, 33272, 33273. When revision of a skin pocket involves incision and drainage of a hematoma or complex wound infection, see 10140, 10180, 11042, 11043, 11044, 11045, 11046, 11047 as appropriate.

Relocation of a skin pocket for a pacemaker (33222) or implantable defibrillator (33223) is necessary for various clinical situations such as infection or erosion. Relocation of an existing pulse generator may be performed as a stand-alone procedure or

---

at the time of a pulse generator or electrode insertion, replacement or repositioning. When skin pocket relocation is performed as part of an explant of an existing generator followed by replacement with a new generator, the pocket relocation is reported separately. Skin pocket relocation includes all work associated with the initial pocket (eg, opening the pocket, incision and drainage of hematoma or abscess if performed, and any closure performed) in addition to the creation of a new pocket for the new generator to be placed.

Repositioning of a pacemaker electrode, implantable defibrillator electrode(s), or a left ventricular pacing electrode is reported using 33215, 33226, or 33273 as appropriate.

Procedure	System	
	Pacemaker	Implantable Defibrillator
Insert transvenous single lead only without pulse generator	33216	33216
Insert transvenous dual leads without pulse generator	33217	33217
Insert transvenous multiple leads without pulse generator	33217 + 33224	33217 + 33224
Insert subcutaneous defibrillator electrode only without pulse generator	N/A	33271
Initial pulse generator insertion only with existing single lead, includes transvenous or subcutaneous defibrillator lead	33212	33240
Initial pulse generator insertion only with existing dual leads	33213	33230
Initial pulse generator insertion only with existing multiple leads	33221	33231
Initial pulse generator insertion or replacement plus insertion of transvenous single lead	33206 (atrial) or 33207 (ventricular)	33249
Initial pulse generator insertion or replacement plus insertion of transvenous dual leads	33208	33249
Initial pulse generator insertion or replacement plus insertion of transvenous multiple leads	33208 + 33225	33249 + 33225
Initial pulse generator insertion or replacement plus insertion of subcutaneous defibrillator electrode	N/A	33270
Insertion, replacement, or removal and replacement of permanent leadless pacemaker	33274	N/A
Upgrade single chamber system to dual chamber system	33214 (incl. removal of existing pulse generator)	33241 + 33249
Removal pulse generator only (without replacement)	33233	33241
Removal pulse generator with replacement pulse generator only single lead system (applies to transvenous or subcutaneous defibrillator lead systems)	33227	33262
Removal pulse generator with replacement pulse generator only dual lead system (transvenous)	33228	33263
Removal pulse generator with replacement pulse generator only multiple lead system (transvenous)	33229	33264
Removal transvenous electrode only single lead system	33234	33244
Removal transvenous electrode only dual lead system	33235	33244
Removal subcutaenous defibrillator lead only	N/A	33272
Removal and replacement of pulse generator and transvenous electrodes	33233 + (33234 or 33235) + (33206, 33207, or 33208) and 33225, when appropriate	33241 + 33244 + 33249 and 33225, when appropriate
Removal and replacement of implantable defibrillator pulse generator and subcutaneous electrode	N/A	33272 + 33241 + 33270
Removal of permanent leadless pacemaker	33275	N/A
Conversion of existing system to bi-ventricular system (addition of LV lead and removal of current pulse generator with insertion of new pulse generator with bi-ventricular pacing capabilities)	33225 + 33228 or 33229	33225 + 33263 or 33264

● New Code   ▲ Revised Code   ✚ Add-On Code   ⊘ Modifier -51 Exempt   ★ Telemedicine

Device evaluation codes 93260, 93261, 93279-93298 for pacemaker system with lead(s) may not be reported in conjunction with pulse generator and lead insertion or revision codes 33206-33249, 33262, 33263, 33264, 33270, 33271, 33272, 33273. For leadless pacemaker systems, device evaluation codes 93279, 93286, 93288, 93294, 93296 may not be reported in conjunction with leadless pacemaker insertion and removal codes 33274, 33275. Defibrillator threshold testing (DFT) during transvenous implantable defibrillator insertion or replacement may be separately reported using 93640, 93641. DFT testing during subcutaneous implantable defibrillator system insertion is not separately reportable. DFT testing for transvenous or subcutaneous implantable defibrillator in follow-up or at the time of replacement may be separately reported using 93642 or 93644.

Radiological supervision and interpretation related to the pacemaker or implantable defibrillator procedure is included in 33206-33249, 33262, 33263, 33264, 33270, 33271, 33272, 33273, 33274, 33275. Fluoroscopy (76000, 77002), ultrasound guidance for vascular access (76937), right ventriculography (93566), and femoral venography (75820) are included in 33274, 33275, when performed). To report fluoroscopic guidance for diagnostic lead evaluation without lead insertion, replacement, or revision procedures, use 76000.

The following definitions apply to 33206-33249, 33262, 33263, 33264, 33270, 33271, 33272, 33273:

Single lead: a pacemaker or implantable defibrillator with pacing and sensing function in only one chamber of the heart or a subcutaneous electrode

Dual lead: a pacemaker or implantable defibrillator with pacing and sensing function in only two chambers of the heart.

Multiple lead: a pacemaker or implantable defibrillator with pacing and sensing function in three or more chambers of the heart.

33202   Insertion of epicardial electrode(s); open incision (eg, thoracotomy, median sternotomy, subxiphoid approach)

33203   endoscopic approach (eg, thoracoscopy, pericardioscopy)

(When epicardial lead placement is performed with insertion of the generator, report 33202, 33203 in conjunction with 33212, 33213, 33221, 33230, 33231, 33240)

33206   Insertion of new or replacement of permanent pacemaker with transvenous electrode(s); atrial

33207   ventricular

33208   atrial and ventricular

(Do not report 33206-33208 in conjunction with 33227-33229)

(Do not report 33206, 33207, 33208 in conjunction with 33216, 33217)

(Codes 33206-33208 include subcutaneous insertion of the pulse generator and transvenous placement of electrode[s])

(For removal and replacement of pacemaker pulse generator and transvenous electrode(s), use 33233 in conjunction with either 33234 or 33235 and 33206-33208)

33210   Insertion or replacement of temporary transvenous single chamber cardiac electrode or pacemaker catheter (separate procedure)

33211   Insertion or replacement of temporary transvenous dual chamber pacing electrodes (separate procedure)

33212   Insertion of pacemaker pulse generator only; with existing single lead

33213   with existing dual leads

33221   with existing multiple leads

(Do not report 33212, 33213, 33221 in conjunction with 33216, 33217)

(Do not report 33212, 33213, 33221 in conjunction with 33233 for removal and replacement of the pacemaker pulse generator. Use 33227-33229, as appropriate, when pulse generator replacment is indicated.)

(When epicardial lead placement is performed with insertion of generator, report 33202, 33203 in conjunction with 33212, 33213, 33221)

33214 Upgrade of implanted pacemaker system, conversion of single chamber system to dual chamber system (includes removal of previously placed pulse generator, testing of existing lead, insertion of new lead, insertion of new pulse generator)

(Do not report 33214 in conjunction with 33216, 33217, 33227, 33228, 33229)

33215 Repositioning of previously implanted transvenous pacemaker or implantable defibillator (right atrial or right ventricular) electrode

33216 Insertion of a single transvenous electrode, permanent pacemaker or implantable defibrillator

(Do not report 33216 in conjunction with 33206, 33207, 33208, 33212, 33213, 33214, 33221, 33227, 33228, 33229, 33230, 33231, 33240, 33249, 33262, 33263, 33264)

33217 Insertion of 2 transvenous electrodes, permanent pacemaker or implantable defibrillator

(Do not report 33217 in conjunction with 33206, 33207, 33208, 33212, 33213, 33214, 33221, 33227, 33228, 33229, 33230, 33231, 33240, 33249, 33262, 33263, 33264)

(For insertion or replacement of cardiac venous system lead, see 33224, 33225)

33218 Repair of single transvenous electrode, permanent pacemaker or implantable defibrillator

(For repair of single permanent pacemaker or implantable defibrillator electrode with replacement of pulse generator, see 33227, 33228, 33229 or 33262, 33263, 33264 and 33218)

33220 Repair of 2 transvenous electrodes for permanent pacemaker or implantable defibrillator

(For repair of 2 tranvenous electrodes for permanent pacemaker or implantable defibrillator with replacement of pulse generator, use 33220 in conjunction with 33228, 33229, 33263, 33264)

33221 Code out of order. See page 373

33222 Relocation of skin pocket for pacemaker

(Do not report 33222 in conjunction with 10140, 10180, 11042, 11043, 11044, 11045, 11046, 11047, 13100, 13101, 13102)

33223 Relocation of skin pocket for implantable defibrillator

(Do not report 33223 in conjunction with 10140, 10180, 11042, 11043, 11044, 11045, 11046, 11047, 13100, 13101, 13102)

33224 Insertion of pacing electrode, cardiac venous system, for left ventricular pacing, with attachment to previously placed pacemaker or implantable defibrillator pulse generator (including revision of pocket, removal, insertion and/or replacement of existing generator)

(When epicardial electrode placement is performed, report 33224 in conjunction with 33202, 33203)

+ 33225 Insertion of pacing electrode, cardiac venous system, for left ventricular pacing, at time of insertion of implantable defibrillator or pacemaker pulse generator (eg, for upgrade to dual chamber system) (List separately in addition to code for primary procedure)

(Use 33225 in conjunction with 33206, 33207, 33208, 33212, 33213, 33214, 33216, 33217, 33221, 33223, 33228, 33229, 33230, 33231, 33233, 33234, 33235, 33240, 33249, 33263, 33264)

(Use 33225 in conjunction with 33222 only with pacemaker pulse generator pocket relocation and with 33223 only with implantable defibrillator [ICD] pocket relocation)

● New Code ▲ Revised Code + Add-On Code ⊘ Modifier -51 Exempt ★ Telemedicine

33226 Repositioning of previously implanted cardiac venous system (left ventricular) electrode (including removal, insertion and/or replacement of existing generator)

33227 Code out of order. See page 375

33228 Code out of order. See page 375

33229 Code out of order. See page 375

33230 Code out of order. See page 375

33231 Code out of order. See page 375

33233 Removal of permanent pacemaker pulse generator only

33227 Removal of permanent pacemaker pulse generator with replacement of pacemaker pulse generator; single lead system

33228 dual lead system

33229 multiple lead system

(Do not report 33227, 33228, 33229 in conjunction with 33214, 33216, 33217, 33233)

(For removal and replacement of pacemaker pulse generator and transvenous electrode[s], use 33233 in conjunction with either 33234 or 33235 and 33206-33208)

33234 Removal of transvenous pacemaker electrode(s); single lead system, atrial or ventricular

33235 dual lead system

33236 Removal of permanent epicardial pacemaker and electrodes by thoracotomy; single lead system, atrial or ventricular

33237 dual lead system

33238 Removal of permanent transvenous electrode(s) by thoracotomy

33240 Insertion of implantable defibrillator pulse generator only; with existing single lead

(Do not report 33240 in conjunction with 33271, 93260, 93261)

(Use 33240, as appropriate, in addition to the epicardial lead placement codes to report the insertion of the generator when done by the same physician during the same session)

33230 with existing dual leads

33231 with existing multiple leads

(Do not report 33230, 33231, 33240 in conjunction with 33216, 33217)

(Do not report 33230, 33231, 33240 in conjunction with 33241 for removal and replacement of the implantable defibrillator pulse generator. Use 33262, 33263, 33264, as appropriate, when pulse generator replacement is indicated)

(When epicardial lead placement if performed with insertion of generator, report 33202, 33203 in conjunction with 33230, 33231, 33240)

33241 Removal of implantable defibrillator pulse generator only

(Do not report 33241 in conjunction with 93260, 93261)

(Do not report 33241 in conjunction with 33230, 33231, 33240 for removal and replacement of the implantable defibrillator pulse generator. Use 33262, 33263, 33264, as appropriate, when pulse generator replacement is indicated)

(For removal and replacement of an implantable defibrillator pulse generator and electrode(s), use 33241 in conjunction with either 33243 or 33244 and 33249 for transvenous electrode[s] or 33270 and 33272 for subcutaneous electrode)

(For removal of implantable defibrillator with substernal lead, generator only, use 0580T)

33262 Removal of implantable defibrillator pulse generator with replacement of implantable defibrillator pulse generator; single lead system

(Do not report 33262 in conjunction with 33271, 93260, 93261, 0614T)

(For removal and replacement of substernal implantable pulse generator, use 0614T)

33263 dual lead system

33264 multiple lead system

(Do not report 33262, 33263, 33264 in conjunction with 33216, 33217, 33241)

(For removal of electrode[s] by thoracotomy in conjunction with pulse generator removal or replacement, use 33243 in conjunction with 33241 or 33262, 33263, 33264)

(For removal of electrode[s] by tranvenous extraction in conjunction with pulse generator removal or replacement, use 33244 in conjunction with 33241 or 33262, 33263, 33264)

(For repair of implantable defibrillator pulse generator and/or leads, see 33218, 33220)

(For removal of subcutaneous electrode in conjunction with implantable defibrillator pulse generator removal or replacement, use 33272 in conjunction with 33241 or 33262)

33243 Removal of single or dual chamber implantable defibrillator electrode(s); by thoracotomy

33244 by transvenous extraction

33249 Insertion or replacement of permanent implantable defibrillator system, with transvenous lead(s), single or dual chamber

(Do not report 33249 in conjunction with 33216, 33217)

(For removal and replacement of an implantable defibrillator pulse generator and transvenous electrode[s], use 33241 in conjunction with either 33243 or 33244 and 33249)

(For insertion of transvenous implantable defibrillator lead[s], without thoracotomy, use 33216 or 33217)

33270 Insertion or replacement of permanent subcutaneous implantable defibrillator system, with subcutaneous electrode, including defibrillation threshold evaluation, induction of arrhythmia, evaluation of sensing for arrhythmia termination, and programming or reprogramming of sensing or therapeutic parameters, when performed

(Do not report 33270 in conjunction with 33271, 93260, 93261, 93644)

(For removal and replacement of an implantable defibrillator pulse generator and subcutaneous electrode, use 33241 in conjunction with 33270 and 33272)

(For insertion of subcutaneous implantable defibrillator lead[s], use 33271)

(For insertion or replacement of permanent implantable defibrillator system with substernal electrode, use 0571T)

33271 Insertion of subcutaneous implantable defibrillator electrode

(Do not report 33271 in conjunction with 33240, 33262, 33270, 93260, 93261)

---

376 ● New Code ▲ Revised Code + Add-On Code ⊘ Modifier -51 Exempt ★ Telemedicine

(For insertion or replacement of a cardiac venous system lead, see 33224, 33225)

(For insertion of substernal defibrillator electrode, use 0572T)

33272 Removal of subcutaneous implantable defibrillator electrode

(For removal of substernal defibrillator electrode, use 0573T)

33273 Repositioning of previously implanted subcutaneous implantable defibrillator electrode

(Do not report 33272, 33273 in conjunction with 93260, 93261)

(For repositioning of substernal defibrillator electrode, use 0574T)

33274 Transcatheter insertion or replacement of permanent leadless pacemaker, right ventricular, including imaging guidance (eg, fluoroscopy, venous ultrasound, ventriculography, femoral venography) and device evaluation (eg, interrogation or programming), when performed

33275 Transcatheter removal of permanent leadless pacemaker, right ventricular, including imaging guidance (eg, fluoroscopy, venous ultrasound, ventriculography, femoral venography), when performed

(Do not report 33275 in conjunction with 33274)

(Do not report 33274, 33275 in conjunction with femoral venography [75820], fluoroscopy [76000, 77002], ultrasound guidance for vascular access [76937], right ventriculography [93566])

(Do not report 33274, 33275 in conjunction with 93451, 93453, 93456, 93457, 93460, 93461, 93530, 93531, 93532, 93533, unless complete right heart catheterization is performed for indications distinct from the leadless pacemaker procedure)

(For subsequent leadless pacemaker device evaluation, see 93279, 93286, 93288, 93294, 93296)

(For insertion, replacement, repositioning, and removal of pacemaker systems with leads, see 33202, 33203, 33206, 33207, 33208, 33212, 33213, 33214, 33215, 33216, 33217, 33218, 33220, 33221, 33227, 33228, 33229, 33233, 33234, 33235, 33236, 33237)

ELECTROPHYSIOLOGIC OPERATIVE PROCEDURES

If excision or isolation of the left atrial appendage by any method, including stapling, oversewing, ligation, or plication, is performed in conjunction with any of the atrial tissue ablation and reconstruction (maze) procedures (33254-33259, 33265-33266), it is considered part of the procedure. Codes 33254-33256 are only to be reported when there is no concurrently performed procedure that requires median sternotomy or cardiopulmonary bypass. The appropriate atrial tissue ablation add-on code, 33257, 33258, 33259 should be reported in addition to an open cardiac procedure requiring sternotomy or cardiopulmonary bypass if performed concurrently.

Incision

33250 Operative ablation of supraventricular arrhythmogenic focus or pathway (eg, Wolff-Parkinson-White, atrioventricular node re-entry), tract(s) and/or focus (foci); without cardiopulmonary bypass

(For intraoperative pacing and mapping by a separate provider, use 93631)

33251 with cardiopulmonary bypass

33254 Operative tissue ablation and reconstruction of atria, limited (eg, modified maze procedure)

33255 Operative tissue ablation and reconstruction of atria, extensive (eg, maze procedure); without cardiopulmonary bypass

33256 with cardiopulmonary bypass

(Do not report 33254-33256 in conjunction with 32100, 32551, 33120, 33130, 33210, 33211, 33390, 33391, 33404-33507, 33510-33523, 33533-33548, 33600-33853, 33858, 33859, 33863, 33864, 33910-33920)

+ 33257 Operative tissue ablation and reconstruction of atria, performed at the time of other cardiac procedure(s), limited (eg, modified maze procedure) (List separately in addition ot code for primary procedure)

(Use 33257 in conjunction with 33120-33130, 33250, 33251, 33261, 33300-33335, 33365, 33390, 33391, 33404-33417, 33420-33476, 33478, 33496, 33500-33507, 33510-33516, 33533-33548, 33600-33619, 33641-33697, 33702-33732, 33735-33767, 33770, 33877, 33910-33922, 33925, 33926, 33975, 33976, 33977, 33978, 33979, 33980, 33981, 33982, 33983)

+ 33258 Operative tissue ablation and reconstruction of atria, performed at the time of other cardiac procedure(s), extensive (eg, maze procedure), without cardiopulmonary bypass (List separately in addition to code for primary procedure)

(Use 33258 in conjunction with 33130, 33250, 33300, 33310, 33320, 33321, 33330, 33365, 33420, 33470, 33471, 33501-33503, 33510-33516, 33533-33536, 33690, 33735, 33737, 33750, 33755, 33762, 33764, 33766, 33800-33813, 33820, 33822, 33824, 33840, 33845, 33851, 33852, 33875, 33877, 33915, 33925, 33981, 33982, when the procedure is performed without cardiopulmonary bypass)

+ 33259 Operative tissue ablation and reconstruction of atria, performed at the time of other cardiac procedure(s), extensive (eg, maze procedure), with cardiopulmonary bypass (List separately in addition to code for primary procedure)

(Use 33259 in conjunction with 33120, 33251, 33261, 33305, 33315, 33322, 33335, 33390, 33391, 33404, 33405, 33406, 33410, 33411, 33412, 33413, 33414, 33415, 33416, 33417, 33422-33468, 33474, 33475, 33476, 33478, 33496, 33500, 33504-33507, 33510-33516, 33533-33548, 33600-33688, 33692-33726, 33730, 33732, 33736, 33767, 33770, 33783, 33786-33788, 33814, 33853, 33858-33877, 33910, 33916-33922, 33926, 33975-33980, 33983, when the procedure is performed with cardiopulmonary bypass)

(Do not report 33257, 33258 and 33259 inconjunction with 32551, 33210, 33211, 33254-33256, 33265, 33266)

33261 Operative ablation of ventricular arrhythmogenic focus with cardiopulmonary bypass

33262 Code out of order. See page 376

33263 Code out of order. See page 376

33264 Code out of order. See page 376

Endoscopy

33265 Endoscopy, surgical; operative tissue ablation and reconstruction of atria, limited (eg, modified maze procedure), without cardiopulmonary bypass

33266 operative tissue ablation and reconstruction of atria, extensive (eg, maze procedure), without cardiopulmonary bypass

(Do not report 33265-33266 in conjunction with 32551, 33210, 33211)

33270 This code is out of order. See page 376

33271 This code is out of order. See page 376

33272 This code is out of order. See page 377

33273 This code is out of order. See page 377

33274 This code is out of order. See page 377

33275 This code is out of order. See page 377

SUBCUTANEOUS CARDIAC RHYTHM MONITOR

A subcutaneous cardiac rhythm monitor, also known as a cardiac event recorder or implantable/insertable loop recorder (ILR), is a subcutaneously placed device that continuously records the electrocardiographic rhythm, triggered automatically by rapid, irregular and/or slow heart rates or by the patient during a symptomatic episode. A subcutaneous cardiac rhythm monitor is placed using a small parasternal incision followed by insertion of the monitor into a small subcutaneous prepectoralpocket, followed by closure of the incision.

(33282   deleted 2018 [2019 Edition]. To report, see 33285, 33286)

(33284   deleted 2018 [2019 Edition]. To report, see 33285, 33286)

33285   Insertion, subcutaneous cardiac rhythm monitor, including programming

33286   Removal, subcutaneous cardiac rhythm monitor

(Initial insertion includes programming. For subsequent electronic analysis and/or reprogramming, see 93285, 93291, 93298)

IMPLANTABLE HEMODYNAMIC MONITORS

Transcatheter implantation of a wireless pulmonary artery pressure sensor (33289) establishes an intravascular device used for long-term remote monitoring of pulmonary artery pressures (93264). The hemodynamic data derived from this device is used to guide management of patients with heart failure. Code 33289 includes deployment and calibration of the sensor, right heart catheterization, selective pulmonary artery catheterization, radiological supervision and interpretation, and pulmonary artery angiography, when performed.

33289   Transcatheter implantation of wireless pulmonary artery pressure sensor for long-term hemodynamic monitoring, including deployment and calibration of the sensor, right heart catheterization, selective pulmonary catheterization, radiological supervision and interpretation, and pulmonary artery angiography, when performed

(For remote monitoring of an implantable wireless pulmonary artery pressure sensor, use 93264)

(Do not report 33289 in conjunction with 36013, 36014, 36015, 75741, 75743, 75746, 76000, 93451, 93453, 93456, 93457, 93460, 93461, 93530, 93531, 93532, 93533, 93568)

HEART (INCLUDING VALVES) AND GREAT VESSELS

Patients receiving major cardiac procedures may require simultaneous cardiopulmonary bypass insertion of cannulae into the venous and arterial vasculatures with support of circulation and oxygenation by a heart-lung machine. Most services are described by codes in dyad arrangements to allow distinct reporting of procedures with or without cardiopulmonary bypass. Cardiopulmonary bypass is distinct from support of cardiac output using devices (eg, ventricular assist or intra-aortic balloon). For cardiac assist services, see 33946, 33947, 33948, 33949, 33967-33983, 33990, 33991, 33992, 33993, 33995, 33997.

33300   Repair of cardiac wound; without bypass

33305   with cardiopulmonary bypass

33310   Cardiotomy, exploratory (includes removal of foreign body, atrial or ventricular thrombus); without bypass

33315   with cardiopulmonary bypass

(Do not report removal of thrombus (33310-33315) in conjunction with other cardiac procedures unless a separate incision in the heart is required to remove the atrial or ventricular thrombus)

(If removal of thrombus with coronary bypass (33315) is reported in conjunction with 33120, 33130, 33420-33430, 33460-33468, 33496, 33542, 33545, 33641-33647, 33670, 33681, 33975-33980 which requires a separate heart incision, report 33315 with modifier '-59')

33320   Suture repair of aorta or great vessels; without shunt or cardiopulmonary bypass

33321   with shunt bypass

Separate Procedure   Unlisted Procedure   CCI Comp. Code   Non-specific Procedure   **379**

33322 with cardiopulmonary bypass

33330 Insertion of graft, aorta or great vessels; without shunt, or cardiopulmonary bypass

33335 with cardiopulmonary bypass

33340 Percutaneous transcatheter closure of the left atrial appendage with endocardial implant, including fluoroscopy, transseptal puncture, catheter placement(s), left atrial angiography, left atrial appendage angiography, when performed, and radiological supervision and interpretation

  (Do not report 33340 in conjunction with 93462)

  (Do not report 33340 in conjunction with 93452, 93453, 93458, 93459, 93460, 93461, 93531, 93532, 93533, unless catheterization of the left ventricle is performed by a non-transseptal approach for indications distinct from the left atrial appendage closure procedure)

  (Do not report 33340 in conjunction with 93451, 93453, 93456, 93460, 93461, 93530, 93531, 93532, 93533, unless complete right heart catheterization is performed for indications distinct from the left atrial appendage closure procedure)

CARDIAC VALVES

  (For multiple valve procedures, see 33390, 33391, 33404-33478 and add modifier 51 to the secondary valve procedure code)

Aortic Valve

Codes 33361, 33362, 33363, 33364, 33365, 33366 are used to report transcatheter aortic valve replacement (TAVR)/transcatheter aortic valve implantation (TAVI). TAVR/TAVI requires two physician operators and all components of the procedure are reported using modifier 62.

Codes 33361, 33362, 33363, 33364, 33365, 33366 include the work, when performed, of percutaneous access, placing the access sheath, balloon aortic valvuloplasty, advancing the valve delivery system into position, repositioning the valve as needed, deploying the valve, temporary pacemaker insertion for rapid pacing (33210), and closure of the arteriotomy when performed. Codes 33361, 33362, 33363, 33364, 33365, 33366 include open arterial or cardiac approach.

Angiography, radiological supervision, and interpretation performed to guide TAVR/TAVI (eg, guiding valve placement, documenting completion of the intervention, assessing the vascular access site for closure) are included in these codes.

Diagnostic left heart catheterization codes (93452, 93453, 93458-93461) and the supravalvular aortography code (93567) should **not** be used with TAVR/TAVI services (33361, 33362, 33363, 33364, 33365, 33366) to report:

1. Contrast injections, angiography, roadmapping, and/or fluoroscopic guidance for the TAVR/TAVI,

2. Aorta/left ventricular outflow tract measurement for the TAVR/TAVI, or

3. Post-TAVR/TAVI aortic or left ventricular angiography, as this work is captured in the TAVR/TAVI services codes (33361, 33362, 33363, 33364, 33365, 33366).

Diagnostic coronary angiography performed at the time of TAVR/TAVI may be separately reportable if:

1. No prior catheter-based coronary angiography study is available and a full diagnostic study is performed, or

2. A prior study is available, but as documented in the medical record:

 a. The patient's condition with respect to the clinical indication has changed since the prior study, or

 b. There is inadequate visualization of the anatomy and/or pathology, or

 c There is a clinical change during the procedure that requires new evaluation.

 ● New Code ▲ Revised Code ✛ Add-On Code ⊘ Modifier -51 Exempt ★ Telemedicine

d. For same session/same day diagnostic coronary angiography services,
report the appropriate diagnostic cardac catheterization code(s)
appended with modifier 59 indicating separate and distance
procedural service from TAVR/TAVI.

Diagnostic coronary angiography performed at a separate session from an interventional procedure may be separately reportable.

Other cardiac catheterization services may be reported separately when performed for diagnostic purposes not intrinsic to TAVR/TAVI.

Percutaneous coronary interventional procedures are reported separately, when performed.

When transcatheter ventricular support is required in conjunction with TAVR/TAVI, the appropriate code may be reported with the appropriate ventricular assist device (VAD) procedure code (33975, 33976, 33990, 33991, 33992, 33993, 33995, 33997) or balloon pump insertion code (33967, 33970, 33973).

The TAVR/TAVI cardiovascular access and delivery procedures are reported with 33361, 33362, 33363, 33364, 33365, 33366. When cardiopulmonary bypass is performed in conjunction with TAVR/TAVI, codes 33361, 33362, 33363, 33364, 33365, 33366 should be reported with the appropriate add-on code for percutaneous peripheral bypass (33367), open peripheral bypass (33368), or central bypass (33369)

33361 Transcatheter aortic valve replacement (TAVR/TAVI) with prosthetic valve; percutaneous femoral artery approach

33362 open femoral artery approach

33363 open axillary artery approach

33364 open iliac artery approach

33365 transaortic approach (eg, median sternotomy, mediastinotomy)

  (Use 0318T for transapical approach [eg, left thoracotomy])

33366 transapical exposure (eg, thoracotomy)

+ **33367** cardiopulmonary bypass support with percutaneous peripheral arterial and venous cannulation (eg, femoral vessels) (List separately in addition to code for primary procedure)

  (Use 33367 in conjunction with 33361, 33362, 33363, 33364, 33365, 33366, 33418, 33477, 0483T, 0484T, 0544T, 0545T, 0569T, 0570T)

  (Do not report 33367 in conjunction with 33368, 33369)

+ **33368** cardiopulmonary bypass support with open peripheral arterial and venous cannulation (eg, femoral, iliac, axillary vessels) (List separately in addition to code for primary procedure)

  (Use 33368 in conjunction with 33361, 33362, 33363, 33364, 33365, 33366, 33418, 33477, 0483T, 0484T, 0544T, 0545T, 0569T, 0570T)

  (Do not report 33368 in conjunction with 33367, 33369)

+ **33369** cardiopulmonary bypass support with central arterial and venous cannulation (eg, aorta, right atrium, pulmonary artery) (List separately in addition to code for primary procedure)

  (Use 33369 in conjunction with 33361, 33362, 33363, 33364, 33365, 33366, 33418, 33477, 0483T, 0484T, 0544T, 0545T, 0569T, 0570T)

  (Do not report 33369 in conjunction with 33367, 33368)

33390 Valvuloplasty, aortic valve, open, with cardiopulmonary bypass; simple (ie, valvotomy, debridement, debulking, and/or simple commissural resuspension)

33391 complex (eg, leaflet extension, leaflet resection, leaflet reconstruction, or annuloplasty)

Separate Procedure Unlisted Procedure CCI Comp. Code Non-specific Procedure **381**

(Do not report 33391 in conjunction with 33390)

33404 Construction of apical-aortic conduit

33405 Replacement, aortic valve, open, with cardiopulmonary bypass; with prosthetic valve other than homograft or stentless valve

33406   with allograft valve (freehand)

33410   with stentless tissue valve

33440 Replacement, aortic valve; by translocation of autologous pulmonary valve and transventricular aortic annulus enlargement of the left ventricular outflow tract with valved conduit replacement of pulmonary valve (Ross-Konno procedure)

(Do not report 33440 in conjunction with 33405, 33406, 33410, 33411, 33412, 33413, 33414, 33416, 33417, 33475, 33608, 33920)

33411   with aortic annulus enlargement, noncoronary sinus

33412   with transventricular aortic annulus enlargement (Konno procedure)

(Do not report 33412 in conjunction with 33413, 33440)

(For replacement of aortic valve with transventricular aortic annulus enlargement [Konno procedure] in conjunction with translocation of autologous pulmonary valve with allograft replacement of pulmonary valve [Ross procedure], use 33440)

33413   by translocation of autologous pulmonary valve with allograft replacement of pulmonary valve (Ross procedure)

(Do not report 33413 in conjunction with 33412, 33440)

(For replacement of aortic valve with transventricular aortic annulus enlargement [Konno procedure] in conjunction with translocation of autologous pulmonary valve with allograft replacement of pulmonary valve [Ross procedure], use 33440)

33414 Repair of left ventricular outflow tract obstruction by patch enlargement of the outflow tract

33415 Resection or incision of subvalvular tissue for discrete subvalvular aortic stenosis

33416 Ventriculomyotomy (-myectomy) for idiopathic hypertrophic subaortic stenosis (eg, asymmetric septal hypertrophy)

(For percutaneous transcatheter septal reduction therapy, use 93583)

33417 Aortoplasty (gusset) for supravalvular stenosis

Mitral Valve

Codes 33418 and 33419 are used to report transcatheter mitral valve repair TMVR. Code 33419 should only be reported once per session.

Codes 33418 and 33419 include the work, when performed, of percutaneous access, placing the access sheath, transseptal puncture, advancing the repair device delivery system into position, repositioning the device as needed, and deploying the devices.

Angiography, radiological supervision, and interpretation performed to guide TMVR (E.g., guiding device placement and documenting completion of the intervention) are included in these codes.

Diagnostic right and left heart catheterization codes (93451, 93452, 93453, 93456, 93457, 93458, 93459, 93460, 93461, 93530, 93531, 93532, 93533) should not be used with 33418, 33419 to report:

● New Code ▲ Revised Code + Add-On Code ⊘ Modifier -51 Exempt ★ Telemedicine

1. Contrast injections, angiography, road-mapping, and/or fluoroscopic guidance for the transcatheter mitral valve repair (TMVR),

2. Left ventricular angiography to assess mitral regurgitation for guidance of TMVR, or

3. Right and left heart catheterization for hemodynamic measurements before, during, and after TMVR for guidance of TMVR.

Diagnostic right and left heart catheterization codes (93451, 93452, 93453, 93456, 93457, 93458, 93459, 93460, 93461, 93530, 93531, 93532, 93533) and diagnostic coronary angiography codes (93454, 93455, 93456, 93457, 93458, 93459, 93460, 93461, 93563, 93564) May be reported with 33418, 33419, representing separate and distinct services from TMVR, if:

1. No prior study is available and a full diagnostic study is performed, or

2. A prior study is available, but as documented in the medical record:

   a. There is inadequate visualization of the anatomy and/or pathology, or

   b. The patient's condition with respect to the clinical indication has changed since the prior study, or

   c. There is a clinical change during the procedure that requires new evaluation.

Other cardiac catheterization services may be reported separately when performed for diagnostic purposes not intrinsic to TMVR.

For same session/same day diagnostic cardiac catheterization services, report the appropriate diagnostic cardiac catheterization codes appended with modifier 59 indicating separate and distinct procedural service from TMVR.

Diagnostic coronary angiography performed at a separate session from an interventional procedure may be separately reportable.

Percutaneous coronary interventional procedures may be reported separately, when performed.

When transcatheter ventricular support is required in conjunction with TMVR, the appropriate code may be reported with the appropriate ventricular assist device (VAD) procedure code (33990, 33991, 33992, 33993, 33995, 33997) or balloon pump insertion code (33967, 33970, 33973).

When a cardiopulmonary bypass is performed in conjunction with TMVR, 33418, 33419 may be reported with the appropriate add-on code for percutaneous peripheral bypass (33367), open peripheral bypass (33368), or central bypass (33369).

33418   Transcatheter mitral valve repair, percutaneous approach, including transseptal puncture when performed; initial prosthesis

   (Do not report 33418 in conjunction with 93462 unless transapical puncture is performed)

+ 33419   additional prosthesis(es) during same session (list separately in addition to code for primary procedure)

   (Use 33419 in conjunction with 33418)

   (For transcatheter mitral valve repair, percutaneous approach via the coronary sinus, use 0345T)

   (For transcatheter mitral valve implantation/ replacement [TMVI], see 0483T, 0484T)

   (For transcatheter mitral valve annulus reconstruction, use 0544T)

33420   Valvotomy, mitral valve; closed heart

33422   open heart, with cardiopulmonary bypass

33425   Valvuloplasty, mitral valve, with cardiopulmonary bypass;

33426   with prosthetic ring

33427   radical reconstruction, with or without ring

33430   Replacement, mitral valve, with cardiopulmonary bypass

---

33440   This code is out of order. See page 382

Tricuspid Valve

(For transcatheter tricuspid valve repair [TTVr], see 0569T, 0570T)

33460   Valvectomy, tricuspid valve, with cardiopulmonary bypass

33463   Valvuloplasty, tricuspid valve; without ring insertion

33464   with ring insertion

33465   Replacement, tricuspid valve, with cardiopulmonary bypass

33468   Tricuspid valve repositioning and plication for Ebstein anomaly

(For transcatheter tricuspid valve annulus reconstruction, use 0545T)

Pulmonary Valve

Code 33477 is used to report transcatheter pulmonary valve implantation (TPVI). code 33477 should only be reported once per session.

Code 33477 includes the work, when performed, of percutaneous access, placing the access sheath, advancing the repair device delivery system into position, repositioning the device as needed, and deploying the device(s). Angiography, radiological supervision, and interpretation performed to guide TPVI (eg, guiding device placement and documenting completion of the intervention) are included in the code.

Code 33477 includes all cardiac catheterization(s), intraprocedural contrast injection(s), fluoroscopic radiological supervision and interpretation, and imaging guidance performed to complete the pulmonary valve procedure. Do not report 33477 in conjunction with 76000, 93451, 93453, 93454, 93455, 93456, 93457, 93458, 93459, 93460, 93461, 93530, 93531, 93532, 93533, 93563, 93566, 93567, 93568 for angiography intrinsic to the procedure.

Code 33477 includes percutaneous balloon angioplasty of the conduit/treatment zone, valvuloplasty of the pulmonaryt valve conduit, and stent deployment within the pulmonary conduit or an existing bioprosthetic pulmonary vavle, when performed. Do not report 33477 in conjunction with 37236, 37237, 92997, 92998 for pulmonary artery angioplasty/valvuloplasty or stenting within the prosthetic valve delivery site.

Codes 92997, 92998 may be reported separately when pulmonary artery angioplasty is performed at a site separate from the prosthetic valve delivery site. Codes 37236, 37237 may be reported separatey when pulmonary artery stenting is performed at a site separate from the prosthetic valve delivery site.

Diagnostic right heart catheterization and diagnostic coronary angiography codes (93451, 93453, 93454, 93455, 93456, 93457, 93458, 93459, 93460, 93461, 93530, 93531, 93532, 93533, 93563, 93566, 93567, 93568) should NOT be used with 33477 to report:

1. Contrast injections, angiography, roadmapping, and/or fluoroscopic guidance for the TPVI;

2. Pulmonary conduit angiography for guidance of TPVI; OR

3. Right heart catheterization for hemodynamic measurements before, during, and after TPVI for guidance of TPVI.

Diagnostic right and left heart catheterization codes (93451, 93452, 93453, 93456, 93457, 93458, 93459, 93460, 93461, 93530, 93531, 93532, 93533), diagnostic coronary angiography codes (93454, 93455, 93456, 93457, 93458, 93459, 93460, 93461, 93563, 93564), and diagnostic pulmonary angiography code (93568) may be reported with 33477, representing separate and distinct services from TPVI, if:

1. No prior study is available and a full diagnostic study is performed; OR

2. A prior study is available, but as documented in the medical record:

a. There is inadequate visualization of the anatomy and or pathology; or

b. The patient's condition with respect to the clinical indication has changed since the prior study; or

---

● New Code   ▲ Revised Code   ✛ Add-On Code   ⊘ Modifier -51 Exempt   ★ Telemedicine

c. There is a clinical change during the procedure that requires new evaluation.

Other cardiac catheterization services may be reported separately when performed for diagnostic purposes not intrinsic to TPVI.

For same session/same day diagnostic cardiac catheterization services, report the appropriate diagnostic cardiac catheterization code(s) appended with modifier 59 to indicate separate and distinct procedural services from TPVI.

Diagnostic coronary angiography peformed at a separate session from an interventional procedure may be separately reportable, when performed.

Percutaneous coronary interventional procedures may be reported separately, when performed.

Percutaneous pulmonary artery branch interventions may be reported separately, when performed.

When transcatheter ventricular support is required in conjunction with TPVI, the appropriate code may be reported with the appropriate percutaneous ventricular assist device (VAD) procedure codes (33990, 33991, 33992, 33993, 33995, 33997), extracorporeal membrane oxygenation (ECMO) or extracorporeal life support services (ECLS) procedure codes (33946-33989), or balloon pump insertion codes (33967, 33970, 33973)

When cardiopulmonary bypass is performed in conjunction with TPVI, code 33477 may be reported with the appropriate add-on code for percutaneous peripheral bypass (33367), open peripheral bypass (33368), or central bypass (33369).

33470 Valvotomy, pulmonary valve, closed heart; transventricular

(Do not report modifier '-63' in conjunction with 33470)

33471 via pulmonary artery

(To report percutaneous valvuloplasty of pulmonary valve, use 92990)

33474 with cardiopulmonary bypass

33475 Replacement, pulmonary valve

33476 Right ventricular resection for infundibular stenosis, with or without commissurotomy

33477 Transcatheter pulmonary valve implantation, percutaneous approach, including pre-stenting of the valve delivery site, when performed.

33478 Outflow tract augmentation (gusset), with or without commissurotomy or infundibular resection

(Use 33478 in conjunction with 33768 when a cavopulmonary anastomosis to a second superior vena cava is performed)

OTHER VALVULAR PROCEDURES

33496 Repair of non-structural prosthetic valve dysfunction with cardiopulmonary bypass (separate procedure)

(For reoperation, use 33530 in addition to 33496)

CORONARY ARTERY ANOMALIES

Basic procedures include endarterectomy or angioplasty.

33500 Repair of coronary arteriovenous or arteriocardiac chamber fistula; with cardiopulmonary bypass

33501 without cardiopulmonary bypass

33502 Repair of anomalous coronary artery from pulmonary artery origin; by ligation

33503 by graft, without cardiopulmonary bypass

(Do not report modifier '-63' in conjunction with 33502, 33503)

33504　　　by graft, with cardiopulmonary bypass

33505　　　with construction of intrapulmonary artery tunnel (Takeuchi procedure)

33506　　　by translocation from pulmonary artery to aorta

　　　　　(Do not report modifier '-63' in conjunction with 33505, 33506)

33507　　Repair of anomalous (eg, intramural) aortic origin of coronary artery by unroofing or translocation

ENDOSCOPY

Surgical vascular endoscopy always includes diagnostic endoscopy

+ 33508　　Endoscopy, surgical, including video-assisted harvest of vein(s) for coronary artery bypass procedure (List separately in addition to code for primary procedure)

　　　　　(Use 33508 in conjunction with code 33510-33523)

　　　　　(For open harvest of upper extremity vein procedure, use 35500)

VENOUS GRAFTING ONLY FOR CORONARY ARTERY BYPASS

The following codes are used to report coronary artery bypass procedures using venous grafts only. These codes should NOT be used to report the performance of coronary artery bypass procedures using arterial grafts and venous grafts during the same procedure. See 33517-33523 and 33533-33536 for reporting combined arterial-venous grafts.

Procurement of the saphenous vein graft is included in the description of the work for 33510-33516 and should not be reported as a separate service or co-surgery. To report harvesting of an upper extremity vein, use 35500 in addition to the bypass procedure. To report harvesting of a femoropopliteal vein segment, report 35572 in addition to the bypass procedure. When surgical assistant performs graft procurement, add modifier 80 to 33510- 33516. For percutaneous ventricular assist device insertion, removal, repositioning, see 33990, 33991, 33992, 33993, 33995, 33997.

33510　　Coronary artery bypass, vein only; single coronary venous graft

33511　　　2 coronary venous grafts

33512　　　3 coronary venous grafts

33513　　　4 coronary venous grafts

33514　　　5 coronary venous grafts

33516　　　6 or more coronary venous grafts

COMBINED ARTERIAL-VENOUS GRAFTING FOR CORONARY BYPASS

The following codes are used to report coronary artery bypass procedures using venous grafts and arterial grafts during the same procedure. These codes may NOT be reported alone.

To report combined arterial-venous grafts it is necessary to report two codes: 1) the appropriate combined arterial venous graft code (33517-33523); and 2) the appropriate arterial graft code (33533-33536).

Procurement of the saphenous vein graft is included in the description of the work for 33517-33523 and should not be reported as a separate service or co-surgery. Procurement of the artery for grafting is included in the description of the work for 33533-33536 and should not be reported as a separate service or co-surgery, except when an upper extremity artery (eg, radial artery) is procured. To report harvesting of an upper extremity artery, use 35600 in addition to the bypass procedure. To report harvesting of an upper extremity vein, use 35500 in addition to the bypass procedure. To report harvesting of a femoropopliteal vein segment, report 35572 in addition to the bypass procedure. When surgical assistant performs arterial and/or venous graft procurement, add modifier 80 to 33517-33523, 33533-33536, as appropriate. For percutaneous ventricular assist device insertion, removal, repositioning, see 33990, 33991, 33992, 33993, 33995, 33997.

　　● New Code　　　▲ Revised Code　　　+ Add-On Code　　　⊘ Modifier -51 Exempt　　　★ Telemedicine

+ **33517**   Coronary artery bypass, using venous graft(s) and arterial graft(s); single vein graft (List separately in addition to code for primary procedure)

    (Use 33517 in conjunction with 33533-33536)

+ **33518**   2 venous grafts (List separately in addition to code for primary procedure)

    (Use 33518 in conjunction with 33533-33536)

+ **33519**   3 venous grafts (List separately in addition to code for primary procedure)

    (Use 33519 in conjunction with 33533-33536)

+ **33521**   4 venous grafts (List separately in addition to code for primary procedure)

    (Use 33521 in conjunction with 33533-33536)

+ **33522**   5 venous grafts (List separately in addition to code for primary procedure)

    (Use 33522 in conjunction with 33533-33536)

+ **33523**   6 or more venous grafts (List separately in addition to code for primary procedure)

    (Use 33523 in conjunction with 33533-33536)

+ **33530**   Reoperation, coronary artery bypass procedure or valve procedure, more than 1 month after original operation (List separately in addition to code for primary procedure)

    (Use 33530 in conjunction with 33390, 33391, 33404-33496; 33510-33536, 33863)

ARTERIAL GRAFTING FOR CORONARY ARTERY BYPASS

The following codes are used to report coronary artery bypass procedures using either arterial grafts only or a combination of arterial-venous grafts. The codes include the use of the internal mammary artery, gastroepiploic artery, epigastric artery, radial artery, and arterial conduits procured from other sites.

To report combined arterial-venous grafts it is necessary to report two codes: 1) the appropriate arterial graft code (33533-33536); and 2) the appropriate combined arterial-venous graft code (33517-33523).

Procurement of the artery for grafting is included in the description of the work for 33533-33536 and should not be reported as a separate service or co-surgery, except when an upper extremity artery (eg, radial artery) is procured. To report harvesting of an upper extremity artery, use 35600 in addition to the bypass procedure. To report harvesting of an upper extremity vein, use 35500 in addition to the bypass procedure. To report harvesting of a femoropopliteal vein segment, report 35572 in addition to the bypass procedure. When surgical assistant performs arterial and/or venous graft procurement, add modifier 80 to 33517-33523, 33533-33536, as appropriate. For percutaneous ventricular assist device insertion, removal, repositioning, see 33990, 33991, 33992, 33993, 33995, 33997.

33533   Coronary artery bypass, using arterial graft(s); single arterial graft

33534   2 coronary arterial grafts

33535   3 coronary arterial grafts

33536   4 or more coronary arterial grafts

33542   Myocardial resection (eg, ventricular aneurysmectomy)

33545   Repair of postinfarction ventricular septal defect, with or without myocardial resection

33548   Surgical ventricular restoration procedure, includes prosthetic patch, when performed (eg, ventricular remodeling, SVR, SAVER, DOR procedures)

    (Do not report 33548 in conjunction with 32551, 33210, 33211, 33310, 33315)

(For Batista procedure or pachopexy, use 33999)

CORONARY ENDARTERECTOMY

+ 33572 Coronary endarterectomy, open, any method, of left anterior descending, circumflex, or right coronary artery performed in conjunction with coronary artery bypass graft procedure, each vessel (List separately in addition to primary procedure)

(Use 33572 in conjunction with 33510-33516, 33533-33536)

SINGLE VENTRICLE AND OTHER COMPLEX CARDIAC ANOMALIES

33600 Closure of atrioventricular valve (mitral or tricuspid) by suture or patch

33602 Closure of semilunar valve (aortic or pulmonary) by suture or patch

33606 Anastomosis of pulmonary artery to aorta (Damus-Kaye-Stansel procedure)

33608 Repair of complex cardiac anomaly other than pulmonary atresia with ventricular septal defect by construction or replacement of conduit from right or left ventricle to pulmonary artery

(For repair of pulmonary artery arborization anomalies by unifocalization, see 33925-33926)

33610 Repair of complex cardiac anomalies (eg, single ventricle with subaortic obstruction) by surgical enlargement of ventricular septal defect

(Do not report modifier '-63' in conjunction with 33610)

33611 Repair of double outlet right ventricle with intraventricular tunnel repair;

(Do not report modifier '-63' in conjunction with 33611)

33612 with repair of right ventricular outflow tract obstruction

33615 Repair of complex cardiac anomalies (eg, tricuspid atresia) by closure of atrial septal defect and anastomosis of atria or vena cava to pulmonary artery (simple Fontan procedure)

33617 Repair of complex cardiac anomalies (eg, single ventricle) by modified Fontan procedure

(Use 33617 in conjunction with 33768 when a cavopulmonary anastomosis to a second superior vena cava is performed)

33619 Repair of single ventricle with aortic outflow obstruction and aortic arch hypoplasia (hypoplastic left heart syndrome) (eg, Norwood procedure)

(Do not report modifier '-63' in conjunction with 33619)

33620 Application of right and left pulmonary artery bands (eg, hybrid approach stage 1)

(For banding of the main pulmonary artery related to septal defect, use 33690)

33621 Transthoracic insertion of catheter for stent placement with catheter removal and closure (eg, hybrid approach stage 1)

(For placement of stent, use 37236)

(Report both 33620, 33621 if performed in same session)

33622 Reconstruction of complex cardiac anomaly (eg, single ventricle or hypoplastic left heart) with palliation of single ventricle with aortic outflow obstruction and aortic arch hypoplasia, creation of cavopulmonary anastomosis, and removal of right and left pulmonary bands (eg, hybrid approach stage 2, Norwood, bidirectional Glenn, pulmonary artery debanding)

(Do not report 33622 in conjunction with 33619, 33767, 33822, 33840, 33845, 33851, 33853, 33917)

● New Code   ▲ Revised Code   **+** Add-On Code   ⊘ Modifier -51 Exempt   ★ Telemedicine

(For bilateral, bidirectional Glenn procedure, use 33622 in conjunction with 33768)

SEPTAL DEFECT

33641 Repair atrial septal defect, secundum, with cardiopulmonary bypass, with or without patch

33645 Direct or patch closure, sinus venosus, with or without anomalous pulmonary venous drainage

(Do not report 33645 in conjunction with 33724, 33726)

33647 Repair of atrial septal defect and ventricular septal defect, with direct or patch closure

(Do not report modifier -63 in conjunction with 33647)

(For repair of tricuspid atresia (eg., Fontan, Gago procedures), use 33615)

33660 Repair of incomplete or partial atrioventricular canal (ostium primum atrial septal defect), with or without atrioventricular valve repair

33665 Repair of intermediate or transitional atrioventricular canal, with or without atrioventricular valve repair

33670 Repair of complete atrioventricular canal, with or without prosthetic valve

(Do not report modifier -63 in conjunction with 33670)

33675 Closure of multiple ventricular septal defects;

33676   with pulmonary valvotomy or infundibular resection (acyanotic)

33677   with removal of pulmonary artery band, with or without gusset

(Do not report 33675-33677 in conjunction with 32100, 32551, 32554, 32555, 33210, 33681, 33684, 33688)

(For percutaneous closure, use 93581)

33681 Closure of single ventricular septal defect, with or without patch;

33684   with pulmonary valvotomy or infundibular resection (acyanotic)

33688   with removal of pulmonary artery band, with or without gusset

(For pulmonary vein repair requiring creation of atrial septal defect, use 33724)

33690 Banding of pulmonary artery

(For right and left pulmonary artery banding in a single ventricle [eg, hybrid approach stage 1], use 33620)

(Do not report modifier 63 in conjunction with 33690)

33692 Complete repair tetralogy of Fallot without pulmonary atresia;

33694   with transannular patch

(Do not report modifier 63 in conjunction with 33694)

(For ligation and takedown of a systematic-to-pulmonary artery shunt, performed in conjunction with a congenital heart procedure, see 33924)

33697 Complete repair tetralogy of Fallot with pulmonary atresia including construction of conduit from right ventricle to pulmonary artery and closure of ventricular septal defect

---

(For ligation and takedown of a systemic-to-pulmonary artery shunt, performed in conjunction with a congenital heart procedure, see 33924)

SINUS OF VALSALVA

33702 Repair sinus of Valsalva fistula, with cardiopulmonary bypass;

33710   with repair of ventricular septal defect

33720 Repair sinus of Valsalva aneurysm, with cardiopulmonary bypass

33722 Closure of aortico-left ventricular tunnel

VENOUS ANOMALIES

33724 Repair of isolated partial anomalous pulmonary venous return (eg, Scimitar Syndrome)

(Do not report 33724 in conjunction with 32551, 33210, 33211)

33726 Repair of pulmonary venous stenosis

(Do not report 33726 in conjunction with 32551, 33210, 33211)

33730 Complete repair of anomalous venous return (supracardiac, intracardiac, or infracardiac types)

(Do not report modifier '-63' in conjunction with 33730)

(For partial anomalous pulmonary venous return, use 33724; for repair of pulmonary venous stenosis, use 33726)

33732 Repair of cor triatriatum or supravalvular mitral ring by resection of left atrial membrane

(Do not report modifier -63 in conjunction with 33732)

SHUNTING PROCEDURES

Codes 33741, 33745 are used to report creation of effective intracardiac blood flow in the setting of congenital heart defects. Code 33741 (transcatheter atrial septostomy) involves the percutaneous creation of improved atrial blood flow (eg, balloon/blade method), typically in infants =4 kg with congenital heart disease. Code 33745 is typically used for intracardiac shunt creation by stent placement to establish improved intracardiac blood flow (eg, atrial septum, Fontan fenestration, right ventricular outflow tract, Mustard/Senning/Warden baffles). Code 33746 is used to describe each additional intracardiac shunt creation by stent placement at a separate location during the same session as the primary intervention (33745).

Code 33741 includes percutaneous access, placing the access sheath(s), advancement of the transcatheter delivery system, and creation of effective intracardiac atrial blood flow. Codes 33741, 33745 include, when performed, ultrasound guidance for vascular access and fluoroscopic guidance for the intervention. Code 33745 additionally includes intracardiac stent placement, target zone angioplasty preceding or after stent implantation, and complete diagnostic right and left heart catheterization, when performed.

Diagnostic cardiac catheterization is not typically performed at the same session as transcatheter atrial septostomy (33741) and, when performed, may be separately reported. Diagnostic cardiac catheterization is typically performed at the same session with 33745 and the code descriptor includes this work, when performed.

Cardiovascular injection procedures for diagnostic angiography reported using 93563, 93565, 93566, 93567, 93568 are not typically performed at the same session as 33741. Although diagnostic angiography is typically performed during 33745, target vessels and chambers are highly variable and, when performed, for an evaluation separate and distinct from the shunt creation may be reported separately.

Codes 33745, 33746 are used to describe intracardiac stent placement. Multiple stents placed in a single location may only be reported with a single code. When additional, different intracardiac locations are treated in the same session, 33746 may be reported. Codes 33745, 33746 include any and all balloon angioplasty(ies) performed in the target lesion, including any pre-dilation (whether performed as a primary or secondary dilation), post-dilation following stent placement, or use of larger/smaller balloon to achieve therapeutic result. Angioplasty in a separate and distinct intracardiac lesion may be reported separately. Use 33746 in conjunction with 33745.

Diagnostic right and left heart catheterization codes (93451, 93452, 93453, 93456, 93458, 93460, 93530, 93531, 93532, 93533) should not be used in conjunction with 33741, 33745 to report:

1. Fluoroscopic guidance for the intervention, or

2. Limited hemodynamic and angiographic data used solely for purposes of accomplishing the intervention (eg, measurement of atrial pressures before and after septostomy, atrial injections to determine appropriate catheter position)

Diagnostic congenital right and left heart catheterization codes (93530, 93531, 93532, 93533) performed at the same session as 33741, may be separately reported, if:

1. No prior study is available, and a full diagnostic study is performed, or

2. A prior study is aviable, but as documented in the medical record:

a. There is inadequate visualization of the anatomy and/or pathology, or

b. The patient's condition with respect to the clinical indication has changed since the prior study, or

c. There is a clinical change during the procedure that requires a more thorough evaluation.

For same-session diagnostic congenital catheterization services, the appropriate diagnostic cardiac catheterization code(s) for congenital anomalies (93530, 93531, 93532, 93533) may be reported by appending modifier 59, indicating separate and distinct procedural service(s) from 33741. For same-session diagnostic cardiac angiography for an evaluation separate and distinct from the shunt creation, the appropriate contrast injection(s) performed (93563, 93565, 93566, 93567, 93568) may be reported by appending modifier 59, indicating separate and distinct procedural service(s) from 33741, 33745.

33735 Atrial septectomy or septostomy; closed heart (Blalock-Hanlon type operation)

33736 open heart with cardiopulmonary bypass

  (Do not report modifier '-63' in conjunction with 33735, 33736)

33737 open heart, with inflow occlusion

● **33741** Transcatheter atrial septostomy (TAS) for congenital cardiac anomalies to create effective atrial flow, including all imaging guidance by the proceduralist, when performed, any method (eg, Rashkind, Sang-Park, balloon, cutting balloon, blade)

  (Do not report modifier 63 in conjunction with 33741)

  (For transseptal puncture, use 93462)

● **33745** Transcatheter intracardiac shunt (TIS) creation by stent placement for congenital cardiac anomalies to establish effective intracardiac flow, including all imaging guidance by the proceduralist, when performed, left and right heart diagnostic cardiac catherization for congenital cardiac anomalies, and target zone angioplasty, when performed (eg, atrial septum, Fontan fenestration, right ventricular outflow tract, Mustard/Senning/Warden baffles); initial intracardiac shunt

●+**33746** each additional intracardiac shunt location (List separately in addition to code for primary procedure)

  (Use 33746 in conjunction with 33745)

  (Do not report 33745, 33746 in conjunction with 93530, 93531, 93532, 93533)

33750 Shunt; subclavian to pulmonary artery (Blalock-Taussig type operation)

33755 ascending aorta to pulmonary artery (Waterston type operation)

33762 descending aorta to pulmonary artery (Potts-Smith type operation)

  (Do not report modifier -63 in conjunction with 33750, 33755, 33762)

33764 central, with prosthetic graft

  Separate Procedure Unlisted Procedure CCI Comp. Code Non-specific Procedure **391**

33766   superior vena cava to pulmonary artery for flow to 1 lung (classical Glenn procedure)

33767   superior vena cava to pulmonary artery for flow to both lungs (bidirectional Glenn procedure)

+ **33768** Anastomosis, cavopulmonary, second superior vena cava (List separately in addition to primary procedure)

(Use 33768 in conjunction with 33478, 33617, 33622, 33767)

(Do not report 33768 in conjunction with 32551, 33210, 33211)

TRANSPOSITION OF THE GREAT VESSELS

33770 Repair of transposition of the great arteries with ventricular septal defect and subpulmonary stenosis; without surgical enlargement of ventricular septal defect

33771   with surgical enlargement of ventricular septal defect

33774 Repair of transposition of the great arteries, atrial baffle procedure (eg, Mustard or Senning type) with cardiopulmonary bypass;

33775   with removal of pulmonary band

33776   with closure of ventricular septal defect

33777   with repair of subpulmonic obstruction

33778 Repair of transposition of the great arteries, aortic pulmonary artery reconstruction (eg, Jatene type);

(Do not report modifier '-63' in conjunction with 33778)

33779   with removal of pulmonary band

33780   with closure of ventricular septal defect

33781   with repair of subpulmonic obstruction

33782 Aortic root translocation with ventricular septal defect and pulmonary stenosis repair (ie, Nikaidoh procedure); without coronary ostium reimplantation

(Do not report 33782 in conjunction with 33412, 33413, 33608, 33681, 33770, 33771, 33778, 33780, 33920)

33783   with reimplantation of 1 or both coronary ostia

TRUNCUS ARTERIOSUS

33786 Total repair, truncus arteriosus (Rastelli type operation)

(Do not report modifier '-63' in conjunction with 33786)

33788 Reimplantation of an anomalous pulmonary artery

(For pulmonary artery band, use 33690)

AORTIC ANOMALIES

33800 Aortic suspension (aortopexy) for tracheal decompression (eg, for tracheomalacia) (separate procedure)

33802 Division of aberrant vessel (vascular ring);

33803   with reanastomosis

● New Code   ▲ Revised Code   + Add-On Code   ⊘ Modifier -51 Exempt   ★ Telemedicine

33813	Obliteration of aortopulmonary septal defect; without cardiopulmonary bypass
33814	with cardiopulmonary bypass
33820	Repair of patent ductus arteriosus; by ligation
33822	by division, under 18 years
33824	by division, 18 years and older

(For percutaneous transcatheter closure of patent ductus arteriosus, use 93582)

33840	Excision of coarctation of aorta, with or without associated patent ductus arteriosus; with direct anastomosis
33845	with graft
33851	repair using either left subclavian artery or prosthetic material as gusset for enlargement
33852	Repair of hypoplastic or interrupted aortic arch using autogenous or prosthetic material; without cardiopulmonary bypass
33853	with cardiopulmonary bypass

(For repair of hypoplastic left heart syndrome (eg., Norwood type), via excision of coarctation of aorta, use 33619)

THORACIC AORTIC ANEURYSM

When ascending aortic disease involves the aortic arch, an aortic hemiarch graft may be necessary in conjunction with the ascending aortic graft and may be reported with add-on code 33866 in conjunction with the appropriate ascending aortic graft code (33858, 33859, 33863, 33864). Aortic hemiarch graft requires all of the following components:

1. Either total circulatory arrest or isolated cerebral perfusion (retrograde or antegrade);

2. Incision into the transverse arch extending under one or more of the arch vessels (eg, innominate, left common carotid, or left subclavian arteries); and

3. Extension of the ascending aortic graft under the aortic arch by construction of a beveled anastomosis to the distal ascending aorta and aortic arch without a crossclamp (an open anastomosis).

An ascending aortic repair with a beveled anastomosis into the arch with a cross-clamp cannot be reported separately as a hemiarch graft using 33866. Use 33866 for aortic hemiarch graft when performed in conjunction with the ascending aortic graft codes 33858, 33859, 33863, 33864. Code 33871 describes a complete transverse arch graft placement, and is not used to report an aortic hemiarch graft procedure.

33858	Ascending aorta graft, with cardiopulmonary bypass, includes valve suspension, when performed; for aortic dissection
33859	for aortic disease other than dissection (eg, aneurysm)
(**33860**	deleted 2019 [2020 Edition]. To report, see 33858, 33859)
33863	Ascending aorta graft, with cardiopulmonary bypass, with aortic root replacement using valved conduit and coronary reconstruction (eg., Bentall)

(Do not report 33863 in conjunction with 33405, 33406, 33410, 33411, 33412, 33413, 33858, 33859)

33864	Ascending aorta graft, with cardiopulmonary bypass with valve suspension, with coronary reconstruction and valve sparing aortic root remodeling (eg, David Procedure, Yacoub Procedure)

(Do not report 33864 in conjunction with 33858, 33859, 33863)

Separate Procedure	Unlisted Procedure	CCI Comp. Code	Non-specific Procedure	**393**

+ **33866**   Aortic hemiarch graft including isolation and control of the arch vessels, beveled open distal aortic anastomosis extending under one or more of the arch vessels, and total circulatory arrest or isolated cerebral perfusion (List separately in addition to code for primary procedure)

(Use 33866 for aortic hemiarch graft performed in conjunction with ascending aortic graft [33858, 33859, 33863, 33864])

(Do not report 33866 in conjunction with 33871)

(**33870**   deleted 2019 [2020 Edition]. To report, use 33871)

33871   Transverse aortic arch graft, with cardiopulmonary bypass, with profound hypothermia, total circulatory arrest and isolated cerebral perfusion with reimplantation of arch vessel(s) (eg, island pedicle or individual arch vessel reimplantation)

(Do not report 33871 for aortic hemiarch graft)

(Do not report 33871 in conjunction with 33866)

(For aortic hemiarch graft performed in conjunction with ascending aortic graft [33858, 33859, 33863, 33864], use 33866)

33875   Descending thoracic aorta graft, with or without bypass

33877   Repair of thoracoabdominal aortic aneurysm with graft, with or without cardiopulmonary bypass

ENDOVASCULAR REPAIR OF DESCENDING THORACIC AORTA

Codes 33880-33891 represent a family of procedures to report placement of an endovascular graft for repair of the descending thoracic aorta. These codes include all device introduction, manipulation, positioning, and deployment. All balloon angioplasty and/or stent deployment within the target treatment zone for the endoprosthesis, either before or after endograft deployment, are not separately reportable. Open arterial exposure and associated closure of the arteriotomy sites (eg., 34812, 34820, 34833, 34834), introduction of guidewires and catheters (eg., 36140, 36200-36218), and extensive repair or replacement of an artery (eg., 35226, 35286) should be additionally reported. Transposition of subclavian artery to carotid, and carotid-carotid bypass performed in conjunction with endovascular repair of the descending thoracic aorta (eg., 33889, 33891)should be separately reported. The primary codes, 33880 and 33881, include placement of all distal extensions, if required, in the distal thoracic aorta, while proximal extensions, if needed, are reported separately.

Open arterial exposure and associated closure of the arteriotomy sites (eg, 34714, 34715, 34716, 34812, 34820, 34833, 34834), introduction of guidewires and catheters (eg, 36140, 36200-36218), and extensive repair or replacement of an artery (eg, 35226, 35286) may be additionally reported. Transposition of subclavian artery to carotid, and carotid-carotid bypass performed in conjunction with endovascular repair of the descending thoracic aorta (eg, 33889, 33891) may be separately reported. The primary codes, 33880 and 33881, include placement of all distal extensions, if required, in the distal thoracic aorta, while proximal extensions, if needed, may be reported separately.

For fluoroscopic guidance in conjunction with endovascular repair of the thoracic aorta, see codes 75956-75959 as appropriate. Codes 75956 and 75957 include all angiography of the thoracic aorta and its branches for diagnostic imaging prior to deployment of the primary endovascular devices (including all routine components of modular devices), fluoroscopic guidance in the delivery of the endovascular components and intraprocedural arterial angiography (eg., confirm position, detect endoleak, evaluate runoff). Code 75958 includes the analogous services for placement of each proximal thoracic endovascular extension. Code 75959 includes the analogous services for placement of a distal thoracic endovascular extension(s) placed during a procedure after the primary repair.

Other interventional procedures performed at the time of endovascular repair of the descending thoracic aorta should be additionally reported (eg., innominate, carotid, subclavian, visceral, or iliac artery transluminal angioplasty or stenting, arterial embolization, intravascular ultrasound) when performed before or after deployment of the aortic prostheses.

33880   Endovascular repair of descending thoracic aorta (eg, aneurysm, pseudoaneurysm, dissection, penetrating ulcer, intramural hematoma, or traumatic disruption); involving coverage of left subclavian artery origin, initial endoprosthesis plus descending thoracic aortic extension(s), if required, to level of celiac artery origin

(For radiological supervision and interpretation, use 75956 in conjunction with 33880)

   ● New Code   ▲ Revised Code   + Add-On Code   ⊘ Modifier -51 Exempt   ★ Telemedicine

33881   not involving coverage of left subclavian artery origin, initial endoprosthesis plus descending thoracic aortic extension(s), if required, to level of celiac artery origin

(For radiological supervision and interpretation, use 75957 in conjunction with 33881)

33883   Placement of proximal extension prosthesis for endovascular repair of descending thoracic aorta (eg, aneurysm, pseudoaneurysm, dissection, penetrating ulcer, intramural hematoma, or traumatic disruption); initial extension

(For radiological supervision and interpretation, use 75958 in conjunction with 33883)

(Do not report 33881, 33883 when extension placement converts repair to cover left subclavian origin. Use only 33880)

+ 33884   each additional proximal extension (List separately in addition to code for primary procedure)

(Use 33884 in conjunction with 33883)

(For radiological supervision and interpretation, use 75958 in conjunction with 33884)

33886   Placement of distal extension prosthesis(es) delayed after endovascular repair of descending thoracic aorta

(Do not report 33886 in conjunction with 33880, 33881)

(Report 33886 once, regardless of number of modules deployed)

(For radiological supervision and interpretation, use 75959 in conjunction with 33886)

33889   Open subclavian to carotid artery transposition performed in conjunction with endovascular repair of descending thoracic aorta, by neck incision, unilateral

(Do not report 33889 in conjunction with 35694)

33891   Bypass graft, with other than vein, transcervical retropharyngeal carotid-carotid, performed in conjunction with endovascular repair of descending thoracic aorta, by neck incision

(Do not report 33891 in conjunction with 35509, 35601)

PULMONARY ARTERY

33910   Pulmonary artery embolectomy; with cardiopulmonary bypass

33915   without cardiopulmonary bypass

33916   Pulmonary endarterectomy, with or without embolectomy, with cardiopulmonary bypass

33917   Repair of pulmonary artery stenosis by reconstruction with patch or graft

33920   Repair of pulmonary atresia with ventricular septal defect, by construction or replacement of conduit from right or left ventricle to pulmonary artery

(For repair of other complex cardiac anomalies by construction or replacement of right or left ventricle to pulmonary artery conduit, use 33608)

33922   Transection of pulmonary artery with cardiopulmonary bypass

(Do not report modifier '-63' in conjunction with 33922)

+ 33924   Ligation and takedown of a systemic-to-pulmonary artery shunt, performed in conjunction with a congenital heart procedure (List separately in addition to code for primary procedure)

(Use 33924 in conjunction with 33470-33478, 33600-33617, 33622, 33684-33688, 33692-33697, 33735-33767, 33770-33783, 33786, 33917, 33920, 33922, 33925, 33926, 33935, 33945)

33925   Repair of pulmonary artery arborization anomalies by unifocalization; without cardiopulmonary bypass

---

Separate Procedure   Unlisted Procedure   CCI Comp. Code   Non-specific Procedure   **395**

33926	with cardiopulmonary bypass

HEART/LUNG TRANSPLANTATION

Heart with or without lung allotransplantation involves three distinct components of physician work:

1) **Cadaver donor cardiectomy with or without pneumonectomy**, which includes harvesting the allograft and cold preservation of the allograft (perfusing with cold preservation solution and cold maintenance) (see 33930, 33940).

2) **Backbench work**:

Preparation of a cadaver donor heart and lung allograft prior to transplantation, including dissection of the allograft from surrounding soft tissues to prepare the aorta, superior vena cava, inferior vena cava, and trachea for implantation (use 33933).

Preparation of a cadaver donor heart allograft prior to transplantation, including dissection of the allograft from surrounding soft tissues to prepare aorta, superior vena cava, inferior vena cava, pulmonary artery, and left atrium for implantation (use 33944).

3) **Recipient heart with or without lung allotransplantation**, which includes transplantation of allograft and care of the recipient (see 33935, 33945).

(For implantation of a total replacement heart system [artificial heart] with recipient cardiectomy, use 33927)

33927	Implantation of a total replacement heart system (artificial heart) with recipient cardiectomy

(For implantation of ventricular assist device, see 33975, 33976, 33979, 33990, 33991, 33995)

33928	Removal and replacement of total replacement heart system (artificial heart)

(For revision or replacement of components only of a replacement heart system [artificial heart], use 33999)

+ 33929	Removal of a total replacement heart system (artificial heart) for heart transplantation (List separately in addition to code for primary procedure)

(Use 33929 in conjunction with 33945)

33930	Donor cardiectomy-pneumonectomy (including cold preservation)
33933	Backbench standard preparation of cadaver donor heart/lung allograft prior to transplantation, including dissection of allograft from surrounding soft tissues to prepare aorta, superior vena cava, inferior vena cava, and trachea for implantation
33935	Heart-lung transplant with recipient cardiectomy-pneumonectomy
33940	Donor cardiectomy (including cold preservation)
33944	Backbench standard preparation of cadaver donor heart allograft prior to transplantation, including dissection of allograft from surrounding soft tissues to prepare aorta, superior vena cava, inferior vena cava, pulmonary artery, and left atrium for implantation

(For repair or resection procedures on the donor heart, see 33300, 33310, 33320, 33390, 33463, 33464, 33510, 33641, 35216, 35276, 35685)

33945	Heart transplant, with or without recipient cardiectomy

EXTRACORPOREAL MEMBRANE OXYGENATION OR EXTRACORPOREAL LIFE SUPPORT SERVICES

Prolonged extracorporeal membrane oxygenation capital (ECMO) or extracorporeal life-support (ECLS) is a procedure that provides cardiac and/or respiratory support to the heart and or lungs, which allows them to rest and recover when sick or injured. ECMO/ECLS supports the function of the heart and/or lungs by continuously pumping some of the patient's blood out of the body to an oxygenator (membrane lung) where oxygen is added to the blood, carbon dioxide (CO_2) is removed, and the blood is

● New Code ▲ Revised Code ✛ Add-On Code ⊘ Modifier -51 Exempt ★ Telemedicine

warmed before it is returned to the patient. There are two methods that can be used to accomplish ECMO/ ECLS. One method is veno-arterial extracorporeal life-support, which will support both the heart and lungs. Veno-arterial ECMO/ECLS requires that two cannula(e) are placed--one in a large vein and one in a large artery. The other method is veno-venous extracorporeal life support. Veno-venous ECMO/ECLS is used for lung support only and requires one or two cannula(e), which are placed in a vein.

Services directly related to the cannulation, initiation, management, and discontinuation of the ECMO/ECLS circuit and parameters (33946, 33947, 33948, 33949) are distinct from the daily overall management of the patient. The daily overall management of the patient is a factor that will vary greatly depending on the patient's age, disease process, and condition. Daily overall management of the patient may be separately reported using the relevant hospital observation services, hospital inpatient services, or critical care evaluation and management codes (99218, 99219, 99220, 99221, 99222, 99223, 99231, 99232, 99233, 99234, 99235, 99236, 99291, 99292, 99468, 99469, 99471, 99472, 99475, 99476, 99477, 99478, 99479, 99480).

Services directly related to the ECMO/ECLS involve the initial cannulation and repositioning, removing, or adding cannula(e) while the patient is being supported by the ECMO/ECLS. Initiation of the ECMO/ECLS circuit and setting parameters (33946, 33947) is performed by the physician and involves determining the necessary ECMO/ECLS device components, blood flow, gas exchange, and other necessary parameters to manage the circuit. The daily management of the ECMO/ECLS circuit and monitoring parameters, (33948, 33949), requires physician oversight to ensure that specific features of the interaction of the circuit with the patient are met. Daily management of the circuit and parameters includes management of blood flow, oxygenation, CO_2 clearance by the membrane lung, systemic response, anticoagulation and treatment of bleeding, and cannula(e) positioning, alarms and safety. Once the patient's heart and/or lung function has sufficiently recovered, the physician will wean the patient from the ECMO/ECLS circuit and finally decannulate the patient. The basic management of the ECMO/ECLS circuit and parameters are similar, regardless of the patient's condition.

ECMO/ECLS commonly involves multiple physicians and supporting nonphysician personnel to manage each patient. Different physicians may insert the cannula(e) and initiate ECMO/ECLS, manage the ECMO/ECLS circuit, and decannulate the patient. In addition, it would be common for one physician to manage the ECMO/ECLS circuit and patient-related issues (eg., anticoagulation, complications related to the ECMO/ECLS devices), while another physician manages the overall patient medical condition and underlying disorders, all on a daily basis. The physicians involved in the patient's care are commonly of different specialties, and significant physician team interaction may be required. Depending on the type of circuit and the patient's condition, there is substantial nonphysician work by ECMO/ECLS specialists, cardiac perfusionists, respiratory therapists, and specially trained nurses who provide long periods of constant attention.

If the same physician provides any or all of the services for placing a patient on an ECMO/ECLS circuit, they may report the appropriate codes for the services they performed, which may include codes for the cannula(e) insertion (33951, 33952, 33953, 33954, 33955, 33956), ECMO/ECLS initiation (33946 or 33947), and overall patient management (99218, 99219, 99220, 99221, 99222, 99223, 99231, 99232, 99233, 99234, 99235, 99236, 99291, 99292, 99468, 99469, 99471, 99472, 99475, 99476, 99477, 99478, 99479, 99480).

CPT CODES FOR ECMO/ECLS PROCEDURES						
INITIATION						
Management		**Cannula insertion procedures**					
Veno-venous 33946	Veno-arterial 33947	Percutaneous		Open		Sternotomy/thoracotomy	
		Birth-5 yrs 33951	≥ 6 yrs 33952	Birth-5 yrs 33953	≥ 6 yrs 33954	Birth-5 yrs 33955	≥ 6 yrs 33956
SUBSEQUENT						
Management		**Cannula repositioning procedures**				
Veno-venous 33948	Veno-arterial 33949	Percutaneous		Open		Sternotomy/thoracotomy	
		Birth-5 yrs 33957	≥ 6 yrs 33958	Birth-5 yrs 33959	≥ 6 yrs 33962	Birth-5 yrs 33963	≥ 6 yrs 33964
DECANNULATION						
Veno-venous and/or Veno-arterial →		**Decannulation (removal) procedures**				
		Percutaneous		Open		Sternotomy/thoracotomy	
		Birth-5 yrs 33965	≥ 6 yrs 33966	Birth-5 yrs 33969	≥ 6 yrs 33984	Birth-5 yrs 33985	≥ 6 yrs 33986
ADDITIONAL PROCEDURES						
		Other cannula procedures				
		Arterial exposure +33987		Insertion left heart vent 33988		Removal left heart vent 33989	

| | Separate Procedure | | Unlisted Procedure | | CCI Comp. Code | | Non-specific Procedure | **397** |

ECMO/ECLS daily management (33948, 33949), and repositioning services (33957, 33958, 33959, 33962, 33963, 33964), may not be reported on the same day as initiation services (33946, 33947) by the same or different individuals.

If different physicians provide parts of the service, each physician may report the correct code(s) for the service(s) they provided, except as noted.

Repositioning of the ECMO/ECLS cannula(e) (33957, 33958, 33959, 33962, 33963, 33964) at the same session as insertion (33951, 33952, 33953, 33954, 33955, 33956) is not separately reportable. Replacement of ECMO/ECLS cannula(e) in the same vessel should only be reported using the insertion code (33951, 33952, 33953, 33954, 33955, 33956). If cannula(e) are removed from one vessel and new cannula(e) are placed in a different vessel, report the appropriate cannula(e) removal (33965, 33966, 33969, 33984, 33985, 33986) and insertion (33951, 33952, 33953, 33954, 33955, 33956) codes. Expensive repair or replacement of an artery may be additionally reported (eg., 35266, 35286, 35371, and 35665). Fluoroscopic guidance used for cannula(e) repositioning (33957, 33958, 33959, 33962, 33963, 33964) is included in the procedure when performed and should not be separately reported.

Daily management codes (33948 and 33949) should not be reported on the same day as initiation of ECMO (33946 or 33947).

Initiation codes (33946 or 33947) should not be reported on the same day as repositioning codes (33957, 33958, 33959, 33962, 33963, 33964).

33946 Extracorporeal membrane oxygenation (ECMO)/extracorporeal life support (ECLS) provided by physician; initiation, veno-venous

(Do not report modifier 63 in conjunction with 33946, 33947, 33948, 33949)

(For insertion of cannula[e] for extracorporeal circulation, see 33951, 33952, 33953, 33954, 33955, 33956)

33947 initiation, veno-arterial

(Do not report modifier 63 in conjunction with 33946, 33947, 33948, 33949)

(Do not report 33946, 33947 in conjunction with 33948, 33949, 33957, 33958, 33959, 33962, 33963, 33964)

33948 daily management, each day, veno-venous

(Do not report modifier 63 in conjunction with 33946, 33947, 33948, 33949)

33949 daily management, each day, veno-arterial

(Do not report modifier 63 in conjunction with 33946, 33947, 33948, 33949)

(Do not report 33948, 33949 in conjunction with 33946, 33947)

33951 insertion of peripheral (arterial and/or venous) cannula(e), percutaneous, birth through 5 years of age (includes fluoroscopic guidance, when performed)

(For initiation and daily management of extracorporeal circulation, see 33946, 33947, 33948, 33949)

33952 insertion of peripheral (arterial and/or venous) cannula(e), percutaneous, 6 years and older (includes fluoroscopic guidance, when performed)

(For maintenance of extracorporeal circulation, see 33946, 33947, 33948, 33949)

33953 insertion of peripheral (arterial and/or venous) cannula(e), open, birth through 5 years of age

(For maintenance of extracorporeal circulation, see 33946, 33947, 33948, 33949)

33954 insertion of peripheral (arterial and/or venous) cannula(e), open, 6 years and older

(Do not report 33953, 33954 in conjunction with 34714, 34715, 34716, 34812, 34820, 34833, 34834)

(For maintenance of extracorporeal circulation, see 33946, 33947, 33948, 33949)

33955 insertion of central cannula(e) by sternotomy or thoracotomy, birth through 5 years of age

(For maintenance of extracorporeal circulation, see 33946, 33947, 33948, 33949)

33956   insertion of central cannula(e) by sternotomy or thoracotomy, 6 years and older

(Do not report 33955, 33956 in conjunction with 32100, 39010)

(For maintenance of extracorporeal circulation, see 33946, 33947, 33948, 33949)

33957   reposition peripheral (arterial and/or venous) cannula(e), percutaneous, birth through 5 years of age (includes fluoroscopic guidance, when performed)

33958   reposition peripheral (arterial and/or venous) cannula(e), percutaneous, 6 years and older (includes fluoroscopic guidance, when performed)

(Do not report 33957, 33958 in conjunction with 34713)

33959   reposition peripheral (arterial and/or venous) cannula(e), open, birth through 5 years of age (includes fluoroscopic guidance, when performed)

33962   reposition peripheral (arterial and/or venous) cannula(e), open, 6 years and older (includes fluoroscopic guidance, when performed)

(Do not report 33959, 33962 in conjunction with 34714, 34715, 34716, 34812, 34820, 34834)

33963   reposition of central cannula(e) by sternotomy or thoracotomy, birth through 5 years of age (includes fluoroscopic guidance, when performed)

33964   reposition central cannula(e) by sternotomy or thoracotomy, 6 years and older (includes fluoroscopic guidance, when performed)

(Do not report 33963, 33964 in conjunction with 32100, 39010)

(Do not report 33957, 33958, 33959, 33962, 33963, 33964 in conjunction with 33946, 33947)

33965   removal of peripheral (arterial and/or venous) cannula(e), percutaneous, birth through 5 years of age

33966   removal of peripheral (arterial and/or venous) cannula(e), percutaneous, 6 years and older

+ 33969   removal of peripheral (arterial and/or venous) cannula(e), open, birth through 5 years of age

(Do not report 33969 in conjunction with 34714, 34715, 34716, 34812, 34820, 34834, 35201, 35206, 35211, 35226)

33984   removal of peripheral (arterial and/or venous) cannula(e), open, 6 years and older

(Do not report 33984 in conjunction with 34714, 34715, 34716, 34812, 34820, 34834, 35201, 35206, 35211, 35226)

33985   removal of central cannula(e) by sternotomy or thoracotomy, birth through 5 years of age

(Do not report 33985 in conjunction with 35211)

33986   removal of central cannula(e) by sternotomy or thoracotomy, 6 years and older

(Do not report 33986 in conjunction with 35211)

+ 33987   Arterial exposure with creation of graft conduit (eg, chimney graft) to facilitate arterial perfusion for ECMO/ECLS (List separately in addition to code for primary procedure)

(Use 33987 in conjunction with 33953, 33954, 33955, 33956)

(Do not report 33987 in conjunction with 34714, 34716, 34833)

33988   Insertion of left heart vent by thoracic incision (eg, sternotomy, thoracotomy) for ECMO/ECLS

| Separate Procedure | Unlisted Procedure | CCI Comp. Code | Non-specific Procedure | **399** |

33989   Removal of left heart vent by thoracic incision (eg, sternotomy, thoracotomy) for ECMO/ECLS

CARDIAC ASSIST

A ventricular assist device is placed to provide hemodynamic support to the right heart, left heart, or both. The insertion of a ventricular assist device (VAD) can be performed via percutaneous (33990, 33991, 33995) or transthoracic (33975, 33976, 33979) approach. The location of the ventricular assist device may be intracorporeal or extracorporeal.

Removal of a transthoracic ventricular assist device (33977, 33978, 33980) or percutaneous ventricular assist device (33992, 33997) includes removal of the entire device, including the cannulas. Removal of a percutaneous ventricular assist device at the same session as insertion is not separately reportable. For removal of a percutaneous ventricular assist device at a separate and distinct session, but on the same day as insertion, report 33992, 33997 appended with modifier 59 indicating a distinct procedural service.

Repositioning of a percutaneous ventricular assist device at the same session as insertion is not separately reportable. Repositioning of percutaneous ventricular assist device not necessitating imaging guidance is not a reportable service. For repositioning of a percutaneous ventricular assist device necessitating imaging guidance at a separate and distinct session, but on the same day as insertion, report 33993 with modifier 59 indicating a distinct procedural service.

Replacement of a ventricular assist device pump (ie, 33981-33983) includes the removal of the pump and insertion of a new pump, connection, de-airing, and initiation of the new pump.

Replacement of the entire implantable ventricular assist device system, ie, pump(s) and cannulas, is reported using the insertion codes (ie, 33975, 33976, 33979). Removal (ie, 33977, 33978, 33980) of the ventricular assist device system being replaced is not separately reported. Replacement of a percutaneous ventricular assist device is reported using implantation codes (ie, 33990, 33991, 33995). Removal (ie, 33992, 33997) is not reported separately when a device is replaced.

33962   This codes is out of order. See page 399

33963   This codes is out of order. See page 399

33964   This codes is out of order. See page 399

33965   This codes is out of order. See page 399

33966   This codes is out of order. See page 399

33967   Insertion of intra-aortic balloon assist device, percutaneous

33968   Removal of intra-aortic balloon assist device, percutaneous

     (For removal of implantable aortic counterpulsation ventricular assist system, see 0455T, 0456T, 0457T, 0458T)

33969   This codes is out of order. See page 399

33970   Insertion of intra-aortic balloon assist device through the femoral artery, open approach

     (For insertion or replacement of implantable aortic counterpulsation ventricular assist system, see 0451T, 0452T, 0453T, 0454T)

33971   Removal of intra-aortic balloon assist device including repair of femoral artery, with or without graft

     (For removal of implantable aortic counterpulsation ventricular assist system, see 0455T, 0456T, 0457T, 0458T)

33973   Insertion of intra-aortic balloon assist device through the ascending aorta

     (For insertion or replacement of implantable aortic counterpulsation ventricular assist system, see 0451T, 0452T, 0453T, 0454T)

33974   Removal of intra-aortic balloon assist device from the ascending aorta, including repair of the ascending aorta, with or without graft

---

(For removal of implantable aortic counterpulsation ventricular assist system, see 0455T, 0456T, 0457T, 0458T)

33975 Insertion of ventricular assist device; extracorporeal, single ventricle

33976   extracorporeal, biventricular

33977 Removal of ventricular assist device; extracorporeal, single ventricle

33978   extracorporeal, biventricular

33979 Insertion of ventricular assist device, implantable intracorporeal, single ventricle

(For insertion or replacement of implantable aortic counterpulsation ventricular assist system, see 0451T, 0452T, 0453T, 0454T)

33980 Removal of ventricular assist device, implantable intracorporeal, single ventricle

(For removal of implantable aortic counterpulsation ventricular assist system, see 0455T, 0456T, 0457T, 0458T)

33981 Replacement of extracorporeal ventricular assist device, single or biventricular, pump(s), single or each pump

33982 Replacement of ventricular assist device pump(s); implantable intracorporeal, single ventricle, without cardiopulmonary bypass

33983   implantable intracorporeal, single ventricle, with cardiopulmonary bypass

(For insertion or replacement of implantable aortic counterpulsation ventricular assist system, see 0451T, 0452T, 0453T, 0454T)

33984 This codes is out of order. See page 399

33985 This codes is out of order. See page 399

33986 This codes is out of order. See page 399

33987 This codes is out of order. See page 399

33988 This codes is out of order. See page 399

33989 This codes is out of order. See page 400

● **33995** Insertion of ventricular assist device, percutaneous, including radiological supervision and interpretation; right heart, venous access only

▲ **33990**   left heart, arterial access only

▲ **33991**   left heart, both arterial and venous access, with transseptal puncture

(For insertion or replacement of implantable aortic counterpulsation ventricular assist system, see 0451T, 0452T, 0453T, 0454T)

▲ **33992** Removal of percutaneous left heart ventricular assist device, arterial or arterial and venous cannula(s), at separate and distinct session from insertion

(For removal of implantable aortic counterpulsation ventricular assist system, see 0455T, 0456T, 0457T, 0458T)

● **33997** Removal of percutaneous right heart ventricular assist device, venous cannula, at separate and distinct session from insertion

---

| ▨ Separate Procedure | ▨ Unlisted Procedure | ▨ CCI Comp. Code | ▨ Non-specific Procedure | **401** |

(For removal of left or right heart ventricular assist device via open approach, see appropriate vessel repair code [eg, 35206, 35226, 35286, 35371])

▲ **33993** Repositioning of percutaneous right or left heart ventricular assist device with imaging guidance at separate and distinct session from insertion

(For relocating and repositioning of implantable aortic counterpulsation ventricular assist system, see 0459T, 0460T, 0461T)

33995 This code is out of order. See page 401

33997 This code is out of order. See page 401

OTHER PROCEDURES, CARDIAC SURGERY

33999 Unlisted procedure, cardiac surgery

ARTERIES AND VEINS

Primary vascular procedure listings include establishing both inflow and outflow by whatever procedures necessary. Also included is that portion of the operative arteriogram performed by the surgeon, as indicated. Sympathectomy, when done, is included in the listed aortic procedures. For unlisted vascular procedures, use 37799.

EMBOLECTOMY/THROMBECTOMY

Arterial, With or Without Catheter

34001 Embolectomy or thrombectomy, with or without catheter; carotid, subclavian or innominate artery, by neck incision

34051 innominate, subclavian artery, by thoracic incision

34101 axillary, brachial, innominate, subclavian artery, by arm incision

34111 radial or ulnar artery, by arm incision

34151 renal, celiac, mesentery, aortoiliac artery, by abdominal incision

34201 femoropopliteal, aortoiliac artery, by leg incision

34203 popliteal-tibio-peroneal artery, by leg incision

Venous, Direct or With Catheter

34401 Thrombectomy, direct or with catheter; vena cava, iliac vein, by abdominal incision

34421 vena cava, iliac, femoropopliteal vein, by leg incision

34451 vena cava, iliac, femoropopliteal vein, by abdominal and leg incision

34471 subclavian vein, by neck incision

34490 axillary and subclavian vein, by arm incision

VENOUS RECONSTRUCTION

34501 Valvuloplasty, femoral vein

34502 Reconstruction of vena cava, any method

34510 Venous valve transposition, any vein donor

● New Code   ▲ Revised Code   ＋ Add-On Code   ⊘ Modifier -51 Exempt   ★ Telemedicine

34520   Cross-over vein graft to venous system

34530   Saphenopopliteal vein anastomosis

ENDOVASCULAR REPAIR OF ABDOMINAL AORTA AND/OR ILIAC ARTERIES

Codes 34701, 34702, 34703, 34704, 34705, 34706 describe introduction, positioning, and deployment of an endograft for treatment of abdominal aortic pathology (with or without rupture), such as aneurysm, pseudoaneurysm, dissection, penetrating ulcer, or traumatic disruption in the infrarenal abdominal aorta with or without extension into the iliac artery(ies). The terms, endovascular graft, endoprosthesis, endograft, and stentgraft, refer to a covered stent. The infrarenal aortic endograft may be an aortic tube device, a bifurcated unibody device, a modular bifurcated docking system with docking limb(s), or an aorto-uni-iliac device. Codes 34707 and 34708 describe introduction, positioning, and deployment of an ilio-iliac endograft for treatment of isolated arterial pathology (with or without rupture), such as aneurysm, pseudoaneurysm, arteriovenous malformation, or trauma involving the iliac artery. For treatment of atherosclerotic occlusive disease in the iliac artery(ies) with a covered stent(s), see 37221, 37223. For covered stent placement for atherosclerotic occlusive disease in the aorta, see 37236, 37237.

Add-on code 34717 is reported at the time of aortoiliac artery endograft placement (34703, 34704, 34705, 34706) for deployment of a bifurcated endograft in the common iliac artery with extension(s) into both the internal iliac and external iliac arteries, when performed, to maintain perfusion in both vessels for treatment of iliac artery pathology (with or without rupture), such as aneurysm, pseudoaneurysm, dissection, penetrating ulcer, arteriovenous malformation, or traumatic disruption. The iliac branched endograft is a multi-piece system consisting of a bifurcated device that is placed in the common iliac artery and then additional extension(s) are placed into both the internal iliac artery and external iliac/common femoral arteries as needed, as well as a proximal extension that overlaps with an aorto-iliac endograft, when performed. All additional extensions proximally into the common iliac artery or distally into the external iliac and/or common femoral arteries are inherent to these codes. Report 34705 or 34706 for simultaneous bilateral iliac artery aneurysm repairs with aorto-bi-iliac endograft. For isolated bilateral iliac artery repair using iliac artery tube endografts, report 34707 or 34708 with modifier 50 appended.

Decompressive laparotomy for abdominal compartment syndrome after ruptured abdominal aortic and/or iliac artery aneurysm repair may be separately reported with 49000 in addition to 34702, 34704, 34706, or 34708.

The treatment zone for endograft procedures is defined by those vessels that contain an endograft(s) (main body, docking limb[s], and/or extension[s]) deployed during that operative session. Adjunctive procedures outside the treatment zone may be separately reported (eg, angioplasty, endovascular stent placement, embolization). For example, when an endograft terminates in the common iliac artery, any additional treatment performed in the external and/or internal iliac artery may be separately reportable. Placement of a docking limb is inherent to a modular endograft(s), and, therefore, 34709 may not be reported separately if the docking limb extends into the external iliac artery. In addition, any interventions (eg, angioplasty, stenting, additional stent graft extension[s]) in the external iliac artery where the docking limb terminates may not be reported separately. Any catheterization or treatment of the internal iliac artery, such as embolization, may be separately reported. For 34701 and 34702, the abdominal aortic treatment zone is defined as the infrarenal aorta. For 34703 and 34704, the abdominal aortic treatment zone is typically defined as the infrarenal aorta and ipsilateral common iliac artery. For 34705 and 34706, the abdominal aortic treatment zone is typically defined as the infrarenal aorta and both common iliac arteries. For 34707, 34708, 34717, 34718, the treatment zone is defined as the portion of the iliac artery(ies) (eg, common, internal, external iliac arteries) that contains the endograft.

Codes 34702, 34704, 34706, 34708 are reported when endovascular repair is performed on ruptured aneurysm in the aorta or iliac artery(ies). Rupture is defined as clinical and/or radiographic evidence of acute hemorrhage for purposes of reporting these codes. A chronic, contained rupture is considered a pseudoaneurysm, and endovascular treatment of a chronic, contained rupture is reported with 34701, 34703, 34705, or 34707.

Code 34709 is reported for placement of extension prosthesis(es) that terminate(s) either in the internal iliac, external iliac, or common femoral artery(ies) or in the abdominal aorta proximal to the renal artery(ies) in conjunction with 34701, 34702, 34703, 34704, 34705, 34706, 34707, 34708. Code 34709 may only be reported once per vessel treated (ie, multiple endograft extensions placed in a single vessel may only be reported once). Endograft extension(s) that terminate(s) in the common iliac arteries are included in 34703, 34704, 34705, 34706, 34707, 34708 and are not separately reported. Treatment zone angioplasty/stenting, when performed, is included in 34709. In addition, proximal infrarenal abdominal aortic extension prosthesis(es) that terminate(s) in the aorta below the renal artery(ies) are also included in 34701, 34702, 34703, 34704, 34705, 34706 and are not separately reportable.

Codes 34710, 34711 are reported for delayed placement of distal or proximal extension prosthesis(es) for endovascular repair of infrarenal abdominal aortic or iliac aneurysm, false aneurysm, dissection, endoleak, or endograft migration. Pre-procedure sizing and device selection, all nonselective catheterization(s), all associated radiological supervision and interpretation, and treatment zone angioplasty/stenting, when performed, are included in 34710 and 34711. Codes 34710 and 34711 may only be reported once per vessel treated (ie, multiple endograft extensions placed in a single vessel may only be reported once).

| Separate Procedure | Unlisted Procedure | CCI Comp. Code | Non-specific Procedure | **403** |

If an aorto-iliac artery endograft (34703, 34704, 34705, 34706) is not being placed during the same operative session, 34718 may be reported for placement of a bifurcated endograft in the common iliac artery with extension(s) into both the internal iliac and external iliac arteries, to maintain perfusion in both vessels for treatment of iliac artery pathology (without rupture), such as aneurysm, pseudoaneurysm, dissection, arteriovenous malformation. The iliac branched endograft is a multi-piece system consisting of a bifurcated device that is placed in the common iliac artery and then additional extension(s) are placed into both the internal iliac artery and external iliac/common femoral arteries as needed as well as a proximal extension that overlaps with an aorto-iliac endograft, when performed. All additional extensions placed proximally into the common iliac artery or distally into the external iliac and/or common femoral arteries are inherent to these codes. For isolated bilateral iliac artery repair using iliac artery branched endografts, use 34718 with modifier 50 appended.

Codes 34709, 34710, 34711 may not be separately reported with 34717, 34718 for ipsilateral extension prosthesis(es). However, 34709, 34710, 34711 may be reported separately for extension prosthesis(es) in the iliac/femoral arteries contralateral to the iliac branched endograft.

Nonselective catheterization is included in 34701, 34702, 34703, 34704, 34705, 34706, 34707, 34708 and is not separately reported. However, selective catheterization of the hypogastric artery(ies), renal artery(ies), and/or arterial families outside the treatment zone of the endograft may be separately reported. Intravascular ultrasound (37252, 37253) performed during endovascular aneurysm repair may be separately reported. Balloon angioplasty and/or stenting within the treatment zone of the endograft, either before or after endograft deployment, is not separately reported. Fluoroscopic guidance and radiological supervision and interpretation in conjunction with endograft repair is not separately reported, and includes all intraprocedural imaging (eg, angiography, rotational CT) of the aorta and its branches prior to deployment of the endovascular device, fluoroscopic guidance and roadmapping used in the delivery of the endovascular components, and intraprocedural and completion angiography (eg, confirm position, detect endoleak, evaluate runoff) performed at the time of the endovascular infrarenal aorta and/or iliac repair.

Selective arterial catheterization of the internal and external iliac arteries (eg, 36245, 36246, 36247, 36248) ipsilateral to an iliac branched endograft is included in 34717, 34718 and not separately reported. However, selective catheterization of the renal artery(ies), the contralateral hypogastric artery, and/or arterial families outside the treatment zone of the graft may be separately reported. Intravascular ultrasound (37252, 37253) performed during endovascular aneurysm repair may be separately reported. Balloon angioplasty within the target treatment zone of the endograft, either before or after endograft deployment, is not separately reported. Fluoroscopic guidance and radiological supervision and interpretation performed in conjunction with endovascular iliac branched repair is not separately reported. Endovascular iliac branched repair includes all intraprocedural imaging (eg, angiography, rotational CT) of the aorta and its branches prior to deployment of the endovascular device, fluoroscopic guidance in the delivery of the endovascular components, and intraprocedural arterial angiography (eg, confirm position, detect endoleak, evaluate runoff) performed at the time of the endovascular aorto-iliac repair).

Codes 34709, 34710, 34711 include nonselective introduction of guidewires and catheters into the treatment zone from peripheral artery access(es). However, selective catheterization of the hypogastric artery(ies), renal artery(ies), and/or arterial families outside the treatment zone may be separately reported. Codes 34709, 34710, 34711 also include balloon angioplasty and/or stenting within the treatment zone of the endograft extension, either before or after deployment of the endograft, fluoroscopic guidance, and all associated radiological supervision and interpretation performed in conjunction with endovascular endograft extension (eg, angiographic diagnostic imaging of the aorta and its branches prior to deployment of the endovascular device, fluoroscopic guidance in the delivery of the endovascular components, and intraprocedural and completion angiography to confirm endograft position, detect endoleak, and evaluate runoff).

Code 34712 describes transcatheter delivery of accessoryenhanced fixation devices to the endograft (eg, anchor, screw, tack), including all associated radiological supervision and interpretation. Code 34712 may only be reported once per operative session.

Vascular access requiring use of closure devices for large sheaths (ie, 12 French or larger) or access requiring open surgical arterial exposure may be separately reported (eg, 34713, 34714, 34715, 34716, 34812, 34820, 34833, 34834). Code 34713 describes percutaneous access and closure of a femoral arteriotomy for delivery of endovascular prosthesis through a large arterial sheath (ie, 12 French or larger). Ultrasound guidance (ie, 76937), when performed, is included in 34713. (Percutaneous access using a sheath smaller than 12 French is included in 34701-34712 and is not separately reported.)

Code 34812 describes open repair and closure of the femoral artery. Extensive repair of an artery (eg, 35226, 35286, 35371) may also be reported separately. Iliac exposure for device delivery through a retroperitoneal incision, open brachial exposure, or axillary or subclavian exposure through an infraclavicular, or supraclavicular or sternotomy incision during endovascular aneurysm repair may be separately reported (eg, 34715, 34812, 34820, 34834). Endovascular device delivery or establishment of cardiopulmonary bypass that requires creation of a prosthetic conduit utilizing a femoral artery, iliac artery with a retroperitoneal incision, or axillary or subclavian artery exposure through an infraclavicular, supraclavicular, or sternotomy incision (eg, 34714, 34716, 34833) and oversewing of the conduit at the time of procedure completion may be separately reported during endovascular aneurysm repair or cardiac procedures requiring cardiopulmonary bypass. If a conduit is converted to a bypass, report the bypass (eg, 35665) and not the arterial exposure with conduit (ie, 34714, 34716, 34833). Arterial embolization(s) of renal, lumbar, inferior mesenteric, hypogastric or external iliac arteries to facilitate complete endovascular aneurysm exclusion may be separately reported (eg, 37242).

Balloon angioplasty and/or stenting at the sealing zone(s) of an endograft is an integral part of the procedure and is not separately reported. However, balloon angioplasty and/or stent deployment in vessels that do not contain endograft (outside the treatment zone for the endograft), either before or after endograft deployment, may be separately reported (eg, 37220, 37221, 37222, 37223).

Other interventional procedures performed at the time of endovascular abdominal aortic aneurysm repair may be additionally reported (eg, renal transluminal angioplasty, arterial embolization, intravascular ultrasound, balloon angioplasty or stenting of native artery[s] outside the endograft treatment zone, when done before or after deployment of endograft).

(For fenestrated endovascular repair of the visceral aorta, see 34841-34844. For fenestrated endovascular repair of the visceral aorta and concomitant infrarenal abdominal aorta, see 34845-34848)

34701 Endovascular repair of infrarenal aorta by deployment of an aorto-aortic tube endograft including pre-procedure sizing and device selection, all nonselective catheterization(s), all associated radiological supervision and interpretation, all endograft extension(s) placed in the aorta from the level of the renal arteries to the aortic bifurcation, and all angioplasty/stenting performed from the level of the renal arteries to the aortic bifurcation; for other than rupture (eg, for aneurysm, pseudoaneurysm, dissection, penetrating ulcer)

(For covered stent placement[s] for atherosclerotic occlusive disease isolated to the aorta, see 37236, 37237)

34702 for rupture including temporary aortic and/or iliac balloon occlusion, when performed (eg, for aneurysm, pseudoaneurysm, dissection, penetrating ulcer, traumatic disruption)

34703 Endovascular repair of infrarenal aorta and/or iliac artery(ies) by deployment of an aorto-uni-iliac endograft including pre-procedure sizing and device selection, all nonselective catheterization(s), all associated radiological supervision and interpretation, all endograft extension(s) placed in the aorta from the level of the renal arteries to the iliac bifurcation, and all angioplasty/stenting performed from the level of the renal arteries to the iliac bifurcation; for other than rupture (eg, for aneurysm, pseudoaneurysm, dissection, penetrating ulcer)

34704 for rupture including temporary aortic and/or iliac balloon occlusion, when performed (eg, for aneurysm, pseudoaneurysm, dissection, penetrating ulcer, traumatic disruption)

34705 Endovascular repair of infrarenal aorta and/or iliac artery(ies) by deployment of an aorto-bi-iliac endograft including pre-procedure sizing and device selection, all nonselective catheterization(s), all associated radiological supervision and interpretation, all endograft extension(s) placed in the aorta from the level of the renal arteries to the iliac bifurcation, and all angioplasty/stenting performed from the level of the renal arteries to the iliac bifurcation; for other than rupture (eg, for aneurysm, pseudoaneurysm, dissection, penetrating ulcer)

34706 for rupture including temporary aortic and/or iliac balloon occlusion, when performed (eg, for aneurysm, pseudoaneurysm, dissection, penetrating ulcer, traumatic disruption)

34707 Endovascular repair of iliac artery by deployment of an ilio-iliac tube endograft including pre-procedure sizing and device selection, all nonselective catheterization(s), all associated radiological supervision and interpretation, and all endograft extension(s) proximally to the aortic bifurcation and distally to the iliac bifurcation, and treatment zone angioplasty/stenting, when performed, unilateral; for other than rupture (eg, for aneurysm, pseudoaneurysm, dissection, arteriovenous malformation)

(For covered stent placement[s] for atherosclerotic occlusive disease of the abdominal aorta, see 37236, 37237)

(For covered stent placement[s] for atherosclerotic occlusive disease of the iliac artery, see 37221, 37223)

34708 for rupture including temporary aortic and/or iliac balloon occlusion, when performed (eg, for aneurysm, pseudoaneurysm, dissection, arteriovenous malformation, traumatic disruption)

(For endovascular repair of iliac artery by deployment of an iliac branched endograft, see 34717, 34718)

Separate Procedure   Unlisted Procedure   CCI Comp. Code   Non-specific Procedure   **405**

+ 34717   Endovascular repair of iliac artery at the time of aortoiliac artery endograft placement by deployment of an iliac branched endograft including pre-procedure sizing and device selection, all ipsilateral selective iliac artery catheterization(s), all associated radiological supervision and interpretation, and all endograft extension(s) proximally to the aortic bifurcation and distally in the internal iliac, external iliac, and common femoral artery(ies), and treatment zone angioplasty/stenting, when performed, for rupture or other than rupture (eg, for aneurysm, pseudoaneurysm, dissection, arteriovenous malformation, penetrating ulcer, traumatic disruption), unilateral (List separately in addition to code for primary procedure)

(Use 34717 in conjunction with 34703, 34704, 34705, 34706)

(34717 may only be reported once per side. For bilateral procedure, report 34717 twice. Do not report modifier 50 in conjunction with 34717)

(Do not report 34717 in conjunction with 34709 on the same side)

(Do not report 34717 in conjunction with 34710, 34711)

(For placement of an iliac branched endograft at a separate setting than aorto-iliac endograft placement, use 34718)

+ 34709   Placement of extension prosthesis(es) distal to the common iliac artery(ies) or proximal to the renal artery(ies) for endovascular repair of infrarenal abdominal aortic or iliac aneurysm, false aneurysm, dissection, penetrating ulcer, including pre-procedure sizing and device selection, all nonselective catheterization(s), all associated radiological supervision and interpretation, and treatment zone angioplasty/stenting, when performed, per vessel treated (List separately in addition to code for primary procedure)

(Use 34709 in conjunction with 34701, 34702, 34703, 34704, 34705, 34706, 34707, 34708)

(34709 may only be reported once per vessel treated [ie, multiple endograft extensions placed in a single vessel may only be reported once])

(Do not report 34709 for placement of a docking limb that extends into the external iliac artery)

(For placement of an iliac branched endograft, see 34717, 34718)

(For endograft placement into a renal artery that is being covered by a proximal extension, see 37236, 37237)

+ 34718   Endovascular repair of iliac artery, not associated with placement of an aorto-iliac artery endograft at the same session, by deployment of an iliac branched endograft, including pre-procedure sizing and device selection, all ipsilateral selective iliac artery catheterization(s), all associated radiological supervision and interpretation, and all endograft extension(s) proximally to the aortic bifurcation and distally in the internal iliac, external iliac, and common femoral artery(ies), and treatment zone angioplasty/stenting, when performed, for other than rupture (eg, for aneurysm, pseudoaneurysm, dissection, arteriovenous malformation, penetrating ulcer), unilateral

(For bilateral placement of an iliac branched endograft, report modifier 50)

(Do not report 34718 in conjunction with 34701, 34702, 34703, 34704, 34705, 34706, 34707, 34708, 34709, 34717)

(Do not report 34718 in conjunction with 34710, 34711 on the same side)

(For placement of an iliac branched endograft in the same setting as aorto-iliac endograft placement, use 34717)

(For placement of an isolated iliac branched endograft for rupture, use 37799)

34710   Delayed placement of distal or proximal extension prosthesis for endovascular repair of infrarenal abdominal aortic or iliac aneurysm, false aneurysm, dissection, endoleak, or endograft migration, including pre-procedure sizing and device selection, all nonselective catheterization(s), all associated radiological supervision and interpretation, and treatment zone angioplasty/stenting, when performed; initial vessel treated

+ 34711   each additional vessel treated (List separately in addition to code for primary procedure)

(Use 34711 in conjunction with 34710)

● New Code   ▲ Revised Code   + Add-On Code   ⊘ Modifier -51 Exempt   ★ Telemedicine

(34710, 34711 may each be reported only once per operative session [ie, multiple endograft extensions placed in a single vessel may only be reported with a single code])

(For decompressive laparotomy, use 49000 in conjunction with 34702, 34704, 34706, 34708, 34710)

(If the delayed revision is a transcatheter enhanced fixation device [eg, anchors, screws], report 34712)

(Do not report 34710, 34711 in conjunction with 34701, 34702, 34703, 34704, 34705, 34706, 34707, 34708, 34709)

(Do not report 34710, 34711 in conjunction with 34718 on the same side)

(Do not report 34701-34711 in conjunction with 34841, 34842, 34843, 34844, 34845, 34846, 34847, 34848)

(For endovascular repair of iliac artery bifurcation [eg, aneurysm, pseudoaneurysm, arteriovenous malformation, trauma] using bifurcated endograft, see 34717, 34718)

(Report 37252, 37253 for intravascular ultrasound when performed during endovascular aneurysm repair)

(For isolated bilateral iliac artery repair using iliac artery tube endografts, report 34707 or 34708 with modifier 50)

(For open arterial exposure, report 34714, 34715, 34716, 34812, 34820, 34833, 34834 as appropriate, in conjunction with 34701, 34702, 34703, 34704, 34705, 34706, 34707, 34708, 34710, 34712, 34718)

(For percutaneous arterial closure, report 34713 as appropriate, in conjunction with 34701, 34702, 34703, 34704, 34705, 34706, 34707, 34708, 34710, 34712, 34718)

(For simultaneous bilateral iliac artery aneurysm repairs with aorto-biiliac endograft, see 34705, 34706, as appropriate)

34712 Transcatheter delivery of enhanced fixation device(s) to the endograft (eg, anchor, screw, tack) and all associated radiological supervision and interpretation

(Report 34712 only once per operative session)

+ 34713 Percutaneous access and closure of femoral artery for delivery of endograft through a large sheath (12 French or larger), including ultrasound guidance, when performed, unilateral (List separately in addition to code for primary procedure)

(Use 34713 in conjunction with 33880, 33881, 33883, 33884, 33886, 34701, 34702, 34703, 34704, 34705, 34706, 34707, 34708, 34710, 34712, 34718, 34841, 34842, 34843, 34844, 34845, 34846, 34847, 34848, as appropriate. Do not report 34713 in conjunction with 33880, 33881, 33883, 33884, 33886, 34701, 34702, 34703, 34704, 34705, 34706, 34707, 34708, 34710, 34712, 34718, 34841, 34842, 34843, 34844, 34845, 34846, 34847, 34848, for percutaneous closure of femoral artery after delivery of endovascular prosthesis if a sheath smaller than 12 French was used)

(34713 may only be reported once per side. For bilateral procedure, report 34713 twice. Do not report modifier 50 in conjunction with 34713)

(Do not report ultrasound guidance [ie, 76937] for percutaneous vascular access in conjunction with 34713 for the same access)

(Do not report 34713 for percutaneous access and closure of the femoral artery in conjunction with 37221, 37223, 37236, 37237)

(Do not report 34713 in conjunction with 37221, 37223 for covered stent placement[s] for atherosclerotic occlusive disease of the iliac artery[ies])

+ 34812 Open femoral artery exposure for delivery of endovascular prosthesis, by groin incision, unilateral (List separately in addition to code for primary procedure)

(Use 34812 in conjunction with 33880, 33881, 33883, 33884, 33886, 33990, 33991, 34701, 34702, 34703, 34704, 34705, 34706, 34707, 34708, 34710, 34712, 34718, 34841, 34842, 34843, 34844, 34845, 34846, 34847, 34848)

(34812 may only be reported once per side. For bilateral procedure, report 34812 twice. Do not report modifier 50 in conjunction with 34812)

(Do not report 34812 in conjunction with 33953, 33954, 33959, 33962, 33969, 33984, 33987)

+ 34714 Open femoral artery exposure with creation of conduit for delivery of endovascular prosthesis or for establishment of cardiopulmonary bypass, by groin incision, unilateral (List separately in addition to code for primary procedure)

(Use 34714 in conjunction with 32852, 32854, 33031, 33120, 33251, 33256, 33259, 33261, 33305, 33315, 33322, 33335, 33390, 33391, 33404, 33405, 33406, 33410, 33411, 33412, 33413, 33414, 33415, 33416, 33417, 33422, 33425, 33426, 33427, 33430, 33440, 33460, 33463, 33464, 33465, 33468, 33474, 33475, 33476, 33478, 33496, 33500, 33502, 33504, 33505, 33506, 33507, 33510, 33511, 33512, 33513, 33514, 33516, 33533, 33534, 33535, 33536, 33542, 33545, 33548, 33600-33688, 33692, 33694, 33697, 33702, 33710, 33720, 33722, 33724, 33726, 33730, 33732, 33736, 33750, 33755, 33762, 33764, 33766, 33767, 33770-33783, 33786, 33788, 33802, 33803, 33814, 33820, 33822, 33824, 33840, 33845, 33851, 33853, 33858, 33859, 33863, 33864, 33871, 33875, 33877, 33880, 33881, 33883, 33884, 33886, 33910, 33916, 33917, 33920, 33922, 33926, 33935, 33945, 33975, 33976, 33977, 33978, 33979, 33980, 33983, 33990, 33991, 34701, 34702, 34703, 34704, 34705, 34706, 34707, 34708, 34710, 34712, 34718, 34841, 34842, 34843, 34844, 34845, 34846, 34847, 34848)

(34714 may only be reported once per side. For bilateral procedure, report 34714 twice. Do not report modifier 50 in conjunction with 34714)

(Do not report 34714 in conjunction with 33362, 33953, 33954, 33959, 33962, 33969, 33984, 34812 when performed on the same side)

+ 34820 Open iliac artery exposure for delivery of endovascular prosthesis or iliac occlusion during endovascular therapy, by abdominal or retroperitoneal incision, unilateral (List separately in addition to code for primary procedure)

(Use 34820 in conjunction with 33880, 33881, 33883, 33884, 33886, 33990, 33991, 34701, 34702, 34703, 34704, 34705, 34706, 34707, 34708, 34710, 34712, 34718, 34841, 34842, 34843, 34844, 34845, 34846, 34847, 34848)

(34820 may only be reported once per side. For bilateral procedure, report 34820 twice. Do not report modifier 50 in conjunction with 34820)

(Do not report 34820 in conjunction with 33953, 33954, 33959, 33962, 33969, 33984)

+ 34833 Open iliac artery exposure with creation of conduit for delivery of endovascular prosthesis or for establishment of cardiopulmonary bypass, by abdominal or retroperitoneal incision, unilateral (List separately in addition to code for primary procedure)

(Use 34833 in conjunction with 32852, 32854, 33031, 33120, 33251, 33256, 33259, 33261, 33305, 33315, 33322, 33335, 33390, 33391, 33404, 33405, 33406, 33410, 33411, 33412, 33413, 33414, 33415, 33416, 33417, 33422, 33425, 33426, 33427, 33430, 33440, 33460, 33463, 33464, 33465, 33468, 33474, 33475, 33476, 33478, 33496, 33500, 33502, 33504, 33505, 33506, 33507, 33510, 33511, 33512, 33513, 33514, 33516, 33533, 33534, 33535, 33536, 33542, 33545, 33548, 33600-33688, 33692, 33694, 33697, 33702, 33710, 33720, 33722, 33724, 33726, 33730, 33732, 33736, 33750, 33755, 33762, 33764, 33766, 33767, 33770-33783, 33786, 33788, 33802, 33803, 33814, 33820, 33822, 33824, 33840, 33845, 33851, 33853, 33858, 33859, 33863, 33864, 33871, 33875, 33877, 33880, 33881, 33883, 33884, 33886, 33910, 33916, 33917, 33920, 33922, 33926, 33935, 33945, 33975, 33976, 33977, 33978, 33979, 33980, 33983, 33990, 33991, 34701, 34702, 34703, 34704, 34705, 34706, 34707, 34708, 34710, 34712, 34718, 34841, 34842, 34843, 34844, 34845, 34846, 34847, 34848)

(34833 may only be reported once per side. For bilateral procedure, report 34833 twice. Do not report modifier 50 in conjunction with 34833)

(Do not report 34833 in conjunction with 33364, 33953, 33954, 33959, 33962, 33969, 33984, 34820 when performed on the same side)

+ 34834 Open brachial artery exposure for delivery of endovascular prosthesis, unilateral (List separately in addition to code for primary procedure)

(Use 34834 in conjunction with 33880, 33881, 33883, 33884, 33886, 33990, 33991, 34701, 34702, 34703, 34704, 34705, 34706, 34707, 34708, 34710, 34712, 34718, 34841, 34842, 34843, 34844, 34845, 34846, 34847, 34848)

● New Code ▲ Revised Code + Add-On Code ⊘ Modifier -51 Exempt ★ Telemedicine

(34834 may only be reported once per side. For bilateral procedure, report 34834 twice. Do not report modifier 50 in conjunction with 34834)

(Do not report 34834 in conjunction with 33953, 33954, 33959, 33962, 33969, 33984)

+ 34715 Open axillary/subclavian artery exposure for delivery of endovascular prosthesis by infraclavicular or supraclavicular incision, unilateral (List separately in addition to code for primary procedure)

(Use 34715 in conjunction with 33880, 33881, 33883, 33884, 33886, 33990, 33991, 34701, 34702, 34703, 34704, 34705, 34706, 34707, 34708, 34710, 34712, 34718, 34841, 34842, 34843, 34844, 34845, 34846, 34847, 34848)

(34715 may only be reported once per side. For bilateral procedure, report 34715 twice. Do not report modifier 50 in conjunction with 34715)

(Do not report 34715 in conjunction with 33363, 33953, 33954, 33959, 33962, 33969, 33984, 0451T, 0452T, 0455T, 0456T)

+ 34716 Open axillary/subclavian artery exposure with creation of conduit for delivery of endovascular prosthesis or for establishment of cardiopulmonary bypass, by infraclavicular or supraclavicular incision, unilateral (List separately in addition to code for primary procedure)

(Use 34716 in conjunction with 32852, 32854, 33031, 33120, 33251, 33256, 33259-33261, 33305, 33315, 33322, 33335, 33390, 33391, 33404, 33405, 33406, 33410, 33411, 33412, 33413, 33414, 33415, 33416, 33417, 33422, 33425, 33426, 33427, 33430, 33440, 33460, 33463, 33464, 33465, 33468, 33474, 33475, 33476, 33478, 33496, 33500, 33502, 33504, 33505, 33506, 33507, 33510, 33511, 33512, 33513, 33514, 33516, 33533, 33534, 33535, 33536, 33542, 33545, 33548, 33600-33688, 33692, 33694, 33697, 33702-33722, 33724, 33726, 33730, 33732, 33736, 33750, 33755, 33762, 33764, 33766, 33767, 33770-33783, 33786, 33788, 33802, 33803, 33814, 33820, 33822, 33824, 33840, 33845, 33851, 33853, 33858, 33859, 33863, 33864, 33871, 33875, 33877, 33880, 33881, 33883, 33884, 33886, 33910, 33916, 33917, 33920, 33922, 33926, 33935, 33945, 33975, 33976, 33977, 33978, 33979, 33980, 33983, 33990, 33991, 34701, 34702, 34703, 34704, 34705, 34706, 34707, 34708, 34710, 34712, 34718, 34841, 34842, 34843, 34844, 34845, 34846, 34847, 34848)

(34716 may only be reported once per side. For bilateral procedure, report 34716 twice. Do not report modifier 50 in conjunction with 34716)

(Do not report 34716 in conjunction with 33953, 33954, 33959, 33962, 33969, 33984, 0451T, 0452T, 0455T, 0456T)

34717 This code is out of order. See page 406

34718 This code is out of order. See page 406

+ 34808 Endovascular placement of iliac artery occlusion device (List separately in addition to code for primary procedure)

(Use 34808 in conjunction with 34701, 34702, 34703, 34704, 34707, 34708, 34709, 34710, 34813, 34841, 34842, 34843, 34844)

34812 This code is out of order. See page 407

+ 34813 Placement of femoral-femoral prosthetic graft during endovascular aortic aneurysm repair (List separately in addition to code for primary procedure)

(Use 34813 in conjunction with code 34812)

(For femoral artery grafting, see 35521, 35533, 35539, 35540, 35556, 35558, 35566, 35621, 35646, 35654-35661, 35666, 35700)

34820 This code is out of order. See page 408

34830 Open repair of infrarenal aortic aneurysm or dissection, plus repair of associated arterial trauma, following unsuccessful endovascular repair; tube prosthesis

34831 aorto-bi-iliac prosthesis

| 34832 | aorto-bifemoral prosthesis |

34833   This code is out of order. See page 408

34834   This code is out of order. See page 408

FENESTRATED ENDOVASCULAR REPAIR OF THE VISCERAL AND INFRARENAL AORTA

The upper abdominal aorta that contains the celiac, superior mesenteric, and renal arteries is termed the visceral aorta. For reporting purposes, the thoracic aorta extends from the aortic valve to the aortic segment just proximal to the celiac artery.

Code 34839 is used to report the physician planning and sizing for a patient-specific fenestrated visceral aortic endograft. The planning includes review of high-resolution cross-sectional images (eg, CT, CTA, MRI) and utilization of 3D software for iterative modeling of the aorta and device in multiplanar views and center line of flow analysis. Code 34839 may only be reported when the physician spends a minimum of 90 total minutes performing patient-specific fenestrated endograft planning. Physician planning time does not need to be continuous and should be clearly documented in the patient record. Code 34839 is reported on the date that planning work is complete and may not include time spent on the day before or the day of the fenestrated endovascular repair procedure (34841, 34842, 34843, 34844, 34845, 34846, 34847, 34848) nor be reported on the day before or the day of the fenestrated endovascular repair procedure.

Codes 34841, 34842, 34843, 34844, 34845, 34846, 34847, 34848 are used to report placement of a fenestrated endovascular graft in the visceral aorta, either alone or in combination with the infrarenal aorta for aneurysm, pseudoaneurysm, dissection, penetrating ulcer, intramural hematoma, or traumatic disruption. The fenestrated main body endoprosthesis is deployed within the visceral aorta. Fenestrations within the fabric allow for selective catheterization of the visceral and/or renal arteries and subsequent placement of an endoprosthesis (ie, bare metal or covered stent) to maintain flow to the visceral artery. Patient variation in the location and relative orientation of the renal and visceral artery origins requires use of a patient-specific fenestrated endograft for endovascular repair that preserves flow to essential visceral arteries and allows proximal seal and fixation to be achieved above the renal level as well as in the distal aorta or iliac vessel(s).

Fenestrated aortic repair is reported based on the extent of aorta treated. Codes 34841, 34842, 34843, 34844 describe repair using proximal endoprostheses that span from the visceral aortic component to one, two, three, or four visceral artery origins and distal extent limited to the infrarenal aorta. These devices do not extend into the common iliac arteries. Codes 34845, 34846, 34847, 34848 are used to report deployment of a fenestrated endograft that spans from the visceral aorta (including one, two, three, or four visceral artery origins) through the infrarenal aorta into the common iliac arteries. The infrarenal component may be a bifurcated unibody device, a modular bifurcated docking system with docking limb(s), or an aorto-uniiliac device. Codes 34845, 34846, 34847, 34848 include placement of unilateral or bilateral docking limbs (depending on the device). Any additional endograft extensions that terminate in the common iliac arteries are included in 34845, 34846, 34847, 34848. Codes 34709, 34710, 34711 may not be separately reported for proximal abdominal aortic extension prosthesis(es) or for distal extension prosthesis(es) that terminate(s) in the aorta or the common iliac arteries. However, 34709, 34710, 34711 may be reported for distal extension prosthesis(es) that terminate(s) in the internal iliac, external iliac, or common femoral artery(ies).

Codes 34841-34844 and 34845-34848 define the total number of visceral and/or renal arteries (ie, celiac, superior mesenteric, and/or unilateral or bilateral renal artery(s)) requiring placement of an endoprosthesis (ie, bare metal or covered stent) through an aortic endograft fenestration.

Introduction of guide wires and catheters in the aorta and visceral and/or renal arteries is included in the work of 34841-34848 and is not separately reportable. However, catheterization of the hypogastric artery(s) and/or arterial families outside the treatment zone of the graft may be separately reported. Balloon angioplasty within the target treatment zone of the endograft, either before or after endograft deployment, is not separately reportable. Fluoroscopic guidance and radiological supervision and interpretation in conjunction with fenestrated endovascular aortic repair is not separately reportable and includes angiographic diagnostic imaging of the aorta and its branches prior to deployment of the fenestrated endovascular device, fluoroscopic guidance in the delivery of the fenestrated endovascular components, and intraprocedural arterial angiography (eg, confirm position, detect endoleak, evaluate runoff) done at the time of the endovascular aortic repair.

Exposure of the access vessels (eg, 34713, 34714, 34715, 34716, 34812, 34820, 34833, 34834) may be reported separately. Extensive repair of an artery (eg, 35226, 35286) may be reported separately. For concomitant endovascular treatment of the descending thoracic aorta, 33880-33886 and 75956-75959 may be reported with 34841, 34842, 34843, 34844, 34845, 34846, 34847, 34848. For isolated endovascular infrarenal abdominal aortic aneurysm repair that does not require placement of a fenestrated graft to preserve flow to the visceral branch(es), see 34701, 34702, 34703, 34704, 34705, 34706.

Other interventional procedures performed at the time of fenestrated endovascular abdominal aortic aneurysm repair may be reported separately (eg, arterial embolization, intravascular ultrasound, balloon angioplasty or stenting of native artery(s) outside the endoprosthesis target zone, when done before or after deployment of endoprosthesis).

● New Code   ▲ Revised Code   + Add-On Code   ⊘ Modifier -51 Exempt   ★ Telemedicine

34839 Physician planning of a patient-specific fenestrated visceral aortic endograft requiring a minimum of 90 minutes of physician time

(Do not report 34839 in conjunction with 76376, 76377)

(Do not report 34839 in conjunction with 34841, 34842, 34843, 34844, 34845, 34846, 34847, 34848 when performed on the day before or the day of the fenestrated endovascular repair procedure)

34841 Endovascular repair of visceral aorta (eg, aneurysm, pseudoaneurysm, dissection, penetrating ulcer, intramural hematoma, or traumatic disruption) by deployment of a fenestrated visceral aortic endograft and all associated radiological supervision and interpretation, including target zone angioplasty, when performed; including one visceral artery endoprosthesis (superior mesenteric, celiac or renal artery)

34842 including two visceral artery endoprostheses (superior mesenteric, celiac and/or renal artery[s])

34843 including three visceral artery endoprostheses (superior mesenteric, celiac and/or renal artery[s])

34844 including four or more visceral artery endoprostheses (superior mesenteric, celiac and/or renal artery[s])

(Do not report 34841, 34842, 34843, 34844 in conjunction with 34701, 34702, 34703, 34704, 34705, 34706, 34845, 34846, 34847, 34848)

(Do not report 34841, 34842, 34843, 34844 in conjunction with 34839 when planning services are performed on the day before or the day of the fenestrated endovascular repair procedure)

34845 Endovascular repair of visceral aorta and infrarenal abdominal aorta (eg, aneurysm, pseudoaneurysm, dissection, penetrating ulcer, intramural hematoma, or traumatic disruption) with a fenestrated visceral aortic endograft and concomitant unibody or modular infrarenal aortic endograft and all associated radiological supervision and interpretation, including target zone angioplasty, when performed; including one visceral artery endoprosthesis (superior mesenteric, celiac or renal artery)

34846 including two visceral artery endoprostheses (superior mesenteric, celiac and/or renal artery[s])

34847 including three visceral artery endoprostheses (superior mesenteric, celiac and/or renal artery[s])

34848 including four or more visceral artery endoprostheses (superior mesenteric, celiac and/or renal artery[s])

(Do not report 34845, 34846, 34847, 34848 in conjunction with 34701, 34702, 34703, 34704, 34705, 34706, 34841, 34842, 34843, 34844, 35081, 35102)b

(Do not report 34845, 34846, 34847, 34848 in conjunction with 34839 when planning services are performed on the day before or the day of the fenestrated endovascular repair procedure)

(Do not report 34841-34848 in conjunction with 37236, 37237 for bare metal or covered stents placed into visceral branches within the endoprosthesis target zone)

(For placement of distal extension prosthesis[es] terminating in the internal iliac, external iliac, or common femoral artery[ies], see 34709, 34710, 34711, 34718)

(Use 34845, 34846, 34847, 34848 in conjunction with 37220, 37221, 37222, 37223 only when 37220, 37221, 37222, 37223 are performed outside the target treatment zone of the endoprosthesis)

ENDOVASCULAR REPAIR OF ILIAC ANEURYSM

(**34900** deleted 2017 [2018 edition]. To report, see 34707, 34708)

DIRECT REPAIR OF ANEURYSM OR EXCISION (PARTIAL OR TOTAL) AND GRAFT INSERTION FOR ANEURYSM, PSEUDOANEURYSM, RUPTURED ANEURYSM, AND ASSOCIATED OCCLUSIVE DISEASE

Procedures 35001-35152 include preparation of artery for anastomosis including endarterectomy.

(For direct repairs associated with occlusive disease only, see 35201-35286)

(For intracranial aneurysm, see 61700 et seq)

(For endovascular repair of abdominal aortic and/or iliac artery aneurysm, see 34701-34716)

(For thoracic aortic aneurysm, see 33858-33875)

(For endovascular repair of descending thoracic aorta, involving coverage of left subclavian artery origin, use 33880)

35001 Direct repair of aneurysm, pseudoaneurysm, or excision (partial or total) and graft insertion, with or without patch graft; for aneurysm and associated occlusive disease, carotid, subclavian artery, by neck incision

35002 for ruptured aneurysm, carotid, subclavian artery, by neck incision

35005 for aneurysm, pseudoaneurysm, and associated occlusive disease, vertebral artery

35011 for aneurysm and associated occlusive disease, axillary-brachial artery, by arm incision

35013 for ruptured aneurysm, axillary-brachial artery, by arm incision

35021 for aneurysm, pseudoaneurysm, and associated occlusive disease, innominate, subclavian artery, by thoracic incision

35022 for ruptured aneurysm, innominate, subclavian artery, by thoracic incision

35045 for aneurysm, pseudoaneurysm, and associated occlusive disease, radial or ulnar artery

35081 for aneurysm, pseudoaneurysm, and associated occlusive disease, abdominal aorta

35082 for ruptured aneurysm, abdominal aorta

35091 for aneurysm, pseudoaneurysm, and associated occlusive disease, abdominal aorta involving visceral vessels (mesenteric, celiac, renal)

35092 for ruptured aneurysm, abdominal aorta involving visceral vessels (mesenteric, celiac, renal)

35102 for aneurysm, pseudoaneurysm, and associated occlusive disease, abdominal aorta involving iliac vessels (common, hypogastric, external)

35103 for ruptured aneurysm, abdominal aorta involving iliac vessels (common, hypogastric, external)

35111 for aneurysm, pseudoaneurysm, and associated occlusive disease, splenic artery

35112 for ruptured aneurysm, splenic artery

35121 for aneurysm, pseudoaneurysm, and associated occlusive disease, hepatic, celiac, renal, or mesenteric artery

35122 for ruptured aneurysm, hepatic, celiac, renal, or mesenteric artery

35131 for aneurysm, pseudoaneurysm, and associated occlusive disease, iliac artery (common, hypogastric, external)

35132 for ruptured aneurysm, iliac artery (common, hypogastric, external)

35141 for aneurysm, pseudoaneurysm, and associated occlusive disease, common femoral artery (profunda femoris, superficial femoral)

35142 for ruptured aneurysm, common femoral artery (profunda femoris, superficial femoral)

35151 for aneurysm, pseudoaneurysm, and associated occlusive disease, popliteal artery

● New Code ▲ Revised Code ＋ Add-On Code ⃠ Modifier -51 Exempt ★ Telemedicine

| 35152 | for ruptured aneurysm, popliteal artery |

REPAIR ARTERIOVENOUS FISTULA

35180	Repair, congenital arteriovenous fistula; head and neck
35182	thorax and abdomen
35184	extremities
35188	Repair, acquired or traumatic arteriovenous fistula; head and neck
35189	thorax and abdomen
35190	extremities

REPAIR BLOOD VESSEL OTHER THAN FOR FISTULA, WITH OR WITHOUT PATCH ANGIOPLASTY

(For AV fistula repair, see 35180-35190)

| 35201 | Repair blood vessel, direct; neck |

(Do not report 35201 in conjunction with 33969, 33984, 33985, 33986)

| 35206 | upper extremity |

(Do not report 35206 in conjunction with 33969, 33984, 33985, 33986)

| 35207 | hand, finger |
| 35211 | intrathoracic, with bypass |

(Do not report 35211 in conjunction with 33969, 33984, 33985, 33986)

| 35216 | intrathoracic, without bypass |

(Do not report 35216 in conjunction with 33969, 33984, 33985, 33986)

| 35221 | intra-abdominal |
| 35226 | lower extremity |

(Do not report 35226 in conjunction with 33969, 33984, 33985, 33986)

35231	Repair blood vessel with vein graft; neck
35236	upper extremity
35241	intrathoracic, with bypass
35246	intrathoracic, without bypass
35251	intra-abdominal
35256	lower extremity
35261	Repair blood vessel with graft other than vein; neck
35266	upper extremity
35271	intrathoracic, with bypass

35276   intrathoracic, without bypass

35281   intra-abdominal

35286   lower extremity

THROMBOENDARTERECTOMY

(For coronary artery, see 33510-33536 and 33572)

(35301-35372 include harvest of saphenous or upper extremity vein when performed)

35301   Thromboendarterectomy, including patch graft, if performed; carotid, vertebral, subclavian, by neck incision

35302   superficial femoral artery

35303   popliteal artery

(Do not report 35302, 35303 in conjunction with 37225, 37227 when performed in the same vessel)

35304   tibioperoneal trunk artery

35305   tibial or peroneal artery, initial vessel

+ **35306**   each additional tibial or peroneal artery (List separately in addition to code for primary procedure)

(Use 35306 in conjunction with 35305)

(Do not report 35304, 35305, 35306 in conjunction with 37229, 37231, 37233, 37235 when performed in the same vessel)

35311   subclavian, innominate, by thoracic incision

35321   axillary-brachial

35331   abdominal aorta

35341   mesenteric, celiac, or renal

35351   iliac

35355   iliofemoral

35361   combined aortoiliac

35363   combined aortoiliofemoral

35371   common femoral

35372   deep (profunda) femoral

+ **35390**   Reoperation, carotid, thromboendarterectomy, more than 1 month after original operation (List separately in addition to code for primary procedure)

(Use 35390 in conjunction with code 35301)

ANGIOSCOPY

+ **35400**   Angioscopy (non-coronary vessels or grafts) during therapeutic intervention (List separately in addition to code for primary procedure)

● New Code   ▲ Revised Code   ✛ Add-On Code   ⦸ Modifier -51 Exempt   ★ Telemedicine

BYPASS GRAFT

Peripheral vascular bypass CPT codes describe bypass procedures using venous grafts (CPT codes 35500-35587) and using other types of bypass procedures (arterial reconstruction, composite). Because, at a given site of obstruction, only one type of bypass is performed, these groups of codes are mutually exclusive. When different sites are treated with different bypass procedures in the same operative session, the different bypass procedures may be separately reported, using an anatomic modifier or modifier -59.

Procurement of the saphenous vein graft is included in the description of the work for 35501-35587 and should not be reported as a separate service or co-surgery. To report harvesting of an upper extremity vein, use 35500 in addition to the bypass procedure. To report harvesting of a femoropopliteal vein segment, use 35572 in addition to the bypass procedure. To report harvesting and construction of an autogenous composite graft of two segments from two distant locations, report 35682 in addition to the bypass procedure, for autogenous composite of three or more segments from distant sites, report 35683.

Vein

+ **35500**   Harvest of upper extremity vein, 1 segment, for lower extremity or coronary artery bypass procedure (List separately in addition to code for primary procedure)

   (Use 35500 in conjunction with 33510-33536, 35556, 35566, 35570, 35571, 35583-35587)

   (For harvest of more than one vein segment, see 35682, 35683)

   (For endoscopic procedure, use 33508)

35501   Bypass graft, with vein; common carotid-ipsilateral internal carotid

35506   carotid-subclavian or subclavian-carotid

35508   carotid-vertebral

35509   carotid-contralateral carotid

35510   carotid-brachial

35511   subclavian-subclavian

35512   subclavian-brachial

35515   subclavian-vertebral

35516   subclavian-axillary

35518   axillary-axillary

35521   axillary-femoral

   (For bypass graft performed with synthetic graft, use 35621)

35522   axillary-brachial

35523   brachial-ulnar or -radial

   (Do not report 35523 in conjunction with 35206, 35500, 35525, 36838)

   (For bypass graft performed with synthetic conduit, use 37799)

35525   brachial-brachial

35526   aortosubclavian, aortoinnominate, or aortocarotid

   (For bypass graft performed with synthetic graft, use 35626)

35531	aortoceliac or aortomesenteric

35533	axillary-femoral-femoral

(For bypass graft performed with synthetic graft, use 35654)

35535	hepatorenal

(Do not report 35535 in conjunction with 35221, 35251, 35281, 35500, 35536, 35560, 35631, 35636)

35536	splenorenal

35537	aortoiliac

(For bypass graft performed with synthetic graft, use 35637)

(Do not report 35537 in conjunction with 35538)

35538	aortobi-iliac

(For bypass graft performed with synthetic graft, use 35638)

(Do not report 35538 in conjunction with 35537)

35539	aortofemoral

(For bypass graft performed with synthetic graft, use 35647)

(Do not report 35539 in conjunction with 35540)

35540	aortobifemoral

(For bypass graft performed with synthetic graft, use 35646)

(Do not report 35540 in conjunction with 35539)

35556	femoral-popliteal

35558	femoral-femoral

35560	aortorenal

35563	ilioiliac

35565	iliofemoral

35566	femoral-anterior tibial, posterior tibial, peroneal artery or other distal vessels

35570	tibial-tibial, peroneal-tibial, or tibial/peroneal trunk-tibial

(Do not report 35570 in conjunction with 35256, 35286)

35571	popliteal-tibial, -peroneal artery or other distal vessels

+ 35572 Harvest of femoropopliteal vein, 1 segment, for vascular reconstruction procedure (eg, aortic, vena caval, coronary, peripheral artery) (List separately in addition to code for primary procedure)

(Use 35572 in conjunction with codes 33510-33516, 33517-33523, 33533-33536, 34502, 34520, 35001, 35002, 35011-35022, 35102, 35103, 35121-35152, 35231-35256, 35501-35587, 35879-35907)

(For bilateral procedure, report 35572 twice. Do not report modifier 50 in conjunction with 35572)

● New Code   ▲ Revised Code   ✛ Add-On Code   ⊘ Modifier -51 Exempt   ★ Telemedicine

In-Situ Vein

(To report aortobifemoral bypass using synthetic conduit, and femoral-popliteal bypass with vein conduit in situ, use 35646 and 35583. To report aorto(uni)femoral bypass with synthetic conduit, and femoral-popliteal bypass with vein conduit in-situ, use 35647 and 35583. To report aortofemoral bypass using vein conduit, and femoral-popliteal bypass with vein conduit in situ, use 35539 and 35583)

35583 In-situ vein bypass; femoral-popliteal

35585 femoral-anterior tibial, posterior tibial, or peroneal artery

35587 popliteal-tibial, peroneal

Other Than Vein

(For aterial transposition and/or reimplantation, see 35691-35695)

+ 35600 Harvest of upper extremity artery, 1 segment, for coronary artery bypass procedure (List separately in addition to code for primary procedure)

(Use 35600 in conjunction with 33533-33536)

35601 Bypass graft, with other than vein; common carotid-ipsilateral internal carotid

35606 carotid-subclavian

(For open transcervical common carotid-common carotid bypass performed in conjunction with endovascular repair of descending thoracic aorta, use 33891)

(For open subclavian to carotid artery transposition performed in conjunction with endovascular thoracic aneurysm repair by neck incision, use 33889)

35612 subclavian-subclavian

35616 subclavian-axillary

35621 axillary-femoral

35623 axillary-popliteal or -tibial

35626 aortosubclavian, aortoinnominate, or aortocarotid

35631 aortoceliac, aortomesenteric, aortorenal

35632 ilio-celiac

(Do not report 35632 in conjunction with 35221, 35251, 35281, 35531, 35631)

35633 ilio-mesenteric

(Do not report 35633 in conjunction with 35221, 35251, 35281, 35531, 35631)

35634 iliorenal

(Do not report 35634 in conjunction with 35221, 35251, 35281, 35560, 35536, 35631)

35636 splenorenal (splenic to renal arterial anastomosis)

35637 aortoiliac

(Do not report 35637 in conjunction with 35638, 35646)

35638 aortobi-iliac

(Do not report 35638 in conjunction with 35637, 35646)

(For open placement of aorto-bi-iliac prosthesis following unsuccessful endovascular repair, use 34831)

35642   carotid-vertebral

35645   subclavian-vertebral

35646   aortobifemoral

(For bypass graft performed with vein graft, use 35540)

(For open placement of aortobifemoral prosthesis following unsuccessful endovascular repair, use 34832)

35647   aortofemoral

(For bypass graft performed with vein graft, use 35539)

35650   axillary-axillary

35654   axillary-femoral-femoral

35656   femoral-popliteal

35661   femoral-femoral

35663   ilioiliac

35665   iliofemoral

35666   femoral-anterior tibial, posterior tibial, or peroneal artery

35671   popliteal-tibial or -peroneal artery

COMPOSITE GRAFTS

Codes 35682, 35683 are used to report harvest and anastomosis of multiple vein segments from distant sites for use as arterial bypass graft conduits. These codes are intended for use when the two or more vein segments are harvested from a limb other than that undergoing bypass.

+ **35681**   Bypass graft; composite, prosthetic and vein (List separately in addition to code for primary procedure)

        (Do not report 35681 in addition to 35682, 35683)

+ **35682**   autogenous composite, 2 segments of veins from 2 locations (List separately in addition to code for primary procedure)

        (Use 35682 in conjunction with 35556, 35566, 35570, 35571, 35583-35587)

        (Do not report 35682 in addition to 35681, 35683)

+ **35683**   autogenous composite, 3 or more segments of vein from 2 or more locations (List separately in addition to code for primary procedure)

        (Use 35683 in conjunction with 35556, 35566, 35570, 35571, 35583-35587)

        (Do not report 35683 in addition to 35681, 35682)

ADJUVANT TECHNIQUES

Adjuvant (additional) technique(s) may be required at the time a bypass graft is created to improve patency of the lower extremity autogenous or synthetic bypass graft (eg., femoral-popliteal, femoral-tibial, or popliteal-tibial arteries). Code 35685 should be reported in addition to the primary synthetic bypass graft procedure, when an interposition of venous tissue (vein patch or cuff) is placed at the anastomosis between the synthetic bypass conduit and the involved artery (includes harvest).

   ● New Code   ▲ Revised Code   + Add-On Code   ⊘ Modifier -51 Exempt   ★ Telemedicine

Code 35686 should be reported in addition to the primary bypass graft procedure, when autogenous vein is used to create a fistula between the tibial or peroneal artery and vein at or beyond the distal bypass anastomosis site of the involved artery.

(For composite graft(s), see 35681-35683)

+ **35685** Placement of vein patch or cuff at distal anastomosis of bypass graft, synthetic conduit (List separately in addition to code for primary procedure)

(Use 35685 in conjunction with codes 35656, 35666 or 35671)

+ **35686** Creation of distal arteriovenous fistula during lower extremity bypass surgery (non-hemodialysis) (List separately in addition to code for primary procedure)

(Use 35686 in conjunction with 35556, 35566, 35570, 35571, 35583-35587, 35623, 35656, 35666, 35671)

ARTERIAL TRANSPOSITION

35691 Transposition and/or reimplantation; vertebral to carotid artery

35693 vertebral to subclavian artery

35694 subclavian to carotid artery

(For open subclavian to carotid artery transposition performed in conjunction with endovascular repair of descending thoracic aorta, use 33889)

35695 carotid to subclavian artery

+ **35697** Reimplantation, visceral artery to infrarenal aortic prosthesis, each artery (List separately in addition to code for primary procedure)

(Do not report 35697 in conjunction with 33877)

EXCISION, EXPLORATION, REPAIR, REVISION

+ **35700** Reoperation, femoral-popliteal or femoral (popliteal)-anterior tibial, posterior tibial, peroneal artery or other distal vessels, more than 1 month after original operation (List separately in addition to code for primary procedure)

(Use 35700 in conjunction with codes 35556, 35566, 35570, 35571, 35583, 35585, 35587, 35656, 35666, 35671)

35701 Exploration not followed by surgical repair, artery; neck (eg, carotid, subclavian)

(Do not report 35701 in conjunction with 35201, 35231, 35261, 35800, when performed on the same side of the neck)

35702 upper extremity (eg, axillary, brachial, radial, ulnar)

35703 lower extremity (eg, common femoral, deep femoral, superficial femoral, popliteal, tibial, peroneal)

(When additional surgical procedures are performed at the same setting by the same surgeon, 35701, 35702, 35703 may only be reported when a nonvascular surgical procedure is performed and only when the artery exploration is performed through a separate incision)

(Do not report 35702, 35703 in conjunction with 35206, 35207, 35236, 35256, 35266, 35286, 35860 in the same extremity)

(Do not report 35701, 35702, 35703 to explore and identify a recipient artery [eg, external carotid artery] when performed in conjunction with 15756, 15757, 15758, 20955, 20956, 20957, 20962, 20969, 20970, 20972, 20973, 43496, 49906)

(**35721** deleted 2019 [2020 Edition])

(**35741** deleted 2019 [2020 Edition])

(To report exploration of lower extremity artery, use 35703)

(**35761** deleted 2019 [2020 Edition])

(To report vascular exploration not followed by surgical repair, other than neck artery, upper extremity artery, lower extremity artery, chest, abdomen, or retroperitoneal area, use 37799)

(For vascular exploration of the chest not followed by surgical repair, use 32100)

(For vascular exploration of the abdomen not followed by surgical repair, use 49000)

(For vascular exploration of the retroperitoneal area not followed by surgical repair, use 49010)

35800 Exploration for postoperative hemorrhage, thrombosis or infection; neck

35820 chest

35840 abdomen

35860 extremity

35870 Repair of graft-enteric fistula

35875 Thrombectomy of arterial or venous graft (other than hemodialysis graft or fistula);

35876 with revision of arterial or venous graft

(For thrombectomy of hemodialysis graft or fistula, see 36831, 36833)

Codes 35879 and 35881 describe open revision of graft-threatening stenoses of lower extremity arterial bypass graft(s) (previously constructed with autogenous vein conduit) using vein patch angioplasty or segmental vein interposition techniques. For thrombectomy with revision of any non-coronary arterial or venous graft, including those of the lower extremity, (other than hemodialysis graft or fistula), use 35876. For direct repair (other than for fistula) of a lower extremity blood vessel (with or without patch angioplasty), use 35226. For repair (other than for fistula) of a lower extremity blood vessel using a vein graft, use 35256.

35879 Revision, lower extremity arterial bypass, without thrombectomy, open; with vein patch angioplasty

35881 with segmental vein interposition

(For revision or femoral anastomosis of sythetic arterial bypass graft, see 35883, 35884)

(For excision of infected graft, see 35901-35907 and appropriate revascularization code)

35883 Revision, femoral anastomosis of synthetic arterial bypass graft in groin, open; with nonautogenous patch graft (eg, Dacron, ePTFE, bovine pericardium)

(For bilateral procedure, use modifier 50)

(Do not report 35883 in conjunction with 35700, 35875, 35876, 35884)

35884 with autogenous vein patch graft

(For bilateral procedure, use modifier -50)

(Do not report 35884 in conjunction with 35700, 35875, 35876, 35883)

35901 Excision of infected graft; neck

35903 extremity

35905 thorax

35907 abdomen

● New Code ▲ Revised Code + Add-On Code ⊘ Modifier -51 Exempt ★ Telemedicine

VASCULAR INJECTION PROCEDURES

Listed services for injection procedures include necessary local anesthesia, introduction of needles or catheter, injection of contrast media with or without automatic power injection, and/or necessary pre- and post-injection care specifically related to the injection procedure.

Catheters, drugs, and contrast media are not included in the listed service for the injection procedures.

Selective vascular catheterization should be coded to include introduction and all lesser order selective catheterization used in the approach (eg., the description for a selective right middle cerebral artery catheterization includes the introduction and placement catheterization of the right common and internal carotid arteries).

Additional second and/or third order arterial catheterization within the same family of arteries or veins supplied by a single first order vessel should be expressed by 36012, 36218, or 36248.

Additional first order or higher catheterization in vascular families supplied by a first order vessel different from a previously selected and coded family should be separately coded using the conventions described above.

> (For radiological supervision and interpretation, see RADIOLOGY)
>
> (For injection procedures in conjunction with cardiac catheterization, see 93452-93461, 93563-93568)
>
> (For chemotherapy of malignant disease, see 96400-96549)

Intravenous

36000 Introduction of needle or intracatheter, vein

36002 Injection procedures (eg, thrombin) for percutaneous treatment of extremity pseudoaneurysm

> (For imaging guidance, see 76942, 77002, 77012, 77021)
>
> (For ultrasound guided compression repair of pseudoaneurysms, use 76936)
>
> (Do not report 36002 for vascular sealant of an arteriotomy site)

36005 Injection procedure for extremity venography (including introduction of needle or intracatheter)

> (For radiological supervision and interpretation, see 75820, 75822)

36010 Introduction of catheter, superior or inferior vena cava

36011 Selective catheter placement, venous system; first order branch (eg, renal vein, jugular vein)

36012   second order, or more selective, branch (eg, left adrenal vein, petrosal sinus)

36013 Introduction of catheter, right heart or main pulmonary artery

36014 Selective catheter placement, left or right pulmonary artery

36015 Selective catheter placement, segmental or subsegmental pulmonary artery

> (For insertion of flow directed catheter (eg, Swan-Ganz), use 93503)
>
> (For venous catheterization for selective organ blood sampling, use 36500)

Intra-Arterial/Intra-Aortic

> (For radiological supervision and interpretation, see RADIOLOGY)

36100 Introduction of needle or intracatheter, carotid or vertebral artery

> (For bilateral procedure, report 36100 with modifier -50)

(**36120**   deleted 2017 [2018 edition])

36140 Introduction of needle or intracatheter, upper or lower extremity artery

(For insertion of arteriovenous cannula, see 36810-36821)

36160 Introduction of needle or intracatheter, aortic, translumbar

Diagnostic Studies of Cervicocerebral Arteries

Codes 36221-36228 describe non-selective and selective arterial catheter placement and diagnostic imaging of the aortic arch, carotid, and vertebral arterial. Codes 36221-36226 include the work of accessing the vessel, placement of catheter(s), contrast injection(s), fluoroscopy, radiological supervision and interpretation, and closure of the arteriotomy by pressure, or application of an arterial closure device. Codes 36221-36228 describe arterial contrast injections with arterial, capillary, and venous phase imaging, when performed.

Code 36227 is an add-on code to report unilateral selective arterial catheter placement and diagnostic imaging of the ipsilateral external carotid circulation and includes all the work of accessing the additional vessel, placement of catheter(s), contrast injection(s), fluoroscopy, radiological supervision and interpretation. Code 36227 is reported in conjunction with 36222, 36223, or 36224.

Code 36228 is an add-on code to report unilateral selective arterial catheter placement and diagnostic imaging of the initial and each additional intracranial branch of the internal carotid or vertebral arteries. Code 36228 is reported in conjunction with 36223, 36224, 36225 or 36226. This includes any additional second or third order catheter selective placement in the same primary branch of the internal carotid, vertebral, or basilar artery and includes all the work of accessing the additional vessel, placement of catheter(s), contrast injection(s), fluoroscopy, radiological supervision and interpretation. It is not reported more than twice per side regardless of the number of additional branches selectively catheterized.

Codes 36221-36226 are built on progressive hierarchies with more intensive services inclusive of less intensive services. The code inclusive of all the services provided for that vessel should be reported (ie, use the code inclusive of the most intensive services provided). Only one code in the range 36222-36224 may be reported for each ipsilateral carotid territory. Only one code in the range 36225-36226 may be reported for each ipsilateral vertebral territory.

Code 36221 is reported for non-selective arterial catheter placement in the thoracic aorta and diagnostic imaging of the aortic arch and great vessel origins. Codes 36222-36228 are reported for unilateral artery catheterization. Do not report 36221 in conjunction with 36222-36226 as these selective codes include the work of 36221 when performed.

Do not report 36222, 36223, or 36224 together for ipsilateral angiography. Instead, select the code that represents the most comprehensive service using the following hierarchy of complexity (listed in descending order of complexity): 36224>36223>36222.

Do not report 36225 and 36226 together for ipsilateral angiography. Select the code that represents the more comprehensive service using the following hierarchy of complexity (listed in descending order of complexity): 36226>36225.

When bilateral carotid and/or vertebral arterial catheterization and imaging is performed, report 36222, 36223, 36224, 36225, 36226 with modifier 50, and report add-on codes 36227, 36228 twice (do not report modifier 50 in conjunction with 36227, 36228) if the same procedure is performed on both sides. For example, bilateral extracranial carotid angiography with selective catheterization of each common carotid artery would be reported with 36222 and modifier 50. However, when different territory(ies) is studied in the same session on both sides of the body, modifiers may be required to report the imaging performed. Use modifier 59 to denote that different carotid and/or vertebral arteries are being studied. For example, when selective right internal carotid artery catheterization accompanied by right extracranial and intracranial carotid angiography is followed by selective left common carotid artery catheterization with left extracranial carotid angiography, use 36224 to report the right side and 36222-59 to report the left side.

Diagnostic angiography of the cervicocerebral vessels may be followed by an interventional procedure at the same session. Interventional procedure may be separately reportable using standard coding conventions.

Do not report 36218 or 75774 as part of diagnostic angiography of the extracranial and intracranial cervicocerebral vessels. It may be appropriate to report 36218 or 75774 for diagnostic angiography of upper extremities and other vascular beds of the neck and/or shoulder girdle performed in the same session as vertibral angiography (eg, workup of a neck tumor that requires catheterization and angiography of the vertebral artery as well as other brachiocephalic arteries).

Report 76376 or 76377 for 3D rendering when performed in conjunction with 36221-36228.

Report 76937 for ultrasound guidance for vascular access, when performed in conjunction with 36221-36228.

36200 Introduction of catheter, aorta

(For non-selective angiography of the extracranial carotid and/or cerebral vessels adn cervicocerebral arch, when performed, use 36221)

36215 Selective catheter placement, arterial system; each first order thoracic or brachiocephalic branch, within a vascular family

(For catheter placement for coronary angiography, see 93454-93961)

36216 initial second order thoracic or brachiocephalic branch, within a vascular family

36217 initial third order or more selective thoracic or brachiocephalic branch, within a vascular family

+ 36218 additional second order, third order, and beyond, thoracic or brachiocephalic branch, within a vascular family (List in addition to code for initial second or third order vessel as appropriate)

(Use 36218 in conjunction with 36216, 36217, 36225, 36226)

(For angiography, see 36222-36228, 75600-75774)

(For transluminal balloon angioplasty [except lower extremity artery[ies] for occlusive disease, intracranial, coronary, pulmonary, or dialysis circuit], see 37246, 37247)

(For transcatheter therapies, see 37200, 37211, 37213, 37214, 37236, 37237, 37238, 37239, 37241, 37242, 37243, 37244, 61624, 61626)

(When coronary artery, arterial conduit [eg., internal mammary, inferior epigastric or free radical artery] or venous bypass graft angiography is performed in conjunction with cardiac catheterization, see the appropriate cardiac catheterization, injection procedure, and imaging supervision code(s) [93455, 93457, 93459, 93461, 93530-93533, 93564] in the **Medicine** section of CPT. When internal mammary artery angiography only is performed without a concomitant cardiac catheterization, use 36216 or 36217 as appropriate.)

36221 Non-selective catheter placement, thoracic aorta, with angiography of the extracranial carotid, vertebral, and/or intracranial vessels, unilateral or bilateral, and all associated radiological supervision and interpretation, includes angiography of the cervicocerebral arch, when performed

(Do not report 36221 with 36222-36226)

36222 Selective catheter placement, common carotid or innominate artery, unilateral, any approach, with angiography of the ipsilateral extracranial carotid circulation and all associated radiological supervision and interpretation, includes angiography of the cervicocerebral arch, when performed

(Do not report 36222 in conjunction with 37215, 37216, 37218 for the treated carotic artery)

36223 Selective catheter placement, common carotid or innominate artery, unilateral, any approach, with angiography of the ipsilateral intracranial carotid circulation and all associated radiological supervision and interpretation, includes angiography of the extracranial carotid and cervicocerebral arch, when performed

(Do not report 36223 in conjunction with 37215, 37216, 37218 for the treated carotic artery)

36224 Selective catheter placement, internal carotid artery, unilateral, with angiography of the ipsilateral intracranial carotid circulation and all associated radiological supervision and interpretation, includes angiography of the extracranial carotid and cervicocerebral arch, when performed

(Do not report 36224 in conjunction with 37215, 37216, 37218 for the treated carotic artery)

36225 Selective catheter placement, subclavian or innominate artery, unilateal with angiography of the ipsilateral vertebral circulation and allassociated radiological supervision and interpretation, includes angiography of the cervicocerebral arch, when performed

36226 Selective catheter placement, vertebral artery, unilateral, with angiography of the ipsilateral vertebral circulation and all associated radiological supervision and interpretation, includes angiography of the cervicocerebral arch, when performed

+ 36227 Selective catheter placement, external carotid artery, unilateral, with angiography of the ipsilateral external carotid circulation and all associated radiological supervision and interpretation (List separately in addition to code for primary procedure)

(Use 36227 in conjunction with 36222, 36223 or 36224)

(Do not report 36221-36227 in conjunction with 37217 for ipsilateral services)

+ 36228 Selective catheter placement, each intracranial branch of the internal carotid or vertebral arteries, unilateral, with angiography of the selected vessel circulation and all associated radiological supervision adn interpretation (eg, middle cerebral artery, posterior inferior cerebellar artery) (List separately in addition to code for primary procedure)

(Use 36228 in conjunction with 36223, 36224, 36225 or 36226)

(Do not report 36228 more than twice per side)

36245 Selective catheter placement, arterial system; each first order abdominal, pelvic, or lower extremity artery branch, within a vascular family

36246 initial second order abdominal, pelvic, or lower extremity artery branch, within a vascular family

36247 initial third order or more selective abdominal, pelvic, or lower extremity artery branch, within a vascular family

+ 36248 additional second order, third order, and beyond, abdominal, pelvic, or lower extremity artery branch, within a vascular family (List in addition to code for initial second or third order vessel as appropriate)

(Use 36248 in conjunction with codes 36246, 36247)

36251 Selective catheter placement (first-order), main renal artery and any accessory renal artery(s) for renal angiography, including arterial puncture and catheter placement(s), fluoroscopy, contrast injection(s), image postprocessing, permanent recording of images, and radiological supervision and interpretation, including pressure gradient measurements when performed, and flush aortogram when performed; unilateral

36252 bilateral

36253 Superselective catheter placement (one or more second order or higher renal artery branches) renal artery and any accessory renal artery(s) for renal angiography, including arterial puncture, catheterization, fluoroscopy, contrast injection(s), image postprocessing, permanent recording of images, and radiological supervision and interpretation, including pressure gradient measurements when performed, and flush aortogram when performed; unilateral

(Do not report 36253 in conjunction with 36251 when performed for the same kidney)

36254 bilateral

(Do not report 36254 in conjunction with 36252)

(Placement of closure device at the vascular access site is not separately reported with 36251-36254)

(Do not report 36251, 36252, 36253, 36254 in conjunction with 0338T, 0339T)

36260 Insertion of implantable intra-arterial infusion pump (eg, for chemotherapy of liver)

36261 Revision of implanted intra-arterial infusion pump

36262 Removal of implanted intra-arterial infusion pump

36299 Unlisted procedure, vascular injection

● New Code ▲ Revised Code + Add-On Code ⊘ Modifier -51 Exempt ★ Telemedicine

Venous

Venipuncture, needle or catheter for diagnostic study or intravenous therapy, percutaneous. These codes are also used to report the therapy as specified. For collection of a specimen from an established catheter, use 36592. For collection of a specimen from a completely implantable venous access device, use 36591.

36400 Venipuncture, younger than age 3 years, necessitating the skill of a physician or other qualified health care professional, not to be used for routine venipuncture; femoral or jugular vein

36405 scalp vein

36406 other vein

36410 Venipuncture, age 3 years or older, necessitating the skill of a physician or other qualified health care professional (separate procedure), for diagnostic or therapeutic purposes (not to be used for routine venipuncture)

36415 Collection of venous blood by venipuncture

(Do not report modifier 63 in conjunction with 36415)

36416 Collection of capillary blood specimen (eg, finger, heel, ear stick)

36420 Venipuncture, cutdown; under age 1 year

(Do not report modifier 63 in conjunction with 36420)

36425 age 1 or over

(Do not report 36425 in conjunction with 36475, 36476, 36478)

36430 Transfusion, blood or blood components

(When a partial exchange transfusion is performed in a newborn, use 36456)

36440 Push transfusion, blood, 2 years or under

(When a partial exchange transfusion is performed in a newborn, use 36456)

36450 Exchange transfusion, blood; newborn

(When a partial exchange transfusion is performed in a newborn, use 36456)

(Do not report modifier 63 in conjunction with 36450)

(For manual red cell exchange, see 36450, 36455, 36456)

(For automated red cell exchange, use 36512)

36455 other than newborn

36456 Partial exchange transfusion, blood, plasma or crystalloid necessitating the skill of a physician or other qualified health care professional, newborn

(Do not report 36456 in conjunction with 36430, 36440, 36450)

(Do not report modifier 63 in conjunction with 36456)

36460 Transfusion, intrauterine, fetal

(Do not report modifier 63 in conjunction with 36460)

(For radiological supervision and interpretation, use 76941)

Separate Procedure ▪ Unlisted Procedure ▪ CCI Comp. Code ▪ Non-specific Procedure **425**

Codes 36468, 36470, 36471 describe injection(s) of a sclerosant for sclerotherapy of telangiectasia and/or incompetent vein(s). Code 36468 may only be reported once per extremity per session, regardless of the number of needle injections performed. Codes 36466, 36471 may only be reported once per extremity, regardless of the number of veins treated. Ultrasound guidance (76942), when performed, is not included in 36468, 36470, 36471 and may be reported separately.

Codes 36465, 36466 describe injection(s) of a noncompounded foam sclerosant into an extremity truncal vein (eg, great saphenous vein, accessory saphenous vein) using ultrasound-guided compression of the junction of the central vein (saphenofemoral junction or saphenopopliteal junction) to limit the dispersion of injectate. Do not report 36465, 36466 for injection of compounded foam sclerosant(s).

Compounding is a practice in which a qualified health care professional (eg, pharmacist, physician) combines, mixes, or alters ingredients of a drug to create a medication tailored to the needs of an individual patient.

When performed in the office setting, all required supplies and equipment are included in 36465, 36466, 36468, 36470, 36471 and may not be separately reported. In addition, application of compression dressing(s) (eg, compression bandages/stockings) is included in 36465, 36466, 36468, 36470, 36471, when performed, and may not be reported separately.

36465 This code is out of order. See page 426

36466 This code is out of order. See page 426

36468 Injection(s) of sclerosant for spider veins (telangiectasia), limb or trunk

(For ultrasound imaging guidance performed in conjunction with 36468, use 76942)

(Do not report 36468 in conjunction with 29520, 29530, 29540, 29550, 29580, 29581, 29584, for the same extremity)

(Do not report 36468 more than once per extremity)

(Do not report 36468 in conjunction with 37241 in the same surgical field)

36470 Injection of sclerosant; single incompetent vein (other than telangiectasia)

36471 multiple incompetent veins (other than telangiectasia), same leg

(For ultrasound imaging guidance performed in conjunction with 36470, 36471, use 76942)

(Do not report 36470, 36471 in conjunction with 29520, 29530, 29540, 29550, 29580, 29581, 29584, for the same extremity)

(Do not report 36471 more than once per extremity)

(If the targeted vein is an extremity truncal vein and injection of non-compounded foam sclerosant with ultrasound guided compression maneuvers to guide dispersion of the injectate is performed, see 36465, 36466)

(Do not report 36470, 36471 in conjunction with 37241 in the same surgical field)

36465 Injection of non-compounded foam sclerosant with ultrasound compression maneuvers to guide dispersion of the injectate, inclusive of all imaging guidance and monitoring; single incompetent extremity truncal vein (eg, great saphenous vein, accessory saphenous vein)

36466 multiple incompetent truncal veins (eg, great saphenous vein, accessory saphenous vein), same leg

(Do not report 36465, 36466 in conjunction with 29520, 29530, 29540, 29550, 29580, 29581, 29584, for the same extremity)

(Do not report 36465, 36466 in conjunction with 37241 in the same surgical field)

(For extremity truncal vein injection of compounded foam sclerosant[s], see 36470, 36471)

(For injection of a sclerosant into an incompetent vein without compression maneuvers to guide dispersion of the injectate, see 36470, 36471)

(For endovenous ablation therapy of incompetent vein[s] by transcatheter delivery of a chemical adhesive, see 36482, 36483)

(For vascular embolization and occlusion procedures, see 37241, 37242, 37243, 37244)

Codes 36473, 36474, 36475, 36476, 36478, 36479, 36482, 36483 describe endovascular ablation therapy of incompetent extremity vein(s), including all necessary imaging guidance and monitoring. Sclerosant injection(s) of vein(s) by needle or mini-catheter (36468, 36470, 36471) followed by a compression technique is not endovascular ablation therapy. Codes 36473, 36474, 36482, 36483 can be performed under local anesthesia without the need for tumescent (peri-saphenous) anesthesia. Codes 36475, 36476, 36478, 36479 are performed using adjunctive tumescent anesthesia.

Codes 36473, 36474 involve concomitant use of an intraluminal device that mechanically disrupts/abrades the venous intima and infusion of a physician-specified medication in the target vein(s).

Codes 36482, 36483 involve positioning an intravenous catheter the length of an incompetent vein, remote from the percutaneous access site, with subsequent delivery of a chemical adhesive to ablate the incompetent vein. This often includes ultrasound compression of the outflow vein to limit the dispersion of the injected solution.

Codes 36475, 36476 involve advancing a radiofrequency device the length of an incompetent vein, with subsequent delivery of radiofrequency energy to ablate the incompetent vein.

Codes 36478, 36479 involve advancing a laser device the length of an incompetent vein, with subsequent delivery of thermal energy to ablate the incompetent vein.

Codes 36474, 36476, 36479, 36483 for subsequent vein(s) treated in the same extremity may only be reported once per extremity, regardless of the number of additional vein(s) treated.

When performed in the office setting, all required supplies and equipment are included in 36473, 36474, 36475, 36476, 36478, 36479, 36482, 36483 and may not be separately reported. In addition, application of compression dressing(s) (eg, compression bandages/stockings) is included in 36473, 36474, 36475, 36476, 36478, 36479, 36482, 36483, when performed, and may not be reported separately.

36473 Endovenous ablation therapy of incompetent vein, extremity, inclusive of all imaging guidance and monitoring, percutaneous, mechanochemical; first vein treated

+ 36474 subsequent vein(s) treated in a single extremity, each through separate access sites (List separately in addition to code for primary procedure)

(Use 36474 in conjunction with 36473)

(Do not report 36474 more than once per extremity)

(Do not report 36473, 36474 in conjunction with 29520, 29530, 29540, 29550, 29580, 29581, 29584, for the same extremity)

(Do not report 36473, 36474 in conjunction with 36000, 36002, 36005, 36410, 36425, 36475, 36476, 36478, 36479, 37241, 75894, 76000, 76937, 76942, 76998, 77022, 93970, 93971, in the same surgical field)

36475 Endovenous ablation therapy of incompetent vein, extremity, inclusive of all imaging guidance and monitoring, percutaneous, radiofrequency; first vein treated

+ 36476 subsequent vein(s) treated in a single extremity, each through separate access sites (list separately in addition to code for primary procedure)

(Use 36476 in conjunction with 36475)

(Do not report 36476 more than once per extremity)

(Do not report 36475, 36476 in conjunction with 29520, 29530, 29540, 29550, 29580, 29581, 29584, for the same extremity)

(Do not report 36475, 36476 in conjunction with 36000, 36002, 36005, 36410, 36425, 36478, 36479, 36482, 36483, 37241-37244, 75894, 76000, 76937, 76942, 76998, 77022, 93970, 93971, in the same surgical field)

36478 Endovenous ablation therapy of incompetent vein, extremity, inclusive of all imaging guidance and monitoring, percutaneous, laser; first vein treated

+ 36479 subsequent vein(s) treated in a single extremity, each through separate access sites (List separately in addition to code for primary procedure)

(Use 36479 in conjunction with 36478)

(Do not report 36479 more than once per extremity)

(Do not report 36478, 36479 in conjunction with 29520, 29530, 29540, 29550, 29580, 29581, 29584, for the same extremity)

(Do not report 36478, 36479 in conjunction with 36000, 36002, 36005, 36410, 36425, 36475, 36476, 36482, 36483, 37241, 75894, 76000, 76937, 76942, 76998, 77022, 93970, 93971, in the same surgical field)

36482 Endovenous ablation therapy of incompetent vein, extremity, by transcatheter delivery of a chemical adhesive (eg, cyanoacrylate) remote from the access site, inclusive of all imaging guidance and monitoring, percutaneous; first vein treated

+ 36483 subsequent vein(s) treated in a single extremity, each through separate access sites (List separately in addition to code for primary procedure)

(Use 36483 in conjunction with 36482)

(Do not report 36483 more than once per extremity)

(Do not report 36482, 36483 in conjunction with 29520, 29530, 29540, 29550, 29580, 29581, 29584, for the same extremity)

(Do not report 36482, 36483 in conjunction with 36000, 36002, 36005, 36410, 36425, 36475, 36476, 36478, 36479, 37241, 75894, 76000, 76937, 76942, 76998, 77022, 93970, 93971, in the same surgical field)

36481 Percutaneous portal vein catheterization by any method

36482 This code is out of order. See page 428

36483 This code is out of order. See page 428

(For radiological supervision and interpretation, see 75885, 75887)

36500 Venous catheterization for selective organ blood sampling

(For catheterization in superior or inferior vena cava, use 36010)

(For radiological supervision and interpretation, use 75893)

36510 Catheterization of umbilical vein for diagnosis or therapy, newborn

(Do not report modifier '-63' in conjunction with 36510)

36511 Therapeutic apheresis; for white blood cells

36512 for red blood cells

(For manual red cell exchange, see 36450, 36455, 36456)

(For automated red cell exchange, use 36512)

36513 for platelets

(Report 36513 only when platelets are removed by apheresis for treatment of the patient. Do not report 36513 for donor platelet collections)

● New Code   ▲ Revised Code   + Add-On Code   ⊘ Modifier -51 Exempt   ★ Telemedicine

36514   for plasma pheresis

(**36515**   deleted 2017 [2018 edition]. For therapeutic aphaeresis with extracorporeal immunoadsorption and plasma rein fusion, use 36516)

36516   with extracorporeal immunoadsorption, selective adsorption or selective filtration and plasma reinfusion

(For professional evaluation, use modifier -26)

36522   Photopheresis, extracorporeal

(For dialysis services, see 90935-90999)

(For ultrafiltration, use 90999)

(For therapeutic apheresis for white blood cells, red blood cells, platelets and plasma pheresis, see 36511, 36512, 36513, 36514)

(For therapeutic apheresis extracorporeal adsorption procedures, use 36516)

Central Venous Access Procedures

To qualify as a central venous access catheter or device, the tip of the catheter/device must terminate in the subclavian, brachiocephalic (innominate) or iliac veins, the superior or inferior vena cava, or the right atrium. The venous access device may be either centrally inserted (jugular, subclavian, femoral vein or inferior vena cava catheter entry site) or peripherally inserted (eg, basilic, cephalic, or saphenous vein entry site). The device may be accessed for use either via exposed catheter (external to the skin), via a subcutaneous port or via a subcutaneous pump.

The procedures involving these types of devices fall into five categories:

1. **Insertion** (placement of catheter through a newly established venous access)

2. **Repair** (fixing device without replacement of either catheter or port/pump, other than pharmacologic or mechanical correction of intracatheter or pericatheter occlusion [see 36595 or 36596])

3. **Partial replacement** of only the catheter component associated with a port/pump device, but not entire device

4. **Complete replacement** of entire device via same venous access site (complete exchange)

5. **Removal** of entire device.

There is no coding distinction between venous access achieve percutaneously vrsus by cutdown or based on catheter size.

For the repair, partial (catheter only) replacement, complete replacement, or removal of both catheters (placed from separate venous access sites) of a multi-catheter device, with or without subcutaneous ports/pumps, use the appropriate code describing the service with a frequency of two.

If an existing central venous access device is removed and a new one placed via a separate venous access site, appropriate codes for both procedures (removal of old, if code exists, and insertion of new device) should be reported.

When imaging guidance is used for centrally inserted central venous catheters, for gaining access to the venous entry site and/or for manipulating the catheter into final central position, imaging guidance codes (eg, 76937, 77001) may be reported separately. Do not use 76937, 77001 in conjunction with 36568, 36569, 36572, 36573, 36584.

(For refilling and maintenance of an implantable pump or reservoir for intravenous or intra-arterial drug delivery, use 96530)

Insertion of Central Venous Access Device

36555   Insertion of non-tunneled centrally inserted central venous catheter; under 5 years of age

(For peripherally inserted non-tunneled central venous catheter, under 5 years of age, use 36568)

36556   age 5 years or older

(For peripherally inserted non-tunneled central venous catheter, age 5 years or older, use 36569)

36557 Insertion of tunneled centrally inserted central venous catheter, without subcutaneous port or pump; under 5 years of age

36558 age 5 years or older

(For peripherally inserted central venous catheter with port, age 5 years or older, use 36571)

36560 Insertion of tunneled centrally inserted central venous access device, with subcutaneous port; under 5 years of age

(For peripherally inserted central venous access device with subcutaneous port, under 5 years of age, use 36570)

36561 age 5 years or older

(For peripherally inserted central venous catheter with subcutaneous port, 5 years or older, use 36571)

36563 Insertion of tunneled centrally inserted central venous access device with subcutaneous pump

36565 Insertion of tunneled centrally inserted central venous access device, requiring 2 catheters via 2 separate venous access sites; without subcutaneous port or pump (eg, Tesio type catheter)

36566 with subcutaneous port(s)

Peripherally inserted central venous catheters (PICCs) may be placed or replaced with or without imaging guidance. When performed without imaging guidance, report using 36568 or 36569. When imaging guidance (eg, ultrasound, fluoroscopy) is used for PICC placement or repositioning, bundled service codes 36572, 36573, 36584 include all imaging necessary to complete the procedure, image documentation (representative images from all modalities used are stored to patient's permanent record), associated radiological supervision and interpretation, venography performed through the same venous puncture, and documentation of final central position of the catheter with imaging. Ultrasound guidance for PICC placement should include documentation of evaluation of the potential puncture sites, patency of the entry vein, and real-time ultrasound visualization of needle entry into the vein.

Codes 71045, 71046, 71047, 71048 should not be reported for the purpose of documenting the final catheter position on the same day of service as 36572, 36573, 36584. Codes 36572, 36573, 36584 include confirmation of catheter tip location. The physician or other qualified health care professional reporting image-guided PICC insertion cannot report confirmation of catheter tip location separately (eg, via X ray, ultrasound). Report 36572, 36573, 36584 with modifier 52 when performed without confirmation of catheter tip location.

"Midline" catheters by definition terminate in the peripheral venous system. They are not central venous access devices and may not be reported as a PICC service. Midline catheter placement may be reported with 36400, 36405, 36406, or 36410. PICCs placed using magnetic guidance or any other guidance modality that does not include imaging or image documentation are reported with 36568, 36569.

36568 Insertion of peripherally inserted central venous catheter (PICC), without subcutaneous port or pump, without imaging guidance; younger than 5 years of age

(For placement of centrally inserted non-tunneled central venous catheter, without subcutaneous port or pump, under 5 years of age, use 36555)

(For placement of peripherally inserted non-tunneled central venous catheter, without subcutaneous port or pump, with imaging guidance, younger than 5 years of age, use 36572)

36569 age 5 years or older

(Do not report 36568, 36569 in conjunction with 76937, 77001)

(For placement of centrally inserted non-tunneled central venous catheter, without subcutaneous port or pump, age 5 years or older, use 36556)

(For placement of peripherally inserted non-tunneled central venous catheter, without subcutaneous port or pump, with imaging guidance, age 5 years or older, use 36573)

● New Code ▲ Revised Code ✚ Add-On Code ⊘ Modifier -51 Exempt ★ Telemedicine

36572 Insertion of peripherally inserted central venous catheter (PICC), without subcutaneous port or pump, including all imaging guidance, image documentation, and all associated radiological supervision and interpretation required to perform the insertion; younger than 5 years of age

(For placement of centrally inserted non-tunneled central venous catheter, without subcutaneous port or pump, younger than 5 years of age, use 36555)

(For placement of peripherally inserted non-tunneled central venous catheter, without subcutaneous port or pump, without imaging guidance, younger than 5 years of age, use 36568)

36573 age 5 years or older

(For placement of centrally inserted non-tunneled central venous catheter, without subcutaneous port or pump, age 5 years or older, use 36556)

(For placement of peripherally inserted non-tunneled central venous catheter, without subcutaneous port or pump, without imaging guidance, age 5 years or older, use 36569)

(Do not report 36572, 36573 in conjunction with 76937, 77001)

36570 Insertion of peripherally inserted central venous access device, with subcutaneous port; under 5 years of age

(For insertion of tunneled centrally inserted central venous access device with subcutaneous port, under 5 years of age, use 36560)

36571 age 5 years or older

(For insertion of tunneled centrally inserted central venous access device with subcutaneous port, age 5 years or older, use 36561)

36572 This code is out of order. See page 431

36573 This code is out of order. See page 431

Repair of Central Venous Access Device

(For mechanical removal of pericatheter obstructive material, use 36595)

(For mechancial removal of intracatheter obstructive material, use 36596)

36575 Repair of tunneled or non-tunneled central venous access catheter, without subcutaneous port or pump, central or peripheral insertion site

36576 Repair of central venous access device, with subcutaneous port or pump, central or peripheral insertion site

Partial Replacement of Central Venous Access Device (Catheter Only)

36578 Replacement, catheter only, of central venous access device, with subcutaneous port or pump, central or peripheral insertion site

(For complete replacement of entire device through same venous access, use 36582 or 36583)

Complete Replacement of Central Venous Access Device Through Same Venous Access Site

36580 Replacement, complete, of a non-tunneled centrally inserted central venous catheter, without subcutaneous port or pump, through same venous access

36581 Replacement, complete, of a tunneled centrally inserted central venous catheter, without subcutaneous port or pump, through same venous access

36582 Replacement, complete, of a tunneled centrally inserted central venous access device, with subcutaneous port, through same venous access

---

Separate Procedure   Unlisted Procedure   CCI Comp. Code   Non-specific Procedure   **431**

The Central Venous Access Procedures Table

	Non-Tunneled	Tunneled w/o port or pump	Central Tunneled	Tunneled with port	Tunneled with pump	Peripheral	<5 years	≥5 years	Any Age
Insertion									
Catheter	36555						36555		
	36556							36556	
		36557	36557				36557		
		36558	36558					36558	
	36568 (w/o port or pump)					36568 (w/o port or pump)	36568 (w/o port or pump)		
	36569 (w/o port or pump)					36569 (w/o port or pump)		36569 (w/o port or pump)	
Catheter, with bundled imaging guidance						36572 (w/o port or pump)	36572 (w/o port or pump)		
						36573 (w/o port or pump)		36573 (w/o port or pump)	
Device			36560	36560			36560		
			36561	36561				36561	
			36563		36563				36563
		36565	36565						36565
			36566	36566					
	36570 (w port0)			36570 (w port)		36570 (w port)	36570 (w port)		
	36571 (w port)			36571 (w port)		36571 (w port)		36571 (w port)	
Repair									
Catheter	36575 (w/o port or pump)	36575 (w/o port or pump)	36575 (w/o port or pump)			36575 (w/o port or pump)			36575
Device	36576 (w port or pump)					36576 (w port or pump)			36576
Partial Replacement - Central Venous Access Device (Catheter only)									
			36578	36578	36578	36578			36578
Complete Replacement - Central Venous Access Device (through same venous access site)									
Catheter	36580 (w/o port or pump)								36580
		36581	36581						36581
	36584 (w/o port or pump)					36584 (w/o port or pump)			36584
Device			36582	36582					36582
			36583		36583				36583
				36585 (w port)		36585 (w port)			36585
Removal									
Catheter		36589							36589
Device			36590	36590	36590	36590			36590
Removal of Obstructive Material from Device									
	36595 peri-catheter	36595 peri-catheter	36595 peri-catheter	36595 peri-catheter	36595 peri-catheter	36595 peri-catheter			36595 peri-catheter
	36596 intraluminal	36596 intraluminal	36596 intraluminal	36596 intraluminal	36596 intraluminal	36596 intraluminal			36596 intraluminal
Repositioning of Catheter									
	36597	36597	36597	36597	36597	36597	36597	36597	36597

36583 Replacement, complete, of a tunneled centrally inserted central venous access device, with subcutaneous pump, through same venous access

36584 Replacement, complete, of a peripherally inserted central venous catheter (PICC), without subcutaneous port or pump, through same venous access, including all imaging guidance, image documentation, and all associated radiological supervision and interpretation required to perform the replacement

(For replacement of a peripherally inserted central venous catheter [PICC] without subcutaneous port or pump, through same venous access, without imaging guidance, use 37799)

(Do not report 36584 in conjunction with 76937, 77001)

36585 Replacement, complete, of a peripherally inserted central venous access device, with subcutaneous port, through same venous access

Removal of Central Venous Access Device

36589 Removal of tunneled central venous catheter, without subcutaneous port or pump

---

● New Code   ▲ Revised Code   ✚ Add-On Code   ⊘ Modifier -51 Exempt   ★ Telemedicine

36590 Removal of tunneled central venous access device, with subcutaneous port or pump, central or peripheral insertion

(Do not report 36589 or 36590 for removal of non-tunneled central venous catheters)

Other Central Venous Access Procedures

36591 Collection of blood specimen from a completely implantable venous access device

(Do not report 36591 in conjunction with other service except a laboratory service)

(For collection of venous blood specimen by venipuncture, use 36415)

(For collection of capillary blood specimen, use 36416)

36592 Collection of blood specimen using established central or peripheral catheter, venous, not otherwise specified

(For blood collection from an established arterial catheter, use 37799)

(Do not report 36592 in conjunction with other services except a laboratory service)

36593 Declotting by thrombolytic agent of implanted vascular access device or catheter

36595 Mechanical removal of pericatheter obstructive material (eg, fibrin sheath) from central venous device via separate venous access

(Do not report 36595 in conjunction with 36593)

(For venous catheterization, see 36010-36012)

(For radiological supervision and interpretation, use 75901)

36596 Mechanical removal of intraluminal (intracatheter) obstructive material from central venous device through device lumen

(Do not report 365596 in conjunction with 36593)

(For venous catheterization, see 36010-36012)

(For radiological supervision and interpretation, use 75902)

36597 Repositioning of previously placed central venous catheter under fluoroscopic guidance

(For fluoroscopic guidance, use 76000)

36598 Contrast injection(s) for radiologic evaluation of existing central venous access device, including fluoroscopy, image documentation and report

(Do not report 36598 in conjunction with 76000)

(Do not report 36598 in conjunction with 36595, 36596)

(For complete diagnostic studies, see 75820, 75825, 75827)

ARTERIAL

36600 Arterial puncture, withdrawal of blood for diagnosis

36620 Arterial catheterization or cannulation for sampling, monitoring or transfusion (separate procedure); percutaneous

36625 cutdown

36640 Arterial catheterization for prolonged infusion therapy (chemotherapy), cutdown

(See also 96420-96425)

(For arterial catheterization for occlusion therapy, see 75894)

36660 Catheterization, umbilical artery, newborn, for diagnosis or therapy

(Do not report modifier '-63' in conjunction with 36660)

INTRAOSSEOUS

36680 Placement of needle for intraosseous infusion

HEMODIALYSIS ACCESS, INTERVASCULAR CANNULIZATION FOR EXTRACORPOREAL CIRCULATION, OR SHUNT INSERTION

36800 Insertion of cannula for hemodialysis, other purpose (separate procedure); vein to vein

36810 arteriovenous, external (Scribner type)

36815 arteriovenous, external revision, or closure

36818 Arteriovenous anastomosis, open; by upper arm cephalic vein transposition

(Do not report 36818 in conjunction with 36819, 36820, 36821, 36830 during a unilateral upper extremity procedure. For bilateral upper extremity open arteriovenous anastomoses performed at the same operative session, use modifier 50 or 59 as appropriate)

36819 by upper arm basilic vein transposition

(Do not report 36819 in conjunction with 36818, 36820, 36821, 36830 during a unilateral upper extremity procedure. For bilateral upper extremity open arteriovenous anastomoses performed at the same operative session, use modifier 50 or 59 as appropriate)

36820 by forearm vein transposition

36821 direct, any site (eg, Cimino type) (separate procedure)

36823 Insertion of arterial and venous cannula(s) for isolated extracorporeal circulation including regional chemotherapy perfusion to an extremity, with or without hyperthermia, with removal of cannula(s) and repair of arteriotomy and venotomy sites

(36823 includes chemotherapy perfusion supported by a membrane oxygenator/perfusion pump. Do not report 96408-96425 in conjunction with 36823)

36825 Creation of arteriovenous fistula by other than direct arteriovenous anastomosis (separate procedure); autogenous graft

(For direct arteriovenous anastomosis, use 36821)

36830 nonautogenous graft (eg, biological collagen, thermoplastic graft)

(For direct arteriovenous anastomosis, use 36821)

36831 Thrombectomy, open, arteriovenous fistula without revision, autogenous or nonautogenous dialysis graft (separate procedure)

36832 Revision, open, arteriovenous fistula; without thrombectomy, autogenous or nonautogenous dialysis graft (separate procedure)

36833 with thrombectomy, autogenous or nonautogenous dialysis graft (separate procedure)

(For percutaneous thrombectomy within the dialysis circuit, see 36904, 36905, 36906)

(For central dialysis segment angioplasty in conjunction with 36818-36833, use 36907)

(For central dialysis segment stent placement in conjunction with 36818-36833, use 36908)

● New Code ▲ Revised Code + Add-On Code ⊘ Modifier -51 Exempt ★ Telemedicine

(Do not report 36832, 36833 in conjunction with 36901, 36902, 36903, 36904, 36905, 36906 for revision of the dialysis circuit)

36835 Insertion of Thomas shunt (separate procedure)

36838 Distal revascularization and interval ligation (DRIL), upper extremity hemodialysis access (steal syndrome)

(Do not report 36838 in conjunction with 35512, 35522, 35523, 36832, 37607, 37618)

36860 External cannula declotting (separate procedure); without balloon catheter

36861 with balloon catheter

(If imaging guidance is performed, use 76000)

DIALYSIS CIRCUIT

Definitions:

Dialysis circuit: The arteriovenous (AV) dialysis circuit is designed for easy and repetitive access to perform hemodialysis. It begins at the arterial anastomosis and extends to the right atrium. The circuit may be created using either an arterial-venous anastomosis, known as an arteriovenous fistula (AVF), or a prosthetic graft placed between an artery and vein, known as an arteriovenous graft (AVG). The dialysis circuit is comprised of two segments, termed the (1) peripheral dialysis segment and (2) central dialysis segment. Both are defined below.

Peripheral dialysis segment: The peripheral dialysis segment is the portion of the dialysis circuit that begins at the arterial anastomosis and extends to the central dialysis segment. In the upper extremity, the peripheral dialysis segment extends through the axillary vein (or entire cephalic vein in the case of cephalic venous outflow). In the lower extremity, the peripheral dialysis segment extends through the common femoral vein. The peripheral dialysis segment includes the historic "perianastomotic region" (defined below).

Central dialysis segment: The central dialysis segment includes all draining veins central to the peripheral dialysis segment. In the upper extremity, the central dialysis segment includes the veins central to the axillary and cephalic veins, including the subclavian and innominate veins through the superior vena cava. In the lower extremity, the central dialysis segment includes the veins central to the common femoral vein, including the external iliac and common iliac veins through the inferior vena cava.

Peri-anastomotic region: A historic term referring to the region of a dialysis circuit near the arterial anastomosis encompassing a short segment of the parent artery, the anastomosis, and a short segment of the dialysis circuit immediately adjacent to the anastomosis. The perianastomotic region is included within the peripheral segment of the dialysis circuit.

Performed through dialysis circuit: Any diagnostic study or therapeutic intervention within the dialysis circuit that is performed through a direct percutaneous access to the dialysis circuit.

Code 36901 includes direct access and imaging of the entire dialysis circuit. Antegrade and/or retrograde punctures of the dialysis circuit are typically used for imaging, and contrast may be injected directly through a needle or through a catheter placed into the dialysis circuit. All dialysis circuit punctures required to perform the procedure are included in 36901. Occasionally, the catheter needs to be advanced further into the circuit to adequately visualize the arterial anastomosis or the central veins, or selective catheterization of a venous branch may be required. All manipulation(s) of the catheter for diagnostic imaging of the dialysis circuit is included in 36901. Advancement of the catheter to the vena cava to adequately image that segment of the dialysis circuit is included in 36901 and is not separately reported. Code 36901 also includes catheterization of additional venous side branches communicating with the dialysis circuit, known as accessory veins. Advancement of the catheter tip through the arterial anastomosis to adequately visualize the anastomosis is also included in the service described by 36901 and is not separately reported. Evaluation of the peri-anastomotic portion of the inflow is an integral part of the dialysis circuit angiogram and is included in 36901.

For the purposes of reporting dialysis access maintenance services, the arterial inflow to the dialysis circuit is considered a separate vessel. If a more proximal arterial inflow problem separate from the peripheral dialysis segment is suspected, additional catheter placement and imaging required for adequate evaluation of the artery may be separately reported. If a catheter is selectively advanced from the dialysis circuit puncture beyond the peri-anastomotic segment into the inflow artery, an additional catheterization code may be reported. For example, 36215 may be used to report image-guided retrograde catheter placement into the inflow artery and into the aorta, if necessary (36200 is not reported in addition to 36215 in this example). Note that 75710 may also be reported if contrast injection for diagnostic arteriography is performed through this catheter and radiological supervision and interpretation and imaging documentation is performed.

Ultrasound guidance for puncture of the dialysis circuit access is not typically performed and is not included in 36901, 36902, 36903, 36904, 36905, 36906. However, in the case of a new (immature) or failing AVF, ultrasound may be necessary to safely and effectively puncture the dialysis circuit for evaluation, and this may be reported separately with 76937, if all the appropriate elements for reporting 76937 are performed and documented.

For radiological supervision and interpretation of dialysis circuit angiography performed through existing access(es) or catheter-based arterial access, report 36901 with modifier 52.

Dialysis Circuit Interventions (AV Grafts and AV Fistulae): For the purposes of coding interventional procedures in the dialysis circuit (both AVF and AVG), the dialysis circuit is artificially divided into two distinct segments: peripheral dialysis segment and central dialysis segment (see definitions).

Codes 36901, 36902, 36903 and 36904, 36905, 36906 are built on progressive hierarchies that have more intensive services, which include less intensive services. Report only one code (36901, 36902, 36903, 36904, 36905, 36906) for services provided in a dialysis circuit.

Code 36901 describes the diagnostic evaluation of the dialysis circuit, and this service is included in the services described by 36901, 36902, 36903, 36904, 36905, 36906. All catheterizations required to perform diagnostic fistulography are included in 36901. All catheterizations required to perform additional interventional services are included in codes 36902, 36903, 36904, 36905, 36906, 36907, 36908, 36909 and not separately reported. All angiography, fluoroscopic image guidance, roadmapping, and radiological supervision and interpretation required to perform each service are included in each code. Closure of the puncture(s) by any method is included in the service of each individual code.

Code 36902 includes the services in 36901 plus transluminal balloon angioplasty in the peripheral segment of the dialysis circuit. Code 36902 would be reported only once per session to describe all angioplasty services performed in the peripheral segment of the dialysis circuit, regardless of the number of distinct lesions treated within that segment, the number of times the balloon is inflated, or the number of balloon catheters or sizes required to open all lesions, and includes angioplasty of the peri-anastomotic segment when performed. Code 36903 includes the services in 36902 plus transcatheter stent placement in the peripheral segment of the dialysis circuit. Code 36903 is reported only once per session to describe placing stent(s) within the peripheral segment, regardless of the number of stent(s) placed or the number of discrete lesion(s) treated within the peripheral segment. If both angioplasty and stenting are performed in the peripheral segment, including treatment of separate lesions, report 36903 only once.

Code 36904 describes percutaneous transluminal mechanical thrombectomy and/or infusion for thrombolysis in the dialysis circuit (all thrombus treated in both the peripheral and central dialysis circuit segments) and includes diagnostic angiography (36901), fluoroscopic image guidance, catheter placement(s), and all maneuvers required to remove thrombus from the peripheral and/or central segments, including all intraprocedural pharmacological thrombolytic injection(s)/infusion(s). It is never appropriate to report removal of the arterial plug during a declot/thrombectomy procedure as an angioplasty (36905). Removal of the arterial plug is included in a fistula thrombectomy, even if a balloon catheter is used to mechanically dislodge the resistant thrombus. Codes 36905 (angioplasty) and 36906 (stent) describe services in the peripheral circuit when performed in conjunction with thrombolysis/thrombectomy. Code 36905 includes the services in 36904 plus transluminal balloon angioplasty in the peripheral segment of the dialysis circuit. Code 36905 may be reported only once per session to describe all angioplasty performed in the peripheral segment of the dialysis circuit, regardless of the number of distinct lesions treated within that segment, the number of times the balloon is inflated, or the number of balloon catheters required to open all lesions.

Code 36906 includes the services in 36905 plus transcatheter stent placement in the peripheral segment of the dialysis circuit. Code 36906 is reported only once per session to describe placing stent(s) within the peripheral segment, regardless of the number of stent(s) placed or the number of discrete lesion(s) treated within the peripheral segment.

Codes 36907 and 36908 describe procedures performed through puncture(s) in the dialysis circuit. Similar procedures performed from a different access (eg, common femoral vein) may be reported using 37248, 37249 or 37238, 37239. Code 36907 is an add-on code used in conjunction with 36901, 36902, 36903, 36904, 36905, 36906 to report angioplasty within the central dialysis segment when performed through puncture of the dialysis circuit, and is reported once per session independent of the number of discrete lesions treated, the number of balloon inflations, and number of balloon catheters or sizes required. These additional services should be clearly documented in the patient record, including the recorded images. Code 36907 may be reported only once per session with 36901, 36902, 36903, 36904, 36905, 36906, as appropriate. Report 36907 once for all angioplasty performed within the central dialysis segment.

Code 36908 is an add-on code used in conjunction with 36901, 36902, 36903, 36904, 36905, 36906 to report stenting lesion(s) in the central dialysis segment when performed through puncture of the dialysis circuit. It is reported once, regardless of the number of discrete lesions treated or the number of stents placed. Code 36908 includes the services in 36907; therefore, 36908 may not be reported with 36907 in the same session. Code 36908 may be reported only once per session with 36901, 36902, 36903, 36904, 36905, 36906, as appropriate.

Code 36909 is an add-on code used to report endovascular embolization or occlusion of the main vessel or side branches arising from (emptying into) the dialysis circuit. Code 36909 may only be reported once per therapeutic session, irrespective of the number of branches embolized or occluded. Embolization or occlusion of the main vessel or these side branches may not be reported with 37241.

If open dialysis circuit creation, revision, and/or thrombectomy (36818-36833) are performed, completion angiography is bundled, as is peripheral segment angioplasty and/or stent placement (36901, 36902, 36903) and, therefore, not separately reported. However, dialysis circuit central segment angioplasty and/or stent placement may be separately reported (36907, 36908)

36901 Introduction of needle(s) and/or catheter(s), dialysis circuit, with diagnostic angiography of the dialysis circuit, including all direct puncture(s) and catheter placement(s), injection(s) of contrast, all necessary imaging from the arterial anastomosis and adjacent artery through entire venous outflow including the inferior or superior vena cava, fluoroscopic guidance, radiological supervision and interpretation and image documentation and report;

(Do not report 36901 in conjunction with 36833, 36902, 36903, 36904, 36905, 36906)

36902 with transluminal balloon angioplasty, peripheral dialysis segment, including all imaging and radiological supervision and interpretation necessary to perform the angioplasty

(Do not report 36902 in conjunction with 36903)

36903 with transcatheter placement of intravascular stent(s), peripheral dialysis segment, including all imaging and radiological supervision and interpretation necessary to perform the stenting, and all angioplasty within the peripheral dialysis segment

(Do not report 36902, 36903 in conjunction with 36833, 36904, 36905, 36906)

(Do not report 36901, 36902, 36903 more than once per operative session)

(For transluminal balloon angioplasty within central vein(s) when performed through dialysis circuit, use 36907)

(For transcatheter placement of intravascular stent(s) within central vein(s) when performed through dialysis circuit, use 36908)

36904 Percutaneous transluminal mechanical thrombectomy and/or infusion for thrombolysis, dialysis circuit, any method, including all imaging and radiological supervision and interpretation, diagnostic angiography, fluoroscopic guidance, catheter placement(s), and intraprocedural pharmacological thrombolytic injection(s);

(For open thrombectomy within the dialysis circuit, see 36831, 36833)

36905 with transluminal balloon angioplasty, peripheral dialysis segment, including all imaging and radiological supervision and interpretation necessary to perform the angioplasty

(Do not report 36905 in conjunction with 36904)

36906 with transcatheter placement of intravascular stent(s), peripheral dialysis segment, including all imaging and radiological supervision and interpretation necessary to perform the stenting, and all angioplasty within the peripheral dialysis circuit

(Do not report 36906 in conjunction with 36901, 36902, 36903, 36904, 36905)

(Do not report 36904, 36905, 36906 more than once per operative session)

(For transluminal balloon angioplasty within central vein(s) when performed through dialysis circuit, use 36907)

(For transcatheter placement of intravascular stent(s) within central vein(s) when performed through dialysis circuit, use 36908)

+ **36907** Transluminal balloon angioplasty, central dialysis segment, performed through dialysis circuit, including all imaging and radiological supervision and interpretation required to perform the angioplasty (List separately in addition to code for primary procedure)

(Use 36907 in conjunction with 36818-36833, 36901, 36902, 36903, 36904, 36905, 36906)

(Do not report 36907 in conjunction with 36908)

(Report 36907 once for all angioplasty performed within the central dialysis segment)

+ 36908 Transcatheter placement of intravascular stent(s), central dialysis segment, performed through dialysis circuit, including all imaging and radiological supervision and interpretation required to perform the stenting, and all angioplasty in the central dialysis segment (List separately in addition to code for primary procedure)

(Use 36908 in conjunction with 36818-36833, 36901, 36902, 36903, 36904, 36905, 36906)

(Do not report 36908 in conjunction with 36907)

(Report 36908 once for all stenting performed within the central dialysis segment)

+ 36909 Dialysis circuit permanent vascular embolization or occlusion (including main circuit or any accessory veins), endovascular, including all imaging and radiological supervision and interpretation necessary to complete the intervention (List separately in addition to code for primary procedure)

(36909 includes all permanent vascular occlusions within the dialysis circuit and may only be reported once per encounter per day)

(Report 36909 in conjunction with 36901, 36902, 36903, 36904, 36905, 36906)

(For open ligation/occlusion in dialysis access, use 37607)

PORTAL DECOMPRESSION PROCEDURES

37140 Venous anastomosis, open; portocaval

(For peritoneal-venous shunt, use 49425)

37145 renoportal

37160 caval-mesenteric

37180 splenorenal, proximal

37181 splenorenal, distal (selective decompression of esophagogastric varices, any technique)

(For percutaneous procedure, use 37182)

37182 Insertion of transvenous intrahepatic portosystemic shunt(s) (TIPS) (includes venous access, hepatic and portal vein catheterization, portography with hemodynamic evaluation, intrahepatic tract formation/dilatation, stent placement and all associated imaging guidance and documentation)

(Do not report 75885 or 75887 in conjunction with code 37182)

(For open procedure, use 37140)

37183 Revision of transvenous intrahepatic portosystemic shunt(s) (TIPS) (includes venous access, hepatic and portal vein catheterization, portography with hemodynamic evaluation, intrahepatic tract recanulization/dilatation, stent placement and all associated imaging guidance and documentation)

(Do not report 75885 or 75887 in conjunction with code 37183)

(For repair of arteriovenous aneurysm, use 36832)

TRANSCATHETER PROCEDURES

Codes for catheter placement and the radiologic supervision and interpretation should also be reported, in addition to the code(s) for the therapeutic aspect of the procedure.

Mechanical Thrombectomy

Code(s) for catheter placement(s), diagnostic studies, and other percutaneous interventions (eg., transluminal balloon angioplasty, stent placement) provided are separately reportable.

Codes 37184-37188 specifically include intraprocedural fluoroscopic radiological supervision and interpretation services for guidance of the procedure.

Intraprocedural injection(s) of a thrombolytic agent is an included service and not separately reportable in conjunction with mechanical thrombectomy. However, subsequent or prior continuous infusion of a thrombolytic is not an included service and is separately reportable (see 37211-37214).

For coronary mechanical thrombectomy, use 92973.

For intracranial arterial mechanical thrombectomy for dialysis fistula, use 61645.

Transcatheter Thrombolytic Infusion

Codes 37211 or 37212 are used to report the initial day of transcatheter thrombolytic infusion(s) including follow-up arteriography/venography, and catheter position change or exchange, when performed. To report bilateral thrombolytic infusion through a separate access site(s), use modifier 50 in conjunction with 37211, 37212. Code 37213 is used to report continued transcatheter thrombolytic infusion(s) on subsequent day(s), other than initial day and final day of treatment. Code 37214 is used to report final day of transcatheter thrombolytic infusion(s). When initiation and completion of thrombolysis occur on the same day, report only 37211 or 37212.

Code(s) for catheter placement(s), diagnostic studies, and other percutaneous interventions (eg, transluminal balloon angioplasty, stent placement) provided may be separately reportable.

Codes 37211-37214 include fluoroscopic guidance and associated radiological supervision and interpretation.

Ongoing E/M services on the day of the procedure related to thrombolysis are included in 37211-37214. If a significant, separately identifiable E/M service is performed by the same physician on the same day of the procedure, report the appropriate level of E/M service and append modifier 25.

Ultrasound guidance for vascular access is not included in 37211-37214. Code 76937 may be reported separately when performed if all the required elements are performed.

For intracranial arterial mechanical thrombectomy and/or infusion for thrombolysis, use 61645.

Arterial Mechanical Thrombectomy

Arterial mechanical thrombectomy may be performed as a "primary" transcatheter procedure with pretreatment planning, performance of the procedure, and postprocedure evaluation focused on providing this service. Typically, the diagnosis of thrombus has been made prior to the procedure, and a mechanical thrombectomy is planned preoperatively. Primary mechanical thrombectomy is reported per vascular family using 37184 for the initial vessel treated and 37185 for second or all subsequent vessel(s) within the same vascular family. To report mechanical thrombectomy of an additional vascular family treated through a separate access site, use modifier 59 in conjunction with the primary service code (37184) for the mechanical transluminal thrombectomy.

Primary mechanical thrombectomy may precede or follow another percutaneous intervention. Most commonly primary mechanical thrombectomy will precede another percutaneous intervention with the decision regarding the need for other services not made until after mechanical thrombectomy has been performed. Occasionally, the performance of primary mechanical thrombectomy may follow another percutaneous intervention.

Do NOT report 37184-37185 for mechanical thrombectomy performed for the retrieval of short segments of thrombus or embolus evident during other percutaneous interventional procedures. See 37186 for these procedures.

Arterial mechanical thrombectomy is considered a "secondary" transcatheter procedure for removal or retrieval of short segments of thrombus or embolus when performed either before or after another percutaneous intervention (eg, percutaneous transluminal balloon angioplasty, stent placement). Secondary mechanical thrombectomy is reported using 37186. Do NOT report 37186 in conjunction with 37184-37185.

Venous Mechanical Thrombectomy

Use 37187 to report the initial application of venous mechanical thrombectomy. To report bilateral venous mechanical thrombectomy performed through a separate access site(s), use modifier 50 in conjunction with 37187. For repeat treatment on a subsequent day during a course of thrombolytic therapy, use 37188.

Arterial Mechanical Thrombectomy

37184   Primary percutaneous transluminal mechanical thrombectomy, noncoronary, nonintracranial, arterial or arterial bypass graft, including fluoroscopic guidance and intraprocedural pharmacological thrombolytic injection(s); initial vessel

(Do not report 37184 in conjunction with 61645, 76000, 96374)

+ 37185   second and all subsequent vessel(s) within the same vascular family (List separately in addition to code for primary mechanical thrombectomy procedure)

(Do not report 37185 in conjunction with 76000, 96375)

(Do not report 37185 in conjunction with 61645 for treatment of the same vascular territory. See Nervous System Endovascular Therapy)

+ 37186   Secondary percutaneous transluminal thrombectomy (eg, nonprimary mechanical, snare basket, suction technique), noncoronary, non-intracranial, arterial or arterial bypass graft, including fluoroscopic guidance and intraprocedural pharmacological thrombolytic injections, provided in conjunction with another percutaneous intervention other than primary mechanical thrombectomy (List separately in addition to code for primary procedure)

(Do not report 37186 in conjunction with 76000, 96375)

(Do not report 37186 in conjunction with 61645 for treatment of the same vascular territory. See Nervous System Endovascular Therapy)

Venous Mechanical Thrombectomy

37187   Percutaneous transluminal mechanical thrombectomy, vein(s), including intraprocedural pharmacological thrombolytic injections and fluoroscopic guidance

(Do not report 37187 in conjunction with 76000, 96375)

37188   Percutaneous transluminal mechanical thrombectomy, vein(s), including intraprocedural pharmacological thrombolytic injections and fluoroscopic guidance, repeat treatment on subsequent day during course of thrombolytic therapy

(Do not report 37188 in conjunction with 76000, 96375)

Other Procedures

37191   Insertion of intravascular vena cava filter, endovascular approach including vascular access, vessel selection, and radiological supervision and interpretation, intraprocedural roadmapping, and imaging guidance (ultrasound and fluoroscopy), when performed

(For open surgical interruption of the inferior vena cava through a laparotomy or retroperitoneal exposure, use 37619)

37192   Repositioning of intravascular vena cava filter, endovascular approach including vascular access, vessel selection, and radiological supervision and interpretation, intraprocedural roadmapping, and imaging guidance (ultrasound and fluoroscopy), when performed

(Do not report 37192 in conjunction with 37191)

37193   Retrieval (removal) of intravascular vena cava filter, endovascular approach including vascular access, vessel selection, and radiological supervision and interpretation, intraprocedural roadmapping, and imaging guidance (ultrasound and fluoroscopy), when performed

(Do not report 37193 in conjunction with 37197)

37195 Thrombolysis, cerebral, by intravenous infusion

37197 Transcatheter retrieval, percutaneous, of intravascular foreign body (eg, fractured venous or arterial catheter), includes radiological supervision and interpretation, and imaging guidance (ultrasound or fluoroscopy), when performed

(For percutaneous retrieval of a vena cava filter, use 37193)

(For transcatheter removal of permanent leadless pacemaker, use 33275)

37200 Transcatheter biopsy

(For radiological supervision and interpretation, use 75970)

37211 Transcatheter therapy, arterial infusion for thrombolysis other than coronary or intracranial, any method, including radiological supervision and interpretation, initial treatment day

(For intracranial arterial mechanical thrombectomy and/or infujsion for thrombolysis, use 61645)

37212 Transcatheter therapy, venous infusion for thrombolysis, any method, including radiological supervision and interpretation, initial treatment day

37213 Transcatheter therapy, arterial or venous infusion for thrombolysis other than coronary, any method, including radiological supervision and interpretation, continued treatment on subsequent day during course of thrombolytic therapy, including follow-up catheter contrast injection, position change, or exchange, when performed;

37214 cessation of thrombolysis including removal of catheter and vessel closure by any method

(Report 37211-37214 once per date of treatment)

(For declotting by thrombolytic agent of implanted vascular access device or catheter, use 36593)

(Do not report 37211-37214 in conjunction with 75898)

37215 Transcatheter placement of intravascular stent(s), cervical carotid artery, open or percutaneous, including angioplasty, when performed, and radiological supervision and interpretation; with distal embolic protection

37216 without distal embolic protection

(37215 and 37216 include all ipsilateral selective carotid catheterization, all diagnostic imaging for ipsilateral, cervical and cerebral carotid arteriography, and all related radiological supervision and interpretation. When ipsilateral carotid arteriogram (including imaging and selective catheterization) confirms the need for carotid stenting, 37215 and 37216 are inclusive of these services. If carotid stenting is not indicated, then the appropriate codes for carotid catheterization and imaging should be reported in lieu of 37215 and 37216)

(Do not report 37215, 37216 in conjunction with 36222-36224 for the treated carotid artery)

(For open or percutaneous transcatheter placement of extracranial vertebral artery stent[s], see Category III codes 0075T, 0076T)

37217 Transcatheter placement of intravascular stent(s), intrathoracic common carotid artery or innominate artery by retrograde treatment, open ipsilateral cervical carotid artery exposure, including angioplasty, when performed, and radiological supervision and interpretation

(37217 includes open vessel exposure and vascular access closure, all access and selective catheterization of the vessel, traversing the lesion, and any radiological supervision and interpretation directly related to the intervention when performed, standard closure of arteriotomy by suture, and imaging performed to document completion of the intervention in addition to the intervention[s] performed. Carotid artery revascularization services [eg, 33891, 35301, 35509, 35510, 35601, 35606] performed during the same session may be reported separately, when performed)

(Do not report 37217 in conjunction with 35201, 36221-36227, 37246, 37247 for ipsilateral services)

(For open or percutaneous transcatheter placement of intravascular cervical carotid artery stent[s], see 37215, 37216)

(For open or percutaneous antegrade transcatheter placement of innominate and/or intrathoracic carotid artery stent[s], use 37218)

(For open or percutaneous transcatheter placement of extracranial vertebral artery stent[s], see 0075T, 0076T)

(For transcatheter placement of intracranial stent[s], use 61635)

37218 Transcatheter placement of intravascular stent(s), intrathoracic common carotid artery or innominate artery, open or percutaneous antegrade approach, including angioplasty, when performed, and radiological supervision and interpretation

(37218 includes all ipsilateral extracranial intrathoracic selective innominate and carotid catheterization, all diagnostic imaging for ipsilateral extracranial intrathoracic innominate and/or carotid artery stenting, and all related radiologic supervision and interpretation. Report 37218 when the ipsilateral extracranial intrathoracic carotid arteriogram (including imaging and selective catheterization) confirms the need for stenting. If stenting is not indicated, report the appropriate codes for selective catheterization and imaging)

(Do not report 37218 in conjunction with 36222, 36223, 36224 for the treated carotid artery)

(For open or percutaneous transcatheter placement of intravascular cervical carotid artery stent[s], see 37215, 37216)

(For open or percutaneous transcatheter placement of extracranial vertebral artery stent[s], see 0075T, 0076T)

(For transcatheter placement of intracranial stent[s], use 61635)

ENDOVASCULAR REVASCULARIZATION (OPEN OR PERCUTANEOUS, TRANSCATHETER)

Codes 37220-37235 are to be used to describe lower extremity endovascular revascularization services performed for occlusive disease. These lower extremity codes are built on progressive hierarchies with more intensive services inclusive of lesser intensive services. The code inclusive of all of the services provided for that vessel should be reported (ie, use the code inclusive of the most intensive services provided). Only one code from this family (37220-37235) should be reported for each lower extremity vessel treated.

These lower extremity endovascular revascularization codes all include the work of accessing and selectively catheterizing the vessel, traversing the lesion, radiological supervision and interpretation directly related to the intervention(s) performed, embolic protection if used, closure of the arteriotomy by pressureand application of an arterial closure device or standard closure of the puncture by suture, and imaging performed to document completion of the intervention in addition to the intervention(s) performed. Extensive repair or replacement of an artery may be additionally reported (eg, 35226, or 35286). These codes describe endovascular procedures performed percutaneously and/or through an open surgical exposure. These codes include balloon angioplasty (eg, low-profile, cutting balloon, cryoplasty), atherectomy (eg, directional, rotational, laser), and stentin (eg, balloon-expandable, self-expanding, bare metal, covered, drug-eluting). Each code in this family (37220-37235) includes balloon angioplasty, when performed.

These codes describe revascularization therapies (ie, transluminal angioplasty, atherectomy, and stent placement) provided in three arterial vascular territories: iliac, femoral/popliteal, and tibial/peroneal.

When treating multiple vessels within a territory, report each additional vessel using an add-on code, as applicable. Select the base code that represents the most complex service using the following hierarchy of complexity (in descending order of complexity): atherectomy and stent>atherectomy>stent>angioplasty. When treating multiple lesions within the same vessel, report one service that reflects the combined procedures, whether done on one lesion or different lesions, using the same hierarchy.

1. **Iliac Vascular Territory** — The iliac territory is divided into 3 vessels: common iliac, internal iliac, and external iliac.

2. **Femoral/Popliteal Vascular Territory** — The entire femoral/popliteal territory of 1 lower extremity is considered a single vessel for CPT reporting specifically for the endovascular lower extremity revascularization codes 37224-37227.

3. **Tibial/Peroneal Territory** — The tibial/peroneal territory is divided into 3 vessels: anterior, tibial, posterial tibial, and peroneal arteries.

There are specific coding guidelines for each of the 3 vascular territories.

1. **Iliac Vascular Territory** — A single primary code is used for the initial iliac artery treated in each leg (37220 or 37221). If other iliac vessels are also treated in that leg, these interventions are reported with th appropriate add-on code(s) (37222, 37223). Up to 2 add-on codes can be used in a unilateral iliac vascular territory since there are 3 vessels which could be treated. Add-on codes are used for different vessels, not distinct lesions within the same vessel.

2. **Femoral/Popliteal Territory** — A single interventional code is used no matter what combination of angioplasty/stent/atherectomy is applied to all segments, including the common, deep and superficial femoral arteries as well as the popliteal artery (37224, 37225, 37226 or 37227). There are no add-on codes for additional vessels treated within the femoral/popliteal territory. Because only 1 service is reported when 2 lesions are treated in this territory, report the most complex service (eg, use 37227 if a stent is placed for 1 lesion and an atherectomy is performed on a second lesion).

3. **Tibial/Peroneal Territory** — A single primary code is used for the initial tibial/peroneal artery treated in each leg (37228, 37229, 37230, or 37231). If other tibial/peroneal vessels are also treated in the same leg, these interventions are reported with the appropriate add-on code(s) (37232-37235). Up to 2 add-on codes could be used to describe services provided in a single leg since there are 3 tibial/peroneal vessels which could be treated. Add-on codes are used for different vessels, not distinct lesions within the same vessel. The common tibio-peroneal trunk is considered part of the tibial/peroneal territory, but is not considered a separate, fourth segment of vessel in the tibio-peroneal family for CPT reporting of endovascular lower extremity interventions. For instance, if lesions in the common tibio-peroneal trunk are treated in conjunction with lesions in the posterior tibial artery, a single code would be reported for treatment of this segment.

When treating multiple territories in the same leg, one primary lower extremity revascularization code is used for each territory treated. When second or third vessel(s) are treated in the iliac and/or tibial/peroneal territories, add-on codes are used to report the additional services. When more than one stent is placed in the same vessel, the code should be reported only once.

When multiple vessels in multiple territories in a single leg are treated at the same setting, the primary code for the treatment in the initial vessel in each vascular territory is reported. Add-on code(s) are reported when second and third iliac or tibial/peroneal arteries are treated in addition to the initial vessel in that vascular territory.

If a lesion extends across the margins of one vessel vascular territory into another, but can be opened with a single therapy, this intervention should be reported with a single code despite treating more than one vessel and/or vascular territory. For instance, if a stenosis extends from the common iliac artery into the proximal external iliac artery, and a single stent is placed to open the entire lesion, this therapy should be coded as a single stent placement in the iliac artery (37221). In this example, a code for an additional vessel treatment would not be used (do not report both 37221 and 37223).

For bifurcation lesions distal to the common iliac origins which require therapy of 2 distinct branches of the iliac or tibial/peroneal vascular territories, a primary code and an add-on code would be used to describe the intervention. In the femoral/popliteal territory, all branches are included in the primary code, so treatment of a bifurcation lesion would be reported as a single code.

When the same territor(ies) of both legs are treated in the same session, modifiers may be required to describe the interventions. Use modifier 59 to denote that different legs are being treated, even if the mode of therapy is different.

Mechanical thrombectomy and/or thrombolysis in the lower extremity vessels are sometimes necessary to aid in restoring flow to areas of occlusive disease, and are reported separately.

37220 Revascularization, endovascular, open or percutaneous, iliac artery, unilateral, initial vessel, with transluminal angioplasty

37221   with transluminal stent placement(s), includes angioplasty within the same vessel, when performed

(Use 37220, 37221 in conjunction with 34701-34711, 34718, 34845, 34846, 34847, 34848, only when 37220 or 37221 is performed outside the treatment zone of the endograft)

+ **37222** Revascularization, endovascular, open or percutaneous, iliac artery, each additional ipsilateral iliac vessel, with transluminal angioplasty (list separately in addition to code for primary procedure)

(Use 37222 in conjunction with 37220, 37221)

+ **37223**   with transluminal stent placement(s), includes angioplasty within the same vessel, when performed (list separately in addition to code for primary procedure)

Separate Procedure   Unlisted Procedure   CCI Comp. Code   Non-specific Procedure   **443**

(Use 37223 in conjunction with 37221)

(Use 37222, 37223 in conjunction with 34701-34711, 34718, 34845, 34846, 34847, 34848 only when 37222 or 37223 are performed outside the treatment zone of the endograft)

37224   Revascularization, endovascular, open or percutaneous, femoral, popliteal artery(s), unilateral, with transluminal angioplasty

37225   with atherectomy, includes angioplasty within the same vessel, when performed

37226   with transluminal stent placement(s), includes angioplasty within the same vessel, when performed

37227   with transluminal stent placement(s) and atherectomy, includes angioplasty within the same vessel when performed

(Do not report 37224, 37225, 37226, 37227 in conjunction with 0505T, within the femoral-popliteal segment)

37228   Revascularization, endovascular, open or percutaneous, tibial, peroneal artery, unilateral, initial vessel, with transluminal angioplasty

37229   with atherectomy, includes angioplasty within the same vessel, when performed

37230   with transluminal stent placement(s), includes angioplasty within the same vessel, when performed

37231   with transluminal stent placement(s) and atherectomy, includes angioplasty within the same vessel, when performed

+ **37232**   Revascularization, endovascular, open or percutaneous, tibial/peroneal artery, unilateral, each additional vessel, with transluminal angioplasty (list separately in addition to code for primary procedure)

(Use 37232 in conjunction with 37228-37231)

+ **37233**   with atherectomy, includes angioplasty within the same vessel, when performed (list separately in addition to code for primary procedure)

(Use 37233 in conjunction with 37229, 37231)

+ **37234**   with transluminal stent placement(s), includes angioplasty within the same vessel, when performed (list separately in addition to code for primary procedure)

(Use 37234 in conjunction with 37229, 37230, 37231)

+ **37235**   with transluminal stent placement(s) and atherectomy, includes angioplasty within the same vessel, when performed (list separately in addition to code for primary procedure)

(Use 37235 in conjunction with 37231)

Codes 37246, 37247, 37248, 37249 describe open or percutaneous transluminal balloon angioplasty (eg, conventional, low profile, cutting, drug-coated balloon). Codes 37246, 37247 describe transluminal balloon angioplasty in an artery excluding the central nervous system (61630, 61635), coronary (92920-92944), pulmonary (92997, 92998), and lower extremities for occlusive disease (37220-37235). Codes 37248 and 37249 describe transluminal balloon angioplasty in a vein excluding the dialysis circuit (36902, 36905, 36907) when approached through the ipsilateral dialysis access. Transluminal balloon angioplasty is inherent to stenting in the extracranial carotid and innominate arteries (37215, 37216, 37217, 37218), peripheral arteries (37220-37237), and in peripheral veins (37238, 37239) and, therefore, is not separately reportable. Multiple angioplasties performed in a single vessel, including treatment of separate and distinct lesions within a single vessel, are reported with a single code. If a lesion extends across the margins of one vessel into another, but can be treated with a single therapy, the intervention should be reported only once. When additional, separate and distinct ipsilateral or contralateral vessels are treated in the same session, 37247 and/or 37249 may be reported as appropriate.

Non-selective and/or selective catheterization (eg, 36005, 36010, 36011, 36012, 36200, 36215, 36216, 36217, 36218, 36245, 36246, 36247, 36248) is reported separately. Codes 37246, 37247, 37248, 37249 include radiological supervision and interpretation directly related to the intervention performed and imaging performed to document completion of the intervention. Extensive repair or replacement of an artery may be reported separately (eg, 35226, 35286). Intravascular ultrasound may be

---

444   ● New Code   ▲ Revised Code   + Add-On Code   ⊘ Modifier -51 Exempt   ★ Telemedicine

reported separately (ie, 37252, 37253). Mechanical thrombectomy and/or thrombolytic therapy, when performed, may be reported separately (eg, 37184, 37185, 37186, 37187, 37188, 37211, 37212, 37213, 37214).

37246 Transluminal balloon angioplasty (except lower extremity artery(ies) for occlusive disease, intracranial, coronary, pulmonary, or dialysis circuit), open or percutaneous, including all imaging and radiological supervision and interpretation necessary to perform the angioplasty within the same artery; initial artery

+ 37247 each additional artery (List separately in addition to code for primary procedure)

(Use 37247 in conjunction with 37246)

(Do not report 37246, 37247 in conjunction with 37215, 37216, 37217, 37218, 37220-37237 when performed in the same artery during the same operative session)

(Do not report 37246, 37247 in conjunction with 34841, 34842, 34843, 34844, 34845, 34846, 34847, 34848 for angioplasty[ies] performed, when placing bare metal or covered stents into the visceral branches within the endoprosthesis target zone)

37248 Transluminal balloon angioplasty (except dialysis circuit), open or percutaneous, including all imaging and radiological supervision and interpretation necessary to perform the angioplasty within the same vein; initial vein

+ 37249 each additional vein (List separately in addition to code for primary procedure)

(Use 37249 in conjunction with 37248)

(Do not report 37248, 37249 in conjunction with 37238, 37239 when performed in the same vein during the same operative session)

(Do not report 37248, 37249 in conjunction with 0505T, within the femoral-popliteal segment)

(Do not report 37248, 37249 in conjunction with 0620T within the tibial-peroneal segment)

(For transluminal balloon angioplasty in aorta/visceral artery[ies] in conjunction with fenestrated endovascular repair, see 34841, 34842, 34843, 34844, 34845, 34846, 34847, 34848)

(For transluminal balloon angioplasty in iliac, femoral, popliteal, or tibial/peroneal artery[ies] for occlusive disease, see 37220-37235)

(For transluminal balloon angioplasty in a dialysis circuit performed through the circuit, see 36902, 36903, 36904, 36905, 36906, 36907, 36908)

(For transluminal balloon angioplasty in an intracranial artery, see 61630, 61635)

(For transluminal balloon angioplasty in a coronary artery, see 92920-92944)

(For transluminal balloon angioplasty in a pulmonary artery, see 92997, 92998)

Codes 37236-37239 are used to report endovascular revascularization for vessels other than lower extremity artery(ies) for occlusive disease (ie, 37221, 37223, 37226, 37227, 37230, 37231, 37234, 37235), cervical carotid (ie, 37215, 37216), intracranial (ie, 61635), intracoronary (ie, 92928, 92929, 92933, 92934, 92937, 92938, 92941, 92943, 92944), innominate and/or intrathoracic carotid artery through an antegrade approach (37218), extracranial vertebral (ie, 0075T, 0076T) performed percutaneously and/or through an open surgical exposure, open retrograde intrathoracic common carotid or innominate (37217), or dialysis circuit when performed through the dialysis circuit (36903, 36905, 36908).

Codes 37236, 37237 describe transluminal intravascular stent insertion in an artery while 37238, 37239 describe transluminal intravascular stent insertion in a vein. Multiple stents placed in a single vessel may only be reported with a single code. If a lesion extends across the margins of one vessel into another, but can be treated with a single therapy, the intervention should be reported only once. When additional, different vessels are treated in the same session, report 37237 and/or 37239 as appropriate. Each coding in this family (37236-37239) includes any and all balloon angioplasty(s) performed in the treated vessel, including any pre-dilation (whether performed as a primary or secondary angioplasty), post-dilation following stent placement, treatment of a lesion outside the stented segment but in the same vessel, or use of larger/smaller balloon to achieve therapeutic result. Angioplasty in a separate and distinct vessel may be reported separately. Non-selective and/or selective catheterization(s) (eg, 36005, 36010-36015, 36200, 36215-36218, 36245-36248), is reported separately.

Codes 37236-37239 include radiological supervision and interpretation directly related to the intervention(s) performed, closure of the arteriotomy by pressure, application of an arterial closure device or standard closure of the puncture by suture, and imaging performed to document completion of the intervention in addition to the intervention(s) performed. Extensive repair or replacement of an artery may be reported separately (eg, 35226 or 35286). Report 76937 for ultrasound guidance for vascular access, when performed in conjunction with 37236-37239. Intravascular ultrasound may be reported separately (ie, 37252, 37253). For mechanical thrombectomy and/or thrombolytic therapy, when performed, see 37184-37188, 37211-37214.

Intravascular stents, both covered and uncovered, are a class of device that may be used as part of an embolization procedure. As such, there is the potential for overlap among codes used for placement of vascular stents and those use for embolization. When a stent is placed for the purpose of providing a latticework for deployment of embolization coils, such as for embolization of an aneurysm, the embolization code is reported and not the stent code. If a covered stent is deployed as the sole management of an aneurysm, pseudoaneurysm, or vascular extravasation, then the stent deployment code should be reported and not the embolization code.

37236 Transcatheter placement of an intravascular stent(s) (except lower extremity artery(s) for occlusie disease, cervical carotid, extracranial vertebral or intrathoracic carotid, intracranial, or coronary), open or percutaneous, including radiological supervision and interpretation and including all angioplasty within the same vessel, when performed; initial artery

+ 37237 each additional artery (List separately in addition to code for primary procedure)

(Use 37237 in conjunction with 37236)

(Do not report 37236, 37237 in conjunction with 34841-34848 for bare metal or covered stents placed into the visceral branches within the endoprosthesis target zone)

(For stent placement(s) in iliac, femoral, popliteal, or tibial/perineal artery(s) for occlusive disease, see 37221, 37223, 37226, 37227, 37230, 37231, 37234, 37235)

(For transcatheter placement of intravascular cervical carotid artery stent(s), see 37215, 37216)

(For transcatheter placement of intracranial stent(s), use 61635)

(For transcatheter placement of intracoronary stent(s), see 92928, 92929, 92933, 92934, 92937, 92938, 92941, 92943, 92944)

(For stenting of visceral arteries in conjunction with fenestrated endovascular repair, see 34841-34848)

(For open or percutaneous antegrade transcatheter placement of intrathoracic carotid/innominate artery stent[s], use 37218)

(For open or percutaneous transcatheter placement of extracranial vertebral artery stent[s], see Category III codes 0075T, 0076T)

(For open retrograde transcatheter placement of intrathoracic common carotid/innominate artery stent(s), use 37217)

(For placement of a stent at the arterial anastomosis of a dialysis circuit with or without transluminal mechanical thrombectomy and/or infusion for thrombolysis, see 36903, 36906)

37238 Transcatheter placement of an intravascular stent(s), open or percutaneous, including radiological supervision and interpretation and including angioplasty within the same vessel, when performed; initial vein

+ 37239 each additional vein (List separately in addition to code for primary procedure)

(Use 37239 in conjunction with 37238)

(Do not report 37238, 37239 in conjunction with 0505T, within the femoral-popliteal segment)

(Do not report 37238, 37239 in conjunction with 0620T within the tibial-peroneal segment)

(For placement of a stent[s] within the peripheral segment of the dialysis circuit, see 36903, 36906)

(For transcatheter placement of an intravascular stent[s] within central dialysis segment when performed through the dialysis circuit, use 36908)

VASCULAR EMBOLIZATION AND OCCLUSION

Codes 37241-37244 are used to describe vascular embolization and occlusion procedures, excluding the central nervous system and the head and neck, which are reported using 61624, 61626, 61710, and 75894, and excluding the ablation/sclerotherapy procedures for venous insufficiency/telangiectasia of the extremities/skin, which are reported using 36468, 36470, and 36471. Embolization and occlusion procedures are performed for a wide variety of clinical indications and in a range of vascular territories. Arteries, veins, and lymphatics may all be the target of embolization.

The embolization codes include all associated radiological supervision and interpretation, intra-procedural guidance and road-mapping, and imaging necessary to document completion of the procedure. They do not include diagnostic angiography and all necessary catheter placement(s). Code(s) for catheter placement(s) may be separately reportable using selecrive catheter placement code(s), if used consistent with guidelines. Code(s) for diagnostic angiography may also be separately reported, when performed according to guidelines for diagnostic angiography during endovascular procedures. Report these services with an appropriate modifier (eg, modifier 59). Please see the guidelines on the reporting of diagnostic angiography preceding 75600 in the Vascular Procedures, Aorta and Arteries section.

Code 37241 is used to report endovascular embolization or occlusion procedures performed for venous conditions other than hemorrhage or hemodialysis access. Examples include embolization of venous malformations, capillary hemangiomas, varicoceles, and visceral varices. (For endovascular embolization or occlusion of side branch[es] of an outflow vein[s] from a hemodialysis access, use 36909.)

Code 37242 is used report vascular embolization or occlusion performed for arterial conditions other than hemorrhage or tumor such as arteriovenous malformations and arteriovenous fistulas whether congenital or acquired. Embolizations of aneurysms and pseudoaneurysms are also reported with 37242. Tumor embolization is reported with 37243. Note that injection to treat an extremity pseudoaneurysm is correctly reported with 36002. Sometimes, embolization and occlusion of an artery are performed prior to another planned interventional procedure; an example is embolization of the left gastric artery prior to planned implantation of a hepatic artery chemotherapy port. The artery embolization is reported with 37242.

Code 37243 is used report embolization for the purpose of tissue ablation and organ infarction and or ischemia. This can be performed in many clinical circumstances including embolization of benign or malignant tumors of the liver, kidney, uterus, or other organs. When chemotherapy is given as part of an embolization procedure, additional codes (eg, 96420), maybe separately reported. When a radioisotope (eg, Yttrium-90) is injected as part of an embolization, then additional codes (eg, 79445) may be separately reported. Uterine fibroid embolization is reported with 37243.

Code 37244 is used to report embolization for treatment of hemorrhage or vascular or lymphatic extravasation. Examples include embolization for management of gastrointestinal bleed, trauma-induced hemorrhage of the viscera or pelvis, embolization of the thoracic duct for chylous effusion and bronchial artery embolization for hemoptysis. Embolization of the uterine arteries for management of hemorrhage (eg, postpartum hemorrhage), is also reported with 37244.

Intravascular stents, both covered and uncovered, are a class of devices that may be used as part of an embolization procedure. As such, there is the potential for overlap among codes used for placement of vascular stents and those use for embolization. When a stent is placed for the purpose of providing a latticework for deployment of embolization coils, such as for embolization of an aneurysm, the embolization code is reported and not the stent code. If a stent is deployed as the sole management of an aneurysm pseudoaneurysm or vascular extravasation, then the stent deployment code should be reported and not the embolization code.

Only one embolization code should be reported for each surgical field (ie, the area immediately surrounding and directly involved in a treatment/procedure). Embolization procedures performed at a single setting and including multiple surgical fields (eg, a patient with multiple trauma and bleeding from the pelvis and the spleen) may be reported with multiple embolization codes with the appropriate modifier (eg, modifier 59).

There may be overlapping indications for an embolization procedure. The code for the immediate indication for the embolization should be used. For instance, if the immediate cause for embolization is bleeding in a patient with an aneurysm, report 37244.

37241 Vascular embolization or occlusion, inclusive of all radiological supervision and interpretation, intraprocedural roadmapping, and imaging guidance necessary to complete the intervention; venous, other than hemorrhage (eg, congenital or acquired venous malformations, venous and capillary hemangiomas, varices, varioceles)

(Do not report 37241 in conjunction with 36468, 36470, 36471, 36473, 36474, 36475-36479, 75894, 75898 in the same surgical field)

(For sclerosis of veins or endovenous ablation of incompetent extremity veins, see 36468-36479)

(For dialysis circuit permanent endovascular embolization or occlusion, use 36909)

37242   arterial, other than hemorrhage or tumor (eg, congenital or acquired arterial malformations, arteriovenous malformations, arteriovenous fistulas, aneurysms, pseudoaneurysms)

(For percutaneous treatment of extremity pseudoaneurysm, use 36002)

37243   for tumors, organ ischemia, or infarction

37244   for arterial or venous hemorrhage or lymphatic extravasation

(Do not report 37242-37244 in conjunction with 75894, 75898 in the same surgical field)

(For embolization procedures of the central nervous system or head and neck, see 61624, 61626, 61710)

37246   Code out of order. See page 445

37247   Code out of order. See page 445

37248   Code out of order. See page 445

37249   Code out of order. See page 445

INTRAVASCULAR ULTRASOUND SERVICES

Intravascular ultrasound (IVUS) services include all transducer manipulations and repositioning within the specific vessel being examined during a diagnostic procedure or before, during, and/or after therapeutic intervention (eg, stent or stent graft placement, angioplasty, atherectomy, embolization, thrombolysis, transcatheter biopsy).

IVUS is included in the work described by codes 37191, 37192, 37193, 37197 (intravascular vena cava [IVC] filter placement, repositioning and removal, and intravascular foreign body retrieval) and should not be separately reported with those procedures. If a lesion extends across the margins of one vessel into another, this should be reported with a single code despite imaging more than one vessel.

Non-selective and/or selective vascular catheterization may be separately reportable (eg, 36005-36248).

(37250, 37251 have been deleted. To report noncoronary intravascular ultrasound during diagnostic evaluation and/or therapeutic intervention, see 37252, 37253)

+ 37252   Intravascular ultrasound (noncoronary vessel) during diagnostic evaluation and/or therapeutic intervention, including radiological supervision and interpretation; initial noncoronary vessel (List separately in addition to code for primary procedure)

+ 37253   each additional noncoronary vessel (List separately in addition to code for primary procedure)

(Use 37253 in conjunction with 37252)

(Report 37252, 37253 in conjunction with 33361, 33362, 33363, 33364, 33365, 33366, 33367, 33368, 33369, 33477, 33880, 33881, 33883, 33884, 33886, 34701, 34702, 34703, 34704, 34705, 34706, 34707, 34708, 34709, 34710, 34711, 34712, 34718, 34841, 34842, 34843, 34844, 34845, 34846, 34847, 34848, 36010, 36011, 36012, 36013, 36014, 36015, 36100, 36140, 36160, 36200, 36215, 36216, 36217, 36218, 36221, 36222, 36223, 36224, 36225, 36226, 36227, 36228, 36245, 36246, 36247, 36248, 36251, 36252, 36253, 36254, 36481, 36555-36571, 36578, 36580, 36581, 36582, 36583, 36584, 36585, 36595, 36901, 36902, 36903, 36904, 36905, 36906, 36907, 36908, 36909, 37184, 37185, 37186, 37187, 37188, 37200, 37211, 37212, 37213, 37214, 37215, 37216, 37218, 37220, 37221, 37222, 37223, 37224, 37225, 37226, 37227, 37228, 37229, 37230, 37231, 37232, 37233, 37234, 37235, 37236, 37237, 37238, 37239, 37241, 37242, 37243, 37244, 37246, 37247, 37248, 37249, 61623, 75600, 75605, 75625, 75630, 75635, 75705, 75710, 75716, 75726, 75731, 75733, 75736, 75741, 75743, 75746, 75756, 75774, 75805, 75807, 75810, 75820, 75822, 75825, 75827, 75831, 75833, 75860, 75870, 75872, 75885, 75887, 75889, 75891, 75893, 75894, 75898, 75901, 75902, 75956, 75957, 75958, 75959, 75970, 76000, 77001, 0075T, 0076T, 0234T, 0235T, 0236T, 0237T, 0238T, 338T)

(Do not report 37252, 37253 in conjunction with 37191, 37192, 37193, 37197)

ENDOSCOPY

Surgical vascular endoscopy always includes diagnostic endoscopy.

  ●   New Code   ▲   Revised Code   +   Add-On Code   ⊘   Modifier -51 Exempt   ★   Telemedicine

37500 Vascular endoscopy, surgical, with ligation or perforator veins, subfascial (SEPS)

(For open procedure, use 37760)

37501 Unlisted vascular endoscopy procedure

LIGATION

(For phleborraphy and arteriorraphy, see 35201-35286)

37565 Ligation, internal jugular vein

37600 Ligation; external carotid artery

37605 internal or common carotid artery

37606 internal or common carotid artery, with gradual occlusion, as with Selverstone or Crutchfield clamp

(For transcatheter permanent arterial occlusion or embolization, see 61624-61626)

(For endovascular temporary arterial balloon occlusion, use 61623)

(For ligation treatment of intracranial aneurysm, use 61703)

37607 Ligation or banding of angioaccess arteriovenous fistula

37609 Ligation or biopsy, temporal artery

37615 Ligation, major artery (eg, post-traumatic, rupture); neck

37616 chest

37617 abdomen

37618 extremity

37619 Ligation of inferior vena cava

(For endovascular delivery of an inferior vena cava filter, use 37191)

37650 Ligation of femoral vein

(For bilateral procedure, report 37650 with modifier -50)

37660 Ligation of common iliac vein

37700 Ligation and division of long saphenous vein at saphenofemoral junction, or distal interruptions

(Do not report 37700 in conjunction with 37718, 37722)

(For bilateral procedure, report 37700 with modifier -50)

37718 Ligation, division, and stripping, short saphenous vein

(For bilateral procedure, use modifier 50)

(Do not report 37718 in conjunction with 37735, 37780)

37722 Ligation, division, and stripping, long (greater) saphenous veins from saphenofemoral junction to knee or below

(For ligation and stripping of the short saphenous vein, use 37718)

(For bilateral procedure, report 37722 with modifier 50)

Separate Procedure   Unlisted Procedure   CCI Comp. Code   Non-specific Procedure

(Do not report 37722 in conjunction with 37700, 37735)

(For ligation, division, and stripping of the greater saphenous vein, use 37722. For ligation, division, and stripping of the short saphenous vein, use 37718)

37735 Ligation and division and complete stripping of long or short saphenous veins with radical excision of ulcer and skin graft and/or interruption of communicating veins of lower leg, with excision of deep fascia

(Do not report 37735 in conjunction with 37700, 37718, 37722, 37780)

(For bilateral procedure, report 37735 with modifier -50)

37760 Ligation of perforator veins, subfascial, radical (Linton type), including skin graft, when performed, open, 1 leg

(For endoscopic procedure, use 37500)

37761 Ligation of perforator vein(s), subfascial, open, including ultrasound guidance, when performed, 1 leg

(For bilateral procedure, report 37761 with modifier -50)

(Do not report 37760, 37761 in conjunction with 76937, 76942, 76998, 93971)

(For endoscopic ligation of subfascial perforator veins, use 37500)

37765 Stab phlebectomy of varicose veins, 1 extremity; 10-20 stab incisions

(For less than 10 incisions, use 37799)

(For more than 20 incisions, use 37766)

37766 more than 20 incisions

37780 Ligation and division of short saphenous vein at saphenopopliteal junction (separate procedure)

(For bilateral procedure, report 37780 with modifier -50)

37785 Ligation, division, and/or excision of varicose vein cluster(s), 1 leg

(For bilateral procedure, report 37785 with modifier -50)

OTHER PROCEDURES

37788 Penile revascularization, artery, with or without vein graft

37790 Penile venous occlusive procedure

37799 Unlisted procedure, vascular surgery

● New Code ▲ Revised Code ✛ Add-On Code ⊘ Modifier -51 Exempt ★ Telemedicine

HEMIC AND LYMPHATIC SYSTEMS

CPT codes from this section of CPT are used to report invasive and surgical procedures performed on the spleen and lymph nodes. Bone marrow transplants are reported using CPT codes 38230-38241 from this section.

When bone marrow aspiration is performed alone, the appropriate code to report is CPT code 38220. When a bone marrow biopsy is performed, the appropriate code is CPT code 38221 (bone marrow biopsy). This code cannot be reported with CPT code 20220 (bone biopsy). CPT codes 38220 and 38221 may only be reported together if the two procedures are performed at separate sites or at separate patient encounters. Separate sites include bone marrow aspiration and biopsy in different bones or two separate skin incisions over the same bone.

When both a bone marrow biopsy (CPT code 38221) and bone marrow aspiration (CPT code 38220) are performed at the same site through the same skin incision, do not report the bone marrow aspiration, CPT code 38220, in addition to the bone marrow biopsy (CPT code 38221). HCPCS/CPT code G0364 may be reported to describe the bone marrow aspiration performed with bone marrow biopsy through the same skin incision on the same date of service.

SPLEEN

EXCISION

38100   Splenectomy; total (separate procedure)

38101   partial (separate procedure)

+ **38102**   total, en bloc for extensive disease, in conjunction with other procedure (List in addition to code for primary procedure)

REPAIR

38115   Repair of ruptured spleen (splenorrhaphy) with or without partial splenectomy

LAPAROSCOPY

Surgical laparoscopy always includes diagnostic laparoscopy. To report a diagnostic laparoscopy (peritoneoscopy) (separate procedure), use 49320.

38120   Laparoscopy, surgical, splenectomy

38129   Unlisted laparoscopy procedure, spleen

INTRODUCTION

38200   Injection procedure for splenoportography

            (For radiological supervision and interpretation, use 75810)

GENERAL

BONE MARROW OR STEM CELL SERVICES/PROCEDURES

Codes 38207-38215 describe various steps used to preserve, prepare and purify bone marrow/stem cells prior to transplantation or reinfusion. Each code may be reported only once per day regardless of the quantity of bone marrow/stem cells manipulated.

38204   Management of recipient hematopoietic progenitor cell donor search and cell acquisition

38205   Blood-derived hematopoietic progenitor cell harvesting for transplantation, per collection; allogeneic

38206   autologous

38207   Transplant preparation of hematopoietic progenitor cells; cryopreservation and storage

---

| Separate Procedure | Unlisted Procedure | CCI Comp. Code | Non-specific Procedure | **451** |

(For diagnostic cryopreservation and storage, see 88240)

38208   thawing of previously frozen harvest, without washing, per donor

(For diagnostic thawing and expansion of frozen cells, see 88241)

38209   thawing of previously frozen harvest, with washing, per donor

38210   specific cell depletion within harvest, T-cell depletion

38211   tumor cell depletion

38212   red blood cell removal

38213   platelet depletion

38214   plasma (volume) depletion

38215   cell concentration in plasma, mononuclear, or buffy coat layer

(Do not report 38207-38215 in conjunction with 88182, 88184-88189)

38220 Diagnostic bone marrow; aspiration(s)

(Do not report 38220 in conjunction with 38221)

(For diagnostic bone marrow biopsy[ies] and aspiration[s] performed at the same session, use 38222)

(For aspiration of bone marrow for bone graft, spine surgery only, use 20939)

(For bone marrow aspiration[s] for platelet-rich stem cell injection, use 0232T)

38221   biopsy (ies)

(Do not report 38221 in conjunction with 38220)

(For diagnostic bone marrow biopsy[ies] and aspiration[s] performed at the same session, use 38222)

38222   biopsy(ies) and aspiration(s)

(Do not report 38222 in conjunction with 38220 and 38221)

(For bilateral procedure, report 38220, 38221, 38222 with modifier 50)

(For bone marrow biopsy interpretation, use 88305)

38230 Bone marrow harvesting for transplantation; allogenic

38232   autologous

(For autologous and allogeneic blood-derived peripheral stem cell harvesting for transplantation, see 38205, 38206)

(For diagnostic bone marrow aspiration[s], see 38220, 38222)

(For aspiration of bone marrow for bone graft, spine surgery only, use 20939)

(For bone marrow aspiration[s] for platelet-rich stem cell injection, use 0232T)

TRANSPLANTATION AND POST-TRANSPLANTATION CELLULAR INFUSIONS

Hematopoietic cell transplantation (HCT) refers to the infusion of hematopoietic progenitor cells (HPC) obtained from bone marrow, peripheral blood apheresis, and/or umbilical cord blood. These procedure codes (38240-38243) include physician monitoring of multiple physiologic parameters, physician verification of cell processing, evaluation of the patient during as well as immediately before and after the HPC/lymphocyte infusion, physician presence during the HPC/lymphocyte infusion with associated direct physician supervision of clinical staff, and management of uncomplicated adverse events (eg, nausea, urticaria) during the infusion, which is not separately reportable.

HOT may be autologous (when the HPV donor and recipient are the same person) or allogenic (when the HPV donor and recipient are not the same person). Code 38241 is used to report any autologous transplant while 38240 is used to report an allogenic transplant. In some cases allogenic transplants involve more than one donor and cells from each donor are infused sequentially whereby one unit of 38240 is reported for each donor infused. code 38242 is used to report a donor lymphocyte infusion. Code 38243 is used to report a HPC boost from the original allogenic HPC donor. A lymphocyte infusion or HPC boost can occur days, months or even years after the initial hematopoietic cell transplant. The lymphocyte infusion is used to treat relapse, infection, or post-transplant lymphoproliferative syndrome. HPC boost represents an infusion of hematopoietic progenitor cells from the original donor that is being used to treat a relapse or or post-transplant cytopenia(s). Codes 38240, 38242, and 38243 should not be reported together on the same date of service.

If a separately identifiable E/M service is performed on the same date of service, the appropriate E/M service code, including office or other outpatient services, established (99211-99215), hospital observation services (99217-99220, 99224-99226), hospital inpatient services (99221-99223, 99231-99239), and inpatient neonatal and pediatric critical care (99471, 99472, 99475, 99476) may be reported, using modifier 25, in addition to 38240, 38242, or 38243. Post transplant infusion management of adverse reactions is reported separately using the appropriate E/M, prolonged service or critical care code(s). In accordance with place of service and facility reporting guideline, the fluid used to administer the cells and other infusions for incidental hydration (eg, 96360, 96361) are not separately reportable. Similarly, infusions of any medication(s) concurrently with the transplant infusion are not separately reportable. However, hydration or administration of medication (eg, antibiotics, narcotics) unrelated to the transplant are separately reportable using modifier 59.

38240   Hematopoietic progenitor cell (HPC); allogeneic transplantation per donor

38241   autologous transplantation

38243   HPC boost

38242   Allogeneic lymphocyte infusions

(For diagnostic bone marrow aspiration[s], see 38220, 38222)

(For aspiration of bone marrow for bone graft, spine surgery only, use 20939)

(For bone marrow aspiration[s] for platelet-rich stem cell injection, use 0232T)

(For modification, treatment, and processing of hematopoietic progenitor cell specimens for transplantation, see 38210-38215)

(For cryopreservation, freezing and storage of hematopoietic progenitor cells for transplantation, use 38207)

(For thawing and expansion of hematopoietic progenitor cells for transplantation, use 38208, 38209)

(For compatibility studies, see 81379-81383, 86812, 86813, 86816, 86817, 86821)

38243   Code out of order. See page 453

LYMPH NODES AND LYMPHATIC CHANNELS

INCISION

38300   Drainage of lymph node abscess or lymphadenitis; simple

38305   extensive

38308   Lymphangiotomy or other operations on lymphatic channels

38380   Suture and/or ligation of thoracic duct; cervical approach

38381   thoracic approach

38382   abdominal approach

EXCISION

(For injection for sentinel node identification, use 38792)

38500   Biopsy or excision of lymph node(s); open, superficial

(Do not report 38500 with 38700-38780)

38505   by needle, superficial (eg, cervical, inguinal, axillary)

(If imaging guidance is performed, see 76942, 77002, 77012, 77021)

(For fine needle aspiration biopsy, see 10004, 10005, 10006, 10007, 10008, 10009, 10010, 10011, 10012, 10021)

(For evaluation of fine needle aspirate, see 88172, 88173)

38510   open, deep cervical node(s)

38520   open, deep cervical node(s) with excision scalene fat pad

38525   open, deep axillary node(s)

38530   open, internal mammary node(s)

(Do not report 38530 with 38720-38746)

(For percutaneous needle biopsy, retroperitoneal lymph node or mass, use 49180)

(For fine needle aspiration biopsy, retroperitoneal lymph node or mass, see 10005, 10006, 10007, 10008, 10009, 10010, 10011, 10012)

38531   open, inguinofemoral node(s)

(For bilateral procedure, report 38531 with modifier 50)

38542   Dissection, deep jugular node(s)

(For radical cervical neck dissection, use 38720)

38550   Excision of cystic hygroma, axillary or cervical; without deep neurovascular dissection

38555   with deep neurovascular dissection

LIMITED LYMPHADENECTOMY FOR STAGING

38562   Limited lymphadenectomy for staging (separate procedure); pelvic and para-aortic

(When combined with prostatectomy, use 55812 or 55842)

(When combined with insertion of radioactive substance into prostate, use 55862)

38564   retroperitoneal (aortic and/or splenic)

LAPAROSCOPY

Surgical laparoscopy always includes diagnostic laparoscopy. To report a diagnostic laparoscopy (peritoneoscopy), (separate procedure), use 49320.

38570   Laparoscopy, surgical; with retroperitoneal lymph node sampling (biopsy), single or multiple

38571   with bilateral total pelvic lymphadenectomy

38572   with bilateral total pelvic lymphadenectomy and peri-aortic lymph node sampling (biopsy), single or multiple

---

● New Code   ▲ Revised Code   ✛ Add-On Code   ⊘ Modifier -51 Exempt   ★ Telemedicine

(For drainage of lymphocele to peritoneal cavity, use 49323)

38573   with bilateral total pelvic lymphadenectomy and periaortic lymph node sampling, peritoneal washings, peritoneal biopsy(ies), omentectomy, and diaphragmatic washings, including diaphragmatic and other serosal biopsy(ies), when performed

(Do not report 38573 in conjunction with 38562, 38564, 38570, 38571, 38572, 38589, 38770, 38780, 49255, 49320, 49326, 58541, 58542, 58543, 58544, 58548, 58550, 58552, 58553, 58554)

38589   Unlisted laparoscopy procedure, lymphatic system

RADICAL LYMPHADENECTOMY (RADICAL RESECTION OF LYMPH NODES)

(For limited pelvic and retroperitoneal lymphadenectomies, see 38562, 38564)

38700   Suprahyoid lymphadenectomy

(For bilateral procedure, report 38700 with modifier -50)

38720   Cervical lymphadenectomy (complete)

(For bilateral procedure, report 38720 with modifier -50)

38724   Cervical lymphadenectomy (modified radical neck dissection)

38740   Axillary lymphadenectomy; superficial

38745   complete

+ 38746   Thoracic lymphadenectomy by thoracotomy, mediastinal and regional lymphadenectomy (List separately in addition to code for primary procedure)

(On the right, mediastinal lymph nodes include the paratracheal, subcarinal, paraesophageal, and inferior pulmonary ligament)

(On the left, mediastinal lymph nodes include the aortopulmonary window, subcarinal, paraesophageal, and inferior pulmonary ligament)

(Report 38746 in conjunction with 21601, 31760, 31766, 31786, 32096-32200, 32220-32320, 32440-32491, 32503-32505, 33025, 33030, 33050-33130, 39200-39220, 39560, 39561, 43101, 43112, 43117, 43118, 43122, 43123, 43351, 60270, 60505)

(To report mediastinal and regional lymphadenectomy via thoracoscopy [VATS], see 32674)

+ 38747   Abdominal lymphadenectomy, regional, including celiac, gastric, portal, peripancreatic, with or without para-aortic and vena caval nodes (List separately in addition to code for primary procedure)

38760   Inguinofemoral lymphadenectomy, superficial, including Cloquets node (separate procedure)

(For bilateral procedure, report 38760 with modifier -50)

38765   Inguinofemoral lymphadenectomy, superficial, in continuity with pelvic lymphadenectomy, including external iliac, hypogastric, and obturator nodes (separate procedure)

(For bilateral procedure, report 38765 with modifier -50)

38770   Pelvic lymphadenectomy, including external iliac, hypogastric, and obturator nodes (separate procedure)

(For bilateral procedure, report 38770 with modifier -50)

38780   Retroperitoneal transabdominal lymphadenectomy, extensive, including pelvic, aortic, and renal nodes (separate procedure)

(For excision and repair of lymphedematous skin and subcutaneous tissue, see 15004-15005, 15570-15650)

Separate Procedure   Unlisted Procedure   CCI Comp. Code   Non-specific Procedure   **455**

INTRODUCTION

38790 Injection procedure; lymphangiography

(For bilateral procedure, report 38790 with modifier -50)

(For radiological supervision and interpretation, see 75801-75807)

38792 radioactive tracer for identification of sentinel node

(For excision of sentinel node, see 38500-38542)

(For nuclear medicine lymphatics and lymph gland imaging, use 78195)

(For intraoperative identification (eg, mapping) of sentinel lymph node(s) including injection of non-radioactive dye, see 38900)

38794 Cannulation, thoracic duct

OTHER PROCEDURES

+ **38900** Intraoperative identification (eg, mapping) of sentinel lymph node(s) includes injection of non-radioactive dye, when performed (list separately in addition to code for primary procedure)

(Use 38900 in conjunction with 19302, 19307, 38500, 38510, 38520, 38525, 38530, 38531, 38542, 38562, 38564, 38570, 38571, 38572, 38740, 38745, 38760, 38765, 38770, 38780, 56630, 56631, 56632, 56633, 56634, 56637, 56640)

(For injection of radioactive tracer for identification of sentinel node, use 38792)

38999 Unlisted procedure, hemic or lymphatic system

● New Code   ▲ Revised Code   + Add-On Code   ⊘ Modifier -51 Exempt   ★ Telemedicine

MEDIASTINUM AND DIAPHRAGM

MEDIASTINUM

INCISION

39000 Mediastinotomy with exploration, drainage, removal of foreign body, or biopsy; cervical approach

39010 transthoracic approach, including either transthoracic or median sternotomy

(Do not report 39010 in conjunction with 33955, 33956, 33963, 33964)

(For VATS pericardial biopsy, use 32604)

EXCISION/RESECTION

39200 Resection of mediastinal cyst

39220 Resection of mediastinal tumor

(For substernal thyroidectomy, use 60270)

(For thymectomy, use 60520)

(For thoracoscopic [VATS] resection of mediastinal cyst, tumor or mass, use 32662)

ENDOSCOPY

39401 Mediastinoscopy; includes biopsy(ies) of mediastinal mass (eg, lymphoma), when performed

39402 with lymph node biopsy(ies) (eg, lung cancer staging

OTHER PROCEDURES

39499 Unlisted procedure, mediastinum

DIAPHRAGM

REPAIR

(For transabdominal repair of diaphragmatic [esophageal hiatal] hernia, use 43325)

(For laparoscopic repair of diaphragmatic [esophageal hiatal] hernias and fundoplication, see 43280, 43281, 43282)

39501 Repair, laceration of diaphragm, any approach

(For laparoscopic paraesophageal hernia repair, see 43281, 43282)

39503 Repair, neonatal diaphragmatic hernia, with or without chest tube insertion and with or without creation of ventral hernia

(Do not report modifier 63 in conjunction with 39503)

(For laparoscopic paraesophageal hernia repair, see 43281, 43282)

39540 Repair, diaphragmatic hernia (other than neonatal), traumatic; acute

39541 chronic

39545 Imbrication of diaphragm for eventration, transthoracic or transabdominal, paralytic or nonparalytic

39560 Resection, diaphragm; with simple repair (eg, primary suture)

Separate Procedure   Unlisted Procedure   CCI Comp. Code   Non-specific Procedure   **457**

39561   with complex repair (eg, prosthetic material, local muscle flap)

OTHER PROCEDURES

39599   Unlisted procedure, diaphragm

DIGESTIVE SYSTEM

MISCELLANEOUS CODING RULES

Gastrointestinal endoscopy codes should be assigned based on the extent of visualization performed. CMS's official guidelines for excision or destruction of a lesion are:

1. *use only the biopsy code if a single lesion is biopsied but not excised;*

2. *code only for the excision if a lesion is biopsied and the remaining portion is excised;*

3. *use the biopsy code once even if multiple biopsies are performed and none are excised; and*

4. *use both a biopsy and excision code if each lesion is taken from different sites.*

If the phrase "with or without biopsy" appears in the excision code's narrative, do not use a separate biopsy code. Diagnostic endoscopies are included in surgical endoscopies.

For upper gastrointestinal endoscopies, choose the appropriate code from documentation indicating whether the procedure was a simple exam, a diagnostic procedure or surgical procedure. Remember that code selection is based on the procedure(s) performed and the anatomical sites through which the scope passes. For example, if the scope is passed to the esophagus only, the code would be chosen from endoscopy codes beginning with 43200. If the scope is passed through the esophagus to the stomach, duodenum and/or the jejunum, the code selection would begin at 43235.

HERNIA REPAIR

Review the patient's age, the kind of hernia, the clinical presentation of the hernia, and method of repair documented in the medical record before assigning a hernia repair code.

APPENDECTOMY

To code appendectomies appropriately, review the documentation for an indicated purpose for the removal. If there is none, then it is probably incidental to a more serious surgery and should not be coded.

LIPS

(For procedures on skin of lips, see 10040 et seq)

EXCISION

40490 Biopsy of lip

40500 Vermilionectomy (lip shave), with mucosal advancement

40510 Excision of lip; transverse wedge excision with primary closure

40520 V-excision with primary direct linear closure

(For excision of mucous lesions, see 40810-40816)

40525 full thickness, reconstruction with local flap (eg, Estlander or fan)

40527 full thickness, reconstruction with cross lip flap (Abbe-Estlander)

40530 Resection of lip, more than one-fourth, without reconstruction

(For reconstruction, see 13131 et seq)

REPAIR (CHEILOPLASTY)

40650 Repair lip, full thickness; vermilion only

DIGEST 40000

40652   up to half vertical height

40654   over one-half vertical height, or complex

40700   Plastic repair of cleft lip/nasal deformity; primary, partial or complete, unilateral

40701   primary bilateral, 1 stage procedure

40702   primary bilateral, 1 of 2 stages

40720   secondary, by recreation of defect and reclosure

    (For bilateral procedure, report 40720 with modifier -50)

    (To report rhinoplasty only for nasal deformity secondary to congenital cleft lip, see 30460, 30462)

    (For repair of cleft lip, with cross lip pedicle flap (Abbe-Estlander type), use 40527)

40761   with cross lip pedicle flap (Abbe-Estlander type), including sectioning and inserting of pedicle

    (For repair cleft palate, see 42200 et seq)

    (For other reconstructive procedures, see 14060, 14061, 15120-15261, 15574, 15576, 15630)

OTHER PROCEDURES

40799   Unlisted procedure, lips

VESTIBULE OF MOUTH

INCISION

40800   Drainage of abscess, cyst, hematoma, vestibule of mouth; simple

40801   complicated

40804   Removal of embedded foreign body, vestibule of mouth; simple

40805   complicated

40806   Incision of labial frenum (frenotomy)

EXCISION, DESTRUCTION

40808   Biopsy, vestibule of mouth

40810   Excision of lesion of mucosa and submucosa, vestibule of mouth; without repair

40812   with simple repair

40814   with complex repair

40816   complex, with excision of underlying muscle

40818   Excision of mucosa of vestibule of mouth as donor graft

40819   Excision of frenum, labial or buccal (frenumectomy, frenulectomy, frenectomy)

40820   Destruction of lesion or scar of vestibule of mouth by physical methods (eg, laser, thermal, cryo, chemical)

REPAIR

40830 Closure of laceration, vestibule of mouth; 2.5 cm or less

40831   over 2.5 cm or complex

40840 Vestibuloplasty; anterior

40842   posterior, unilateral

40843   posterior, bilateral

40844   entire arch

40845   complex (including ridge extension, muscle repositioning)

       (For skin grafts, see 15002 et seq)

OTHER PROCEDURES

40899 Unlisted procedure, vestibule of mouth

TONGUE AND FLOOR OF MOUTH

INCISION

41000 Intraoral incision and drainage of abscess, cyst, or hematoma of tongue or floor of mouth; lingual

41005   sublingual, superficial

41006   sublingual, deep, supramylohyoid

41007   submental space

41008   submandibular space

41009   masticator space

41010 Incision of lingual frenum (frenotomy)

41015 Extraoral incision and drainage of abscess, cyst, or hematoma of floor of mouth; sublingual

41016   submental

41017   submandibular

41018   masticator space

       (For frenoplasty, use 41520)

41019 Placement of needles, catheters, or other device(s) into the head and/or neck region (percutaneous, transoral, or transnasal) for subsequent interstitial radioelement application

       (For imaging guidance, see 76942, 77002, 77012, 77021)

       (For stereotactic insertion of intracranial brachytherapy radiation sources, use 61770)

       (For interstitial radioelement application, see 77770, 77771, 77772, 77778)

EXCISION

41100 Biopsy of tongue; anterior two-thirds

41105	posterior one-third
41108	Biopsy of floor of mouth
41110	Excision of lesion of tongue without closure
41112	Excision of lesion of tongue with closure; anterior two-thirds
41113	posterior one-third
41114	with local tongue flap

(Do not report 41114 in conjunction with 41112, 41113)

41115	Excision of lingual frenum (frenectomy)
41116	Excision, lesion of floor of mouth
41120	Glossectomy; less than one-half tongue
41130	hemiglossectomy
41135	partial, with unilateral radical neck dissection
41140	complete or total, with or without tracheostomy, without radical neck dissection
41145	complete or total, with or without tracheostomy, with unilateral radical neck dissection
41150	composite procedure with resection floor of mouth and mandibular resection, without radical neck dissection
41153	composite procedure with resection floor of mouth, with suprahyoid neck dissection
41155	composite procedure with resection floor of mouth, mandibular resection, and radical neck dissection (Commando type)

REPAIR

41250	Repair of laceration 2.5 cm or less; floor of mouth and/or anterior two-thirds of tongue
41251	posterior one-third of tongue
41252	Repair of laceration of tongue, floor of mouth, over 2.6 cm or complex

OTHER PROCEDURES

(**41500**	deleted 2018 [2019 Edition])
41510	Suture of tongue to lip for micrognathia (Douglas type procedure)
41512	Tongue base suspension, permanent suture technique

(For fixation of tongue, mechanical, other than suture, use 41500)

(For suture of tongue to lip for micrognathia, use 41510)

41520	Frenoplasty (surgical revision of frenum, eg, with Z-plasty)

(For frenotomy, see 40806, 41010)

41530	Submucosal ablation of the tongue base, radiofrequency, 1 or more sites, per session

---

● New Code ▲ Revised Code + Add-On Code ⊘ Modifier -51 Exempt ★ Telemedicine

41599   Unlisted procedure, tongue, floor of mouth

DENTOALVEOLAR STRUCTURES

INCISION

41800   Drainage of abscess, cyst, hematoma from dentoalveolar structures

41805   Removal of embedded foreign body from dentoalveolar structures; soft tissues

41806   bone

EXCISION, DESTRUCTION

41820   Gingivectomy, excision gingiva, each quadrant

41821   Operculectomy, excision pericoronal tissues

41822   Excision of fibrous tuberosities, dentoalveolar structures

41823   Excision of osseous tuberosities, dentoalveolar structures

41825   Excision of lesion or tumor (except listed above), dentoalveolar structures; without repair

41826   with simple repair

41827   with complex repair

(For nonexcisional destruction, use 41850)

41828   Excision of hyperplastic alveolar mucosa, each quadrant (specify)

41830   Alveolectomy, including curettage of osteitis or sequestrectomy

41850   Destruction of lesion (except excision), dentoalveolar structures

OTHER PROCEDURES

41870   Periodontal mucosal grafting

41872   Gingivoplasty, each quadrant (specify)

41874   Alveoloplasty, each quadrant (specify)

(For closure of lacerations, see 40830, 40831)

(For segmental osteotomy, use 21206)

(For reduction of fractures, see 21421-21490)

41899   Unlisted procedure, dentoalveolar structures

PALATE AND UVULA

INCISION

42000   Drainage of abscess of palate, uvula

EXCISION, DESTRUCTION

42100   Biopsy of palate, uvula

42104 Excision, lesion of palate, uvula; without closure

42106   with simple primary closure

42107   with local flap closure

    (For skin graft, see 14040-14302)

    (For mucosal graft, use 40818)

42120 Resection of palate or extensive resection of lesion

    (For reconstruction of palate with extraoral tissue, see 14040-14302, 15050, 15120, 15240, 15576)

42140 Uvulectomy, excision of uvula

42145 Palatopharyngoplasty (eg, uvulopalatopharyngoplasty, uvulopharyngoplasty)

    (For removal of exostosis of the bony palate, see 21031, 21032)

42160 Destruction of lesion, palate or uvula (thermal, cryo or chemical)

REPAIR

42180 Repair, laceration of palate; up to 2 cm

42182   over 2 cm or complex

42200 Palatoplasty for cleft palate, soft and/or hard palate only

42205 Palatoplasty for cleft palate, with closure of alveolar ridge; soft tissue only

42210   with bone graft to alveolar ridge (includes obtaining graft)

42215 Palatoplasty for cleft palate; major revision

42220   secondary lengthening procedure

42225   attachment pharyngeal flap

42226 Lengthening of palate, and pharyngeal flap

42227 Lengthening of palate, with island flap

42235 Repair of anterior palate, including vomer flap

    (For repair of oronasal fistula, use 30600)

42260 Repair of nasolabial fistula

    (For repair of cleft lip, see 40700 et seq)

42280 Maxillary impression for palatal prosthesis

42281 Insertion of pin-retained palatal prosthesis

OTHER PROCEDURES

42299 Unlisted procedure, palate, uvula

● New Code   ▲ Revised Code   + Add-On Code   ⊘ Modifier -51 Exempt   ★ Telemedicine

SALIVARY GLAND AND DUCTS

INCISION

42300   Drainage of abscess; parotid, simple

42305   parotid, complicated

42310   submaxillary or sublingual, intraoral

42320   submaxillary, external

42330   Sialolithotomy; submandibular (submaxillary), sublingual or parotid, uncomplicated, intraoral

42335   submandibular (submaxillary), complicated, intraoral

42340   parotid, extraoral or complicated intraoral

EXCISION

42400   Biopsy of salivary gland; needle

       (For fine needle aspiration biopsy, see 10004, 10005, 10006, 10007, 10008, 10009, 10010, 10011, 10012, 10021)

       (For evaluation of fine needle aspirate, see 88172, 88173)

       (If imaging guidance, is performed, see 76942, 77002, 77012, 77021)

42405   incisional

       (If imaging guidance is performed, see 76942, 77002, 77012, 77021)

42408   Excision of sublingual salivary cyst (ranula)

42409   Marsupialization of sublingual salivary cyst (ranula)

42410   Excision of parotid tumor or parotid gland; lateral lobe, without nerve dissection

42415   lateral lobe, with dissection and preservation of facial nerve

42420   total, with dissection and preservation of facial nerve

42425   total, en bloc removal with sacrifice of facial nerve

42426   total, with unilateral radical neck dissection

       (For suture or grafting of facial nerve, see 64864, 64865, 69740, 69745)

42440   Excision of submandibular (submaxillary) gland

42450   Excision of sublingual gland

REPAIR

42500   Plastic repair of salivary duct, sialodochoplasty; primary or simple

42505   secondary or complicated

42507   Parotid duct diversion, bilateral (Wilke type procedure);

Separate Procedure   Unlisted Procedure   CCI Comp. Code   Non-specific Procedure   **465**

| 42509 | with excision of both submandibular glands |
| 42510 | with ligation of both submandibular (Wharton's) ducts |

OTHER PROCEDURES

42550	Injection procedure for sialography
	(For radiological supervision and interpretation, use 70390)
42600	Closure salivary fistula
42650	Dilation salivary duct
42660	Dilation and catheterization of salivary duct, with or without injection
42665	Ligation salivary duct, intraoral
42699	Unlisted procedure, salivary glands or ducts

PHARYNX, ADENOIDS, AND TONSILS

INCISION

42700	Incision and drainage abscess; peritonsillar
42720	retropharyngeal or parapharyngeal, intraoral approach
42725	retropharyngeal or parapharyngeal, external approach

EXCISION, DESTRUCTION

42800	Biopsy; oropharynx
42804	nasopharynx, visible lesion, simple
42806	nasopharynx, survey for unknown primary lesion
	(For laryngoscopic biopsy, see 31510, 31535, 31536)
42808	Excision or destruction of lesion of pharynx, any method
42809	Removal of foreign body from pharynx
42810	Excision branchial cleft cyst or vestige, confined to skin and subcutaneous tissues
42815	Excision branchial cleft cyst, vestige, or fistula, extending beneath subcutaneous tissues and/or into pharynx
42820	Tonsillectomy and adenoidectomy; under age 12
42821	age 12 or over
42825	Tonsillectomy, primary or secondary; under age 12
42826	age 12 or over
42830	Adenoidectomy, primary; under age 12
42831	age 12 or over

● New Code   ▲ Revised Code   + Add-On Code   ⃠ Modifier -51 Exempt   ★ Telemedicine

42835 Adenoidectomy, secondary; under age 12

42836   age 12 or over

42842 Radical resection of tonsil, tonsillar pillars, and/or retromolar trigone; without closure

42844   closure with local flap (eg, tongue, buccal)

42845   closure with other flap

(For closure with other flap(s), use appropriate number for flap(s))

(When combined with radical neck dissection, use also 38720)

42860 Excision of tonsil tags

42870 Excision or destruction lingual tonsil, any method (separate procedure)

(For resection of the nasopharynx (eg., juvenile angiofibroma) by bicoronal and/or transzygomatic approach, see 61586 and 61600)

42890 Limited pharyngectomy

42892 Resection of lateral pharyngeal wall or pyriform sinus, direct closure by advancement of lateral and posterior pharyngeal walls

(When combined with radical neck dissection, use also 38720)

42894 Resection of pharyngeal wall requiring closure with myocutaneous or fasciocutaneous flap or free muscle, skin, or fascial flap with microvascular anastamosis

(When combined with radical neck dissection, use also 38720)

(For limited pharyngectomy with radical neck dissection, use 38720 with 42890)

(For flap used for reconstruction, see 15730, 15733, 15734, 15756, 15757, 15758)

REPAIR

42900 Suture pharynx for wound or injury

42950 Pharyngoplasty (plastic or reconstructive operation on pharynx)

(For pharyngeal flap, use 42225)

42953 Pharyngoesophageal repair

(For closure with myocutaneous or other flap, use appropriate number in addition)

OTHER PROCEDURES

42955 Pharyngostomy (fistulization of pharynx, external for feeding)

42960 Control oropharyngeal hemorrhage, primary or secondary (eg, post-tonsillectomy); simple

42961   complicated, requiring hospitalization

42962   with secondary surgical intervention

42970 Control of nasopharyngeal hemorrhage, primary or secondary (eg, postadenoidectomy); simple, with posterior nasal packs, with or without anterior packs and/or cautery

42971   complicated, requiring hospitalization

      Separate Procedure   Unlisted Procedure   CCI Comp. Code   Non-specific Procedure   **467**

42972   with secondary surgical intervention

42999 Unlisted procedure, pharynx, adenoids, or tonsils

ESOPHAGUS

INCISION

(For esophageal intubation with laparotomy, use 43510)

43020 Esophagotomy, cervical approach, with removal of foreign body

43030 Cricopharyngeal myotomy

43045 Esophagotomy, thoracic approach, with removal of foreign body

EXCISION

(For gastrointestinal reconstruction for previous esophagectomy, see 43360, 43361)

43100 Excision of lesion, esophagus, with primary repair; cervical approach

43101   thoracic or abdominal approach

(For wide excision of malignant lesion of cervical esophagus, with total laryngectomy without radical neck dissection, see 43107, 43116, 43124 and 31360)

(For wide excision of malignant lesion of cervical esophagus, with total laryngectomy with radical neck dissection, see 43107, 43116, 43124, and 31365)

43107 Total or near total esophagectomy, without thoracotomy; with pharyngogastrostomy or cervical esophagogastrostomy, with or without pyloroplasty (transhiatal)

43108   with colon interposition or small intestine reconstruction, including intestine mobilization, preparation and anastomosis(es)

43112 Total or near total esophagectomy, with thoracotomy; with pharyngogastrostomy or cervical esophagogastrostomy, with or without pyloroplasty (ie, McKeown esophagectomy or tri-incisional esophagectomy)

43113   with colon interposition or small intestine reconstruction, including intestine mobilization, preparation, and anastomosis(es)

43116 Partial esophagectomy, cervical, with free intestinal graft, including microvascular anastomosis, obtaining the graft and intestinal reconstruction

(Do not report 43116 in conjunction with 69990)

(Report 43116 with the modifier -52 appended if intestinal or free jejunal graft with microvascular anastomosis is performed by another physician)

(For free jejunal graft with microvascular anastomosis performed by another physician, use 43496)

43117 Partial esophagectomy, distal two-thirds, with thoracotomy and separate abdominal incision, with or without proximal gastrectomy; with thoracic esophagogastrostomy, with or without pyloroplasty (Ivor Lewis)

43118   with colon interposition or small intestine reconstruction, including intestine mobilization, preparation, and anastomosis(es)

(For total esophagectomy with gastropharyngostomy, see 43107, 43124)

(For esophagogastrectomy (lower third) and vagotomy, use 43122)

43121 Partial esophagectomy, distal two-thirds, with thoracotomy only, with or without proximal gastrectomy, with thoracic esophagogastrostomy, with or without pyloroplasty

43122 Partial esophagectomy, thoracoabdominal or abdominal approach, with or without proximal gastrectomy; with esophagogastrostomy, with or without pyloroplasty

43123 with colon interposition or small intestine reconstruction, including intestine mobilization, preparation, and anastomosis(es)

43124 Total or partial esophagectomy, without reconstruction (any approach), with cervical esophagostomy

43130 Diverticulectomy of hypopharynx or esophagus, with or without myotomy; cervical approach

43135 thoracic approach

(For endoscopic diverticulectomy of hypopharynx or cervical esophagus, use 43180)

ENDOSCOPY

When bleeding occurs as a result of an endoscopic procedure, control of bleeding is not reported separately during the same operative session.

Esophagoscopy includes examination from the cricopharyngeus muscle (upper esophageal sphincter) to and including the gastroesophageal junction. It may also include examination of the proximal region of the stomach via retroflexion when performed.

Esophagoscopy

43180 Esophagoscopy, rigid, transoral with diverticulectomy of hypopharynx or cervical esophagus (eg, Zenker's diverticulum), with cricopharyngeal myotomy, includes use of telescope or operating microscope and repair, when performed

(Do not report 43180 in conjunction with 43210, 69990)

(For diverticulectomy of hypopharynx or esophagus [open], see 43130, 43135)

43191 Esophagoscopy, rigid, transoral; diagnostic, including collection of specimen(s) by brushing or washing when performed (separate procedure)

(Do not report 43191 in conjunction with 43192, 43193, 43194, 43195, 43196, 43197, 43198, 43210)

(For diagnostic transnasal esophagoscopy, see 43197, 43198)

(For diagnostic flexible transoral esophagoscopy, use 43200)

43192 with directed submucosal injection(s), any substance

(Do not report 43192 in conjunction with 43191, 43197, 43198)

(For flexible transoral esophagoscopy with directed submucosal injection(s), use 43201)

(For flexible transoral esophagoscopy with injection sclerosis of esophageal varices, use 43204)

(For rigid transoral esophagoscopy with injection sclerosis of esophageal varices, use 43499)

43193 with biopsy, single or multiple

(Do not report 43193 in conjunction with 43191, 43197, 43198)

(For flexible transoral esophagoscopy with biopsy, use 43202)

43194 with removal of foreign body(s)

(Do not report 43194 in conjunction with 43191, 43197, 43198)

(If fluoroscopic guidance is performed, use 76000)

Separate Procedure   Unlisted Procedure   CCI Comp. Code   Non-specific Procedure   **469**

(For flexible transoral esophagoscopy with removal of foreign body(s), use 43215)

43195   with balloon dilation (less than 30 mm diameter)

(Do not report 43195 in conjunction with 43191, 43197, 43198)

(If fluoroscopic guidance is performed, use 74360)

(For esophageal dilation with balloon 30 mm diameter or larger, see 43214, 43233)

(For dilation without endoscopic visualization, see 43450, 43453)

(For flexible transoral esophagoscopy with balloon dilation [less than 30 mm diameter], use 43220)

43196   with insertion of guide wire followed by dilation over guide wire

(Do not report 43196 in conjunction with 43191, 43197, 43198)

(If fluoroscopic guidance is performed, use 74360)

(For flexible transoral esophagoscopy with insertion of guide wire followed by dilation over guide wire, use 43226)

43197   Esophagoscopy, flexible, transnasal; diagnostic, including collection of specimen(s) by brushing or washing, when performed (separate procedure)

(Do not report 43197 in conjunction with 31575, 43191, 43192, 43193, 43194, 43195, 43196, 43198, 43200-43232, 43235-43259, 43266, 43270, 92511)

(For transoral esophagoscopy, see 43191, 43200)

(Do not report 43197 in conjunction with 31231 unless separate type of endoscope [eg, rigid endoscope] is used)

43198   with biopsy, single or multiple

(Do not report 43198 in conjunction with 31575, 43191, 43192, 43193, 43194, 43195, 43196, 43197, 43200-43232, 43235-43259, 43266, 43270, 92511)

(For transoral esophagoscopy with biopsy, see 43193, 43202)

(Do not report 43198 in conjunction with 31231 unless separate type of endoscope [eg, rigid endoscope] is used)

43200   Esophagoscopy, flexible, transoral; diagnostic, including collection of specimen(s) by brushing or washing, when performed (separate procedure)

(Do not report 43200 in conjunction with 43197, 43198, 43201-43232)

(For diagnostic rigid transoral esophagoscopy, use 43191)

(For diagnostic flexible transnasal esophacoscopy, use 43197)

(For diagnostic flexible esophagogastroduodenoscopy, use 43235)

43201   with directed submucosal injection(s), any substance

(Do not report 43201 in conjunction with 43204, 43211, 43227 for the same lesion)

(Do not report 43201 in conjunction with 43197, 43198, 43200)

(For rigid transoral esophagoscopy with directed submucosal injection[s], use 43192)

(For flexible transoral esophagoscopy with injection sclerosis of esophageal varices, use 43204)

(For rigid transoral esophagoscopy with injection sclerosis of esophageal varices, use 43499)

43202   with biopsy, single or multiple

(Do not report 43202 in conjunction with 43211 for the same lesion)

(Do not report 43202 in conjunction with 43197, 43198, 43200)

(For rigid transoral esophagoscopy with biopsy, use 43193)

(For flexible transnasal esophagoscopy with biopsy, use 43198)

43204   with injection sclerosis of esophageal varices

(Do not report 43204 in conjunction with 43201, 43227 for the same lesion)

(Do not report 43204 in conjunction with 43197, 43198, 43200)

(For rigid transoral esophagoscopy with injection sclerosisk of esophageal varices, use 43499)

43205   with band ligation of esophageal varices

(Do not report 43205 in conjunction with 43227 for the same lesion)

(Do not report 43205 in conjunction with 43197, 43198, 43200)

(To report control of nonvariceal bleeding with band ligation, use 43227)

43206   with optial endomicroscopy

(Report supply of contrast agent separately)

(Do not report 43206 in conjunction with 43197, 43198, 43200, 88375)

43210   This code is out of order. See page 476

43211   This code is out of order. See page 471

43212   This code is out of order. See page 472

43213   This code is out of order. See page 472

43214   This code is out of order. See page 472

43215   with removal of foreign body(s)

(Do not report 43215 in conjunction with 43197, 43198, 43200)

(If fluoroscopic guidance is performed, use 76000)

(For rigid transoral esophagoscopy with removal of foreign body(s), use 43194)

43216   with removal of tumor(s), polyp(s), or other lesion(s) by hot biopsy forceps or bipolar cautery

(Do not report 43216 in conjunction with 43197, 43198, 43200)

43217   with removal of tumor(s), polyp(s), or other lesion(s) by snare technique

(Do not report 43217 in conjunction with 43211 for the same lesion)

(Do not report 43217 in conjunction with 43197, 43198, 43200)

(For esophagogastroduodenoscopy with removal of tumor[s], polyp[s], or other lesion[s] by snare technique, use 43251)

(For endoscopic mucosal resection, use 43211)

43211   with endoscopic mucosal resection

(Do not report 43211 in conjunction with 43201, 43202, 43217 for the same lesion)

(Do not report 43211 in conjunction with 43197, 43198, 43200)

Separate Procedure   Unlisted Procedure   CCI Comp. Code   Non-specific Procedure   **471**

43212   with placement of endoscopic stent (includes pre- and post-dilation and guide wire passage, when performed)

(Do not report 43212 in conjunction with 43197, 43198, 43200, 43220, 43226, 43241)

(If fluoroscopic guidance is performed, use 74360)

43220   with transendoscopic balloon dilation (less than 30 mm diameter)

(Do not report 43220 in conjunction with 43197, 43198, 43200, 43212, 43226, 43229)

(If fluoroscopic guidance is performed, use 74360)

(For rigid transoral esophagoscopy with balloon dilation [less than 30 mm diameter], use 43195)

(For esophageal dilation with balloon 30 mm diameter or larger, use 43214)

(For dilation without endoscopic visualization, see 43450, 43453)

43213   with dilation of esophagus, by balloon or dilator, retrograde (includes fluoroscopic guidance, when performed)

(Do not report 43213 in conjunction with 43197, 43198, 43200, 74360, 76000)

(For transendoscopic balloon dilation of multiple strictures during the same session, report 43213 with modifier 59 for each additiional stricture dilated)

43214   with dilation of esophagus with balloon (30 mm diameter or larger) (includes fluoroscopic guidance, when performed)

(Do not report 43214 in conjunction with 43197, 43198, 43200, 74360, 76000)

43226   with insertion of guide wire followed by passage of dilator(s) over guide wire

(Do not report 43226 in conjunction with 43229 for the same lesion)

(Do not report 43226 in conjunction with 43197, 43198, 43200, 43212, 43220)

(If fluoroscopic guidance is performed, use 74360)

(For rigid transoral esophagoscopy wit insertion of guide wire followed by dilation over guide wire, use 43196)

43227   with control of bleeding, any method

(Do not report 43227 in conunction with 43201, 43204, 43205 for the same lesion)

(Do not report 43227 in conjunction with 43197, 43198, 43200)

43229   with ablation of tumor(s), polyp(s), or other lesion(s) (includes pre- and post-dilation and guide wire passage, when performed)

(Do not report 43229 in conjunction with 43220, 43226 for the same lesion)

(Do not report 43229 in conjunction with 43197, 43198, 43200)

(For esophagoscopic photodynamic therapy, report 43229 in conjunction with 96570, 96571 as appropriate)

43231   with endoscopic ultrasound examination

(Do not report 43231 in conjunction with 43197, 43198, 43200, 43232, 76975)

(Do not report 43231 more than once per session)

43232   with transendoscopic ultrasound-guided intramural or transmural fine needle aspiration/biopsy(s)

(Do not report 43232 in conjunction with 43197, 43198, 43200, 43231, 76942, 76975)

● New Code   ▲ Revised Code   + Add-On Code   ⊘ Modifier -51 Exempt   ★ Telemedicine

(Do not report 43232 more than once per session)

43233   This code is out of order. See page 475

Esophagogastroduodenoscopy

(For examination of the esophagus from the cricopharyngeus muscle [upper esophageal sphincter] to and including the gastroesophageal junction, including examination of the proximal region of the stomach via retroflexion when perofrmed, see 43197, 43198, 43200, 43201, 43202, 43204, 43205, 43206, 43211, 43212, 43213, 43214, 43215, 43216, 43217, 43220, 43226, 43227, 43229, 43231, 43232)

(Use 43233, 43235-43259, 43266, 43270 for examination of a surgically altered stomach where the jejunum is examined distal to the anastomosis [eg, gastric bypass, gastroenterostomy{BillrothII}])

To report esophagogastroscopy where the duodenum is deliberately not examined (eg, judged clinically not pertinent), or because the clinical situation precludes such exam (eg, significant gastric retention precludes safe exam of duodenum], append modifier 52 if repeat examination is not planned, or modifier 53 if repeat examiniation is planned.

43235   Esophagogastroduodenoscopy, flexible, transoral; diagnostic, including collection of specimen(s) by brushing or washing, when performed (separate procedure)

(Do not report 43235 in conjunction with 43197, 43198, 43210, 43236-43259, 43266, 43270, 44360, 44361, 44363, 44364, 44365, 44366, 44369, 44370, 44372, 44373, 44376, 44377, 44378, 44379)

43236   with directed submucosal injection(s), any substance

(Do not report 43236 in conjunction with 43243, 43254, 43255 for the same lesion)

(Do not report 43236 in conjunction with 43197, 43198, 43235, 44360, 44361, 44363, 44364, 44365, 44366, 44369, 44370, 44372, 44373, 44376, 44377, 44378, 44379)

(For flexible, transoral esophagogastroduodenoscopy with injection sclerosis of esophageal and/or gastric varicies, use 43243)

43237   with endoscopic ultrasound examination limited to the esophagus, stomach or duodenum, and adjacent structures

(Do not report 43237 in conjunction with 43197, 43198, 43235, 43238, 43242, 43253, 43259, 44360, 44361, 44363, 44364, 44365, 44366, 44369, 44370, 44372, 44373, 44376, 44377, 44378, 44379, 76975)

(Do not report 43237 more than once per session)

43238   with transendoscopic ultrasound-guided intramural or transmural fine needle aspiration/biopsy(s), esophagus (includes endoscopic ultrasound examination limited to the esophagus, stomach or duodenum, and adjacent structures)

(Do not report 43238 in conjunction with 43197, 43198, 43235, 43237, 43242, 44360, 44361, 44363, 44364, 44365, 44366, 44369, 44370, 44372, 44373, 44376, 44377, 44378, 44379, 76942, 76975)

(Do not report 43238 more than once per session)

43239   with biopsy, single or multiple

(Do not report 43239 in conjunction with 43254 for the same lesion)

(Do not report 43238 in conjunction with 43197, 43198, 43235, 44360, 44361, 44363, 44364, 44365, 44366, 44369, 44370, 44372, 44373, 44376, 44377, 44378, 44379)

43240   with transmural drainage of pseudocyst (includes placement of transmural drainage catheter[s]/stent[s], when performed, and endoscopic ultrasound, when performed

(Do not report 43240 in conjunction with 43253 for the same lesion)

(Do not report 43240 in conjunction with 43197, 43198, 43235, 43242, 43259, 43266, 44360, 44361, 44363, 44364, 44365, 44366, 44369, 44370, 44372, 44373, 44376, 44377, 44378, 44379)

(Do not report 43240 more than once per session)

(For endoscopic pancreatic necrosectomy, use 48999)

43241   with insertion of intraluminal tube or catheter

(Do not report 43241 in conjunction with 43197, 43198, 43212, 43235, 43266, 44360, 44361, 44363, 44364, 44365, 44366, 44369, 44370, 44372, 44373, 44376, 44377, 44378, 44379)

(For naso- or oro-gastric tube placement requiring physician's or other qualified health care professional's skill and fluoroscopic guidance, use 43752)

(For nonendoscopic enteric tube placement, see 44500, 74340)

43242   with transendoscopic ultrasound-guided intramural or transmural fine needle aspiration/biopsy(s) (includes endoscopic ultrasound examination of the esophagus, stomach, and either the duodenum or a surgically latered stomach where the jejunum is examined distal to the anastomosis)

(Do not report 43242 in conjunction with 43197, 43198, 43235, 43237, 43238, 43240, 43259, 44360, 44361, 44363, 44364, 44365, 44366, 44369, 44370, 44372, 44373, 44376, 44377, 44378, 44379, 76942, 76975)

(Do not report 43242 more than once per session)

(For transendoscopic ultrasound-guided transmural fine needle aspiration/biopsy limited to the esophagus, stomach, duodenum, or adjacent structure, use 43238)

43243   with injection sclerosis of esophagea/gastric varices

(Do not report 43243 in conjunction with 43236, 43255 for the same lesion)

(Do not report 43243 in conjunction with 43197, 43198, 43235, 44360, 44361, 44363, 44364, 44365, 44366, 44369, 44370, 44372, 44373, 44376, 44377, 44378, 44379)

43244   with band ligation of esophageal/gastric varices

(Do not report 43244 in conjunction with 43197, 43198, 43235, 43255, 44360, 44361, 44363, 44364, 44365, 44366, 44369, 44370, 44372, 44373, 44376, 44377, 44378, 44379)

(To report control of noninvasive bleeding with band ligation, use 43255)

43245   with dilation of gastric/duodenal stricture(s) (eg, balloon, bougie)

(Do not report 43245 in conjunction with 43197, 43198, 43235, 43266, 44360, 44361, 44363, 44364, 44365, 44366, 44369, 44370, 44372, 44373, 44376, 44377, 44378, 44379)

(If fluoroscopic guidance is performed, use 74360)

43246   with directed placement of percutaneous gastrostomy tube

(Do not report 43246 in conjunction with 43197, 43198, 43235, 44360, 44361, 44363, 44364, 44365, 44366, 44369, 44370, 44372, 44376, 44377, 44378, 44379)

(For percutaneous insertion of gastrostomy tube under fluoroscopic guidance, use 49440)

(For percutaneous replacement of gastrostomy tube without imaging or endoscopy, see 43762, 43763)

43247   with removal of foreign body(s)

(Do not report 43247 in conjunction with 43197, 43198, 43235, 44360, 44361, 44363, 44364, 44365, 44366, 44369, 44370, 44372, 44373, 44376, 44377, 44378, 44379)

(If fluoroscopic guidance is performed, use 76000)

43248   with insertion of guide wire followed by passage of dilator(s) through esophagus over guide wire

(Do not report 43248 in conjunction with 43197, 43198, 43235, 43266, 43270, 44360, 44361, 44363, 44364, 44365, 44366, 44369, 44370, 44372, 44373, 44376, 44377, 44378, 44379)

(If fluoroscopic guidance is performed, use 74360)

43249   with transendoscopic balloon dilation of esophagus (less than 30 mm diameter)

(Do not report 43249 in conjunction with 43197, 43198, 43235, 43266, 43270, 44360, 44361, 44363, 44364, 44365, 44366, 44369, 44370, 44372, 44373, 44376, 44377, 44378, 44379)

(If fluoroscopic guidance is performed, use 74360)

43233   with dilation of esophagus with balloon (30 mm diameter or larger) (includes fluoroscopic guidance, when performed)

(Do not report 43233 in conjunction with 43197, 43198, 43235, 44360, 44361, 44363, 44364, 44365, 44366, 44369, 44370, 44372, 44373, 44376, 44377, 44378, 44379, 74360, 76000)

43250   with removal of tumor(s), polyp(s), or other lesion(s) by hot biopsy forceps

(Do not report 43250 in conjunction with 43197, 43198, 43235, 44360, 44361, 44363, 44364, 44365, 44366, 44369, 44370, 44372, 44373, 44376, 44377, 44378, 44379)

43251   with removal of tumor(s), polyp(s), or other lesion(s) by snare technique

(Do not report 43251 in conjunction with 43254 for the same lesion)

(Do not report 43251 in conjunction with 43197, 43198, 43235, 44360, 44361, 44363, 44364, 44365, 44366, 44369, 44370, 44372, 44373, 44376, 44377, 44378, 44379)

(For endoscopic mucosal resection, use 43254)

43252   with optical endomicroscopy

(Report supply of contrast agent separately)

(Do not report 43252 in conjunction with 43197, 43198, 43235, 44360, 44361, 44363, 44364, 44365, 44366, 44369, 44370, 44372, 44373, 44376, 44377, 44378, 44379, 88375)

43253   with transendoscopic ultrasound-guided transmural injection of diagnostic or therapeutic substance(s) (eg, anesthetic, neurolytic agent) or fiducial marker(s) (includes endoscopic ultrasound examination of the esophagus, stomach, and either the duodenum or a surgically altered stomach where the jejunum is examined distal to the anastomosis)

(Do not report 43253 in conjunction with 43240 for the same lesion)

(Do not report 43253 in conjunction with 43197, 43198, 43235, 43237, 43259, 44360, 44361, 44363, 44364, 44365, 44366, 44369, 44370, 44372, 44373, 44376, 44377, 44378, 44379, 76942, 76975)

(Do not report 43253 more than once per session)

(For transendoscopic ultrasound-guided transmural fine needle aspiration/biopsy, see 43238, 43242)

43254   with endoscopic mucoal resection

(Do not report 43254 in conjunction with 43236, 43239, 43251 for the same lesion)

(Do not report 43254 in conjunction with 43197, 43198, 43235, 44360, 44361, 44363, 44364, 44365, 44366, 44369, 44370, 44372, 44373, 44376, 44377, 44378, 44379)

43255   with control of bleeding, any method

(Do not report 43255 in conjunction with 43236, 43243, 43244 for the same lesion)

(Do not report 43255 in conjunction with 43197, 43198, 43235, 44360, 44361, 44363, 44364, 44365, 44366, 44369, 44370, 44372, 44373, 44376, 44377, 44378, 44379)

43266   with placement of endoscopic stent (includes pre- and post-dilation and guide wire passage, when performed)

(Do not report 43266 in conjunction with 43197, 43198, 43235, 43240, 43241, 43245, 43248, 43249, 44360, 44361, 44363, 44364, 44365, 44366, 44369, 44370, 44372, 44373, 44376, 44377, 44378, 44379)

| | Separate Procedure | | Unlisted Procedure | | CCI Comp. Code | | Non-specific Procedure | **475** |

(If fluoroscopic guidance is performed, use 74360)

43257   with delivery of thermal energy to the muscle of lower esophageal sphincter and/or gastric cardia, for treatment of gastroesophageal reflux disease

(Do not report 43257 in conjunction with 43197, 43198, 43235, 44360, 44361, 44363, 44364, 44365, 44366, 44369, 44370, 44372, 44373, 44376, 44377, 44378, 44379)

(For ablation of metaplastic/dysplastic esophageal lesion [eg., Barrett's esophagus], see 43229, 43270)

43270   with ablation of tumor(s), polyp(s), or other lesion(s) (includes pre-and post-dilation and guide wire passage, when performed)

(Do not report 43270 in conjunction with 43248, 43249 for the same lesion)

(Do not report 43270 in conjunction with 43197, 43198, 43235, 44360, 44361, 44363, 44364, 44365, 44366, 44369, 44370, 44372, 44373, 44376, 44377, 44378, 44379)

(For esophagoscopic photodynamic therapy, use 43270 in conjunction with 96570, 96571 as appropriate)

43259   with endoscopic ultrasound examination, including the esophagus, stomach, and either the duodenum or a surgically altered stomach where the jejunum is examined distal to the anastomosis

(Do not report 43259 in conjunction with 43197, 43198, 43235, 43237, 43240, 43242, 43253, 44360, 44361, 44363, 44364, 44365, 44366, 44369, 44370, 44372, 44373, 44376, 44377, 44378, 44379, 76975)

(Do not report 43259 more than once per session)

43210   with esophagogastric fundoplasty, partial or complete, includes duodenoscopy when performed

(Do not report 43210 in conjunction with 43180, 43191, 43197, 43200, 43235)

Endoscopic Retrograde Cholangiopancreatography (ERCP)

Report the appropriate code(s) for each service performed. Therapeutic ERCP (43261, 43262, 43263, 43264, 43265, 43274, 43275, 43276, 43277, 43278) includes diagnostic ERCP (43260). ERCP includes guide wire passage when performed. An ERCP is considered complete if one or more of the ductal system(s), (pancreatic/biliary) is visualized. To report ERCP attempted but with unsuccessful cannulation of any ductal system, see 43235-43259, 43266, 43270.

(For percutaneous biliary catheter procedures, see 47490-47544)

Codes 43274, 43275, 43276 and 43277 describe ERCP with stent placement, removal or replacement (exchange) of stent(s), and balloon dilation within the pancreatico-biliary system. For reporting purposes, ducts that may be reported as stented or subject to stent repalcement (exchange) or to balloon dilation include:

Pancreas: major and minor ducts.

Biliary tree: common bile duct, right hepatic duct, left hepatic duct, cystic duct/gallbladder

ERCP with stent placement includes any balloon dilation performed in that duct. ERCP with more than one stent placement (eg, different ducts or side-by-side in the same duct) performed during the same day/session may be reported with 43274 more than once with modifier 59 appended to the subsequent procedure(s). For ERCP with more than one stent exchanged during the same day/session, 43276 may be reported for the initial stent exchange, and 43276 with modifier 59 for each additional stent exchange. ERCP with balloon dilation of more than one duct during the same day/session may be reported with modifier 59 appended to the subsequent procedure(s). Sphincteroplasty, which is balloon dilation of the ampulla (sphincter of Oddi), is reported with 43277, and includes sphincterotomy (43262) when performed.

To report ERCP via altered postoperative anatomy, see 43260, 43262, 43263, 43264, 43265, 43273, 43274, 43275, 43276, 43277, 43278, for Billroth II gastroenterostomy. See 47999 (Unlisted procedure, biliary tract), or 48999 (Unlisted procedure, pancreas) for ERCP via gastrostomy (laparoscopic or open) or via Roux-en-Y anatomy (eg, post-bariatric gastric bypass, post-total gastrectomy).

To report optical endomicroscopy of the biliary tract and pancreas, use 0397T. Do not report optical endomicroscopy more than once per session

   ● New Code   ▲ Revised Code   + Add-On Code   ⃠ Modifier -51 Exempt   ★ Telemedicine

Stone destruction includes any stone removal in the same ductal system (biliary/pancreatic). Code 43277 may be separately reported if sphincteroplasty or dilation of the ductal stricture is required before proceeding to remove stones/debris from the duct during the same session. Dilation that is incidental to the passage of an instrument to clear stones or debris is not separately reported.

(Do not report 43277 for use of a balloon catheter to clear stones/debris from a duct. Any dilation of the duct that may occur during this maneuver is considered inherent to the work of 43264 and 43265)

(If imaging of the ductal systems is performed, including images saved to the permanent record and report of the imaging, see 74328, 74329, 74330)

43260 Endoscopic retrograde cholangiopancreatography (ERCP); diagnostic, including collection of specimen(s) by brushing or washing, when performed (separate procedure)

(Do not report 43260 in conjunction with 43261, 43262, 43263, 43264, 43265, 43274, 43275, 43276, 43277, 43278)

43261 with biopsy, single or multiple

(Do not report 43261 in conjunction with 43260)

(For percutaneous endoluminal biopsy of biliary tree, use 47543)

43262 with sphincterotomy/papillotomy

(43262 may be reported when sphincterotomy is performed in addition to 43261, 43263, 43264, 43265, 43275, 43278)

(Do not report 43262 in conjunction with 43274 for stent placement or with 43276 for stent replacement [exhange] in the same location)

(Do not report 43262 in conjunction with 43260, 43277)

(For percutaneous balloon dilation of biliary duct(s) or of ampulla, use 47542)

43263 with pressure measurement of sphincter of Oddi

(Do not report 43263 in conjunction with 43260)

(Do not report 43263 more than once per session)

43264 with removal of calculi/debris from biliary/pancreatic duct(s)

(Do not report 43264 if no calculi or debris are found, even if balloon catheter is deployed)

(Do note report 43264 in conjunction with 43260, 43265)

(For percutaneous removal of calculi/debris, use 47544)

43265 with destruction of calculi, any method (eg, mechanical, electrohydraulic, lithotripsy)

(Do not report 43265 in conjunction with 43260, 43264)

(For percutaneous removal of calculi/debris, use 47544)

43266 This code is out of order. See page 475

43270 This code is out of order. See page 476

43274 with placement of endoscopic stent into biliary or pancreatic duct, including lpre- and post-dilation and guide wire passage, when performed, including sphincterotomy, when performed, each stent

(Do not report 43274 in conjunction with 43262, 43275, 43276, 43277 for stent placement or replacement [exchange] in the same duct)

(For stent placement in both the pancreatic duct and the common bile duct during the same operative session, placement of separate stents in both the right and left hepatic ducts, or placement of two side-by-side stents in the same duct 43274 may be reported for each additional stent placed, using modifier 59 with the subsequent procedure[s])

(To report naso-biliary or naso-pancreatic drainage tube placement, use 43274)

(For percutaneous placement of biliary stent(s), see 47538, 47539, 47540)

43275 with removal of foreign body(s) or stent(s) from biliary/pancreatic duct(s)

(Do not report 43275 in conjunction with 43260, 43274, 43276)

(For removal of stent from biliary or pancreatic duct without ERCP, use 43247)

(Report 43275 only once for removal of one or more stents or foreign bodies from biliary/pancreatic ducts during the same session)

(For percutaneous removal of calculi/debris, use 47544)

43276 with removal and exchange of stent(s), biliary or pancreatic duct, including pre- and post-dilation and guide wire passage, when performed, including sphincterotomy, when performed, each stent exchanged

(43276 includes removal and replacement [exchange] of one stent. For replacement [exchange] of additional stent[s] during the same session, report 43276 with modifier 59 for each additional replacement [exchange])

(Do not report 43276 in conjunction with 43260, 43275)

(Do not report 43276 in conjunction with 43262, 43274 for stent placement or exchange in the same duct)

43277 with trans-endoscopic balloon dilation of biliary/pancreatic duct(s) or of ampulla (sphincteroplasty), including sphincterotomy, when performed, each duct

(Do not report 43277 in conjunction with 43278 for the same lesion)

(Do not report 43277 in conjunction with 43260, 43262)

(Do not report 43277 for incidental dilation using balloon for stone/debris removal reported with 43264, 43265)

(If sphincterotomy without sphincteroplasty is performed on a separate pancreatic duct orifice during the same session [ie, pancreas divisum], report 43262 with modifier 59)

(Do not report 43277 in conjunction with 43274, 43276 for dilation and stent placement/replacement [exchange] in the same duct)

(For transendoscopic balloon dilation of multiple strictures during the same session, use 43277 with modifier 59 for each additional stricture dilated)

(For bilateral balloon dilation [both right and left hepatic ducts], 43277 may be reported twice with modifier 59 appended to the second procedure)

(For percutaneous balloon dilation of biliary duct(s) or of ampulla (sphincteroplasty), use 47542)

43278 with ablation of tumor(s), polyp(s), or other lesion(s), including pre- and post-dilation and guide wire passage, when performed

(Do not report 43278 in conjunction with 43277 for the same lesion)

(Do not report 43278 in conjunction with 43260)

(For ampullectomy, use 43254)

+ 43273 Endoscopic cannulation of papilla with direct visualization of pancreatic/common bile duct(s) (List separately in addition to code(s) for primary procedure)

(Report 43273 once per procedure)

(Use 43273 in conjunction with 43260, 43261, 43262, 43263, 43264, 43265, 43274, 43275, 43276, 43277, 43278)

43274   This code is out of order. See page 477

43275   This code is out of order. See page 478

43276   This code is out of order. See page 478

43277   This code is out of order. See page 478

43278   This code is out of order. See page 478

LAPAROSCOPY

Surgical laparoscopy always includes diagnostic laparoscopy. To report a diagnostic laparoscopy (peritoneoscopy) (separate procedure), use 49320.

43279   Laparoscopy, surgical, esophagomyotomy (Heller type), with fundoplasty, when performed

(For open approach, see 43330, 43331)

(Do not report 43279 in conjunction with 43280)

43280   Laparoscopy, surgical, esophagogastric fundoplasty (eg, Nissen, Toupet procedures)

(Do not report 43280 in conjunction with 43279, 43281, 43282)

(For open esophagogastric fundoplasty, see 43327, 43328)

(For laparoscopy, surgical, esophageal sphincter augmentation procedure, placement of sphincter augmentation device, see 43284, 43285)

(For esophagogastroduodenoscopy fundoplasty, partial or complete, transoral approach, use 43210)

43281   Laparoscopy, surgical, repair of paraesophageal hernia, includes fundoplasty, when performed; without implantation of mesh

43282   with implantation of mesh

(To report transabdominal paraesophageal hiatal hernia repair, see 43332, 43333)

(To report transthoracic diaphragmatic hernia repair, see 43334, 43335)

(Do not report 43281, 43282 in conjunction with 43280, 43450, 43453)

+ **43283**   Laparoscopy, surgical, esophageal lengthening procedure (eg, Collis gastroplasty or wedge gastroplasty) (list separately in addition to code for primary procedure)

(Use 43283 in conjunction with 43280, 43281, 43282)

43284   Laparoscopy, surgical, esophageal sphincter augmentation procedure, placement of sphincter augmentation device (ie, magnetic band), including cruroplasty when performed

(Do not report 43284 in conjunction with 43279, 43280, 43281, 43282)

43285   Removal of esophageal sphincter augmentation device

43286   Esophagectomy, total or near total, with laparoscopic mobilization of the abdominal and mediastinal esophagus and proximal gastrectomy, with laparoscopic pyloric drainage procedure if performed, with open cervical pharyngogastrostomy or esophagogastrostomy (ie, laparoscopic transhiatal esophagectomy)

43287   Esophagectomy, distal two-thirds, with laparoscopic mobilization of the abdominal and lower mediastinal esophagus and proximal gastrectomy, with laparoscopic pyloric drainage procedure if performed, with separate thoracoscopic mobilization of the middle and upper mediastinal esophagus and thoracic esophagogastrostomy (ie, laparoscopic thoracoscopic esophagectomy, Ivor Lewis esophagectomy)

(Do not report 43287 in conjunction with 32551 for right tube thoracostomy)

43288 Esophagectomy, total or near total, with thoracoscopic mobilization of the upper, middle, and lower mediastinal esophagus, with separate laparoscopic proximal gastrectomy, with laparoscopic pyloric drainage procedure if performed, with open cervical pharyngogastrostomy or esophagogastrostomy (ie, thoracoscopic, laparoscopic and cervical incision esophagectomy, McKeown esophagectomy, tri-incisional esophagectomy)

(Do not report 43288 in conjunction with 32551 for right tube thoracostomy)

43289 Unlisted laparoscopy procedure, esophagus

REPAIR

43300 Esophagoplasty, (plastic repair or reconstruction), cervical approach; without repair of tracheoesophageal fistula

43305 with repair of tracheoesophageal fistula

43310 Esophagoplasty, (plastic repair or reconstruction), thoracic approach; without repair of tracheoesophageal fistula

43312 with repair of tracheoesophageal fistula

43313 Esophagoplasty for congenital defect, (plastic repair or reconstruction), thoracic approach; without repair of congenital tracheoesophageal fistula

43314 with repair of congenital tracheoesophageal fistula

(Do not report modifier 63 in conjunction with 43313, 43314)

43320 Esophagogastrostomy (cardioplasty), with or without vagotomy and pyloroplasty, transabdominal or transthoracic approach

(For laparoscopic procedure, use 43280)

43325 Esophagogastric fundoplasty; with fundic patch (Thal-Nissen procedure)

(For cricopharyngeal myotomy, use 43030)

43327 Esophagogastric fundoplasty, partial or complete; laparotomy

43328 thoracotomy

(For esophagogastroduodenoscopy fundoplasty, partial or complete, transoral approach, use 43210)

43330 Esophagomyotomy (Heller type); abdominal approach

(For laparoscopic esophagomyotomy procedure, use 43279)

43331 thoracic approach

(For thoracoscopic esophagomyotomy, use 32665)

43332 Repair, paraesophageal hiatal hernia (including fundoplication), via laparotomy, except neonatal; without implantation of mesh or other prosthesis

43333 with implantation of mesh or other prosthesis

(For neonatal diaphragmatic hernia repair, use 39503)

43334 Repair, paraesophageal hiatal hernia (including fundoplication), via thoracotomy, except neonatal; without implantation of mesh or other prosthesis

43335 with implantation of mesh or other prosthesis

● New Code ▲ Revised Code ✛ Add-On Code ⃠ Modifier -51 Exempt ★ Telemedicine

(For neonatal diaphragmatic hernia repair, use 39503)

43336   Repair, paraesophageal hiatal hernia (including fundoplication), via thoracoabdominal incision, except neonatal; without implantation of mesh or other prosthesis

43337   with implantation of mesh or other prosthesis

(For neonatal diaphragmatic hernia repair, use 39503)

+ 43338   Esophageal lengthening procedure (eg, Collis gastroplasty or wedge gastroplasty) (List separately in addition to code for primary procedure)

(Use 43338 in conjunction with 43280, 43327-43337)

43340   Esophagojejunostomy (without total gastrectomy); abdominal approach

43341   thoracic approach

43351   Esophagostomy, fistulization of esophagus, external; thoracic approach

43352   cervical approach

43360   Gastrointestinal reconstruction for previous esophagectomy, for obstructing esophageal lesion or fistula, or for previous esophageal exclusion; with stomach, with or without pyloroplasty

43361   with colon interposition or small intestine reconstruction, including intestine mobilization, preparation, and anastomosis(es)

43400   Ligation, direct, esophageal varices

(43401   deleted 2019 [2020 Edition])

43405   Ligation or stapling at gastroesophageal junction for pre-existing esophageal perforation

43410   Suture of esophageal wound or injury; cervical approach

43415   transthoracic or transabdominal approach

43420   Closure of esophagostomy or fistula; cervical approach

43425   transthoracic or transabdominal approach

(To report transabdominal paraesophageal hiatal hernia repair, see 43332, 43333. To report transthoracic diaphragmatic hernia repair, see 43334, 43335.)

MANIPULATION

(For associated esophagogram, use 74220)

43450   Dilation of esophagus, by unguided sound or bougie, single or multiple passes

(For radiological supervision and interpretation, use 74360)

43453   Dilation of esophagus, over guide wire

(For dilation with endoscopic visualization, see 43195, 43226)

(For dilation of esophagus, by balloon or dilator, see 43214, 43220, 43233, 43249)

(For radiological supervision and interpretation, use 74360)

(For endoscopic dilation of esophagus with balloon less than 30 mm diameter, see 43195, 43220, 43249)

(For endoscopic dilation of esophagus with balloon 30 mm diameter or larger, see 43214, 43233)

Separate Procedure   Unlisted Procedure   CCI Comp. Code   Non-specific Procedure   **481**

43460 Esophagogastric tamponade, with balloon (Sengstaken type)

(For removal of esophageal foreign body by balloon catheter, see 43499, 74235)

OTHER PROCEDURES

43496 Free jejunum transfer with microvascular anastomosis

(Do not report code 69990 in addition to code 43496)

43499 Unlisted procedure, esophagus

STOMACH

INCISION

43500 Gastrotomy; with exploration or foreign body removal

43501 with suture repair of bleeding ulcer

43502 with suture repair of pre-existing esophagogastric laceration (eg, Mallory-Weiss)

43510 with esophageal dilation and insertion of permanent intraluminal tube (eg, Celestin or Mousseaux-Barbin)

43520 Pyloromyotomy, cutting of pyloric muscle (Fredet-Ramstedt type operation)

(Do not report modifier '-63' in conjunction with 43520)

EXCISION

43605 Biopsy of stomach by laparotomy

43610 Excision, local; ulcer or benign tumor of stomach

43611 malignant tumor of stomach

43620 Gastrectomy, total; with esophagoenterostomy

43621 with Roux-en-Y reconstruction

43622 with formation of intestinal pouch, any type

43631 Gastrectomy, partial, distal; with gastroduodenostomy

43632 with gastrojejunostomy

43633 with Roux-en-Y reconstruction

43634 with formation of intestinal pouch

+ **43635** Vagotomy when performed with partial distal gastrectomy (List separately in addition to code(s) for primary procedure)

(Use 43635 in conjunction with codes 43631, 43632, 43633, 43634)

43640 Vagotomy including pyloroplasty, with or without gastrostomy; truncal or selective

(For pyloroplasty, use 43800)

(For vagotomy, see 64755, 64760)

43641 parietal cell (highly selective)

● New Code   ▲ Revised Code   + Add-On Code   ⊘ Modifier -51 Exempt   ★ Telemedicine

(For upper gastrointestinal endoscopy, see 43235-43259)

LAPAROSCOPY

Surgical laparoscopy always includes diagnostic laparoscopy. To report a diagnostic laparoscopy (peritoneoscopy) (separate procedure), use 49320.

> (For upper gastrointestinal endoscopy including esophagus, stomach, and either the duodenum and/or jejunum, see 43235-43259)

43644 Laparoscopy, surgical, gastric restrictive procedure; with gastric bypass and Roux-en-Y gastroenterostomy (Roux limb 150 cm or less)

> (Do not report 43644 in conjunction with 43846, 49320)

> (Esophagogastroduodenoscopy (EGD) performed for a separate condition should be reported with modifier 59)

> (For greater than 150 cm, use 43645)

> (For open procedure, use 43846)

43645 with gastric bypass and small intestine reconstruction to limit absorption

> (Do not report 43645 in conjunction with 49320, 43847)

43647 Laparoscopy, surgical; implantation or replacement of gastric neurostimulator electrodes, antrum

43648 revision or removal of gastric neurostimulator electrodes, antrum

> (For open approach, see 43881, 43882)

> (For insertion of gastric neruostimulator pulse generator, use 64590)

> (For revision or removal of gastric neurostimulator pulse generator, use 64595)

> (For electronic analaysis and programming of gastric neurostimulator pulse generator, see 95980-95982)

> (For laparoscopic implantation, revision, or removal of gastric neurostimulator electrodes, lesser curvature [morbid obesity], use 43659)

> (For laparoscopic implantation, revision, replacement, or removal of vagus nerve blocking neurostimulator electrode array and/or pulse generator at the esophagogastric junction, see 0312T-0317T)

43651 Laparoscopy, surgical; transection of vagus nerves, truncal

43652 transection of vagus nerves, selective or highly selective

43653 gastrostomy, without construction of gastric tube (eg, Stamm procedure) (separate procedure)

43659 Unlisted laparoscopy procedure, stomach

INTRODUCTION

43752 Naso- or oro-gastric tube placement, requiring physician's skill and fluoroscopic guidance (includes fluoroscopy, image documentation and report)

> (Do not report 43752 in conjunction with critical care codes 99291-99292, neonatal critical care codes 99468, pediatric critical care codes 99471, 99472 or low birth weight intensive care service codes 99478, 99479)

> (For percutaneous placement of gastrostomy tube, use 49440)

> (For enteric tube placement, see 44500, 74340)

43753 Gastric intubation and aspiration(s), therapeutic, necessitating physician's skill (eg, for gastrointestinal hemorrhage), including lavage if performed

43754 Gastric intubation and aspiration, diagnostic; single specimen (eg, acid analysis)

43755 collection of multiple fractional specimens with gastric stimulation, single or double lumen tube (gastric secretory study) (eg, histamine, insulin, pentagastrin, calcium, secretin), includes drug administration

(For gastric acid analysis, use 82930)

(For naso- or oro-gastric tube placement by physician with fluoroscopic guidance, use 43752)

(Report the drug(s) or substance(s) administered. The fluid used to administer the drug(s) is not separately reported)

43756 Duodenal intubation and aspiration, diagnostic, includes image guidance; single specimen (eg, bile study for crystals or afferent loop culture)

43757 collection of multiple fractional specimens with pancreatic or gallbladder stimulation, single or double lumen tube, includes drug administration

(For appropriate chemical analysis procedures, see 89049-89240)

(Report the substance(s) or drug(s) administered. The fluid used to administer the drug(s) is not separately reported)

(**43760** deleted 2018 [2019 edition]. To report replacement of gastrostomy tube without imaging or endoscopy, see 43762, 43763)

(To report fluoroscopically guided replacement of gastrostomy tube, use 49450)

(For endoscopic placement of gastrostomy tube, use 43246)

43761 Repositioning of a naso- or oro-gastric feeding tube, through the duodenum for enteric nutrition

(Do not report 43761 in conjunction with 44500, 49446)

(If imaging guidance is performed, use 76000)

(For endoscopic conversion of a gastrostomy tube to jejunostomy tube, use 44373)

(For placement of a long gastrointestinal tube into the duodenum, use 44500)

43762 Replacement of gastrostomy tube, percutaneous, includes removal, when performed, without imaging or endoscopic guidance; not requiring revision of gastrostomy tract

43763 requiring revision of gastrostomy tract

(For percutaneous replacement of gastrostomy tube under fluoroscopic guidance, use 49450)

(For endoscopically directed placement of gastrostomy tube, use 43246)

BARIATRIC SURGERY

Laparoscopy

Surgical laparoscopy always includes diagnostic laparoscopy. To report a diagnostic laparoscopy (separate procedure), use 49320.

Typical postoperative follow-up care after gastric restriction using the adjustable gastric restrictive device includes subsequent restrictive device adjustment(s) through the postoperative period for the typcial patient. Adjustment consists of changing the gastric restrictive device component diameter by injection or aspiration of fluid through the subcutaneous port component.

43770 Laparoscopy, surgical, gastric restrictive procedure; placement of adjustable gastric restrictive device (eg, gastric band and subcutaneous port components)

(For individual component placement, report 43770 with modifier 52)

43771   revision of adjustable gastric restrictive device component only

43772   removal of adjustable gastric restrictive device component only

43773   removal and replacement of adjustable gastric restrictive device component only

(Do not report 43773 in conjunction with 43772)

43774   removal of adjustable gastric restrictive device and subcutaneous port components

(For removal and replacement of both gastric band and subcutaneous port components, use 43659)

43775   longitudinal gastrectomy (ie, sleeve gastrectomy)

(For open gastric restrictive procedure, without gastric bypass, for morbid obesity, other than vertical-banded gastroplasty, use 43843)

(For laparoscopic implantation, revision, replacement, removal or reprogramming of vagus nerve blocking neurostimulator electrode array and/or pulse generator at the esophagogastric junction, see 0312T-0317T)

OTHER PROCEDURES

43800   Pyloroplasty

(For pyloroplasty and vagotomy, use 43640)

43810   Gastroduodenostomy

43820   Gastrojejunostomy; without vagotomy

43825   with vagotomy, any type

43830   Gastrostomy, open; without construction of gastric tube (eg, Stamm procedure) (separate procedure)

43831   neonatal, for feeding

(For percutaneous replacement of gastrostomy tube with removal when performed without imaging or endoscopy, see 43762, 43763)

(For percutaneous replacement of gastrostomy tube under fluoroscopic guidance, use 49450)

(Do not report modifier '-63' in conjunction with 43831)

43832   with construction of gastric tube (eg, Janeway procedure)

(For percutaneous endoscopic gastrostomy, use 43246)

43840   Gastrorrhaphy, suture of perforated duodenal or gastric ulcer, wound, or injury

43842   Gastric restrictive procedure, without gastric bypass, for morbid obesity; vertical-banded gastroplasty

43843   other than vertical-banded gastroplasty

(For laparoscopic longitudinal gastrectomy [ie, sleeve gastrectomy], use 43775)

43845   Gastric restrictive procedure with partial gastrectomy, pylorus- preserving duodenoileostomy and ileoileostomy (50 to 100 cm common channel) to limit absorption (biliopancreatic diversion with duodenal switch)

(Do not report 43845 in conjunction with 43633, 43847, 44130, 49000)

Separate Procedure   Unlisted Procedure   CCI Comp. Code   Non-specific Procedure   **485**

43846 Gastric restrictive procedure, with gastric bypass for morbid obesity; with short limb (150 cm or less) Roux-en-Y gastroenterostomy

(For greater than 150 cm, use 43847)

(For laparoscopic procedure, use 43644)

43847 with small intestine reconstruction to limit absorption

43848 Revision, open, of gastric restrictive procedure for morbid obesity, other than adjustable gastric restrictive device (separate procedure)

(For laparoscopic adjustable gastric restrictive procedures, see 43770-43774)

(For gastric restrictive port procedures, see 43886-43888)

43850 Revision of gastroduodenal anastomosis (gastroduodenostomy) with reconstruction; without vagotomy

43855 with vagotomy

43860 Revision of gastrojejunal anastomosis (gastrojejunostomy) with reconstruction, with or without partial gastrectomy or intestine resection; without vagotomy

43865 with vagotomy

43870 Closure of gastrostomy, surgical

43880 Closure of gastrocolic fistula

43881 Implantation or replacement of gastric neurostimulator electrodes, antrum, open

43882 Revision or removal of gastric neurostimulator electrodes, antrum, open

(For laparoscopic approach, see 43647, 43648)

(For insertion of gastric neurostimulator pulse generator, use 64590)

(For revision or removal of gastric neurostimulator pulse generator, use 64595)

(For electronic analysis and programming of gastric neurostimulator pulse generator, use 95980-95982)

(For open implantation, revision, or removal of gastric neurostimulator electrodes, lesser curvature [morbid obesity], use 43999)

(For laparaoscopic implantation, revision, replacement, removal or reprogramming of vagus nerve blocking neurostimulator electrode array and/or pulse generator at the esophagogastric junction, see 0312T-0317T)

(For open implantation, revision, or removal of gastric lesser curvature or vagal trunk (EGJ) neurostimulator electrodes, [morbid obesity], use 43999)

43886 Gastric restrictive procedure, open; revision of subcutaneous port component only

43887 removal of subcutaneous port component only

43888 removal and replacement of subcutaneous port component only

(Do not report 43888 in conjunction with 43774, 43887)

(For laparoscopic removal of both gastric restrictive device and subcutaneous port components, use 43774)

(For removal and replacement of both gastric restrictive device and subcutaneous port components, use 43659)

43999 Unlisted procedure, stomach

● New Code ▲ Revised Code + Add-On Code ⊘ Modifier -51 Exempt ★ Telemedicine

INTESTINES (EXCEPT RECTUM)

INCISION

44005   Enterolysis (freeing of intestinal adhesion) (separate procedure)

        (Do not report 44005 in addition to 45136)

        (For laparoscopic approach, use 44180)

44010   Duodenotomy, for exploration, biopsy(s), or foreign body removal

+ 44015   Tube or needle catheter jejunostomy for enteral alimentation, intraoperative, any method (List separately in addition to primary procedure)

44020   Enterotomy, small intestine, other than duodenum; for exploration, biopsy(s), or foreign body removal

44021   for decompression (eg, Baker tube)

44025   Colotomy, for exploration, biopsy(s), or foreign body removal

        (For exteriorization of intestine (Mikulicz resection with crushing of spur), see 44602-44605)

44050   Reduction of volvulus, intussusception, internal hernia, by laparotomy

44055   Correction of malrotation by lysis of duodenal bands and/or reduction of midgut volvulus (eg, Ladd procedure)

        (Do not report modifier '-63' in conjunction with 44055)

EXCISION

Intestinal allotransplantation involves three distinct components of physician work:

1) **Cadaver donor enterectomy**, which includes harvesting the intestine graft and cold preservation of the graft (perfusing with cold preservation solution and cold maintenance) (use 44132). **Living donor enterectomy**, which includes harvesting the intestine graft, cold preservation of the graft (perfusing with cold preservation solution and cold maintenance), and care of the donor (use 44133).

2) **Backbench work**:

Standard preparation of an intestine allograft prior to transplantation includes mobilization and fashioning of the superior mesenteric artery and vein (see 44715).

Additional reconstruction of an intestine allograft prior to transplantation may include venous and/or arterial anastomosis(es) (see 44720-44721).

3) **Recipient intestinal allotransplantation with or without recipient enterectomy**, which includes transplantation of allograft and care of the recipient (see 44135, 44136)

44100   Biopsy of intestine by capsule, tube, peroral (1 or more specimens)

44110   Excision of 1 or more lesions of small or large intestine not requiring anastomosis, exteriorization, or fistulization; single enterotomy

44111   multiple enterotomies

44120   Enterectomy, resection of small intestine; single resection and anastomosis

        (Do not report 44120 in addition to 45136)

+ 44121   each additional resection and anastomosis (List separately in addition to code for primary procedure)

(Use 44121 in conjunction with code 44120)

44125   with enterostomy

44126   Enterectomy, resection of small intestine for congenital atresia, single resection and anastomosis of proximal segment of intestine; without tapering

44127   with tapering

+ **44128**   each additional resection and anastomosis (List separately in addition to code for primary procedure)

(Use 44128 in conjunction with codes 44126, 44127)

(Do not report modifier '-63' in conjunction with 44126, 44127, 44128)

44130   Enteroenterostomy, anastomosis of intestine, with or without cutaneous enterostomy (separate procedure)

44132   Donor enterectomy (including cold preservation), open; from cadaver donor

44133   partial, from living donor

(For backbench intestinal graft preparation or reconstruction, see 44715, 44720, 44721)

44135   Intestinal allotransplantation; from cadaver donor

44136   from living donor

44137   Removal of transplanted intestinal allograft, complete

(For partial removal of transplant allograft, see 44120, 44121, 44140)

+ **44139**   Mobilization (take-down) of splenic flexure performed in conjunction with partial colectomy (List separately in addition to primary procedure)

(Use 44139 in conjunction with codes 44140-44147)

44140   Colectomy, partial; with anastomosis

(For laparoscopic procedure, use 44204)

44141   with skin level cecostomy or colostomy

44143   with end colostomy and closure of distal segment (Hartmann type procedure)

(For laparoscopic procedure, use 44206)

44144   with resection, with colostomy or ileostomy and creation of mucofistula

44145   with coloproctostomy (low pelvic anastomosis)

(For laparoscopic procedure, use 44207)

44146   with coloproctostomy (low pelvic anastomosis), with colostomy

(For laparoscopic procedure, use 44208)

44147   abdominal and transanal approach

44150   Colectomy, total, abdominal, without proctectomy; with ileostomy or ileoproctostomy

(For laparoscopic procedure, use 44210)

44151   with continent ileostomy

44155   Colectomy, total, abdominal, with proctectomy; with ileostomy

(For laparoscopic procedure, use 44212)

44156   with continent ileostomy

44157   with ileoanal anastomosis, includes loop ileostomy, and rectal mucosectomy, when performed

44158   with ileoanal anastomosis, creation of ileal reservoir (S or J), includes loop ileostomy, and rectal mucosectomy, when performed

(For laparoscopic procedure, use 44211)

44160   Colectomy, partial, with removal of terminal ileum and ileocolostomy

(For laparoscopic procedure, use 44205)

LAPAROSCOPY

Surgical laparoscopy always includes diagnostic laparoscopy. To report a diagnostic laparoscopy (peritoneoscopy) (separate procedure), use 49320.

Incision

44180   Laparoscopy, surgical, enterolysis (freeing of intestinal adhesion) (separate procedure)

(For laparoscopy with salpingolysis, ovariolysis, use 58660)

Enterostomy—External Fistulization of Intestines

44186   Laparoscopy, surgical; jejunostomy (eg, for decompression or feeding)

44187   ileostomy or jejunostomy, non-tube

(For open procedure, use 44310)

44188   Laparoscopy, surgical, colostomy or skin level cecostomy

(For open procedure, use 44320)

(Do not report 44188 in conjunction with 44970)

Excision

44202   Laparoscopy, surgical; enterectomy, resection of small intestine, single resection and anastomosis

+ 44203   each additional small intestine resection and anastomosis (List separately in addition to code for primary procedure)

(Use 44203 in conjunction with code 44202)

(For open procedure, see 44120, 44121)

44204   colectomy, partial, with anastomosis

(For open procedure, use 44140)

44205   colectomy, partial, with removal of terminal ileum with ileocolostomy

(For open procedure, use 44160)

44206   colectomy, partial, with end colostomy and closure of distal segment (Hartmann type procedure)

(For open procedure, use 44143)

44207   colectomy, partial, with anastomosis, with coloproctostomy (low pelvic anastomosis)

(For open procedure, use 44145)

44208   colectomy, partial, with anastomosis, with coloproctostomy (low pelvic anastomosis) with colostomy

(For open procedure, use 44146)

44210   colectomy, total, abdominal, without proctectomy, with ileostomy or ileoproctostomy

(For open procedure, use 44150)

44211   colectomy, total, abdominal, with proctectomy, with ileoanal anastomosis, creation of ileal reservoir (S or J), with loop ileostomy, includes rectal mucosectomy, when performed

(For open procedure, see 44157, 44158)

44212   colectomy, total, abdominal, with proctectomy, with ileostomy

(For open procedure, use 44155)

+ 44213   Laparoscopy, surgical, mobilization (take-down) of splenic flexure performed in conjunction with partial colectomy (List separately in addition to primary procedure)

(Use 44213 in conjunction with 44204-44208)

(For open procedure, use 44139)

Repair

44227   Laparoscopy, surgical, closure of enterostomy, large or small intestine, with resection and anastomosis

(For open procedure, see 44625, 44626)

Other Procedures

44238   Unlisted laparoscopy procedure, intestine (except rectum)

ENTEROSTOMY—EXTERNAL FISTULIZATION OF INTESTINES

44300   Placement, enterostomy or cecostomy, tube open (eg, for feeding or decompression) (separate procedure)

(Do not report 44300 in conjunction with 44701 for cannulation of the colon for intraoperative colonic lavage)

(For percutaneous placement of duodenostomy, jejunostomy, gastro-jejunostomy or cecostomy [or other colonic] tube including fluoroscopic imaging guidance, see 49441-49442)

44310   Ileostomy or jejunostomy, non-tube

(For laparoscopic procedure, use 44187)

(Do not report 44310 in conjunction with 44144, 44150-44153, 44155, 44156, 45113, 45119, 45136)

44312   Revision of ileostomy; simple (release of superficial scar) (separate procedure)

44314   complicated (reconstruction in-depth) (separate procedure)

44316   Continent ileostomy (Kock procedure) (separate procedure)

(For fiberoptic evaluation, use 44385)

44320   Colostomy or skin level cecostomy

(For laparoscopic procedure, use 44188)

● New Code   ▲ Revised Code   + Add-On Code   ⊘ Modifier -51 Exempt   ★ Telemedicine

(Do not report 44320 in conjunction with 44141, 44144, 44146, 44605, 45110, 45119, 45126, 45563, 45805, 45825, 50810, 51597, 57307, or 58240)

44322   with multiple biopsies (eg, for congenital megacolon) (separate procedure)

44340   Revision of colostomy; simple (release of superficial scar) (separate procedure)

44345   complicated (reconstruction in-depth) (separate procedure)

44346   with repair of paracolostomy hernia (separate procedure)

ENDOSCOPY, SMALL INTESTINE AND STOMAL

When bleeding occurs as the result of an endoscopic procedure, control of bleeding is not reported separately during the same operative session.

Antegrade transoral small intestinal endoscopy (enteroscopy) is defined by the most distal segment of small intestine that is examined. Codes 44360, 44361, 44363, 44364, 44365, 44366, 44369, 44370, 44372, 44373 are endoscopic procedures to visualize the esophagus through the jejunum using an antegrade approach. Codes 44376, 44377, 44378, 44379 are endscopic procedures to visualize the esophagus through the ileum using an antegrade approach. If an endscope cannot be advanced at least 50cm beyond the pylorus, see 43233, 43235-43259, 43266, 43270; if an endoscope can be passed at least 50cm beyond pylorus but only into jejunum, see 44360, 44361, 44363, 44364, 44365, 44366, 44369, 44370, 44372, 44373.

To report retrograde examination of small intestine via anus or colon stoma, use 44799, unlisted procedure, intestine.

(Do not report 44360, 44361, 44363, 44364, 44365, 44366, 44369, 44370, 44372, 44373 in conjunction with 43233, 43235-43259, 43266, 43270, 44376, 44377, 44378, 44379)

(Do not report 44376, 44377, 44378, 44379 in conjunction with 43233, 43235-43259, 43266, 43270, 44360, 44361, 44363, 44364, 44365, 44366, 44369, 44370, 44372, 44373)

(For esophagogastroduodenoscopy, see 43233, 43235-43259, 43266, 43270)

44360   Small intestinal endoscopy, enteroscopy beyond second portion of duodenum, not including ileum; diagnostic, including collection of specimen(s) by brushing or washing, when performed (separate procedure)

44361   with biopsy, single or multiple

44363   with removal of foreign body(s)

44364   with removal of tumor(s), polyp(s), or other lesion(s) by snare technique

44365   with removal of tumor(s), polyp(s), or other lesion(s) by hot biopsy forceps or bipolar cautery

44366   with control of bleeding (eg, injection, bipolar cautery, unipolar cautery, laser, heater probe, stapler, plasma coagulator)

44369   with ablation of tumor(s), polyp(s), or other lesion(s) not amenable to removal by hot biopsy forceps, bipolar cautery or snare technique

44370   with transendoscopic stent placement (includes predilation)

44372   with placement of percutaneous jejunostomy tube

44373   with conversion of percutaneous gastrostomy tube to percutaneous jejunostomy tube

(For fiberoptic jejunostomy through stoma, use 43235)

44376   Small intestinal endoscopy, enteroscopy beyond second portion of duodenum, including ileum; diagnostic, with or without collection of specimen(s) by brushing or washing (separate procedure)

(Do not report 44376 in conjunction with 44360, 44361, 44363, 44364, 44365, 44366, 44369, 44370, 44372, 44373)

44377   with biopsy, single or multiple

(Do not report 44377 in conjunction with 44360, 44361, 44363, 44364, 44365, 44366, 44369, 44370, 44372, 44373)

44378   with control of bleeding (eg, injection, bipolar cautery, unipolar cautery, laser, heater probe, stapler, plasma coagulator)

(Do not report 44378 in conjunction with 44360, 44361, 44363, 44364, 44365, 44366, 44369, 44370, 44372, 44373)

44379   with transendoscopic stent placement (includes predilation)

(Do not report 44379 in conjunction with 44360, 44361, 44363, 44364, 44365, 44366, 44369, 44370, 44372, 44373)

ENDOSCOPY, STOMAL

Definitions:

Proctosigmoidoscopy is the examination of the rectum and may include examination of a portion of the sigmoid colon.

Sigmoidoscopy is the examination of the entire rectum, sigmoid colon and may include examination of a portion of the descending colon.

Colonoscopy is the examination of the entire colon, from the rectum to the cecum, and may include examination of the terminal ileum or small intestine proximal to an anastomosis.

Colonoscopy through stoma is the examination of the colon, from the colostomy stoma to the cecum or colon-small intestine anastomosis, and may include examination of the terminal ileum or small instestine proximal to an anastomosis.

When performing a disgnostic or screening endoscopic procedure on a patient who is scheduled and prepared for a total colonoscopy, if the physician is unable to advance the colonscope to the cecum or colon-small intestine anastomosis due to unforeseen circumstances, report 45378 (colonoscopy) or 44388 (colonoscopy through stoma) with modifier 53 and provide appropriate documentation.

If a therapeutic colonoscopy (44389-44407, 45379, 45380, 45381, 45382, 45384, 45388, 45398) is performed and does not reach the cecum or colon-small intestine anastomosis, report the approprite therapeutic colonoscopy code with modifier 52 and provide appropriate documentation.

Report ileoscopy through stoma (44380, 44381, 44382, 44384) for endoscopic examination of a patient who has an ileostomy.

Report colonoscopy through stoma (44388-44408) for endoscopic examination of a patient who has undergone segmental resection of the colon (eg, hemicolectomy, sigmoid colectomy, low anterior resection) and has a colostomy.

For colonoscopy per rectum, see 45378, 45390, 45392, 45393, 45398.

Report proctosigmoidoscopy (45300-45327), flexible sigmoidoscopy (45330- 45347), or anoscopy (46600, 46604, 46606, 46608, 46610, 46611, 46612, 46614, 46615), as appropriate for endoscopic examination of the defunctionalized rectum or distal colon in a patient who has undergone colectomy, in addition to colonoscopy through stoma (44388-44408) or ileoscopy through stoma (44380, 44381, 44382, 44384) if appropriate.

When bleeding occurs as the result of an endoscopic procedure, control of bleeding is not reported separately during the same operative session.

For computed tomographic colonography, see 74261, 74262, 74263.

  ● New Code   ▲ Revised Code   ✛ Add-On Code   ⊘ Modifier -51 Exempt   ★ Telemedicine

44380   Ileoscopy, through stoma; diagnostic, including collection of specimen(s) by brushing or washing, when performed (separate procedure)

(Do not report 44380 in conjunction with 44381, 44382, 44384)

44381   This code is out of order. See page 493

44382   with biopsy, single or multiple

(Do not report 44382 in conjunction with 44380)

44381   with transendoscopic balloon dilation

(Do not report 44381 in conjunction with 44380, 44384)

(If fluoroscoic guidance is performed, use 74360)

(For transendoscopic balloon dilation of multiple strictures during the same session, report 44381 with modifier 59 for each additional stricture dilated)

44384   with placement of endoscopic stent (includes pre- and post-dilation and guide wire passage, when performed)

(Do not report 44384 in conjunction with 44380, 44381)

(If fluoroscopic guidance is performed, use 74360)

44385   Endoscopic evaluation of small intestinal pouch (eg, Kock pouch, ileal reservoir [S or J]); diagnostic, including collection of specimen(s) by brushing or washing, when performed (separate procedure)

(Do not report 44385 in conjunction with 44386)

44386   with biopsy, single or multiple

(Do not report 44386 in conjunction with 44385)

44388   Colonoscopy through stoma; diagnostic, including collection of specimen(s) by brushing or washing, when performed (separate procedure)

(Do not report 44388 in conjunction with 44389-44408)

44389   with biopsy, single or multiple

(Do not report 44389 in conjunction with 44403 for the same lesion)

(Do not report 44389 in conjunction with 44388)

44390   with removal of foreign body(s)

(Do not report 44390 in conjunction with 44388)

(If fluoroscopic guidance is performed, use 76000)

44391   with control of bleeding, any method

(Do not report 44391 in conjunction with 44404 for the same lesion)

(Do not report 44391 in conjunction with 44388)

44392   with removal of tumor(s), polyp(s), or other lesion(s) by hot biopsy forceps

(Do not report 44392 in conjunction with 44388)

44401   with ablation of tumor(s), polyp(s), or other lesion(s) (includes pre- and post-dilation and guide wire passage, when performed)

(Do not report 44401 in conjunction with 44405 for the same lesion)

(Do not report 44401 in conjunction with 44388)

44394   with removal of tumor(s), polyp(s), or other lesion(s) by snare technique

(Do not report 44394 in conjunction with 44403 for the same lesion)

(Do not report 44394 in conjunction with 44388)

(For endoscopic mucosal resection, use 44403)

44401   This code is out of order. See page 493

44402   with endoscopic stent placement (including pre- and post-dilation and guide wire passage, when performed)

(Do not report 44402 in conjunction with 44388, 44405)

(If fluoroscopic guidance is performed, use 74360)

44403   with endoscopic mucosal resection

(Do not report 44403 in conjunction with 44389, 44394, 44404 for the same lesion)

(Do not report 44403 in conjunction with 44388)

44404   with directed submucosal injection(s), any substance

(Do not report 44404 in conjunction with 44391, 44403 for the same lesion)

(Do not report 44404 in conjunction with 44388)

44405   with transendoscopic balloon dilation

(Do not report 44405 in conjunction with 44388, 44401, 44402)

(If fluorscopic guidance is performed, use 74360)

(For transendoscopic balloon dilation of multiple strictures during the same session, report 44405 with modifier 59 for each additional stricture dilated)

44406   with endoscopic ultrasound examination, limited to the sigmoid, descending, transverse, or ascending colon and cecum and adjacent structures

(Do not report 44406 in conjunction with 44388, 44407, 76975)

(Do not report 44406 more than once per session)

44407   with transendoscopic ultrasound guided intramural or transmural fine needle aspiration/biopsy(s), includes endoscopic ultrasound examination limited to the sigmoid, descending, transverse, or ascending colon and cecum and adjacent structures

(Do not report 44407 in conjunction with 44388, 44406, 76942, 76975)

(Do not report 44407 more than once per session)

44408   with decompression (for pathologic distention) (eg, volvulus, megacolon), including placement of decompression tube, when performed

(Do not report 44408 in conjunction with 44388)

(Do not report 44408 more than once per session)

INTRODUCTION

⊘ **44500**   Introduction of long gastrointestinal tube (eg, Miller-Abbott) (separate procedure)

(For radiological supervision and interpretation, use 74340)

(For naso- or oro-gastric tube placement, use 43752)

REPAIR

44602 Suture of small intestine (enterorrhaphy) for perforated ulcer, diverticulum, wound, injury or rupture; single perforation

44603   multiple perforations

44604 Suture of large intestine (colorrhaphy) for perforated ulcer, diverticulum, wound, injury, or rupture (single or multiple perforations); without colostomy

44605   with colostomy

44615 Intestinal stricturoplasty (enterotomy and enterorrhaphy) with or without dilation, for intestinal obstruction

44620 Closure of enterostomy, large or small intestine;

44625   with resection and anastomosis other than colorectal

44626   with resection and colorectal anastomosis (eg, closure of Hartmann type procedure)

(For laparoscopic procedure, use 44227)

44640 Closure of intestinal cutaneous fistula

44650 Closure of enteroenteric or enterocolic fistula

44660 Closure of enterovesical fistula; without intestinal or bladder resection

44661   with intestine and/or bladder resection

(For closure of renocolic fistula, see 50525, 50526)

(For closure of gastrocolic fistula, use 43880)

(For closure of rectovesical fistula, see 45800, 45805)

44680 Intestinal plication (separate procedure)

OTHER PROCEDURES

44700 Exclusion of small intestine from pelvis by mesh or other prosthesis, or native tissue (eg, bladder or omentum)

(For therapeutic radiation clinical treatment, see Radiation Oncology section)

+ **44701** Intraoperative colonic lavage (List separately in addition to code for primary procedure)

(Use 44701 in conjunction with codes 44140, 44145, 44150, or 44604 as appropriate)

(Do not report 44701 in conjunction with 44950- 44960)

44705 Preparation of fecal microbiota for instillation, including assessment of donor specimen

(Do not report 44705 in conjunction with 74283)

(For fecal instillation by oro-nasogastric tube or enema, use 44799)

44715 Backbench standard preparation of cadaver or living donor intestine allograft prior to transplantation, including mobilization and fashioning of the superior mesenteric artery and vein

44720   Backbench reconstruction of cadaver or living donor intestine allograft prior to transplantation; venous anastomosis, each

44721   arterial anastomosis, each

44799   Unlisted procedure, small intestine

(For unlisted laparoscopic procedure, intestine except rectum, use 44238)

(For unlisted procedure, colon, use 45399)

MECKEL'S DIVERTICULUM AND THE MESENTERY

EXCISION

44800   Excision of Meckel's diverticulum (diverticulectomy) or omphalomesenteric duct

44820   Excision of lesion of mesentery (separate procedure)

(With intestine resection, see 44120 or 44140 et seq)

SUTURE

44850   Suture of mesentery (separate procedure)

(For reduction and repair of internal hernia, use 44050)

OTHER PROCEDURES

44899   Unlisted procedure, Meckel's diverticulum and the mesentery

APPENDIX

INCISION

44900   Incision and drainage of appendiceal abscess; open

(For percutaneous image-guided drainage by catheter of appendiceal abscess, use 49406)

EXCISION

44950   Appendectomy;

(Incidental appendectomy during intra-abdominal surgery does not usually warrant a separate identification. If necessary to report, add modifier -52)

+ **44955**   when done for indicated purpose at time of other major procedure (not as separate procedure) (List separately in addition to code for primary procedure)

44960   for ruptured appendix with abscess or generalized peritonitis

LAPAROSCOPY

Surgical laparoscopy always includes diagnostic laparoscopy. To report a diagnostic laparoscopy (peritoneoscopy) (separate procedure), use 49320.

44970   Laparoscopy, surgical, appendectomy

44979   Unlisted laparoscopy procedure, appendix

● New Code   ▲ Revised Code   ✚ Add-On Code   ⊘ Modifier -51 Exempt   ★ Telemedicine

COLONOSCOPY DECISION TREE					
Decision to Undergo Colonoscopy					
Diagnostic Procedure			**Therapeutic Procedure**		
Does not reach splenic flexure:	Beyond splenic flexure, but not to the cecum:	To cecum:	Does not reach splenic flexure:	Beyond splenic flexure, but not to the cecum:	To cecum:
Flexible Sigmoidoscopy (45330)	Colonoscopy (45378; modifer 53)	Colonoscopy (45378; no modifier)	Flexible Sigmoidoscopy (45331-45347)	Colonoscopy (45379-45398; modifier 52)	Colonoscopy (45379-45398; no modifier)

COLON AND RECTUM

INCISION

45000 Transrectal drainage of pelvic abscess

(For transrectal image-guided fluid collection drainage by catheter of pelvic abscess, use 49407)

45005 Incision and drainage of submucosal abscess, rectum

45020 Incision and drainage of deep supralevator, pelvirectal, or retrorectal abscess

(See also 46050, 46060)

EXCISION

45100 Biopsy of anorectal wall, anal approach (eg, congenital megacolon)

(For endoscopic biopsy, use 45305)

45108 Anorectal myomectomy

45110 Proctectomy; complete, combined abdominoperineal, with colostomy

(For laparoscopic procedure, use 45395)

45111   partial resection of rectum, transabdominal approach

45112 Proctectomy, combined abdominoperineal, pull-through procedure (eg, colo-anal anastomosis)

(For colo-anal anastomosis with colonic reservoir or pouch, use 45119)

45113 Proctectomy, partial, with rectal mucosectomy, ileoanal anastomosis, creation of ileal reservoir (S or J), with or without loop ileostomy

45114 Proctectomy, partial, with anastomosis; abdominal and transsacral approach

45116   transsacral approach only (Kraske type)

45119 Proctectomy, combined abdominoperineal pull-through procedure (eg, colo-anal anastomosis), with creation of colonic reservoir (eg, J-pouch), with diverting enterostomy when performed

(For laparoscopic procedure, use 45397)

45120 Proctectomy, complete (for congenital megacolon), abdominal and perineal approach; with pull-through procedure and anastomosis (eg, Swenson, Duhamel, or Soave type operation)

45121   with subtotal or total colectomy, with multiple biopsies

45123 Proctectomy, partial, without anastomosis, perineal approach

	Separate Procedure		Unlisted Procedure		CCI Comp. Code		Non-specific Procedure	**497**

45126 Pelvic exenteration for colorectal malignancy, with proctectomy (with or without colostomy), with removal of bladder and ureteral transplantations, and/or hysterectomy, or cervicectomy, with or without removal of tube(s), with or without removal of ovary(s), or any combination thereof

45130 Excision of rectal procidentia, with anastomosis; perineal approach

45135 abdominal and perineal approach

45136 Excision of ileoanal reservoir with ileostomy

(Do not report 45136 in conjunction with 44005, 44310)

45150 Division of stricture of rectum

45160 Excision of rectal tumor by proctotomy, transsacral or transcoccygeal approach

45171 Excision of rectal tumor, transanal approach; not including muscularis propria (ie, partial thickness)

45172 including muscularis propria (ie, full thickness)

(For destruction of rectal tumor, transanal approach, use 45190)

(For transanal endoscopic microsurgical [ie, TEMS] excision of rectal tumor, including muscularis propria [ie., full thickness], use 0184T)

DESTRUCTION

45190 Destruction of rectal tumor (eg, electrodesiccation, electrosurgery, laser ablation, laser resection, cryosurgery) transanal approach

(For excision of rectal tumor, transanal approach, see 45171, 45172)

(For transanal endoscopic microsurgical [ie, TEMS] excision of rectal tumor, including muscularis propria [ie., full thickness], use 0184T)

ENDOSCOPY

When performing a diagnostic or screening endoscopic procedure on a patient who is scheduled and prepared for a total colonoscopy, if the physician is unable to advance the colonoscope to the cecum or colon-small intestine anastomosis due to unforseen circumstances, report 45378 (colonoscopy) or 44388 (colonoscopy through stoma) with modifier 53 and provide appropriate documentation.

If therapeutic colonoscopy (44389-44407, 45379, 45380, 45381, 45382, 45384, 45388, 45389) is performed and does not reach the cecum or colon-small intestine anastomosis, report the appropriate therapeutic colonoscopy code with modifier 52 and provide appropriate documentation.

Report flexible sigmoidoscopy (45330-45347) for endoscopic examination during which the endoscope is not advanced beyond the splenic flexure.

Report flexible sigmoidoscopy (45330-45347) for endoscopic examination of a patient who has undergone resection of the colon proximal to the sigmoid (eg, subtotal colectomy) and has an ileo-sigmoid or ileo-rectal anastomosis. Report pouch endoscopy codes (44385, 44386) for endoscopic examination of a patient who has undergone resection of colon with ileo-anal anastomosis (eg., J-pouch).

Report colonoscopy (45378-45398) for endoscopic examination of a patient who has undergone segmental resection of the colon (eg., hemicolectomy, sigmoid colectomy, low anterior resection).

For colonoscopy through stoma, see 44388-44408.

Report proctosigmoidoscopy (45300-45327), flexible sigmoidoscopy (45330- 45347), or anoscopy (46600, 46604, 46606, 46608, 46610, 46611, 46612, 46614, 46615) as appropriate for endoscopic examination of the defunctionalized rectum or distal colon in a patient who has undergone colectomy, in addition to colonoscopy through stoma (44388-44408) or ileoscopy through stoma (44380, 44381, 44382, 44384) if appropriate.

● New Code   ▲ Revised Code   ✚ Add-On Code   ⊘ Modifier -51 Exempt   ★ Telemedicine

When bleeding occurs as a result of an endoscopic procedure, control of bleeding is not reported separately during the same operative session.

For computed tomographic colonography, see 74261-74263.

45300 Proctosigmoidoscopy, rigid; diagnostic, with or without collection of specimen(s) by brushing or washing (separate procedure)

45303 with dilation (eg, balloon, guide wire, bougie)

(For radiological supervision and interpretation, use 74360)

45305 with biopsy, single or multiple

45307 with removal of foreign body

45308 with removal of single tumor, polyp, or other lesion by hot biopsy forceps or bipolar cautery

45309 with removal of single tumor, polyp, or other lesion by snare technique

45315 with removal of multiple tumors, polyps, or other lesions by hot biopsy forceps, bipolar cautery or snare technique

45317 with control of bleeding (eg, injection, bipolar cautery, unipolar cautery, laser, heater probe, stapler, plasma coagulator)

45320 with ablation of tumor(s), polyp(s), or other lesion(s) not amenable to removal by hot biopsy forceps, bipolar cautery or snare technique (eg, laser)

45321 with decompression of volvulus

45327 with transendoscopic stent placement (includes predilation)

45330 Sigmoidoscopy, flexible; diagnostic, including collection of specimen(s) by brushing or washing, when performed (separate procedure)

(Do not report 45330 in conjunction with 45331-45342, 45346, 45347, 45349, 45350)

45331 with biopsy, single or multiple

(Do not report 45331 in conjunction with 45349 for the same lesion)

45332 with removal of foreign body(s)

(Do not report 45332 in conjunction with 45330)

(If fluoroscopic guidance is performed, use 76000)

45333 with removal of tumor(s), polyp(s), or other lesion(s) by hot biopsy forceps

(Do not report 45333 in conjunction with 45330)

45334 with control of bleeding, any method

(Do not report 45334 in conjunction with 45335, 45350 for the same lesion)

(Do not report 45334 in conjunction with 45330)

45335 with directed submucosal injection(s), any substance

(Do not report 45335 in conjunction with 45334, 45349 for the same lesion)

(Do not report 45335 in conjunction with 45330)

Separate Procedure   Unlisted Procedure   CCI Comp. Code   Non-specific Procedure   **499**

45337   with decompression (for pathologic distention) (eg, volvulus, megacolon), including placement of decompression tube, when performed

(Do not report 45337 in conjunction with 45330)

(Do not report 45337 more than once per session)

45338   with removal of tumor(s), polyp(s), or other lesion(s) by snare technique

(Do not report 45338 in conjunction with 45349 for the same lesion)

(Do not report 45338 in conjunction with 45330)

(For endoscopic mucosal resection, use 45349)

45346   with ablation of tumor(s), polyp(s), or other lesion(s) (includes pre- and post-dilation and guide wire passage, when performed)

(Do not report 45346 in conjunction with 45330)

(Do not report 45346 in conjunction with 45340 for the same lesion)

45340   with transendoscopic balloon dilation

(Do not report 45340 in conjunction with 45330, 45346, 45347)

(If fluoroscopic guidance is performed, use 74360)

(For transendoscopic balloon dilation of multiple strictures during the same session, use 45340 with modifier 59 for each additional stricture dilated)

45341   with endoscopic ultrasound examination

(Do not report 45341 in conjunction with 45330, 45342, 76872, 76975)

(Do not report 45341 more than once per session)

45342   with transendoscopic ultrasound guided intramural or transmural fine needle aspiration/biopsy(s)

(Do not report 45342 in conjunction with 45330, 45341, 76872, 76942, 76975)

(Do not report 45342 more than once per session)

45346   This code is out of order. See page 500

45347   with placement of endoscopic stent (includes pre- and post-dilation and guide wire passage, when performed)

(Do not report 45347 in conjunction with 45330, 45340)

(If fluoroscopic guidance is performed, use 74360)

45349   with endoscopic mucosal resection

(Do not report 45349 in conjunction with 45331, 45335, 45338, 45350 for the same lesion)

(Do not report 45349 in conjunction with 45330)

45350   with band ligation(s) (eg, hemorrhoids)

(Do not report 45350 in conjunction with 45334 for the same lesion)

(Do not report 45350 in conjunction with 45330, 45349, 46221)

(Do not report 45350 more than once per session)

(To report control of active bleeding with band ligation[s], use 45334)

● New Code   ▲ Revised Code   + Add-On Code   ⊘ Modifier -51 Exempt   ★ Telemedicine

45378 Colonoscopy, flexible; diagnostic, including collection of specimen(s) by brushing or washing, when performed (separate procedure)

(Do not report 45378 in conjunction with 45379-45393, 45398)

(For colonoscopy with decompression [pathologic distention], use 45393)

45379 with removal of foreign body(s)

(Do not report 45379 in conjunction with 45378)

(If fluoroscopic guidance is performed, use 76000)

45380 with biopsy, single or multiple

(Do not report 45380 in conjunction with 45390 for the same lesion)

(Do not report 45380 in conjunction with 45378)

45381 with directed submucosal injection(s), any substance

(Do not report 45381 in conjunction with 45382, 45390 for the same lesion)

(Do not report 45381 in conjunction with 45378)

45382 with control of bleeding, any method

(Do not report 45382 in conjunction with 45381, 45398 for the same lesion)

(Do not report 45382 in conjunction with 45378)

45388 with ablation of tumor(s), polyp(s), or other lesion(s) (includes pre- and post-dilation and guide wire passage, when performed)

(Do not report 45388 in conjunction with 45386 for the same lesion)

(Do not report 45388 in conjunction with 45378)

45384 with removal of tumor(s), polyp(s), or other lesion(s) by hot biopsy forceps

(Do not report 45384 in conjunction with 45378)

45385 with removal of tumor(s), polyp(s), or other lesion(s) by snare technique

(Do not report 45385 in conjunction with 45390 for the same lesion)

(Do not report 45385 in conjunction with 45378)

(For endoscopic mucosal resection, use 45390)

45386 with transendoscopic balloon dilation

(Do not report 45386 in conjunction with 45378, 45388, 45389)

(If fluoroscopic guidance is performed, use 74360)

(For transendoscopic balloon dilation of multiple strictures during the same session, report 45386 with modifier 59 for each additional stricture dilated)

45388 This code is out of order. See page 501

45389 with endoscopic stent placement (includes pre- and post-dilation and guide wire passage, when performed)

(Do not report 45389 in conjunction with 45378, 45386)

(If fluoroscopic guidance is performed, use 74360)

45390   This code is out of order. See page 502

45391   with endoscopic ultrasound examination limited to the rectum, sigmoid, descending, transverse, or ascending colon and cecum, and adjacent structures

       (Do not report 45391 in conjunction with 45378, 45392, 76872, 76975)

       (Do not report 45391 more than once per session)

45392   with transendoscopic ultrasound guided intramural or transmural fine needle aspiration/biopsy(s), includes endoscopic ultrasound examination limited to the rectum, sigmoid, descending, transverse, or ascending colon and cecum, and adjacent structures

       (Do not report 45392 in conjunction with 45378, 45391, 76872, 76942, 76975)

       (Do not report 45392 more than once per session)

45390   with endoscopic mucosal resection

       (Do not report 45390 in conjunction with 45380, 45381, 45385, 45398 for the same lesion)

       (Do not report 45390 in conjunction with 45378)

45393   with decompression (for pathologic distention) (eg, volvulus, megacolon), including placement of decompression tube, when performed

       (Do not report 45393 in conjunction with 45378)

       (Do not report 45393 more than once per session)

45398   with band ligation(s) (eg, hemorrhoids)

       (Do not report 45398 in conjunction with 45382 for the same lesion)

       (Do not report 45398 in conjunction with 45378, 45390, 46221)

       (Do not report 45398 more than once per session)

       (To report control of active bleeding with band ligation[s], use 45382)

LAPAROSCOPY

Surgical laparoscopy always includes diagnostic laparoscopy. To report a diagnostic laparoscopy (peritoneoscopy) (separate procedure), use 49320.

Excision

45395   Laparoscopy, surgical; proctectomy, complete, combined abdominoperineal, with colostomy

       (For open procedure, use 45110)

45397   proctectomy, combined abdominoperineal pull-through procedure (eg, colo-anal anastomosis), with creation of colonic reservoir (eg, J-pouch), with diverting enterostomy, when performed

       (For open procedure, use 45119)

45398   This code is out of order. See page 502

45399   This code is out of order. See page 503

Repair

45400   Laparoscopy, surgical; proctopexy (for prolapse)

       (For open procedure, use 45540, 45541)

45402   proctopexy (for prolapse), with sigmoid resection

(For open procedure, use 45550)

45499 Unlisted laparoscopy procedure, rectum

REPAIR

45500 Proctoplasty; for stenosis

45505   for prolapse of mucous membrane

45520 Perirectal injection of sclerosing solution for prolapse

45540 Proctopexy (eg, for prolapse); abdominal approach

(For laparoscopic procedure, use 45400)

45541   perineal approach

45550   with sigmoid resection, abdominal approach

(For laparoscopic procedure, use 45402)

45560 Repair of rectocele (separate procedure)

(For repair of rectocele with posterior colporrhaphy, use 57250)

45562 Exploration, repair, and presacral drainage for rectal injury;

45563   with colostomy

45800 Closure of rectovesical fistula;

45805   with colostomy

45820 Closure of rectourethral fistula;

45825   with colostomy

(For rectovaginal fistula closure, see 57300-57308)

MANIPULATION

45900 Reduction of procidentia (separate procedure) under anesthesia

45905 Dilation of anal sphincter (separate procedure) under anesthesia other than local

45910 Dilation of rectal stricture (separate procedure) under anesthesia other than local

45915 Removal of fecal impaction or foreign body (separate procedure) under anesthesia

OTHER PROCEDURES

Surgical diagnostic anorectal exam (45990) includes the following elements: external perineal exam, digital rectal exam, pelvic exam (when performed), diagnostic anoscopy, and diagnostic rigid proctoscopy.

45399 Unlisted procedure, colon

45990 Anorectal exam, surgical, requiring anesthesia (general, spinal, or epidural), diagnostic

(Do not report 45990 in conjunction with 45300-45327, 46600, 57410, 99170)

▭ Separate Procedure   ▭ Unlisted Procedure   ▭ CCI Comp. Code   ▭ Non-specific Procedure   **503**

45999 Unlisted procedure, rectum

(For unlisted laparoscopic procedure, rectum, use 45499)

ANUS

For incision of thrombosed external hemorrhoid, use 46083. For ligation of internal hemorrhoid(s), see 46221, 46945, 46946. For excision of internal and/or external hemorrhoid(s), see 46250-46262, 46320. For injection of hemorrhoid(s), use 46500. For destruction of internal hemorrhoid(s) by thermal energy, use 46930. For destruction of hemorrhoid(s) by cryosurgery, use 46999.

For transanal hemorrhoidal dearterialization, including ultrasound guidance, with mucopexy, when performed, use 46948. For hemorrhoidopexy, use 46947. Do not report 46600 in conjunction with 46020-46947, 0184T, during the same operative session.

INCISION

(For subcutaneous fistulotomy, use 46270)

46020 Placement of seton

(Do not report 46020 in conjunction with 46060, 46280, 46600)

46030 Removal of anal seton, other marker

46040 Incision and drainage of ischiorectal and/or perirectal abscess (separate procedure)

46045 Incision and drainage of intramural, intramuscular, or submucosal abscess, transanal, under anesthesia

46050 Incision and drainage, perianal abscess, superficial

(See also 45020, 46060)

46060 Incision and drainage of ischiorectal or intramural abscess, with fistulectomy or fistulotomy, submuscular, with or without placement of seton

(Do not report 46060 in addition to 46020)

(See also 45020)

46070 Incision, anal septum (infant)

(For anoplasty, see 46700-46705)

(Do not report modifier '-63' in conjunction with 46070)

46080 Sphincterotomy, anal, division of sphincter (separate procedure)

46083 Incision of thrombosed hemorrhoid, external

EXCISION

46200 Fissurectomy, including sphincterotomy when performed

46220 This code is out of order. See page 505

46221 Hemorrhoidectomy, internal, by rubber band ligation(s)

(Do not report 46221 in conjunction with 45350, 45398)

(For ligation, hemorrhoidal vascular bundle(s), including ultrasound guidance, use 0249T)

46945 Hemorrhoidectomy, internal, by ligation other than rubber band; single hemorrhoid column/group, without imagaing guidance

46946 2 or more hemorrhoid columns/groups, without imaging guidance

---

● New Code ▲ Revised Code + Add-On Code ⊘ Modifier -51 Exempt ★ Telemedicine

(Do not report 46221, 46945, 46946 in conjunction with 46948)

(Do not report 46945, 46946 in conjunction with 76872, 76942, 76998)

46948 Hemorrhoidectomy, internal, by transanal hemorrhoidal dearterialization, 2 or more hemorrhoid columns/groups, including ultrasound guidance, with mucopexy, when performed

(Do not report 46948 in conjunction with 76872, 76942, 76998)

(For transanal hemorrhoidal dearterialization, single hemorrhoid column/group, use 46999)

46220 Excision of single external papilla or tag, anus

46230 Excision of multiple external papillae or tags, anus

46320 Excision of thrombosed hemorrhoid, external

46250 Hemorrhoidectomy, external, 2 or more columns/groups

(For hemorrhoidectomy, external, single column/group, use 46999)

46255 Hemorrhoidectomy, internal and external, single column/group;

46257 with fissurectomy

46258 with fistulectomy, including fissurectomy, when performed

46260 Hemorrhoidectomy, internal and external, 2 or more columns/groups;

46261 with fissurectomy

46262 with fistulectomy, including fissurectomy, when performed

(Do not report 46250-46262 in conjunction with 46948)

46270 Surgical treatment of anal fistula (fistulectomy/fistulotomy); subcutaneous

46275 intersphincteric

46280 transsphincteric, suprasphincteric, extrasphincteric or multiple, including placement of seton, when performed

(Do not report 46280 in addition to 46020)

46285 second stage

46288 Closure of anal fistula with rectal advancement flap

46320 This code is out of order. See page 505

INTRODUCTION

46500 Injection of sclerosing solution, hemorrhoids

(For anoscopy with directed submucosal injection of bulking agent for fecal incontinence, use 0377T)

46505 Chemodenervation of internal anal sphincter

(For chemodenervation of other muscles, see 64612, 64616, 64617, 64642, 64643, 64644, 64645, 64646, 64647. For destruction of nerve by neurolytic agent, use 64630)

(Report the specific service in conjunction with the specific substance(s) or drug(s) provided)

ENDOSCOPY

Surgical endoscopy always includes diagnostic endoscopy.

46600   Anoscopy; diagnostic, including collection of specimen(s) by brushing or washing, when performed (separate procedure)

(Do not report 46600 in conjunction with 46020-46947, 0184T, during the same operative session)

(For diagnostic high-resolution anoscopy [HRA], use 46601)

46601   diagnostic, with high-resolution magnification (hra) (eg, colposcope, operating microscope) and chemical agent enhancement, including collection of specimen(s) by brushing or washing, when performed

(Do not report 46601 in conjunction with 69990)

46604   with dilation (eg, balloon, guide wire, bougie)

46606   with biopsy, single or multiple

(For high-resolution anoscopy [HRA] with biopsy, use 46607)

46607   with high-resolution magnification (hra) (eg, colposcope, operating microscope) and chemical agent enhancement, with biopsy, single or multiple

(Do not report 46607 in conjunction with 69990)

46608   with removal of foreign body

46610   with removal of single tumor, polyp, or other lesion by hot biopsy forceps or bipolar cautery

46611   with removal of single tumor, polyp, or other lesion by snare technique

46612   with removal of multiple tumors, polyps, or other lesions by hot biopsy forceps, bipolar cautery or snare technique

46614   with control of bleeding (eg, injection, bipolar cautery, unipolar cautery, laser, heater probe, stapler, plasma coagulator)

46615   with ablation of tumor(s), polyp(s), or other lesion(s) not amenable to removal by hot biopsy forceps, bipolar cautery or snare technique

(For delivery of thermal energy to the muscle of the anal canal, use 0288T)

REPAIR

46700   Anoplasty, plastic operation for stricture; adult

46705   infant

(Do not report modifier '-63' in conjunction with 46705)

(For simple incision of anal septum, use 46070)

46706   Repair of anal fistula with fibrin glue

46707   Repair of anorectal fistula with plug (eg, porcine small intestine submucosa [SIS])

46710   Repair of ileoanal pouch fistula/sinus (eg, perineal or vaginal), pouch advancement; transperineal approach

46712   combined transperineal and transabdominal approach

46715 Repair of low imperforate anus; with anoperineal fistula (cut-back procedure)

46716   with transposition of anoperineal or anovestibular fistula

(Do not report modifier 63 in conjunction with 46715, 46716)

46730 Repair of high imperforate anus without fistula; perineal or sacroperineal approach

46735   combined transabdominal and sacroperineal approaches

(Do not report modifier 63 in conjunction with 46730, 46735)

46740 Repair of high imperforate anus with rectourethral or rectovaginal fistula; perineal or sacroperineal approach

46742   combined transabdominal and sacroperineal approaches

(Do not report modifier 63 in conjunction with 46740, 46742)

46744 Repair of cloacal anomaly by anorectovaginoplasty and urethroplasty, sacroperineal approach

(Do not report modifier 63 in conjunction with 46744)

46746 Repair of cloacal anomaly by anorectovaginoplasty and urethroplasty, combined abdominal and sacroperineal approach;

46748   with vaginal lengthening by intestinal graft or pedicle flaps

46750 Sphincteroplasty, anal, for incontinence or prolapse; adult

46751   child

46753 Graft (Thiersch operation) for rectal incontinence and/or prolapse

46754 Removal of Thiersch wire or suture, anal canal

46760 Sphincteroplasty, anal, for incontinence, adult; muscle transplant

46761   levator muscle imbrication (Park posterior anal repair)

(**46762** deleted 2018 [2019 Edition])

(For anoscopy with directed submucosal injection of bulking agent for fecal incontinence, use 0377T)

46947 Hemorrhoidopexy (eg, for prolapsing internal hemorrhoids) by stapling

DESTRUCTION

46900 Destruction of lesion(s), anus (eg, condyloma, papilloma, molluscum contagiosum, herpetic vesicle), simple; chemical

46910   electrodesiccation

46916   cryosurgery

46917   laser surgery

46922   surgical excision

46924 Destruction of lesion(s), anus (eg, condyloma, papilloma, molluscum contagiosum, herpetic vesicle), extensive (eg, laser surgery, electrosurgery, cryosurgery, chemosurgery)

| 46930 | Destruction of internal hemorrhoid(s) by thermal energy (eg, infrared coagulation, cautery, radiofrequency) |

| 46940 | Curettage or cautery of anal fissure, including dilation of anal sphincter (separate procedure); initial |

| 46942 | subsequent |

| 46945 | This code is out of order. See page 504 |

| 46946 | This code is out of order. See page 504 |

| 46947 | This code is out of order. See page 507 |

| 46948 | This code is out of order. See page 505 |

OTHER PROCEDURES

| 46999 | Unlisted procedure, anus |

LIVER

INCISION

| 47000 | Biopsy of liver, needle; percutaneous |

(If imaging guidance is performed, see 76942, 77002, 77012, 77021)

| + 47001 | when done for indicated purpose at time of other major procedure (List separately in addition to code for primary procedure) |

(If imaging guidance is performed, see 76942, 77002)

(For fine needle aspiration biopsy in conjunction with 47000, 47001, see 10004, 10005, 10006, 10007, 10008, 10009, 10010, 10011, 10012, 10021)

(For evaluation of fine needle aspirate in conjunction with 47000, 47001, see 88172, 88173)

| 47010 | Hepatotomy; for open drainage of abscess or cyst, 1 or 2 stages |

(For percutaneous image-guided fluid collection drainage by catheter of hepatic abscess or cyst, use 49405)

| 47015 | Laparotomy, with aspiration and/or injection of hepatic parasitic (eg, amoebic or echinococcal) cyst(s) or abscess(es) |

EXCISION

| 47100 | Biopsy of liver, wedge |

| 47120 | Hepatectomy, resection of liver; partial lobectomy |

| 47122 | trisegmentectomy |

| 47125 | total left lobectomy |

| 47130 | total right lobectomy |

LIVER TRANSPLANTATION

Liver allotransplantation involves three distinct components of physician work:

1) **Cadaver donor hepatectomy**, which includes harvesting the graft and cold preservation of the graft (perfusing with cold preservation solution and cold maintenance) (use 47133). **Living donor hepatectomy**, which includes harvesting the graft, cold preservation of the graft (perfusing with cold preservation solution and cold maintenance), and care of the donor (see 47140-47142).

● New Code ▲ Revised Code + Add-On Code ⊘ Modifier -51 Exempt ★ Telemedicine

2) Backbench work:

Standard preparation of the whole liver graft will include one of the following:

Preparation of whole liver graft (including cholecystectomy, if necessary, and dissection and removal of surrounding soft tissues to prepare vena cava, portal vein, hepatic artery, and common bile duct for implantation) (use 47143).

Preparation as described for whole liver graft, plus trisegment split into two partial grafts (use 47144).

Preparation as described for whole liver graft, plus lobe split into two partial grafts (use 47145).

Additional reconstruction of the liver graft may include venous and/or arterial anastomosis(es) (see 47146, 47147).

3) Recipient liver allotransplantation, which includes recipient hepatectomy (partial or whole), transplantation of the allograft (partial or whole), and care of the recipient (see 47135).

47133	Donor hepatectomy (including cold preservation), from cadaver donor
47135	Liver allotransplantation; orthotopic, partial or whole, from cadaver or living donor, any age
47140	Donor hepatectomy (including cold preservation), from living donor; left lateral segment only (segments II and III)
47141	total left lobectomy (segments II, III, and IV)
47142	total right lobectomy (segments V, VI, VII, and VIII)
47143	Backbench standard preparation of cadaver donor whole liver graft prior to allotransplantation, including cholecystectomy, if necessary, and dissection and removal of surrounding soft tissues to prepare the vena cava, portal vein, hepatic artery, and common bile duct for implantation; without trisegment or lobe split
47144	with trisegment split of whole liver graft into 2 partial liver grafts (ie, left lateral segment [segments II and III] and right trisegment [segments I and IV through VIII])
47145	with lobe split of whole liver graft into 2 partial liver grafts (ie, left lobe (segments II, III, and IV) and right lobe (segments I and V through VIII))
47146	Backbench reconstruction of cadaver or living donor liver graft prior to allotransplantation; venous anastomosis, each
47147	arterial anastomosis, each

(Do not report 47143-47147 in conjunction with 47120-47125, 47600, 47610)

REPAIR

47300	Marsupialization of cyst or abscess of liver
47350	Management of liver hemorrhage; simple suture of liver wound or injury
47360	complex suture of liver wound or injury, with or without hepatic artery ligation
47361	exploration of hepatic wound, extensive debridement, coagulation and/or suture, with or without packing of liver
47362	re-exploration of hepatic wound for removal of packing

LAPAROSCOPY

Surgical laparoscopy always include diagnostic laparoscopy. To report a diagnostic laparoscopy (peritneoscopy) (separate procedure), use 49320.

47370 Laparoscopy, surgical, ablation of 1 or more liver tumor(s); radiofrequency

(For imaging guidance, use 76490)

47371 cryosurgical

(For imaging guidance, use 76490)

47379 Unlisted laparoscopic procedure, liver

OTHER PROCEDURES

47380 Ablation, open, of 1 or more liver tumor(s); radiofrequency

(For imaging guidance, use 76490)

47381 cryosurgical

(For imaging guidance, use 76490)

47382 Ablation, 1 or more liver tumor(s), percutaneous, radiofrequency

(For imaging guidance and monitoring, see 76490, 77013, 77022)

47383 Ablation, 1 or more liver tumor[s], percutaneous, cryoablation

(For imaging guidance and monitoring, see 76940, 77013, 77022)

47399 Unlisted procedure, liver

BILIARY TRACT

INCISION

47400 Hepaticotomy or hepaticostomy with exploration, drainage, or removal of calculus

47420 Choledochotomy or choledochostomy with exploration, drainage, or removal of calculus, with or without cholecystotomy; without transduodenal sphincterotomy or sphincteroplasty

47425 with transduodenal sphincterotomy or sphincteroplasty

47460 Transduodenal sphincterotomy or sphincteroplasty, with or without transduodenal extraction of calculus (separate procedure)

47480 Cholecystotomy or cholecystostomy, open, with exploration, drainage, or removal of calculus (separate procedure)

(For percutaneous cholecystostomy, use 47490)

INTRODUCTION

Percutaneous biliary procedures (eg, transhepatic, transcholecystic) are described by 47490 and 47531-47544, and are performed with imaging guidance. They are differentiated from endoscopic procedures that utilize an access to the biliary tree from a hollow viscus for diagnosis and therapy. Diagnostic cholangiography is typically performed with percutaneous biliary procedures, and is included in 47490, 47533, 47534, 47535, 47536, 47537, 47538, 47539, 47540, and 47541.

Codes 47531 and 47532 describe percutaneous diagnostic cholangiography that includes injection(s) of contrast material, all associated radiological supervision and interpretation, and procedural imaging guidance (eg, ultrasound and/or fluoroscopy). Code 47532 also includes accessing the biliary system with a needle or catheter. Codes 47531 and 47532 may not be reported with codes 47533, 47534, 47535, 47536, 47537, 47538, 47539, 47540, and 47541.

An external biliary drainage catheter is a catheter placed into a bile duct that does not terminate in bowel, and that drains bile externally only. An internal-external biliary drainage catheter is a single, externally accessible catheter that terminates in the small

● New Code   ▲ Revised Code   + Add-On Code   ⊘ Modifier -51 Exempt   ★ Telemedicine

intestine, and may drain bile into the small intestine and/or externally. A "stent," as used in this code set, is a percutaneously placed device (eg, self-expanding metallic mesh stent, plastic tube) that is positioned within the biliary tree and is completely internal, with no portion extending outside the patient.

Codes 47533, 47534, 47535, 47536, 47537, 47538, 47539, and 47540 describe percutaneous therapeutic biliary procedures that include catheter or stent placement, catheter removal and replacement (exchange), and/or catheter removal. These codes include the elements of access, drainage catheter manipulations, diagnostic cholangiography, imaging guidance (eg, ultrasonography and/or fluoroscopy), and all associated radiological supervision and interpretation. Codes 47533, 47534, 47538, 47539, 47540 may be reported once for each catheter or stent placed (eg, bilobar placement, multi-segmental placement). Codes 47535, 47536, and 47537 may be reported once for each catheter conversion, exchange, or removal (eg, bilobar, bisegmental).

Codes 47538, 47539, 47540 may be reported only once per session to describe one or more overlapping or serial stent(s) placed within a single bile duct, or bridging more than one ductal segment (eg, left hepatic duct and common bile duct) through a single percutaneous access. Codes 47538, 47539, 47540 may be reported more than once in the same session using modifier 59 for the additional procedures in the following circumstances: (i) placement of side-by-side (double-barrel) stents within a single bile duct; (ii) placement of two or more stents into separate bile ducts through a single percutaneous access; or (iii) placement of stents through two or more percutaneous access sites (eg, placement of one stent through the interstices of another stent). Code 47538 describes biliary stent placement through an existing access. Therefore, 47538 should not be reported together with 47536 if a biliary drainage catheter (eg, external or internal-external) is replaced after the biliary stent is placed. Code 47540 describes biliary stent placement with the additional service of placing a biliary drainage catheter (eg, external or internal-external). Therefore, 47540 should not be reported with 47533, 47534 for the same ductal system.

Code 47541 describes a procedure to assist with endoscopic procedures performed in conjunction with other physician specialists. Access placed may include wire and/or catheter. Code 47541 may not be reported if a wire is placed through existing percutaneous access.

Codes 47542, 47543, and 47544 describe procedures that may be performed in conjunction with other codes in this family, are add-on codes and do not include access, catheter placement, or diagnostic imaging. Do not report 47542 with 47538, 47539, 47540 because balloon dilation is included in 47538, 47539, and 47540. Code 47544 should not be reported with 47531-47543 for incidental removal of debris. Code 47542 should not be reported with 47544, if a balloon is used for removal of calculi or debris rather than for dilation.

EXCHANGES/CONVERSIONS				
(Existing Access)		**To**		
Do not report exchange with stent for same percutaneous access		**Internal-External**	**External**	**Stent**
From	External Drain	47535 Conversion	47536 Exchange	47538 Stent
	Internal-External Drain	47536 Exchange	47536 Exchange	47538 Stent

47490 Cholecystostomy, percutaneous, complete procedure, including imaging guidance, catheter placement, cholecystogram when performed, and radiological supervision and interpretation

(Do not report 47490 in conjunction with 47531, 47532, 75989, 76942, 77002, 77012, 77021)

47531 Injection procedure for cholangiography, percutaneous, complete diagnostic procedure including imaging guidance (eg, ultrasound and/or fluoroscopy) and all associated radiological supervision and interpretation; existing access

47532 new access (eg, percutaneous transhepatic cholangiogram)

(Do not report 47531, 47532 in conjunction with 47490, 47533, 47534, 47535, 47536, 47537, 47538, 47539, 47540, 47541 for procedures performed through the same percutaneous access)

(For intraoperative cholangiography, see 74300, 74301)

47533 Placement of biliary drainage catheter, percutaneous, including diagnostic cholangiography when performed, imaging guidance (eg, ultrasound and/or fluoroscopy), and all associated radiological supervision and interpretation; external

47534 internal-external

47535   Conversion of external biliary drainage catheter to internal-external biliary drainage catheter, percutaneous, including diagnostic cholangiography when performed, imaging guidance (eg, fluoroscopy), and all associated radiological supervision and interpretation

47536   Exchange of biliary drainage catheter (eg, external, internal-external, or conversion of internal-external to external only), percutaneous, including diagnostic cholangiography when performed, imaging guidance (eg, fluoroscopy), and all associated radiological supervision and interpretation

(Do not report 47536 in conjunction with 47538 for the same access)

(47536 includes exchange of one catheter. For exchange of additional catheter[s] during the same session, report 47536 with modifier 59 for each additional exchange)

47537   Removal of biliary drainage catheter, percutaneous, requiring fluoroscopic guidance (eg, with concurrent indwelling biliary stents), including diagnostic cholangiography when performed, imaging guidance (eg, fluoroscopy), and all associated radiological supervision and interpretation

(Do not report 47537 in conjunction with 47538 for the same access)

(For removal of biliary drainage catheter not requiring fluoroscopic guidance, see E/M services and report the appropriate level of service provided [eg, 99202-99215, 99217, 99218, 99219, 99220, 99221, 99222, 99223, 99224, 99225, 99226, 99231, 99232, 99233])

47538   Placement of stent(s) into a bile duct, percutaneous, including diagnostic cholangiography, imaging guidance (eg, fluoroscopy and/or ultrasound), balloon dilation, catheter exchange(s) and catheter removal(s) when performed, and all associated radiological supervision and interpretation; existing access

(Do not report 47538 in conjunction with 47536, 47537 for the same percutaneous access)

47539   new access, without placement of separate biliary drainage catheter

47540   new access, with placement of separate biliary drainage catheter (eg, external or internal-external)

(Do not report 47538, 47539, 47540 in conjunction with 43277, 47542, 47555, 47556 for the same lesion in the same session)

(Do not report 47540 in conjunction with 47533, 47534 for the same percutaneous access)

(47538, 47539, 47540 may be reported more than once per session, when specific conditions described in the Introduction within the Biliary Tract subsection guidelines are met)

47541   Placement of access through the biliary tree and into small bowel to assist with an endoscopic biliary procedure (eg, rendezvous procedure), percutaneous, including diagnostic cholangiography when performed, imaging guidance (eg, ultrasound and/or fluoroscopy), and all associated radiological supervision and interpretation, new access

(Do not report 47541 in conjunction with 47531, 47532, 47533, 47534, 47535, 47536, 47537, 47538, 47539, 47540)

(Do not report 47541 when there is existing catheter access)

(For use of existing access through the biliary tree into small bowel to assist with an endoscopic biliary procedure, see 47535, 47536, 47537)

+ 47542   Balloon dilation of biliary duct(s) or of ampulla (sphincteroplasty), percutaneous, including imaging guidance (eg, fluoroscopy), and all associated radiological supervision and interpretation, each duct (List separately in addition to code for primary procedure)

(Use 47542 in conjunction with 47531, 47532, 47533, 47534, 47535, 47536, 47537, 47541)

(Do not report 47542 in conjunction with 43262, 43277, 47538, 47539, 47540, 47555, 47556)

(Do not report 47542 in conjunction with 47544 if a balloon is used for removal of calculi, debris, and/or sludge rather than for dilation)

(For percutaneous balloon dilation of multiple ducts during the same session, report an additional dilation once with 47542 and modifier 59, regardless of the number of additional ducts dilated)

(For endoscopic balloon dilation, see 43277, 47555, 47556)

+ **47543**   Endoluminal biopsy(ies) of biliary tree, percutaneous, any method(s) (eg, brush, forceps, and/or needle), including imaging guidance (eg, fluoroscopy), and all associated radiological supervision and interpretation, single or multiple (List separately in addition to code for primary procedure)

(Use 47543 in conjunction with 47531, 47532, 47533, 47534, 47535, 47536, 47537, 47538, 47539, 47540)

(Report 47543 once per session)

(For endoscopic brushings, see 43260, 47552)

(For endoscopic biopsy, see 43261, 47553)

+ **47544**   Removal of calculi/debris from biliary duct(s) and/or gallbladder, percutaneous, including destruction of calculi by any method (eg, mechanical, electrohydraulic, lithotripsy) when performed, imaging guidance (eg, fluoroscopy), and all associated radiological supervision and interpretation (List separately in addition to code for primary procedure)

(Use 47544 in conjunction with 47531, 47532, 47533, 47534, 47535, 47536, 47537, 47538, 47539, 47540)

(Do not report 47544 if no calculi or debris are found, even if removal device is deployed)

(Do not report 47544 in conjunction with 43264, 47554)

(Do not report 47544 in conjunction with 47531-47543 for incidental removal of debris)

(For endoscopic removal of calculi, see 43264, 47554)

(For endoscopic destruction of calculi, use 43265)

ENDOSCOPY

Surgical endoscopy always includes diagnostic endoscopy.

+ **47550**   Biliary endoscopy, intraoperative (choledochoscopy) (List separately in addition to code for primary procedure)

47552   Biliary endoscopy, percutaneous via T-tube or other tract; diagnostic, with collection of specimen(s) by brushing and/or washing, when performed (separate procedure)

47553   with biopsy, single or multiple

47554   with removal of calculus/calculi

47555   with dilation of biliary duct stricture(s) without stent

47556   with dilation of biliary duct stricture(s) with stent

(For ERCP, see 43260-43278, 74328, 74329, 74330, 74363)

(If imaging guidance is performed, see 74363)

LAPAROSCOPY

Surgical laparoscopy always include diagnostic laparoscopy. To report a diagnostic laparoscopy (peritneoscopy) (separate procedure), use 49320.

47562   Laparoscopy, surgical; cholecystectomy

47563   cholecystectomy with cholangiography

(For intraoperative cholangiography radiological supervision and interpretation, see 74300, 74301)

(For percutaneous cholangiography, see 47531, 47532)

47564   cholecystectomy with exploration of common duct

47570   cholecystoenterostomy

47579   Unlisted laparoscopy procedure, biliary tract

EXCISION

47600   Cholecystectomy;

47605   with cholangiography

(For laparoscopic approach, see 47562-47564)

47610   Cholecystectomy with exploration of common duct;

(For cholecystectomy with exploration of common duct with biliary endoscopy, use 47610 with 47550)

47612   with choledochoenterostomy

47620   with transduodenal sphincterotomy or sphincteroplasty, with or without cholangiography

47700   Exploration for congenital atresia of bile ducts, without repair, with or without liver biopsy, with or without cholangiography

(Do not report modifier 63 in conjunction with 47700)

47701   Portoenterostomy (eg, Kasai procedure)

(Do not report modifier 63 in conjunction with 47701)

47711   Excision of bile duct tumor, with or without primary repair of bile duct; extrahepatic

47712   intrahepatic

(For anastomosis, see 47760-47800)

47715   Excision of choledochal cyst

REPAIR

47720   Cholecystoenterostomy; direct

(For laparoscopic approach, use 47570)

47721   with gastroenterostomy

47740   Roux-en-Y

47741   Roux-en-Y with gastroenterostomy

47760   Anastomosis, of extrahepatic biliary ducts and gastrointestinal tract

47765   Anastomosis, of intrahepatic ducts and gastrointestinal tract

47780   Anastomosis, Roux-en-Y, of extrahepatic biliary ducts and gastrointestinal tract

47785   Anastomosis, Roux-en-Y, of intrahepatic biliary ducts and gastrointestinal tract

47800   Reconstruction, plastic, of extrahepatic biliary ducts with end-to-end anastomosis

47801   Placement of choledochal stent

47802 U-tube hepaticoenterostomy

47900 Suture of extrahepatic biliary duct for pre-existing injury (separate procedure)

OTHER PROCEDURES

47999 Unlisted procedure, biliary tract

PANCREAS

(For peroral pancreatic endoscopic procedures, see 43260-43265, 43274-43278)

INCISION

48000 Placement of drains, peripancreatic, for acute pancreatitis;

48001   with cholecystostomy, gastrostomy, and jejunostomy

48020 Removal of pancreatic calculus

EXCISION

48100 Biopsy of pancreas, open (eg, fine needle aspiration, needle core biopsy, wedge biopsy)

48102 Biopsy of pancreas, percutaneous needle

(For radiological supervision and interpretation, see 76942, 77002, 77012, 77021)

(For fine needle aspiration biopsy, see 10005, 10006, 10007, 10008, 10009, 10010, 10011, 10012)

(For evaluation of fine needle aspirate, see 88172, 88173)

48105 Resection or debridement of pancreas and peripancreatic tissue for acute necrotizing pancreatitis

48120 Excision of lesion of pancreas (eg, cyst, adenoma)

48140 Pancreatectomy, distal subtotal, with or without splenectomy; without pancreaticojejunostomy

48145   with pancreaticojejunostomy

48146 Pancreatectomy, distal, near-total with preservation of duodenum (Child-type procedure)

48148 Excision of ampulla of Vater

48150 Pancreatectomy, proximal subtotal with total duodenectomy, partial gastrectomy, choledochoenterostomy and gastrojejunostomy (Whipple-type procedure); with pancreatojejunostomy

48152   without pancreatojejunostomy

48153 Pancreatectomy, proximal subtotal with near-total duodenectomy, choledochoenterostomy, and duodenojejunostomy (pylorus-sparing, whipple-type procedure); with pancreatojejunostomy

48154   without pancreatojejunostomy

48155 Pancreatectomy, total

48160 Pancreatectomy, total or subtotal, with autologous transplantation of pancreas or pancreatic islet cells

(To report pancreatic islet cell transplantation via portal vein catheterization and infusion, see 0584T, 0585T, 0586T)

Separate Procedure   Unlisted Procedure   CCI Comp. Code   Non-specific Procedure   **515**

INTRODUCTION

+ **48400**   Injection procedure for intraoperative pancreatography (List separately in addition to code for primary procedure)

(For radiological supervision and interpretation, see 74300, 74301)

(For intraoperative pancreatography radiological supervision and interpretation, see 74300, 74301)

REPAIR

48500   Marsupialization of pancreatic cyst

48510   External drainage, pseudocyst of pancreas; open

(For percutaneous image-guided fluid collection drainage by catheter of pancreatic pseudocyst, use 49405)

48520   Internal anastomosis of pancreatic cyst to gastrointestinal tract; direct

48540   Roux-en-Y

48545   Pancreatorrhaphy for injury

48547   Duodenal exclusion with gastrojejunostomy for pancreatic injury

48548   Pancreaticojejunostomy, side-to-side anastomosis (Puestow-type operation)

PANCREAS TRANSPLANTATION

Pancreas allotransplantation involves three distinct components of physician work:

1) **Cadaver donor pancreatectomy**, which includes harvesting the pancreas graft, with or without duodenal segment, and cold preservation of the graft (perfusing with cold preservation solution and cold maintenance) (use 48550).

2) **Backbench work**:

Standard preparation of a cadaver donor pancreas allograft prior to transplantation includes dissection of the allograft from surrounding soft tissues, splenectomy, duodenotomy, ligation of bile duct, ligation of mesenteric vessels, and Y-graft arterial anastomoses from the iliac artery to the superior mesenteric artery and to the splenic artery (use 48551).

Additional reconstruction of a cadaver donor pancreas allograft prior to transplantation may include venous anastomosis(es) (use 48552).

3) **Recipient pancreas allotransplantation**, which includes transplantation of allograft, and care of the recipient (use 48554).

48550   Donor pancreatectomy (including cold preservation), with or without duodenal segment for transplantation

48551   Backbench standard preparation of cadaver donor pancreas allograft prior to transplantation, including dissection of allograft from surrounding soft tissues, splenectomy, duodenotomy, ligation of bile duct, ligation of mesenteric vessels, and Y-graft arterial anastomoses from iliac artery to superior mesenteric artery and to splenic artery

48552   Backbench reconstruction of cadaver donor pancreas allograft prior to transplantation, venous anastomosis, each

(Do not report 48551 and 48552 in conjunction with 35531, 35563, 35685, 38100-38102, 44010, 44820, 44850, 47460, 47550-47556, 48100-48120, 48545)

48554   Transplantation of pancreatic allograft

48556   Removal of transplanted pancreatic allograft

OTHER PROCEDURES

48999   Unlisted procedure, pancreas

ABDOMEN, PERITONEUM, AND OMENTUM

INCISION

49000   Exploratory laparotomy, exploratory celiotomy with or without biopsy(s) (separate procedure)

(To report wound exploration due to penetrating trauma without laparatomy, use 20102)

49002   Reopening of recent laparotomy

(To report re-exploration of hepatic wound for removal of packing, use 47362)

(To report re-exploration of pelvic wound for removal, including repacking, when performed, use 49014)

49010   Exploration, retroperitoneal area with or without biopsy(s) (separate procedure)

(To report wound exploration due to penetrating trauma without laparotomy, use 20102)

49013   Preperitoneal pelvic packing for hemorrhage associated with pelvic trauma, including local exploration

49014   Re-exploration of pelvic wound with removal of preperitoneal pelvic packing, including repacking, when performed

49020   Drainage of peritoneal abscess or localized peritonitis, exclusive of appendiceal abscess; open

(For appendiceal abscess, use 44900)

(For percutaneous image-guided drainage of peritoneal abscess or localized peritonitis by catheter, use 49406)

(For transrectal or transvaginal image-guided drainage of peritoneal abscess by catheter, use 49407)

49040   Drainage of subdiaphragmatic or subphrenic abscess; open

(For percutaneous image-guided drainage of subdiaphragmatic or subphrenic abscess by catheter, use 49406)

49060   Drainage of retroperitoneal abscess; open

(For percutaneous image-guided drainage of retroperitoneal abscess by catheter, use 49406)

(For transrectal or transvaginal image-guided drainage of retroperitoneal abscess by catheter, use 49407)

49062   Drainage of extraperitoneal lymphocele to peritoneal cavity, open

(For laparoscopic drainage of lymphocele to peritoneal cavity, use 49323)

(for percutaneous image-guided drainage of peritoneal or retroperitoneal lymphocele by catheter, use 49406)

49082   Abdominal paracentesis (diagnostic or therapeutic); without imaging guidance

49083   with imaging guidance

(Do not report 49083 in conjunction with 76942, 77002, 77012, 77021)

(For percutaneous image-guided drainage of retroperitoneal abscess by catheter, use 49406)

49084   Peritoneal lavage, including imaging guidance, when performed

(Do not report 49084 in conjunction with 76942, 77002, 77012, 77021)

(For percutaneous image-guided drainage of retroperitoneal abscess by cathete, use 49406)

EXCISION, DESTRUCTION

Code 49185 describes sclerotherapy of a fluid collection (eg, lymphocele, cyst, or seroma) through a percutaneous access. It includes contrast injection(s), sclerosant injection(s), sclerosant dwell time, diagnostic study, imaging guidance (eg, ultrasound, fluoroscopy), and radiological supervision and interpretation, when performed. Code 49185 may be reported once per day for each lesion treated through a separate catheter. Do not report 49185 more than once if treating multiple lesions through the same catheter. Codes for access to and drainage of the collection may be separately reportable according to location (eg, 10030, 10160, 49405, 49406, 49407, 50390).

(For lysis of intestinal adhesions, use 44005)

49180   Biopsy, abdominal or retroperitoneal mass, percutaneous needle

(If imaging guidance is performed, see 76942, 77002, 77012, 77021)

(For fine needle aspiration biopsy, see 10004, 10005, 10006, 10007, 10008, 10009, 10010, 10011, 10012, 10021)

(For evaluation of fine needle aspirate, see 88172, 88173)

49185   Sclerotherapy of a fluid collection (eg, lymphocele, cyst, or seroma), percutaneous, including contrast injection(s), sclerosant injection(s), diagnostic study, imaging guidance (eg, ultrasound, fluoroscopy) and radiological supervision and interpretation when performed

(For treatment of multiple lesions in a single day requiring separate access, use modifier 59 for each additional treated lesion)

(For treatment of multiple interconnected lesions treated through a single access, report 49185 once)

(For access/drainage with needle, see 10160, 50390)

(For access/drainage with catheter, see 10030, 49405, 49406, 49407, 50390)

(For exchange of existing catheter, before or after injection of sclerosant, see 49423, 75984)

(For sclerotherapy of a lymphatic/vascular malformation, use 37241)

(For sclerosis of veins or endovenous ablation of incompetent extremity veins, see 36468, 36470, 36471, 36475, 36476, 36478, 36479)

(For pleurodesis, use 32560)

(Do not report 49185 in conjunction with 49424, 76080)

49203   Excision or destruction, open, intra-abdominal tumors, cysts or endometriomas, 1 or more peritoneal, mesenteric, or retroperitoneal primary or secondary tumors; largest tumor 5 cm diameter or less

49204   largest tumor 5.1-10.0 cm diameter

49205   largest tumor greater than 10.0 cm diameter

(Do not report 49203-49205 in conjunction with 38770, 38780, 49000, 49010, 49215, 50010, 50205, 50225, 50236, 50250, 50290, 58920, 58925, 58940, 58943, 58951, 58952, 58953, 58954, 58956, 58957, 58958, 58960)

(For partial or total nephrectomy, use 50220 or 50240 in conjunction with 49203-49205)

(For colectomy, use 44140 in conjunction with 49203-49205)

(For small bowel resection, use 44120 in conjunction with 49203-49205)

(For vena caval resection with reconstruction, use 49203-49205 in conjunction with 37799)

(For resection of recurrent ovarian, tubal, primary peritoneal, or uterine malignancy, see 58957, 58958)

(For cryoablation of renal tumors, see 50250, 50593)

49215   Excision of presacral or sacrococcygeal tumor

(Do not report modifier 63 in conjunction with 49215)

(**49220**   deleted 2020 [2021 edition])

49250   Umbilectomy, omphalectomy, excision of umbilicus (separate procedure)

49255   Omentectomy, epiploectomy, resection of omentum (separate procedure)

LAPAROSCOPY

Surgical laparoscopy always includes diagnostic laparoscopy. To report a diagnostic laparoscopy (peritneoscopy) (separate procedure), use 49320.

For laparoscopic fulguration or excision of lesions of the ovary, pelvic viscera, or peritoneal surface, use 58662.

49320   Laparoscopy, abdomen, peritoneum, and omentum; diagnostic, with or without collection of specimen(s) by brushing or washing (separate procedure)

49321   Laparoscopy, surgical; with biopsy (single or multiple)

49322   with aspiration of cavity or cyst (eg, ovarian cyst) (single or multiple)

49323   with drainage of lymphocele to peritoneal cavity

(For open drainage of lymphocele to peritoneal cavity, use 49062)

49324   with insertion of tunneled intraperitoneal catheter

(For subcutaneous extension of intraperitoneal catheter with remote chest exit site, use 49435 in conjunction with 49324)

(For open insertion of tunneled intraperitoneal catheter, use 49421)

49325   with revision of previously placed intraperitoneal cannula or catheter, with removal of intraluminal obstructive material if performed

+ **49326**   with omentopexy (omental tacking procedure) (List separately in addition to code for primary procedure)

(Use 49326 in conjunction with 49324, 49325)

+ **49327**   with placement of interstitial device(s) for radiation therapy guidance (eg, fiducial markers, dosimeter), intra-abdominal, intrapelvic, and/or retroperitoneum, including imaging guidance, if performed, single or multiple (List separately in addition to code for primary procedure)

(Use 49327 in conjunction with laparoscopic abdominal, pelvic, or retroperitoneal procedure[s] performed concurrently)

(For placement of interstitial device[s] for intra-abdominal, intrapelvic, and/or retroperitoneal radiation therapy guidance concurrent with open procedure, use 49412)

(For percutaneous placement of interstitial device[s] for intra-abdominal, intrapelvic, and/or retroperitoneal radiation therapy guidance, use 49411)

49329   Unlisted laparoscopy procedure, abdomen, peritoneum and omentum

INTRODUCTION, REVISION, REMOVAL

49400   Injection of air or contrast into peritoneal cavity (separate procedure)

(For radiological supervision and interpretation, use 74190)

49402   Removal of peritoneal foreign body from peritoneal cavity

(For lysis of intestinal adhesions, use 44005)

(For open or percutaneous peritoneal drainage or lavage, see 49406, 49020, 49040, 49082-49084, as appropriate)

(For percutaneous insertion of a tunneled intraperitoneal catheter without subcutaneous port, use 49418)

49405   Image-guided fluid collection drainage by catheter (eg, abscess, hematoma, seroma, lymphocele, cyst); visceral (eg, kidney, liver, spleen, lung/mediastinum), percutaneous

(Do not report 49405 in conjunction with 75989, 76942, 77002, 77003, 77012, 77021)

(For percutaneous cholecystostomy, use 47490)

(For pneumonostomy, use 32200)

(For thoracentesis, see 32554, 32555)

(For pleural drainage, see 32556, 32557)

(For percutaneous pleural drainage, see 32556, 32557)

(For open visceral drainage, see 32200 [lung abscess or cyst], 47010 [liver abscess or cyst], 48510 [pseudocyst of pancreas], 50020 [perirenal or renal abscess])

49406   peritoneal or retroperitoneal, percutaneous

(Do not report 49406 in conjunction with 75989, 76942, 77002, 77003, 77012, 77021)

(For abdominal paracentesis [diagnostic or therapeutic], see 49082, 49083)

(For transrectal or transvaginal image-guided peritoneal or retroperitoneal fluid collection drainage by catheter, use 49407)

(For open transrectal drainage of pelvic abscess, use 45000)

(For open peritoneal or retroperitoneal drainage, see 44900 [appendiceal abscess], 49020 [subdiaphragmatic or subphrenic abscess], 49060 [retroperitoneal abscess], 49062 [extraperitoneal lymphocele], 49084 [peritoneal lavage], 50020 [perirenal or renal abscess], 58805 [ovarian cyst], 58822 [ovarian abscess])

(For percutaneous paracentesis, see 49082, 49083)

(For percutaneous insertion of a tunneled intraperitoneal catheter without subcutaneous port, use 49418)

49407   peritoneal or retroperitoneal, transvaginal or transrectal

(Do not report 49407 in conjunction with 75989, 76942, 77002, 77003, 77012, 77021)

(Report 49405, 49406, 49407 separately for each individual collection drained with a separate catheter)

(For open transrectal or transvaginal drainage, see 45000 [pelvic abscess], 58800 [ovarian cyst], 58820 [ovarian abscess])

(For percutaneous image-guided fluid collection drainage by catheter [eg, abscess, hematoma, seroma, lymphocele, cyst] for soft tissue [eg, extremity, abdominal wall, neck], use 10030)

49411   Placement of interstitial device(s) for radiation therapy guidance (eg, fiducial markers, dosimeter), percutaneous, intra abdominal, intra-pelvic (except prostate), and/or retroperitoneum, single or multiple

(Report supply of device separately)

(For imaging guidance, see 76942, 77002, 77012, 77021)

(For percutaneous placement of interstitial device[s] for intra-thoracic radiation therapy guidance, use 32553)

+ 49412 Placement of interstitial device(s) for radiation therapy guidance (eg, fiducial markers, dosimeter), open, intra-abdominal, intrapelvic and/or retroperitoneum, including imaging guidance, if performed, single or multiple (List separately in addition to code for primary procedure)

(Use 49412 in conjunction with open abdominal, pelvic, or retroperitoneal procedure[s] performed concurrently)

(For placement of interstitial device[s] for intra-abdominal, intrapelvic, and/or retroperitoneal radiation therapy guidance concurrent with laparoscopic procedure, use 49327)

(For percutaneous placement of interstitial device[s] for intra-abdominal, intrapelvic, and/or retroperitoneal radiation therapy guidance, use 49411)

49418 Insertion of tunneled intraperitoneal catheter (eg, dialysis, intraperitoneal chemotherapy instillation, management of ascites), complete procedure, including imaging guidance, catheter placement, contrast injection when performed, and radiological supervision and interpretation, percutaneous

49419 Insertion of tunneled intraperitoneal catheter, with subcutaneous port (ie, totally implantable)

(For removal, use 49422)

49421 Insertion of tunneled intraperitoneal catheter for dialysis, open

(For laparoscopic insertion of tunneled intraperitoneal catheter, use 49324)

(For subcutaneous extension of intraperitoneal catheter with remote chest exit site, use 49435 in conjunction with 49421)

49422 Removal of tunneled intraperitoneal catheter

(For removal of a non-tunneled catheter, use appropriate E/M code)

49423 Exchange of previously placed abscess or cyst drainage catheter under radiological guidance (separate procedure)

(For radiological supervision and interpretation, use 75984)

49424 Contrast injection for assessment of abscess or cyst via previously placed drainage catheter or tube (separate procedure)

(For radiological supervision and interpretation, use 76080)

49425 Insertion of peritoneal-venous shunt

49426 Revision of peritoneal-venous shunt

(For shunt patency test, use 78291)

49427 Injection procedure (eg, contrast media) for evaluation of previously placed peritoneal-venous shunt

(For radiological supervision and interpretation, see 75809, 78291)

49428 Ligation of peritoneal-venous shunt

49429 Removal of peritoneal-venous shunt

+ 49435 Insertion of subcutaneous extension to intraperitoneal cannula or catheter with remote chest exit site (List separately in addition to code for primary procedure)

(Use 49435 in conjunction with 49324, 49421)

49436 Delayed creation of exit site from embedded subcutaneous segment of intraperitoneal cannula or catheter

---

Separate Procedure	Unlisted Procedure	CCI Comp. Code	Non-specific Procedure

Initial Placement

Do not additionally report 43752 for placement of a nasogastric (NG) or orogastric (OG) tube to insufflate the stomach prior to percutaneous gastrointestinal tube placement. NG or OG tube placement is considered part of the procedure in this family of codes.

49440   Insertion of gastrostomy tube, percutaneous, under fluoroscopic guidance including contrast injection(s), image documentation and report

(For conversion to a gastro-jejunostomy tube at the time of initial gastrostomy tube placement, use 49440 in conjunction with 49446)

49441   Insertion of duodenostomy or jejunostomy tube, percutaneous, under fluoroscopic guidance including contrast injection(s), image documentation and report

(For conversion of gastrostomy tube to gastro-jejunostomry tube, use 49446)

49442   Insertion of cecostomy or other colonic, tube, percutaneous, under fluoroscopic guidance including contrast injection(s), image documentation and report

Conversion

49446   Conversion of gastrostomy tube to gastro-jejunostomy tube, percutaneous, under fluoroscopic guidance including contrast injection(s), image documentation and report

(For conversion to a gastro-jejunostomy tube at the time of initial gastrostomy tube placement, use 49446 in conjunction with 49440)

Replacement

If an existing gastrostomy, duodenostomy, jejunostomy, gastro-jejunostomy, or cecostomy (or other colonic) tube is removed and a new tube is placed via a separate percutaneous access site, the placement of the new tube is not considered a replacement and would be reported using the appropriate initial placement codes 49440-49442.

49450   Replacement of gastrostomy or cecostomy (or other colonic) tube, percutaneous, under fluoroscopic guidance including contrast injection(s), image documentation and report

(For percutaneous replacement of gastrostomy tube with removal when performed without imaging or endoscopy, see 43762, 43763)

49451   Replacement of duodenostomy or jejunostormy tube, percutaneous, under fluoroscopic guidance including contrast injection(s), image documentation and report

49452   Replacement of gastro-jejunostomy tube, percutaneous, under fluoroscopic guidance including contrast injection(s), image documentation and report

Mechanical Removal Of Obstructive Material

49460   Mechanical removal of obstructive material from gastrostomy, duodenostomy, jejunostomy, gastro-jejunostomy, or cecostomy (or other colonic) tube, any method, under fluoroscopic guidance including contrast injection(s), if performed, image documentation and report

(Do not report 49460 in conjunction with 49450-49452, 49465)

Other

49465   Contrast injection(s) for radiological evaluation of existing gastrostomy, duodenostomy, jejunostomy, gastro-jejunostomy, or cecostomy (or other colonic) tube, from a percutaneous approach including image documentation and report

(Do not report 49465 in conjunction with 49450-49460)

REPAIR

Hernioplasty, Herniorrhaphy, Herniotomy

The hernia repair codes in this section are categorized primarily by the type of hernia (inguinal, femoral, incisional, etc.).

Some types of herias are further categorized as initial or recurrent based on whether or not the hernia has required previous repairs.

Additional variables accounted for by some of the codes include patient age and clinical presentation (reducible vs. incarcerated or strangulated).

With the exception of the incisional hernia repairs (see 49560-49566) the use of mesh or other prostheses is not separately reported.

The excision/repair of strangulated organs or structures such as testicle(s), intestine, ovaries are reported by using the appropriate code for the excision/repair (eg., 44120, 54520, and 58940) in addition to the appropriate code for the repair of the strangulated hernia.

(For reduction and repair of intra-abdominal hernia, use 44050)

(For debridement of abdominal wall, see 11042, 11043)

(Codes 49491-49651 are unilateral procedures. For bilateral procedure, report 49491-49566, 49570-49651 with modifier 50. Report add-on code 49568 twice, when performed bilaterally. Do not report modifier 50 in conjunction with 49568)

49491 Repair, initial inguinal hernia, preterm infant (less than 37 weeks gestation at birth), performed from birth up to 50 weeks postconception age, with or without hydrocelectomy; reducible

49492 incarcerated or strangulated

(Do not report modifier -63 in conjunction with 49491, 49492)

(Post-conception age equals gestational age at birth plus age of infant in weeks at the time of the hernia repair. Initial inguinal hernia repairs that are performed on preterm infants who are over 50 weeks postconceptual age and under age 6 months at the time of surgery, should be reported using codes 49495, 49496)

49495 Repair, initial inguinal hernia, full term infant under age 6 months, or preterm infant over 50 weeks postconception age and under age 6 months at the time of surgery, with or without hydrocelectomy; reducible

49496 incarcerated or strangulated

(Do not report modifier -63 in conjunction with 49491, 49492)

(Post-conception age equals gestational age at birth plus age in weeks at the time of the hernia repair. Initial inguinal hernia repairs that are performed on preterm infants who are under or up to 50 weeks postconceptual age but under 6 months of age since birth, should be reported using codes 49491, 49492. Inguinal hernia repairs on infants age 6 months to under 5 years should be reported using codes 49500-49501)

49500 Repair initial inguinal hernia, age 6 months to under 5 years, with or without hydrocelectomy; reducible

49501 incarcerated or strangulated

49505 Repair initial inguinal hernia, age 5 years or over; reducible

49507 incarcerated or strangulated

(For inguinal hernia repair, with simple orchiectomy, see 49505 or 49507 and 54520)

(For inguinal hernia repair, with excision of hydrocele or spermatocele, see 49505 or 49507 and 54840 or 55040)

49520   Repair recurrent inguinal hernia, any age; reducible

49521   incarcerated or strangulated

49525   Repair inguinal hernia, sliding, any age

(For incarcerated or strangulated inguinal hernia repair, see 49496, 49501, 49507, 49521)

49540   Repair lumbar hernia

49550   Repair initial femoral hernia, any age; reducible

49553   incarcerated or strangulated

49555   Repair recurrent femoral hernia; reducible

49557   incarcerated or strangulated

49560   Repair initial incisional or ventral hernia; reducible

49561   incarcerated or strangulated

49565   Repair recurrent incisional or ventral hernia; reducible

49566   incarcerated or strangulated

+ **49568**   Implantation of mesh or other prosthesis for open incisional or ventral hernia repair or mesh for closure of debridement for necrotizing soft tissue infection (List separately in addition to code for the incisional or ventral hernia repair)

(Use 49568 in conjunction with 11004-11006, 49560-49566)

49570   Repair epigastric hernia (eg, preperitoneal fat); reducible (separate procedure)

49572   incarcerated or strangulated

49580   Repair umbilical hernia, under age 5 years; reducible

49582   incarcerated or strangulated

49585   Repair umbilical hernia, age 5 years or over; reducible

49587   incarcerated or strangulated

49590   Repair spigelian hernia

49600   Repair of small omphalocele, with primary closure

(Do not report modifier -63 in conjunction with 49600)

49605   Repair of large omphalocele or gastroschisis; with or without prosthesis

49606   with removal of prosthesis, final reduction and closure, in operating room

(Do not report modifier -63 in conjunction with 49605, 49606)

49610   Repair of omphalocele (Gross type operation); first stage

49611   second stage

(Do not report modifier -63 in conjunction with 49610, 49611)

● New Code   ▲ Revised Code   + Add-On Code   ⊘ Modifier -51 Exempt   ★ Telemedicine

(For diaphragmatic or hiatal hernia repair, see 39503, 43332)

(For surgical repair of omentum, use 49999)

LAPAROSCOPY

Surgical laparoscopy always includes diagnostic laparoscopy. To report a diagnostic laparoscopy (peritoneoscopy) (separate procedure), use 49320.

49650   Laparoscopy, surgical; repair initial inguinal hernia

49651   repair recurrent inguinal hernia

49652   Laparoscopy, surgical, repair, ventral, umbilical, spigelian or epigastric hernia (includes mesh insertion, when performed); reducible

(Do not report 49652 in conjunction with 44180, 49568)

49653   incarcerated or strangulated

(Do not report 49653 in conjunction with 44180, 49568)

49654   Laparoscopy, surgical, repair, incisional hernia (includes mesh insertion, when performed); reducible

(Do not report 49654 in conjunction with 44180, 49568)

49655   incarcerated or strangulated

(Do not report 49655 in conjunction with 44180, 49568)

49656   Laparoscopy, surgical, repair, recurrent incisional hernia (includes mesh insertion, when performed); reducible

(Do not report 49656 in conjunction with 44180, 49568)

49657   incarcerated or strangulated

(Do not report 49657 in conjunction with 44180, 49568)

49659   Unlisted laparoscopy procedure, hernioplasty, herniorrhaphy, herniotomy

SUTURE

49900   Suture, secondary, of abdominal wall for evisceration or dehiscence

(For suture of ruptured diaphragm, see 39540, 39541)

(For debridement of abdominal wall, see 11042, 11043)

OTHER PROCEDURES

49904   Omental flap, extra-abdominal (eg, for reconstruction of sternal and chest wall defects)

(Code 49904 includes harvest and transfer. If a second surgeon harvests the omental flap, then the two surgeons should code 49904 as co-surgeons, using modifier -62)

+ **49905**   Omental flap, intra-abdominal (List separately in addition to code for primary procedure)

(Do not report 49905 in conjunction with 44700)

49906   Free omental flap with microvascular anastomosis

(Do not report code 69990 in addition to code 49906)

49999   Unlisted procedure, abdomen, peritoneum and omentum

This page intentionally left blank.

● New Code   ▲ Revised Code   ✚ Add-On Code   ⊘ Modifier -51 Exempt   ★ Telemedicine

URINARY SYSTEM

CPT codes from this section are used to report invasive and surgical procedures performed on the kidney; ureter; bladder; prostate (resection); and urethra.

URODYNAMICS

CPT codes in this section may be used separately or in various combinations. When multiple procedures are performed in the same session, modifier -51 should be added .to the second and all subsequent CPT codes. Procedures in this section are performed by, or under the direct supervision of, a physician.

In addition, all materials and supplies, used in the provision of these services, such as instruments, equipment, fluids, gases, probes, catheters, technician's fees, medications, gloves, trays, tubing and other sterile supplies are considered to be included in the base code. Use modifier -26 to code and report interpretation of results or operation of equipment only.

CYSTOSCOPY, URETHROSCOPY, and CYSTOURETHROSCOPY

The descriptions of CPT codes in this section are listed so that the main procedure can be identified without having to list all of the minor related procedures performed at the same time. For example:

52601   Transurethral electrosurgical resection of prostate, including control of postoperative bleeding, complete (vasectomy, meatotomy, cystourethroscopy, urethral calibration and/or dilation, and internal urethrotomy are included)

All of the secondary procedures are included in the single code 52601. If any of the secondary procedures requires significant additional time and effort, to the point of making the procedure "unusual", modifier -22 should be added with an appropriate increase in fee and a report explaining what made the procedure unusual.

(For provision of chemotherapeutic agents, report both the specific service in addition to code(s) for the specific substance(s) or drug(s) provided)

KIDNEY

INCISION

(For retroperitoneal exploration, abscess, tumor, or cyst, see 49010, 49060, 49203-49205)

50010   Renal exploration, not necessitating other specific procedures

(For laparoscopic ablation of renal mass lesion(s), use 50542)

50020   Drainage of perirenal or renal abscess; open

(For percutaneous image-guided fluid collection drainage by catheter of perirenal/renal abscess, use 49405)

50040   Nephrostomy, nephrotomy with drainage

50045   Nephrotomy, with exploration

(For renal endoscopy performed in conjunction with this procedure, see 50570-50580)

50060   Nephrolithotomy; removal of calculus

50065   secondary surgical operation for calculus

50070   complicated by congenital kidney abnormality

50075   removal of large staghorn calculus filling renal pelvis and calyces (including anatrophic pyelolithotomy)

50080   Percutaneous nephrostolithotomy or pyelostolithotomy, with or without dilation, endoscopy, lithotripsy, stenting, or basket extraction; up to 2 cm

---

50081 over 2cm

(For establishment of nephrostomy without nephrostolithotomy, see 50040, 50432, 50433, 52334)

(For fluoroscopic guidance, use 76000)

(Do not report 50080, 50081 in conjunction with 50436, 50437, when performed by the same physician or other qualified health care professional)

50100 Transection or repositioning of aberrant renal vessels (separate procedure)

50120 Pyelotomy; with exploration

(For renal endoscopy performed in conjunction with this procedure, see 50570-50580)

50125 with drainage, pyelostomy

50130 with removal of calculus (pyelolithotomy, pelviolithotomy, including coagulum pyelolithotomy)

50135 complicated (eg, secondary operation, congenital kidney abnormality)

(For supply of anticarcinogenic agents, use 99070 in addition to code for primary procedure)

EXCISION

(For excision of retroperitoneal tumor or cyst, see 49203-49205)

(For laparoscopic ablation of renal mass lesion(s), use 50542)

50200 Renal biopsy; percutaneous, by trocar or needle

(For radiological supervision and interpretation, see 76942, 77002, 77012, 77021)

(For fine needle aspiration biopsy, see 10005, 10006, 10007, 10008, 10009, 10010, 10011, 10012)

(For evaluation of fine needle aspirate, see 88172, 88173)

50205 by surgical exposure of kidney

50220 Nephrectomy, including partial ureterectomy, any open approach including rib resection;

50225 complicated because of previous surgery on same kidney

50230 radical, with regional lymphadenectomy and/or vena caval thrombectomy

(When vena caval resection with reconstruction is necessary, use 37799)

50234 Nephrectomy with total ureterectomy and bladder cuff; through same incision

50236 through separate incision

50240 Nephrectomy, partial

(For laparoscopic partial nephrectomy, use 50543)

50250 Ablation, open, 1 or more renal mass lesion(s), cryosurgical, including intraoperative ultrasound guidance and monitoring, if performed

(For laparoscopic ablation of renal mass lesions, use 50542)

(For percutaneous ablation of renal tumors, see 50592, 50593)

50280 Excision or unroofing of cyst(s) of kidney

(For laparoscopic ablation of renal cysts, use 50541)

● New Code ▲ Revised Code + Add-On Code ⊘ Modifier -51 Exempt ★ Telemedicine

50290 Excision of perinephric cyst

RENAL TRANSPLANTATION

Renal *auto*transplantation includes reimplantation of the autograft as the primary procedure, along with secondary extra-corporeal procedure(s) (eg., partial nephrectomy, nephrolithotomy) reported with modifier 51 (see 50380 and applicable secondary procedure[s]).

Renal *allo*transplantation involves three distinct components of physician work:

1. **Cadaver donor nephrectomy**, unilateral or bilateral, which includes harvesting the graft(s) and cols preservation of the graft(s) (perfusing with cold preservation solution and cold maintenance) (use 50300). **Living donor nephrectomy**, which includes harvesting the graft, cold preservation of the graft (perfusing with cold preservation solution and cold maintenance), and care of the donor (see 50320, 50547).

2. **Backbench work**:

    Standard preparation of a cadaver donor renal allograft prior to transplantation including dissection and removal of perinephric fat, diaphragmatic and retroperitoneal attachments; excision of adrenal gland; and preparation of ureter(s), renal vein(s), and renal artery(s), ligating branches as necessary (use 50325).

    Standard preparation of a living donor renal allograft (open or laparoscopic) prior to transplantation including dissection and removal of perinephric fat and preparation of ureter(s), renal vein(s), and renal artery(s), ligating branches as necessary (use 50325).

    Additional reconstruction of a cadaver or living donor renal allograft prior to transplantation may include venous, arterial, and/or ureteral anastomosis(es) necessary for implantation (see 50327-50329)

3. **Recipient renal allotransplantation,** which includes transplantation of the allograft (with or without recipient nephrectomy) and care of the recipient (see 50360, 50365).

    (For dialysis, see 90935-90999)

    (For laparoscopic donor nephrectomy, use 50547)

    (For laparoscopic drainage of lymphocele to peritoneal cavity, use 49323)

50300 Donor nephrectomy (including cold preservation); from cadaver donor, unilateral or bilateral

50320 open, from living donor

50323 Backbench standard preparation of cadaver donor renal allograft prior to transplantation, including dissection and removal of perinephric fat, diaphragmatic and retroperitoneal attachments, excision of adrenal gland, and preparation of ureter(s), renal vein(s), and renal artery(s), ligating branches, as necessary

(Do not report 50323 in conjunction with 60540, 60545)

50325 Backbench standard preparation of living donor renal allograft (open or laparoscopic) prior to transplantation, including dissection and removal of perinephric fat and preparation of ureter(s), renal vein(s), and renal artery(s), ligating branches, as necessary

50327 Backbench reconstruction of cadaver or living donor renal allograft prior to transplantation; venous anastomosis, each

50328 arterial anastomosis, each

50329 ureteral anastomosis, each

50340 Recipient nephrectomy (separate procedure)

(For bilateral procedure, report 50340 with modifier -50)

50360   Renal allotransplantation, implantation of graft; without recipient nephrectomy

50365   with recipient nephrectomy

(For bilateral procedure, report 50365 with modifier -50)

50370   Removal of transplanted renal allograft

50380   Renal autotransplantation, reimplantation of kidney

(For renal autotransplantation extra-corporeal (bench) surgery, use autotransplantation as the primary procedure and report secondary procedure(s) (eg, partial nephrectomy, nephrolithotomy) with modifier -51)

INTRODUCTION

Renal Pelvis Catheter Procedures

Internally Dwelling

50382   Removal (via snare/capture) and replacement of internally dwelling ureteral stent via percutaneous approach, including radiological supervision and interpretation

(For bilateral procedure, use modifier -50)

(For removal and replacement of an internally dwelling ureteral stent via a transurethral approach, use 50385)

50384   Removal (via snare/capture) of internally dwelling ureteral stent via percutaneous approach, including radiological supervision and interpretation

(For bilateral procedure, use modifier 50)

(Do not report 50382, 50384 in conjunction with 50436, 50437)

(For removal of an internally dwelling ureteral stent via a transurethral approach, use 50386)

50385   Removal (via snare/capture) and replacement of internally dwelling ureteral stent via transurethral approach, without use of cystoscopy, including radiological supervision and interpretation

50386   Removal (via snare/capture) of internally dwelling ureteral stent via transurethral approach, without use of cystoscopy, including radiological supervision and interpretation

Externally Accessible

50387   Removal and replacement of externally accessible nephroureteral catheter (eg, external/internal stent) requiring fluoroscopic guidance, including radiological supervision and interpretation

(For bilateral procedure, use modifier 50)

(For removal and replacement of externally accessible ureteral stent via ureterostomy or ileal conduit, use 50688)

(For removal without replacement of an externally accessible ureteral stent not requiring fluoroscopic guidance, see Evaluation and Management services codes)

50389   Removal of nephrostomy tube, requiring fluoroscopic guidance (eg, with concurrent indwelling ureteral stent)

(Removal of nephrostomy tube not requiring fluoroscopic guidance is considered inherent to E/M services. Report the appropriate level of E/M service provided)

Other Introduction (Injection/Change/Removal) Procedures

Percutaneous genitourinary procedures are performed with imaging guidance (eg, fluoroscopy and/or ultrasound). Diagnostic nephrostogram and/or ureterogram are typically performed with percutaneous genitourinary procedures and are included in 50432, 50433, 50434, 50435, 50436, 50437, 50693, 50694, 50695.

   ● New Code   ▲ Revised Code   ✛ Add-On Code   ⊘ Modifier -51 Exempt   ★ Telemedicine

Code 50436 describes enlargement of an existing percutaneous tract to the renal collecting system to accommodate large instruments used in an endourologic procedure. Code 50436 includes predilation urinary tract imaging, postprocedure nephrostomy tube placement, when performed, and includes all radiological supervision and interpretation and imaging guidance (eg, ultrasound, fluoroscopy). Code 50436 may not be reported with 50432, 50433, 52334 for basic dilation of a percutaneous tract during initial placement of a catheter or device.

Code 50437 includes all elements of 50436, but also includes new access into the renal collecting system performed in the same session when a pre-existing tract is not present.

Codes 50430 and 50431 are diagnostic procedure codes that include injection(s) of contrast material, all associated radiological supervision and interpretation, and procedural imaging guidance (eg, ultrasound and/or fluoroscopy). Code 50430 also includes accessing the collecting system and/or associated ureter with a needle and/or catheter. Code 50430 or 50431 may not be reported together with 50432, 50433, 50434, 50435, 50693, 50694, 50695.

Codes 50432, 50433, 50434, 50435 represent therapeutic procedures describing catheter placement or exchange, and include the elements of access, drainage catheter manipulations, and imaging guidance (eg, ultrasonography and/or fluoroscopy), as well as diagnostic imaging supervision and interpretation, when performed.

Code 50433 describes percutaneous nephrostomy with the additional accessing of the ureter/bladder to ultimately place a nephroureteral catheter (a single transnephric catheter with nephrostomy and ureteral components that allows drainage internally, externally, or both).

For codes 50430, 50431, 50432, 50433, 50434, 50435, 50606, 50693, 50694, 50695, 50705, and 50706, the renal pelvis and its associated ureter are considered a single entity for reporting purposes. Codes 50430, 50431, 50432, 50433, 50434, 50435, 50606, 50693, 50694, 50695, 50705, and 50706 may be reported once for each renal collecting system/ureter accessed (eg, two separate codes would be reported for bilateral nephrostomy tube placement or for unilateral duplicated collecting system/ureter requiring two separate procedures.

50390   Aspiration and/or injection of renal cyst or pelvis by needle, percutaneous

(For radiological supervision and interpretation, see 74425, 74470, 76942, 77002, 77012, 77021)

(For antegrade nephrostogram and/or antegrade pyelogram, see 50430, 50431)

50391   Instillation(s) of therapeutic agent into renal pelvis and/or ureter through established nephrostomy, pyelostomy or ureterostomy tube (eg, anticarcinogenic or antifungal agent)

(**50395**   deleted 2018 [2019 Edition]. To report, see 50436, 50437)

50436   Dilation of existing tract, percutaneous, for an endourologic procedure including imaging guidance (eg, ultrasound and/or fluoroscopy) and all associated radiological supervision and interpretation, with postprocedure tube placement, when performed;

50437   including new access into the renal collecting system

(For nephrostolithotomy, see 50080, 50081)

(For retrograde percutaneous nephrostomy, use 52334)

(For endoscopic surgery, see 50551-50561)

(Do not report 50436, 50437 in conjunction with 50080, 50081, 50382, 50384, 50430, 50431, 50432, 50433, 52334, 74485)

50396   Manometric studies through nephrostomy or pyelostomy tube, or indwelling ureteral catheter

(For radiological supervision and interpretation, use 74425)

50430   Injection procedure for antegrade nephrostogram and/or ureterogram, complete diagnostic procedure including imaging guidance (eg, ultrasound and fluoroscopy) and all associated radiological supervision and interpretation; new access

50431   existing access

(Do not report 50430, 50431 in conjunction with 50432, 50433, 50434, 50435, 50693, 50694, 50695, 74425 for the same renal collecting system and/or associated ureter)

50432 Placement of nephrostomy catheter, percutaneous, including diagnostic nephrostogram and/or ureterogram when performed, imaging guidance (eg, ultrasound and/or fluoroscopy) and all associated radiological supervision and interpretation

(Do not report 50432 in conjunction with 50430, 50431, 50433, 50436, 50437, 50694, 50695, 74425, for the same renal collecting system and/or associated ureter)

(Do not report 50432 in conjunction with 50436, 50437, for dilation of the nephrostomy tube tract)

50433 Placement of nephroureteral catheter, percutaneous, including diagnostic nephrostogram and/or ureterogram when performed, imaging guidance (eg, ultrasound and/or fluoroscopy) and all associated radiological supervision and interpretation, new access

(Do not report 50433 in conjunction with 50430, 50431, 50432, 50693, 50694, 50695, 74425 for the same renal collecting system and/or associated ureter)

(Do not report 50433 in conjunction with 50436, 50437, for dilation of the nephroureteral catheter tract)

(For nephroureteral catheter removal and replacement, use 50387)

50434 Convert nephrostomy catheter to nephroureteral catheter, percutaneous, including diagnostic nephrostogram and/or ureterogram when performed, imaging guidance (eg, ultrasound and/or fluoroscopy) and all associated radiological supervision and interpretation, via preexisting nephrostomy tract

(Do not report 50434 in conjunction with 50430, 50431, 50435, 50684, 50693, 74425 for the same renal collecting system and/or associated ureter)

50435 Exchange nephrostomy catheter, percutaneous, including diagnostic nephrostogram and/or ureterogram when performed, imaging guidance (eg, ultrasound and/or fluoroscopy) and all associated radiological supervision and interpretation

(Do not report 50435 in conjunction with 50430, 50431, 50434, 50693, 74425 for the same renal collecting system and/or associated ureter)

(For removal of nephrostomy catheter requiring fluoroscopic guidance, use 50389)

REPAIR

50400 Pyeloplasty (Foley Y-pyeloplasty), plastic operation on renal pelvis, with or without plastic operation on ureter, nephropexy, nephrostomy, pyelostomy, or ureteral splinting; simple

50405 complicated (congenital kidney abnormality, secondary pyeloplasty, solitary kidney, calycoplasty)

(For laparoscopic approach, use 50544)

50430 This code is out of order. See page 531

50431 This code is out of order. See page 531

50432 This code is out of order. See page 532

50433 This code is out of order. See page 532

50434 This code is out of order. See page 532

50435 This code is out of order. See page 532

50436 This code is out of order. See page 531

50437 This code is out of order. See page 531

50500 Nephrorrhaphy, suture of kidney wound or injury

● New Code ▲ Revised Code ✚ Add-On Code ⊘ Modifier -51 Exempt ★ Telemedicine

50520   Closure of nephrocutaneous or pyelocutaneous fistula

50525   Closure of nephrovisceral fistula (eg, renocolic), including visceral repair; abdominal approach

50526   thoracic approach

50540   Symphysiotomy for horseshoe kidney with or without pyeloplasty and/or other plastic procedure, unilateral or bilateral (1 operation)

LAPAROSCOPY

Surgical laparoscopy always includes diagnostic laparoscopy. To report a diagnostic laparoscopy (peritoneoscopy) (separate procedure), use 49320.

50541   Laparoscopy, surgical; ablation of renal cysts

50542   ablation of renal mass lesion(s), including intraoperative ultrasound guidance and monitoring, when performed

(For open procedure, see 50250)

(For percutaneous ablation of renal tumors, see 50592, 50593)

50543   partial nephrectomy

(For open procedure, use 50240)

50544   pyeloplasty

50545   radical nephrectomy (includes removal of Gerota's fascia and surrounding fatty tissue, removal of regional lymph nodes, and adrenalectomy

(For open procedure, use 50230)

50546   nephrectomy including partial ureterectomy

50547   donor nephrectomy (including cold preservation), from living donor

(For open procedure, use 50320)

(For backbench renal allograft standard preparation prior to transplantation, use 50325)

(For backbench renal allograft reconstruction prior to transplantation, see 50327-50329)

50548   nephrectomy with total ureterectomy

(For open procedure, see 50234, 50236)

50549   Unlisted laparoscopy procedure, renal

(For laparoscopic drainage of lymphocele to peritoneal cavity, use 49323)

ENDOSCOPY

(For supplies and materials, use 99070)

50551   Renal endoscopy through established nephrostomy or pyelostomy, with or without irrigation, instillation, or ureteropyelography, exclusive of radiologic service;

50553   with ureteral catheterization, with or without dilation of ureter

(For image-guided dilation of ureter without endoscopic guidance, use 50706)

50555   with biopsy

(For image-guided biopsy of ureter and/or renal pelvis without endoscopic guidance, use 50606)

50557   with fulguration and/or incision, with or without biopsy

50561   with removal of foreign body or calculus

50562   with resection of tumor

(When procedures 50570-50580 provide a significant identifiable service, they may be added to 50045 and 50120)

50570   Renal endoscopy through nephrotomy or pyelotomy, with or without irrigation, instillation, or ureteropyelography, exclusive of radiologic service;

(For nephrotomy, use 50045)

(For pyelotomy, use 50120)

50572   with ureteral catheterization, with or without dilation of ureter

(For image-guided dilation of ureter without endoscopic guidance, use 50706)

50574   with biopsy

(For image-guided biopsy of ureter and/or renal pelvis without endoscopic guidance, use 50606)

50575   with endopyelotomy (includes cystoscopy, ureteroscopy, dilation of ureter and ureteral pelvic junction, incision of ureteral pelvic junction and insertion of endopyelotomy stent)

50576   with fulguration and/or incision, with or without biopsy

50580   with removal of foreign body or calculus

OTHER PROCEDURES

50590   Lithotripsy, extracorporeal shock wave

50592   Ablation, one or more renal tumor(s), percutaneous, unilateral, radiofrequency

(50592 is a unilateral procedure. For bilateral procedure, report 50592 with modifier 50)

(For imaging guidance and monitoring, see 76940, 77013, 77022)

50593   Ablation, renal tumor(s), unilateral, percutaneous, cryotherapy

(50593 is a unilatral procedure. For bilateral procedure, report 50593 with modifier -50)

(For imaging guidance and monitoring, see codes 76940, 77013, 77022)

URETER

INCISION/BIOPSY

Code 50606 is an add-on code describing endoluminal biopsy (eg, brush) using non-endoscopic imaging guidance, which may be reported once per ureter per day. This code includes the work of the biopsy and the imaging guidance and radiological supervision and interpretation required to accomplish the biopsy. The biopsy may be performed through de novo transrenal access, an existing renal/ureteral access, transurethral access, an ileal conduit, or ureterostomy. The service of gaining access may be reported separately. Diagnostic pyelography/ureterography is not included in the work of 50606 and may be reported separately. Other interventions or catheter placements performed at the same setting as the biopsy may be reported separately. For codes 50430, 50431, 50432, 50433, 50434, 50435, 50606, 50693, 50694, 50695, 50705, and 50706, the renal pelvis and its associated ureter are considered a single entity for reporting purposes. Codes 50430, 50431, 50432, 50433, 50434, 50435, 50606, 50693, 50694, 50695, 50705, and 50706 may be reported once for each renal collecting system/ureter accessed (eg, two separate codes would be reported for bilateral nephrostomy tube placement or for unilateral duplicated collecting system/ureter requiring two separate procedures.

50600   Ureterotomy with exploration or drainage (separate procedure)

(For ureteral endoscopy performed in conjunction with this procedure, see 50970-50980)

50605 Ureterotomy for insertion of indwelling stent, all types

+ 50606 Endoluminal biopsy of ureter and/or renal pelvis, nonendoscopic, including imaging guidance (eg, ultrasound and/or fluoroscopy) and all associated radiological supervision and interpretation (List separately in addition to code for primary procedure)

(Use 50606 in conjunction with 50382, 50384, 50385, 50386, 50387, 50389, 50430, 50431, 50432, 50433, 50434, 50435, 50684, 50688, 50690, 50693, 50694, 50695, 51610)

(Do not report 50606 in conjunction with 50555, 50574, 50955, 50974, 52007, 74425 for the same renal collecting system and/or associated ureter)

50610 Ureterolithotomy; upper one-third of ureter

50620 middle one-third of ureter

50630 lower one-third of ureter

(For laparoscopic approach, use 50945)

(For transvesical ureterolithotomy, use 51060)

(For cystotomy with stone basket extraction of ureteral calculus, use 51065)

(For endoscopic extraction or manipulation of ureteral calculus, see 50080, 50081, 50561, 50961, 50980, 52320-52330, 52352, 52353, 52356)

EXCISION

(For ureterocele, see 51535, 52300)

50650 Ureterectomy, with bladder cuff (separate procedure)

50660 Ureterectomy, total, ectopic ureter, combination abdominal, vaginal and/or perineal approach

INTRODUCTION

Other Introduction (Injection/Change/Removal) Procedures

Codes 50693, 50694, 50695 are therapeutic procedure codes describing percutaneous placement of ureteral stents. These codes include access, drainage, catheter manipulations, diagnostic nephrostogram and/or ureterogram, when performed, imaging guidance (eg, ultrasonography and/or fluoroscopy), and all associated radiological supervision and interpretation. When a separate ureteral stent and a nephrostomy catheter are placed into a ureter and its associated renal pelvis during the same session through a new percutaneous renal access, use 50695 to report the procedure.

50684 Injection procedure for ureterography or ureteropyelography through ureterostomy or indwelling ureteral catheter

(Do not report 50684 in conjunction with 50433, 50434, 50693, 50694, 50695)

(For radiological supervision and interpretation, use 74425)

50686 Manometric studies through ureterostomy or indwelling ureteral catheter

50688 Change of ureterostomy tube or externally accessible ureteral stent via ileal conduit

(If imaging guidance is performed, use 75984)

50690 Injection procedure for visualization of ileal conduit and/or ureteropyelography, exclusive of radiologic service

(For radiological supervision and interpretation, see 74420 for retrograde or 74425 for antegrade injection)

50693 Placement of ureteral stent, percutaneous, including diagnostic nephrostogram and/or ureterogram when performed, imaging guidance (eg, ultrasound and/or fluoroscopy), and all associated radiological supervision and interpretation; pre-existing nephrostomy tract

50694   new access, without separate nephrostomy catheter

50695   new access, with separate nephrostomy catheter

(Do not report 50693, 50694, 50695 in conjunction with 50430, 50431, 50432, 50433, 50434, 50435, 50684, 74425 for the same renal collecting system and/or associated ureter)

REPAIR

Codes 50705, 50706 are add-on codes describing embolization and balloon dilation of the ureter using non-endoscopic imaging guidance, and each may be reported once per ureter per day. These codes include embolization or dilation plus imaging guidance and radiological supervision and interpretation required to accomplish the embolization or dilation. These procedures may be performed through de novo transrenal access, an existing renal/ureteral access, transurethral access, an ileal conduit, or ureterostomy. The service of gaining access may be reported separately. Diagnostic pyelography/ureterography is not included in 50705 and 50706 and may be reported separately. Other interventions or catheter placements performed at the same setting as the embolization/dilation may be reported separately.

50700 Ureteroplasty, plastic operation on ureter (eg, stricture)

+ 50705 Ureteral embolization or occlusion, including imaging guidance (eg, ultrasound and/or fluoroscopy) and all associated radiological supervision and interpretation (List separately in addition to code for primary procedure)

(Use 50705 in conjunction with 50382, 50384, 50385, 50386, 50387, 50389, 50430, 50431, 50432, 50433, 50434, 50435, 50684, 50688, 50690, 50693, 50694, 50695, 51610)

+ 50706 Balloon dilation, ureteral stricture, including imaging guidance (eg, ultrasound and/or fluoroscopy) and all associated radiological supervision and interpretation (List separately in addition to code for primary procedure)

(Use 50706 in conjunction with 50382, 50384, 50385, 50386, 50387, 50389, 50430, 50431, 50432, 50433, 50434, 50435, 50684, 50688, 50690, 50693, 50694, 50695, 51610)

(Do not report 50706 in conjunction with 50553, 50572, 50953, 50972, 52341, 52344, 52345, 74485)

(For percutaneous nephrostomy, nephroureteral catheter, and/or ureteral catheter placement use 50385, 50387, 50432, 50433, 50434, 50435, 50693, 50694, 50695)

50715 Ureterolysis, with or without repositioning of ureter for retroperitoneal fibrosis

(For bilateral procedure, report 50715 with modifier -50)

50722 Ureterolysis for ovarian vein syndrome

50725 Ureterolysis for retrocaval ureter, with reanastomosis of upper urinary tract or vena cava

50727 Revision of urinary-cutaneous anastomosis (any type urostomy);

50728   with repair of fascial defect and hernia

50740 Ureteropyelostomy, anastomosis of ureter and renal pelvis

50750 Ureterocalycostomy, anastomosis of ureter to renal calyx

50760 Ureteroureterostomy

50770 Transureteroureterostomy, anastomosis of ureter to contralateral ureter

(Codes 50780-50785 include minor procedures to prevent vesicoureteral reflux)

50780 Ureteroneocystostomy; anastomosis of single ureter to bladder

(For bilateral procedure, report 50780 with modifier -50)

(When combined with cystourethroplasty or vesical neck revision, use 51820)

50782 anastomosis of duplicated ureter to bladder

50783 with extensive ureteral tailoring

50785 with vesico-psoas hitch or bladder flap

(For bilateral procedure, report 50785 with modifier -50)

50800 Ureteroenterostomy, direct anastomosis of ureter to intestine

(For bilateral procedure, report 50800 with modifier -50)

50810 Ureterosigmoidostomy, with creation of sigmoid bladder and establishment of abdominal or perineal colostomy, including intestine anastomosis

50815 Ureterocolon conduit, including intestine anastomosis

(For bilateral procedure, report 50815 with modifier -50)

50820 Ureteroileal conduit (ileal bladder), including intestine anastomosis (Bricker operation)

(For bilateral procedure, report 50820 with modifier -50)

(For combination of 50800-50820 with cystectomy, see 51580-51595)

50825 Continent diversion, including intestine anastomosis using any segment of small and/or large intestine (Kock pouch or Camey enterocystoplasty)

50830 Urinary undiversion (eg, taking down of ureteroileal conduit, ureterosigmoidostomy or ureteroenterostomy with ureteroureterostomy or ureteroneocystostomy)

50840 Replacement of all or part of ureter by intestine segment, including intestine anastomosis

(For bilateral procedure, report 50840 with modifier -50)

50845 Cutaneous appendico-vesicostomy

50860 Ureterostomy, transplantation of ureter to skin

(For bilateral procedure, report 50860 with modifier -50)

50900 Ureterorrhaphy, suture of ureter (separate procedure)

50920 Closure of ureterocutaneous fistula

50930 Closure of ureterovisceral fistula (including visceral repair)

50940 Deligation of ureter

(For ureteroplasty, ureterolysis, see 50700-50860)

LAPAROSCOPY

Surgical laparoscopy always includes diagnostic laparoscopy. To report a diagnostic laparoscopy (peritoneoscopy) (separate procedure), use 49320.

50945 Laparoscopy, surgical; ureterolithotomy

| ■ Separate Procedure | ■ Unlisted Procedure | ■ CCI Comp. Code | ■ Non-specific Procedure | **537** |

50947   ureteroneocystostomy with cystoscopy and ureteral stent placement

50948   ureteroneocystostomy without cystoscopy and ureteral stent placement

    (For open ureteroneocystostomy, see 50780-50785)

50949 Unlisted laparoscopy procedure, ureter

ENDOSCOPY

50951 Ureteral endoscopy through established ureterostomy, with or without irrigation, instillation, or ureteropyelography, exclusive of radiologic service;

50953   with ureteral catheterization, with or without dilation of ureter

    (For image-guided dilation of ureter without endoscopic guidance, use 50706)

50955   with biopsy

    (For image-guided biopsy of ureter and/or renal pelvis without endoscopic guidance, use 50606)

50957   with fulguration and/or incision, with or without biopsy

50961   with removal of foreign body or calculus

50970 Ureteral endoscopy through ureterotomy, with or without irrigation, instillation, or ureteropyelography, exclusive of radiologic service;

    (For ureterotomy, use 50600)

50972   with ureteral catheterization, with or without dilation of ureter

    (For image-guided dilation of ureter without endoscopic guidance, use 50706)

50974   with biopsy

    (For image-guided biopsy of ureter and/or renal pelvis without endoscopic guidance, use 50606)

50976   with fulguration and/or incision, with or without biopsy

50980   with removal of foreign body or calculus

BLADDER

INCISION

51020 Cystotomy or cystostomy; with fulguration and/or insertion of radioactive material

51030   with cryosurgical destruction of intravesical lesion

51040 Cystostomy, cystotomy with drainage

51045 Cystotomy, with insertion of ureteral catheter or stent (separate procedure)

51050 Cystolithotomy, cystotomy with removal of calculus, without vesical neck resection

51060 Transvesical ureterolithotomy

51065 Cystotomy, with calculus basket extraction and/or ultrasonic or electrohydraulic fragmentation of ureteral calculus

51080 Drainage of perivesical or prevesical space abscess

(For percutaneous image-guided fluid collection drainage by catheter of perivesicular or prevesicular space abscess, use 49406)

REMOVAL

51100 Aspiration of bladder; by needle

51101 by trocar or intracatheter

51102 with insertion of suprapubic catheter

(For imaging guidance, see 76942, 77002, 77012)

EXCISION

51500 Excision of urachal cyst or sinus, with or without umbilical hernia repair

51520 Cystotomy; for simple excision of vesical neck (separate procedure)

51525 for excision of bladder diverticulum, single or multiple (separate procedure)

51530 for excision of bladder tumor

(For transurethral resection, see 52234-52240, 52305)

51535 Cystotomy for excision, incision, or repair of ureterocele

(For bilateral procedure, report 51535 with modifier -50)

(For transurethral excision, use 52300)

51550 Cystectomy, partial; simple

51555 complicated (eg, postradiation, previous surgery, difficult location)

51565 Cystectomy, partial, with reimplantation of ureter(s) into bladder (ureteroneocystostomy)

51570 Cystectomy, complete; (separate procedure)

51575 with bilateral pelvic lymphadenectomy, including external iliac, hypogastric, and obturator nodes

51580 Cystectomy, complete, with ureterosigmoidostomy or ureterocutaneous transplantations;

51585 with bilateral pelvic lymphadenectomy, including external iliac, hypogastric, and obturator nodes

51590 Cystectomy, complete, with ureteroileal conduit or sigmoid bladder, including intestine anastomosis;

51595 with bilateral pelvic lymphadenectomy, including external iliac, hypogastric, and obturator nodes

51596 Cystectomy, complete, with continent diversion, any open technique, using any segment of small and/or large intestine to construct neobladder

51597 Pelvic exenteration, complete, for vesical, prostatic or urethral malignancy, with removal of bladder and ureteral transplantations, with or without hysterectomy and/or abdominoperineal resection of rectum and colon and colostomy, or any combination thereof

(For pelvic exenteration for gynecologic malignancy, use 58240)

INTRODUCTION

51600 Injection procedure for cystography or voiding urethrocystography

---

(For radiological supervision and interpretation, see 74430, 74455)

51605 Injection procedure and placement of chain for contrast and/or chain urethrocystography

(For radiological supervision and interpretation, use 74430)

51610 Injection procedure for retrograde urethrocystography

(For radiological supervision and interpretation, use 74450)

51700 Bladder irrigation, simple, lavage and/or instillation

(Codes 51701-51702 are reported only when performed independently. Do not report 51701-51702 when catheter insertion is an inclusive component of another procedure.)

51701 Insertion of non-indwelling bladder catheter (eg, straight catheterization of residual urine)

51702 Insertion of temporary indwelling bladder catheter; simple (eg, Foley)

(Do not report 51702 in conjunction with 0071T, 0072T)

51703 complicated (eg, altered anatomy, fractured catheter/balloon)

51705 Change of cystostomy tube; simple

51710 complicated

(If imaging guidance is performed, use 75984)

51715 Endoscopic injection of implant material into the submucosal tissues of the urethra and/or bladder neck

(For anoscopy with directed submucosal injection of bulking agent for fecal incontinence, use 0377T)

51720 Bladder instillation of anticarcinogenic agent (including retention time)

URODYNAMICS

The following section (51725-51798) lists procedures that may be used separately or in many and varied combinations.

When multiple procedures are performed in the same investigative session, modifier -51 should be employed.

All procedures in this section imply that these services are performed by, or are under the direct supervision of, a physician or other qualified health care professional and that all instruments, equipment, fluids, gases, probes, catheters, technician's fees, medications, gloves, trays, tubing and other sterile supplies be provided by that individual. When the individual only interprets the results and/or operates the equipment, a professional component, modifier -26 should be used to identify physcians' services.

51725 Simple cystometrogram (CMG) (eg, spinal manometer)

51726 Complex cystometrogram (ie, calibrated electronic equipment)

51727 with urethral pressure profile studies (ie, urethral closure pressure profile), any technique

51728 with voiding pressure studies (ie, bladder voiding pressure), any technique

51729 with voiding pressure studies (ie, bladder voiding pressure) and urethral closure pressure profile studies (ie, urethral closure pressure profile), any technique

+ **51797** Voiding pressure studies, intra-abdominal (ie, rectal, gastric, intraperitoneal) (List separately in addition to code for primary procedure)

(Use 51797 in conjunction with 51728, 51729)

51736 Simple uroflowmetry (UFR) (eg, stop-watch flow rate, mechanical uroflowmeter)

● New Code   ▲ Revised Code   + Add-On Code   ⊘ Modifier -51 Exempt   ★ Telemedicine

51741 Complex uroflowmetry (eg, calibrated electronic equipment)

51784 Electromyography studies (EMG) of anal or urethral sphincter, other than needle, any technique

(Do not report 51784 in conjunction with 51792)

51785 Needle electromyography studies (EMG) of anal or urethral sphincter, any technique

51792 Stimulus evoked response (eg, measurement of bulbocavernosus reflex latency time)

(Do not report 51792 in conjunction with 51784)

51797 This code is out of order. See page 540

51798 Measurement of post-voiding residual urine and/or bladder capacity by ultrasound, non-imaging

REPAIR

51800 Cystoplasty or cystourethroplasty, plastic operation on bladder and/or vesical neck (anterior Y-plasty, vesical fundus resection), any procedure, with or without wedge resection of posterior vesical neck

51820 Cystourethroplasty with unilateral or bilateral ureteroneocystostomy

51840 Anterior vesicourethropexy, or urethropexy (eg, Marshall-Marchetti-Krantz, Burch); simple

51841 complicated (eg, secondary repair)

(For urethropexy (Pereyra type), use 57289)

51845 Abdomino-vaginal vesical neck suspension, with or without endoscopic control (eg, Stamey, Raz, modified Pereyra)

51860 Cystorrhaphy, suture of bladder wound, injury or rupture; simple

51865 complicated

51880 Closure of cystostomy (separate procedure)

51900 Closure of vesicovaginal fistula, abdominal approach

(For vaginal approach, see 57320-57330)

51920 Closure of vesicouterine fistula;

51925 with hysterectomy

(For closure of vesicoenteric fistula, see 44660, 44661)

(For closure of rectovesical fistula, see 45800-45805)

51940 Closure, exstrophy of bladder

(See also 54390)

51960 Enterocystoplasty, including intestinal anastomosis

51980 Cutaneous vesicostomy

LAPAROSCOPY

Surgical laparoscopy always includes diagnostic laparoscopy. To report a diagnostic laparoscopy (peritoneoscopy) (separate procedure), use 49320.

| Separate Procedure | Unlisted Procedure | CCI Comp. Code | Non-specific Procedure | **541** |

51990 Laparoscopy, surgical; urethral suspension for stress incontinence

51992   sling operation for stress incontinence (eg, fascia or synthetic)

(For open sling operation for stress incontinence, use 57288)

(For reversal or removal of sling operation for stress incontinence, use 57287)

51999 Unlisted laparoscopy procedure, bladder

ENDOSCOPY—CYSTOSCOPY, URETHROSCOPY, CYSTOURETHROSCOPY

Endoscopic descriptions are listed so that the main procedure can be identified without having to list all the minor related functions performed at the same time. For example, meatotomy, urethral calibration and/or dilation, urethroscopy, and cystoscopy prior to a transurethral resection of prostate; ureteral catheterization following extraction of ureteral calculus; internal urethrotomy and bladder neck fulguration when performing a cystourethroscopy for the female urethral syndrome. When the secondary procedure requires significant additional time and effort, it may be identified by the addition of modifier 22.

For example, urethrotomy performed for a documented pre-existing stricture or bladder neck contracture.

Because cutaneous urinary diversions utilizing ileum or colon serve as functional replacements of a native bladder, endoscopy of such bowel segments, as well as performance of secondary procedures can be captured by using the cystourethroscopy codes. For example, endoscopy of an ileal loop with removal of ureteral calculus would be coded as cystourethroscopy (including ureteral catheterization); with removal of ureteral calculus (52320).

52000 Cystourethroscopy (separate procedure)

(Do not report 52000 in conjunction with 52001, 52320, 52325, 52327, 52330, 52332, 52334, 52341, 52342, 52343, 52356)

(Do not report 52000 in conjunction with 57240, 57260, 57265)

52001 Cystourethroscopy with irrigation and evacuation of multiple obstructing clots

(Do not report 52001 in addition to 52000)

52005 Cystourethroscopy, with ureteral catheterization, with or without irrigation, instillation, or ureteropyelography, exclusive of radiologic service;

52007   with brush biopsy of ureter and/or renal pelvis

(For image-guided biopsy of ureter and/or renal pelvis without endoscopic guidance, use 50606)

52010 Cystourethroscopy, with ejaculatory duct catheterization, with or without irrigation, instillation, or duct radiography, exclusive of radiologic service

(For radiological supervision and interpretation, use 74440)

TRANSURETHRAL SURGERY

Urethra and Bladder

52204 Cystourethroscopy, with biopsy(s)

52214 Cystourethroscopy, with fulguration (including cryosurgery or laser surgery) of trigone, bladder neck, prostatic fossa, urethra, or periurethral glands

(For transurethral fulguration of prostate tissue performed within the postoperative period of 52601 or 52630 performed by the same physician, append modifier 78)

(For transurethral fulguration of prostate tissue performed within the postoperative period of a related procedure performed by the same physician, append modifier 78)

(For transurethral fulguration of prostate for postoperative bleeding performed by the same physician, append modifier 78)

52224 Cystourethroscopy, with fulguration (including cryosurgery or laser surgery) or treatment of MINOR (less than 0.5 cm) lesion(s) with or without biopsy

52234 Cystourethroscopy, with fulguration (including cryosurgery or laser surgery) and/or resection of; SMALL bladder tumor(s) (0.5 up to 2.0 cm)

52235   MEDIUM bladder tumor(s) (2.0 to 5.0 cm)

52240   LARGE bladder tumor(s)

52250 Cystourethroscopy with insertion of radioactive substance, with or without biopsy or fulguration

52260 Cystourethroscopy, with dilation of bladder for interstitial cystitis; general or conduction (spinal) anesthesia

52265   local anesthesia

52270 Cystourethroscopy, with internal urethrotomy; female

52275   male

52276 Cystourethroscopy with direct vision internal urethrotomy

52277 Cystourethroscopy, with resection of external sphincter (sphincterotomy)

52281 Cystourethroscopy, with calibration and/or dilation of urethral stricture or stenosis, with or without meatotomy, with or without injection procedure for cystography, male or female

(To report cystourethroscopy with urethral therapeutic drug delivery, use 0499T)

52282 Cystourethroscopy, with insertion of permanent urethral stent

(For placement of temporary prostatic urethral stent, use 53855)

52283 Cystourethroscopy, with steroid injection into stricture

52285 Cystourethroscopy for treatment of the female urethral syndrome with any or all of the following: urethral meatotomy, urethral dilation, internal urethrotomy, lysis of urethrovaginal septal fibrosis, lateral incisions of the bladder neck, and fulguration of polyp(s) of urethra, bladder neck, and/or trigone

52287 Cystourethroscopy, with injection(s) for chemodenervation of the bladder

(The suppy of the chemodenervation agent is reported separately)

52290 Cystourethroscopy; with ureteral meatotomy, unilateral or bilateral

52300   with resection or fulguration of orthotopic ureterocele(s), unilateral or bilateral

52301   with resection or fulguration of ectopic ureterocele(s), unilateral or bilateral

52305   with incision or resection of orifice of bladder diverticulum, single or multiple

52310 Cystourethroscopy, with removal of foreign body, calculus, or ureteral stent from urethra or bladder (separate procedure); simple

52315   complicated

52317 Litholapaxy: crushing or fragmentation of calculus by any means in bladder and removal of fragments; simple or small (less than 2.5 cm)

52318   complicated or large (over 2.5 cm)

URETER AND PELVIS

Therapeutic cystourethroscopy always includes diagnostic cystourethroscopy. To report diagnostic cystourethroscopy, use 52000. Therapeutic cystourethroscopy with ureteroscopy and/or pyeloscopy always includes diagnostic cystourethroscopy with ureteroscopy and/or pyeloscopy. To report a diagnostic cystourethroscopy with ureteroscopy and/or pyeloscopy, use 52351.

Do not report 52000 in conjunction with 52320-52343, 52356.

Do not report 52351 in conjunction with 52344-52346, 52352-52356.

The insertion and removal of a temporary ureteral catheter (52005) during diagnostic or therapeutic cystourethroscopy with ureteroscopy and/or pyeloscopy is included in 52320-52356 and should not be reported separately.

To report insertion of a self-retaining, indwelling stent performed during diagnostic or therapeutic cystourethroscopy with ureteroscopy and/or pyeloscopy, report 52332 in addition to primary procedure(s) performed (52320-52330, 52334-52352, 52354, 52355) and append modifier 51. Code 52332 is used to report a unilateral procedure unless otherwise specified.

For bilateral insertion of self-retaining, indwelling ureteral stents, use code 52332, and append modifier 50.

To report cystourethroscopic removal of a self-retaining indwelling ureteral stent, see 52310, 52315, and append modifier 58 if appropriate

52320 Cystourethroscopy (including ureteral catheterization); with removal of ureteral calculus

52325 with fragmentation of ureteral calculus (eg, ultrasonic or electro-hydraulic technique)

52327 with subureteric injection of implant material

52330 with manipulation, without removal of ureteral calculus

(Do not report 52320, 52325, 52327, 52330 in conjunction with 52000)

52332 Cystourethroscopy, with insertion of indwelling ureteral stent (eg, Gibbons or double-J type)

(Do not report 52332 in conjunction with 52000, 52353, 52356 when performed together on the same side)

52334 Cystourethroscopy with insertion of ureteral guide wire through kidney to establish a percutaneous nephrostomy, retrograde

(For percutaneous nephrostolithotomy, see 50080, 50081; for establishment of percutaneous nephrostomy, see 50432, 50433)

(For cystourethroscopy, with ureteroscopy and/or pyeloscopy, see 52351-52356)

(For cystourethroscopy with incision, fulguration, or resection of congenital posterior urethral valves or obstructive hypertrophic mucosal folds, use 52400)

(Do not report 52334 in conjunction with 50437, 52000, 52351)

52341 Cystourethroscopy; with treatment of ureteral stricture (eg, balloon dilation, laser, electrocautery, and incision)

52342 with treatment of ureteropelvic junction stricture (eg, balloon dilation, laser, electrocautery, and incision)

52343 with treatment of intra-renal stricture (eg, balloon dilation, laser, electrocautery, and incision)

(Do note report 52341, 52342, 52343 in conjunction with 52000, 52351)

(For image-guided dilation of ureter, ureteropelvic junction stricture without endoscopic guidance, use 50706)

52344 Cystourethroscopy with ureteroscopy; with treatment of ureteral stricture (eg, balloon dilation, laser, electrocautery, and incision)

52345 with treatment of ureteropelvic junction stricture (eg, balloon dilation, laser, electrocautery, and incision)

52346 with treatment of intra-renal stricture (eg, balloon dilation, laser, electrocautery, and incision)

(For transurethral resection or incision of ejaculatory ducts, use 52402)

(Do not report 52344, 52345, 52346 in conjunction with 52351)

(For image-guided dilation of ureter, ureteropelvic junction stricture without endoscopic guidance, use 50706)

52351 Cystourethroscopy, with ureteroscopy and/or pyeloscopy; diagnostic

(For radiological supervision and interpretation, use 74485)

(Do not report 52351 in conjunction with 52341, 52342, 52343, 52344, 52345, 52346, 52352-52356)

52352 with removal or manipulation of calculus (ureteral catheterization is included)

52353 with lithotripsy (ureteral catheterization is included)

(Do not report 52353 in conjunction with 52332, 52356 when performed together on the same side)

52356 with lithotripsy including insertion of indwelling ureteral stent (eg, Gibbons or double-J type)

(Do not report 52356 in conjunction with 52332, 52353 when performed together on the same side)

52354 with biopsy and/or fulguration of ureteral or renal pelvic lesion

(For image-guided biopsy of ureter and/or renal pelvic without endoscopic guidance, use 50606)

52355 with resection of ureteral or renal pelvic tumor

52356 This code is out of order. See page 545

VESICAL NECK AND PROSTATE

52400 Cystourethroscopy with incision, fulguration, or resection of congenital posterior urethral valves, or congenital obstructive hypertrophic mucosal folds

52402 Cystourethroscopy with transurethral resection or incision of ejaculatory ducts

52441 Cystourethroscopy, with insertion of permanent adjustable transprostatic implant; single implant

+ **52442** each additional permanent adjustable transprostatic implant (list separately in addition to code for primary procedure)

(Use 52442 in conjunction with 52441)

(To report removal of implant[s], use 52310)

(For insertion of a permanent urethral stent, use 52282. For insertion of a temporary prostatic urethral stent, use 53855)

52450 Transurethral incision of prostate

52500 Transurethral resection of bladder neck (separate procedure)

52601 Transurethral electrosurgical resection of prostate, including control of postoperative bleeding, complete (vasectomy, meatotomy, cystourethroscopy, urethral calibration and/or dilation, and internal urethrotomy are included)

(For transurethral waterjet ablation of prostate, use 0421T)

(For other approaches, see 55801-55845)

(52612, 52614, 52620 have been deleted. For first stage transurethral partial resectin of prostate, use 52601. For second stage partial resection of prostate, use 52601 with modifier 58. For transurethral resection of residual or regrowth of obstructive prostate tissue, use 52630)

52630 Transurethral resection; residual or regrowth of obstructive prostate tissue including control of postoperative bleeding, complete (vasectomy, meatotomy, cystourethroscopy, urethral calibration and/or dilation, and internal urethrotomy are included)

(For resection of residual prostate tissue performed within the postoperative period of a related procedure performed by the same physician, append modifier 78)

(For transurethral waterjet ablation of prostate, use 0421T)

52640 of postoperative bladder neck contracture

52647 Laser coagulation of prostate, including control of postoperative bleeding, complete (vasectomy, meatotomy, cystourethroscopy, urethral calibration and/or dilation, and internal urethrotomy are included if performed)

52648 Laser vaporization of prostate, including control of postoperative bleeding, complete (vasectomy, meatotomy, cystourethroscopy, urethral calibration and/or dilation, internal urethrotomy and transurethral resection of prostate are included if performed)

52649 Laser enucleation of the prostate with morcellation, including control of postoperative bleeding, complete (vasectomy, meatotomy, cystourethroscopy, urethral calibration and/or dilation, internal urethrotomy and transurethral resection of prostate are included if performed)

(Do not report 52649 in conjunction with 52000, 52276, 52281, 52601, 52647, 52648, 53020, 55250)

52700 Transurethral drainage of prostatic abscess

(For litholapaxy, use 52317, 52318)

URETHRA

(For endoscopy, see cystoscopy, urethroscopy, cystourethroscopy, 52000-52700)

(For injection procedure for urethrocystography, see 51600-51610)

INCISION

53000 Urethrotomy or urethrostomy, external (separate procedure); pendulous urethra

53010 perineal urethra, external

53020 Meatotomy, cutting of meatus (separate procedure); except infant

53025 infant

(Do not report modifier '-63' in conjunction with 53025)

53040 Drainage of deep periurethral abscess

(For subcutaneous abscess, see 10060, 10061)

53060 Drainage of Skene's gland abscess or cyst

● New Code   ▲ Revised Code   ✛ Add-On Code   ⊘ Modifier -51 Exempt   ★ Telemedicine

53080 Drainage of perineal urinary extravasation; uncomplicated (separate procedure)

53085   complicated

EXCISION

53200 Biopsy of urethra

53210 Urethrectomy, total, including cystostomy; female

53215   male

53220 Excision or fulguration of carcinoma of urethra

53230 Excision of urethral diverticulum (separate procedure); female

53235   male

53240 Marsupialization of urethral diverticulum, male or female

53250 Excision of bulbourethral gland (Cowper's gland)

53260 Excision or fulguration; urethral polyp(s), distal urethra

(For endoscopic approach, see 52214, 52224)

53265   urethral caruncle

53270   Skene's glands

53275   urethral prolapse

REPAIR

(For hypospadias, see 54300-54352)

53400 Urethroplasty; first stage, for fistula, diverticulum, or stricture (eg, Johannsen type)

53405   second stage (formation of urethra), including urinary diversion

53410 Urethroplasty, 1-stage reconstruction of male anterior urethra

53415 Urethroplasty, transpubic or perineal, one stage, for reconstruction or repair of prostatic or membranous urethra

53420 Urethroplasty, 2-stage reconstruction or repair of prostatic or membranous urethra; first stage

53425   second stage

53430 Urethroplasty, reconstruction of female urethra

53431 Urethroplasty with tubularization of posterior urethra and/or lower bladder for incontinence (eg, Tenago, Leadbetter procedure)

53440 Sling operation for correction of male urinary incontinence (eg, fascia or synthetic)

53442 Removal or revision of sling for male urinary incontinence (eg, fascia or synthetic)

53444 Insertion of tandem cuff (dual cuff)

53445 Insertion of inflatable urethral/bladder neck sphincter, including placement of pump, reservoir, and cuff

53446 Removal of inflatable urethral/bladder neck sphincter, including pump, reservoir, and cuff

53447 Removal and replacement of inflatable urethral/bladder neck sphincter including pump, reservoir, and cuff at the same operative session

53448 Removal and replacement of inflatable urethral/bladder neck sphincter including pump, reservoir, and cuff through an infected field at the same operative session including irrigation and debridement of infected tissue

(Do not report 11042, 11043 in addition to 53448)

53449 Repair of inflatable urethral/bladder neck sphincter, including pump, reservoir, and cuff

53450 Urethromeatoplasty, with mucosal advancement

(For meatotomy, see 53020, 53025)

53460 Urethromeatoplasty, with partial excision of distal urethral segment (Richardson type procedure)

53500 Urethrolysis, transvaginal, secondary, open, including cystourethroscopy (eg, postsurgical obstruction, scarring)

(For urethrolysis by retropubic approach, use 53899)

(Do not report 53500 in conjunction with 52000)

53502 Urethrorrhaphy, suture of urethral wound or injury; female

53505 penile

53510 perineal

53515 prostatomembranous

53520 Closure of urethrostomy or urethrocutaneous fistula, male (separate procedure)

(For closure of urethrovaginal fistula, use 57310)

(For closure of urethrorectal fistula, see 45820, 45825)

MANIPULATION

(For radiological supervision and interpretation, use 74485)

53600 Dilation of urethral stricture by passage of sound or urethral dilator, male; initial

53601 subsequent

53605 Dilation of urethral stricture or vesical neck by passage of sound or urethral dilator, male, general or conduction (spinal) anesthesia

(For dilation of urethral stricture, male, performed under local anesthesia, see 53600, 53601, 53620, 53621)

53620 Dilation of urethral stricture by passage of filiform and follower, male; initial

53621 subsequent

53660 Dilation of female urethra including suppository and/or instillation; initial

53661 subsequent

● New Code   ▲ Revised Code   ✛ Add-On Code   ⊘ Modifier -51 Exempt   ★ Telemedicine

53665   Dilation of female urethra, general or conduction (spinal) anesthesia

(For urethral catheterization, see 51701-51703)

(For dilation of urethra performed under local anesthesia, female, see 53660, 53661)

OTHER PROCEDURES

(For two or three glass urinalysis, use 81020)

53850   Transurethral destruction of prostate tissue; by microwave thermotherapy

53852   by radiofrequency thermotherapy

53854   by radiofrequency generated water vapor thermotherapy

(For transurethral ablation of malignant prostate tissue by high-energy water vapor thermotherapy, including intraoperative imaging and needle guidance, use 0582T)

53855   Insertion of a temporary prostatic urethral stent, including urethral measurement

(For insertion of permanent urethral stent, use 52282)

53860   Transurethral radiofrequency micro-remodeling of the female bladder neck and proximal urethra for stress urinary incontinence

53899   Unlisted procedure, urinary system

This page intentionally left blank

● New Code ▲ Revised Code ✚ Add-On Code ⊘ Modifier -51 Exempt ★ Telemedicine

MALE GENITAL SYSTEM

CPT codes from this section of CPT are used to report invasive and surgical procedures performed on the penis; testis; epididymis; scrotum; spermatic cord and prostate.

Transurethral drainage of a prostatic abscess (e.g. CPT code 52700) is included in male transurethral prostatic procedures and is not reported separately.

Urethral catheterization (e.g. CPT codes 51701, 51702, and 51703), when medically necessary to successfully accomplish a procedure, should not be separately reported.

The puncture aspiration of a hydrocele (e.g. CPT code 55000) is included in services involving the tunica vaginalis and proximate anatomy (scrotum, vas deferens) and in inguinal hernia repairs.

A number of codes describe surgical procedures of a progressively more comprehensive nature or with different approaches to accomplish similar services. In general, these groups of codes are not to be reported together (see mutually exclusive policy). While a number of these groups of codes exist in CPT, a specific example includes the series of codes describing prostate procedures (CPT codes 55801-55845). In addition, all prostatectomy procedures (e.g. CPT codes 52601-52648 and 55801-55845) are also mutually exclusive of one another.

PENIS

INCISION

(For abdominal perineal gangrene debridement, see 11004-11006)

54000 Slitting of prepuce, dorsal or lateral (separate procedure); newborn

(Do not report modifier '-63' in conjunction with 54000)

54001 except newborn

54015 Incision and drainage of penis, deep

(For skin and subcutaneous abscess, see 10060-10160)

DESTRUCTION

54050 Destruction of lesion(s), penis (eg, condyloma, papilloma, molluscum contagiosum, herpetic vesicle), simple; chemical

54055 electrodesiccation

54056 cryosurgery

54057 laser surgery

54060 surgical excision

54065 Destruction of lesion(s), penis (eg, condyloma, papilloma, molluscum contagiosum, herpetic vesicle), extensive (eg, laser surgery, electosurgery, cryosurgery, chemosurgery)

(For destruction or excision of other lesions, see Integumentary System)

EXCISION

54100 Biopsy of penis; (separate procedure)

54105 deep structures

54110 Excision of penile plaque (Peyronie disease);

| Separate Procedure | Unlisted Procedure | CCI Comp. Code | Non-specific Procedure | **551** |

54111	with graft to 5 cm in length

54112	with graft greater than 5 cm in length

54115	Removal foreign body from deep penile tissue (eg, plastic implant)

54120	Amputation of penis; partial

54125	complete

54130	Amputation of penis, radical; with bilateral inguinofemoral lymphadenectomy

54135	in continuity with bilateral pelvic lymphadenectomy, including external iliac, hypogastric and obturator nodes

(For lymphadenectomy (separate procedure) see 38760-38770)

54150	Circumcision, using clamp or other device with regional dorsal penile or ring block

(Do not report modifier -63 in conjunction with 54150)

(Report 54150 with modifier 52 when performed without dorsal penile or ring block)

54160	Circumcision, surgical excision other than clamp, device or dorsal slit; neonate (28 days of age or less)

(Do not report modifier -63 in conjunction with 54160)

54161	older than 28 days of age

54162	Lysis or excision of penile post-circumcision adhesions

54163	Repair incomplete circumcision

54164	Frenulotomy of penis

(Do not report with circumcision codes 54150-54161, 54162, 54163)

INTRODUCTION

54200	Injection procedure for Peyronie disease;

54205	with surgical exposure of plaque

54220	Irrigation of corpora cavernosa for priapism

54230	Injection procedure for corpora cavernosography

(For radiological supervision and interpretation, use 74445)

54231	Dynamic cavernosometry, including intracavernosal injection of vasoactive drugs (eg, papaverine, phentolamine)

54235	Injection of corpora cavernosa with pharmacologic agent(s) (eg, papaverine, phentolamine)

54240	Penile plethysmography

54250	Nocturnal penile tumescence and/or rigidity test

REPAIR

(For other urethroplasties, see 53400-53430)

● New Code   ▲ Revised Code   + Add-On Code   ⊘ Modifier -51 Exempt   ★ Telemedicine

(For penile revascularization, use 37788)

54300 Plastic operation of penis for straightening of chordee (eg, hypospadias), with or without mobilization of urethra

54304 Plastic operation on penis for correction of chordee or for first stage hypospadias repair with or without transplantation of prepuce and/or skin flaps

54308 Urethroplasty for second stage hypospadias repair (including urinary diversion); less than 3 cm

54312   greater than 3 cm

54316 Urethroplasty for second stage hypospadias repair (including urinary diversion) with free skin graft obtained from site other than genitalia

54318 Urethroplasty for third stage hypospadias repair to release penis from scrotum (eg, third stage Cecil repair)

54322 1 stage distal hypospadias repair (with or without chordee or circumcision); with simple meatal advancement (eg, Magpi, V-flap)

54324   with urethroplasty by local skin flaps (eg, flip-flap, prepucial flap)

54326   with urethroplasty by local skin flaps and mobilization of urethra

54328   with extensive dissection to correct chordee and urethroplasty with local skin flaps, skin graft patch, and/or island flap

(For urethroplasty and straightening of chordee, use 54308)

54332 1 stage proximal penile or penoscrotal hypospadias repair requiring extensive dissection to correct chordee and urethroplasty by use of skin graft tube and/or island flap

54336 1 stage perineal hypospadias repair requiring extensive dissection to correct chordee and urethroplasty by use of skin graft tube and/or island flap

54340 Repair of hypospadias complications (ie, fistula, stricture, diverticula); by closure, incision, or excision, simple

54344   requiring mobilization of skin flaps and urethroplasty with flap or patch graft

54348   requiring extensive dissection and urethroplasty with flap, patch or tubed graft (includes urinary diversion)

54352 Repair of hypospadias cripple requiring extensive dissection and excision of previously constructed structures including re-release of chordee and reconstruction of urethra and penis by use of local skin as grafts and island flaps and skin brought in as flaps or grafts

54360 Plastic operation on penis to correct angulation

54380 Plastic operation on penis for epispadias distal to external sphincter;

54385   with incontinence

54390   with exstrophy of bladder

54400 Insertion of penile prosthesis; non-inflatable (semi-rigid)

54401   inflatable (self-contained)

(For removal or replacement of penile prosthesis, see 54415, 54416)

Separate Procedure   Unlisted Procedure   CCI Comp. Code   Non-specific Procedure   **553**

54405 Insertion of multi-component inflatable penile prosthesis, including placement of pump, cylinders, and reservoir

(For reduced services, report 54405 with modifier -52)

54406 Removal of all components of a multi-component inflatable penile prosthesis without replacement of prosthesis

(For reduced services, report 54406 with modifier -52)

54408 Repair of component(s) of a multi-component, inflatable penile prosthesis

54410 Removal and replacement of all component(s) of a multi-component inflatable penile prosthesis at the same operative session

54411 Removal and replacement of all components of a multi-component inflatable penile prosthesis through an infected field at the same operative session, including irrigation and debridement of infected tissue

(For reduced services, report 54411 with modifier -52)

(Do not report 11042, 11043 in addition to 54411)

54415 Removal of non-inflatable (semi-rigid) or inflatable (self-contained) penile prosthesis, without replacement of prosthesis

54416 Removal and replacement of non-inflatable (semi-rigid) or inflatable (self-contained) penile prosthesis at the same operative session

54417 Removal and replacement of non-inflatable (semi-rigid) or inflatable (self-contained) penile prosthesis through an infected field at the same operative session, including irrigation and debridement of infected tissue

(Do not report 11042, 11043 in addition to 54417)

54420 Corpora cavernosa-saphenous vein shunt (priapism operation), unilateral or bilateral

54430 Corpora cavernosa-corpus spongiosum shunt (priapism operation), unilateral or bilateral

54435 Corpora cavernosa-glans penis fistulization (eg, biopsy needle, Winter procedure, rongeur, or punch) for priapism

54437 Repair of traumatic corporeal tear(s)

(For repair of urethra, see 53410, 53415)

54438 Replantation, penis, complete amputation including urethral repair

(To report replantation of incomplete penile amputation, see 54437 for repair of corporeal tear[s], and 53410, 53415 for repair of the urethra)

54440 Plastic operation of penis for injury

MANIPULATION

54450 Foreskin manipulation including lysis of preputial adhesions and stretching

TESTIS

EXCISION

(For abdominal perineal gangrene debridement, see 11004-11006)

54500 Biopsy of testis, needle (separate procedure)

● New Code ▲ Revised Code + Add-On Code ⊘ Modifier -51 Exempt ★ Telemedicine

(For fine needle aspiration biopsy, see 10004, 10005, 10006, 10007, 10008, 10009, 10010, 10011, 10012, 10021)

(For evaluation of fine needle aspirate, see 88172, 88173)

54505 Biopsy of testis, incisional (separate procedure)

(For bilateral procedure, report 54505 with modifier -50)

(When combined with vasogram, seminal vesiculogram, or epididymogram, use 55300)

54512 Excision of extraparenchymal lesion of testis

54520 Orchiectomy, simple (including subcapsular), with or without testicular prosthesis, scrotal or inguinal approach

(For bilateral procedure, report 54520 with modifier -50)

54522 Orchiectomy, partial

54530 Orchiectomy, radical, for tumor; inguinal approach

54535   with abdominal exploration

(For orchiectomy with repair of hernia, see 49505 or 49507 and 54520)

(For radical retroperitoneal lymphadenectomy, use 38780)

EXPLORATION

54550 Exploration for undescended testis (inguinal or scrotal area)

(For bilateral procedure, report 54550 with modifier -50)

54560 Exploration for undescended testis with abdominal exploration

(For bilateral procedure, report 54560 with modifier -50)

REPAIR

54600 Reduction of torsion of testis, surgical, with or without fixation of contralateral testis

54620 Fixation of contralateral testis (separate procedure)

54640 Orchiopexy, inguinal or scrotal approach

(For bilateral procedure, report 54640 with modifier -50)

(For inguinal hernia repair performed in conjunction with inguinal orchiopexy, see 49495-49525)

54650 Orchiopexy, abdominal approach, for intra-abdominal testis (eg, Fowler-Stephens)

(For laparoscopic approach, use 54692)

54660 Insertion of testicular prosthesis (separate procedure)

(For bilateral procedure, report 54660 with modifier -50)

54670 Suture or repair of testicular injury

54680 Transplantation of testis(es) to thigh (because of scrotal destruction)

LAPAROSCOPY

Surgical laparoscopy always includes diagnostic laparoscopy. To report a diagnostic laparoscopy (peritoneoscopy) (separate procedure), use 49320.

54690 Laparoscopy, surgical; orchiectomy

54692 orchiopexy for intra-abdominal testis

54699 Unlisted laparoscopy procedure, testis

EPIDIDYMIS
INCISION

54700 Incision and drainage of epididymis, testis and/or scrotal space (eg, abscess or hematoma)

(For debridement of necrotizing soft tissue infection of external genitalia, see 11004-11006)

EXCISION

54800 Biopsy of epididymis, needle

(For fine needle aspiration biopsy, see 10004, 10005, 10006, 10007, 10008, 10009, 10010, 10011, 10012, 10021)

(For evaluation of fine needle aspirate, see 88172, 88173)

54830 Excision of local lesion of epididymis

54840 Excision of spermatocele, with or without epididymectomy

54860 Epididymectomy; unilateral

54861 bilateral

EXPLORATION

54865 Exploration of epididymis, with or without biopsy

REPAIR

54900 Epididymovasostomy, anastomosis of epididymis to vas deferens; unilateral

54901 bilateral

(For operating microscope, use 69990)

TUNICA VAGINALIS
INCISION

55000 Puncture aspiration of hydrocele, tunica vaginalis, with or without injection of medication

EXCISION

55040 Excision of hydrocele; unilateral

55041 bilateral

(With hernia repair, see 49495-49501)

● New Code ▲ Revised Code ✚ Add-On Code ⊘ Modifier -51 Exempt ★ Telemedicine

REPAIR

55060 Repair of tunica vaginalis hydrocele (Bottle type)

SCROTUM

INCISION

55100 Drainage of scrotal wall abscess

(See also 54700)

(For debridement of necrotizing soft tissue infection of external genitalia, see 11004-11006)

55110 Scrotal exploration

55120 Removal of foreign body in scrotum

EXCISION

(For excision of local lesion of skin of scrotum, see Integumentary System)

55150 Resection of scrotum

REPAIR

55175 Scrotoplasty; simple

55180   complicated

VAS DEFERENS

INCISION

55200 Vasotomy, cannulization with or without incision of vas, unilateral or bilateral (separate procedure)

EXCISION

55250 Vasectomy, unilateral or bilateral (separate procedure), including postoperative semen examination(s)

INTRODUCTION

55300 Vasotomy for vasograms, seminal vesiculograms, or epididymograms, unilateral or bilateral

(For radiological supervision and interpretation, use 74440)

(When combined with biopsy of testis, see 54505 and use modifier -51)

REPAIR

55400 Vasovasostomy, vasovasorrhaphy

(For bilateral procedure, report 55400 with modifier -50)

(For operating microscope, use 69990)

SUTURE

(**55450** deleted 2017 [2018 edition]. To report, use 55250)

SPERMATIC CORD

EXCISION

55500 Excision of hydrocele of spermatic cord, unilateral (separate procedure)

55520   Excision of lesion of spermatic cord (separate procedure)

55530   Excision of varicocele or ligation of spermatic veins for varicocele; (separate procedure)

55535   abdominal approach

55540   with hernia repair

LAPAROSCOPY

Surgical laparoscopy always includes diagnostic laparoscopy. To report a diagnostic laparoscopy (peritoneoscopy) (separate procedure), use 49320.

55550   Laparoscopy, surgical, with ligation of spermatic veins for varicocele

55559   Unlisted laparoscopy procedure, spermatic cord

SEMINAL VESICLES

INCISION

55600   Vesiculotomy;

            (For bilateral procedure, report 55600 with modifier -50)

55605   complicated

EXCISION

55650   Vesiculectomy, any approach

            (For bilateral procedure, report 55650 with modifier -50)

55680   Excision of Mullerian duct cyst

            (For injection procedure, see 52010, 55300)

PROSTATE

INCISION

55700   Biopsy, prostate; needle or punch, single or multiple, any approach

            (If imaging guidance is performed, see 76942, 77002, 77012, 77021)

            (For fine needle aspiration biopsy, see 10004, 10005, 10006, 10007, 10008, 10009, 10010, 10011, 10012, 10021)

            (For evaluation of fine needle aspirate, see 88172, 88173)

            (For transperineal stereotactic template guided saturation prostate biopsies, use 55706)

55705   incisional, any approach

55706   Biopsies, prostate, needle, transperineal, stereotactic template guided saturation sampling, including imaging guidance

            (Do not report 55706 in conjunction with 55700)

55720   Prostatotomy, external drainage of prostatic abscess, any approach; simple

55725   complicated

            (For transurethral drainage, use 52700)

● New Code   ▲ Revised Code   + Add-On Code   ⊘ Modifier -51 Exempt   ★ Telemedicine

EXCISION

    (For transurethral removal of prostate, see 52601-52640)

    (For transurethral destruction of prostate, see 53850-53852)

    (For limited pelvic lymphadenectomy for staging (separate procedure), use 38562)

    (For independent node dissection, see 38770-38780)

55801 Prostatectomy, perineal, subtotal (including control of postoperative bleeding, vasectomy, meatotomy, urethral calibration and/or dilation, and internal urethrotomy)

55810 Prostatectomy, perineal radical;

55812   with lymph node biopsy(s) (limited pelvic lymphadenectomy)

55815   with bilateral pelvic lymphadenectomy, including external iliac, hypogastric and obturator nodes

    (If 55815 is carried out on separate days, use 38770 with modifier -50 and 55810)

55821 Prostatectomy (including control of postoperative bleeding, vasectomy, meatotomy, urethral calibration and/or dilation, and internal urethrotomy); suprapubic, subtotal, one or two stages

55831   retropubic, subtotal

55840 Prostatectomy, retropubic radical, with or without nerve sparing;

55842   with lymph node biopsy(s) (limited pelvic lymphadenectomy)

55845   with bilateral pelvic lymphadenectomy, including external iliac, hypogastric, and obturator nodes

    (If 55845 is carried out on separate days, use 38770 with modifier -50 and 55840)

    (For laparoscopic retropubic radical prostatectomy, use 55866)

55860 Exposure of prostate, any approach, for insertion of radioactive substance;

    (For application of interstitial radioelement, see 77770, 77771, 77772, 77778)

55862   with lymph node biopsy(s) (limited pelvic lymphadenectomy)

55865   with bilateral pelvic lymphadenectomy, including external iliac, hypogastric and obturator nodes

LAPAROSCOPY

Surgical laparoscopy always includes diagnostic laparoscopy. To report a diagnostic laparoscopy (peritoneoscopy) (separate procedure), use 49320.

55866 Laparoscopy, surgical prostatectomy, retropubic radical, including nerve sparing, includes robotic assistance, when performed

    (For open procedure, use 55840)

OTHER PROCEDURES

    (For artificial insemination, see 58321, 58322)

55870 Electroejaculation

55873 Cryosurgical ablation of the prostate (includes ultrasonic guidance and monitoring)

55874 Transperineal placement of biodegradable material, periprostatic, single or multiple injection(s), including image guidance, when performed

---

Separate Procedure   Unlisted Procedure   CCI Comp. Code   Non-specific Procedure   **559**

(Do not report 55874 in conjunction with 76942)

55875 Transperineal placement of needles or catheters into prostate for interstitial radioelement application, with or without cystoscopy

(For placement of needles or catheters into pelvic organs and/or genitalia [except prostate] for interstitial radioelement application, use 55920)

(For interstitial radioelement application, see 77770, 77771, 77772, 77778)

(For ultrasonic guidance for interstitial radioelement application, use 76965)

55876 Placement of interstitial device(s) for radiation therapy guidance (eg, fiducial markers, dosimeter), prostate (via needle, any approach), single or multiple

(Report supply of device separately)

(For imaging guidance, see 76942, 77002, 77012, 77021)

● **55880** Ablation of malignant prostate tissue, transrectal, with high intensity-focused ultrasound (HIFU), including ultrasound guidance

55899 Unlisted procedure, male genital system

● New Code ▲ Revised Code ✚ Add-On Code ⊘ Modifier -51 Exempt ★ Telemedicine

REPRODUCTIVE SYSTEM PROCEDURES

55920   Placement of needles or catheters into pelvic organs and/or genitalia (except prostate) for subsequent interstitial radioelement application

(For placement of needles or catheters into prostate, use 55875)

. (For insertion of uterine tandems and/or vaginal ovoids for clinical brachytherapy, use 57155)

(For insertion of Heyman capsules for clinical brachytherapy, us 58346)

INTERSEX SURGERY

55970   Intersex surgery; male to female

55980   female to male

This page intentionally left blank.

● New Code ▲ Revised Code ✚ Add-On Code ⊘ Modifier -51 Exempt ★ Telemedicine

FEMALE GENITAL SYSTEM

When a pelvic examination is performed in conjunction with a gynecologic procedure, either as a necessary part of the procedure or as a confirmatory examination, the pelvic examination is not separately reported. A diagnostic pelvic examination may be performed for the purposes of deciding to perform a procedure; however, this examination is included in the evaluation and management service at the time the decision to perform the procedure is made.

All surgical laparoscopic, hysteroscopic or peritoneoscopic procedures include diagnostic procedures. Therefore, CPT code 49320 is included in 38120, 38570- 38572, 43280, 43651-43653, 44200- 44202, 44970, 47560-47570, 49321- 49323, 49650-49651, 54690-54692, 55550, 58545-58554, 58660-58673, 60650; and 58555 is included in 58558- 58563.

Lysis of adhesions (CPT code 58660) is not to be reported separately when done in conjunction with other surgical laparoscopic procedures.

Pelvic exam under anesthesia indicated by CPT code 57410, is included in all major and most minor gynecological procedures and is not to be reported separately. This procedure represents routine evaluation of the surgical field.

Dilation of vagina or cervix (CPT codes 57400 or 57800), when done in conjunction with vaginal approach procedures, is not to be reported separately unless the CPT code descriptor states "without cervical dilation." 6. Administration of anesthesia, when necessary, is included in every surgical procedure code, when performed by the surgeon.

Colposcopy (CPT codes 56820, 57420, 57452) should not be reported separately when performed as a "scout" procedure to confirm the lesion or to assess the surgical field prior to a surgical procedure. A diagnostic colposcopy resulting in the decision to perform a non-colposcopic procedure may be reported with modifier - 58. Diagnostic colposcopies (56820, 57420, 57452) are not separately reported with other colposcopic procedures.

(For pelvic laparotomy, use 49000)

(For excision or destruction of endometriomas, open method, see 49203-49205, 58957, 58958)

(For paracentesis, see 49082, 49083, 49084)

(For secondary closure of abdominal wall evisceration or disruption, use 49900)

(For fulguration or excision of lesions, laparoscopic approach, use 58662)

(For chemotherapy, see 96401-96549)

VULVA, PERINEUM AND INTROITUS

The following definitions apply to the vulvectomy codes (56620-56640):

A **simple** procedure is the removal of skin and superficial subcutaneous tissues.

A **radical** procedure is the removal of skin and deep subcutaneous tissues.

A **partial** procedure is the removal of less than 80% of the vulvar area.

A **complete** procedure is the removal of greater than 80% of the vulvar area.

INCISION

(For incision and drainage of sebaceous cyst, furuncle, or abscess, see 10040, 10060, 10061)

56405   Incision and drainage of vulva or perineal abscess

56420   Incision and drainage of Bartholin's gland abscess

(For incision and drainage of Skene's gland abscess or cyst, use 53060)

56440   Marsupialization of Bartholin's gland cyst

56441   Lysis of labial adhesions

56442   Hymenotomy, simple incision

DESTRUCTION

56501   Destruction of lesion(s), vulva; simple (eg, laser surgery, electrosurgery, cryosurgery, chemosurgery)

56515   extensive (eg, laser surgery, electrosurgery, cryosurgery, chemosurgery)

(For destruction of Skene's gland cyst or abscess, use 53270)

(For cautery destruction of urethral caruncle, use 53265)

EXCISION

56605   Biopsy of vulva or perineum (separate procedure); 1 lesion

+ 56606   each separate additional lesion (List separately in addition to code for primary procedure)

(Use 56606 in conjunction with code 56605)

(For excision of local lesion, see 11420-11426, 11620-11626)

56620   Vulvectomy simple; partial

56625   complete

(For skin graft, see 15002 et seq)

56630   Vulvectomy, radical, partial;

(For skin graft, if used, see 15004-15005, 15120, 15121, 15240, 15241)

56631   with unilateral inguinofemoral lymphadenectomy

56632   with bilateral inguinofemoral lymphadenectomy

(For partial radical vulvectomy with inguinofemoral lymph node biopsy without complete inguinofemoral lymphadenectomy, use 56630 in conjunction with 38531)

56633   Vulvectomy, radical, complete;

56634   with unilateral inguinofemoral lymphadenectomy

56637   with bilateral inguinofemoral lymphadenectomy

(For complete radical vulvectomy with inguinofemoral lymph node biopsy without complete inguinofemoral lymphadenectomy, use 56633 in conjunction with 38531)

56640   Vulvectomy, radical, complete, with inguinofemoral, iliac, and pelvic lymphadenectomy

(For bilateral procedure, report 56640 with modifier -50)

(For lymphadenectomy, see 38760-38780)

56700   Partial hymenectomy or revision of hymenal ring

56740   Excision of Bartholin's gland or cyst

(For excision of Skene's gland, use 53270)

(For excision of urethral caruncle, use 53265)

(For excision or fulguration of urethral carcinoma, use 53220)

(For excision or marsupialization of urethral diverticulum, see 53230, 53240)

   ● New Code   ▲ Revised Code   + Add-On Code   ⊘ Modifier -51 Exempt   ★ Telemedicine

REPAIR

(For repair of urethra for mucosal prolapse, use 53275)

56800 Plastic repair of introitus

56805 Clitoroplasty for intersex state

56810 Perineoplasty, repair of perineum, nonobstetrical (separate procedure)

(See also 56800)

(For repair of wounds to genitalia, see 12001-12007, 12041-12047, 13131-13133)

(For repair of recent injury of vagina and perineum, nonobstetrical, use 57210)

(For anal sphincteroplasty, see 46750, 46751)

(For episiorrhaphy, episioperineorrhaphy for recent injury of vulva and/or perineum, nonobstetrical, use 57210)

ENDOSCOPY

56820 Colposcopy of the vulva

56821 with biopsy(s)

(For colposcopic examinations/procedures involving the vagina, see 57420, 57421; cervix, see 57452-57461)

VAGINA

INCISION

57000 Colpotomy; with exploration

57010 with drainage of pelvic abscess

57020 Colpocentesis (separate procedure)

57022 Incision and drainage of vaginal hematoma; obstetrical/ postpartum

57023 non-obstetrical (eg, post-trauma, spontaneous bleeding)

DESTRUCTION

57061 Destruction of vaginal lesion(s); simple (eg, laser surgery, electrosurgery, cryosurgery, chemosurgery)

57065 extensive (eg, laser surgery, electrosurgery, cryosurgery, chemosurgery)

EXCISION

57100 Biopsy of vaginal mucosa; simple (separate procedure)

57105 extensive, requiring suture (including cysts)

57106 Vaginectomy, partial removal of vaginal wall;

57107 with removal of paravaginal tissue (radical vaginectomy)

57109 with removal of paravaginal tissue (radical vaginectomy) with bilateral total pelvic lymphadenectomy and para-aortic lymph node sampling (biopsy)

57110 Vaginectomy, complete removal of vaginal wall;

57111   with removal of paravaginal tissue (radical vaginectomy)

(57112 deleted 2020 [2021 Edition})

57120 Colpocleisis (Le Fort type)

57130 Excision of vaginal septum

57135 Excision of vaginal cyst or tumor

INTRODUCTION

57150 Irrigation of vagina and/or application of medicament for treatment of bacterial, parasitic, or fungoid disease

57155 Insertion of uterine tandem and/or vaginal ovoids for clinical brachytherapy

(For placement of needles or catheters into pelvic organs and/or genitalia [except prostate] for interstitial radioelement application, use 55920)

(For insertion of radioelement sources or ribbons, see 77761-77763, 77770, 77771, 77772)

57156 Insertion of a vaginal radiation afterloading apparatus for clinical brachytherapy

57160 Fitting and insertion of pessary or other intravaginal support device

57170 Diaphragm or cervical cap fitting with instructions

57180 Introduction of any hemostatic agent or pack for spontaneous or traumatic nonobstetrical vaginal hemorrhage (separate procedure)

REPAIR

(For urethral suspension, Marshall-Marchetti-Krantz type, abdominal approach, see 51840, 51841)

(For laparoscopic suspension, use 51990)

57200 Colporrhaphy, suture of injury of vagina (nonobstetrical)

57210 Colpoperineorrhaphy, suture of injury of vagina and/or perineum (nonobstetrical)

57220 Plastic operation on urethral sphincter, vaginal approach (eg, Kelly urethral plication)

57230 Plastic repair of urethrocele

57240 Anterior colporrhaphy, repair of cystocele with or without repair of urethrocele, including cystourethroscopy, when performed

(Do not report 57240 in conjunction with 52000)

57250 Posterior colporrhaphy, repair of rectocele with or without perineorrhaphy

(For repair of rectocele (separate procedure) without posterior colporrhaphy, use 45560)

57260 Combined anteroposterior colporrhaphy, including cystourethroscopy, when performed;

(Do not report 57260 in conjunction with 52000)

57265   with enterocele repair

(Do not report 57265 in conjunction with 52000)

● New Code   ▲ Revised Code   ✛ Add-On Code   ⊘ Modifier -51 Exempt   ★ Telemedicine

+ **57267** Insertion of mesh or other prosthesis for repair of pelvic floor defect, each site (anterior, posterior compartment), vaginal approach (List separately in addition to code for primary procedure)

(Use 57267 in addition to 45560, 57240-57265, 57285)

57268 Repair of enterocele, vaginal approach (separate procedure)

57270 Repair of enterocele, abdominal approach (separate procedure)

57280 Colpopexy, abdominal approach

57282 Colpopexy, vaginal; extra-peritoneal approach (sacrospinous, iliococcygeus)

57283   intra-peritoneal approach (uterosacral, levator myorrhaphy)

(Do not report 57283 in conjunction with 58263, 57556, 58270, 58280, 58292, 58294)

57284 Paravaginal defect repair (including repair of cystocele, if performed); open abdominal approach

(Do not report 57284 in conjunction with 51840, 51841, 51990, 57240, 57260, 57265, 58152, 58267)

57285   vaginal approach

(Do not report 57285 in conjunction with 51990, 57240, 57260, 57265, 58267)

57287 Removal or revision of sling for stress incontinence (eg, fascia or synthetic)

57288 Sling operation for stress incontinence (eg, fascia or synthetic)

(For laparoscopic approach, use 51992)

57289 Pereyra procedure, including anterior colporrhaphy

57291 Construction of artificial vagina; without graft

57292   with graft

57295 Revision (including removal) of prosthetic vaginal graft, vaginal approach

57296   open abdominal approach

(For laparoscopic approach, use 57426)

57300 Closure of rectovaginal fistula; vaginal or transanal approach

57305   abdominal approach

57307   abdominal approach, with concomitant colostomy

57308   transperineal approach, with perineal body reconstruction, with or without levator plication

57310 Closure of urethrovaginal fistula;

57311   with bulbocavernosus transplant

57320 Closure of vesicovaginal fistula; vaginal approach

(For concomitant cystostomy, see 51020-51040, 51101, 51102)

57330   transvesical and vaginal approach

(For abdominal approach, use 51900)

57335 Vaginoplasty for intersex state

MANIPULATION

57400 Dilation of vagina under anesthesia (other than local)

57410 Pelvic examination under anesthesia (other than local)

57415 Removal of impacted vaginal foreign body (separate procedure) under anesthesia (other than local)

(For removal without anesthesia of an impacted vaginal foreign body, use the appropriate E/M code)

ENDOSCOPY/LAPAROSCOPY

57420 Colposcopy of the entire vagina, with cervix if present;

57421   with biopsy(s) of vagina/cervix

(For colposcopic visualization of cervix and adjacent upper vagina, use 57452)

(When reporting colposcopies of multiple sites, use modifier -51 as appropriate. For colposcopic examinations/procedures involving the vulva, see 56820, 56821; cervix, see 57452-57461)

(For computer-aided mapping of cervix uteri during colposcopy, use 57465)

(For endometrial sampling (biopsy) performed in conjunction with colposcopy, use 58110)

57423 Paravaginal defect repair (including repair of cystocele, if performed), laparoscopic approach

(Do not report 57423 in conjunction with 49320, 51840, 51841, 51990, 57240, 57260, 58152, 58267)

57425 Laparoscopy, surgical, colpopexy (suspension of vaginal apex)

57426 Revision (including removal) of prosthetic vaginal graft, laparoscopic approach

(For vaginal approach, see 57295. For open abdominal approach, see 57296)

CERVIX UTERI

(For cervicography, see Category III code 0003T)

ENDOSCOPY

(For colposcopic examinations/procedures involving the vulva, see 56820, 56821; vagina, see 57420, 57421)

57452 Colposcopy of the cervix including upper/adjacent vagina

(Do not report 57452 in addition to 57454-57461)

57454   with biopsy(s) of the cervix and endocervical curettage

57455   with biopsy(s) of the cervix

57456   with endocervical curettage

57460   with loop electrode biopsy(s) of the cervix

57461   with loop electrode conization of the cervix

(Do not report 57456 in addition to 57461)

(For computer-aided mapping of cervix uteri during colposcopy, use 57465)

(For endometrial sampling [biopsy] performed in conjunction with colposcopy, use 58110)

●+57465 Computer-aided mapping of cervix uteri during colposcopy, including optical dynamic spectral imaging and algorithmic quantification of the acetowhitening effect (List separately in addition to code for primary procedure)

(Use 57465 in conjunction with 57420, 57421, 57452, 57454, 57455, 57456, 57460, 57461)

EXCISION

(For radical surgical procedures, see 58200-58240)

57500 Biopsy of cervix, single or multiple, or local excision of lesion, with or without fulguration (separate procedure)

57505 Endocervical curettage (not done as part of a dilation and curettage)

57510 Cautery of cervix; electro or thermal

57511   cryocautery, initial or repeat

57513   laser ablation

57520 Conization of cervix, with or without fulguration, with or without dilation and curettage, with or without repair; cold knife or laser

(See also 58120)

57522   loop electrode excision

57530 Trachelectomy (cervicectomy), amputation of cervix (separate procedure)

57531 Radical trachelectomy, with bilateral total pelvic lymphadenectomy and para-aortic lymph node sampling biopsy, with or without removal of tube(s), with or without removal of ovary(s)

(For radical abdominal hysterectomy, use 58210)

57540 Excision of cervical stump, abdominal approach;

57545   with pelvic floor repair

57550 Excision of cervical stump, vaginal approach;

57555   with anterior and/or posterior repair

57556   with repair of enterocele

(For insertion of intrauterine device, use 58300)

(For insertion of any hemostatic agent or pack for control of spontaneous non-obstetrical hemorrhage, see 57180)

57558 Dilation and curettage of cervical stump

REPAIR

57700 Cerclage of uterine cervix, nonobstetrical

57720 Trachelorrhaphy, plastic repair of uterine cervix, vaginal approach

MANIPULATION

57800 Dilation of cervical canal, instrumental (separate procedure)

Separate Procedure   Unlisted Procedure   CCI Comp. Code   Non-specific Procedure   **569**

CORPUS UTERI

EXCISION

58100 Endometrial sampling (biopsy) with or without endocervical sampling (biopsy), without cervical dilation, any method (separate procedure)

(For endocervical curettage only, use 57505)

(For endometrial sampling (biopsy) performed in conjunction with colposcopy (57420, 57421, 57452-57461), use 58110)

+ 58110 Endometrial sampling (biopsy) performed in conjunction with colposcopy (List separately in addition to code for primary procedure)

(Use 58110 in conjunction with 57420, 57421, 57452-57461)

58120 Dilation and curettage, diagnostic and/or therapeutic (nonobstetrical)

(For postpartum hemorrhage, use 59160)

58140 Myomectomy, excision of fibroid tumor(s) of uterus, 1 to 4 intramural myoma(s) with total weight of 250 grams or less and/or removal of surface myomas; abdominal approach

58145 vaginal approach

58146 Myomectomy, excision of fibroid tumor(s) of uterus, 5 or more intramural myomas and/or intramural myomas with total weight greater than 250 grams, abdominal approach

(Do not report 58146 in addition to 58140-58145, 58150-58240)

Hysterectomy Procedures

58150 Total abdominal hysterectomy (corpus and cervix), with or without removal of tube(s), with or without removal of ovary(s);

58152 with colpo-urethrocystopexy (eg, Marshall-Marchetti-Krantz, Burch)

(For urethrocystopexy without hysterectomy, see 51840, 51841)

58180 Supracervical abdominal hysterectomy (subtotal hysterectomy), with or without removal of tube(s), with or without removal of ovary(s)

58200 Total abdominal hysterectomy, including partial vaginectomy, with para-aortic and pelvic lymph node sampling, with or without removal of tube(s), with or without removal of ovary(s)

58210 Radical abdominal hysterectomy, with bilateral total pelvic lymphadenectomy and para-aortic lymph node sampling (biopsy), with or without removal of tube(s), with or without removal of ovary(s)

(For radical hysterectomy with ovarian transposition, use also 58825)

58240 Pelvic exenteration for gynecologic malignancy, with total abdominal hysterectomy or cervicectomy, with or without removal of tube(s), with or without removal of ovary(s), with removal of bladder and ureteral transplantations, and/or abdominoperineal resection of rectum and colon and colostomy, or any combination thereof

(For pelvic exenteration for lower urinary tract or male genital malignancy, use 51597)

58260 Vaginal hysterectomy, for uterus 250 grams or less;

58262 with removal of tube(s), and/or ovary(s)

58263 with removal of tube(s), and/or ovary(s), with repair of enterocele

---

● New Code   ▲ Revised Code   ✚ Add-On Code   ⊘ Modifier -51 Exempt   ★ Telemedicine

58267 with colpo-urethrocystopexy (Marshall-Marchetti-Krantz type, Pereyra type) with or without endoscopic control

58270 with repair of enterocele

(For repair of enterocele with removal of tubes and/or ovaries, use 58263)

58275 Vaginal hysterectomy, with total or partial vaginectomy;

58280 with repair of enterocele

58285 Vaginal hysterectomy, radical (Schauta type operation)

58290 Vaginal hysterectomy, for uterus greater than 250 grams;

58291 with removal of tube(s) and/or ovary(s)

58292 with removal of tube(s) and/or ovary(s), with repair of enterocele

(58293 deleted 2020 [2021 Edition])

58294 with repair of enterocele

INTRODUCTION

(To report insertion of non-biodegradable drug delivery implant for contraception, use 11981. To report removal of implantable contraceptive capsules with subsequent insertion of non-biodegradable drug delivery implant, use 11976 and 11981)

58300 Insertion of intrauterine device (IUD)

58301 Removal of intrauterine device (IUD)

58321 Artificial insemination; intra-cervical

58322 intra-uterine

58323 Sperm washing for artificial insemination

58340 Catheterization and introduction of saline or contrast material for saline infusion sonohysterography (SIS) or hysterosalpingography

(For radiological supervision and interpretation of saline infusion sonohysterography, use 76831)

(For radiological supervision and interpretation of hysterosalpingography, use 74740)

58345 Transcervical introduction of fallopian tube catheter for diagnosis and/or re-establishing patency (any method), with or without hysterosalpingography

(For radiological supervision and interpretation, use 74742)

58346 Insertion of Heyman capsules for clinical brachytherapy

(For placement of needles or catheters into pelvic organs and/or genitalia [except prostate] for interstitial radioelement application, use 55920)

(For insertion of radioelement sources or ribbons, see 77761-77763, 77770, 77771, 77772)

58350 Chromotubation of oviduct, including materials

(To report the supply of any materials, use 99070)

58353 Endometrial ablation, thermal, without hysteroscopic guidance

---

Separate Procedure   Unlisted Procedure   CCI Comp. Code   Non-specific Procedure   **571**

(For hysteroscopic procedure, use 58563)

58356 Endometrial cryoablation with ultrasonic guidance, including endometrial curettage, when performed

(Do not report 58356 in conjunction with 58100, 58120, 58340, 76700, 76856)

REPAIR

58400 Uterine suspension, with or without shortening of round ligaments, with or without shortening of sacrouterine ligaments; (separate procedure)

58410   with presacral sympathectomy

(For anastomosis of tubes to uterus, use 58752)

58520 Hysterorrhaphy, repair of ruptured uterus (nonobstetrical)

58540 Hysteroplasty, repair of uterine anomaly (Strassman type)

(For closure of vesicouterine fistula, use 51920)

LAPAROSCOPY/HYSTEROSCOPY

Surgical laparoscopy always includes diagnostic laparoscopy. To report diagnostic laparoscopy (peritoneoscopy) (separate procedure), use 49320. To report a diagnostic hysteroscopy (separate procedure), use 58555.

58674 Laparoscopy, surgical, ablation of uterine fibroid(s) including intraoperative ultrasound guidance and monitoring, radiofrequency

(Do not report 58674 in conjunction with 49320, 58541- 58554, 58570, 58571, 58572, 58573, 76998)

58541 Laparoscopy, surgical, supracervical hysterectomy, for uterus 250 g or less;

58542   with removal of tube(s) and/or ovary(s)

(Do not report 58541-58542 in conjunction with 49320, 57000, 57180, 57410, 58140-58146, 58545, 58546, 58561, 58661, 58670, 58671)

58543 Laparoscopy, surgical, supracervical hysterectomy, for uterus greater than 250 g;

58544   with removal of tube(s) and/or ovary(s)

(Do not report 58543-58544 in conjunction with 49320, 57000, 57180, 57410, 58140-58146, 58545, 58546, 58561, 58661, 58670, 58671)

58545 Laparoscopy, surgical, myomectomy, excision; 1 to 4 intramural myomas with total weight of 250 g or less and/or removal of surface myomas

58546   5 or more intramural myomas and/or intramural myomas with total weight greater than 250 g

58548 Laparoscopy, surgical, with radical hysterectomy, with bilateral total pelvic lymphadenectomy and para-aortic lymph node sampling (biopsy), with removal of tube(s) and ovary(s), if performed

(Do not report 58548 in conjunction with 38570-38572, 58210 58285, 58550-58554)

58550 Laparoscopy, surgical with vaginal hysterectomy, for uterus 250 grams or less;

58552   with removal of tube(s) and/or ovary(s)

(Do not report 58550-58552 in conjunction with 49320, 57000, 57180, 57410, 58140-58146, 58545, 58546, 58561, 58661, 58670, 58671)

58553 Laparoscopy, surgical, with vaginal hysterectomy, for uterus greater than 250 grams;

58554   with removal of tube(s) and/or ovary(s)

(Do not report 58553-58554 in conjunction with 49320, 57000, 57180, 57410, 58140-58146, 58545, 58546, 58561, 58661, 58670, 58671)

58555   Hysteroscopy, diagnostic (separate procedure)

58558   Hysteroscopy, surgical; with sampling (biopsy) of endometrium and/or polypectomy, with or without D & C

58559   with lysis of intrauterine adhesions (any method)

58560   with division or resection of intrauterine septum (any method)

58561   with removal of leiomyomata

58562   with removal of impacted foreign body

58563   with endometrial ablation (eg, endometrial resection, electrosurgical ablation, thermoablation)

58565   with bilateral fallopian tube cannulation to induce occlusion by placement of permanent implants

(Do not report 58565 in conjunction with 58555 or 57800)

(For unilateral procedure, use modifier -52)

58570   Laparoscopy, surgical, with total hysterectomy, for uterus 250g or less;

58571   with removal of tube(s) and/or ovary(s)

58572   Laparoscopy, surgical, with total hysterectomy, for uterus greater than 250g;

58573   with removal of tube(s) and/or ovary(s)

(Do not report 58570-58573 in conjunction with 49320, 57000, 57180, 57410, 58140-58146, 58150, 58545, 58546, 58561, 58661, 58670, 58671)

58575   Laparoscopy, surgical, total hysterectomy for resection of malignancy (tumor debulking), with omentectomy including salpingo-oophorectomy, unilateral or bilateral, when performed

(Do not report 58575 in conjunction with 49255, 49320, 49321, 58570, 58571, 58572, 58573, 58661)

58578   Unlisted laparoscopy procedure, uterus

58579   Unlisted hysteroscopy procedure, uterus

OVIDUCT/OVARY

INCISION

58600   Ligation or transection of fallopian tube(s), abdominal or vaginal approach, unilateral or bilateral

58605   Ligation or transection of fallopian tube(s), abdominal or vaginal approach, postpartum, unilateral or bilateral, during same hospitalization (separate procedure)

(For laparoscopic procedures, use 58670, 58671)

+ 58611   Ligation or transection of fallopian tube(s) when done at the time of cesarean delivery or intra-abdominal surgery (not a separate procedure) (List separately in addition to code for primary procedure)

58615   Occlusion of fallopian tube(s) by device (eg, band, clip, Falope ring) vaginal or suprapubic approach

---

(For laparoscopic approach, use 58671)

(For lysis of adnexal adhesions, use 58740)

LAPAROSCOPY

Surgical laparoscopy always includes diagnostic laparoscopy. To report diagnostic laparoscopy (peritoneoscopy) (separate procedure), use 49320.

58660 Laparoscopy, surgical; with lysis of adhesions (salpingolysis, ovariolysis) (separate procedure)

58661 with removal of adnexal structures (partial or total oophorectomy and/or salpingectomy)

58662 with fulguration or excision of lesions of the ovary, pelvic viscera, or peritoneal surface by any method

58670 with fulguration of oviducts (with or without transection)

58671 with occlusion of oviducts by device (eg, band, clip, or Falope ring)

58672 with fimbrioplasty

58673 with salpingostomy (salpingoneostomy)

(Codes 58672 and 58673 are used to report unilateral procedures. For bilateral procedure, use modifier -50)

58674 This code is out of order. See page 572

58679 Unlisted laparoscopy procedure, oviduct, ovary

(For laparoscopic aspiration of ovarian cyst, use 49322)

(For laparoscopic biopsy of the ovary or fallopian tube, use 49321)

EXCISION

58700 Salpingectomy, complete or partial, unilateral or bilateral (separate procedure)

58720 Salpingo-oophorectomy, complete or partial, unilateral or bilateral (separate procedure)

REPAIR

58740 Lysis of adhesions (salpingolysis, ovariolysis)

(For laparoscopic approach, use 58660)

(For excision or destruction of endometriomas, open method, see 49203-49205, 58957, 58958)

(For fulguration or excision of lesions, laparscopic approach, use 58662)

58750 Tubotubal anastomosis

58752 Tubouterine implantation

58760 Fimbrioplasty

(For laparoscopic approach, use 58672)

58770 Salpingostomy (salpingoneostomy)

(For laparscopic approach, use 58673)

● New Code   ▲ Revised Code   ✛ Add-On Code   ⊘ Modifier -51 Exempt   ★ Telemedicine

OVARY

INCISION

58800 Drainage of ovarian cyst(s), unilateral or bilateral, (separate procedure); vaginal approach

58805 abdominal approach

58820 Drainage of ovarian abscess; vaginal approach, open

58822 abdominal approach

(For transrectal image-guided fluid collection drainage by catheter of pelvic abscess, use 49407)

58825 Transposition, ovary(s)

EXCISION

58900 Biopsy of ovary, unilateral or bilateral (separate procedure)

(For laparoscopic biopsy of the ovary or fallopian tube, use 49321)

58920 Wedge resection or bisection of ovary, unilateral or bilateral

58925 Ovarian cystectomy, unilateral or bilateral

58940 Oophorectomy, partial or total, unilateral or bilateral;

(For oophorectomy with concomitant debulking for ovarian malignancy, use 58952)

58943 for ovarian, tubal or primary peritoneal malignancy, with para-aortic and pelvic lymph node biopsies, peritoneal washings, peritoneal biopsies, diaphragmatic assessments, with or without salpingectomy(s), with or without omentectomy

58950 Resection (initial) of ovarian, tubal or primary peritoneal malignancy with bilateral salpingo-oophorectomy and omentectomy;

58951 with total abdominal hysterectomy, pelvic and limited para-aortic lymphadenectomy

58952 with radical dissection for debulking (ie, radical excision or destruction, intra-abdominal or retroperitoneal tumors)

(For resection of recurrent ovarian, tubal, primary peritoneal, or uterine malignancy, see 58957, 58958)

58953 Bilateral salpingo-oophorectomy with omentectomy, total abdominal hysterectomy and radical dissection for debulking;

58954 with pelvic lymphadenectomy and limited para-aortic lymphadenectomy

58956 Bilateral salpingo-oophorectomy with total omentectomy, total abdominal hysterectomy for malignancy

(Do not report 58956 in conjunction with 49255, 58150, 58180, 58262, 58263, 58550, 58661, 58700, 58720, 58900, 58925, 58940, 58957, 58958)

58957 Resection (tumor debulking) of recurrent ovarian, tubal, primary peritoneal, uterine malignancy (intra-abdominal, retroperitoneal tumors), with omentectomy, if performed;

58958 with pelvic lymphadenectomy and limited para-aortic lymphadenectomy

(Do not report 58957, 58958 in conjunction with 38770, 38780, 44005, 49000, 49203-49215, 49255, 58900-58960)

58960   Laparotomy, for staging or restaging of ovarian, tubal or primary peritoneal malignancy (second look), with or without omentectomy, peritoneal washing, biopsy of abdominal and pelvic peritoneum, diaphragmatic assessment with pelvic and limited para-aortic lymphadenectomy

(Do not report 58960 in conjunction with 58957, 58958)

IN VITRO FERTILIZATION

58970   Follicle puncture for oocyte retrieval, any method

(For radiological supervision and interpretation, use 76948)

58974   Embryo transfer, intrauterine

58976   Gamete, zygote, or embryo intrafallopian transfer, any method

(For laparoscopic adnexal procedures, see 58660-58673)

OTHER PROCEDURES

58999   Unlisted procedure, female genital system (nonobstetrical)

   ● New Code   ▲ Revised Code   + Add-On Code   ⊘ Modifier -51 Exempt   ★ Telemedicine

MATERNITY CARE AND DELIVERY

The services normally provided in uncomplicated maternity cases include antepartum care, delivery, and postpartum care. Pregnancy confirmation during a problem oriented or preventive visit is not considered a part of antepartum care and should be reported using the appropriate E/M service codes 99202, 99203, 99204, 99205, 99211, 99212, 99213, 99214, 99215, 99241, 99242, 99243, 99244, 99245, 99281, 99282, 99283, 99284, 99285, 99384, 99385, 99386, 99394, 99395, 99396 for that visit.

Antepartum care includes the initial prenatal history and physical examination; subsequent prenatal history and physical examinations; recording of weight, blood pressures, fetal heart tones, routine chemical urinalysis, and monthly visits up to 28 weeks gestation; biweekly visits to 36 weeks gestation; and weekly visits until delivery. Any other visits or services within this time period should be coded separately.

Delivery services inlcude admission to the hospital, the admission history and physical examination, management of uncomplicated labor, vaginal delivery (with or without episiotomy, with or without forceps), or cesarean delivery. When reporting delivery only services (59409, 59514, 59612, 59620), report inpatient postdelivery management and discharge services using Evaluation and Management Services codes 99217-99239. Delivery and postpartum services (59410, 59515, 59614, 59622) include delivery services and all inpatient and outpatient postpartum services. Medical complications of pregnancy (eg, cardiac problems, neurological problems, diabetes, hypertension, toxemia, hyperemesis, preterm labor, premature rupture of membranes, trauma) and medical problems complicating labor and delivery management may require additional resources and may be reported separately.

Postpartum care only services (59430) include office or other outpatient visits following vaginal or cesarean section delivery.

For surgical complications of pregnancy (eg., appendectomy, hernia, ovarian cyst, Bartholin cyst), see services in the Surgery section.

If all or part of the antepartum and/or postpartum patient care is provided except delivery due to termination of pregnancy by abortion or referral to another physician or other qualified health care professional for delivery, see the antepartum and postpartum care codes 59425, 59426 and 59430.

(For circumcision of newborn, see 54150, 54160)

ANTEPARTUM AND FETAL INVASIVE SERVICES

(For fetal intrauterine transfusion, use 36460)

(For unlisted fetal invasive procedure, use 59897)

59000 Amniocentesis, diagnostic
(For radiological supervision and interpretation, use 76946)

59001 therapeutic amniotic fluid reduction (includes ultrasound guidance)

59012 Cordocentesis (intrauterine), any method
(For radiological supervision and interpretation, use 76941)

59015 Chorionic villus sampling, any method
(For radiological supervision and interpretation, use 76945)

59020 Fetal contraction stress test

59025 Fetal non-stress test

59030 Fetal scalp blood sampling
(For repeat fetal scalp blood sampling, use 59030 and see modifiers -76 and -77)

59050 Fetal monitoring during labor by consulting physician (ie, non-attending physician) with written report; supervision and interpretation

Separate Procedure　　Unlisted Procedure　　CCI Comp. Code　　Non-specific Procedure　　**577**

59051	interpretation only
59070	Transabdominal amnioinfusion, including ultrasound guidance
59072	Fetal umbilical cord occlusion, including ultrasound guidance
59074	Fetal fluid drainage (eg, vesicocentesis, thoracocentesis, paracentesis), including ultrasound guidance
59076	Fetal shunt placement, including ultrasound guidance

EXCISION

59100	Hysterotomy, abdominal (eg, for hydatidiform mole, abortion)
	(When tubal ligation is performed at the same time as hysterotomy, use 58611 in addition to 59100)
59120	Surgical treatment of ectopic pregnancy; tubal or ovarian, requiring salpingectomy and/or oophorectomy, abdominal or vaginal approach
59121	tubal or ovarian, without salpingectomy and/or oophorectomy
59130	abdominal pregnancy
59135	interstitial, uterine pregnancy requiring total hysterectomy
59136	interstitial, uterine pregnancy with partial resection of uterus
59140	cervical, with evacuation
59150	Laparoscopic treatment of ectopic pregnancy; without salpingectomy and/or oophorectomy
59151	with salpingectomy and/or oophorectomy
59160	Curettage, postpartum

INTRODUCTION

	(For intrauterine fetal transfusion, use 36460)
	(For introduction of hypertonic solution and/or prostaglandins to initiate labor, see 59850-59857)
59200	Insertion of cervical dilator (eg, laminaria, prostaglandin) (separate procedure)

REPAIR

	(For tracheoplasty, use 57700)
59300	Episiotomy or vaginal repair, by other than attending
59320	Cerclage of cervix, during pregnancy; vaginal
59325	abdominal
59350	Hysterorrhaphy of ruptured uterus

VAGINAL DELIVERY, ANTEPARTUM AND POSTPARTUM CARE

59400	Routine obstetric care including antepartum care, vaginal delivery (with or without episiotomy, and/or forceps) and postpartum care
59409	Vaginal delivery only (with or without episiotomy and/or forceps);

● New Code   ▲ Revised Code   + Add-On Code   ⊘ Modifier -51 Exempt   ★ Telemedicine

59410   including postpartum care

59412   External cephalic version, with or without tocolysis

(Use 59412 in addition to code(s) for delivery)

59414   Delivery of placenta (separate procedure)

(For antepartum care only, see 59425, 59426 or appropriate E/M code(s))

(For 1-3 antepartum care visits, see appropriate E/M code(s))

59425   Antepartum care only; 4-6 visits

59426   7 or more visits

59430   Postpartum care only (separate procedure)

CESAREAN DELIVERY

(For standby attendance for infant, use 99360)

(For low cervical cesarean section, see 59510, 59515, 59525)

59510   Routine obstetric care including antepartum care, cesarean delivery, and postpartum care

59514   Cesarean delivery only;

59515   including postpartum care

(For classic cesarean section, see 59510, 59515, 59525)

+ 59525   Subtotal or total hysterectomy after cesarean delivery (List separately in addition to code for primary procedure)

(Use 59525 in conjunction with codes 59510, 59514, 59515, 59618, 59620, 59622)

(For extraperitoneal cesarean section, or cesarean section with subtotal or total hysterectomy, see 59510, 59515, 59525)

DELIVERY AFTER PREVIOUS CESAREAN DELIVERY

Patients who have had a previous cesarean delivery and now present with the expectation of a vaginal delivery are coded using codes 59610-59622. If the patient has a successful vaginal delivery after a previous cesarean delivery (VBAC), use codes 59610-59614. If the attempt is unsuccessful and another cesarean delivery is carried out, use codes 59618-59622. To report elective cesarean deliveries use code 59510, 59514 or 59515.

59610   Routine obstetric care including antepartum care, vaginal delivery (with or without episiotomy, and/or forceps) and postpartum care, after previous cesarean delivery

59612   Vaginal delivery only, after previous cesarean delivery (with or without episiotomy and/or forceps);

59614   including postpartum care

59618   Routine obstetric care including antepartum care, cesarean delivery, and postpartum care, following attempted vaginal delivery after previous cesarean delivery

59620   Cesarean delivery only, following attempted vaginal delivery after previous cesarean delivery;

59622   including postpartum care

Separate Procedure   Unlisted Procedure   CCI Comp. Code   Non-specific Procedure   **579**

ABORTION

(For medical treatment of spontaneous complete abortion, any trimester, use E/M codes 99202-99233)

(For surgical treatment of spontaneous abortion, use 59812)

59812 Treatment of incomplete abortion, any trimester, completed surgically

59820 Treatment of missed abortion, completed surgically; first trimester

59821 second trimester

59830 Treatment of septic abortion, completed surgically

59840 Induced abortion, by dilation and curettage

59841 Induced abortion, by dilation and evacuation

59850 Induced abortion, by 1 or more intra-amniotic injections (amniocentesis-injections), including hospital admission and visits, delivery of fetus and secundines;

59851 with dilation and curettage and/or evacuation

59852 with hysterotomy (failed intra-amniotic injection)

(For insertion of cervical dilator, use 59200)

59855 Induced abortion, by 1 or more vaginal suppositories (eg, prostaglandin) with or without cervical dilation (eg, laminaria), including hospital admission and visits, delivery of fetus and secundines;

59856 with dilation and curettage and/or evacuation

59857 with hysterotomy (failed medical evacuation)

OTHER PROCEDURES

59866 Multifetal pregnancy reduction(s) (MPR)

59870 Uterine evacuation and curettage for hydatidiform mole

59871 Removal of cerclage suture under anesthesia (other than local)

59897 Unlisted fetal invasive procedure, including ultrasound guidance, when performed

59898 Unlisted laparoscopy procedure, maternity care and delivery

59899 Unlisted procedure, maternity care and delivery

● New Code ▲ Revised Code ✚ Add-On Code ⊘ Modifier -51 Exempt ★ Telemedicine

ENDOCRINE SYSTEM

(For pituitary and pineal surgery, see Nervous System)

THYROID GLAND

INCISION

60000 Incision and drainage of thyroglossal duct cyst, infected

EXCISION

60100 Biopsy thyroid, percutaneous core needle

(If imaging guidance is performed, see 76942, 77002, 77012, 77021)

(For fine needle aspiration biopsy, see 10004, 10005, 10006, 10007, 10008, 10009, 10010, 10011, 10012, 10021)

(For evaluation of fine needle aspirate, see 88172, 88173)

60200 Excision of cyst or adenoma of thyroid, or transection of isthmus

60210 Partial thyroid lobectomy, unilateral; with or without isthmusectomy

60212   with contralateral subtotal lobectomy, including isthmusectomy

60220 Total thyroid lobectomy, unilateral; with or without isthmusectomy

60225   with contralateral subtotal lobectomy, including isthmusectomy

60240 Thyroidectomy, total or complete

(For thyroidectomy, subtotal or partial, use 60271)

60252 Thyroidectomy, total or subtotal for malignancy; with limited neck dissection

60254   with radical neck dissection

60260 Thyroidectomy, removal of all remaining thyroid tissue following previous removal of a portion of thyroid

(For bilateral procedure, report 60260 with modifier -50)

60270 Thyroidectomy, including substernal thyroid; sternal split or transthoracic approach

60271   cervical approach

60280 Excision of thyroglossal duct cyst or sinus;

60281   recurrent

(For thyroid ultrasonography, use 76536)

REMOVAL

60300 Aspiration and/or injection, thyroid cyst

(For fine needle aspiration biopsy, see 10004, 10005, 10006, 10007, 10008, 10009, 10010, 10011, 10012, 10021)

(If imaging guidance is performed, see 76942, 77012)

Separate Procedure   Unlisted Procedure   CCI Comp. Code   •   Non-specific Procedure   **581**

PARATHYROID, THYMUS, ADRENAL GLANDS, PANCREAS, AND CAROTID BODY

EXCISION

(For pituitary and pineal surgery, see Nervous System)

60500 Parathyroidectomy or exploration of parathyroid(s);

60502 re-exploration

60505 with mediastinal exploration, sternal split or transthoracic approach

+ 60512 Parathyroid autotransplantation (List separately in addition to code for primary procedure)

(Use 60512 in conjunction with codes 60500, 60502, 60505, 60212, 60225, 60240, 60252, 60254, 60260, 60270, 60271)

60520 Thymectomy, partial or total; transcervical approach (separate procedure)

60521 sternal split or transthoracic approach, without radical mediastinal dissection (separate procedure)

60522 sternal split or transthoracic approach, with radical mediastinal dissection (separate procedure)

(For thoracoscopic [VATS] thymectomy, see 32673)

60540 Adrenalectomy, partial or complete, or exploration of adrenal gland with or without biopsy, transabdominal, lumbar or dorsal (separate procedure);

60545 with excision of adjacent retroperitoneal tumor

(Do not report 60540, 60545 in conjunction with 50323)

(For bilateral procedure, report 60540 with modifier 50)

(For excision of remote or disseminated pheochromocytoma, see 49203-49205)

(For laparoscopic approach, use 56321)

60600 Excision of carotid body tumor; without excision of carotid artery

60605 with excision of carotid artery

LAPAROSCOPY

Surgical laparoscopy always includes diagnostic laparoscopy. To report a diagnostic laparoscopy (peritoneoscopy) (separate procedure), use 49320.

60650 Laparoscopy, surgical, with adrenalectomy, partial or complete, or exploration of adrenal gland with or without biopsy, transabdominal, lumbar or dorsal

60659 Unlisted laparoscopy procedure, endocrine system

OTHER PROCEDURES

60699 Unlisted procedure, endocrine system

● New Code ▲ Revised Code + Add-On Code ⊘ Modifier -51 Exempt ★ Telemedicine

NERVOUS SYSTEM

There are numerous codes for spinal injections found in this section. Review documentation for whether the injection is a single one, differential one or continuous. Also determine the number of levels involved when a regional block is administered.

SKULL, MENINGES, AND BRAIN

(For injection procedure for cerebral angiography, see 36100-36218)

(For injection procedure for ventriculography, see 61026, 61120, 61130)

(For injection procedure for pneumoencephalography, use 61055)

INJECTION, DRAINAGE OR ASPIRATION

61000 Subdural tap through fontanelle, or suture, infant, unilateral or bilateral; initial

61001 subsequent taps

61020 Ventricular puncture through previous burr hole, fontanelle, suture, or implanted ventricular catheter/reservoir; without injection

61026 with injection of medication or other substance for diagnosis or treatment

61050 Cisternal or lateral cervical (C1-C2) puncture; without injection (separate procedure)

61055 with injection of medication or other substance for diagnosis or treatment

(Do not report 61055 in conjunction with 62302, 62303, 62304, 62305)

(For radiological supervision and interpretation by a different physician or qualified health care professional, see Radiology)

61070 Puncture of shunt tubing or reservoir for aspiration or injection procedure

(For radiological supervision and interpretation, use 75809)

TWIST DRILL, BURR HOLE(S), OR TREPHINE

61105 Twist drill hole(s) for subdural or ventricular puncture;

⊘ **61107** Twist drill hole(s) for subdural, intracerebral or ventricular puncture; for implanting ventricular catheter, pressure recording device, or other intracerebral monitoring device

(For intracranial neuroendoscopic ventricular catheter placement, use 62160)

61108 for evacuation and/or drainage of subdural hematoma

61120 Burr hole(s) for ventricular puncture (including injection of gas, contrast media, dye, or radioactive material)

61140 Burr hole(s) or trephine; with biopsy of brain or intracranial lesion

61150 with drainage of brain abscess or cyst

61151 with subsequent tapping (aspiration) of intracranial abscess or cyst

61154 Burr hole(s) with evacuation and/or drainage of hematoma, extradural or subdural

(For bilateral procedure, report 61154 with modifier -50)

61156 Burr hole(s); with aspiration of hematoma or cyst, intracerebral

---

Separate Procedure   Unlisted Procedure   CCI Comp. Code   Non-specific Procedure   **583**

61210 for implanting ventricular catheter, reservoir, EEG electrode(s), pressure recording device, or other cerebral monitoring device (separate procedure)

(For intracranial neuroendoscopic ventricular catheter placement, use 62160)

61215 Insertion of subcutaneous reservoir, pump or continuous infusion system for connection to ventricular catheter

(For refilling and maintenance of an implantable infusion pump for spinal or brain drug therapy, use 95990)

(For chemotherapy, use 96450)

61250 Burr hole(s) or trephine, supratentorial, exploratory, not followed by other surgery

(For bilateral procedure, report 61250 with modifier -50)

61253 Burr hole(s) or trephine, infratentorial, unilateral or bilateral

(If burr hole(s) or trephine are followed by craniotomy at same operative session, use 61304-61321; do not use 61250 or 61253)

CRANIECTOMY OR CRANIOTOMY

61304 Craniectomy or craniotomy, exploratory; supratentorial

61305 infratentorial (posterior fossa)

61312 Craniectomy or craniotomy for evacuation of hematoma, supratentorial; extradural or subdural

61313 intracerebral

61314 Craniectomy or craniotomy for evacuation of hematoma, infratentorial; extradural or subdural

61315 intracerebellar

+ **61316** Incision and subcutaneous placement of cranial bone graft (List separately in addition to code for primary procedure)

(Use 61316 in conjunction with codes 61304, 61312, 61313, 61322, 61323, 61340, 61570, 61571, 61680-61705)

61320 Craniectomy or craniotomy, drainage of intracranial abscess; supratentorial

61321 infratentorial

61322 Craniectomy or craniotomy, decompressive, with or without duraplasty, for treatment of intracranial hypertension, without evacuation of associated intraparenchymal hematoma; without lobectomy

(Do not report 61313 in addition to 61322)

(For subtemporal decompression, use 61340)

61323 with lobectomy

(Do not report 61313 in addition to 61323)

(For subtemporal decompression, use 61340)

61330 Decompression of orbit only, transcranial approach

(For bilateral procedure, report 61330 with modifier -50)

(**61332** deleted 2018 [2019 Edition])

● New Code ▲ Revised Code + Add-On Code ⊘ Modifier -51 Exempt ★ Telemedicine

61333   with removal of lesion

61340   Subtemporal cranial decompression (pseudotumor cerebri, slit ventricle syndrome)

      (For bilateral procedure, report 61340 with modifier -50)

      (For decompressive craniotomy or craniectomy for intracranial hypertension, without hematoma evacuation, see 61322, 61323)

61343   Craniectomy, suboccipital with cervical laminectomy for decompression of medulla and spinal cord, with or without dural graft (eg, Arnold-Chiari malformation)

61345   Other cranial decompression, posterior fossa

      (For orbital decompression by lateral wall approach, Kroenlein type, use 67445)

61450   Craniectomy, subtemporal, for section, compression, or decompression of sensory root of gasserian ganglion

61458   Craniectomy, suboccipital; for exploration or decompression of cranial nerves

61460   for section of 1 or more cranial nerves

(**61480**   deleted 2018 [2019 Edition])

61500   Craniectomy; with excision of tumor or other bone lesion of skull

61501   for osteomyelitis

61510   Craniectomy, trephination, bone flap craniotomy; for excision of brain tumor, supratentorial, except meningioma

61512   for excision of meningioma, supratentorial

61514   for excision of brain abscess, supratentorial

61516   for excision or fenestration of cyst, supratentorial

      (For excision of pituitary tumor or craniopharyngioma, see 61545, 61546, 61548)

+ **61517**   Implantation of brain intracavitary chemotherapy agent (List separately in addition to code for primary procedure)

      (Use 61517 only in conjunction with codes 61510 or 61518)

      (Do not report 61517 for brachytherapy insertion. For intracavitary insertion of radioelement sources or ribbons, see 77770, 77771, 77772)

61518   Craniectomy for excision of brain tumor, infratentorial or posterior fossa; except meningioma, cerebellopontine angle tumor, or midline tumor at base of skull

61519   meningioma

61520   cerebellopontine angle tumor

61521   midline tumor at base of skull

61522   Craniectomy, infratentorial or posterior fossa; for excision of brain abscess

61524   for excision or fenestration of cyst

61526   Craniectomy, bone flap craniotomy, transtemporal (mastoid) for excision of cerebellopontine angle tumor;

61530   combined with middle/posterior fossa craniotomy/ craniectomy

61531   Subdural implantation of strip electrodes through 1 or more burr or trephine hole(s) for long term seizure monitoring

     (For stereotactic implantation of electrodes, use 61760)

     (For craniotomy for excision of intracranial arteriovenous malformation, see 61680-61692)

61533   Craniotomy with elevation of bone flap; for subdural implantation of an electrode array, for long term seizure monitoring

     (For continuous EEG monitoring, see 95700-95726)

61534   for excision of epileptogenic focus without electrocorticography during surgery

61535   for removal of epidural or subdural electrode array, without excision of cerebral tissue (separate procedure)

61536   for excision of cerebral epileptogenic focus, with electrocorticography during surgery (includes removal of electrode array)

61537   for lobectomy, temporal lobe, without electrocorticography during surgery

61538   for lobectomy, temporal lobe, with electrocorticography during surgery

61539   for lobectomy, other than temporal lobe, partial or total, with electrocorticography during surgery

61540   for lobectomy, other than temporal lobe, partial or total, without electrocorticography during surgery

61541   for transection of corpus callosum

61543   for partial or subtotal (functional) hemispherectomy

61544   for excision or coagulation of choroid plexus

61545   for excision of craniopharyngioma

     (For craniotomy for selective amygdalohippocampectomy, use 61566)

     (For craniotomy for multiple subpial transections during surgery, use 61567)

61546   Craniotomy for hypophysectomy or excision of pituitary tumor, intracranial approach

61548   Hypophysectomy or excision of pituitary tumor, transnasal or transseptal approach, nonstereotactic

     (Do not report code 69990 in addition to code 61548)

61550   Craniectomy for craniosynostosis; single cranial suture

61552   multiple cranial sutures

     (For cranial reconstruction for orbital hypertelorism, see 21260-21263)

     (For reconstruction, see 21172-21180)

61556   Craniotomy for craniosynostosis; frontal or parietal bone flap

61557   bifrontal bone flap

61558   Extensive craniectomy for multiple cranial suture craniosynostosis (eg, cloverleaf skull); not requiring bone grafts

---

   ● New Code   ▲ Revised Code   + Add-On Code   ⊘ Modifier -51 Exempt   ★ Telemedicine

61559   recontouring with multiple osteotomies and bone autografts (eg, barrel-stave procedure) (includes obtaining grafts)

(For reconstruction, see 21172-21180)

61563   Excision, intra and extracranial, benign tumor of cranial bone (eg, fibrous dysplasia); without optic nerve decompression

61564   with optic nerve decompression

(For reconstruction, see 21181-21183)

61566   Craniotomy with elevation of bone flap; for selective amygdalohippocampectomy

61567   for multiple subpial transections, with electrocorticography during surgery

61570   Craniectomy or craniotomy; with excision of foreign body from brain

61571   with treatment of penetrating wound of brain

(For sequestrectomy for osteomyelitis, use 61501)

61575   Transoral approach to skull base, brain stem or upper spinal cord for biopsy, decompression or excision of lesion;

61576   requiring splitting of tongue and/or mandible (including tracheostomy)

(For arthrodesis, use 22548)

SURGERY OF SKULL BASE

The surgical management of lesions involving the skull base (base of anterior, middle, and posterior cranial fossae) often requires the skills of several surgeons of different surgical specialties working together or in tandem during the operative session. These operations are usually not staged because of the need for definitive closure of dura, subcutaneous tissues, and skin to avoid serious infections such as osteomyelitis and/or meningitis.

For primary closure, see the appropriate codes (ie, 15730, 15733, 15756, 15757, 15758).

When one surgeon performs the approach procedure, another surgeon performs the definitive procedure, and another surgeon performs the repair/reconstruction procedure, each surgeon reports only the code for the specific procedure performed.

If one surgeon performs more than one procedure (ie, approach procedure and definitive procedure), then both codes are reported, adding modifier -51 to the seondary, additional procedure(s).

APPROACH PROCEDURES

Anterior Cranial Fossa

61580   Craniofacial approach to anterior cranial fossa; extradural, including lateral rhinotomy, ethmoidectomy, sphenoidectomy, without maxillectomy or orbital exenteration

61581   extradural, including lateral rhinotomy, orbital exenteration, ethmoidectomy, sphenoidectomy and/or maxillectomy

61582   extradural, including unilateral or bifrontal craniotomy, elevation of frontal lobe(s), osteotomy of base of anterior cranial fossa

61583   intradural, including unilateral or bifrontal craniotomy, elevation or resection of frontal lobe, osteotomy of base of anterior cranial fossa

61584   Orbitocranial approach to anterior cranial fossa, extradural, including supraorbital ridge osteotomy and elevation of frontal and/or temporal lobe(s); without orbital exenteration

---

61585   with orbital exenteration

61586   Bicoronal, transzygomatic and/or LeFort I osteotomy approach to anterior cranial fossa with or without internal fixation, without bone graft

Middle Cranial Fossa

61590   Infratemporal pre-auricular approach to middle cranial fossa (parapharyngeal space, infratemporal and midline skull base, nasopharynx), with or without disarticulation of the mandible, including parotidectomy, craniotomy, decompression and/or mobilization of the facial nerve and/or petrous carotid artery

61591   Infratemporal post-auricular approach to middle cranial fossa (internal auditory meatus, petrous apex, tentorium, cavernous sinus, parasellar area, infratemporal fossa) including mastoidectomy, resection of sigmoid sinus, with or without decompression and/or mobilization of contents of auditory canal or petrous carotid artery

61592   Orbitocranial zygomatic approach to middle cranial fossa (cavernous sinus and carotid artery, clivus, basilar artery or petrous apex) including osteotomy of zygoma, craniotomy, extra- or intradural elevation of temporal lobe

Posterior Cranial Fossa

61595   Transtemporal approach to posterior cranial fossa, jugular foramen or midline skull base, including mastoidectomy, decompression of sigmoid sinus and/or facial nerve, with or without mobilization

61596   Transcochlear approach to posterior cranial fossa, jugular foramen or midline skull base, including labyrinthectomy, decompression, with or without mobilization of facial nerve and/or petrous carotid artery

61597   Transcondylar (far lateral) approach to posterior cranial fossa, jugular foramen or midline skull base, including occipital condylectomy, mastoidectomy, resection of C1-C3 vertebral body(s), decompression of vertebral artery, with or without mobilization

61598   Transpetrosal approach to posterior cranial fossa, clivus or foramen magnum, including ligation of superior petrosal sinus and/or sigmoid sinus

DEFINITIVE PROCEDURES

Base of Anterior Cranial Fossa

61600   Resection or excision of neoplastic, vascular or infectious lesion of base of anterior cranial fossa; extradural

61601   intradural, including dural repair, with or without graft

Base of Middle Cranial Fossa

61605   Resection or excision of neoplastic, vascular or infectious lesion of infratemporal fossa, parapharyngeal space, petrous apex; extradural

61606   intradural, including dural repair, with or without graft

61607   Resection or excision of neoplastic, vascular or infectious lesion of parasellar area, cavernous sinus, clivus or midline skull base; extradural

61608   intradural, including dural repair, with or without graft

(**61610**   deleted 2018 [2019 Edition])

Code 61611 is reported in addition to code(s) for primary procedure(s) 61605-61608. Report only one transection or ligation of carotid artery code per operative session.

   ● New Code   ▲ Revised Code   ✛ Add-On Code   ⊘ Modifier -51 Exempt   ★ Telemedicine

+ 61611 Transection or ligation, carotid artery in petrous canal; without repair (List separately in addition to code for primary procedure)

(61612 deleted 2018 [2019 Edition])

61613 Obliteration of carotid aneurysm, arteriovenous malformation, or carotid-cavernous fistula by dissection within cavernous sinus

Base of Posterior Cranial Fossa

61615 Resection or excision of neoplastic, vascular or infectious lesion of base of posterior cranial fossa, jugular foramen, foramen magnum, or C1-C3 vertebral bodies; extradural

61616   intradural, including dural repair, with or without graft

REPAIR AND/OR RECONSTRUCTION OF SURGICAL DEFECTS OF SKULL BASE

61618 Secondary repair of dura for cerebrospinal fluid leak, anterior, middle or posterior cranial fossa following surgery of the skull base; by free tissue graft (eg, pericranium, fascia, tensor fascia lata, adipose tissue, homologous or synthetic grafts)

61619   by local or regionalized vascularized pedicle flap or myocutaneous flap (including galea, temporalis, frontalis or occipitalis muscle)

ENDOVASCULAR THERAPY

61623 Endovascular temporary balloon arterial occlusion, head or neck (extracranial/intracranial) including selective catheterization of vessel to be occluded, positioning and inflation of occlusion balloon, concomitant neurological monitoring, and radiologic supervision and interpretation of all angiography required for balloon occlusion and to exclude vascular injury post occlusion

(If selective catheterization and angiography of arteries other than artery to be occluded is performed, use appropriate catheterization and radiologic supervision and interpretation codes)

(If complete diagnostic angiography of the artery to be occluded is performed immediately prior to temporary occlusion, use appropriate radiologic supervision and interpretation codes only)

61624 Transcatheter permanent occlusion or embolization (eg, for tumor destruction, to achieve hemostasis, to occlude a vascular malformation), percutaneous, any method; central nervous system (intracranial, spinal cord)

(For non-central nervous system and non-head or neck embolization, see 37241-37244)

(For radiological supervision and interpretation, use 75894)

61626   non-central nervous system, head or neck (extracranial, brachiocephalic branch)

(For non-central nervous system and non-head or neck embolization, see 37241-37244)

(For radiological supervision and interpretation, use 75894)

61630 Balloon angioplasty, intracranial (eg, atherosclerotic stenosis), percutaneous

61635 Transcatheter placement of intravascular stent(s), intracranial (eg, atherosclerotic stenosis), including balloon angioplasty, if performed

(61630 and 61635 include all selective vascular catheterization of the target vascular territory, all diagnostic imaging for arteriography of the target vascular territory, and all related radiological supervision and interpretation. When diagnostic arteriogram (including imaging and selective catheterization) confirms the need for angioplasty or stent placement, 61630 and 61635 are inclusive of these services. If angioplasty or stenting are not indicated, then the appropriate codes for selective catheterization and imaging should be reported in lieu of 61630 and 61635)

(Do not report 61630 or 61635 in conjunction with 61645 for the same vascular territory)

(For definition of vascular territory, see the Nervous System Endovascular Therapy guidelines)

61640 Balloon dilatation of intracranial vasospasm, percutaneous; initial vessel

+ 61641 each additional vessel in same vascular territory (List separately in addition to code for primary procedure)

+ 61642 each additional vessel in different vascular territory (List separately in addition to code for primary procedure)

(Use 61641 and 61642 in conjunction with 61640)

(61640, 61641, 61642 include all selective vascular catheterization of the target vessel, contrast injection(s), vessel measurement, roadmapping, postdilatation angiography, and fluoroscopic guidance for the balloon dilatation)

(Do not report 61640, 61642 in conjunction with 61650 ir 61651 for the same vascular territory)

(For definition of vascular territory, see the Nervous System Endovascular Therapy guidelines)

Codes 61645, 61650, 61651 describe cerebral endovascular therapeutic interventions in any intracranial artery. They include selective catheterization, diagnostic angiographpy, and all subsequent angiography including associated radiological supervision and interpretation within the treated vascular territory, fluoroscopic guidance, neurologic and hemodynamic monitoring of the patient, and closure of the arteriotomy by manual pressure, an arterial closure device, or suture.

For purposes of reporting services described by 61645, 61650, 61651, the intracranial arteries are divided into three vascular territories: 1) right carotid circulation; 2) left carotid circulation; 3) vertebro basilar circulation. Code 61645 may be reported once for each intracranial vascular territory treated. Code 61650 is reported once for the first intracranial vascular territory treated with intra-arterial prolonged administration of pharmacologic agent(s). If additional intracranial vascular territory(ies) is also treated with intra-arterial prolonged administration of pharmacologic agent(s) during the same session, the treatment of each additional vascular territory(ies) is reported using 61651 (may be reported maximally two times per day).

Code 61645 describes endovascular revascularization of thrombotic/embolic occlusion of intracranial arterial vessel(s) via any method, including mechanical thrombectomy (eg, mechanical retrieval device, aspiration catheter) and/or the administration of any agent(s) for the purpose of revascularization, such as thrombolytics or IIB/IIIA inhibitors.

Code 61650, 61651 describe the cerebral endovascular continuous or intermittent therapeutic prolonged administration of any non-thrombolytic agent(s) (eg, spasmolytics or chemotherapy) into an artery to treat non-iatrogenic central nervous system diseases or sequelae thereof. These code should not be used to report administration of agents (eg, heparin, nitroglycerin, saline) usually administered during endovascular interventions. These codes are used for prolonged administrations, ie, of at least 10 minutes continuous or intermittent duration.

Do not report 61645, 61650, or 61651 in conjunction with 36221, 36226, 36228, 37184, or 37186 for the treated vascular territory. Do not report 61645 in conjunction with 61650 or 61651 for the same vascular distribution. Diagnostic angiography of a non-treated vascular territory may be reported separately. For example, angiography of the left carotid and/or the vertebral circulations may be reported if the intervention is performed in the right carotid circulation.

61645 Percutaneous arterial transluminal mechanical thrombectomy and/or infusion for thrombolysis, intracranial, any method, including diagnostic angiography, fluoroscopic guidance, catheter placement, and intraprocedural pharmacological thrombolytic injection(s)

(Do not report 61645 in conjunction with, 37184, 61630, 61635, 61650, 61651 for the same vascular territory)

(To report venous mechanical thrombectomy and/or thrombolysis, see 37187, 37188, 37212, 37214)

61650 Endovascular intracranial prolonged administration of pharmacologic agent(s) other than for thrombolysis, arterial, including catheter placement, diagnostic angiography, and imaging guidance; initial vascular territory

+ 61651 each additional vascular territory (List separately in addition to code for primary procedure)

(Use 61651 in conjunction with 61650)

(Do not report 61650 or 61651 in conjunction with 36221, 36222, 36223, 36224, 36225, 36226, 61640, 61641, 61642, 61645 for the same vascular territory)

(Do not report 61650 or 61651 in conjunction with 96420, 96422, 96423, 96425 for the same vascular territory)

SURGERY FOR ANEURYSM, ARTERIOVENOUS MALFORMATION OR VASCULAR DISEASE

Includes craniotomy when appropriate for procedure.

61680 Surgery of intracranial arteriovenous malformation; supratentorial, simple

61682 supratentorial, complex

61684 infratentorial, simple

61686 infratentorial, complex

61690 dural, simple

61692 dural, complex

61697 Surgery of complex intracranial aneurysm, intracranial approach; carotid circulation

61698 vertebrobasilar circulation

(61697, 61698 involve aneurysms that are larger than 15 mm or with calcification of the aneurysm neck, or with incorporation of normal vessels into the aneurysm neck, or a procedure requiring temporary vessel occlusion, trapping or cardiopulmonary bypass to successfully treat the aneurysm)

61700 Surgery of simple intracranial aneurysm, intracranial approach; carotid circulation

61702 vertebrobasilar circulation

61703 Surgery of intracranial aneurysm, cervical approach by application of occluding clamp to cervical carotid artery (Selverstone-Crutchfield type)

(For cervical approach for direct ligation of carotid artery, see 37600-37606)

61705 Surgery of aneurysm, vascular malformation or carotid-cavernous fistula; by intracranial and cervical occlusion of carotid artery

61708 by intracranial electrothrombosis

(For ligation or gradual occlusion of internal/common carotid artery, see 37605, 37606)

61710 by intra-arterial embolization, injection procedure, or balloon catheter

61711 Anastomosis, arterial, extracranial-intracranial (eg, middle cerebral/cortical) arteries

(For carotid or vertebral thromboendarterectomy, use 35301)

(Use 69990 when the surgical microscope is employed for the microsurgical procedure. Do not use 69990 for visualization with magnifying loupes or corrected vision)

STEREOTAXIS

61720 Creation of lesion by stereotactic method, including burr hole(s) and localizing and recording techniques, single or multiple stages; globus pallidus or thalamus

61735 subcortical structure(s) other than globus pallidus or thalamus

61750 Stereotactic biopsy, aspiration, or excision, including burr hole(s), for intracranial lesion;

| Separate Procedure | Unlisted Procedure | CCI Comp. Code | Non-specific Procedure | **591** |

61751   with computed tomography and/or magnetic resonance guidance

(For radiological supervision and interpretation of computerized tomography, see 70450, 70460, or 70470 as appropriate)

(For radiological supervision and interpretation of magnetic resonance imaging, see 70551, 70552, or 70553 as appropriate)

61760   Stereotactic implantation of depth electrodes into the cerebrum for long term seizure monitoring

61770   Stereotactic localization, including burr hole(s), with insertion of catheter(s) or probe(s) for placement of radiation source

+ 61781   Stereotactic computer-assisted (navigational) procedure; cranial, intradural (list separately in addition to code for primary procedure)

(Do not report 61781 in conjunction with 61720-61791, 61796-61799, 61863-61868, 62201, 77371-77373, 77432)

+ 61782   cranial, extradural (list separately in addition to code for primary procedure)

(Do not report 61781, 61782 by the same individual during the same surgical session)

+ 61783   spinal (list separately in addition to code for primary procedure)

(Do not report 61783 in conjunction with 63620, 63621)

61790   Creation of lesion by stereotactic method, percutaneous, by neurolytic agent (eg, alcohol, thermal, electrical, radiofrequency); gasserian ganglion

61791   trigeminal medullary tract

STEREOTACTIC RADIOSURGERY (CRANIAL)

Cranial stereotactic radiosurgery is a distinct procedure that utilizes externally generated ionizing radiation to inactivate or eradicate defined target(s) in the head without the need to make an incision. The target is defined by and the treatment is delivered using high-resolution stereotactic imaging. Stereotactic radiosurgery codes and headframe application procedures are reported by the neurosurgeon. The radiation oncologist reports the appropriate code(s) for clinical treatment planning, physics and dosimetry, treatment delivery, and management from the Radiation Oncology section (77261-77790). Any necessary planning, dosimetry, targeting, positioning, or blocking by the neurosurgeon is included in the stereotactic radiation surgery services. The same individual should not report stereotactic radiosurgery services with radiation treatment management codes (77427-77435).

Do not report stereotactic radiosurgery more than once per lesion per course of treatment when the treatment requires more than one session.

Codes 61796 and 61797 involve stereotactic radiosurgery for simple cranial lesions. Simple cranial lesions are lesions less than 3.5 cm in maximum dimension that do not meet the definition of a complex lesion provided below. Report code 61796 when all lesions are simple.

Codes 61798 and 61799 involve stereotactic radiosurgery for complex cranial lesions and procedures that create therapeutic lesions (eg., thalamotomy or pallidotomy). All lesions 3.5 cm in maximum dimension or greater are complex. When performing therapeutic lesion creation procedures, report code 61798 only once regardless of the number of lesions created. Schwannomas, arterio-venous malformations, pituitary tumors, glomus tumors, pineal region tumors and cavernous sinus/parasellar/petroclival tumors are complex. Any lesion that is adjacent (5 mm or less) to the optic nerve/optic chasm/optic tract or within the brainstem is complex. If treating multiple lesions, and any single lesion treated is complex, use 61798.

Do not report 61796-61800 in conjunction with code 20660.

Codes 61796-61799 include computer-assisted planning. Do not report codes 61796-61799 in conjunction with 61795.

(For intensity modulated beam delivery plan and treatment, see 77301, 77385, 77386. For stereotactic body radiation therapy, see 77373, 77435)

   ●   New Code   ▲   Revised Code   +   Add-On Code   ⊘   Modifier -51 Exempt   ★   Telemedicine

61796 Stereotactic radiosurgery (particle beam, gamma ray, or linear accelerator); 1 simple cranial lesion

(Do not report 61796 more than once per course of treatment)

(Do not report 61796 in conjunction with 61798)

+ **61797** each additional cranial lesion, simple (list separately in addition to code for primary procedure)

(Use 61797 in conjunction with 61796, 61798)

(For each course of treatment, 61797 and 61799 may be reported no more than once per lesion. Do not report any combination of 61797 and 61799 more than 4 times for entire course of treatment regardless of number of lesions treated)

61798 1 complex cranial lesion

(Do not report 61798 more than once per course of treatment)

(Do not report 61798 in conjunction with 61796)

+ **61799** each additional cranial lesion, complex (list separately in addition to code for primary procedure)

(Use 61799 in conjunction with 61798)

(For each course of treatment, 61797 and 61799 may be reported no more than once per lesion. Do not report any combination of 61797 and 61799 more than 4 times for entire course of treatment regardless of number of lesions treated)

+ **61800** Application of stereotactic headframe for stereotactic radiosurgery (list separately in addition to code for primary procedure)

(Use 61800 in conjunction with 61796, 61798)

NEUROSTIMULATORS (INTRACRANIAL)

For electronic analysis with programming, when performed, of cranial nerve and brain neurostimulator pulse generator/transmitters, see codes 95970, 95976, 95977, 95983, 95984. Test stimulation to confirm correct target site placement of the electrode array(s) and/or to confirm the functional status of the system is inherent to placement and is not separately reported as electronic analysis or programming of the neurostimulator system. Electronic analysis (95970) at the time of implantation is not separately reported.

Microelectrode recording, when performed by the operating surgeon in association with implantation of neurostimulator electrode arrays, is an inclusive service and should not be reported separately. If another individual participates in neurophysiological mapping during a deep brain stimulator implantation procedure, this service may be reported by the second individual with codes 95961-95962.

61850 Twist drill or burr hole(s) for implantation of neurostimulator electrodes, cortical

61860 Craniectomy or craniotomy for implantation of neurostimulator electrodes, cerebral, cortical

61863 Twist drill, burr hole, craniotomy, or craniectomy with stereotactic implantation of neurostimulator electrode array in subcortical site (eg, thalamus, globus pallidus, subthalamic nucleus, periventricular, periaqueductal gray), without use of intraoperative microelectrode recording; first array

+ **61864** each additional array (List separately in addition to primary procedure)

(Use 61864 in conjunction with 61863)

61867 Twist drill, burr hole, craniotomy, or craniectomy with stereotactic implantation of neurostimulator electrode array in subcortical site (eg, thalamus, globus pallidus, subthalamic nucleus, periventricular, periaqueductal gray), with use of intraoperative microelectrode recording; first array

+ **61868** each additional array (List separately in addition to primary procedure)

(Use 61868 in conjunction with 61867)

(**61870** deleted 2020 [2021 Edition])

61880 Revision or removal of intracranial neurostimulator electrodes

61885 Insertion or replacement of cranial neurostimulator pulse generator or receiver, direct or inductive coupling; with connection to a single electrode array

61886 with connection to 2 or more electrode arrays

(For percutaneous placement of cranial nerve (eg, vagus, trigeminal) neurostimulator electrode(s), use 64553)

(For revision or removal of cranial nerve (eg, vagus, trigeminal) neurostimulator electrode array, use 64569)

61888 Revision or removal of cranial neurostimulator pulse generator or receiver

(Do not report 61888 in conjunction with 61885 or 61886 for the same pulse generator)

REPAIR

62000 Elevation of depressed skull fracture; simple, extradural

62005 compound or comminuted, extradural

62010 with repair of dura and/or debridement of brain

62100 Craniotomy for repair of dural/cerebrospinal fluid leak, including surgery for rhinorrhea/otorrhea

(For repair of spinal dural/CSF leak, see 63707, 63709)

62115 Reduction of craniomegalic skull (eg, treated hydrocephalus); not requiring bone grafts or cranioplasty

62117 requiring craniotomy and reconstruction with or without bone graft (includes obtaining grafts)

62120 Repair of encephalocele, skull vault, including cranioplasty

62121 Craniotomy for repair of encephalocele, skull base

62140 Cranioplasty for skull defect; up to 5 cm diameter

62141 larger than 5 cm diameter

62142 Removal of bone flap or prosthetic plate of skull

62143 Replacement of bone flap or prosthetic plate of skull

62145 Cranioplasty for skull defect with reparative brain surgery

62146 Cranioplasty with autograft (includes obtaining bone grafts); up to 5 cm diameter

62147 larger than 5 cm diameter

+ **62148** Incision and retrieval of subcutaneous cranial bone graft for cranioplasty (List separately in addition to code for primary procedure)

(Use 62148 in conjunction with codes 62140-62147)

NEUROENDOSCOPY

Surgical endoscopy always includes diagnostic endoscopy

+ **62160** Neuroendoscopy, intracranial, for placement or replacement of ventricular catheter and attachment to shunt system or external drainage (List separately in addition to code for primary procedure)

   (Use 62160 only in conjunction with codes 61107, 61210, 62220-62230, 62258)

62161 Neuroendoscopy, intracranial; with dissection of adhesions, fenestration of septum pellucidum or intraventricular cysts (including placement, replacement, or removal of ventricular catheter)

62162 with fenestration or excision of colloid cyst, including placement of external ventricular catheter for drainage

(**62163** deleted 2020 [2021 Edition])

62164 with excision of brain tumor, including placement of external ventricular catheter for drainage

62165 with excision of pituitary tumor, transnasal or transsphenoidal approach

CEREBROSPINAL FLUID (CSF) SHUNT

62180 Ventriculocisternostomy (Torkildsen type operation)

62190 Creation of shunt; subarachnoid/subdural-atrial, -jugular, -auricular

62192 subarachnoid/subdural-peritoneal, -pleural, other terminus

62194 Replacement or irrigation, subarachnoid/subdural catheter

62200 Ventriculocisternostomy, third ventricle;

62201 stereotactic, neuroendoscopic method

   (For intracranial neuroendoscopic procedures, see 62161-62165)

62220 Creation of shunt; ventriculo-atrial, -jugular, -auricular

   (For intracranial neuroendoscopic ventricular catheter placement, use 62160)

62223 ventriculo-peritoneal, -pleural, other terminus

   (For intracranial neuroendoscopic ventricular catheter placement, use 62160)

62225 Replacement or irrigation, ventricular catheter

   (For intracranial neuroendoscopic ventricular catheter placement, use 62160)

62230 Replacement or revision of cerebrospinal fluid shunt, obstructed valve, or distal catheter in shunt system

   (For intracranial neuroendoscopic ventricular catheter placement, use 62160)

   (For replacement of **only** the valve and proximal catheter, use 62230 in conjunction with 62225)

62252 Reprogramming of programmable cerebrospinal shunt

62256 Removal of complete cerebrospinal fluid shunt system; without replacement

62258 with replacement by similar or other shunt at same operation

   (For percutaneous irrigation or aspiration of shunt reservoir, use 61070)

(For reprogramming of programmable CSF shunt, use 62252)

(For intracranial neuroendoscopic ventricular catheter placement, use 62160)

SPINE AND SPINAL CORD

(For application of caliper or tongs, use 20660)

(For treatment of fracture or dislocation of spine, see 22310-22327)

INJECTION, DRAINAGE, OR ASPIRATION

Injection of contrast during fluoroscopic guidance and localization is an inclusive component of 62263, 62264, 62267, 62273, 62280, 62281, 62282, 62302, 62303, 62304, 62305, 62321, 62323, 62325, 62327, 62328, 62329. Fluoroscopic guidance and localization is reported with 77003, unless a formal contrast study (myelography, epidurography, or arthrography) is performed, in which case the use of fluoroscopy is included in the supervision and interpretation codes or the myelography via lumbar injection code. Image guidance and the injection of contrast are inclusive components and are required for the performance of myelography, as described by codes 62302, 62303, 62304, 62305.

For radiologic supervision and interpretation of epidurography, use 72275. Code 72275 is only to be used when an epidurogram is performed, images documented, and a formal radiologic report is issued.

Code 62263 describes a catheter-based treatment involving targeted injection of various substances (eg., hypertonic saline, steroid, anesthetic) via an indwelling epidural catheter. Code 62263 includes percutaneous insertion and removal of an epidural catheter (remaining in place over a several-day period), for the administration of multiple injections of a neurolytic agent(s) performed during serial treatment sessions (ie., spanning two or more treatment days). If required, adhesions or scarring may also be lysed by mechanical means. Code 62263 is NOT reported for each adhesiolysis treatment, but should be reported ONCE to describe the entire series of injections/infusions spanning two or more treatment days.

Code 62264 describes multiple adhesiolysis treatment sessions performed on the same day. Adhesions or scarring may be lysed by injections of neurolytic agent(s). If required, adhesions or scarring may also be lysed mechanically using a percutaneously-deployed catheter.

Codes 62263 and 62264 include the procedure of injections of contrast for epidurography (72275) and fluoroscopic guidance and localization (77003) during initial or subsequent sessions.

Fluoroscopy or CT and any injection of contrast are inclusive components of 62321, 62323, 62325, 62327. For epidurography, use 72275.

The placement and use of a catheter to administer one or more epidural or subarachnoid injections on a single calendar day should be reported in the same manner as if a needle had been used, ie, as a single injection using either 62320, 62321, 62322, or 62323. Such injections should not be reported with 62324, 62325, 62326, or 62327.

Threading a catheter into the epidural space, injecting substances at one or more levels and then removing the catheter should be treated as a single injection (62320, 62321, 62322, 62323). If the catheter is left in place to deliver substance(s) over a prolonged period (ie, more than a single calendar day) either continuously or via intermittent bolus, use 62324, 62325, 62326, 62327 as appropriate.

When reporting 62320, 62321, 62322, 62323, 62324, 62325, 62326, 62327 code choice is based on the region at which the needle or catheter entered the body (eg, lumbar). Codes 62320, 62321, 62322, 62323, 62324, 62325, 62326, 62327 should be reported only once, when the substance injected spreads or catheter tip insertion moves into another spinal region (eg, 62322 is reported only once for injection or catheter insertion at L3-4 with spread of the substance or placement of the catheter tip to the thoracic region).

Percutaneous spinal procedures are done with indirect visualization (eg, image guidance) (eg, 62287). Endoscopic assistance during an open procedure with continuous and direct visualization (light-based) is reported using excision codes (eg, 63020-63035).

(For transforaminal epidural injection, see 64479- 64484)

(Report 01996 for daily hospital management of continuous epidural or subarachnoid drug administration performed in conjunction with 62324, 62325, 62326, 62327)

● New Code   ▲ Revised Code   + Add-On Code   ⊘ Modifier -51 Exempt   ★ Telemedicine

Definitions

For purposes of CPT coding, the following definitions of approach and visualization apply. The primary approach and visualization define the service, whether another method is incidentally applied. Surgical services are presumed open, unless otherwise specified.

Percutaneous: Image-guided procedures (eg, computer tomography [CT] or fluoroscopy) performed with indirect visualization of the spine without the use of any device that allows visualization through a surgical incision.

Endoscopic: Spinal procedures performed with continuous direct visualization of the spine through an endoscope.

Open: Spinal procedures performed with continuous direct visualization of the spine through a surgical opening.

Indirect visualization: Image-guided (eg, CT or fluoroscopy), not light-based visualization.

Direct visualization: Light-based visualization; can be performed by eye, or with surgical loupes, microscope, or endoscope.

(For the techniques of microsurgery and/or use of microscope, use 69990)

62263   Percutaneous lysis of epidural adhesions using solution injection (eg, hypertonic saline, enzyme) or mechanical means (eg, catheter) including radiologic localization (includes contrast when administered), multiple adhesiolysis sessions; 2 or more days

(62263 includes codes 72275 and 77003)

62264   1 day

(Do not report 62264 with 62263)

(62264 includes codes 72275 and 77003)

62267   Percutaneous aspiration within the nucleus pulposus, intervertebral, disc, or paravertebral tissue for diagnostic purposes

(For imaging, use 77003)

(Do not report 62267 in conjunction with 10005, 10006, 10007, 10008, 10009, 10010, 10011, 10012, 20225, 62287, 62290, 62291)

62268   Percutaneous aspiration, spinal cord cyst or syrinx

(For radiological supervision and interpretation, see 76942, 77002, 77012)

62269   Biopsy of spinal cord, percutaneous needle

(For radiological supervision and interpretation, see 76942, 77002, 77012)

(For fine needle aspiration biopsy, see 10004, 10005, 10006, 10007, 10008, 10009, 10010, 10011, 10012, 10021)

(For evaluation of fine needle aspirate, see 88172, 88173)

62270   Spinal puncture, lumbar, diagnostic;

62328   with fluoroscopic or CT guidance

(Do not report 62270, 62328 in conjunction with 77003, 77012)

(If ultrasound or MRI guidance is performed, see 76942, 77021)

62272   Spinal puncture, therapeutic, for drainage of cerebrospinal fluid (by needle or catheter);

62329   with fluoroscopic or CT guidance

(Do not report 62272, 62329 in conjunction with 77003, 77012)

(If ultrasound or MRI guidance is performed, see 76942, 77021)

62273 Injection, epidural, of blood or clot patch

(For injection of diagnostic or therapeutic substance[s], see 62320, 62321, 62322, 62323, 62324, 62325, 62326, 62327)

62280 Injection/infusion of neurolytic substance (eg, alcohol, phenol, iced saline solutions), with or without other therapeutic substance; subarachnoid

62281 epidural, cervical or thoracic

62282 epidural, lumbar, sacral (caudal)

62284 Injection procedure for myelography and/or computed tomography, lumbar

(Do not report 62284 in conjunction with 62302, 62303, 62304, 62305, 72240, 72255, 72265, 72270)

(When both 62284 and 72240, 72255, 72265, 72270 are performed by the same physician or other qualified health care professional for myelography, see 62302, 62303, 62304, 62305)

(For injection procedure at C1-C2, use 61055)

(For radiological supervision and interpretation, see Radiology)

62287 Decompression procedure, percutaneous, of nucleus pulposus of intervertebral disc, any method utilizing needle based technique to remove disc material under fluoroscopic imaging or other form of indirect visualization, with discography and/or epidural injection(s) at the treated level(s), when performed, single or multiple levels, lumbar

(Do not report 62287 in conjunction with 62267, 62290, 62322, 77003, 77012, 72295, when performed at same level)

(For non-needle based technique for percutaneous decompression of nucleus pulposus of intervertebral disc, see codes 0274T, 0275T)

62290 Injection procedure for diskography, each level; lumbar

62291 cervical or thoracic

(For radiological supervision or interpretation, see 72285, 72295)

62292 Injection procedure for chemonucleolysis, including diskography, intervertebral disk, single or multiple levels, lumbar

62294 Injection procedure, arterial, for occlusion of arteriovenous malformation, spinal

62302 Myelography via lumbar injection, including radiological supervision and interpretation; cervical

(Do not report 62302 in conjunction with 62284, 62303, 62304, 62305, 72240, 72255, 72265, 72270)

62303 thoracic

(Do not report 62303 in conjunction with 62284, 62302, 62304, 62305, 72240, 72255, 72265, 72270)

62304 lumbosacral

(Do not report 62304 in conjunction with 62284, 62302, 62303, 62305, 72240, 72255, 72265, 72270)

62305 2 or more regions (eg, lumbar/thoracic, cervical/thoracic, lumbar/cervical, lumbar/thoracic/cervical)

(Do not report 62305 in conjunction with 62284, 62302, 62303, 62304, 72240, 72255, 72265, 72270)

(For myelography lumbar injection and imaging performed by different physicians or other qualified health care professionals, see 62284 or 72240, 72255, 72265, 72270)

(For injection procedure at C1-C2, use 61055)

62320 Injection(s), of diagnostic or therapeutic substance(s) (eg, anesthetic, antispasmodic, opioid, steroid, other solution), not including neurolytic substances, including needle or catheter placement, interlaminar epidural or subarachnoid, cervical or thoracic; without imaging guidance

62321 with imaging guidance (ie, fluoroscopy or CT)

(Do not report 62321 in conjunction with 77003, 77012, 76942)

62322 Injection(s), of diagnostic or therapeutic substance(s) (eg, anesthetic, antispasmodic, opioid, steroid, other solution), not including neurolytic substances, including needle or catheter placement, interlaminar epidural or subarachnoid, lumbar or sacral (caudal); without imaging guidance

62323 with imaging guidance (ie, fluoroscopy or CT)

(Do not report 62323 in conjunction with 77003, 77012, 76942)

62324 Injection(s), including indwelling catheter placement, continuous infusion or intermittent bolus, of diagnostic or therapeutic substance(s) (eg, anesthetic, antispasmodic, opioid, steroid, other solution), not including neurolytic substances, interlaminar epidural or subarachnoid, cervical or thoracic; without imaging guidance

62325 with imaging guidance (ie, fluoroscopy or CT)

(Do not report 62325 in conjunction with 77003, 77012, 76942)

62326 Injection(s), including indwelling catheter placement, continuous infusion or intermittent bolus, of diagnostic or therapeutic substance(s) (eg, anesthetic, antispasmodic, opioid, steroid, other solution), not including neurolytic substances, interlaminar epidural or subarachnoid, lumbar or sacral (caudal); without imaging guidance

62327 with imaging guidance (ie, fluoroscopy or CT)

(Do not report 62327 in conjunction with 77003, 77012, 76942)

(Report 01996 for daily hospital management of continuous epidural or subarachnoid drug administration performed in conjunction with 62324, 62325, 62326, 62327)

62328 This code is out of order. See page 597

62329 This code is out of order. See page 597

CATHETER IMPLANTATION

(For percutaneous placement of intrathecal or epidural catheter, see 62270, 62272, 62273, 62280, 62281, 62282, 62284, 62320, 62321, 62322, 62323, 62324, 62325, 62326, 62327, 62328, 62329)

62350 Implantation, revision or repositioning of tunneled intrathecal or epidural catheter, for long-term medication administration via an external pump or implantable reservoir/infusion pump; without laminectomy

62351 with laminectomy

(For refilling and maintenance of an implantable infusion pump for spinal or brain drug therapy, use 95990)

62355 Removal of previously implanted intrathecal or epidural catheter

RESERVOIR/PUMP IMPLANTATION

62360 Implantation or replacement of device for intrathecal or epidural drug infusion; subcutaneous reservoir

62361 non-programmable pump

62362 programmable pump, including preparation of pump, with or without programming

62365 Removal of subcutaneous reservoir or pump, previously implanted for intrathecal or epidural infusion

62367 Electronic analysis of programmable, implanted pump for intrathecal or epidural drug infusion (includes evaluation of reservoir status, alarm status, drug prescription status); without reprogramming or refill

62368 with reprogramming

(For refilling and maintenance of an implantable infusion pump for spinal or brain drug therapy, use 95990)

62369 with reprogramming and refill

62370 with reprogramming and refill (requiring skill of a physician or other qualified health care professional)

(Do not report 62367-62370 in conjunction with 95990, 95991. For refilling and maintenance of a reservoir or an implantable infusion pump for spinal or brain drug delivery without reprogramming, see 95990, 95991)

Endoscopic Decompression of Neural Elements and/or Excision of Herniated Intervertebral Discs

Definitions

For purposes of CPT coding, the following definitions of approach and visualization apply. The primary approach and visualization define the service, whether another method is incidentally applied. Surgical services are presumed open, unless otherwise specified. Percutaneous: Image-guided procedures (eg, computer tomography [CT] or fluoroscopy) performed with indirect visualization of the spine without the use of any device that allows visualization through a surgical incision.

Endoscopic: Spinal procedures performed with continuous direct visualization of the spine through an endoscope.

Open: Spinal procedures performed with continuous direct visualization of the spine through a surgical opening.

Indirect visualization: Image-guided (eg, CT or fluoroscopy), not light-based visualization.

Direct visualization: Light-based visualization; can be performed by eye, or with surgical loupes, microscope, or endoscope.

(For the techniques of microsurgery and/or use of microscope, use 69990)

(For percutaneous decompression, see 62287, 0274T, 0275T)

62380 Endoscopic decompression of spinal cord, nerve root(s), including laminotomy, partial facetectomy, foraminotomy, discectomy and/or excision of herniated intervertebral disc, 1 interspace, lumbar

(For open procedures, see 63030, 63056)

(For bilateral procedure, report 62380 with modifier 50)

POSTERIOR EXTRADURAL LAMINOTOMY OR LAMINECTOMY FOR EXPLORATION/DECOMPRESSION OF NEURAL ELEMENTS OR EXCISION OF HERNIATED INTERVERTEBRAL DISKS

Definitions

For purposes of CPT coding, the following definitions of approach and visualization apply. The primary approach and visualization define the service, whether another method is incidentally applied. Surgical services are presumed open, unless otherwise specified. Percutaneous: Image-guided procedures (eg, computer tomography [CT] or fluoroscopy) performed with indirect visualization of the spine without the use of any device that allows visualization through a surgical incision.

Endoscopic: Spinal procedures performed with continuous direct visualization of the spine through an endoscope.

Open: Spinal procedures performed with continuous direct visualization of the spine through a surgical opening.

Indirect visualization: Image-guided (eg, CT or fluoroscopy), not light-based visualization.

● New Code ▲ Revised Code ✛ Add-On Code ⊘ Modifier -51 Exempt ★ Telemedicine

Direct visualization: Light-based visualization; can be performed by eye, or with surgical loupes, microscope, or endoscope.

(When 63001-63048 are followed by arthrodesis, see 22590-22614)

(For open procedures, see 63030, 63056)

(For bilateral procedure, report 62380 with modifier 50)

63001 Laminectomy with exploration and/or decompression of spinal cord and/or cauda equina, without facetectomy, foraminotomy or diskectomy, (eg, spinal stenosis), one or two vertebral segments; cervical

63003 thoracic

63005 lumbar, except for spondylolisthesis

63011 sacral

63012 Laminectomy with removal of abnormal facets and/or pars inter-articularis with decompression of cauda equina and nerve roots for spondylolisthesis, lumbar (Gill type procedure)

63015 Laminectomy with exploration and/or decompression of spinal cord and/or cauda equina, without facetectomy, foraminotomy or diskectomy, (eg, spinal stenosis), more than 2 vertebral segments; cervical

63016 thoracic

63017 lumbar

63020 Laminotomy (hemilaminectomy), with decompression of nerve root(s), including partial facetectomy, foraminotomy and/or excision of herniated intervertebral disc; 1 interspace, cervical

(For bilateral procedure, report 63020 with modifier -50)

63030 1 interspace, lumbar

(For bilateral procedure, report 63030 with modifier -50)

+ 63035 each additional interspace, cervical or lumbar (List separately in addition to code for primary procedure)

(Use 63035 in conjunction with codes 63020-63030)

(For bilateral procedure, report 63035 twice. Do not report modifier 50 in conjunction with 63035)

(For percutaneous endoscopic approach, see 0274T, 0275T)

63040 Laminotomy (hemilaminectomy), with decompression of nerve root(s), including partial facetectomy, foraminotomy and/or excision of herniated intervertebral disk, reexploration, single interspace; cervical

(For bilateral procedure, report 63040 with modifier -50)

63042 lumbar

(For bilateral procedure, report 63042 with modifier -50)

+ 63043 each additional cervical interspace (List separately in addition to code for primary procedure)

(Use 63043 in conjunction with code 63040)

(For bilateral procedure, report 63043 twice. Do not report modifier 50 in conjunction with 63043)

+ 63044 each additional lumbar interspace (List separately in addition to code for primary procedure)

(Use 63044 in conjunction with code 63042)

(For bilateral procedure, report 63044 twice. Do not report modifier 50 in conjunction with 63044)

Separate Procedure   Unlisted Procedure   CCI Comp. Code   Non-specific Procedure   **601**

63045 Laminectomy, facetectomy and foraminotomy (unilateral or bilateral with decompression of spinal cord, cauda equina and/or nerve root(s), (eg, spinal or lateral recess stenosis)), single vertebral segment; cervical

63046 thoracic

63047 lumbar

+ 63048 each additional segment, cervical, thoracic, or lumbar (List separately in addition to code for primary procedure)

(Use 63048 in conjunction with codes 63045-63047)

63050 Laminoplasty, cervical, with decompression of the spinal cord, 2 or more vertebral segments;

63051 with reconstruction of the posterior bony elements (including the application of bridging bone graft and non-segmental fixation devices (eg, wire, suture, mini-plates), when performed)

(Do not report 63050 or 63051 in conjunction with 22600, 22614, 22840-22842, 63001, 63015, 63045, 63048, 63295 for the same vertebral segment(s))

TRANSPEDICULAR OR COSTOVERTEBRAL APPROACH FOR POSTEROLATERAL EXTRADURAL EXPLORATION/ DECOMPRESSION

63055 Transpedicular approach with decompression of spinal cord, equina and/or nerve root(s) (eg, herniated intervertebral disk), single segment; thoracic

63056 lumbar (including transfacet, or lateral extraforaminal approach) (eg, far lateral herniated intervertebral disk)

+ 63057 each additional segment, thoracic or lumbar (List separately in addition to code for primary procedure)

(Use 63057 in conjunction with codes 63055, 63056)

63064 Costovertebral approach with decompression of spinal cord or nerve root(s), (eg, herniated intervertebral disk), thoracic; single segment

+ 63066 each additional segment (List separately in addition to code for primary procedure)

(Use 63066 in conjunction with code 63064)

(For excision of thoracic intraspinal lesions by laminectomy, see 63266, 63271, 63276, 63281, 63286)

ANTERIOR OR ANTEROLATERAL APPROACH FOR EXTRADURAL EXPLORATION/DECOMPRESSION

For the following codes, when two surgeons work together as primary surgeons performing distinct part(s) of spinal cord exploration/decompression operation, each surgeon should report his/her distinct operative work by appending modifier 62 to the procedure code (and any associated add-on codes for that procedure code as long as both surgeons continue to work together as primary surgeons). In this situation, modifier 62 may be appended to the definitive procedure code(s) 63075, 63077, 63081, 63085, 63087, 63090 and, as appropriate, to associated additional interspace add-on code(s) 63076, 63078 or additional segment add-on codes 63082, 63086, 63088, 63091 as long as both surgeons continue to work together as primary surgeons.

For vertebral corpectomy, the term **partial** is used to describe removal of a substantial portion of the body of the vertebra. In the cervical spine, the amount of bone removed is defined as at least one-half of the vertebral body. In the thoracic and lumbar spine, the amount of bone removed is defined as at least one-third of the vertebral body.

63075 Diskectomy, anterior, with decompression of spinal cord and/or nerve root(s), including osteophytectomy; cervical, single interspace

(Do not report 63075 in conjunction with 22554, even if performed by separate individuals. To report anterior cervical discectomy and interbody fusion at the same level during the same session, use 22551)

+ 63076 cervical, each additional interspace (List separately in addition to code for primary procedure)

● New Code   ▲ Revised Code   + Add-On Code   ⊘ Modifier -51 Exempt   ★ Telemedicine

(Do not report 63076 in conjunction with 22554, even if performed by separate individuals. To report anterior cervical discectomy and interbody fusion at the same level during the same session, use 22552)

(Use 63076 in conjunction with code 63075)

63077   thoracic, single interspace

+ 63078   thoracic, each additional interspace (List separately in addition to code for primary procedure)

(Use 63078 in conjunction with code 63077)

(Do not report code 69990 in addition to codes 63075-63078)

63081   Vertebral corpectomy (vertebral body resection), partial or complete, anterior approach with decompression of spinal cord and/or nerve root(s); cervical, single segment

+ 63082   cervical, each additional segment (List separately in addition to code for primary procedure)

(Use 63082 in conjunction with code 63081)

(For transoral approach, see 61575, 61576)

63085   Vertebral corpectomy (vertebral body resection), partial or complete, transthoracic approach with decompression of spinal cord and/or nerve root(s); thoracic, single segment

+ 63086   thoracic, each additional segment (List separately in addition to code for primary procedure)

(Use 63086 in conjunction with code 63085)

63087   Vertebral corpectomy (vertebral body resection), partial or complete, combined thoracolumbar approach with decompression of spinal cord, cauda equina or nerve root(s), lower thoracic or lumbar; single segment

+ 63088   each additional segment (List separately in addition to code for primary procedure)

(Use 63088 in conjunction with code 63087)

63090   Vertebral corpectomy (vertebral body resection), partial or complete, transperitoneal or retroperitoneal approach with decompression of spinal cord, cauda equina or nerve root(s), lower thoracic, lumbar, or sacral; single segment

+ 63091   each additional segment (List separately in addition to code for primary procedure)

(Use 63091 in conjunction with code 63090)

(Procedures 63081-63091 include diskectomy above and/or below vertebral segment)

(If followed by arthrodesis, see 22548-22812)

(For reconstruction of spine, use appropriate vertebral corpectomy codes 63081-63091, bone graft codes 20930-20938, arthrodesis codes 22548-22812, and spinal instrumentation codes 22840-22855, 22859)

LATERAL EXTRACAVITARY APPROACH FOR EXTRADURAL EXPLORATION/DECOMPRESSION

For vertebral corpectomy, the term partial is used to describe removal of a substantial portion of the body of the vertebra. In the cervical spine, the amount of bone removed is defined as at least one-half of the vertebral body. In the thoracic and lumbar spine, the amount of bone removed is defined as at least one-third of the vertebral body

63101   Vertebral corpectomy (vertebral body resection), partial or complete, lateral extracavitary approach with decompression of spinal cord and/or nerve root(s) (eg, for tumor or retropulsed bone fragments); thoracic, single segment

63102   lumbar, single segment

+ 63103   thoracic or lumbar, each additional segment (List separately in addition to code for primary procedure)

(Use 63103 in conjunction with 63101 and 63102)

INCISION

63170 Laminectomy with myelotomy (eg, Bischof or DREZ type), cervical, thoracic, or thoracolumbar

63172 Laminectomy with drainage of intramedullary cyst/syrinx; to subarachnoid space

63173   to peritoneal or pleural space

(**63180** deleted 2020 [2021 Edition])

(**63182** deleted 2020 [2021 Edition])

63185 Laminectomy with rhizotomy; 1 or 2 segments

63190   more than 2 segments

63191 Laminectomy with section of spinal accessory nerve

(For bilateral procedure, report 63191 with modifier -50)

(For resection of sternocleidomastoid muscle, use 21720)

63194 Laminectomy with cordotomy, with section of one spinothalamic tract, 1 stage; cervical

63195   thoracic

63196 Laminectomy with cordotomy, with section of both spinothalamic tracts, 1 stage; cervical

63197   thoracic

63198 Laminectomy with cordotomy with section of both spinothalamic tracts, 2 stages within 14 days; cervical

63199   thoracic

63200 Laminectomy, with release of tethered spinal cord, lumbar

EXCISION BY LAMINECTOMY OF LESION OTHER THAN HERNIATED DISC

63250 Laminectomy for excision or occlusion of arteriovenous malformation of spinal cord; cervical

63251   thoracic

63252   thoracolumbar

63265 Laminectomy for excision or evacuation of intraspinal lesion other than neoplasm, extradural; cervical

63266   thoracic

63267   lumbar

63268   sacral

63270 Laminectomy for excision of intraspinal lesion other than neoplasm, intradural; cervical

63271   thoracic

63272   lumbar

63273   sacral

● New Code   ▲ Revised Code   ✛ Add-On Code   ⊘ Modifier -51 Exempt   ★ Telemedicine

63275   Laminectomy for biopsy/excision of intraspinal neoplasm; extradural, cervical

63276   extradural, thoracic

63277   extradural, lumbar

63278   extradural, sacral

63280   intradural, extramedullary, cervical

63281   intradural, extramedullary, thoracic

63282   intradural, extramedullary, lumbar

63283   intradural, sacral

63285   intradural, intramedullary, cervical

63286   intradural, intramedullary, thoracic

63287   intradural, intramedullary, thoracolumbar

63290   combined extradural-intradural lesion, any level

(For drainage of intramedullary cyst/syrinx, use 63172, 63173)

+ 63295   Osteoplastic reconstruction of dorsal spinal elements, following primary intraspinal procedure (List separately in addition to code for primary procedure)

(Use 63295 in conjunction with 63172, 63173, 63185, 63190, 63200-63290)

(Do not report 63295 in conjunction with 22590-22614, 22840-22844, 63050, 63051 for the same vertebral segment(s))

EXCISION, ANTERIOR OR ANTEROLATERAL APPROACH, INTRASPINAL LESION

For the following codes, when two surgeons work together as primary surgeons performing distinct part(s) of an anterior approach for an intraspinal excision, each surgeon should report his/her distinct operative work by appending modifier 62 to the single definitive procedure code. In this situation, modifier 62 may be appended to the definitive procedure code(s) 63300-63307 and, as appropriate, to the associated additional segment add-on code 63308 as long as both surgeons continue to work together as primary surgeons.

For vertebral corpectomy, the term partial is used to describe removal of a substantial portion of the body of the vertebra. In the cervical spine, the amount of bone removed is defined as at least one-half of the vertebral body. In the thoracic and lumbar spine, the amount of bone removed is defined as at least one-third of the vertebral body.

(For arthrodesis, see 22548-22585)

(For reconstruction of spine, see 20930-20938)

63300   Vertebral corpectomy (vertebral body resection), partial or complete, for excision of intraspinal lesion, single segment; extradural, cervical

63301   extradural, thoracic by transthoracic approach

63302   extradural, thoracic by thoracolumbar approach

63303   extradural, lumbar or sacral by transperitoneal or retroperitoneal approach

63304   intradural, cervical

63305   intradural, thoracic by transthoracic approach

| 63306 | intradural, thoracic by thoracolumbar approach |

| 63307 | intradural, lumbar or sacral by transperitoneal or retroperitoneal approach |

+ 63308   each additional segment (List separately in addition to codes for single segment)

(Use 63308 in conjunction with codes 63300-63307)

STEREOTAXIS

| 63600 | Creation of lesion of spinal cord by stereotactic method, percutaneous, any modality (including stimulation and/or recording) |

| 63610 | Stereotactic stimulation of spinal cord, percutaneous, separate procedure not followed by other surgery |

(63615   deleted 2018 [2019 Edition])

STEREOTACTIC RADIOSURGERY (SPINAL)

Spinal stereotactic radiosurgery is a distinct procedure that utilizes externally generated ionizing radiation to inactivate or eradicate defined target(s) in the spine without the need to make an incision. The target is defined by and the treatment is delivered using high-resolution stereotactic imaging. These codes are reported by the surgeon. The radiation oncologist reports the appropriate code(s) for clinical treatment planning, physics and dosimetry, treatment delivery and management from the Radiation Oncology section (77261-77790). Any necessary planning, dosimetry, targeting, positioning, or blocking by the neurosurgeon is included in the stereotactic radiation surgery services. The same individual should not report stereotactic radiosurgery services with radiation treatment management codes (77427-77432).

Spinal stereotactic radiosurgery is typically performed in a single planning and treatment session using a stereotactic image-guidance system, but can be performed with a planning session and in a limited number of treatment sessions, up to a maximum of five sessions. Do not report stereotactic radiosurgery more than once per lesion per course of treatment when the treatment requires greater than one session.

Stereotactic spinal surgery is only used when the tumor being treated affects spinal neural tissue or abuts the dura mater. Arteriovenous malformations must be subdural. For other radiation services of the spine, see Radiation Oncology Services.

Codes 63620, 63621 include computer-assisted planning. Do not report 63620, 63621 in conjunction with 61781-61783.

(For intensity modulated beam delivery plan and treatment, see 77301, 77385, 77386. For stereotactic body radiation therapy, see 77373, 77435)

| 63620 | Stereotactic radiosurgery (particle beam, gamma ray, or linear accelerator); 1 spinal lesion |

(Do not report 63620 more than once per course of treatment)

+ 63621   each additional spinal lesion (list separately in addition to code for primary procedure)

(Report 63621 in conjunction with 63620)

(For each course of treatment, 63621 may be reported no more than once per lesion. Do not report 63621 more than 2 times for entire course of treatment regardless of number of lesions treated)

NEUROSTIMULATORS (SPINAL)

For electronic analysis with programming, when performed, of spinal cord neurostimulator pulse generator/transmitters, see codes 95970, 95971, 95972. Test stimulation to confirm correct target site placement of the electrode array(s) and/or to confirm the functional status of the system is inherent to placement, and is not separately reported as electronic analysis or programming of the neurostimulator system. Electronic analysis (95970) at the time of implantation is not separately reported.

Codes 63650, 63655, and 63661-63664 describe the operative placement, revision, replacement, or removal of the spinal neurostimulator system components to provide spinal electrical stimulation. A neurostimulator system includes an implanted neurostimulator, external controller, extension, and collection of contacts. Multiple contacts or electrodes (4 or more) provide the actual electrical stimulation in the epidural space.

● New Code   ▲ Revised Code   + Add-On Code   ⊘ Modifier -51 Exempt   ★ Telemedicine

For percutaneously placed neurostimulator systems (63650, 63661, 63663), the contacts are on a catheter-like lead. An array defines the collection of contacts that are on one catheter.

For systems placed via an open surgical exposure (63655, 63662, 63664), the contacts are on a plate or paddle-shaped surface.

Do not report 63661 or 63663 when removing or replacing a temporary percutaneously placed array for an external generator.

63650 Percutaneous implantation of neurostimulator electrode array, epidural

63655 Laminectomy for implantation of neurostimulator electrodes, plate/paddle, epidural

63661 Removal of spinal neurostimulator electrode percutaneous array(s), including fluoroscopy, when performed

63662 Removal of spinal neurostimulator electrode plate/paddle(s) placed via laminotomy or laminectomy, including fluoroscopy, when performed

63663 Revision including replacement, when performed, of spinal neurostimulator electrode percutaneous array(s), including fluoroscopy, when performed

(Do not report 63663 in conjunction with 63661, 63662 for the same spinal level)

63664 Revision including replacement, when performed, of spinal neurostimulator electrode plate/paddle(s) placed via laminotomy or laminectomy, including fluoroscopy, when performed

(Do not report 63664 in conjunction with 63661, 63662 for the same spinal level)

63685 Insertion or replacement of spinal neurostimulator pulse generator or receiver, direct or inductive coupling

(Do not report 63685 in conjunction with 63688 for the same pulse generator or receiver)

63688 Revision or removal of implanted spinal neurostimulator pulse generator or receiver

(For electronic analysis with programming, when performed, of implanted spinal cord neurostimulator pulse generator/transmitter, see 95970, 95971, 95972)

REPAIR

63700 Repair of meningocele; less than 5 cm diameter

63702 larger than 5 cm diameter

(Do not use modifier -63 in conjunction with 63700, 63702)

63704 Repair of myelomeningocele; less than 5 cm diameter

63706 larger than 5 cm diameter

(Do not use modifier -63 in conjunction with 63704, 63706)

(For complex skin closure, see Integumentary System)

63707 Repair of dural/cerebrospinal fluid leak, not requiring laminectomy

63709 Repair of dural/cerebrospinal fluid leak or pseudomeningocele, with laminectomy

63710 Dural graft, spinal

(For laminectomy and section of dentate ligaments, with or without dural graft, cervical, see 63180, 63182)

SHUNT, SPINAL CSF

63740 Creation of shunt, lumbar, subarachnoid-peritoneal, -pleural, or other; including laminectomy

---

Separate Procedure   Unlisted Procedure   CCI Comp. Code   Non-specific Procedure   **607**

63741   percutaneous, not requiring laminectomy

63744   Replacement, irrigation or revision of lumbosubarachnoid shunt

63746   Removal of entire lumbosubarachnoid shunt system without replacement

(For insertion of subarachnoid catheter with reservoir and/or pump for intermittent or continuous infusion of drug including laminectomy, see 62351 and 62360, 62361 or 62362)

(For insertion or replacement of subarachnoid or epidural catheter, with reservoir and/or pump for drug infusion without laminectomy, see 62350 and 62360, 62361 or 62362)

EXTRACRANIAL NERVES, PERIPHERAL NERVES, AND AUTONOMIC NERVOUS SYSTEM

(For intracranial surgery on cranial nerves, see 61450, 61460, 61790)

INTRODUCTION/INJECTION OF ANESTHETIC AGENT (NERVE BLOCK), DIAGNOSTIC OR THERAPEUTIC

(For destruction by neurolytic agent or chemodenervation, see 62280-62282, 64600-64681)

(For epidural or subarachnoid injection, see 62320, 62321, 62322, 62323, 62324, 62325, 62326, 62327)

(64400-64455, 64461, 64462, 64463, 64479, 64480, 64483, 64484, 64490-64495 are unilateral procedures. For bilateral procedures, report 64400, 64405, 64408, 64415, 64416, 64417, 64418, 64420, 64425-64455, 64461, 64463, 64479, 64483, 64490, 64493 with modifier 50. Report add-on codes 64421, 64462, 64480, 64484, 64491, 64492, 64494, 64495 twice, when performed bilaterally. Do not report modifier 50 in conjunction with 64421, 64462, 64480, 64484, 64491, 64492, 64494, 64495)

Somatic Nerves

Codes 64400-64489 describe the introduction/injection of an anesthetic agent and/or steroid into the somatic nervous system for diagnostic or therapeutic purposes. For injection or destruction of genicular nerve branches, see 64454, 64624, respectively.

Codes 64400-64450, 64454 describe the injection of an anesthetic agent(s) and/or steroid into a nerve plexus, nerve, or branch. These codes are reported once per nerve plexus, nerve, or branch as described in the descriptor regardless of the number of injections performed along the nerve plexus, nerve, or branch described by the code.

Imaging guidance and localization may be reported separately for 64400-64450. Imaging guidance and any injection of contrast are inclusive components of 64451 and 64454.

Codes 64455, 64479, 64480, 64483, 64484 are reported for single or multiple injections on the same site. For 64479, 64480, 64483, 64484, imaging guidance (fluoroscopy or CT) and any injection of contrast are inclusive components and are not reported separately. For 64455, imaging guidance (ultrasound, fluoroscopy, CT) and localization may be reported separately.

Codes 64461, 64462, 64463 describe injection of a paravertebral block (PVB). Codes 64486, 64487, 64488, 64489 describe injection of a transversus abdominis plane (TAP) block. Imaging guidance and any injection of contrast are inclusive components of 64461, 64462, 64463, 64486, 64487, 64488, 64489 and are not reported separately.

64400   Injection(s), anesthetic agent(s) and/or steroid; trigeminal nerve, each branch (ie, ophthalmic, maxillary, mandibular)

(**64402**   deleted 2019 [2020 Edition]. To report injection of anesthetic agent and/or steroid to the facial nerve, use 64999)

64405   greater occipital nerve

64408   vagus nerve

(**64410**   deleted 2019 [2020 Edition]. To report injection of anesthetic agent and/or steroid to the phrenic nerve, cervical plexus, use 64999)

● New Code   ▲ Revised Code   + Add-On Code   ⊘ Modifier -51 Exempt   ★ Telemedicine

(**64413** deleted 2019 [2020 Edition]. To report injection of anesthetic agent and/or steroid to the phrenic nerve, cervical plexus, use 64999)

64415 brachial plexus, single

64416 brachial plexus, continuous infusion by catheter (including catheter placement)

(Do not report 64416 in conjunction with 01996)

64417 axillary nerve

64418 suprascapular nerve

64420 intercostal nerve, single

+ 64421 intercostal nerve, each additional level (List separately in addition to code for primary procedure)

(Use 64421 in conjunction with 64420)

64425 ilioinguinal, iliohypogastric nerves

64430 pudendal nerve

64435 paracervical (uterine) nerve

64445 sciatic nerve

64446 sciatic nerve, continuous infusion by catheter, (including catheter placement)

(Do not report 64446 in conjuction with 01996)

64447 femoral nerve

(Do not report 64447 in conjunction with 01996)

64448 femoral nerve, continuous infusion by catheter (including catheter placement)

(Do not report 64448 in conjunction with 01996)

64449 lumbar plexus, posterior approach, continuous infusion by catheter (including catheter placement)

(Do not report 64449 in conjunction with 01996)

64450 other peripheral nerve or branch

(For injection, anesthetic agent, nerves innervating the sacroiliac joint, use 64451)

64451 nerves innervating the sacroiliac joint, with image guidance (ie, fluoroscopy or computed tomography)

(Do not report 64451 in conjunction with 64493, 64494, 64495, 77002, 77003, 77012, 95873, 95874)

(For injection, anesthetic agent, nerves innervating the sacroiliac joint, with ultrasound, use 76999)

(For bilateral procedure, report 64451 with modifier 50)

64454 genicular nerve branches, including imaging guidance, when performed

(Do not report 64454 in conjunction with 64624)

(64454 requires injecting all of the following genicular nerve branches: superolateral, superomedial, and inferomedial. If all 3 of these genicular nerve branches are not injected, report 64454 with modifier 52)

Code(s)	Unit	Image Guidance Included	Image Guidance Separately Reported, When Performed
	Extracranial Nerves, Peripheral Nerves, and Autonomic Nervous System		
	Introduction/Injection of Anesthetic Agent (Nerve Block), Diagnostic or Therapeutic Nerve		
	Somatic Nerve		
64400-64450	1 unit per plexus, nerve, or branch injected regardless of the number of injections		X
64451	1 unit for any number of nerves innervating the sacroiliac joint injected regardless of the number of injections	X	
64454	1 unit for any number of genicular nerve branches, with a required minimum of three nerve branches	X	
64455	1 or more injections per level		X
64479	1 or more injections per level	X	
+64480	1 or more additional injections per level (add-on)	X	
64483	1 or more injections per level	X	
+64484	1 or more additional injections per level (add-on)	X	
64461	1 injection site	X	
+64462	1 or more additional injections per code (add-on)	X	
64463	1 or more injections per code	X	
64486-64489	By injection site	X	
	Destruction by Neurolytic Agent (eg, Chemical, Thermal, Electrical, or Radiofrequency), Chemodenervation		
Code(s)	**Unit**	**Image Guidance Included**	**Image Guidance Separately Reported, When Performed**
	Somatic Nerves		
64624	1 unit for any number of genicular nerve branches, with a required minimum of three nerve branches	X	

▲ **64455**   plantar common digital nerve(s) (eg, Morton's neuroma)

(Do note report 64455 in conjunction with 64632)

(Imaging guidance (fluoroscopy or CT) and any injection of contrast are inclusive components of 64479-64484. Imaging guidance and localization are required for the performance of 64479-64484.)

(Codes 64470-64476 have been deleted. To report, see 64490-64495)

64461   Code is out of order. See page 611

64462   Code is out of order. See page 611

64463   Code is out of order. See page 611

▲ **64479**   transforaminal epidural, with imaging guidance (fluoroscopy or CT), cervical or thoracic, single level

▲ +**64480**   transforaminal epidural, with imaging guidance (fluoroscopy or CT), cervical or thoracic, each additional level (List separately in addition to code for primary procedure)

(Use 64480 in conjunction with code 64479)

(For transforaminal epidural injection at the T12-L1 level, use 64479)

▲ **64483**   transforaminal epidural, with imaging guidance (fluoroscopy or CT), lumbar or sacral, single level

▲ +**64484**   transforaminal epidural, with imaging guidance (fluoroscopy or CT), lumbar or sacral, each additional level (List separately in addition to code for primary procedure)

(Use 64484 in conjunction with code 64483)

● New Code   ▲ Revised Code   ✚ Add-On Code   ⊘ Modifier -51 Exempt   ★ Telemedicine

(64479-64484 are unilateral procedures. For bilateral procedures, report 64479, 64483 with modifier 50. Report add-on codes 64480, 64484 twice, when performed bilaterally. Do not report modifier 50 in conjunction with 64480, 64484)

64461 Paravertebral block (PVB) (paraspinous block), thoracic; single injection site (includes imaging guidance, when performed)

+ **64462** second and any additional injection site(s) (includes imaging guidance, when performed) (List separately in addition to code for primary procedure)

(Use 64462 in conjunction with 64461)

(Do not report 64462 more than once per day)

64463 thoracic; continuous infusion by catheter (includes imaging guidance, when performed)

(Do not report 64461, 64462, 64463 in conjunction with 62320, 62324, 64420, 64421, 64479, 64480, 64490, 64491, 64492, 76942, 77002, 77003)

64486 Transversus abdominis plane (tap) block (abdominal plane block, rectus sheath block) unilateral; by injection(s) (includes imaging guidance, when performed)

64487 by continuous infusion(s) (includes imaging guidance, when performed)

64488 Transversus abdominis plane (tap) block (abdominal plane block, rectus sheath block) bilateral; by injections (includes imaging guidance, when performed)

64489 by continuous infusions (includes imaging guidance, when performed)

Paravertebral Spinal Nerves and Branches

(Image guidance [fluoroscopy or CT] and any injection of contrast are inclusive components of 64490-64495. Imaging guidance and localization are required for the performance of paravertebral facet joint injections described by codes 64490-64495. If imaging is not used, report 20552-20553. If ultrasound guidance is used, report 0213T-0218T)

(For bilateral paravertebral facet injection procedures, report 64490, 64493 with modifier 50. Report add-on codes 64491, 64492, 64494, 64495 twice, when performed bilaterally. Do not report modifier 50 in conjunction with 64491, 64492, 64494, 64495)

(For paravertebral facet injection of the T12-L1 joint, or nerves innervating that joint, use 64490)

64490 Injection(s), diagnostic or therapeutic agent, paravertebral facet (zygapophyseal) joint (or nerves innervating that joint) with image guidance (fluoroscopy or CT), cervical or thoracic; single level

+ **64491** second level (List separately in addition to code for primary procedure)

(Use 64491 in conjunction with 64490)

+ **64492** third and any additional level(s) (List separately in addition to code for primary procedure)

(Do not report 64492 more than once per day)

(Use 64492 in conjunction with 64490, 64491)

64493 Injection(s), diagnostic or therapeutic agent, paravertebral facet (zygapophyseal) joint (or nerves innervating that joint) with image guidance (fluoroscopy or CT), lumbar or sacral; single level

(For injection, anesthetic agent, nerves innervating the sacroiliac joint, use 64451)

+ **64494** second level (List separately in addition to code for primary procedure)

(Use 64494 in conjunction with 64493)

+ **64495** third and any additional level(s) (List separately in addition to code for primary procedure)

(Do not report 64495 more than once per day)

(Use 64495 in conjunction with 64493, 64494)

Autonomic Nerves

64505   Injection, anesthetic agent; sphenopalatine ganglion

(**64508**   deleted 2018 [2019 Edition])

64510   stellate ganglion (cervical sympathetic)

64517   superior hypogastric plexus

64520   lumbar or thoracic (paravertebral sympathetic)

64530   celiac plexus, with or without radiologic monitoring

(For transendoscopic ultrasound-guided transmural injection, anesthetic, celiac plexus, use 43253)

NEUROSTIMULATORS (PERIPHERAL NERVE)

For electronic analysis with programming, when performed, of peripheral nerve neurostimulator pulse generator/transmitters, see codes 95970, 95971, 95972. An electrode array is a catheter or other device with more than one contact. The function of each contact may be capable of being adjusted during programming services. Test stimulation to confirm correct target site placement of the electrode array(s) and/or to confirm the functional status of the system is inherent to placement, and is not separately reported as electronic analysis or programming of the neurostimulator system. Electronic analysis (95970) at the time of implantation is not separately reported.

Codes 64553, 64555, and 64561 may be used to report both temporary and permanent placement of percutaneous electrode arrays.

(**64550**   deleted 2018 [2019 Edition])

(For transcutaneous nerve stimulation [TENS], use 97014 for electrical stimulation requiring supervision only or use 97032 for electrical stimulation requiring constant attendance)

(For percutaneous implantation or replacement of integrated neurostimulation system, posterior tibial nerve, use 0587T)

64553   Percutaneous implantation of neurostimulator electrode array; cranial nerve

(For percutaneous electrical stimulation of a cranial nerve using needle[s] or needle electrode[s] [eg, PENS, PNT], use 64999)

(For open placement of cranial nerve (eg, vagus, trigeminal) neurostimulator pulse generator or receiver, see 61885, 61886, as appropriate)

64555   peripheral nerve (excludes sacral nerve)

(Do not report 64555 in conjunction with 64566)

(For percutaneous electrical stimulation of a peripheral nerve using needle[s] or needle electrode[s] [eg, PENS, PNT], use 64999)

64561   sacral nerve (transforaminal placement) including image guidance, if performed

(**64565**   deleted 2017 [2018 edition.])

(For percutaneous electrical neuromuscular stimulation or neuromodulation using needle[s] or needle electrode[s] [eg, PENS, PNT], use 64999)

64566   Posterior tibial neurostimulation, percutaneous needle electrode, single treatment, includes programming

(Do not report 64566 in conjunction with 64555, 95970-95972)

● New Code   ▲ Revised Code   ＋ Add-On Code   ⊘ Modifier -51 Exempt   ★ Telemedicine

64568 Incision for implantation of cranial nerve (eg, vagus nerve) neurostimulator electrode array and pulse generator

(Do not report 64568 in conjunction with 61885, 61886, 64570)

(For insertion of chest wall respiratory sensor electrode or electrode array, including connection to pulse generator, use 0466T)

64569 Revision or replacement of cranial nerve (eg, vagus nerve) neurostimulator electrode array, including connection to existing pulse generator

(Do not report 64569 in conjunction with 64570 or 61888)

(For replacement of pulse generator, use 61885)

(For revision or replacement of chest wall respiratory sensor electrode or electrode array, including connection to existing pulse generator, use 0467T)

64570 Removal of cranial nerve (eg, vagus nerve) neurostimulator electrode array and pulse generator

(Do not report 64570 in conjunction with 61888)

(For laparoscopic implantation, revision, replacement, or removal of vagus nerve blocking neurostimulator electrode array and/or pulse generator at the esophagogastric junction, see 0312T-0317T)

(For removal of chest wall respiratory sensor electrode or electrode array, use 0468T)

64575 Incision for implantation of neurostimulator electrode array; peripheral nerve (excludes sacral nerve)

64580   neuromuscular

64581   sacral nerve (transforaminal placement)

64585 Revision or removal of peripheral neurostimulator electrode array

64590 Insertion or replacement of peripheral or gastric neurostimulator pulse generator or receiver, direct or inductive coupling

(Do not report 64590 in conjunction with 64595)

64595 Revision or removal of peripheral or gastric neurostimulator pulse generator or receiver

DESTRUCTION BY NEUROLYTIC AGENT (eg, CHEMICAL, THERMAL, ELECTRICAL, OR RADIOFREQUENCY), CHEMODENERVATION

Codes 64600-64681 include the injection of other therapeutic agents (eg., corticosteroids). Do not report diagnostic/therapeutic injections separately. Do not report a code labeled as destruction when using theraies that are not destructive of the target nerve (eg, pulsed radiofrequency), use 64999. For codes labeled as chemodenervation, the supply of the chemodenervation agent is reported separately.

(For chemodenervation of internal anal sphincter, use 46505)

(For chemodenervation of the bladder, use 52287)

(For chemodenervation for strabismus involving the extraocular muscles, use 67345)

(For chemodenervation guided by needle electromyography or muscle electrical stimulation, see 95873, 95874)

Somatic Nerves

64600 Destruction by neurolytic agent, trigeminal nerve; supraorbital, infraorbital, mental, or inferior alveolar branch

64605   second and third division branches at foramen ovale

64610   second and third division branches at foramen ovale under radiologic monitoring

64624   Destruction by neurolytic agent, genicular nerve branches including imaging guidance, when performed

(Do not report 64624 in conjunction with 64454)

(64624 requires the destruction of each of the following genicular nerve branches: superolateral, superomedial, and inferomedial. If a neurolytic agent for the purposes of destruction is not applied to all of these nerve branches, report 64624 with modifier 52)

64625   Radiofrequency ablation, nerves innervating the sacroiliac joint, with image guidance (ie, fluoroscopy or computed tomography)

(Do not report 64625 in conjunction with 64635, 77002, 77003, 77012, 95873, 95874)

(For radiofrequency ablation, nerves innervating the sacroiliac joint, with ultrasound, use 76999)

(For bilateral procedure, report 64625 with modifier 50)

64611   Chemodenervation of parotid and submandibular salivary glands, bilateral

(Report 64611 with modifier 52 if fewer than four salivary glands are injected)

64612   Chemodenervation of muscle(s); muscle(s) innervated by facial nerve, unilateral (eg, for blepharospasm, hemifacial spasm)

(For bilateral procedure, report 64612 with modifier 50)

64615   muscle(s) innervated by facial, trigeminal, cervical spinal and accessory nerves, bilateral (eg, for chronic migraine)

(Report 64615 only once per session)

(Do not report 64615 in conjunction with 64612, 64616, 64617, 64642, 64643, 64644, 64645, 64646, 64647)

(For guidance see 95873, 95874. Do not report more than one guidance code for 64615)

64616   neck muscle(s), excluding muscles of the larynx, unilateral (eg, for cervical dystonia, spasmodic torticollis)

(For bilateral procedure, report 64616 with modifier 50)

(For chemodenervation guided by needle electromyography or muscle electrical stimulation, see 95873, 95874. Do not report more than one guidance code for any unit of 64616)

64617   larynx, unilateral, percutaneous (eg, for spasmodic dysphonia), includes guidance by needle electromyography, when performed

(For bilateral procedure, report 64617 with modifier 50)

(Do not report 64617 in conjunction with 95873, 95874)

(For diagnostic needle electromyography of the larynx, use 95865)

(For chemodenervation of the larynx performed with direct laryngoscopy, see 31570, 31571)

64620   Destruction by neurolytic agent, intercostal nerve

(Imaging guidance [fluoroscopy, CT] are inclusive components of 64633-64636)

(Imaging guidance [fluoroscopy, CT] and any injection of contrast are inclusive components of 64633-64636. Image guidance and localization are required for the performance of paravertebral facet joint nerve destruction by neurolytic agent described by 64633-64636. If CT or fluoroscopic imaging is not used, report 64999)

  ●   New Code   ▲   Revised Code   ✛   Add-On Code   ⊘   Modifier -51 Exempt   ★   Telemedicine

Report 64633, 64634, 64635, 64636 per joint, not per nerve. Although two nerves innervate each facet joint, only one code may be reported for each joint denervated, regardless of the number of nerves treated. Use 64634 or 64636 to report each additional facet joint at a different vertebral level in the same spinal region.

For neurolytic destruction of the nerves innervating the T12-L1 paravertebral facet joint, use 64633.

Do not report 64633, 64634, 64635, 64636 for non-thermal facet joint denervation including chemical, low-grade thermal energy (<80 degrees Celsius), or any form of pulsed radiofrequency. To appropriately report any of these modalities, use 64999.

64624	This code is out of order. See page 614
64625	This code is out of order. See page 614

64633 Destruction by neurolytic agent, paravertebral facet joint nerve(s), with imaging guidance (fluoroscopy or CT); cervical or thoracic, single facet joint

(For bilateral procedure, report 64633 with modifier 50)

+ **64634** cervical or thoracic, each additional facet joint (List separately in addition to code for primary procedure)

(Use 64634 in conjunction with 64633)

(For bilateral procedure, report 64634 twice. Do not report modifier 50 in conjunction with 64634)

64635 lumbar or sacral, single facet joint

(For bilateral procedure, report 64635 with modifier 50)

+ **64636** lumbar or sacral, each additional facet joint (List separately in addition to code for primary procedure)

(Use 64636 in conjunction with 64635)

(For bilateral procedure, report 64636 twice. Do not report modifier 50 in conjunction with 64636)

(Do not report 64633-64636 in conjunction with 77003, 77012)

(For destruction by neurolytic agent, individual nerves, sacroiliac joint, use 64640)

64630 Destruction by neurolytic agent; pudendal nerve

64632 plantar common digital nerve

(Do not report 64632 in conjunction with 64455)

64633	Code out of order. See page 615
64634	Code out of order. See page 615
64635	Code out of order. See page 615
64636	Code out of order. See page 615

64640 other peripheral nerve or branch

Report 64642, 64643, 64644, 64645 once per extremity. Codes 64642, 64643, 64644, 64645 can be reported together up to a combined total of four units of service per patient when all four extremities are injected. Report only one base code (64642 or 64644) per session. Report one or more units of additional extremity code(s) (64643 or 64645) for each additional extremity injected.

Report 64646 or 64647 for chemodenervation of muscles of the trunk.

Trunk muscles include the erector spinae and paraspinal muscles, rectus abdominus and obliques. All other somatic muscles are extremity muscles, head muscles, or neck muscles.

(For chemodenervation guided by needle electromyography or muscle electrical stimulation, see 95873, 95874. Do not report more than one guidance code for each corresponding chemodenervation of extremity or trunk code)

(Do not report modifier 50 in conjunction with 64642, 64643, 64644, 64645, 64646, 64647)

64642 Chemodenervation of one extremity; 1-4 muscle(s)

+ 64643 each additional extremity, 1-4 muscle(s) (List separately in addition to code for primary procedure)

(Use 64643 in conjunction with 64642, 64644)

64644 Chemodenercvation of one extremity; 5 or more muscles

+ 64645 each additional extremity, 5 or more muscles (List separately in addition to code for primary procedure)

(Use 64645 in conjunction with 64644)

64646 Chemodenervation of trunk muscle(s); 1-5 muscle(s)

64647 6 or more muscles

(Report either 64646 or 64647 only once per session)

Sympathetic Nerves

64650 Chemodenervation of eccrine glands; both axillae

64653 other area(s) (eg, scalp, face, neck), per day

(Report the specific service in conjunction with code(s) for the specific substance(s) or drug(s) provided)

(For chemodenervation of extremities (eg, hands or feet), use 64999)

(For chemodenervation of bladder, use 52287)

64680 Destruction by neurolytic agent, with or without radiologic monitoring; celiac plexus

(For transendoscopic ultrasound-guided transmural injection, neurolytic agent, celiac plexus, use 43253)

64681 superior hypogastric plexus

NEUROPLASTY (EXPLORATION, NEUROLYSIS OR NERVE DECOMPRESSION)

Neuroplasty is the surgical decompression or freeing of intact nerve from scar tissue, including extrenal neurolysis and/or transposition to repair or restore the nerve.

(For percutaneous neurolysis, see 62263, 62264, 62280-62282)

(For internal neurolysis requiring use of operating microscope, use 64727)

(For facial nerve decompression, use 69720)

(For neuroplasty with nerve wrapping, see 64702-64727, 64999)

64702 Neuroplasty; digital, 1 or both, same digit

64704 nerve of hand or foot

(Do not report 64702, 64704 in conjunction with 11960)

64708 Neuroplasty, major peripheral nerve, arm or leg, open; other than specified

64712 sciatic nerve

64713   brachial plexus

64714   lumbar plexus

(Do not report 64708, 64712, 64713, 64714 in conjunction with 11960)

64716   Neuroplasty and/or transposition; cranial nerve (specify)

64718   ulnar nerve at elbow

64719   ulnar nerve at wrist

64721   median nerve at carpal tunnel

(Do not report 64716, 64718, 64719, 64721 in conjunction with 11960)

(For endoscopic procedure, use 29848)

64722   Decompression; unspecified nerve(s) (specify)

64726   plantar digital nerve

(Do not report 64722, 64726 in conjunction with 11960)

+ 64727   Internal neurolysis, requiring use of operating microscope (List separately in addition to code for neuroplasty) (Neuroplasty includes external neurolysis)

(Do not report code 69990 in addition to code 64727)

TRANSECTION OR AVULSION

(For stereotactic lesion of gasserian ganglion, use 61790)

64732   Transection or avulsion of; supraorbital nerve

64734   infraorbital nerve

64736   mental nerve

64738   inferior alveolar nerve by osteotomy

64740   lingual nerve

64742   facial nerve, differential or complete

64744   greater occipital nerve

64746   phrenic nerve

(For section of recurrent laryngeal nerve, use 31595)

64755   vagus nerves limited to proximal stomach (selective proximal vagotomy, proximal gastric vagotomy, parietal cell vagotomy, supra- or highly selective vagotomy)

(For laparoscopic approach, use 43652)

64760   vagus nerve (vagotomy), abdominal

(For laparoscopic approach, use 43651)

64763   Transection or avulsion of obturator nerve, extrapelvic, with or without adductor tenotomy

(For bilateral procedure, report 64763 with modifier -50)

64766   Transection or avulsion of obturator nerve, intrapelvic, with or without adductor tenotomy

(For bilateral procedure, report 64766 with modifier -50)

64771   Transection or avulsion of other cranial nerve, extradural

64772   Transection or avulsion of other spinal nerve, extradural

(For excision of tender scar, skin and subcutaneous tissue, with or without tiny neuroma, see 11400-11446, 13100-13153)

EXCISION

Somatic Nerves

(For Morton neurectomy, use 28080)

64774   Excision of neuroma; cutaneous nerve, surgically identifiable

64776   digital nerve, 1 or both, same digit

+ 64778   digital nerve, each additional digit (List separately in addition to code for primary procedure)

(Use 64778 in conjunction with code 64776)

64782   hand or foot, except digital nerve

+ 64783   hand or foot, each additional nerve, except same digit (List separately in addition to code for primary procedure)

(Use 64783 in conjunction with code 64782)

64784   major peripheral nerve, except sciatic

64786   sciatic nerve

+ 64787   Implantation of nerve end into bone or muscle (List separately in addition to neuroma excision)

(Use 64787 in conjunction with codes 64774-64786)

64788   Excision of neurofibroma or neurolemmoma; cutaneous nerve

64790   major peripheral nerve

64792   extensive (including malignant type)

(For destruction of extensive cutaneous neurofibroma, see 0419T, 0420T)

64795   Biopsy of nerve

Sympathetic Nerves

64802   Sympathectomy, cervical

(For bilateral procedure, report 64802 with modifier -50)

64804   Sympathectomy, cervicothoracic

(For bilateral procedure, report 64804 with modifier -50)

64809   Sympathectomy, thoracolumbar

(For bilateral procedure, report 64809 with modifier -50)

   ●   New Code   ▲   Revised Code   +   Add-On Code   ⦸   Modifier -51 Exempt   ★   Telemedicine

64818 Sympathectomy, lumbar

(For bilateral procedure, report 64818 with modifier -50)

64820 Sympathectomy; digital arteries, each digit

(Do not report 69990 in addition to code 64820)

64821 radial artery

(Do not report 69990 in addition to code 64821)

64822 ulnar artery

(Do not report 69990 in addition to code 64822)

64823 superficial palmar arch

(Do not report 69990 in addition to code 64823)

NEURORRHAPHY

64831 Suture of digital nerve, hand or foot; 1 nerve

+ **64832** each additional digital nerve (List separately in addition to code for primary procedure)

(Use 64832 in conjunction with code 64831)

64834 Suture of 1 nerve; hand or foot, common sensory nerve

64835 median motor thenar

64836 ulnar motor

+ **64837** Suture of each additional nerve, hand or foot (List separately in addition to code for primary procedure)

(Use 64837 in conjunction with codes 64834-64836)

64840 Suture of posterior tibial nerve

64856 Suture of major peripheral nerve, arm or leg, except sciatic; including transposition

64857 without transposition

64858 Suture of sciatic nerve

+ **64859** Suture of each additional major peripheral nerve (List separately in addition to code for primary procedure)

(Use 64859 in conjunction with codes 64856, 64857)

64861 Suture of; brachial plexus

64862 lumbar plexus

64864 Suture of facial nerve; extracranial

64865 infratemporal, with or without grafting

64866 Anastomosis; facial-spinal accessory

64868 facial-hypoglossal

+ 64872   Suture of nerve; requiring secondary or delayed suture (List separately in addition to code for primary neurorrhaphy)

(Use 64872 in conjunction with codes 64831-64865)

+ 64874   requiring extensive mobilization, or transposition of nerve (List separately in addition to code for nerve suture)

(Use 64874 in conjunction with codes 64831-64865)

+ 64876   requiring shortening of bone of extremity (List separately in addition to code for nerve suture)

(Use 64876 in conjunction with codes 64831-64865)

NEURORRHAPHY WITH NERVE GRAFT, VEIN GRAFT, OR CONDUIT

64885   Nerve graft (includes obtaining graft), head or neck; up to 4 cm in length

64886   more than 4 cm length

64890   Nerve graft (includes obtaining graft), single strand, hand or foot; up to 4 cm length

64891   more than 4 cm length

64892   Nerve graft (includes obtaining graft), single strand, arm or leg; up to 4 cm length

64893   more than 4 cm length

64895   Nerve graft (includes obtaining graft), multiple strands (cable), hand or foot; up to 4 cm length

64896   more than 4 cm length

64897   Nerve graft (includes obtaining graft), multiple strands (cable), arm or leg; up to 4 cm length

64898   more than 4 cm length

+ 64901   Nerve graft, each additional nerve; single strand (List separately in addition to code for primary procedure)

(Use 64901 in conjunction with codes 64885-64893)

+ 64902   multiple strands (cable) (List separately in addition to code for primary procedure)

(Use 64902 in conjunction with codes 64885, 64886, 64895-64898)

64905   Nerve pedicle transfer; first stage

64907   second stage

64910   Nerve repair; with synthetic conduit or vein allograft (eg, nerve tube), each nerve

64911   with autogenous vein graft (includes harvest of vein graft), each nerve

(Do not report 69990 in addition to 64910, 64911)

64912   with nerve allograft, each nerve, first strand (cable)

+ 64913   with nerve allograft, each additional strand (List separately in addition to code for primary procedure)

(Use 64913 in conjunction with 64912)

(Do not report 64912, 64913 in conjunction with 69990)

   ● New Code   ▲ Revised Code   + Add-On Code   ⃠ Modifier -51 Exempt   ★ Telemedicine

OTHER PROCEDURES

64999 Unlisted procedure, nervous system

This page intentionally left blank.

EYE AND OCULAR ADNEXA

CPT codes from this section of the CPT coding system are used to report surgical procedures on the eye and ocular adnexa. Diagnostic services and medical treatment of the eye are defined in the Medicine Section of the CPT manual.

If surgical procedures are performed only on the eyelid, code from the Integumentary System subsection of the CPT coding system. Cataract codes are selected on the type of procedure performed. Whenever injections are performed during cataract surgery, do not report them separately.

When a subconjunctival injection (e.g. CPT code 68200) with a local anesthetic is performed as part of a more extensive anesthetic procedure (e.g. peribulbar or retrobulbar block), a separate service for this procedure is not to be reported. This is a routine part of the anesthetic procedure and does not represent a separate service.

Iridectomy, trabeculectomy, and anterior vitrectomy may be performed in conjunction with cataract removal. When an iridectomy is performed in order to accomplish the cataract extraction, it is an integral part of the procedure; it does not represent a separate service, and is not separately reported. Similarly, the minimal vitreous loss occurring during routine cataract extraction does not represent a vitrectomy and is not to be separately reported unless it is medically necessary for a different diagnosis.

While a trabeculectomy is not performed as a part of a cataract extraction, it may be performed to control glaucoma at the same time as a cataract extraction. If the procedure is medically necessary at the same time as a cataract extraction, it can be reported under a different diagnosis (e.g. glaucoma). The codes describing iridectomies, trabeculectomies, and anterior vitrectomies, when performed with a cataract extraction under a separate diagnosis, must be reported with modifier - 59. This indicates that the procedure was performed as a different service for a separate situation. The medical record should reflect the medical necessity of the service if separately reported.

For example, if a patient presents with a cataract and has evidence of glaucoma, (i.e. elevated intraocular pressure preoperatively) and a trabeculectomy represents the appropriate treatment for the glaucoma, a separate service for the trabeculectomy would be separately reported. Performance of a trabeculectomy as a preventative service for an expected transient increase in intraocular pressure postoperatively, without other evidence for glaucoma, is not to be separately reported.

The various approaches to removing a cataract are mutually exclusive of one another when performed on the same eye.

Some retinal detachment repair procedures include some vitreous procedures (e.g. CPT code 67108 includes 67015, 67025, 67028, 67031, 67036, 67039, and 67040). Certain retinal detachment repairs are mutually exclusive to anterior procedures such as focal endolaser photocoagulation (e.g. CPT codes 67110 and 67112 are mutually exclusive to CPT code 67108).

CPT codes 68020-68200 (incision, drainage, excision of the conjunctiva) are included in all conjunctivoplasties (CPT codes 68320-68362).

CPT code 67950 (canthoplasty) is included in repair procedures such as blepharoplasties (CPT codes 67917, 67924, 67961, 67966).

Correction of lid retraction (CPT code 67911) includes full thickness graft (e.g. CPT code 15260) as part of the total service performed.

In the circumstance that it is medically necessary and reasonable to inject sclerosing agents in the same session as surgery to correct glaucoma, the service is included in the glaucoma surgery. Accordingly, codes such as CPT codes 67500, 67515, and 68200 for injection of sclerosing agents (e.g. 5-FU, HCPCS/CPT code J9190) should not be reported with other pressure-reducing or glaucoma procedures.

(For diagnostic and treatment ophthalmological services, see Medicine, Ophthalmology, and 92002 et seq)

(Do not report code 69990 in addition to codes 65091-68850)

EYEBALL

REMOVAL OF EYE

65091 Evisceration of ocular contents; without implant

65093 with implant

65101	Enucleation of eye; without implant
65103	with implant, muscles not attached to implant
65105	with implant, muscles attached to implant

(For conjunctivoplasty after enucleation, see 68320 et seq)

65110	Exenteration of orbit (does not include skin graft), removal of orbital contents; only
65112	with therapeutic removal of bone
65114	with muscle or myocutaneous flap

(For skin graft to orbit (split skin), see 15120, 15121; free, full thickness, see 15260, 15261)

(For eyelid repair involving more than skin, see 67930 et seq)

SECONDARY IMPLANT(S) PROCEDURES

65125	Modification of ocular implant with placement or replacement of pegs (eg, drilling receptacle for prosthesis appendage) (separate procedure)
65130	Insertion of ocular implant secondary; after evisceration, in scleral shell
65135	after enucleation, muscles not attached to implant
65140	after enucleation, muscles attached to implant
65150	Reinsertion of ocular implant; with or without conjunctival graft
65155	with use of foreign material for reinforcement and/or attachment of muscles to implant
65175	Removal of ocular implant

(For orbital implant (implant outside muscle cone) insertion, use 67550; removal, use 67560)

REMOVAL OF FOREIGN BODY

(For removal of implanted material: ocular implant, use 65175; anterior segment implant, use 65920; posterior segment implant, use 67120; orbital implant, use 67560)

(For diagnostic x-ray for foreign body, use 70030)

(For diagnostic echography for foreign body, use 76529)

(For removal of foreign body from orbit: frontal approach, use 67413; lateral approach, use 67430)

(For removal of foreign body from eyelid, embedded, use 67938)

(For removal of foreign body from lacrimal system, use 68530)

65205	Removal of foreign body, external eye; conjunctival superficial
65210	conjunctival embedded (includes concretions), subconjunctival, or scleral nonperforating
65220	corneal, without slit lamp
65222	corneal, with slit lamp

(For repair of corneal laceration with foreign body, use 65275)

| 65235 | Removal of foreign body, intraocular; from anterior chamber of eye or lens |

(For removal of implanted material from anterior segment, use 65920)

65260   from posterior segment, magnetic extraction, anterior or posterior route

65265   from posterior segment, nonmagnetic extraction

(For removal of implanted material from posterior segment, use 67120)

REPAIR OF LACERATION

(For fracture of orbit, see 21385 et seq)

(For repair of wound of eyelid, skin, linear, simple, see 12011-12018; intermediate, layered closure, see 12051-12057; linear, complex, see 13151-13160; other, see 67930, 67935)

(For repair of wound of lacrimal system, use 68700)

(For repair of operative wound, use 66250)

65270   Repair of laceration; conjunctiva, with or without nonperforating laceration sclera, direct closure

65272   conjunctiva, by mobilization and rearrangement, without hospitalization

65273   conjunctiva, by mobilization and rearrangement, with hospitalization

65275   cornea, nonperforating, with or without removal foreign body

65280   cornea and/or sclera, perforating, not involving uveal tissue

65285   cornea and/or sclera, perforating, with reposition or resection of uveal tissue

(65280 amd 65285 are not used for repair of a surgical wound)

65286   application of tissue glue, wounds of cornea and/or sclera

(Repair of laceration includes use of conjunctival flap and restoration of anterior chamber, by air or saline injection when indicated)

(For repair of iris or ciliary body, use 66680)

65290   Repair of wound, extraocular muscle, tendon and/or Tenon's capsule

ANTERIOR SEGMENT

CORNEA

Excision

65400   Excision of lesion, cornea (keratectomy, lamellar, partial), except pterygium

65410   Biopsy of cornea

65420   Excision or transposition of pterygium; without graft

65426   with graft

Removal or Destruction

65430   Scraping of cornea, diagnostic, for smear and/or culture

65435   Removal of corneal epithelium; with or without chemocauterization (abrasion, curettage)

(Do not report 65435 in conjunction with 0402T)

65436	with application of chelating agent (eg, EDTA)
65450	Destruction of lesion of cornea by cryotherapy, photocoagulation or thermocauterization
65600	Multiple punctures of anterior cornea (eg, for corneal erosion, tattoo)

Keratoplasty

Corneal transplant includes use of fresh or preserved grafts. The preparation of donor material is included for penetrating or anterior lamellar keratoplasty, but reported separately for endothelial keratoplasty. Do not report 65710-65757 in conjunction with 92025.

(Keratoplasty excludes refractive keratoplasty procedures, 65760, 65765, and 65767)

65710	Keratoplasty (corneal transplant); anterior lamellar
65730	penetrating (except in aphakia or pseudoaphakia)
65750	penetrating (in aphakia)
65755	penetrating (in pseudophakia)
65756	endothelial
+ 65757	Backbench preparation of corneal endothelial allograft prior to transplantation (list separately in addition to code for primary procedure)

(Use 65757 in conjunction with 65756)

Other Procedures

Do not report 65760-65771 in conjunction with 92025.

65760	Keratomileusis
65765	Keratophakia
65767	Epikeratoplasty
65770	Keratoprosthesis
65771	Radial keratotomy
65772	Corneal relaxing incision for correction of surgically induced astigmatism
65775	Corneal wedge resection for correction of surgically induced astigmatism

(For fitting of contact lens for treatment of disease, use 92071, 92072)

(For unlisted procedures on cornea, use 66999)

| 65778 | Placement of amniotic membrane on the ocular surface; without sutures |
| 65779 | single layer, sutured |

(Do not report 65778, 65779 in conjunction with 65430, 65435, 65780)

(For placement of amniotic membrane using tissue glue, use 66999)

| 65780 | Ocular surface reconstruction; amniotic membrane transplantation, multiple layers |

(For placement of amniotic membrane without reconstruction using no sutures or single layer suture technique, see 65778, 65779)

● New Code ▲ Revised Code + Add-On Code ⊘ Modifier -51 Exempt ★ Telemedicine

65781   limbal stem cell allograft (eg, cadaveric or living donor)

65782   limbal conjunctival autograft (includes obtaining graft)

(For harvesting conjunctival allograft, living donor, use 68371)

65785   Implantation of intrastromal corneal ring segments

ANTERIOR CHAMBER

Incision

65800   Paracentesis of anterior chamber of eye (separate procedure); with removal of aqueous

65810   with removal of vitreous and/or discission of anterior hyaloid membrane, with or without air injection

65815   with removal of blood, with or without irrigation and/or air injection

(For injection, see 66020-66030)

(For removal of blood clot, use 65930)

65820   Goniotomy

(Do not report modifier -63 in conjunction with 65820)

(For use of ophthalmic endoscope with 65820, use 66990)

65850   Trabeculotomy ab externo

65855   Trabeculoplasty by laser surgery

(Do not report 65855 in conjunction with 65860, 65865, 65870, 65875, 65880)

(For trabeculectomy, use 66170)

65860   Severing adhesions of anterior segment, laser technique (separate procedure)

65865   Severing adhesions of anterior segment of eye, incisional technique (with or without injection of air or liquid) (separate procedure); goniosynechiae

(For trabeculoplasty by laser surgery, use 65855)

65870   anterior synechiae, except goniosynechiae

65875   posterior synechiae

(For use of ophthalmic endoscope with 65875, use 66990)

65880   corneovitreal adhesions

(For laser surgery, use 66821)

Removal

65900   Removal of epithelial downgrowth, anterior chamber of eye

65920   Removal of implanted material, anterior segment of eye

(For use of ophthalmic endoscope with 65920, use 66990)

65930   Removal of blood clot, anterior segment of eye

Separate Procedure   Unlisted Procedure   CCI Comp. Code   Non-specific Procedure   **627**

Introduction

66020   Injection, anterior chamber of eye (separate procedure); air or liquid

66030   medication

(For unlisted procedures on anterior segment, use 66999)

ANTERIOR SCLERA

Excision

(For removal of intraocular foreign body, use 65235)

(For operations on posterior sclera, use 67250, 67255)

66130   Excision of lesion, sclera

66150   Fistulization of sclera for glaucoma; trephination with iridectomy

66155   thermocauterization with iridectomy

66160   sclerectomy with punch or scissors, with iridectomy

66170   trabeculectomy ab externo in absence of previous surgery

(For trabeculotomy ab externo, use 65850)

(For repair of operative wound, use 66250)

66172   trabeculectomy ab externo with scarring from previous ocular surgery or trauma (includes injection of antifibrotic agents)

66174   Transluminal dilation of aqueous outflow canal; without retention of device or stent

66175   with retention of device or stent

Aqueous Shunt

66179   Aqueous shunt to extraocular equatorial plate reservois, external approach; without graft

66180   with graft

(Do not report 66180 in conjunction with 67255)

66183   Insertion of anterior segment aqueous drainage device, without extraocular reservoir, external approach

66184   Revision of aqueous shunt to extraocular equatorial plate reservoir; without graft

66185   with graft

(Do not report 66185 in conjunction with 67255)

(For removal of implanted shunt, use 67120)

Repair or Revision

(For scleral procedures in retinal surgery, see 67101 et seq)

(**66220**   deleted 2018 [2019 Edition])

66225   Repair of scleral staphyloma with graft

(For scleral reinforcement, see 67250, 67255)

66250   Revision or repair of operative wound of anterior segment, any type, early or late, major or minor procedure

(For unlisted procedures on anterior sclera, use 66999)

IRIS, CILIARY BODY

Incision

66500   Iridotomy by stab incision (separate procedure); except transfixion

66505   with transfixion as for iris bombe

(For iridotomy by photocoagulation, use 66761)

Excision

66600   Iridectomy, with corneoscleral or corneal section; for removal of lesion

66605   with cyclectomy

66625   peripheral for glaucoma (separate procedure)

66630   sector for glaucoma (separate procedure)

66635   optical (separate procedure)

(For coreoplasty by photocoagulation, use 66762)

Repair

66680   Repair of iris, ciliary body (as for iridodialysis)

(For reposition or resection of uveal tissue with perforating wound of cornea or sclera, use 65285)

66682   Suture of iris, ciliary body (separate procedure) with retrieval of suture through small incision (eg, McCannel suture)

Destruction

66700   Ciliary body destruction; diathermy

66710   cyclophotocoagulation, transscleral

66711   cyclophotocoagulation, endoscopic, without concomitant removal of crystalline lens

(For endoscopic cyclophotocoagulation performed at same encounter as extracapsular cataract removal with intraocular lens insertion, see 66987, 66988)

(Do not report 66711 in conjunction with 66990)

66720   cryotherapy

66740   cyclodialysis

66761   Iridotomy/iridectomy by laser surgery (eg, for glaucoma) (per session)

66762   Iridoplasty by photocoagulation (1 or more sessions) (eg, for improvement of vision, for widening of anterior chamber angle)

66770   Destruction of cyst or lesion iris or ciliary body (nonexcisional procedure)

(For excision lesion iris, ciliary body, see 66600, 66605; for removal of epithelial downgrowth, use 65900)

(For unlisted procedures on iris, ciliary body, use 66999)

LENS

Incision

66820   Discission of secondary membranous cataract (opacified posterior lens capsule and/or anterior hyaloid); stab incision technique (Ziegler or Wheeler knife)

66821   laser surgery (eg, YAG laser) (1 or more stages)

66825   Repositioning of intraocular lens prosthesis, requiring an incision (separate procedure)

Removal

Lateral canthotomy, iridectomy, iridotomy, anterior capsulotomy, posterior capsulotomy, the use of viscoelastic agents, enzymatic zonulysis, use of other pharmacologic agents, and subconjunctival or sub-tenon injections are included as part of the code for the extraction of lens.

66830   Removal of secondary membranous cataract (opacified posterior lens capsule and/or anterior hyaloid) with corneo-scleral section, with or without iridectomy (iridocapsulotomy, iridocapsulectomy)

66840   Removal of lens material; aspiration technique, 1 or more stages

66850   phacofragmentation technique (mechanical or ultrasonic) (eg, phacoemulsification), with aspiration

66852   pars plana approach, with or without vitrectomy

66920   intracapsular

66930   intracapsular, for dislocated lens

66940   extracapsular (other than 66840, 66850, 66852)

(For removal of intralenticular foreign body without lens extraction, use 65235)

(For repair of operative wound, use 66250)

INTRAOCULAR LENS PROCEDURES

66982   Extracapsular cataract removal with insertion of intraocular lens prosthesis (1-stage procedure), manual or mechanical technique (eg, irrigation and aspiration or phacoemulsification), complex, requiring devices or techniques not generally used in routine cataract surgery (eg, iris expansion device, suture support for intraocular lens, or primary posterior capsulorrhexis) or performed on patients in the amblyogenic developmental stage; without endoscopic cyclophotocoagulation

(For complex extracapsular cataract removal with concomitant endoscopic cyclophotocoagulation, use 66987)

(For insertion of ocular telescope prosthesis including removal of crystalline lens, use 0308T)

66987   with endoscopic cyclophotocoagulation

(For complex extracapsular cataract removal without endoscopic cyclophotocoagulation, use 66982)

(For insertion of ocular telescope prosthesis including removal of crystalline lens, use 0308T)

66983   Intracapsular cataract extraction with insertion of intraocular lens prosthesis (1 stage procedure)

(Do not report 66983 in conjunction with 0308T)

66984   Extracapsular cataract removal with insertion of intraocular lens prosthesis (1 stage procedure), manual or mechanical technique (eg, irrigation and aspiration or phacoemulsification); without endoscopic cyclophotocoagulation

---

   ● New Code   ▲ Revised Code   + Add-On Code   ⊘ Modifier -51 Exempt   ★ Telemedicine

(For complex extracapsular cataract removal, use 66982)

(For extracapsular cataract removal with concomitant endoscopic cyclophotocoagulation, use 66988)

(For insertion of ocular telescope prosthesis including removal of crystalline lens, use 0308T)

66988   with endoscopic cyclophotocoagulation

(For extracapsular cataract removal without endoscopic cyclophotocoagulation, use 66984)

(For complex extracapsular cataract removal with endoscopic cyclophotocoagulation, use 66987)

(For insertion of ocular telescope prosthesis, including removal of crystalline lens, use 0308T)

66985   Insertion of intraocular lens prosthesis (secondary implant), not associated with concurrent cataract removal

(To code implant at time of concurrent cataract surgery, see 66982, 66983, 66984)

(To report supply of intraocular lens prosthesis, use 99070)

(For ultrasonic determination of intraocular lens power, use 76519)

(For removal of implanted material from anterior segment, use 65920)

(For secondary fixation (separate procedure), use 66682)

(For use of ophthalmic endoscope with 66985, use 66990)

66986   Exchange of intraocular lens

(For use of ophthalmic endoscope with 66986, use 66990)

66987   This code is out of order. See page 630

66988   This code is out of order. See page 631

OTHER PROCEDURES

+ 66990   Use of ophthalmic endoscope (List separately in addition to code for primary procedure)

(66990 may be used only with codes 65820, 65875, 65920, 66985, 66986, 67036, 67039, 67040, 67041, 67042, 67043, 67113)

66999   Unlisted procedure, anterior segment of eye

POSTERIOR SEGMENT

VITREOUS

67005   Removal of vitreous, anterior approach (open sky technique or limbal incision); partial removal

67010   subtotal removal with mechanical vitrectomy

(For removal of vitreous by paracentesis of anterior chamber, use 65810)

(For removal of corneovitreal adhesions, use 65880)

67015   Aspiration or release of vitreous, subretinal or choroidal fluid, pars plana approach (posterior sclerotomy)

67025   Injection of vitreous substitute, pars plana or limbal approach, (fluid-gas exchange), with or without aspiration (separate procedure)

67027   Implantation of intravitreal drug delivery system (eg, ganciclovir implant), includes concomitant removal of vitreous

(For removal, use 67121)

67028   Intravitreal injection of a pharmacologic agent (separate procedure)

67030   Discission of vitreous strands (without removal), pars plana approach

67031   Severing of vitreous strands, vitreous face adhesions, sheets, membranes or opacities, laser surgery (1 or more stages)

67036   Vitrectomy, mechanical, pars plana approach;

(For application of intraocular epiretinal radiation with 67036, use 0190T)

67039   with focal endolaser photocoagulation

67040   with endolaser panretinal photocoagulation

67041   with removal of preretinal cellular membrane (eg, macular pucker)

67042   with removal of internal limiting membrane of retina (eg, for repair of macular hole, diabetic macular edema), includes, if performed, intraocular tamponade (ie, air, gas or silicone oil)

67043   with removal of subretinal membrane (eg, choroidal neovascularization), includes, if performed, intraocular tamponade (ie, air, gas or silicone oil) and laser photocoagulation

(For use of ophthalmic endoscope with 67036, 67039, 67040-67043, use 66990)

(For associated lensectomy, use 66850)

(For use of vitrectomy in retinal detachment surgery, see 67108, 67113)

(For associated removal of foreign body, see 65260, 65265)

(For unlisted procedures on vitreous, use 67299)

RETINA OR CHOROID

Repair

(If diathermy, cryotherapy and/or photocoagulation are combined, report under principal modality used)

67101   Repair of retinal detachment, including drainage of subretinal fluid when performed; cryotherapy

67105   photocoagulation

67107   Repair of retinal detachment; scleral buckling (such as lamellar scleral dissection, imbrication or encircling procedure), including, when performed, implant, cryotherapy, photocoagulation, and drainage of subretinal fluid

67108   with vitrectomy, any method, including, when performed, air or gas tamponade, focal endolaser photocoagulation, cryotherapy, drainage of subretinal fluid, scleral buckling, and/or removal of lens by same technique

67110   by injection of air or other gas (eg, pneumatic retinopexy)

(For aspiration of drainage of subretinal or subchoroidal fluid, use 67015)

67113   Repair of complex retinal detachment (eg, proliferative vitreoretinopathy, stage C-1 or greater, diabetic traction retinal detachment, retinopathy of prematurity, retinal tear of greater than 90 degrees), with vitrectomy and membrane peeling, including, when performed, air, gas, or silicone oil tamponade, cryotherapy, endolaser photocoagulation, drainage of subretinal fluid, scleral buckling, and/or removal of lens

(To report vitrectomy, pars plana approach, other than in retinal detachment surgery, see 67036-67043)

(For use of ophthalmic endoscope with 67113, use 66990)

67115	Release of encircling material (posterior segment)
67120	Removal of implanted material, posterior segment; extraocular
67121	intraocular

(For removal from anterior segment, use 65920)

(For removal of foreign body, see 65260, 65265)

Prophylaxis

Codes 67141, 67145 include treatment at one or more sessions that may occur at different encounters. These codes should be reported once during a defined treatment period.

Repetitive services. The services listed below are often performed in multiple sessions or groups of sessions. The methods of reporting vary. The following descriptors are intended to include all sessions in a defined treatment period.

67141	Prophylaxis of retinal detachment (eg, retinal break, lattice degeneration) without drainage, 1 or more sessions; cryotherapy, diathermy
67145	photocoagulation (laser or xenon arc)

Destruction

Codes 67208, 67210, 67218, 67220, 67229 include treatment at one or more sessions that may occur at different encounters. These codes should be reported once during a defined treatment period.

67208	Destruction of localized lesion of retina (eg, macular edema, tumors), 1 or more sessions; cryotherapy, diathermy
67210	photocoagulation
67218	radiation by implantation of source (includes removal of source)
67220	Destruction of localized lesion of choroid (eg, choroidal neovascularization); photocoagulation (eg, laser), 1 or more sessions
67221	photodynamic therapy (includes intravenous infusion)
+ **67225**	photodynamic therapy, second eye, at single session (List separately in addition to code for primary eye treatment)

(Use 67225 in conjunction with code 67221)

67227	Destruction of extensive or progressive retinopathy (eg, diabetic retinopathy), cryotherapy, diathermy
67228	Treatment of extensive or progressive retinopathy (eg, diabetic retinopathy), photocoagulation
67229	preterm infant (less than 37 weeks gestation at birth), performed from birth up to 1 year of age (eg, retinopathy of prematurity), photocoagulation or cryotherapy

(For bilateral procedure, use modifier 50 with 67208, 67210, 67218, 67220, 67227, 67228, 67229)

(For unlisted procedures on retina, use 67299)

POSTERIOR SCLERA

Repair

(For excision lesion sclera, use 66130)

67250	Scleral reinforcement (separate procedure); without graft

67255   with graft

(Do not report 67255 in conjunction with 66180, 66185)

(For repair scleral staphyloma, see 66225)

OTHER PROCEDURES

67299   Unlisted procedure, posterior segment

OCULAR ADNEXA

EXTRAOCULAR MUSCLES

67311   Strabismus surgery, recession or resection procedure; 1 horizontal muscle

67312   2 horizontal muscles

67314   1 vertical muscle (excluding superior oblique)

67316   2 or more vertical muscles (excluding superior oblique)

(For adjustable sutures, use 67335 in addition to codes 67311-67334 for primary procedure reflecting number of muscles operated on)

67318   Strabismus surgery, any procedure, superior oblique muscle

+ **67320**   Transposition procedure (eg, for paretic extraocular muscle), any extraocular muscle (specify) (List separately in addition to code for primary procedure)

(Use 67320 in conjunction with codes 67311-67318)

+ **67331**   Strabismus surgery on patient with previous eye surgery or injury that did not involve the extraocular muscles (List separately in addition to code for primary procedure)

(Use 67331 in conjunction with codes 67311-67318)

+ **67332**   Strabismus surgery on patient with scarring of extraocular muscles (eg, prior ocular injury, strabismus or retinal detachment surgery) or restrictive myopathy (eg, dysthyroid ophthalmopathy) (List separately in addition to code for primary procedure)

(Use 67332 in conjunction with codes 67311-67318)

+ **67334**   Strabismus surgery by posterior fixation suture technique, with or without muscle recession (List separately in addition to code for primary procedure)

(Use 67334 in conjunction with codes 67311-67318)

+ **67335**   Placement of adjustable suture(s) during strabismus surgery, including postoperative adjustment(s) of suture(s) (List separately in addition to code for specific strabismus surgery)

(Use 67335 in conjunction with codes 67311-67334)

+ **67340**   Strabismus surgery involving exploration and/or repair of detached extraocular muscle(s) (List separately in addition to code for primary procedure)

(Use 67340 in conjunction with codes 67311-67334)

67343   Release of extensive scar tissue without detaching extraocular muscle (separate procedure)

(Use 67343 in conjunction with codes 67311-67340, when such procedures are performed other than on the affected muscle)

67345   Chemodenervation of extraocular muscle

● New Code   ▲ Revised Code   + Add-On Code   ⊘ Modifier -51 Exempt   ★ Telemedicine

(For chemodenervation for blepharospasm and other neurological disorders, see 64612 and 64616)

67346 Biopsy of extraocular muscle

(For repair of wound, extraocular muscle, tendon or Tenon's capsule, use 65290)

Other Procedures

67399 Unlisted procedure, extraocular muscle

ORBIT

Exploration, Excision, Decompression

67400 Orbitotomy without bone flap (frontal or transconjunctival approach); for exploration, with or without biopsy

67405 with drainage only

67412 with removal of lesion

67413 with removal of foreign body

67414 with removal of bone for decompression

67415 Fine needle aspiration of orbital contents

(For exenteration, enucleation, and repair, see 65101 et seq; for optic nerve decompression, use 67570)

67420 Orbitotomy with bone flap or window, lateral approach (eg, Kroenlein); with removal of lesion

67430 with removal of foreign body

67440 with drainage

67445 with removal of bone for decompression

(For optic nerve sheath decompression, use 67570)

67450 for exploration, with or without biopsy

(For orbitotomy, transcranial approach, see 61330, 61333)

(For orbital implant, see 67550, 67560)

(For removal of eyeball or for repair after removal, see 65091-65175)

Other Procedures

67500 Retrobulbar injection; medication (separate procedure, does not include supply of medication)

67505 alcohol

67515 Injection of medication or other substance into Tenon's capsule

(For subconjunctival injection, use 68200)

67550 Orbital implant (implant outside muscle cone); insertion

67560 removal or revision

(For ocular implant (implant inside muscle cone), see 65093-65105, 65130-65175)

(For treatment of fractures of malar area, orbit, see 21355 et seq)

67570   Optic nerve decompression (eg, incision or fenestration of optic nerve sheath)

67599   Unlisted procedure, orbit

EYELIDS

Incision

67700   Blepharotomy, drainage of abscess, eyelid

67710   Severing of tarsorrhaphy

67715   Canthotomy (separate procedure)

(For canthoplasty, use 67950)

(For division of symblepharon, use 68340)

67810   Incisional biopsy of eyelid skin includnig lid margin

(For biopsy of skin of eyelid, see 11102, 11103, 11104, 11105, 11106, 11107)

Excision, Destruction

Codes for removal of lesions include more than skin (ie., involving lid margin, tarsus, and/or palpebral conjunctiva).

(For removal of lesion, involving mainly skin of eyelid, see 11310-11313; 11440-11446, 11640-11646; 17000-17004)

(For repair of wounds, blepharoplasty, grafts, reconstructive surgery, see 67930-67975)

67800   Excision of chalazion; single

67801   multiple, same lid

67805   multiple, different lids

67808   under general anesthesia and/or requiring hospitalization, single or multiple

67810   Code out of order. See page 636

67820   Correction of trichiasis; epilation, by forceps only

67825   epilation by other than forceps (eg, by electrosurgery, cryotherapy, laser surgery)

67830   incision of lid margin

67835   incision of lid margin, with free mucous membrane graft

67840   Excision of lesion of eyelid (except chalazion) without closure or with simple direct closure

(For excision and repair of eyelid by reconstructive surgery, see 67961, 67966)

67850   Destruction of lesion of lid margin (up to 1 cm)

(For Mohs micrographic surgery, see 17311-17315)

(For initiation or follow-up care of topical chemotherapy (eg, 5-FU or similar agents), see appropriate office visits)

   ● New Code   ▲ Revised Code   + Add-On Code   ⊘ Modifier -51 Exempt   ★ Telemedicine

Tarsorrhaphy

67875 Temporary closure of eyelids by suture (eg, Frost suture)

67880 Construction of intermarginal adhesions, median tarsorrhaphy, or canthorrhaphy;

67882   with transposition of tarsal plate

(For severing of tarsorrhaphy, use 67710)

(For canthoplasty, reconstruction canthus, use 67950)

(For canthotomy, use 67715)

Repair (Brow Ptosis, Blepharoptosis, Lid Retraction, Ectropion, Entropion)

67900 Repair of brow ptosis (supraciliary, mid-forehead or coronal approach)

(For forehead rhytidectomy, use 15824)

67901 Repair of blepharoptosis; frontalis muscle technique with suture or other material (eg, banked fascia)

67902   frontalis muscle technique with autologous fascial sling (includes obtaining fascia)

67903   (tarso) levator resection or advancement, internal approach

67904   (tarso) levator resection or advancement, external approach

67906   superior rectus technique with fascial sling (includes obtaining fascia)

67908   conjunctivo-tarso-Muller's muscle-levator resection (eg, Fasanella-Servat type)

67909 Reduction of overcorrection of ptosis

67911 Correction of lid retraction

(For obtaining autologous graft materials, see 15769, 20920, 20922)

(For correction of lid defects using fat harvested via liposuction technique, see 15773, 15774)

(For correction of trichiasis by mucous membrane graft, use 67835)

67912 Correction of lagophthalmos, with implantation of upper eyelid load (eg, gold weight)

67914 Repair of ectropion; suture

67915   thermocauterization

67916   excision tarsal wedge

67917   extensive (eg, tarsal strip operations)

(For correction of everted punctum, use 68705)

67921 Repair of entropion; suture

67922   thermocauterization

67923   excision tarsal wedge

67924   extensive (eg, tarsal strip or capsulopalpebral fascia repairs operation)

(For repair of cicatricial ectropion or entropion requiring scar excision or skin graft, see also 67961 et seq)

| Separate Procedure | Unlisted Procedure | CCI Comp. Code | Non-specific Procedure | **637** |

Reconstruction

Codes for blepharoplasty involve more than skin (ie., involving lid margin, tarsus, and/or palpebral conjunctiva).

67930 Suture of recent wound, eyelid, involving lid margin, tarsus, and/or palpebral conjunctiva direct closure; partial thickness

67935 full thickness

67938 Removal of embedded foreign body, eyelid

(For repair of skin of eyelid, see 12011-12018; 12051-12057; 13151-13153)

(For tarsorrhaphy, canthorrhaphy, see 67880, 67882)

(For repair of blepharoptosis and lid retraction, see 67901-67911)

(For blepharoplasty for entropion, ectropion, see 67916, 67917, 67923, 67924)

(For correction of blepharochalasis (blepharorhytidectomy), see 15820-15823)

(For repair of skin of eyelid, adjacent tissue transfer, see 14060, 14061; preparation for graft, use 15004; free graft, see 15120, 15121, 15260, 15261)

(For excision of lesion of eyelid, use 67800 et seq)

(For repair of lacrimal canaliculi, use 68700)

67950 Canthoplasty (reconstruction of canthus)

67961 Excision and repair of eyelid, involving lid margin, tarsus, conjunctiva, canthus, or full thickness, may include preparation for skin graft or pedicle flap with adjacent tissue transfer or rearrangement; up to one-fourth of lid margin

67966 over one-fourth of lid margin

(For canthoplasty, use 67950)

(For free skin grafts, see 15120, 15121, 15260, 15261)

(For tubed pedicle flap preparation, use 15576; for delay, use 15630; for attachment, use 15650)

67971 Reconstruction of eyelid, full thickness by transfer of tarsoconjunctival flap from opposing eyelid; up to two-thirds of eyelid, 1 stage or first stage

67973 total eyelid, lower, 1 stage or first stage

67974 total eyelid, upper, 1 stage or first stage

67975 second stage

Other Procedures

67999 Unlisted procedure, eyelids

CONJUNCTIVA

(For removal of foreign body, see 65205 et seq)

INCISION AND DRAINAGE

68020 Incision of conjunctiva, drainage of cyst

68040 Expression of conjunctival follicles (eg, for trachoma)

● New Code   ▲ Revised Code   ＋ Add-On Code   ⊘ Modifier -51 Exempt   ★ Telemedicine

(To report automated evacuation of Meibomian glands, use 0207T)

(For manual evacuation of meibomian glands, use 0563T)

EXCISION AND/OR DESTRUCTION

68100 Biopsy of conjunctiva

68110 Excision of lesion, conjunctiva; up to 1 cm

68115   over 1 cm

68130   with adjacent sclera

68135 Destruction of lesion, conjunctiva

INJECTION

(For injection into Tenon's capsule or retrobulbar injection, see 67500-67515)

68200 Subconjunctival injection

CONJUNCTIVOPLASTY

(For wound repair, see 65270-65273)

68320 Conjunctivoplasty; with conjunctival graft or extensive rearrangement

68325   with buccal mucous membrane graft (includes obtaining graft)

68326 Conjunctivoplasty, reconstruction cul-de-sac; with conjunctival graft or extensive rearrangement

68328   with buccal mucous membrane graft (includes obtaining graft)

68330 Repair of symblepharon; conjunctivoplasty, without graft

68335   with free graft conjunctiva or buccal mucous membrane (includes obtaining graft)

68340   division of symblepharon, with or without insertion of conformer or contact lens

OTHER PROCEDURES

68360 Conjunctival flap; bridge or partial (separate procedure)

68362   total (such as Gunderson thin flap or purse string flap)

(For conjunctival flap for perforating injury, see 65280, 65285)

(For repair of operative wound, use 66250)

(For removal of conjunctival foreign body, see 65205, 65210)

68371 Harvesting conjunctival allograft, living donor

68399 Unlisted procedure, conjunctiva

LACRIMAL SYSTEM

Incision

68400 Incision, drainage of lacrimal gland

68420 Incision, drainage of lacrimal sac (dacryocystotomy or dacryocystostomy)

68440   Snip incision of lacrimal punctum

Excision

68500   Excision of lacrimal gland (dacryoadenectomy), except for tumor; total

68505   partial

68510   Biopsy of lacrimal gland

68520   Excision of lacrimal sac (dacryocystectomy)

68525   Biopsy of lacrimal sac

68530   Removal of foreign body or dacryolith, lacrimal passages

68540   Excision of lacrimal gland tumor; frontal approach

68550   involving osteotomy

Repair

68700   Plastic repair of canaliculi

68705   Correction of everted punctum, cautery

68720   Dacryocystorhinostomy (fistulization of lacrimal sac to nasal cavity)

68745   Conjunctivorhinostomy (fistulization of conjunctiva to nasal cavity); without tube

68750   with insertion of tube or stent

68760   Closure of the lacrimal punctum; by thermocauterization, ligation, or laser surgery

68761   by plug, each

(For insertion and removal of drug-eluting implant into lacrimal canaliculus for intra-ocular pressure, use 0356T)

(For placement of drug-eluting insert under the eyelid[s], see 0444T, 0445T)

68770   Closure of lacrimal fistula (separate procedure)

Probing and/or Related Procedures

68801   Dilation of lacrimal punctum, with or without irrigation

(To report a bilateral procedure, use 68801 with modifier -50)

68810   Probing of nasolacrimal duct, with or without irrigation;

(For bilateral procedure, report 68810 with modifier -50)

68811   requiring general anesthesia

(For bilateral procedure, report 68811 with modifier -50)

68815   with insertion of tube or stent

(See also 92018)

(For bilateral procedure, report 68815 with modifier -50)

---

640   ● New Code   ▲ Revised Code   + Add-On Code   ⊘ Modifier -51 Exempt   ★ Telemedicine

(For insertion and removal of drug-eluting implant into lacrimal canaliculus for intra-ocular pressure, use 0356T)

(For placement of drug-eluting insert under the eyelid[s], see 0444T, 0445T)

68816   with transluminal balloon catheter dilation

(Do not report 68816 in conjunction with 68810, 68811, 68815)

(For bilateral procedure, report 68816 with modifier -50)

68840 Probing of lacrimal canaliculi, with or without irrigation

68850 Injection of contrast medium for dacryocystography

(For radiological supervision and interpretation, see 70170, 78660)

Other Procedures

68899 Unlisted procedure, lacrimal system

This page intentionally left blank.

● New Code ▲ Revised Code ＋ Add-On Code ⊘ Modifier -51 Exempt ★ Telemedicine

AUDITORY SYSTEM

CPT codes from this subsection of the CPT coding system are used to report invasive and surgical procedures performed on the external ear; middle ear; inner ear and temporal bone. Includes procedures performed on the inner, outer and middle ear and to the temporal bone.

Diagnostic services, such as otoscopy under general anesthesia, audiometry and vestibular tests, are defined in the Medicine Section of the CPT manual.

Wound repairs to the external ear are located in the Integumentary Subsection of the CPT coding system.

When a mastoidectomy is included in the description of an auditory procedure (e.g. CPT codes 69530, 69910), separate codes describing mastoidectomy are not reported.

Myringotomies (e.g. CPT codes 69420 and 69421) are included in tympanoplasties and tympanostomies.

(For diagnostic services (eg, audiometry, vestibular tests), see 92502 et seq)

EXTERNAL EAR

INCISION

69000 Drainage external ear, abscess or hematoma; simple

69005 complicated

69020 Drainage external auditory canal, abscess

69090 Ear piercing

EXCISION

69100 Biopsy external ear

69105 Biopsy external auditory canal

69110 Excision external ear; partial, simple repair

69120 complete amputation

(For reconstruction of ear, see 15120 et seq)

69140 Excision exostosis(es), external auditory canal

69145 Excision soft tissue lesion, external auditory canal

69150 Radical excision external auditory canal lesion; without neck dissection

69155 with neck dissection

(For resection of temporal bone, use 69535)

(For skin grafting, see 15004-15261)

REMOVAL

69200 Removal foreign body from external auditory canal; without general anesthesia

69205 with general anesthesia

69209 Removal impacted cerumen using irrigation/lavage, unilateral

(Do not report 69209 in conjunction with 69210 when performed on the same ear)

(For bilateral procedure, report 69209 with modifier 50)

(For removal of impacted cerumen requiring instrumentation, use 69210)

(For cerumen removal that is not impacted, see E/M service code, which may include new or established patient office or other outpatient services [99202-99215], hospital observation services [99217-99220, 99224-99226], hospital care [99221-99223, 99231-99233], consultations [99241-99255], emergency department services [99281-99285], nursing facility services [99304-99318], domiciliary, rest home, or custodial care services [99324-99337], home services [99341-99350])

69210 Removal impacted cerumen requiring instrumentation, unilateral

(Do not report 69210 in conjunction with 69209 when performed on the same ear)

(For bilateral procedure, report 69210 with modifier 50)

(For removal of impacted cerumen achieved with irrigation and/or lavage but without instrumentation, use 69209)

(For cerumen removal that is not impacted, see E/M service code, which may include new or established patient office or other outpatient services [99202-99215], hospital observation services [99217-99220, 99224-99226], hospital care [99221-99223, 99231-99233], consultations [99241-99255], emergency department services [99281-99285], nursing facility services [99304-99318], domiciliary, rest home, or custodial care services [99324-99337], home services [99341-99350])

69220 Debridement, mastoidectomy cavity, simple (eg, routine cleaning)

(For bilateral procedure, report 9220 with modifier -50)

69222 Debridement, mastoidectomy cavity, complex (eg, with anesthesia or more than routine cleaning)

(For bilateral procedure, report 69222 with modifier -50)

REPAIR

(For suture of wound or injury of external ear, see 12011-14302)

69300 Otoplasty, protruding ear, with or without size reduction

(For bilateral procedure, report 69300 with modifier -50)

69310 Reconstruction of external auditory canal (meatoplasty) (eg, for stenosis due to injury, infection) (separate procedure)

69320 Reconstruction external auditory canal for congenital atresia, single stage

(For combination with middle ear reconstruction, see 69631, 69641)

(For other reconstructive procedures with grafts (eg, skin, cartilage, bone), see 13151-15760, 21230-21235)

OTHER PROCEDURES

(For otoscopy under general anesthesia, use 92502)

69399 Unlisted procedure, external ear

MIDDLE EAR

INCISION

69420 Myringotomy including aspiration and/or eustachian tube inflation

69421 Myringotomy including aspiration and/or eustachian tube inflation requiring general anesthesia

69424 Ventilating tube removal requiring general anesthesia

(For bilateral procedure, report 69424 with modifier -50)

(Do not report code 69424 in conjunction with codes 69205, 69210, 69420, 69421, 69433-69676, 69710-69745, 69801-69930)

69433 Tympanostomy (requiring insertion of ventilating tube), local or topical anesthesia

(For bilateral procedure, report 69433 with modifier -50)

(For tympanostomy requiring insertion of ventilating tube, with iontophoresis, using an automated tube delivery system, use 0583T)

69436 Tympanostomy (requiring insertion of ventilating tube), general anesthesia

(For bilateral procedure, report 69436 with modifier -50)

69440 Middle ear exploration through postauricular or ear canal incision

(For atticotomy, see 69601 et seq)

69450 Tympanolysis, transcanal

EXCISION

69501 Transmastoid antrotomy (simple mastoidectomy)

69502 Mastoidectomy; complete

69505 modified radical

69511 radical

(For skin graft, see 15004 et seq)

(For mastoidectomy cavity debridement, see 69220, 69222)

69530 Petrous apicectomy including radical mastoidectomy

69535 Resection temporal bone, external approach

(For middle fossa approach, see 69950-69970)

69540 Excision aural polyp

69550 Excision aural glomus tumor; transcanal

69552 transmastoid

69554 extended (extratemporal)

REPAIR

69601 Revision mastoidectomy; resulting in complete mastoidectomy

69602 resulting in modified radical mastoidectomy

69603 resulting in radical mastoidectomy

69604 resulting in tympanoplasty

(For planned secondary tympanoplasty after mastoidectomy, see 69631, 69632)

(For skin graft, see 15120, 15121, 15260, 15261)

(**69605**   deleted 2020 [2021 Edition])

69610   Tympanic membrane repair, with or without site preparation or perforation for closure, with or without patch

69620   Myringoplasty (surgery confined to drumhead and donor area)

69631   Tympanoplasty without mastoidectomy (including canalplasty, atticotomy and/or middle ear surgery), initial or revision; without ossicular chain reconstruction

69632   with ossicular chain reconstruction (eg, postfenestration)

69633   with ossicular chain reconstruction and synthetic prosthesis (eg, partial ossicular replacement prosthesis [PORP], total ossicular replacement prosthesis [TORP])

69635   Tympanoplasty with antrotomy or mastoidotomy (including canalplasty, atticotomy, middle ear surgery, and/or tympanic membrane repair); without ossicular chain reconstruction

69636   with ossicular chain reconstruction

69637   with ossicular chain reconstruction and synthetic prosthesis (eg, partial ossicular replacement prosthesis [PORP], total ossicular replacement prosthesis [TORP])

69641   Tympanoplasty with mastoidectomy (including canalplasty, middle ear surgery, tympanic membrane repair); without ossicular chain reconstruction

69642   with ossicular chain reconstruction

69643   with intact or reconstructed wall, without ossicular chain reconstruction

69644   with intact or reconstructed canal wall, with ossicular chain reconstruction

69645   radical or complete, without ossicular chain reconstruction

69646   radical or complete, with ossicular chain reconstruction

69650   Stapes mobilization

69660   Stapedectomy or stapedotomy with reestablishment of ossicular continuity, with or without use of foreign material;

69661   with footplate drill out

69662   Revision of stapedectomy or stapedotomy

69666   Repair oval window fistula

69667   Repair round window fistula

69670   Mastoid obliteration (separate procedure)

69676   Tympanic neurectomy

(For bilateral procedure, report 69676 with modifier -50)

OTHER PROCEDURES

69700   Closure postauricular fistula, mastoid (separate procedure)

● **69705**   Nasopharyngoscopy, surgical, with dilation of eustachian tube (ie, balloon dilation); unilateral

● **69706**   bilateral

       (Do not report 69705, 69706 in conjunction with 31231, 92511)

69710   Implantation or replacement of electromagnetic bone conduction hearing device in temporal bone

       (Replacement procedure includes removal of old device)

69711   Removal or repair of electromagnetic bone conduction hearing device in temporal bone

69714   Implantation, osseointegrated implant, temporal bone, with percutaneous attachment to external speech processor/cochlear stimulator; without mastoidectomy

69715   with mastoidectomy

69717   Replacement (including removal of existing device), osseointegrated implant, temporal bone, with percutaneous attachment to external speech processor/cochlear stimulator; without mastoidectomy

69718   with mastoidectomy

69720   Decompression facial nerve, intratemporal; lateral to geniculate ganglion

69725   including medial to geniculate ganglion

69740   Suture facial nerve, intratemporal, with or without graft or decompression; lateral to geniculate ganglion

69745   including medial to geniculate ganglion

       (For extracranial suture of facial nerve, use 64864)

69799   Unlisted procedure, middle ear

INNER EAR

INCISION AND/OR DESTRUCTION

69801   Labyrinthotomy, with perfusion of vestibuloactive drug(s); transcanal

       (Do not report 69801 more than once per day)

       (Do not report 69801 in conjunction with 69420, 69421, 69433, 69436 when performed on the same ear)

69805   Endolymphatic sac operation; without shunt

69806   with shunt

(**69820**   deleted 2017 [2018 edition])

(**69840**   deleted 2017 [2018 edition])

EXCISION

69905   Labyrinthectomy; transcanal

69910   with mastoidectomy

69915   Vestibular nerve section, translabyrinthine approach

       (For transcranial approach, use 69950)

INTRODUCTION

69930 Cochlear device implantation, with or without mastoidectomy

OTHER PROCEDURES

69949 Unlisted procedure, inner ear

TEMPORAL BONE, MIDDLE FOSSA APPROACH

(For external approach, use 69535)

69950 Vestibular nerve section, transcranial approach

69955 Total facial nerve decompression and/or repair (may include graft)

69960 Decompression internal auditory canal

69970 Removal of tumor, temporal bone

OTHER PROCEDURES

69979 Unlisted procedure, temporal bone, middle fossa approach

● . New Code   ▲ Revised Code   ✛ Add-On Code   ⊘ Modifier -51 Exempt   ★ Telemedicine

OPERATING MICROSCOPE

The surgical microscope is employed when the surgical services are performed using the techniques of microsurgery. Code 69990 should be reported (without modifier 51 appended) in addition to the code for the primary procedure performed. Do not use 69990 for visualization with magnifying loupes or corrected vision. Do not report 69990 in addition to procedures where use of the operating microscope is an inclusive component (15756-15758, 15842, 19364, 19368, 20955-20962, 20969-20973, 22551, 22552, 22856-22861, 26551-26554, 26556, 31526, 31531, 31536, 31541, 31545, 31546, 31561, 31571, 43116, 43180, 43496, 46601, 46607, 49906, 61548, 63075-63078, 64727, 64820- 64823, 64912, 64913, 65091-68850, 0184T, 0308T, 0402T, 0583T).

+ **69990**   Microsurgical techniques, requiring use of operating microscope (List separately in addition to code for primary procedure)

This page intentionally left blank.

● New Code ▲ Revised Code ＋ Add-On Code ⊘ Modifier -51 Exempt ★ Telemedicine

RADIOLOGY

RADIOLOGY SECTION OVERVIEW

The fourth section of the CPT coding system is the radiology section, which includes diagnostic and therapeutic radiology, nuclear medicine and diagnostic ultrasound services. Within each subsection, the CPT codes are arranged by anatomical site.

Diagnostic radiology uses all modalities of radiant energy in medical diagnosis and therapeutic procedures requiring radiologic guidance. This includes imaging techniques and methodologies using radiation emitted by x-ray tubes, radionuclides, ultrasonographic devices, and radiofrequency electromagnetic radiation.

RADIOLOGY SUBSECTIONS

The RADIOLOGY section of the CPT coding system is divided into 7 subsections; namely:

Diagnostic Radiology (Diagnostic Imaging)	70010-76499
Diagnostic Ultrasound	76506-76999
Radiologic Guidance	77001-77022
Breast, Mammography	77046-77067
Bone/Joint Studies	77071-77086
Radiation Oncology	77261-77799
Nuclear Medicine	78012-79999

COMPLETE PROCEDURES

Interventional radiologic procedures or diagnostic studies involving injection of contrast media include all usual preinjection and postinjection services, for example, necessary local anesthesia, placement of needle or catheter, injection of contrast media, supervision of the study, and interpretation of results. When one of these procedures is performed in full by a single physician, it is designated as a "complete procedure."

SUPERVISION AND INTERPRETATION ONLY

When a procedure is performed by a radiologist-clinician team, it is designated as "supervision and interpretation only" and the separate injection procedure is listed in the appropriate section of the SURGERY section of the CPT coding system. These CPT codes are used only when a procedure is performed by more than one physician, for example, a radiologist-clinician team.

RADIOLOGY SERVICE MODIFIERS

Listed surgical services and procedures may be modified under certain circumstances. When applicable, the modifying circumstance is identified by adding the appropriate two digit modifier to the base procedure code(s). Modifiers commonly used to report RADIOLOGY services include:

-22 Unusual services

-26 Professional component

-32 Mandated services

-51 Multiple procedures

-52 Reduced services

-62 Two surgeons

-66 Surgical team

-76 Repeat procedure by same physician

-77 Repeat procedure by another physician

XRAY
70000

-78   Return to the operating room for a related procedure during the postoperative period

-79   Unrelated procedure or service by the same physician during the postoperative period

-80   Assistant surgeon

-90   Reference (outside) laboratory

-99   Multiple modifiers

-LT   Left side of body

-RT   Right side of body

BILATERAL PROCEDURE CODES

The RADIOLOGY section includes some CPT codes which include the term "bilateral" in the definition. When reporting these services, do not add the modifier -50, because the procedure is already defined as "bilateral."

RADIOLOGY SERVICES MEDICARE CONSIDERATIONS

Most of the CPT codes in this section are subject to Medicare Purchased Diagnostic Services guidelines. Coding and reporting should be as instructed by your local Medicare carrier.

SEPARATE PROCEDURES

Some procedures or services listed in the CPT coding system that are usually provided as an integral component of another total service or procedure are identified by the inclusion of the term (separate procedure). Codes designated as (separate procedure) should not be reported in addition to the code for the total procedure or service of which it is considered an integral component.

However, when a procedure or service designated as a (separate procedure) is provided independently or is considered to be unrelated or distinct from other procedures/services provided at the same time, the CPT code may be reported by itself. If the (separate procedure) is provided in addition to other procedures or services, the modifier -59 should be added to the (separate procedure) code to indicate that it is a distinct, independent procedure.

UNLISTED SERVICE OR PROCEDURE

A service or procedure may be provided that is not listed in this edition of the CPT codebook. When reporting such a service, the appropriate "Unlisted Procedure" code may be used to indicate the service, identifying it by "Special Report" as discussed below. The "Unlisted Procedures" and accompanying codes for Radiology (Including Nuclear Medicine and Diagnostic Ultrasound) are as follows:

76496   Unlisted fluoroscopic procedure (eg, diagnostic, interventional)

76497   Unlisted computed tomography procedure (eg, diagnostic, interventional)

76498   Unlisted magnetic resonance procedure (eg, diagnostic, interventional)

76499   Unlisted diagnostic radiographic procedure

76999   Unlisted ultrasound procedure (eg, diagnostic, interventional)

77299   Unlisted procedure, therapeutic radiology clinical treatment planning

77399   Unlisted procedure, medical radiation physics, dosimetry and treatment devices, and special services

77499   Unlisted procedure, therapeutic radiology treatment management

77799   Unlisted procedure, clinical brachytherapy

78099   Unlisted endocrine procedure, diagnostic nuclear medicine

78199   Unlisted hematopoietic, reticuloendothelial and lymphatic procedure, diagnostic nuclear medicine

78299   Unlisted gastrointestinal procedure, diagnostic nuclear medicine

78399   Unlisted musculoskeletal procedure, diagnostic nuclear medicine

78499   Unlisted cardiovascular procedure, diagnostic nuclear medicine

78599   Unlisted respiratory procedure, diagnostic nuclear medicine

78699   Unlisted nervous system procedure, diagnostic nuclear Medicine

78799   Unlisted genitourinary procedure, diagnostic nuclear medicine

78999   Unlisted miscellaneous procedure, diagnostic nuclear medicine

79999   Radiopharmaceutical therapy, unlisted procedure

SUPERVISION AND INTERPRETATION, IMAGING GUIDANCE

Radiologic imaging may be required during the performance of certain procedures and/or certain diagnostic imaging procedures may require surgical procedures in order to access the imaged area. Many procedures and services include image guidance, and imaging guidance is not separately reportable when it is included in the base service.

the CPT coding system typically defines in descriptors and/or guidelines when imaging guidance is included in a procedure. When imaging is not included in a surgical procedure or procedure from the Medicine section, image guidance codes or codes labeled "radiological supervision and interpretation" may be reported for the portion of the service that requires imaging.

All imaging guidance codes require image documentation in the medical record. All radiological superviaion and interpretation codes require image documentation in the medical record and a report of findings.

Radiological supervision and interpretation codes do not apply to the Radiation Oncology subsection.

This page intentionally left blank.

● New Code ▲ Revised Code ✚ Add-On Code ⊘ Modifier -51 Exempt ★ Telemedicine

RADIOLOGY CODES

DIAGNOSTIC RADIOLOGY (DIAGNOSTIC IMAGING)

HEAD AND NECK

70010 Myelography, posterior fossa, radiological supervision and interpretation

70015 Cisternography, positive contrast, radiological supervision and interpretation

70030 Radiologic examination, eye, for detection of foreign body

70100 Radiologic examination, mandible; partial, less than 4 views

70110 complete, minimum of 4 views

70120 Radiologic examination, mastoids; less than 3 views per side

70130 complete, minimum of 3 views per side

70134 Radiologic examination, internal auditory meati, complete

70140 Radiologic examination, facial bones; less than3e views

70150 complete, minimum of 3 views

70160 Radiologic examination, nasal bones, complete, minimum of 3 views

70170 Dacryocystography, nasolacrimal duct, radiological supervision and interpretation

70190 Radiologic examination; optic foramina

70200 orbits, complete, minimum of 4 views

70210 Radiologic examination, sinuses, paranasal, less than 3 views

70220 Radiologic examination, sinuses, paranasal, complete, minimum of 3 views

70240 Radiologic examination, sella turcica

70250 Radiologic examination, skull; less than 4 views

70260 complete, minimum of 4 views

70300 Radiologic examination, teeth; single view

70310 partial examination, less than full mouth

70320 complete, full mouth

70328 Radiologic examination, temporomandibular joint, open and closed mouth; unilateral

70330 bilateral

70332 Temporomandibular joint arthrography, radiological supervision and interpretation

(Do not report 70332 in conjunction with 77002)

| | Separate Procedure | Unlisted Procedure | CCI Comp. Code | Non-specific Procedure | **655** |

70336 Magnetic resonance (eg, proton) imaging, temporomandibular joint(s)

70350 Cephalogram, orthodontic

70355 Orthopantogram (eg, panoramic x-ray)

70360 Radiologic examination; neck, soft tissue

70370 pharynx or larynx, including fluoroscopy and/or magnification technique

70371 Complex dynamic pharyngeal and speech evaluation by cine or video recording

(For laryngeal computed tomography, see 70490, 70491, 70492)

70380 Radiologic examination, salivary gland for calculus

70390 Sialography, radiological supervision and interpretation

70450 Computed tomography, head or brain; without contrast material

70460 with contrast material(s)

70470 without contrast material, followed by contrast material(s) and further sections

(To report 3D rendering, see 76376, 76377)

70480 Computed tomography, orbit, sella, or posterior fossa or outer, middle, or inner ear; without contrast material

70481 with contrast material(s)

70482 without contrast material, followed by contrast material(s) and further sections

(To report 3D rendering, see 76376, 76377)

70486 Computed tomography, maxillofacial area; without contrast material

70487 with contrast material(s)

70488 without contrast material, followed by contrast material(s) and further sections

(To report 3D rendering, see 76376, 76377)

70490 Computed tomography, soft tissue neck; without contrast material

70491 with contrast material(s)

70492 without contrast material followed by contrast material(s) and further sections

(To report 3D rendering, see 76376, 76377)

(For cervical spine, see 72125, 72126)

70496 Computed tomographic angiography, head, with contrast material(s), including noncontrast images, if performed, and image post-processing

70498 Computed tomographic angiography, neck, with contrast material(s), including noncontrast images, if performed, and image post-processing

70540 Magnetic resonance (eg, proton) imaging, orbit, face, and/or neck; without contrast material(s)

(For head or neck magnetic resonance angiography studies, see 70544-70546, 70547-70549)

● New Code ▲ Revised Code + Add-On Code ⊘ Modifier -51 Exempt ★ Telemedicine

70542 with contrast material(s)

70543 without contrast material(s), followed by contrast material(s) and further sequences

(Report 70540-70543 once per imaging session)

70544 Magnetic resonance angiography, head; without contrast materials

70545 with contrast materials

70546 without contrast material(s), followed by contrast material(s) and further sequences

70547 Magnetic resonance angiography, neck; without contrast materials

70548 with contrast materials

70549 without contrast material(s), followed by contrast material(s) and further sequences

70551 Magnetic resonance (eg, proton) imaging, brain (including brain stem); without contrast material

70552 with contrast material(s)

70553 without contrast material, followed by contrast material(s) and further sequences

(For magnetic spectroscopy, use 76390)

Functional MRI involves identification and mapping of stimulation of brain function. When neurofunctional tests are administered by a technologist or other non-physician or non-physiologist, use 70554. When neurofunctional tests are entirely administered by a physician or psychologist, use 70555.

70554 Magnetic resonance imaging, brain, functional MRI; including test selection and administration of repetitive body part movement and/or visual stimulation, not requiring physician or psychologist administration

(Do not report 70554 in conjunction with 96020)

70555 requiring physician or psychologist administration of entire neurofunctional testing

(Do not report 70555 unless 96020 is performed)

(Do not report 70554, 70555 in conjunction with 70551-70553 unless a separate diagnostic MRI is performed)

70557 Magnetic resonance (eg, proton) imaging, brain (including brain stem and skull base), during open intracranial procedure (eg, to assess for residual tumor or residual vascular malformation); without contrast material

70558 with contrast material(s)

70559 without contrast material(s), followed by contrast material(s) and further sequences

(For stereotactic biopsy of intracranial lesion with magnetic resonance guidance, use 61751. 70557, 70558 or 70559 may be reported only if a separate report is generated. Report only one of the above codes once per operative session. Do not use these codes in conjunction with 61751, 77021, 77022)

CHEST

(For fluoroscopic or ultrasonic guidance for needle placement procedures (eg., biopsy, aspiration, injection, localization device) of the thorax, see 76942, 77002)

(**71010** deleted 2017 [2018 edition]. To report, use 71045)

(**71015** deleted 2017 [2018 edition]. To report, use 71045)

Separate Procedure   Unlisted Procedure   CCI Comp. Code   Non-specific Procedure   **657**

(**71020**   deleted 2017 [2018 edition]. To report, use 71046)

(**71021**   deleted 2017 [2018 edition]. To report, use 71047)

(**71022**   deleted 2017 [2018 edition]. To report, see 71047, 71048)

(**71023**   deleted 2017 [2018 edition]. To report, see 71046, 76000)

(**71030**   deleted 2017 [2018 edition]. To report, use 71048)

(**71034**   deleted 2017 [2018 edition]. To report, see 71048, 76000)

(**71035**   deleted 2017 [2018 edition]. To report, see 71046, 71047, 71048)

71045   Radiologic examination, chest; single view

71046   2 views

71047   3 views

71048   4 or more views

(For complete acute abdomen series that includes 2 or more views of the abdomen [eg, supine, erect, decubitus], and a single view chest, use 74022)

(For concurrent computer-aided detection [CAD] performed in addition to 71045, 71046, 71047, 71048, use 0174T)

(Do not report 71045, 71046, 71047, 71048 in conjunction with 0175T for computer-aided detection [CAD] performed remotely from the primary interpretation)

71100   Radiologic examination, ribs, unilateral; 2 views

71101   including posteroanterior chest, minimum of 3 views

71110   Radiologic examination, ribs, bilateral; 3 views

71111   including posteroanterior chest, minimum of 4 views

71120   Radiologic examination; sternum, minimum of 2 views

71130   sternoclavicular joint or joints, minimum of 3 views

▲ **71250**   Computed tomography, thorax diagnostic; without contrast material

▲ **71260**   with contrast material(s)

▲ **71270**   without contrast material, followed by contrast material(s) and further sections

(Do not report 71270 in conjunction with 71250, 71260, 71271)

(Do not report 71250, 71260, 71270 for breast CT procedures)

(For cardiac computed tomography of the heart, see 75571-75574)

(To report 3D rendering, see 76376, 76377)

● **71271**   Computed tomography, thorax, low dose for lung cancer screening, without contrast material(s)

(Do not report 71271 in conjunction with 71250, 71260, 71270)

(Do not report 71271 for breast CT procedures)

(For cardiac computed tomography of the heart, see 75571, 75572, 75573, 75574)

71275 Computed tomographic angiography, chest (noncoronary), with contrast material(s), including noncontrast images, if performed, and image post-processing

(For coronary artery computed tomographic angiography including calcification score and/or cardiac morphology, use 75574)

71550 Magnetic resonance (eg, proton) imaging, chest (eg, for evaluation of hilar and mediastinal lymphadenopathy); without contrast material(s)

71551 with contrast material(s)

71552 without contrast material(s), followed by contrast material(s) and further sequences

(For breast MRI, see 77046, 77047, 77048, 77049)

71555 Magnetic resonance angiography, chest (excluding myocardium), with or without contrast material(s)

SPINE AND PELVIS

72020 Radiologic examination, spine, single view, specify level

(For a single view that includes the entire thoracic and lumbar spine, use 72081)

72040 Radiologic examination, spine, cervical; 2 or 3 views

72050 of 4 or 5 views

72052 6 or more views

72070 Radiologic examination, spine; thoracic, 2 views

72072 thoracic, 3 views

72074 thoracic, minimum of 4 views

72080 thoracolumbar, junction, minimum of 2 views

(For a single view examination of the thoracolumbar junction, use 72020)

72081 Radiologic examination, spine, entire thoracic and lumbar, including skull, cervical and sacral spine if performed (eg, scoliosis evaluation); one view

72082 2 or 3 views

72083 4 or 5 views

72084 minimum of 6 views

72100 Radiologic examination, spine, lumbosacral; 2 or 3 views

72110 minimum of 4 views

72114 complete, including bending views, minimum of 6 views

72120 bending views only, 2 or 3 views

(Contrast material in CT of spine is either by intrathecal or intravenous injection. For intrathecal injection, use also 61055 or 62284. IV injection of contrast material is part of the CT procedure)

72125   Computed tomography, cervical spine; without contrast material

72126   with contrast material

72127   without contrast material, followed by contrast material(s) and further sections

     (For intrathecal injection procedure, see 61055, 62284)

72128   Computed tomography, thoracic spine; without contrast material

72129   with contrast material

     (For intrathecal injection procedure, see 61055, 62284)

72130   without contrast material, followed by contrast material(s) and further sections

     (For intrathecal injection procedure, see 61055, 62284)

72131   Computed tomography, lumbar spine; without contrast material

72132   with contrast material

72133   without contrast material, followed by contrast material(s) and further sections

     (For intrathecal injection procedure, see 61055, 62284)

     (To report 3D rendering, see 76376, 76377)

72141   Magnetic resonance (eg, proton) imaging, spinal canal and contents, cervical; without contrast material

72142   with contrast material(s)

     (For cervical spinal canal imaging without contrast material followed by contrast material, use 72156)

     (For magnetic resonance spectroscopy, determination and localization of discogenic pain, see 0609T, 0610T)

72146   Magnetic resonance (eg, proton) imaging, spinal canal and contents, thoracic; without contrast material

72147   with contrast material(s)

     (For thoracic spinal canal imaging without contrast material followed by contrast material, use 72157)

     (For magnetic resonance spectroscopy, determination and localization of discogenic pain, see 0609T, 0610T)

72148   Magnetic resonance (eg, proton) imaging, spinal canal and contents, lumbar; without contrast material

72149   with contrast material(s)

     (For lumbar spinal canal imaging without contrast material followed by contrast material, use 72158)

     (For magnetic resonance spectroscopy, determination and localization of discogenic pain, see 0609T, 0610T)

72156   Magnetic resonance (eg, proton) imaging, spinal canal and contents, without contrast material, followed by contrast material(s) and further sequences; cervical

72157   thoracic

72158   lumbar

     (For magnetic resonance spectroscopy, determination and localization of discogenic pain, see 0609T, 0610T)

   ● New Code   ▲ Revised Code   + Add-On Code   ⊘ Modifier -51 Exempt   ★ Telemedicine

72159 Magnetic resonance angiography, spinal canal and contents, with or without contrast material(s)

72170 Radiologic examination, pelvis; 1 or 2 views

72190 complete, minimum of 3 views

(For pelvimetry, use 74710)

(For a combined computed tomography (CT) or computed tomographic angiography abdomen and pelvis study, see 74174, 74176-74178)

72191 Computed tomographic angiography, pelvis; with contrast material(s), including noncontrast images, if performed, and image post-processing

(Do not report 72191 in conjunction with 73706 or 75635. For CTA aorto-iliofemoral runoff, use 75635)

(Do not report 72191 in conjunction with 74175. For a combined computed tomographic angiography abdomen and pelvis study, use 74174)

72192 Computed tomography, pelvis; without contrast material

72193 with contrast material(s)

72194 without contrast material, followed by contrast material(s) and further sections

(For a combined CT abdomen and pelvis study, see 74176-74178)

(To report 3D rendering, see 76376, 76377)

(For computed tomographic colonography, diagnostic, see 74261-74262. For computed tomographic colonography, screening, use 74263)

(Do not report 72192-72194 in conjunction with 74261-74263)

72195 Magnetic resonance (eg, proton) imaging, pelvis; without contrast material(s)

72196 with contrast material(s)

72197 without contrast material(s), followed by contrast material(s) and further sequences

(Do not report 72195, 72196, 72197 in conjunction with 74712, 74713)

(For magnetic resonance imaging of a fetus[es], see 74712, 74713)

72198 Magnetic resonance angiography, pelvis, with or without contrast material(s)

72200 Radiologic examination, sacroiliac joints; less than3e views

72202 3 or more views

72220 Radiologic examination, sacrum and coccyx, minimum of 2 views

72240 Myelography, cervical, radiological supervision and interpretation

(Do not report 72240 in conjunction with 62284, 62302, 62303, 62304, 62305)

(When both 62284 and 72240 are performed by the same physician or other qualified health care professional for cervical myelography, use 62302)

(For complete cervical myelography via injection procedure at C1-C2, see 61055, 72240)

72255 Myelography, thoracic, radiological supervision and interpretation

(Do not report 72255 in conjunction with 62284, 62302, 62303, 62304, 62305)

(When both 62284 and 72255 are performed by the same physician or other qualified health care professional for cervical myelography, use 62303)

(For complete thoracic myelography via injection procedure at C1-C2, see 61055, 72255)

72265 Myelography, lumbosacral, radiological supervision and interpretation

(Do not report 72265 in conjunction with 62284, 62302, 62303, 62304, 62305)

(When both 62284 and 72265 are performed by the same physician or other qualified health care professional for cervical myelography, use 62304)

(For complete lumbosacral myelography via injection procedure at C1-C2, see 61055, 72265)

72270 Myelography, 2 or more regions (eg, lumbar/thoracic, cervical/thoracic, lumbar/cervical, lumbar/thoracic/cervical), radiological supervision and interpretation

(Do not report 72270 in conjunction with 62284, 62302, 62303, 62304, 62305)

(When both 62284 and 72270 are performed by the same physician or other qualified health care professional for cervical myelography, use 62305)

(For complete myelography of 2 or more regions via injection procedure at C1-C2, see 61055, 72270)

72275 Epidurography, radiological supervision and interpretation

(72275 includes 77003)

(For injection procedure, see 62280, 62281, 62282, 62320, 62321, 62322, 62323, 62324, 62325, 62326, 62327, 64479, 64480, 64483, 64484)

(Use 72275 only when an epidurogram is performed, images documented, and a formal radiologic report is issued)

(Do not report 72275 in conjunction with 22586)

72285 Discography, cervical or thoracic, radiological supervision and interpretation

72295 Discography, lumbar, radiological supervision and interpretation

UPPER EXTREMITIES

(For stress views, any joint, use 77071)

73000 Radiologic examination; clavicle, complete

73010 scapula, complete

73020 Radiologic examination, shoulder; 1 view

73030 complete, minimum of 2 views

73040 Radiologic examination, shoulder, arthrography, radiological supervision and interpretation

(Do not report 77002 in conjunction with 73040)

73050 Radiologic examination; acromioclavicular joints, bilateral, with or without weighted distraction

73060 humerus, minimum of 2 views

73070 Radiologic examination, elbow; 2 views

73080 complete, minimum of 3 views

73085 Radiologic examination, elbow, arthrography, radiological supervision and interpretation

(Do not report 77002 in conjunction with 73085)

73090 Radiologic examination; forearm, 2 views

73092 upper extremity, infant, minimum of 2 views

73100 Radiologic examination, wrist; 2 views

73110 complete, minimum of 3 views

73115 Radiologic examination, wrist, arthrography, radiological supervision and interpretation

(Do not report 77002 in conjunction with 73115)

73120 Radiologic examination, hand; 2 views

73130 minimum of 3 views

73140 Radiologic examination, finger(s), minimum of 2 views

73200 Computed tomography, upper extremity; without contrast material

73201 with contrast material(s)

73202 without contrast material, followed by contrast material(s) and further sections

(To report 3D rendering, see 76376, 76377)

73206 Computed tomographic angiography, upper extremity, with contrast material(s), including noncontrast images, if performed, and image post-processing

73218 Magnetic resonance (eg, proton) imaging, upper extremity, other than joint; without contrast material(s)

73219 with contrast material(s)

73220 without contrast material(s), followed by contrast material(s) and further sequences

73221 Magnetic resonance (eg, proton) imaging, any joint of upper extremity; without contrast material(s)

73222 with contrast material(s)

73223 without contrast material(s), followed by contrast material(s) and further sequences

73225 Magnetic resonance angiography, upper extremity, with or without contrast material(s)

LOWER EXTREMITIES

(For stress views, any joint, use 77071)

73501 Radiologic examination, hip, unilateral, with pelvis when performed; 1 view

73502 2-3 views

73503 minimum of 4 views

73521 Radiologic examination, hips, bilateral, with pelvis when performed; 2 views

73522 3-4 views

73523	minimum of 5 views
73525	Radiologic examination, hip, arthrography, radiological supervision and interpretation
	(Do not report 73525 in conjunction with 77002)
73551	Radiologic examination, femur; 1 view
73552	minimum 2 views
73560	Radiologic examination, knee; 1 or 2 views
73562	3 views
73564	complete, 4 or more views
73565	both knees, standing, anteroposterior
73580	Radiologic examination, knee, arthrography, radiological supervision and interpretation
	(Do not report 73580 in conjunction with 77002)
73590	Radiologic examination; tibia and fibula, 2 views
73592	lower extremity, infant, minimum of 2 views
73600	Radiologic examination, ankle; 2 views
73610	complete, minimum of 3 views
73615	Radiologic examination, ankle, arthrography, radiological supervision and interpretation
	(Do not report 73615 in conjunction with 77002)
73620	Radiologic examination, foot; 2 views
73630	complete, minimum of 3 views
73650	Radiologic examination; calcaneus, minimum of 2 views
73660	toe(s), minimum of 2 views
73700	Computed tomography, lower extremity; without contrast material
73701	with contrast material(s)
73702	without contrast material, followed by contrast material(s) and further sections
	(To report 3D rendering, see 76376, 76377)
73706	Computed tomographic angiography, lower extremity, with contrast material(s), including noncontrast images, if performed, and image post-processing
	(For CTA aorto-iliofemoral runoff, use 75635)
73718	Magnetic resonance (eg, proton) imaging, lower extremity, other than joint; without contrast material(s)
73719	with contrast material(s)
73720	without contrast material(s), followed by contrast material(s) and further sequences

● New Code   ▲ Revised Code   + Add-On Code   ⊘ Modifier -51 Exempt   ★ Telemedicine

73721 Magnetic resonance (eg, proton) imaging, any joint of lower extremity; without contrast material

73722 with contrast material

73723 without contrast material followed by contrast material(s) and further sequences

73725 Magnetic resonance angiography, lower extremity, with or without contrast material(s)

ABDOMEN

(**74000** deleted 2017 [2018 edition]. To report, use 74018)

(**74010** deleted 2017 [2018 edition]. To report, see 74019, 74021)

(**74020** deleted 2017 [2018 edition]. To report, see 74019, 74021)

74018 Radiologic examination, abdomen; 1 view

74019 2 views

74021 3 or more views

74022 Radiologic examination, complete acute abdomen series, including 2 or more views of the abdomen (eg, supine, erect, decubitus), and a single view chest

74150 Computed tomography, abdomen; without contrast material

74160 with contrast material(s)

74170 without contrast material, followed by contrast material(s) and further sections

(For a combined CT abdomen and pelvis study, see 74176-74178)

(To report 3D rendering, see 76376, 76377)

(For computed tomographic colonography, diagnostic, see 74261-74262. For computed tomographic colonography, screening, use 74263)

(Do not report 74150-74170 in conjunction with 74261-74263)

74174 Computed tomographic angiography, abdomen and pelvis, with contrast material(s), including noncontrast images, if performed, and image postprocessing

(Do not report 74174 in conjunction with 72191, 73706, 74175, 75635, 76376, 76377)

(For CTA aorto-iliofemoral runoff, use 75635

For combinations of CT of the abdomen with CT of the pelvis performed at the same session, use the following table. Do not report more than one CT of the abdomen or CT of the pelvis for any session.

Stand Alone Code	74150 CT Abdomen WO Contrast	74160 CT Abdomen W Contrast	74170 CT Abdomen WO/W Contrast
72192 CT Pelvis WO Contrast	74176	74178	74178
72193 CT Pelvis W Contrast	74178	74177	74178
72194 CT Pelvis WO/W Contrast	74178	74178	74178

74175 Computed tomographic angiography, abdomen, with contrast material(s), including noncontrast images, if performed, and image post-processing

(Do not report 74175 in conjunction with 73706 or 75635. For CTA aorto-iliofemoral runoff, use 75635)

(Do not report 74175 in conjunction with 72191. For a combined computed tomographic angiography abdomen and pelvis study, use 74174)

74176 Computed tomography, abdomen and pelvis; without contrast material

74177 with contrast material(s)

74178 without contrast material in one or both body regions, followed by contrast material(s) and further sections in one or both body regions

(Do not report 74176-74178 in conjunction with 72192-72194, 74150-74170)

(Report 74176, 74177, or 74178 only once per CT abdomen and pelvis examination)

74181 Magnetic resonance (eg, proton) imaging, abdomen; without contrast material(s)

74182 with contrast material(s)

74183 without contrast material, followed by contrast material(s) and further sequences

74185 Magnetic resonance angiography, abdomen, with or without contrast material(s)

74190 Peritoneogram (eg, after injection of air or contrast), radiological supervision and interpretation

(For procedure, use 49400)

(For computerized axial tomography, see 72192 or 74150)

GASTROINTESTINAL TRACT

(For percutaneous placement of gastrostomy tube, use 43246)

74210 Radiologic examination, pharynx and/or cervical esophagus, including scout neck radiograph(s) and delayed image(s), when performed, contrast (eg, barium) study

74220 Radiologic examination, esophagus, including scout chest radiograph(s) and delayed image(s), when performed; single-contrast (eg, barium) study

(Do not report 74220 in conjunction with 74221, 74240, 74246, 74248)

74221 double-contrast (eg, high-density barium and effervescent agent) study

(Do not report 74221 in conjunction with 74220, 74240, 74246, 74248)

74230 Radiologic examination, swallowing function, with cineradiography/videoradiography, including scout neck radiograph(s) and delayed image(s), when performed, contrast (eg, barium) study

(For otorhinolaryngologic services fluoroscopic evaluation of swallowing function, use 92611)

74235 Removal of foreign body(s), esophageal, with use of balloon catheter, radiological supervision and interpretation

(For procedure, see 43499)

74240 Radiologic examination, upper gastrointestinal tract, including scout abdominal radiograph(s) and delayed image(s), when performed; single-contrast (eg, barium) study

(Do not report 74240 in conjunction with 74220, 74221, 74246)

(**74241**   deleted 2019 [2020 edition]. To report, use 74240)

(**74245**   deleted 2019 [2020 edition]. To report, use 74240, 74248)

74246   double-contrast (eg, high-density barium and effervescent agent) study, including glucagon, when administered

(Do not report 74246 in conjunction with 74220, 74221, 74240)

(**74247**   deleted 2019 [2020 edition]. To report, use 74246)

+ **74248**   Radiologic small intestine follow-through study, including multiple serial images (List separately in addition to code for primary procedure for upper GI radiologic examination)

(Use 74248 in conjunction with 74240, 74246)

(Do not report 74248 in conjunction with 74250, 74251)

(**74249**   deleted 2019 [2020 edition]. To report, use 74246, 74248)

74250   Radiologic examination, small intestine, including multiple serial images and scout abdominal radiograph(s), when performed; single-contrast (eg, barium) study

(Do not report 74250 in conjunction with 74248, 74251)

74251   double-contrast (eg, high-density barium and air via enteroclysis tube) study, including glucagon, when administered

(For placement of enteroclysis tube, see 44500, 74340)

(Do not report 74251 in conjunction with 74248, 74250)

(**74260**   deleted 2019 [2020 edition]. To report, use 74251)

74261   Computed tomographic (CT) colonography, diagnostic, including image postprocessing; without contrast material

74262   with contrast material(s) including non contrast images, if performed

(Do not report 74261, 74262 in conjunction with 72192-72194, 74150-74170, 74263, 76376, 76377)

74263   Computed tomographic (CT) colonography, screening, including image postprocessing

(Do not report 74263 in conjunction with 72192-72194, 74150-74170, 74261, 74262, 76376, 76377)

74270   Radiologic examination, colon, including scout abdominal radiograph(s) and delayed image(s), when performed; single-contrast (eg, barium) study

(Do not report 74270 in conjunction with 74280)

74280   double-contrast (eg, high density barium and air) study, including glucagon, when administered

(Do not report 74280 in conjunction with 74270)

74283   Therapeutic enema, contrast or air, for reduction of intussusception or other intraluminal obstruction (eg, meconium ileus)

74290   Cholecystography, oral contrast

74300   Cholangiography and/or pancreatography; intraoperative, radiological supervision and interpretation

+ **74301**   additional set intraoperative, radiological supervision and interpretation (List separately in addition to code for primary procedure)

(Use 74301 in conjunction with code 74300)

74328   Endoscopic catheterization of the biliary ductal system, radiological supervision and interpretation

(For procedure, see 43260-43278 as appropriate)

74329   Endoscopic catheterization of the pancreatic ductal system, radiological supervision and interpretation

(For procedure, see 43260-43278 as appropriate)

74330   Combined endoscopic catheterization of the biliary and pancreatic ductal systems, radiological supervision and interpretation

(For procedure, see 43260-43278 as appropriate)

74340   Introduction of long gastrointestinal tube (eg, Miller-Abbott), including multiple fluoroscopies and images, radiological supervision and interpretation

(For tube placement, use 44500)

74355   Percutaneous placement of enteroclysis tube, radiological supervision and interpretation

74360   Intraluminal dilation of strictures and/or obstructions (eg, esophagus), radiological supervision and interpretation

(Do not report 74360 in conjunction with 43213, 43214, 43233)

74363   Percutaneous transhepatic dilation of biliary duct stricture with or without placement of stent, radiological supervision and interpretation

(For procedure, see 47555, 47556)

URINARY TRACT

74400   Urography (pyelography), intravenous, with or without KUB, with or without tomography

74410   Urography, infusion, drip technique and/or bolus technique;

74415   with nephrotomography

74420   Urography, retrograde, with or without KUB

74425   Urography, antegrade, radiological supervision and interpretation

(Use 74425 in conjunction with 50390, 50396, 50684, 50690)

(Do not report 74425 in conjunction with 50430, 50431, 50432, 50433, 50434, 50435, 50693, 50694, 50695)

74430   Cystography, minimum of three views, radiological supervision and interpretation

74440   Vasography, vesiculography, or epididymography, radiological supervision and interpretation

74445   Corpora cavernosography, radiological supervision and interpretation

74450   Urethrocystography, retrograde, radiological supervision and interpretation

74455   Urethrocystography, voiding, radiological supervision and interpretation

74470   Radiologic examination, renal cyst study, translumbar, contrast visualization, radiological supervision and interpretation

---

74485   Dilation of ureter(s) or urethra, radiological supervision and interpretation

(Do not report 74485 in conjunction with 50436, 50437)

(For dilation of ureter without radiologic guidance, use 52341, 52344)

(For change of nephrostomy or pyelostomy tube, use 50435)

(For dilation of a nephrostomy tract for endourologic procedure, see 50436, 50437)

GYNECOLOGICAL AND OBSTETRICAL

(For abdomen and pelvis, see 72170-72190, 74018, 74019, 74021, 74022, 74150, 74160, 74170)

74710   Pelvimetry, with or without placental localization

74712   Magnetic resonance (eg, proton) imaging, fetal, including placental and maternal pelvic imaging when performed; single or first gestation

+ 74713   each additional gestation (List separately in adddition to code for primary procedure)

(Use 74713 in conjunction with 74712)

(Do not report 74712, 74713 in conjunction with 72195, 72196, 72197)

(If only placenta or maternal pelvis is imaged without fetal imaging, see 72195, 72196, 72197)

74740   Hysterosalpingography, radiological supervision and interpretation

(For introduction of saline or contrast for hysterosalpingography, see 58340)

74742   Transcervical catheterization of fallopian tube, radiological supervision and interpretation

(For procedure, use 58345)

74775   Perineogram (eg, vaginogram, for sex determination or extent of anomalies)

HEART

Cardiac magnetic imaging differs from traditional magnetic resonance imaging (MRI) in its ability to provide a physiologic evaluation of cardiac function. Traditional MRI relies on static images to obtain clinical diagnoses based upon anatomic information. Improvement in spatial and temporal resolution has expanded the application from an anatomic test and includes physiologic evaluation of cardiac function. Flow and velocity assessment for valves and intracardiac shunts is performed in addition to a function and morphologic evaluation. Use 75559 with 75565 to report flow with pharmacologic wall motion stress evaluation without contrast. Use 75563 with 75565 to report flow with pharmacologic perfusion stress with contrast.

Cardiac MRI for velocity flow mapping can be reported in conjunction with 75557, 75559, 75561, or 75563.

Listed procedures may be performed independently or in the course of overall medical care. If the individual providing these services is also responsible for diagnostic workup and/or follow-up care of the patient, see appropriate sections also. Only one procedure in the series 75557-75563 is appropriately reported per session. Only one add-on code for flow velocity can be reported per session.

Cardiac MRI studies may be performed at rest and/or during pharmacologic stress. Therefore, the appropriate stress testing code from the 93015-93018 series should be reported in addition to 75559 or 75563.

Cardiac computed tomography (CT) and coronary computed tomographic angiography (CTA) include the axial source images of the pre-contrast, arterial phase sequence, and venous phase sequence (if performed), as well as the two-dimensional and three-dimensional reformatted images resulting from the study, including cine review. Each of the contrast enhanced cardiac CT and coronary CTA codes (75572, 75573, 75574) includes conventional quantitative assessment(s) intrinsic to the service listed in the code descriptor (ie, quantification of coronary percentage stenosis, ventricular volume[s], ejection fraction[s], and stroke volume[s]), when performed. Report only one computed tomography heart service per encounter (75571, 75572, 75573, 75574).

(For separate injection procedures for vascular radiology, see Surgery section, 36000-36299)

(For cardiac catheterization procedures, see 93451-93572)

(75552-75556 have been deleted. To report, see 75557, 75559, 75561, 75563, 75565)

75557 Cardiac magnetic resonance imaging for morphology and function without contrast material;

75559 with stress imaging

75561 Cardiac magnetic resonance imaging for morphology and function without contrast material(s), followed by contrast material(s) and further sequences;

75563 with stress imaging

(75558, 75560, 75562, 75564 have been deleted. To report flow velocity, use 75565)

+ **75565** Cardiac magnetic resonance imaging for velocity flow mapping (List separately in addition to code for primary procedure)

(Use 75565 in conjunction with 75557, 75559, 75561, 75563)

(Do not report 75557, 75559, 75561, 75563, 75565 in conjunction with 76376, 76377)

75571 Computed tomography, heart, without contrast material, with quantitative evaluation of coronary calcium

75572 Computed tomography, heart, with contrast material, for evaluation of cardiac structure and morphology (including 3D image postprocessing, assessment of cardiac function, and evaluation of venous structures, if performed)

75573 Computed tomography, heart, with contrast material, for evaluation of cardiac structure and morphology in the setting of congenital heart disease (including 3D image postprocessing, assessment of LV cardiac function, RV structure and function and evaluation of venous structures, if performed)

75574 Computed tomographic angiography, heart, coronary arteries and bypass grafts (when present), with contrast material, including 3D image postprocessing (including evaluation of cardiac structure and morphology, assessment of cardiac function, and evaluation of venous structures, if performed)

(For noninvasive estimated coronary fractional flow reserve [FFR] derived from coronary computed tomography angiography data, see 0501T, 0502T, 0503T, 0504T)

(For automated quantification and characterization of coronary atherosclerotic plaque, see 0623T, 0624T, 0625T, 0626T)

VASCULAR PROCEDURES

AORTA AND ARTERIES

Selective vascular catheterizations should be coded to include introduction and all lesser order selective catheterizations used in the approach (eg., the description for a selective right middle cerebral artery catheterization includes the introduction and placement catheterization of the right common and internal carotid arteries).

Additional second and/or third order arterial catheterizations within the same family of arteries supplied by a single first order artery should be expressed by 36218 or 36248. Additional first order or higher catheterizations in vascular families supplied by a first order vessel different from a previously selected and coded family should be separately coded using the conventions described above.

The lower extremity endovascular revascularization codes describing services performed for occlusive disease (37220-37235) include catheterization (36200, 36240, 36245-36248) in the work described by the codes. Catheterization codes are not additionally reported for diagnostic lower extremity angiography when performed through the same access site as the therapy (37220-37235) performed in the same session. However, catheterization for the diagnostic lower extremity angiogram may be reported separately if a different arterial puncture site is necessary.

For angiography performed in conjunction with therapeutic transcatheter radiological supervision and interpretation services, see the Radiology Transcatheter Procedures guidelines.

Diagnostic angiography (radiological supervision and interpretation) codes should NOT be used with interventional procedures for:

1. Contrast injections, angiography, roadmapping, and/or fluoroscopic guidance for the intervention;

2. Vessel measurement; AND

3. Post-angioplasty/stent/atherectomy angiography, as this work is captured in the radiological supervision and interpretation code(s). In those therapeutic codes that include radiological supervision and interpretation, this work is captured in the therapeutic code.

Diagnostic angiography performed at the time of an interventional procedure is separately reportable if:

1. No prior catheter-based angiographic study is available and a full diagnostic study is performed, and the decision to intervene is based on the diagnostic study, OR

2. A prior study is available, but as documented in the medical record:

   a. The patient's condition with respect to the clinical indication has changed since the prior study; OR

   b. There is inadequate visualization of the anatomy and/or pathology; OR

   c. There is a clinical change during the procedure that requires new evaluation outside the target area of intervention.

Diagnostic angiography performed at a separate session from an interventional procedure is separately reported.

If diagnostic angiography is necessary, is performed at the same session as the interventional procedure, and meets the above criteria, modifier 59 must be appended to the diagnostic radiological supervision and interpretation code(s) to denote that diagnostic work has been done following these guidelines.

Diagnostic angiography performed at the time of an interventional procedure is NOT separately reportable if it is specifically included in the interventional code descriptor.

   (For intravenous procedure, see 36000, 36005-36015, and for intra-arterial procedure, see 36100-36248)

   (For radiological supervision and interpretation, see 75600-75893)

75600   Aortography, thoracic, without serialography, radiological supervision and interpretation

   (For isupravalvular aortography performed at the time of cardiac catheterization, use 93567, which includes imaging supervision, interpretation and report)

75605   Aortography, thoracic, by serialography, radiological supervision and interpretation

   (For supravalvular aortography performed at the time of cardiac catheterization, use 93567, which includes imaging supervision, interpretation and report)

75625   Aortography, abdominal, by serialography, radiological supervision and interpretation

75630   Aortography, abdominal plus bilateral iliofemoral lower extremity, catheter, by serialography, radiological supervision and interpretation

75635   Computed tomographic angiography, abdominal aorta and bilateral iliofemoral lower extremity runoff, with contrast material(s), including noncontrast images, if performed, and image post-processing

   (Do not report 75635 in conjunction with 72191, 73706, 74175, or 74174)

(**75658**   deleted 2017 [2018 edition]. To report, use 75710)

75705   Angiography, spinal, selective, radiological supervision and interpretation

75710   Angiography, extremity, unilateral, radiological supervision and interpretation

75716   Angiography, extremity, bilateral, radiological supervision and interpretation

75726 Angiography, visceral, selective or supraselective, (with or without flush aortogram), radiological supervision and interpretation

(For selective angiography, each additional visceral vessel studied after basic examination, use 75774)

75731 Angiography, adrenal, unilateral, selective, radiological supervision and interpretation

75733 Angiography, adrenal, bilateral, selective, radiological supervision and interpretation

75736 Angiography, pelvic, selective or supraselective, radiological supervision and interpretation

75741 Angiography, pulmonary, unilateral, selective, radiological supervision and interpretation

75743 Angiography, pulmonary, bilateral, selective, radiological supervision and interpretation

75746 Angiography, pulmonary, by nonselective catheter or venous injection, radiological supervision and interpretation

(For pulmonary angiography by nonselective catheter or venous injuection performed at the time of cardiac catheterization, use 93568, which includes imaging supervision, interpretation and report)

75756 Angiography, internal mammary, radiological supervision and interpretation

(For internal mammary angiography performed at the time of cardiac catheterization, see 93455, 93457, 93459, 93461, 93564 which include imaging supervision, interpretation and report)

+ **75774** Angiography, selective, each additional vessel studied after basic examination, radiological supervision and interpretation (List separately in addition to code for primary procedure)

(Use 75774 in addition to code for specific initial vessel studied)

(Do not report 75774 as part of diagnostic angiography of the extracranial and intracranial cervicocerebral vessels. It may be appropriate to reort 75774 for diagnostic angiography of upper extremities and other vascular beds performed in the same session)

(For angiography, see 75600-75756)

(For catheterizations, see codes 36215-36248)

(For cardiac catheterization procedures, see 93452-93462, 93531-93533, 93563-93568)

(For radiological supervision and interpretation of dialysis circuit angiography performed through existing access[es] or catheter-based arterial access, use 36901 with modifier 52)

VEINS AND LYMPHATICS

For venography performed in conjunction with therapeutic transcatheter radiological supervision and interpretation services, see the Radiology Transcatheter Procedures guidelines.

Diagnostic venography (radiological supervision and interpretation) codes should NOT be used with interventional procedures for:

(1) Contrast injections, venography, roadmapping, and/or fluoroscopic guidance for intervention;

(2) Vessel measurement; and

(3) Post-angioplasty/stent venography, as this work is captured in the radiological supervision and interpretation code(s).

Diagnostic venography performed at the time of an interventional procedure is separately reportable if:

1. No prior catheter-based venographic study is available and a full diagnostic study is performed, and decision to intervene is based on the diagnostic study, OR

2. A prior study is available, but as documented in the medical record:

a. The patient's condition with respect to the clinical indication has changed since the prior study, OR

● New Code ▲ Revised Code + Add-On Code ⊘ Modifier -51 Exempt ★ Telemedicine

b. There is inadequate visualization of the anatomy and/or pathology, OR

c. There is a clinical change during the procedure that requires new evaluation outside the target area of intervention.

Diagnostic venography performed at a separate setting from an interventional procedure is separately reported.

Diagnostic venography performed at the time of an interventional procedure is NOT separately reportable if it is specifically included in the interventional code descriptor.

(For injection procedure for venous system, see 36000-36015, 36400-36510)

(For injection procedure for lymphatic system, use 38790)

75801 Lymphangiography, extremity only, unilateral, radiological supervision and interpretation

75803 Lymphangiography, extremity only, bilateral, radiological supervision and interpretation

75805 Lymphangiography, pelvic/abdominal, unilateral, radiological supervision and interpretation

75807 Lymphangiography, pelvic/abdominal, bilateral, radiological supervision and interpretation

75809 Shuntogram for investigation of previously placed indwelling nonvascular shunt (eg, LeVeen shunt, ventriculoperitoneal shunt, indwelling infusion pump), radiological supervision and interpretation

(For procedure, see 49427 or 61070)

75810 Splenoportography, radiological supervision and interpretation

75820 Venography, extremity, unilateral, radiological supervision and interpretation

75822 Venography, extremity, bilateral, radiological supervision and interpretation

75825 Venography, caval, inferior, with serialography, radiological supervision and interpretation

75827 Venography, caval, superior, with serialography, radiological supervision and interpretation

75831 Venography, renal, unilateral, selective, radiological supervision and interpretation

75833 Venography, renal, bilateral, selective, radiological supervision and interpretation

75840 Venography, adrenal, unilateral, selective, radiological supervision and interpretation

75842 Venography, adrenal, bilateral, selective, radiological supervision and interpretation

75860 Venography, venous sinus (eg, petrosal and inferior sagittal) or jugular, catheter, radiological supervision and interpretation

75870 Venography, superior sagittal sinus, radiological supervision and interpretation

75872 Venography, epidural, radiological supervision and interpretation

75880 Venography, orbital, radiological supervision and interpretation

75885 Percutaneous transhepatic portography with hemodynamic evaluation, radiological supervision and interpretation

75887 Percutaneous transhepatic portography without hemodynamic evaluation, radiological supervision and interpretation

75889 Hepatic venography, wedged or free, with hemodynamic evaluation, radiological supervision and interpretation

---

75891 Hepatic venography, wedged or free, without hemodynamic evaluation, radiological supervision and interpretation

75893 Venous sampling through catheter, with or without angiography (eg, for parathyroid hormone, renin), radiological supervision and interpretation

(For procedure, use 36500)

TRANSCATHETER PROCEDURES

Therapeutic transcatheter radiological supervision and interpretation code(s) include the following services associated with that intervention:

1. Contrast injections, angiography/venography, roadmapping, and fluoroscopic guidance for the intervention;

2. Vessel measurement; and

3. Completion angiography/venography (except for those uses permitted by 75898).

Unless specifically included in the code descriptor, diagnostic angiography/venography performed at the time of transcatheter service(s) is separately reportable (eg., no prior catheter-based diagnostic angiography/ venography study of the target vessel is available, prior diagnostic study is inadequate, patient's condition with respect to the clinical indication has changed since the prior study or during the intervention). See 75600-75893.

Codes 75956 and 75957 include all angiography of the thoracic aorta and its branches for diagnostic imaging prior to deployment of the primary endovascular devices (including all routine components of modular devices), fluoroscopic guidance in the delivery of the endovascular components, and intraprocedural arterial angiography (eg., confirm position, detect endoleak, evaluate runoff).

Code 75958 includes the analogous services for placement of each proximal thoracic endovascular extension. Code 75959 includes the analogous services for placement of a distal thoracic endovascular extension(s) placed during a procedure after the primary repair.

75894 Transcatheter therapy, embolization, any method, radiological supervision and interpretation

(Do not report 75894 in conunction with 36475, 36476, 36478, 36479, 37241-37244)

75898 Angiography through existing catheter for follow-up study for transcatheter therapy, embolization or infusion, other than for thrombolysis

(For thrombolysis infusion management other than coronary, see 37211-37214, 61645)

(For non-thrombolysis infusion management other than coronary, see 61650, 61651)

(Do not report 75898 in conjunction with 37211-37214, 37241-37244, 61645, 61650, 61651)

75901 Mechanical removal of pericatheter obstructive material (eg., fibrin sheath) from central venous device via separate venous access, radiologic supervision and interpretation

(For procedure, use 36595)

(For venous catheterization, see 36010-36012)

75902 Mechanical removal of intraluminal (intracatheter) obstructive material from central venous device through device lumen, radiologic supervision and interpretation

(For procedure, use 36596)

(For venous catheterization, see 36010-36012)

(**75952** have been deleted. To report, see 34701-34711, 34718)

(**75953** have been deleted. To report, see 34701-34711, 34718)

(**75954** have been deleted. To report, see 34701-34711, 34718)

● New Code   ▲ Revised Code   + Add-On Code   ⊘ Modifier -51 Exempt   ★ Telemedicine

75956 Endovascular repair of descending thoracic aorta (eg, aneurysm, pseudoaneurysm, dissection, penetrating ulcer, intramural hematoma, or traumatic disruption); involving coverage of left subclavian artery origin, initial endoprosthesis plus descending thoracic aortic extension(s), if required, to level of celiac artery origin, radiological supervision and interpretation

(For implantation of endovascular graft, use 33880)

75957 not involving coverage of left subclavian artery origin, initial endoprosthesis plus descending thoracic aortic extension(s), if required, to level of celiac artery origin, radiological supervision and interpretation

(For implantation of endovascular graft, use 33881)

75958 Placement of proximal extension prosthesis for endovascular repair of descending thoracic aorta (eg, aneurysm, pseudoaneurysm, dissection, penetrating ulcer, intramural hematoma, or traumatic disruption), radiological supervision and interpretation

(Report 75958 for each proximal extension)

(For implantation of proximal endovascular extension, see 33883, 33884)

75959 Placement of distal extension prosthesis(es) (delayed) after endovascular repair of descending thoracic aorta, as needed, to level of celiac origin, radiological supervision and interpretation

(Do not report 75959 in conjunction with 75956, 75957)

(Report 75959 once, regardless of number of modules deployed)

(For implantation of distal endovascular extension, use 33886)

(Radiologic supervision for transcatheter placement of stent(s) is included in the therapeutic service codes)

(For removal of a vena cava filter, use 37193)

75970 Transcatheter biopsy, radiological supervision and interpretation

(For injection procedure only for transcatheter therapy or biopsy, see 36100-36299)

(For transcatheter renal and ureteral biopsy, use 52007)

(For percutaneous needle biopsy of pancreas, use 48102; of retroperitoneal lymph node or mass, use 49180)

(For radiological supervision and interpretation of transluminal balloon angioplasty within the peripheral and/or central segments of a dialysis circuit performed through the dialysis circuit, see 36902, 36905, 36907)

75984 Change of percutaneous tube or drainage catheter with contrast monitoring (eg, genitourinary system, abscess), radiological supervision and interpretation

(For percutaneous replacement of gastrostomy, duodenostomy, jejunostomy, gastro-jejunostomy, or cecostomy [or other colonic] tube including fluoroscopic imaging guidance, see 49450-49452)

(To report exchange of a percutaneous nephrostomy catheter, use 50435)

(For percutaneous choloecystostomy, use 47490)

(For percutaneous biliary procedures, including radiological supervision and interpretation, see 47531-47544)

(For percutaneous nephrostolithotomy or pyelostolithotomy, see 50080, 50081)

(For removal and/or replacement of an internally dwelling ureteral stent via a transurethral approach, see 50385-50386)

75989 Radiological guidance (ie, fluoroscopy, ultrasound, or computed tomography), for percutaneous drainage (eg., abscess, specimen collection), with placement of catheter, radiological supervision and interpretation

---

Separate Procedure   Unlisted Procedure   CCI Comp. Code   Non-specific Procedure   **675**

(Do not report 75989 in conjunction with 10030, 32554, 32555, 32556, 32557, 33017, 33018, 33019, 47490, 49405, 49406, 49407)

OTHER PROCEDURES

(For computed tomography cerebral perfusion analysis, see Category III code 0042T)

(For arthrography of shoulder, use 73040; elbow, use 73085; wrist, use 73115; hip, use 73525; knee, use 73580; ankle, use 73615)

76000 Fluoroscopy (separate procedure), up to 1 hour physician or other qualified health care professional time

(Do not report 76000 in conjunction with 33274, 33275, 33957, 33958, 33959, 33962, 33963, 33964, 0515T, 0516T, 0517T, 0518T, 0519T, 0520T)

(76001 deleted 2018 [2019 Edition])

76010 Radiologic examination from nose to rectum for foreign body, single view, child

76080 Radiologic examination, abscess, fistula or sinus tract study, radiological supervision and interpretation

(For contrast injection[s] and radiological assessment of gastrostomy, duodenostomy, jejunostomy, gastro-jejunostomy, or cecostomy [or other colonic] tube including fluoroscopic imaging guidance, use 49465)

76098 Radiological examination, surgical specimen

(Do not report 76098 in conjunction with 19081-19086)

76100 Radiologic examination, single plane body section (eg, tomography), other than with urography

76101 Radiologic examination, complex motion (ie, hypercycloidal) body section (eg, mastoid polytomography), other than with urography; unilateral

76102   bilateral

(Do not report 76101, 76102 more than once per day)

(For panoramic X-ray, use 70355)

(For nephrotomography, use 74415)

76120 Cineradiography/videoradiography, except where specifically included

+ 76125 Cineradiography/videoradiography to complement routine examination (List separately in addition to code for primary procedure)

76140 Consultation on x-ray examination made elsewhere, written report

(2D reformatting is no longer separately reported. To report 3D rendering, see 76376, 76377)

● 76145 Medical physics dose evaluation for radiation exposure that exceeds institutional review threshold, including report

76376 3D rendering with interpretation and reporting of computed tomography, magnetic resonance imaging, ultrasound, or other tomographic modality with image post processing under concurrent supervision; not requiring image postprocessing on an independent workstation

(Use 76376 in conjunction with code(s) for base imaging procedure(s))

(Do not report 76376 in conjunction with 31627, 34839, 70496, 70498, 70544, 70545, 70546, 70547, 70548, 70549, 71275, 71555, 72159, 72191, 72198, 73206, 73225, 73706, 73725, 74174, 74175, 74185, 74261, 74262, 74263, 75557, 75559, 75561, 75563, 75565, 75571, 75572, 75573, 75574, 75635, 76377, 77046, 77047, 77048, 77049, 77061, 77062, 77063, 78012-78999, 93355, 0523T, 0559T, 0560T, 0561T, 0562T, 0623T, 0624T, 0625T, 0626T, 0633T, 0634T, 0635T, 0636T, 0637T, 0638T)

● New Code   ▲ Revised Code   ✛ Add-On Code   ⊘ Modifier -51 Exempt   ★ Telemedicine

76377 requiring image postprocessing on an independent workstation

(Use 76377 in conjunction with code(s) for base imaging procedure(s))

(Do not report 76377 in conjunction with 34839, 70496, 70498, 70544, 70545, 70546, 70547, 70548, 70549, 71275, 71555, 72159, 72191, 72198, 73206, 73225, 73706, 73725, 74174, 74175, 74185, 74261, 74262, 74263, 75557, 75559, 75561, 75563, 75565, 75571, 75572, 75573, 75574, 75635, 76376, 77046, 77047, 77048, 77049, 77061, 77062, 77063, 78012-78999, 93355, 0523T, 0559T, 0560T, 0561T, 0562T, 0623T, 0624T, 0625T, 0626T, 0633T, 0634T, 0635T, 0636T, 0637T, 0638T)

(76376, 76377 require concurrent supervision of image post processing 3D manipulation of volumetric data set and image rendering)

76380 Computed tomography, limited or localized follow-up study

76390 Magnetic resonance spectroscopy

(For magnetic resonance imaging, use appropriate MRI body site code)

(For magnetic resonance spectroscopy, determination and localization of discogenic pain, see 0609T, 0610T)

76391 Magnetic resonance (eg, vibration) elastography

76496 Unlisted fluoroscopic procedure (eg., diagnostic, interventional)

76497 Unlisted computed tomography procedure (eg., diagnostic, interventional)

76498 Unlisted magnetic resonance procedure (eg., diagnostic, interventional)

76499 Unlisted diagnostic radiographic procedure

DIAGNOSTIC ULTRASOUND

Diagnostic ultrasound is a non-invasive medical imaging technology that uses high frequency sound waves to form an image of body tissues. Ultrasound, when compared to other imaging modalities like MRI (Magnetic Resonance Imaging) and CT (Computed Tomography), is a relatively low cost non-invasive procedure that does not utilize either magnetic fields or ionizing radiation (x-rays).

All diagnostic ultrasound examinations require permanently recorded images with measurements, when such measurements are clinically indicated. For those codes whose sole diagnostic goal is a biometric measure (ie., 76514, 76516, 76519), permanently recorded images are not required. A final, written report should be issued for inclusion in the patient's medical record. The prescription form for the intraocular lens satisfies the written report requirement for 76519. For those anatomic regions that have "complete" and "limited" ultrasound codes, note the elements that comprise a "complete"exam. The report should contain a description of these elements or the reason that an element could not be visualized (eg., obscured by bowel gas, surgically absent).

If less than the required elements for a "complete" exam are reported (eg., limited number of organs or limited portion of region evaluated), the "limited" code for that anatomic region should be used once per patient exam session. A "limited" exam of an anatomic region should not be reported for the same exam session as a "complete" exam of the same region.

Evaluation of vascular structures using both color and spectral Doppler is separately reportable. To report, see Noninvasive Vascular Diagnostic Studies (93875-93990). However, color Doppler alone, when performed for anatomic structure identification in conjunction with a real-time ultrasound examination, is not reported separately.

Ultrasound guidance procedures also require permanently recorded images of the site to be localized, as well as a documented description of the localization process, either separately or within the report of the procedure for which the guidance is utilized.

Use of ultrasound, without thorough evaluation of organ(s) or anatomic region, image documentation, and final written report, is not separately reportable.

Ultrasound Modes

A-mode   *Now obsolete in medical imaging. Wave spikes are represented when a single beam passes through objects of different consistency and hardness. The distance between these spikes (for example A and B) can be measured accurately by dividing the speed of sound in tissue (1540 m/sec) by half the sound travel time.*

B-mode   *Same as A-mode, but one-dimensional graphical display, with brightness corresponding to amplitude of reflected sound.*

M-mode   *A single beam in an ultrasound scan can be used to produce an M-mode picture, where movement of a structure such as a heart valve can be depicted in a wave-like manner. Because of its high sampling frequency (up to 1000 pulses per second), this is useful in assessing rates and motion and is still used extensively in cardiac and fetal cardiac imaging.*

Real time   *Most modern ultrasound devices are 2D-real time imaging systems. Multiple crystals (linear, curved or phased-array) or moving crystal. Sequential B-mode pulses sweeping across a plane to display the image in either a linear or 'sector' format. Displayed as real time imaging with up to 100 images per second.*

(To report diagnostic vascular ultrasound studies, see 93880-93990)

(For focused ultrasound ablation treatment of uterine leiomyomata, see Category III codes 0071T, 0072T)

HEAD AND NECK

76506   Echoencephalography, real time with image documentation (gray scale) (for determination of ventricular size, delineation of cerebral contents and detection of fluid masses or other intracranial abnormalities), including A-mode encephalography as secondary component where indicated

76510   Ophthalmic ultrasound, diagnostic; B-scan and quantitative A-scan performed during the same patient encounter

76511   quantitative A-scan only

76512   B-scan (with or without superimposed non-quantitative A-scan)

▲ **76513**   anterior segment ultrasound, immersion (water bath) B-scan or high resolution biomicroscopy, unilateral or bilateral

(For scanning computerized ophthalmic diagnostic imaging of the anterior and posterior segments using technology other than ultrasound, see 92132, 92133, 92134)

76514   corneal pachymetry, unilateral or bilateral (determination of corneal thickness)

(Do not report 76514 in conjunction with 0402T)

76516   Ophthalmic biometry by ultrasound echography, A-scan;

76519   with intraocular lens power calculation

(For partial coherence interferometry, use 92136)

76529   Ophthalmic ultrasonic foreign body localization

76536   Ultrasound, soft tissues of head and neck (eg, thyroid, parathyroid, parotid), real time with image documentation

CHEST

Code 76641 represents a complete ultrasound examination of the breast. Code 76641 consists of an ultrasound examination of all four quadrants of the breast and the retroareolar region. It also includes ultrasound examination of the axilla, if performed.

Code 76642 consists of a focused ultrasound examination of the breast limited to the assessment of one or more, but not all of the elements listed in code 76641. It also includes ultrasound examination of the axilla, if performed.

Use of ultrasound, without thorough evaluation of organ(s) or anatomic region, image documentation, and final written report, is not separately reportable.

76604 Ultrasound, chest, (includes mediastinum) real time with image documentation

76641 Ultrasound, breast, unilateral, real time with image documentation, including axilla when performed; complete

76642 limited

(Report 76641, 76442 only once per breast, per session)

(For axillary ultrasound only, use 76882)

ABDOMEN AND PERITONEUM

A complete ultrasound examination of the abdomen (76700) consists of real-time scans of the liver, gall bladder, common bile duct, pancreas, spleen, kidneys, and the upper abdominal aorta and inferior vena cava including any demonstrated abdominal abnormality.

A complete ultrasound examination of the retroperitoneum (76770) consists of real-time scans of the kidneys, abdominal aorta, common iliac artery origins, and inferior vena cava, including any demonstrated retroperitoneal abnormality. Alternatively, if clinical history suggests urinary tract pathology, complete evaluation of the kidneys and urinary bladder also comprises a complete retroperitoneal ultrasound.

Use of ultrasound, without thorough evaluation of organ(s) or anatomic region, image documentation and final, written report, is not separately reportable.

76700 Ultrasound, abdominal, real time with image documentation; complete

76705 limited (eg, single organ, quadrant, follow-up)

76706 Ultrasound, abdominal aorta, real time with image documentation, screening study for abdominal aortic aneurysm (AAA)

(For ultrasound or duplex ultrasound of the abdominal aorta other than screening, see 76770, 76775, 93978, 93979)

76770 Ultrasound, retroperitoneal (eg, renal, aorta, nodes), real time with image documentation; complete

76775 limited

76776 Ultrasound, transplanted kidney, real time and duplex Doppler with image documentation

(For ultrasound or transplanted kidney without duplex Doppler, use 76775)

(For ultrasound and duplex Doppler of a transplanted kidney, do not report 76776 in conjunction with 93975, 93976)

SPINAL CANAL

76800 Ultrasound, spinal canal and contents

PELVIS

OBSTETRICAL

Codes 76801 and 76802 include determination of the number of gestational sacs and fetuses, gestational sac/fetal measurements appropriate for gestation (younger than 14 weeks 0 days), survey of visible fetal and placental anatomic structure, qualitative assessment of amniotic fluid volume/gestational sac shape and examination of the maternal uterus and adnexa.

Codes 76805 and 76810 include determination of number of fetuses and amniotic/chorionic sacs, measurements appropriate for gestational age (older than or equal to 14 weeks 0 days), survey of intracranial/spinal/abdominal anatomy, 4 chambered heart, umbilical cord insertion site, placenta location and amniotic fluid assessment, and when visible, examination of maternal adnexa.

Codes 76811 and 76812 include all elements of codes 76805 and 76810 plus detailed anatomic evaluation of the fetal brain/ventricles, face, heart/outflow tracts and chest anatomy, abdominal organ specific anatomy, number/length/architecture of limbs and detailed evaluation of the umbilical cord and placenta and other fetal anatomy as clinically indicated.

Report should document the results of the evaluation of each element described above or the reason for non-visualization.

Code 76815 represents a focused "quick look" exam limited to the assessment of one or more of the elements listed in code 76815.

Code 76816 describes an examination designed to reassess fetal size and interval growth or reevaluate one or more anatomic abnormalities of a fetus previously demonstrated on ultrasound, and should be coded once for each fetus requiring reevaluation using modifier 59 for each fetus after the first.

Code 76817 describes a transvaginal obstetric ultrasound performed separately or in addition to one of the transabdominal examinations described above. For transvaginal examinations performed for non-obstetrical purposes, use code 76830

76801   Ultrasound, pregnant uterus, real time with image documentation, fetal and maternal evaluation, first trimester (>14 weeks 0 days), transabdominal approach; single or first gestation

   (To report first trimester fetal nuchal translucency measurement, use 76813)

+ **76802**   each additional gestation (List separately in addition to code for primary procedure)

   (Use 76802 in conjunction with code 76801)

   (To report first trimester fetal nuchal translucency measurement, use 76814)

76805   Ultrasound, pregnant uterus, real time with image documentation, fetal and maternal evaluation, after first trimester (>or = 14 weeks 0 days), transabdominal approach; single or first gestation

+ **76810**   each additional gestation (List separately in addition to code for primary procedure)

   (Use 76810 in conjunction with code 76805)

76811   Ultrasound, pregnant uterus, real time with image documentation, fetal and maternal evaluation plus detailed fetal anatomic examination, transabdominal approach; single or first gestation

+ **76812**   each additional gestation (List separately in addition to code for primary procedure)

   (Use 76812 in conjunction with code 76811)

76813   Ultrasound, pregnant uterus, real time with image documentation, first trimester fetal nuchal translucency measurement, transabdominal or transvaginal approach; single or first gestation

+ **76814**   each additional gestation (List separately in addition to code for primary procedure)

   (Use 76814 in conjunction with 76813)

76815   Ultrasound, pregnant uterus, real time with image documentation, limited (eg., fetal heart beat, placental location, fetal position, and/or qualitative amniotic fluid volume), 1 or more fetuses

   (Use 76815 only once per exam and not per element)

   (To report first trimester fetal nuchal translucency measurement, see 76813, 76814)

76816   Ultrasound, pregnant uterus, real time with image documentation, follow-up (eg., re-evaluation of fetal size by measuring standard growth parameters and amniotic fluid volume, re-evaluation of organ system(s) suspected or confirmed to be abnormal on a previous scan), transabdominal approach, per fetus

   (Report 76816 with modifier -59 for each additional fetus examined in a multiple pregnancy)

76817 Ultrasound, pregnant uterus, real time with image documentation, transvaginal

(For non-obstetrical transvaginal ultrasound, use 76830)

(If transvaginal examination is done in addition to transabdominal obstetrical ultrasound exam, use 76817 in addition to appropriate transabdominal exam code)

76818 Fetal biophysical profile; with non-stress testing

76819 without non-stress testing

(Fetal biophysical profile assessments for the second and any additional fetuses, should be reported separately by code 76818 or 76819 with the modifier -59 appended)

(For amniotic fluid index without non-stress test, use 76815)

76820 Doppler velocimetry, fetal; umbilical artery

76821 middle cerebral artery

76825 Echocardiography, fetal, cardiovascular system, real time with image documentation (2D), with or without M-mode recording;

76826 follow-up or repeat study

76827 Doppler echocardiography, fetal, pulsed wave and/or continuous wave with spectral display; complete

76828 follow-up or repeat study

(To report the use of color mapping, use 93325)

NON-OBSTETRICAL

Code 76856 includes the complete evaluation of the female pelvic anatomy. Elements of this examination include a description and measurements of the uterus and adnexal structures, measurement of the endometrium, measurement of the bladder (when applicable) and a description of any pelvic pathology (eg., ovarian cysts, uterine leiomyomata, free pelvic fluid).

Code 76856 is also applicable to a complete evaluation of the male pelvis. Elements of the examination include evaluation and measurement (when applicable) of the urinary bladder, evaluation of the prostate and seminal vesicles to the extent that they are visualized transabdominally, and any pelvic pathology (eg., bladder tumor, enlarged prostate, free pelvic fluid, pelvic abscess).

Code 76857 represents a focused examination limited to the assessment of one or more elements listed in code 76856 and/or the reevaluation of one or more pelvic abnormalities previously demonstrated on ultrasound. Code 76857, rather than 76770, should be utilized if the urinary bladder alone (ie., not including the kidneys) is imaged, whereas code 51798 should be utilized if a bladder volume or post-void residual measurement is obtained without imaging the bladder.

Use of ultrasound, without thorough evaluation of organ(s) or anatomic region, image documentation, and final, written report, is not separately reportable.

76830 Ultrasound, transvaginal

(For obstetrical transvaginal ultrasound, use 76817)

(If transvaginal examination is done in addition to transabdominal non-obstetrical ultrasound exam, use 76830 in addition to appropriate transabdominal exam code)

76831 Saline infusion sonohysterography (SIS), including color flow Doppler, when performed

(For introduction of saline for saline infusion sonohysterography, use 58340)

76856 Ultrasound, pelvic (nonobstetric), real time with image documentation; complete

76857 limited or follow-up (eg, for follicles)

GENITALIA

76870   Ultrasound, scrotum and contents

76872   Ultrasound, transrectal;

(Do not report 76872 in conjunction with 45341, 45342, 45391, 45392, 46948, 0421T, 0619T)

76873   prostate volume study for brachytherapy treatment planning (separate procedure)

EXTREMITIES

Code 76881 represents a complete evaluation of a specific joint in an extremity. Code 76881 requires ultrasound examination of all of the following joint elements: joint space (eg, effusion), peri-articular softtissue structures that surround the joint (ie, muscles, tendons, other soft-tissue structures), and any identifiable abnormality. In some circumstances, additional evaluations such as dynamic imaging or stress maneuvers may be performed as part of the complete evaluation. Code 76881 also requires permanently recorded images and a written report containing a description of each of the required elements or reason that an element(s) could not be visualized (eg, absent secondary to surgery or trauma).

When fewer than all of the required elements for a "complete" exam (76881) are performed, report the "limited" code (76882).

Code 76882 represents a limited evaluation of a joint or an evaluation of a structure(s) in an extremity other than a joint (eg, soft-tissue mass, fluid collection, or nerve[s]). Limited evaluation of a joint includes assessment of a specific anatomic structure(s) (eg, joint space only [effusion] or tendon, muscle, and/or other soft-tissue structure[s] that surround the joint) that does not assess all of the required elements included in 76881. Code 76882 also requires permanently recorded images and a written report containing a description of each of the elements evaluated.

For spectral and color Doppler evaluation of the extremities, use 93925, 93926, 93930, 93931, 93970, or 93971 as appropriate.

76881   Ultrasound, complete joint (ie, joint space and periarticular soft-tissue structures), real-time with image documentation

76882   Ultrasound, limited, joint or other nonvascular extremity structure(s) (eg, joint space, peri-articular tendon[s], muscle[s], nerve[s], other soft-tissue structure[s], or softtissue mass[es]), real-time with image documentation

76885   Ultrasound, infant hips, real time with imaging documentation; dynamic (requiring physician or other qualified health care professional manipulation)

76886   limited, static (not requiring physician or other qualified health care professional manipulation)

ULTRASONIC GUIDANCE PROCEDURES

(76930   deleted 2019 [2020 Edition]. To report, see 33016, 33017, 33018)

76932   Ultrasonic guidance for endomyocardial biopsy, imaging supervision and interpretation

76936   Ultrasound guided compression repair of arterial pseudoaneurysm or arteriovenous fistulae (includes diagnostic ultrasound evaluation, compression of lesion and imaging)

+ **76937**   Ultrasound guidance for vascular access requiring ultrasound evaluation of potential access sites, documentation of selected vessel patency, concurrent realtime ultrasound visualization of vascular needle entry, with permanent recording and reporting (List separately in addition to code for primary procedure)

(Do not report 76937 in conjunction with 33274, 33275, 36568, 36569, 36572, 36573, 36584, 37191, 37192, 37193, 37760, 37761, 76942)

(Do not report 76937 in conjunction with 0505T, 0620T for ultrasound guidance for vascular access)

(If extremity venous non-invasive vascular diagnostic study is performed separate from venous access guidance, see 93970, 93971)

76940 Ultrasound guidance for, and monitoring of, parenchymal tissue ablation

(Do not report 76940 in conjunction with 20982, 20983, 32994, 32998, 50250, 50542, 76942, 76998, 0582T, 0600T, 0601T)

(For ablation, see 47370-47382, 47383, 50592, 50593)

76941 Ultrasonic guidance for intrauterine fetal transfusion or cordocentesis, imaging supervision and interpretation

(For procedure, see 36460, 59012)

76942 Ultrasonic guidance for needle placement (eg, biopsy, aspiration, injection, localization device) imaging supervision and interpretation

(Do not report 76942 in conjunction with 10004, 10005, 10006, 10021, 10030, 19083, 19285, 20604, 20606, 20611, 27096, 32408, 32554, 32555, 32556, 32557, 37760, 37761, 43232, 43237, 43242, 45341, 45342, 46948, 55874, 64479, 64480, 64483, 64484, 64490, 64491, 64493, 64494, 64495, 76975, 0213T, 0214T, 0215T, 0216T, 0217T, 0218T, 0232T, 0481T, 0582T)

(For harvesting, preparation, and injection[s] of platelet-rich plasma, use 0232T)

76945 Ultrasonic guidance for chorionic villus sampling, imaging supervision and interpretation

(For procedure, use 59015)

76946 Ultrasonic guidance for amniocentesis, imaging supervision and interpretation

76948 Ultrasonic guidance for aspiration of ova, imaging supervision and interpretation

(For placement of interstitial device[s] for radiation therapy guidance, see 31627, 32553, 49411, 55876)

76965 Ultrasonic guidance for interstitial radioelement application

OTHER PROCEDURES

(**76970** deleted 2020 [2021 Edition])

76975 Gastrointestinal endoscopic ultrasound, imaging supervision and interpretation

(Do not report 76975 in conjunction with 43231, 43232, 43237, 43238, 43240, 43242, 43259, 44406, 44407, 45341, 45342, 45391, 45392, 76942)

76977 Ultrasound bone density measurement and interpretation, peripheral site(s), any method

76978 Ultrasound, targeted dynamic microbubble sonographic contrast characterization (non-cardiac); initial lesion

+ **76979** each additional lesion with separate injection (List separately in addition to code for primary procedure)

(Use 76979 in conjunction with 76978)

(Do not report 76978, 76979 in conjunction with 96374)

76981 Ultrasound, elastography; parenchyma (eg, organ)

76982 first target lesion

+ **76983** each additional target lesion (List separately in addition to code for primary procedure)

(Use 76983 in conjunction with 76982)

(Report 76981 only once per session for evaluation of the same parenchymal organ)

(To report shear wave liver elastography without imaging, use 91200)

(For evaluation of a parenchymal organ and lesion[s] in the same parenchymal organ at the same session, report only 76981)

(Do not report 76983 more than two times per organ)

76998   Ultrasonic guidance, intraoperative

(Do not report 76998 in conjunction with 36475, 36479, 37760, 37761, 46948, 47370, 47371, 47380, 47381, 47382, 0515T, 0516T, 0517T, 0518T, 0519T, 0520T)

(For ultrasound guidance for open and laparoscopic radiofrequency tissue ablation, use 76940)

76999   Unlisted ultrasound procedure (eg., diagnostic, interventional)

RADIOLOGIC GUIDANCE

FLUOROSCOPIC GUIDANCE

(Do not report guidance codes 77001, 77002, 77003 for services in which fluoroscopic guidance is included in the descriptor)

+ **77001**   Fluoroscopic guidance for central venous access device placement, replacement (catheter only or complete), or removal (includes fluoroscopic guidance for vascular access and catheter manipulation, any necessary contrast injections through access site or catheter with related venography radiologic supervision and interpretation, and radiographic documentation of final catheter position) (List separately in addition to code for primary procedure)

(Do not report 77001 in conjunction with 33957, 33958, 33959, 33962, 33963, 33964, 36568, 36569, 36572, 36573, 36584, 77002)

(If formal extremity venography is performed from separate venous access and separately interpreted, use 36005 and 75820, 75822, 75825 or 75827)

+ **77002**   Fluoroscopic guidance for needle placement (eg, biopsy, aspiration, injection, localization device) (List separately in addition to code for primary procedure)

(Use 77002 in conjunction with 10160, 20206, 20220, 20225, 20520, 20525, 20526, 20550, 20551, 20552, 20553, 20555, 20600, 20605, 20610, 20612, 20615, 21116, 21550, 23350, 24220, 25246, 27093, 27095, 27369, 27648, 32400, 32553, 36002, 38220, 38221, 38222, 38505, 38794, 41019, 42400, 42405, 47000, 47001, 48102, 49180, 49411, 50200, 50390, 51100, 51101, 51102, 55700, 55876, 60100, 62268, 62269, 64400-64448, 64450, 64455, 64505, 64600, 64605)

(77002 is included in allarthrography radiological supervision and interpretation codes. See Administration of Contrast Material[s] introductory guidelines for reporting of arthrography procedures)

+ **77003**   Fluoroscopic guidance and localization of needle or catheter tip for spine or paraspinous diagnostic or therapeutic injection procedures (epidural or subarachnoid) (List separately in addition to code for primary procedure)

(Use 77003 in conjunction with 61050, 61055, 62267, 62273, 62280, 62281, 62282, 62284, 64510, 64517, 64520, 64610, 96450)

(Do not report 77003 in conjunction with 62270, 62272, 62320, 62321, 62322, 62323, 62324, 62325, 62326, 62327, 62328, 62329, 0627T, 0628T)

COMPUTED TOMOGRAPHY GUIDANCE

77011   Computed tomography guidance for stereotactic localization

77012   Computed tomography guidance for needle placement (eg, biopsy, aspiration, injection, localization device), radiological supervision and interpretation

(Do not report 77011, 77012 in conjunction with 22586)

(Do not report 77012 in conjunction with 10009, 10010, 10030, 27096, 32408, 32554, 32555, 32556, 32557, 62270, 62272, 62328, 62329, 64479, 64480, 64483, 64484, 64490, 64491, 64492, 64493, 64494, 64495, 64633, 64634, 64635, 64636, 0232T, 0481T, 0629T, 0630T)

(For harvesting, preparation, and injection[s] of platelet-rich plasma, use 0232T)

77013 Computerized tomography guidance for, and monitoring of, parenchymal tissue ablation

(Do not report 77013 in conjunction with 20982, 20983, 32994, 32998, 0600T)

(For percutaneous ablation, see 47382, 47383, 50592, 50593)

77014 Computed tomography guidance for placement of radiation therapy fields

(For placement of interstitial device(s) for radiation therapy guidance, see 31627, 32553, 49411, 55876)

MAGNETIC RESONANCE IMAGING GUIDANCE

77021 Magnetic resonance imaging guidance for needle placement (eg, for biopsy, needle aspiration, injection, or placement of localization device) radiological supervision and interpretation

(For procedure, see appropriate organ or site)

(Do not report 77021 in conjunction with 10011, 10012, 10030, 19085, 19287, 32408, 32554, 32555, 32556, 32557, 0232T, 0481T)

(For harvesting, preparation, and injection[s] of platelet-rich plasma, use 0232T)

77022 Magnetic resonance imaging guidance for, and monitoring of, parenchymal tissue ablation

(Do not report 77022 in conjunction with 20982, 20983, 32994, 32998, 0071T, 0072T, 0600T)

(For percutaneous ablation, see 47382, 47383, 50592, 50593)

(For focused ultrasound ablation treatment of uterine leiomyomata, see Category III codes 0071T, 0072T)

(To report stereotactic localization guidance for breast biopsy or for placement of breast localization device[s], see 19081, 19283)

(To report mammographic guidance for placement of breast localization device[s], use 19281)

BREAST, MAMMOGRAPHY

77046 Magnetic resonance imaging, breast, without contrast material; unilateral

77047 bilateral

77048 Magnetic resonance imaging, breast, without and with contrast material(s), including computer-aided detection (CAD real-time lesion detection, characterization and pharmacokinetic analysis), when performed; unilateral

77049 bilateral

77053 Mammary ductogram or galactogram, single duct, radiological supervision and interpretation

(For mammary ductogram or galactogram injection, use 19030)

77054 Mammary ductogram or galactogram, multiple ducts, radiological supervision and interpretation

(**77058** deleted 2018 [2019 Edition]. To report, see 77046, 77048)

(**77059** deleted 2018 [2019 Edition]. To report, see 77047, 77049)

77061 Digital breast tomosynthesis; unilateral

77062   bilateral

(Do not report 77061, 77062 in conjunction with 76376, 76377, 77067)

+ 77063   Screening digital breast tomosynthesis, bilateral (list separately in addition to code for primary procedure)

(Do not report 77063 in conjunction with 76376, 76377, 77065, 77066)

(Use 77063 in conjunction with 77067)

77065   Diagnostic mammography, including computer-aided detection (CAD) when performed; unilateral

77066   bilateral

77067   Screening mammography, bilateral (2-view study of each breast), including computer-aided detection (CAD) when performed

(For electrical impedance breast scan, use 76499)

BONE/JOINT STUDIES

77071   Manual application of stress performed by physician or other qualified health care professional for joint radiography, including contralateral joint if indicated

(For radiographic interpretation of stressed images, see appropriate anatomic site and number of views)

77072   Bone age studies

77073   Bone length studies (orthoroentgenogram, scanogram)

77074   Radiologic examination, osseous survey; limited (eg, for metastases)

77075   complete (axial and appendicular skeleton)

77076   Radiologic examination, osseous survey, infant

77077   Joint survey, single view, 2 or more joints (specify)

77078   Computed tomography, bone mineral density study, 1 or more sites; axial skeleton (eg, hips, pelvis, spine)

77080   Dual-energy X-ray absorptiometry (DXA), bone density study, 1 or more sites; axial skeleton (eg, hips, pelvis, spine)

(Do not report 77080 in conjunction with 77085, 77086)

77081   appendicular skeleton (peripheral) (eg, radius, wrist, heel)

(For dual-energy X-ray absorptiometry [DEXA] body composition study, use 76499)

77085   axial skeleton (eg, hips, pelvis, spine), including vertebral fracture assessment

(Do not report 77085 in conjunction with 77080, 77086)

77086   Vertebral fracture assessment via dual-energy X-ray absorptiometry (DXA)

(Do not report 77086 in conjunction with 77080, 77085)

77084   Magnetic resonance (eg, proton) imaging, bone marrow blood supply

77085   This code is out of order. See page 686

77086   This code is out of order. See page 686

RADIATION ONCOLOGY

Listings for Radiation Oncology provide for teletherapy and brachytherapy to include initial consultation, clinical treatment planning, simulation, medical radiation physics, dosimetry, treatment devices, special services, and clinical treatment management procedures. They include normal follow-up care during course of treatment and for three months following its completion.

When a service or procedure is provided that is not listed in this edition of CPT, it should be identified by a Special Report and one of the following unlisted procedure codes: **77299** Unlisted procedure, therapeutic radiology clinical treatment planning; or **77399** Unlisted procedure, medical radiation physics, dosimetry and treatment devices, and special services; or **77499** Unlisted procedure, therapeutic radiology treatment management; or **77799** Unlisted procedure, clinical brachytherapy.

For treatment by injectable or ingestible isotopes, see subsection Nuclear Medicine.

CONSULTATION: CLINICAL MANAGEMENT

Preliminary consultation, evaluation of patient prior to decision to treat, or full medical care (in addition to treatment management) when provided by the therapeutic radiologist may be identified by the appropriate procedure codes from Evaluation and Management, Medicine, or Surgery sections.

CLINICAL TREATMENT PLANNING (EXTERNAL AND INTERNAL SOURCES)

The clinical treatment planning process is a complex service including interpretation of special testing, tumor localization, treatment volume determination, treatment time/dosage determination, choice of treatment modality, determination of number and size of treatment ports, selection of appropriate treatment devices, and other procedures.

Definitions

Simple planning requires a single treatment area of interest encompassed in a single port or simple parallel opposed ports with simple or no blocking.

Intermediate planning requires 3 or more converging ports, 2 separate treatment areas, multiple blocks, or special time dose constraints.

Complex planning requires highly complex blocking, custom shielding blocks, tangential ports, special wedges or compensators, 3 or more separate treatment areas, rotational or special beam considerations, combination of therapeutic modalities.

77261   Therapeutic radiology treatment planning; simple

77262   intermediate

77263   complex

Simulation is the process of defining relevant normal and abnormal target anatomy, and acquiring the images and data necessary to develop the optimal radiation treatment process for the patient. A simulation is defined as complex if any of these criteria are met: particle, rotation or arc therapy, complex or custom blocking, brachytherapy simulation, hyperthermia probe verification, or any use of contrast material. If a simulation does not meet any of these criteria, the complexity is defined by the number of treatment areas: one treatment area is simple, two treatment areas are intermediate, and three or more treatment areas are complex.

A treatment area is a contiguous anatomic location that will be treated with radiation therapy. Generally, this includes the primary tumor organ or the resection bed and the draining lymph node chains, if indicated. An example is a breast cancer patient for whom a single treatment area could be the breast alone or the breast, adjacent supraclavicular fossa, and internal mammary nodes. In some cases, a patient might receive radiation therapy to more than one discontinuous anatomic location. An example would be a patient with multiple bone metastases in separate sites (eg, femur and cervical spine); in this case, each distinct and separate anatomic site to be irradiated is a separate treatment area.

Definitions.

Simple: simulation of a single treatment area.

Intermediate: two separate treatment areas.

Complex: three or more treatment areas, or any number of treatment areas if any of the following are involved: particle, rotation or arc therapy, complex blocking, custom shielding blocks, brachytherapy simulation, hyperthermia probe verification, any use of contrast materials.

77280	Therapeutic radiology simulation-aided field setting; simple
77285	intermediate
77290	complex
+ 77293	Respiratory motion management simulation (List separately in addition to code for primary procedure)

(Use 77293 in conjunction with 77295, 77301)

77295 This code is out of order. See page 688

77299 Unlisted procedure, therapeutic radiology clinical treatment planning

MEDICAL RADIATION PHYSICS, DOSIMETRY, TREATMENT DEVICES, AND SPECIAL SERVICES

77295 3-dimensional radiotherapy plan, including dose-volume histograms

77300 Basic radiation dosimetry calculation, central axis depth dose calculation, TDF, NSD, gap calculation, off axis factor, tissue inhomogeneity factors, calculation of non-ionizing radiation surface and depth dose, as required during course of treatment, only when prescribed by the treating physician

(Do not report 77300 in conjunction with 77306, 77307, 77316, 77317, 77318, 77321, 77767, 77768, 77770, 77771, 77772, 0394T, 0395T)

77301 Intensity modulated radiotherapy plan, including dose-volume histograms for target and critical structure partial tolerance specifications

(Dose plan is optimized using inverse or forward planning technique for modulated beam delivery (eg, binary, dynamic MLC) to create highly conformal dose distribution. Computer plan distribution must be verified for positional accuracy based on dosimetric verification of the intensity map with verification of treatment set up and interpretation of verification methodology)

77306 Teletherapy isodose plan; simple (1 or 2 unmodified ports directed to a single area of interest), includes basic dosimetry calculation(s)

77307 complex (multiple treatment areas, tangential ports, the use of wedges, blocking, rotational beam, or special beam considerations), includes basic dosimetry calculation(s)

(Only one teletherapy isodose plan may be reported for a given course of therapy to a specific treatment area)

(Do not report 77306, 77307 in conjunction with 77300)

77316 Brachytherapy isodose plan; simple (calculation[s] made from 1 to 4 sources, or remote afterloading brachytherapy, 1 channel), includes basic dosimetry calculation(s)

(For definition of source, see clinical brachytherapy introductory guidelines)

77317 intermediate (calculation[s] made from 5 to 10 sources, or remote afterloading brachytherapy, 2-12 channels), includes basic dosimetry calculation(s)

77318 complex (calculation[s] made from over 10 sources, or remote afterloading brachytherapy, over 12 channels), includes basic dosimetry calculation(s)

(Do not report 77316, 77317, 77318 in conjunction with 77300)

77321 Special teletherapy port plan, particles, hemibody, total body

● New Code ▲ Revised Code + Add-On Code ⊘ Modifier -51 Exempt ★ Telemedicine

77331 Special dosimetry (eg, TLD, microdosimetry) (specify), only when prescribed by the treating physician

77332 Treatment devices, design and construction; simple (simple block, simple bolus)

77333 intermediate (multiple blocks, stents, bite blocks, special bolus)

77334 complex (irregular blocks, special shields, compensators, wedges, molds or casts)

77336 Continuing medical physics consultation, including assessment of treatment parameters, quality assurance of dose delivery, and review of patient treatment documentation in support of the radiation oncologist, reported per week of therapy

77338 Multi leaf collimator (MLC) device(s) for intensity modulated radiation therapy (IMRT), design and construction per IMRT plan

(Do not report 77338 in conjunction with 77385 for compensator based IMRT)

(Do not report 77338 more than once per IMRT plan)

(For immobilization in IMRT treatment, see 77332-77334)

77370 Special medical radiation physics consultation

STEREOTACTIC RADIATION TREATMENT DELIVERY

77371 Radiation treatment delivery, stereotactic radiosurgery (SRS), complete course of treatment of cranial lesion(s) consisting of 1 session; multi-source Cobalt 60 based

77372 linear accelerator based

(For radiation treatment management, use 77432)

77373 Stereotactic body radiation therapy, treatment delivery, per fraction to 1 or more lesions, including image guidance, entire course not to exceed 5 fractions

(Do not report 77373 in conjunction with 77385, 77386, 77401, 77402, 77407, 77412)

(For single fraction cranial lesions(s), see 77371, 77372)

77385 This code is out of order. See page 691

77386 This code is out of order. See page 691

77387 This code is out of order. See page 691

OTHER PROCEDURES

77399 Unlisted procedure, medical radiation physics, dosimetry and treatment devices, and special services

RADIATION TREATMENT DELIVERY

Following dosimetry calculations, there are a number of alternative methods to deliver external radiation treatments, which are described with specific CPT codes:

X-ray (photon), including conventional and intensity modulated radiation therapy IMRT beams;

Electron beams;

Neutron beams;

Proton beams.

All treatment delivery codes are reported once per treatment session. The treatment delivery codes recognize technical-only services and contain no physician work (the professional component). In contrast, the treatment management codes contain only the professional component.

Radiation treatment delivery with conventional X-ray or electron beams is assigned levels of complexity based on the number of treatment sites and complexity of the treatment fields, blocking, wedges, and physical or virtual tissue compensators. A simple block is straight-edged or an approximation of a straight edge created by a multileaf collimator (MLC). Energy of the megavoltage less than or equal to 1MEV beam does not contribute to complexity. Techniques such as treating a field-in-field to ensure dose homogeneity reflect added complexity.

Energies below the megavoltage range maybe used in the treatment of skin lesions. Superficial radiation energies (up to 200 kV) may be generated by a variety of technologies and should not be reported with megavoltage (77402, 77407, 77412) for surface application. Do not report clinical treatment planning (77261, 77262, 77263), treatment devices (77332, 77333, 77334), isodose planning (77306, 77307, 77316, 77317, 77318), physics consultation (77336), or radiation treatment management (77427, 77431, 77432, 77435, 77469, 77470, 77499), with 77401, 0394T, or 0395T. When reporting 77401 alone, evaluation and management, when performed, may be reported with the appropriate E/M codes.

Intensity modulated radiation therapy (IMRT) uses computer-based optimization techniques with non-uniform radiation beam intensities to create highly conformal dose distributions that can be delivered by a radiotherapy treatment machine. A number of technologies, including spatially and temporally modulated beams, cylindrical beamlets, dynamic MLC, single or multiple fields or arcs, or compensators, may be used to generate IMRT. The complexity of IMRT may vary depending on the area being treated or the technique being used.

Image guided radiation therapy (IGRT) may be used to direct the radiation beam and to reflect motion during treatment. A variety of techniques may be used to perform this guidance including imaging (eg., ultrasound, CT, MRI, stereoscopic imaging) and non-imaging (eg., electromagnetic or infrared) techniques. Guidance may be used with any radiation treatment delivery technique and is typically used with IMRT delivery. IMRT delivery codes include the technical component of guidance or tracking, if performed. Because only the technical portion of IGRT is bundled into IMRT, the physician involvement in guidance or tracking may be reported separately. When guidance is required with conventional radiation treatment delivery, both the professional and technical components are reported because neither component of guidance is bundled into conventional radiation treatment delivery services.

The technical and professional components of guidance are handled differently with each radiation delivery code depending on the type of radiation being administered. The Radiation Management and Treatment Table is provided for clarity.

Definitions

Radiation Treatment Delivery, megavoltage (less than or equal to 1MeV, any energy.

Simple: all of the following criteria are met and none of the complex or intermediate criteria are met: single treatment area, one or two ports, and two or fewer simple blocks.

Intermediate: any of the following criteria are met and none of the complex criteria are met: two separate treatment areas, three or more ports on a single treatment area, or three or more simple blocks.

Complex: any of the following criteria are met: three or more separate treatment areas, custom blocking, tangential ports, wedges, rotational beam, field-in-field or other tissue compensation that does not meet IMRT guidelines, or electron beam.

Intensity Modulated Radiation Therapy (IMRT), any energy, includes the technical services for guidance

Simple: any of the following: prostate, breast, and all sites using physical compensator based IMRT.

Complex: includes all other sites if not using physical compensator based IMRT

77401 Radiation treatment delivery, superficial and/or ortho voltage, per day

(Do not report 77401 in conjunction with 77373)

77402 Radiation treatment delivery, ≥ 1 MeV; simple

(Do not report 77402 in conjunction with 77373)

77407 intermediate

(Do not report 77407 in conjunction with 77373)

77412   complex

(Do not report 77412 in conjunction with 77373)

77417   Therapeutic radiology port image(s)

(For intensity modulated treatment planning, use 77301)

77385   Intensity modulated radiation treatment delivery (IMRT), includes guidance and tracking, when performed; simple

(To report professional component [PC] of guidance and tracking, use 77387 with modifier 26)

77386   complex

(To report professional component [PC] of guidance and tracking, use 77387 with modifier 26)

(Do not report 77385, 77386 in conjunction with 77371, 77372, 77373)

77387   Guidance for localization of target volume for delivery of radiation treatment, includes intrafraction tracking, when performed

(Do not report technical component [TC] with 77385, 77386, 77371, 77372, 77373)

(For placement of interstitial device(s) for radiation therapy guidance, see 31627, 32553, 49411, 55876)

77424   Intraoperative radiation treatment delivery, x-ray, single treatment session

77425   Intraoperative radiation treatment delivery, electrons, single treatment session

NEUTRON BEAM TREATMENT DELIVERY

(**77422**   deleted 2017 [2018 edition])

77423   High energy neutron radiation treatment delivery, 1 or more isocenter(s) with coplanar or non-coplanar geometry with blocking and/or wedge, and/or compensator(s)

77424   Code out of order. See page 691

77425   Code out of order. See page 691

RADIATION TREATMENT MANAGEMENT

CPT codes in this section presume treatment on a daily basis (4 or 5 fractions per week) with the use of megavoltage photon or high energy particle sources. Daily and weekly clinical treatment management are mutually exclusive for the same dates. CPT defines three distinct levels of clinical treatment management: simple, intermediate and complex. Review this section of CPT for detailed definitions of these levels of service.

Radiation treatment management is reported in units of five fractions or treatment sessions, regardless of the actual time period in which the services are furnished. The services need not be furnished on consecutive days. Multiple fractions representing two or more treatment sessions furnished on the same day may be counted separately as long as there has been a distinct break in therapy sessions, and the fractions are of the character usually furnished on different days. Code 77427 is also reported if there are three or four fractions beyond a multiple of five at the end of a course of treatment; one or two fractions beyond a multiple of five at the end of a course of treatment are not reported separately.

Radiation treatment management requires **and includes** a minimum of one examination of the patient by the physician for medical evaluation and management (eg., assessment of the patient's response to treatment, coordination of care and treatment, review of imaging and/or lab test results with doumentation) for each reporting of the radiation treatment management service. Code 77469 represents only the intraoperative session management and does not include medical evaluation and management outside of that session. The professional services furnished during treatment management typically include:

• Review of port images;

- Review of dosimetry, dose delivery, and treatment parameters;
- Review of patient treatment set-up.

Stereotactic radiosurgery (SRS [77432]) and stereotactic body radiation treatment (SBRT [77435]) management also include the professional component of guidance for localization of target volume for the delivery of radiation therapy (77387). See also the Radiation Management and Treatment Table.

77427 Radiation treatment management, 5 treatments

77431 Radiation therapy management with complete course of therapy consisting of 1 or 2 fractions only

(77431 is not to be used to fill in the last week of a long course of therapy)

77432 Stereotactic radiation treatment management of cranial lesion(s) (complete course of treatment consisting of 1 session)

(The same physician should not report both stereotactic radiosurgery services [61796-61800] and radiation treatment management [77432 or 77435] for cranial lesions)

(For stereotactic body radiation therapy treatment, use 77435)

(To report the technical component of guidance for localization of target volume, use 77387 with a technical component modifier [TC])

RADIATION MANAGEMENT AND TREATMENT TABLE

Category	Code	Descriptor	IGRT TC (77387-TC) Bundled into code?	IGRT PC (77387-PC) Bundled into code?	Code Type (Technical/ Professional)
Radiation Treatment Management	77427	Treatment management, 1-5 treatments	N	N	Professional
	77431	Treatment management, 1-2 fractions	N	N	Professional
	77432	SRS management, cranial lesion(s)	N	Y	Professional
	77435	SBRT management	N	Y	Professional
SRS Treatment Delivery	77371	SRS Multisource 60 Based	Y	N	Technical
	77372	SRS Linear Based	Y	N	Technical
SBRT Treatment Delivery	77373	SBRT, 1 or more lesions, 1-5 fractions	Y	N	Technical
Radiation Treatment Delivery	77401	Superficial and/or Ortho Voltage	N	N	Technical
	77402	Radiation treatment delivery, simple	N	N	Technical
	77407	Radiation treatment delivery, intermediate	N	N	Technical
	77412	Radiation treatment delivery, complex	N	N	Technical
IMRT Treatment Delivery	77385	IMRT treatment delivery, simple	Y	N	Technical
	77386	IMRT treatment delivery, complex	Y	N	Technical
Neutron Beam Treatment Delivery	77423	Neutron beam treatment, complex	N	N	Technical
Proton Treatment Delivery	77520	Proton treatment, simple	N	N	Technical
	77522	Proton treatment, simple	N	N	Technical
	77523	Proton treatment, intermediate	N	N	Technical
	77525	Proton treatment, complex	N	N	Technical

KEY:
SRS - Stereotactic radiosurgery
SBRT - Stereotactic body radiation therapy
IMRT - Intensity modulated radiation therapy
IGRT - Image guided radiation therapy
TC - Technical component
PC - Professional component

● New Code   ▲ Revised Code   + Add-On Code   ⊘ Modifier -51 Exempt   ★ Telemedicine

77435   Stereotactic body radiation therapy, treatment management, per treatment course, to 1 or more lesions, including image guidance, entire course not to exceed 5 fractions

(Do not report 77435 in conjunction with 77427-77432)

(The same physician should not report both stereotactic radiosurgery services [32701, 63620, 63621] and radiation treatment management [77435])

(To report the technical component of guidance for localization of target volume, use 77387 with a technical component modifier [TC])

77469   Intraoperative radiation treatment management

77470   Special treatment procedure (eg, total body irradiation, hemibody irradiation, per oral or endocavitary irradiation)

(77470 assumes that the procedure is performed one or more times during the course of therapy, in addition to daily or weekly patient management)

(For intraoperative radiation treatment delivery and management, see 77424, 77425, 77469)

77499   Unlisted procedure, therapeutic radiology treatment management

PROTON BEAM TREATMENT DELIVERY

Definitions

Simple proton treatment delivery to a single treatment area utilizing a single non-tangential/oblique port, custom block with compensation (77522) and without compensation (77520).

Intermediate proton treatment delivery to one or more treatment areas utilizing two or more ports or one or more tangential/oblique ports, with custom blocks and compensators.

Complex proton treatment delivery to one or more treatment areas utilizing two or more ports per treatment area with matching or patching fields and/or multiple isocenters, with custom blocks and compensators.

77520   Proton treatment delivery; simple, without compensation

77522   simple, with compensation

77523   intermediate

77525   complex

HYPERTHERMIA

Hyperthermia treatments as listed in this section include external (superficial and deep), interstitial, and intracavitary. Radiation therapy when given concurrently is listed separately.

Hyperthermia is used only as an adjunct to radiation therapy or chemotherapy. It may be induced by a variety of sources (eg, microwave, ultrasound, low energy radiofrequency conduction, or by probe).

The listed treatments include management during the course of therapy and follow-up care for three months after completion.

Preliminary consultation is not included (see Evaluation and Management 99241-99255). Physics planning and interstitial insertion of temperature sensors, and use of external or interstitial heat generating sources are included.

The following descriptors are included in the treatment schedule:

77600   Hyperthermia, externally generated; superficial (ie, heating to a depth of 4 cm or less)

77605   deep (ie, heating to depths greater than 4 cm)

(For focused microwave thermotherapy of the breast, use 0301T)

77610 Hyperthermia generated by interstitial probe(s); 5 or fewer interstitial applicators

77615 more than 5 interstitial applicators

CLINICAL INTRACAVITARY HYPERTHERMIA

77620 Hyperthermia generated by intracavitary probe(s)

CLINICAL BRACHYTHERAPY

Services 77750-77799 include admission to the hospital and daily visits.

For insertion of ovoids and tandems, use 57155.

For insertion of Heyman capsules, use 58346.

Definitions

A *simple* application has 1 to 4 sources/ribbons.

An *intermediate* application has 5 to 10 sources/ribbons.

A *complex* application has greater than 10 sources/ribbons.

High dose-rate brachytherapy involves treatment with radiation sources that cannot safely be handled manually. These systems are remotely controlled and place a radionuclide source (radioelement or radioisotope) within an applicator placed in or near the target. These applicators may be placed in the body or on the skin surface.

Small electronic X-ray sources placed into an applicator within or close to the target may also be used to generate radiation at high-dose rates. This is referred to as high dose-rate electronic brachytherapy.

To report high dose-rate electronic brachytherapy, see 0394T, 0395T.

77750 Infusion or instillation of radioelement solution (includes 3 months follow-up care)

(For administration of radiolabeled monoclonal antibodies, use 79403)

(For non-antibody radiopharmaceutical therapy by intravenous administration only, not including three month follow-up care, use 79101)

77761 Intracavitary radiation source application; simple

77762 intermediate

77763 complex

(Do not report 77761-77763 in conjunction with Category III codes 0394T, 0395T)

77767 Remote afterloading high dose rate radionuclide skin surface brachytherapy, includes basic dosimetry, when performed; lesion diameter up to 2.0 cm or 1 channel

77768 lesion diameter over 2.0 cm and 2 or more channels, or multiple lesions

77770 Remote afterloading high dose rate radionuclide interstitial or intracavitary brachytherapy, includes basic dosimetry, when performed; 1 channel

77771 2-12 channels

77772 over 12 channels

(Do not report 77767, 77768, 77770, 77771, 77772 in conjunction with 77300, 0394T, 0395T)

(For non-brachytherapy superficial [eg, ≤200kV] radiation treatment delivery, use 77401)

77778 Interstitial radiation source application, complex, includes supervision, handling, loading of radiation source, when performed

(Do not report 77778 in conjunction with Category III codes 0394T, 0395T)

(Do not report 77778 in conjunction with 77790)

(77782-77784 have been deleted. To report, see 77767, 77768, 77770, 77771, 77772)

77789 Surface application of low dose rate radionuclide source

(Do not report 77789 in conjunction with 77401, 77767, 77768, 0394T, 0395T)

77790 Supervision, handling, loading of radiation source

(Do not report 77790 in conjunction with 77778)

77799 Unlisted procedure, clinical brachytherapy

NUCLEAR MEDICINE

Introduction

Nuclear medicine is used in the diagnosis, management, treatment, and prevention of serious disease. Nuclear medicine imaging procedures often identify abnormalities very early in the progression of a disease. This early detection allows a disease to be treated early in its course when there may be a more successful prognosis.

Nuclear medicine uses very small amounts of radioactive materials or radiopharmaceuticals to diagnose and treat disease. Radiopharmaceuticals are substances that are attracted to specific organs, bones, or tissues. The radiopharmaceuticals used in nuclear medicine emit gamma rays that can be detected externally by special types of cameras: gamma or PET cameras. These cameras work in conjunction with computers used to form images that provide data and information about the area of body being imaged. The amount of radiation from a nuclear medicine procedure is comparable to that received during a diagnostic x-ray.

Nuclear medicine procedures may be performed independently or in the course of overall medical care. If the physician providing nuclear medicine services is also responsible for the diagnostic work-up and/or follow-up care of the patient, evaluation and management service codes should be coded in addition to the nuclear medicine procedures.

Radioimmunoassay tests are located in the Clinical Pathology section (codes 82000-84999). These CPT codes can be appropriately used by any specialist performing such tests in a laboratory licensed and/or certified for radioimmunoassays. The reporting of these tests is not confined to clinical pathology laboratories alone.

The injection of a radiopharmaceutical is included as an inherent component of the procedure. Separate vascular access and injection codes (e.g. 36000, 90783 (90773 in 2006), G0345-G0354 (90760-90772, 90774-90775 in 2006) should not be reported. However, the services do not include the actual radiopharmaceutical or drug used. Diagnostic and therapeutic radiopharmaceuticals and drugs supplied by the physician should be reported separately using the appropriate supply code(s), in addition to the procedure code.

Single photon emission computed tomography (SPECT) studies represent an enhanced methodology over standard planar nuclear imaging. When a limited anatomic area is studied, there is no additional information procured by obtaining both planar and SPECT studies. While both represent medically acceptable imaging studies, when a SPECT study of a limited area is performed, a planar study is not to be separately reported. When vascular flow studies are obtained using planar technology in addition to SPECT studies, the appropriate CPT code for the vascular flow study should be reported, not the flow, planar and SPECT studies. In cases where planar images must be procured because of the extent of the scanned area (e.g. bone imaging), both planar and SPECT scans may be necessary and reported separately.

Myocardial perfusion imaging (CPT codes 78451-78454) are not reportable with cardiac blood pool imaging by gated equilibrium (CPT codes 78472-78473) because the two types of tests utilize different radiopharmaceuticals.

| ▮ Separate Procedure | ▮ Unlisted Procedure | ▮ CCI Comp. Code | ▮ Non-specific Procedure | **695** |

CPT codes 76376, 76377 (3-D rendering) are not separately reportable for nuclear medicine procedures (CPT codes 78000-78999). However, they may be separately reported with modifier - 59 on the same date of service as a nuclear medicine procedure if the 3D rendering procedure is performed in association with a third procedure (other than nuclear medicine) for which 3D rendering is appropriately reported.

Nuclear Medicine Notes

Listed procedures may be performed independently or in the course of overall medical care. If the individual providing these services is also responsible for diagnostic work-up and/or follow-up care of patient, see appropriate sections also.

Radioimmunoassay tests are found in the Clinical Pathology section (codes 82009-84999). These codes can be appropriately used by any specialist performing such tests in a laboratory licensed and/or certified for radioimmunoassays. The reporting of these tests is not confined to clinical pathology laboratories alone.

The services listed do not include the radiopharmaceutical or drug. To separately report supply of diagnostic and therapeutic radiopharmaceuticals and drugs, use the appropriate supply code(s), in addition to the procedure code..

DIAGNOSTIC NUCLEAR MEDICINE

ENDOCRINE SYSTEM

78012 Thyroid uptake, single or multiple quantitative measurement(s) (including stimulation, suppression, or discharge, when performed)

78013 Thyroid imaging (including vascular flow, when performed);

78014 with single or multiple uptake(s) quantitative measurement(s) (including stimulation, suppression, or discharge, when performed)

78015 Thyroid carcinoma metastases imaging; limited area (eg, neck and chest only)

78016 with additional studies (eg, urinary recovery)

78018 whole body

+ **78020** Thyroid carcinoma metastases uptake (List separately in addition to code for primary procedure)

(Use 78020 in conjunction with code 78018 only)

78070 Parathyroid planar imaging (including subtraction, when performed);

78071 with tomographic (SPECT)

78072 with tomographic (SPECT), and concurrently acquired computed tomography (CT) for anatomical localization

(Do not report 78070, 78071, 78072 in conjunction with 78800, 78801, 78802, 78803, 78804, 78830, 78831, 78832, 78835)

78075 Adrenal imaging, cortex and/or medulla

78099 Unlisted endocrine procedure, diagnostic nuclear medicine

(For chemical analysis, see Chemistry section)

HEMATOPOIETIC, RETICULOENDOTHELIAL AND LYMPHATIC SYSTEM

78102 Bone marrow imaging; limited area

78103 multiple areas

78104 whole body

78110	Plasma volume, radiopharmaceutical volume-dilution technique (separate procedure); single sampling
78111	multiple samplings
78120	Red cell volume determination (separate procedure); single sampling
78121	multiple samplings
78122	Whole blood volume determination, including separate measurement of plasma volume and red cell volume (radiopharmaceutical volume-dilution technique)
▲ **78130**	Red cell survival study
(**78135**	deleted 2020 [2021 Edition])
78140	Labeled red cell sequestration, differential organ/tissue, (eg, splenic and/or hepatic)
78185	Spleen imaging only, with or without vascular flow

(If combined with liver study, use procedures 78215 and 78216)

(**78190**	deleted 2017 [2018 edition])
78191	Platelet survival study
78195	Lymphatics and lymph nodes imaging

(For sentinel node identification without scintigraphy imaging, use 38792)

(For sentinal node excision, see 38500-38542)

78199	Unlisted hematopoietic, reticuloendothelial and lymphatic procedure, diagnostic nuclear medicine

(For chemical analysis, see Chemistry section)

GASTROINTESTINAL SYSTEM

78201	Liver imaging; static only
78202	with vascular flow

(For spleen imaging only, use 78185)

(**78205**	deleted 2019 [2020 Edition]. To report, use 78803)
(**78206**	deleted 2019 [2020 Edition]. To report, use 78803)
78215	Liver and spleen imaging; static only
78216	with vascular flow
78226	Hepatobiliary system imaging, including gallbladder when present;
78227	with pharmacologic intervention, including quantitative measurement(s) when performed.=
78230	Salivary gland imaging;
78231	with serial images
78232	Salivary gland function study

78258	Esophageal motility
78261	Gastric mucosa imaging
78262	Gastroesophageal reflux study
78264	Gastric emptying imaging study (eg, solid, liquid, or both);
78265	with small bowel transit
78266	with small bowel and colon transit, multiple days

(Report 78264, 78265, or 78266 only once per imaging study)

| 78267 | Urea breath test, C-14 (isotopic); acquisition for analysis |
| 78268 | analysis |

(For breath hydrogen or methane testing and analysis, use 91065)

(78270   deleted 2018 [2019 Edition])

(78271   deleted 2018 [2019 Edition])

(78272   deleted 2018 [2019 Edition])

78278	Acute gastrointestinal blood loss imaging
78282	Gastrointestinal protein loss
78290	Intestine imaging (eg, ectopic gastric mucosa, Meckels localization, volvulus)
78291	Peritoneal-venous shunt patency test (eg, for LeVeen, Denver shunt)

(For injection procedure, use 49427)

| 78299 | Unlisted gastrointestinal procedure, diagnostic nuclear medicine |

MUSCULOSKELETAL SYSTEM

Bone and joint imaging can be used in the diagnosis of a variety of inflammatory processes (eg, osteomyelitis), as well as for localization of primary and/or metastatic neoplasms.

78300	Bone and/or joint imaging; limited area
78305	multiple areas
78306	whole body
78315	3 phase study

(78320   deleted 2019 [2020 Edition]. To report, use 78803)

78350	Bone density (bone mineral content) study, 1 or more sites; single photon absorptiometry
78351	dual photon absorptiometry, 1 or more sites
78399	Unlisted musculoskeletal procedure, diagnostic nuclear medicine

● New Code   ▲ Revised Code   ✚ Add-On Code   ⊘ Modifier -51 Exempt   ★ Telemedicine

CARDIOVASCULAR SYSTEM

Myocardial perfusion (SPECT and PET) and cardiac blood pool imaging studies may be performed at rest and/or during stress. When performed during exercise and/or pharmacologic stress, the appropriate stress testing code from the 93015-93018 series may be reported in addition to 78430, 78431, 78432, 78433, 78451-78454, 78472, 78491, 78492. PET can be performed on either a dedicated PET machine (which uses a PET source for attenuation correction) or a combination PET/CT camera (78429, 78430, 78431, 78433). A cardiac PET study performed on a PET/CT camera includes examination of the CT transmission images for review of anatomy in the field of view.

78414   Determination of central c-v hemodynamics (non-imaging) (eg, ejection fraction with probe technique) with or without pharmacologic intervention or exercise, single or multiple determinations

78428   Cardiac shunt detection

78429   This code is out of order. See page 699

78430   This code is out of order. See page 700

78431   This code is out of order. See page 700

78432   This code is out of order. See page 700

78433   This code is out of order. See page 700

78434   This code is out of order. See page 700

78445   Non-cardiac vascular flow imaging (ie, angiography, venography)

78451   Myocardial perfusion imaging, tomographic (SPECT) (including attenuation correction, qualitative or quantitative wall motion, ejection fraction by first pass or gated technique, additional quantification, when performed); single study, at rest or stress (exercise or pharmacologic)

   (Do not report 78451 in conjunction with 78800, 78801, 78802, 78803, 78804, 78830, 78831, 78832, 78835)

78452   multiple studies, at rest and/or stress (exercise or pharmacologic) and/or redistribution and/or rest reinjection

   (Do not report 78452 in conjunction with 78800, 78801, 78802, 78803, 78804, 78830, 78831, 78832, 78835)

78453   Myocardial perfusion imaging, planar (including qualitative or quantitative wall motion, ejection fraction by first pass or gated technique, additional quantification, when performed); single study, at rest or stress (exercise or pharmacologic)

78454   multiple studies, at rest and/or stress (exercise or pharmacologic) and/or redistribution and/or rest reinjection

78456   Acute venous thrombosis imaging, peptide

78457   Venous thrombosis imaging, venogram; unilateral

78458   bilateral

78459   Myocardial imaging, positron emission tomography (PET), metabolic evaluation study (including ventricular wall motion[s] and/or ejection fraction[s], when performed), single study;

78429   with concurrently acquired computed tomography transmission scan

   (For CT coronary calcium scoring, use 75571)

(CT performed for other than attenuation correction and anatomical localization is reported using the appropriate site specific CT code with modifier 59)

78466 Myocardial imaging, infarct avid, planar; qualitative or quantitative

78468   with ejection fraction by first pass technique

78469   tomographic SPECT with or without quantification

(For myocardial sympathetic innervation imaging, see 0331T, 0332T)

(Do not report 78469 in conjunction with 78800, 78801, 78802, 78803, 78804, 78830, 78831, 78832, 78835)

78472 Cardiac blood pool imaging, gated equilibrium; planar, single study at rest or stress (exercise and/or pharmacologic), wall motion study plus ejection fraction, with or without additional quantitative processing

(For assessment of right ventricular ejection fraction by first pass technique, use 78496)

78473   multiple studies, wall motion study plus ejection fraction, at rest and stress (exercise and/or pharmacologic), with or without additional quantification

(Do not report 78472, 78473 in conjunction with 78451-78454, 78481, 78483, 78494)

(78478, 78480 have been deleted. To report, see 78451-78454)

78481 Cardiac blood pool imaging, (planar), first pass technique; single study, at rest or with stress (exercise and/or pharmacologic), wall motion study plus ejection fraction, with or without quantification

78483   multiple studies, at rest and with stress (exercise and/or pharmacologic), wall motion study plus ejection fraction, with or without quantification

(For cerebral blood flow study, use 78610)

(Do not report 78481-78483 in conjunction with 78451-78454)

78491 Myocardial imaging, positron emission tomography (PET), perfusion study (including ventricular wall motion[s] and/or ejection fraction[s], when performed); single study, at rest or stress (exercise or pharmacologic)

78430   single study, at rest or stress (exercise or pharmacologic), with concurrently acquired computed tomography transmission scan

78492   multiple studies at rest and stress (exercise or pharmacologic)

78431   multiple studies at rest and stress (exercise or pharmacologic), with concurrently acquired computed tomography transmission scan

78432 Myocardial imaging, positron emission tomography (PET), combined perfusion with metabolic evaluation study (including ventricular wall motion[s] and/or ejection fraction[s], when performed), dual radiotracer (eg, myocardial viability);

78433   with concurrently acquired computed tomography transmission scan

(CT performed for other than attenuation correction and anatomical localization is reported using the appropriate site specific CT code with modifier 59)

+ **78434** Absolute quantitation of myocardial blood flow (AQMBF), positron emission tomography (PET), rest and pharmacologic stress (List separately in addition to code for primary procedure)

(Use 78434 in conjunction with 78431, 78492)

(For CT coronary calcium scoring, use 75571)

(For myocardial imaging by planar or SPECT, see 78451, 78452, 78453, 78454)

  ● New Code   ▲ Revised Code   + Add-On Code   ⊘ Modifier -51 Exempt   ★ Telemedicine

78494 Cardiac blood pool imaging, gated equilibrium, SPECT, at rest, wall motion study plus ejection fraction, with or without quantitative processing

(Do not report 78494 in conjunction with 78800, 78801, 78802, 78803, 78804, 78830, 78831, 78832, 78835)

+ **78496** Cardiac blood pool imaging, gated equilibrium, single study, at rest, with right ventricular ejection fraction by first pass technique (List separately in addition to code for primary procedure)

(Use 78496 in conjunction with code 78472)

78499 Unlisted cardiovascular procedure, diagnostic nuclear medicine

RESPIRATORY SYSTEM

78579 Pulmonary ventilation imaging (eg, aerosol or gas)

78580 Pulmonary perfusion imaging (eg, particulate)

78582 Pulmonary ventilation (eg, aerosol or gas) and perfusion imaging

78597 Quantitative differential pulmonary perfusion, including imaging when performed

78598 Quantitative differential pulmonary perfusion and ventilation (eg, aerosol or gas), including imaging when performed

(Report 78579, 78580, 78582-78598 only once per imaging session)

(Do not report 78580, 78582-78598 in conjunction with 78451-78454)

78599 Unlisted respiratory procedure, diagnostic nuclear medicine

NERVOUS SYSTEM

78600 Brain imaging, less than 4 static views;

78601   with vascular flow

78605 Brain imaging, minimum 4 static views;

78606   with vascular flow

(**78607** deleted 2019 [2020 Edition]. To report, use 78803)

78608 Brain imaging, positron emission tomography (PET); metabolic evaluation

78609   perfusion evaluation

78610 Brain imaging, vascular flow only

78630 Cerebrospinal fluid flow, imaging (not including introduction of material); cisternography

(For injection procedure, see 61000-61070, 62270-62319)

78635   ventriculography

(For injection procedure, see 61000-61070, 62270-62294)

78645   shunt evaluation

(For injection procedure, see 61000-61070, 62270-62294)

(**78647** deleted 2019 [2020 Edition]. To report, use 78803)

78650 Cerebrospinal fluid leakage detection and localization

(For injection procedure, see 61000-61070, 62270-62294)

78660 Radiopharmaceutical dacryocystography

78699 Unlisted nervous system procedure, diagnostic nuclear medicine

GENITOURINARY SYSTEM

78700 Kidney imaging morphology;

78701 with vascular flow

78707 with vascular flow and function, single study without pharmacological intervention

78708 with vascular flow and function, single study, with pharmacological intervention (eg, angiotensin converting enzyme inhibitor and/or diuretic)

78709 with vascular flow and function, multiple studies, with and without pharmacological intervention (eg, angiotensin converting enzyme inhibitor and/or diuretic)

(For introduction of radioactive substance in association with renal endoscopy, see 77778)

(**78710** deleted 2019 [2020 Edition]. To report, use 78803)

78725 Kidney function study, non-imaging radioisotopic study

+ **78730** Urinary bladder residual study (List separately in addition to code for primary procedure)

(Use 78730 in conjunction with 78740)

(For measurement of postvoid residual urine and/or bladder capacity by ultrasound, nonimaging, use 51798)

(For ultrasound imaging of the bladder only, with measurement of postvoid residual urine when performed, use 76857)

78740 Ureteral reflux study (radiopharmaceutical voiding cystogram)

(Use 78740 in conjunction with 78730 for urinary bladder residual study)

(For catheterization, see 51701-51703)

78761 Testicular imaging with vascular flow

78799 Unlisted genitourinary procedure, diagnostic nuclear medicine

(For chemical analysis, see Chemistry section)

OTHER PROCEDURES

(For specific organ, see appropriate heading)

78800 Radiopharmaceutical localization of tumor, inflammatory process or distribution of radiopharmaceutical agent(s) (includes vascular flow and blood pool imaging, when performed); planar, single area (eg, head, neck, chest, pelvis), single day imaging

(For specific organ, see appropriate heading)

78801 planar, 2 or more areas (eg, abdomen and pelvis, head and chest), 1 or more days imaging or single area imaging over 2 or more days

78802	planar, whole body, single day imaging
78804	planar, whole body, requiring 2 or more days imaging
78803	tomographic (SPECT), single area (eg, head, neck, chest, pelvis), single day imaging

78804   This code is out of order. See page 703

(78805   deleted 2019 [2020 Edition]. To report, see 78300, 78305, 78306, 78315, 78800, 78801, 78802, 78803, 78830, 78831, 78832)

(78806   deleted 2019 [2020 Edition]. To report, see 78300, 78305, 78306, 78315, 78800, 78801, 78802, 78803, 78830, 78831, 78832)

(78807   deleted 2019 [2020 Edition]. To report, see 78300, 78305, 78306, 78315, 78800, 78801, 78802, 78803, 78830, 78831, 78832)

(For imaging bone infectious or inflammatory disease with a bone imaging radiopharmaceutical, see 78300, 78305, 78306, 78315)

78830	tomographic (SPECT) with concurrently acquired computed tomography (CT) transmission scan for anatomical review, localization and determination/detection of pathology, single area (eg, head, neck, chest, pelvis), single day imaging
78831	tomographic (SPECT), minimum 2 areas (eg, pelvis and knees, abdomen and pelvis), single day imaging, or single area imaging over 2 or more days
78832	tomographic (SPECT) with concurrently acquired computed tomography (CT) transmission scan for anatomical review, localization and determination/detection of pathology, minimum 2 areas (eg, pelvis and knees, abdomen and pelvis), single day imaging, or single area imaging over 2 or more days

(For cerebrospinal fluid studies that require injection procedure, see 61055, 61070, 62320, 62321, 62322, 62323)

| 78835 | Radiopharmaceutical quantification measurement(s) single area (List separately in addition to code for primary procedure) |

(Use 78835 in conjunction with 78830, 78832)

(Report multiple units of 78835 if quantitation is more than 1 area or more than 1 day imaging)

(Report myocardial SPECT imaging with 78451, 78452, 78469, 78494)

(For all nuclear medicine codes, select the organ/system-specific code[s] first; if there is no organ/systemspecific code[s], see 78800, 78801, 78802, 78803, 78830, 78831, 78832)

(For parathyroid imaging, see 78070, 78071, 78072)

| 78808 | Injection procedure for radiopharmaceutical localization by non-imaging probe study, intravenous (eg, parathyroid adenoma) |

(For sentinel lymph node identification, use 38792)

(For PET of brain, see 78608, 78609)

(For PET myocardial imaging, see 78459, 78491, 78492)

78811	Positron emission tomography (PET) imaging; limited area (eg, chest, head/neck)
78812	skull base to mid-thigh
78813	whole body

78814 Positron emission tomography (PET) with concurrently acquired computed tomography (CT) for attenuation correction and anatomical localization imaging; limited area (eg, chest, head/neck)

78815 skull base to mid-thigh

78816 whole body

(Report 78811-78816 only once per imaging session)

(Computed tomography (CT) performed for other than attenuation correction and anatomical localization is reported using the appropriate site specific CT code with modifier 59)

78830 This code is out of order. See page 703

78831 This code is out of order. See page 703

78832 This code is out of order. See page 703

78835 This code is out of order. See page 703

78999 Unlisted miscellaneous procedure, diagnostic nuclear medicine

THERAPEUTIC

The oral and intravenous administration codes in this section are inclusive of the mode of administration. For intra-arterial, intra-cavitary, and intra-articular administration, also use the appropriate injection and/or procedure code, as well as imaging guidance and radiological supervision and interpretation codes, when appropriate.

79005 Radiopharmaceutical therapy, by oral administration

(For monoclonal antibody therapy, use 79403)

79101 Radiopharmaceutical therapy, by intravenous administration

(Do not report 79101 in conjunction with 36400, 36410, 79403, 96360, 96374 or 96375, 96409)

(For radiolabeled monoclonal antibody by intravenous infusion, use 79403)

(For infusion or instillation of non-antibody radioelement solution that includes three months follow-up care, use 77750)

79200 Radiopharmaceutical therapy, by intracavitary administration

79300 Radiopharmaceutical therapy, by interstitial radioactive colloid administration

79403 Radiopharmaceutical therapy, radiolabeled monocloanl antibody by intravenous infusion

(For pre-treatment imaging, see 78802, 78804)

(Do not report 79403 in conjunction with 79101)

79440 Radiopharmaceutical therapy, by intra-articular administration

79445 Radiopharmaceutical therapy, by intra-arterial particulate administration

(Do not report 79445 in conjunction with 96373, 96420)

(Use appropriate procedural and radiological supervision and interpretation codes for the angiographic and interventional procedures provided pre-requisite to intra-arterial radiopharmaceutical therapy)

79999 Radiopharmaceutical therapy, unlisted procedure

● New Code   ▲ Revised Code   + Add-On Code   ⊘ Modifier -51 Exempt   ★ Telemedicine

PATHOLOGY/ LABORATORY

LABORATORY SECTION OVERVIEW

The fifth section of the CPT coding system is the laboratory section, which includes codes for pathology and laboratory services. Within each subsection, the CPT codes are arranged by the type of testing or service.

SEPARATE OR MULTIPLE PROCEDURES

When multiple surgical procedures are performed during a single anesthetic administration, the anesthesia code representing the most complex procedure is reported. The anesthesia time reported is the combined total for all surgical procedures.

UNLISTED SERVICE OR PROCEDURE

A pathology or laboratory service or procedure may be provided that is not listed in the CPT codebook. When reporting such service(s), the appropriate "Unlisted Procedure" code should be used to indicate the service, identifying it by "Special Report" as discussed below. The "Unlisted Procedures" and accompanying code for Pathology and Laboratory is as follows:

81099 Unlisted urinalysis procedure

81479 Unlisted molecular pathology procedure

81599 Unlisted multianalyte assay with algorithmic analysis

84999 Unlisted chemistry procedure

85999 Unlisted hematology and coagulation procedure

86486 unlisted antigen, each

86849 Unlisted immunology procedure

86999 Unlisted transfusion medicine procedure

87999 Unlisted microbiology procedure

88099 Unlisted necropsy (autopsy) procedure

88199 Unlisted cytopathology procedure

88299 Unlisted cytogenetic study

88399 Unlisted surgical pathology procedure

88749 Unlisted in vivo (eg, transcutaneous) laboratory service

89240 Unlisted miscellaneous pathology test

89398 Unlisted reproductive medicine laboratory procedure

SPECIAL REPORT

A service that is rarely provided, unusual, variable, or new may require a special report. Pertinent information should include an adequate definition or description of the nature, extent, and need for the procedure and the time, effort, and equipment necessary to provide the service.

LAB 80000

| | Separate Procedure | | Unlisted Procedure | | CCI Comp. Code | | Non-specific Procedure | **705** |

LABORATORY SUBSECTIONS

The PATHOLOGY AND LABORATORY section of CPT is divided into the following subsections:

Organ or Disease Oriented Panels	80047-80081
Drug Assay	80305-80377, 83992
Therapeutic Drug Assays	80143-80299
Evocative/Suppression Testing	80400-80439
Consultations (Clinical Pathology)	80500-80502
Urinalysis	81000-81099
Molecular Pathology	81105-81408, 81479
Genomic Sequencing Procedures and Other Molecular Mutlianalyte Assays	81410-81471
Multianalyte Assays with Algorithmic Assays	81490-81599
Chemistry	82009-84999
Hematology and Coagulation	85002-85999
Immunology	86000-86849
Transfusion Medicine	86850-86999
Microbiology	87003-87999
Anatomic Pathology	88000-88099
Cytopathology	88104-88199
Cytogenetic Studies	88230-88299
Surgical Pathology	88300-88399
In Vivo (eg. Transcutaneous) Laboratory Procedures	88720-88749
Other Procedures	89049-89240
Reproductive Medicine Procedures	89250-89398
Proprietary Laboratory Analyses	0001U-0222U

LABORATORY SERVICE MODIFIERS

Pathology and laboratory services and procedures may be modified under certain circumstances. When applicable, the modifying circumstances should be identified by adding the appropriate modifier to the basic service code. The addition of modifier -22 requires a special report. Modifiers commonly used to report PATHOLOGY and LABORATORY procedures include:

-22   unusual services

-26   professional component

-32   mandated services

-52   reduced services

-90   reference (outside) laboratory

PATHOLOGY

Pathology is that discipline of the practice of medicine that deals with the causes and nature of disease. It contributes to diagnosis, prognosis, and treatment through knowledge gained by the laboratory application of the biologic, chemical, and physical sciences to man, or materials obtained from man. Pathologists diagnose, exclude, and monitor disease by means of information gathered from the microscopic examination of tissue specimens, cells, and body fluids, and from clinical laboratory tests on body fluids and secretions. Pathologists are involved with the management of laboratories and in data processing and with new developments in high technology.

CLINICAL PATHOLOGY

Clinical Pathology focuses on microbiology (including bacteriology, mycology, parasitology, and virology), immunopathology, blood banking/transfusion medicine, chemical pathology, cytogenetics, hematology, coagulation, toxicology, medical microscopy (including urinalysis), molecular biologic techniques, and other advanced diagnostic techniques as they become available.

● New Code   ▲ Revised Code   ✛ Add-On Code   ⊘ Modifier -51 Exempt   ★ Telemedicine

MOLECULAR PATHOLOGY GENE TABLE

Claim Designation	Abbreviated Gene Name	Full Gene Name	Commonly Associated Proteins/Disease	CPT Code(s)
ABCA4	ABCA4	ATP-binding cassette, sub-family A [ABC1], member 4	Stargardt disease, age-related macular degeneration, hereditary retinal disorders	81408, 81434
ABCC8	ABCC8	ATP-binding cassette, sub-family C [CFTR/MRP], member 8	Familial hyperinsulinism	81401, 81407
ABCD1	ABCD1	ATP-binding cassette, sub-family D [ALD], member 1	Adrenoleukodystrophy	81405
	ABL1	ABL proto-oncogene 1, non-receptor tyrosine kinase	Acquired imatinib tyrosine kinase inhibitor resistance	81170
ABL1	ABL1	ABL proto-oncogene 1, non-receptor tyrosine kinase	Acquired imatinib resistance	81401
ACADM	ACADM	Acyl-CoA dehydrogenase, C-4 to C-12 straight chain, MCAD	Medium chain acyl dehydrogenase deficiency, severe inherited condition	81400, 81401, 81433
ACADS	ACADS	Acyl-CoA dehydrogenase, C-2 to C-3 short chain	Short chain acyl-CoA dehydrogenase deficiency	81404, 81405
ACADVL	ACADVL	Acyl-CoA dehydrogenase, very long chain	Very long chain acyl-coenzyme A dehydrogenase deficiency	81406
ACE	ACE	Angiotensin converting enzyme	Hereditary blood pressure regulation	81400
ACTA2	ACTA2	Actin, alpha 2, smooth muscle, aorta	Thoracic aortic aneurysms and aortic dissections, aortic dysfunction or dilation	81405, 81410
ACTC1	ACTC1	Actin, alpha, cardiac muscle 1	Familial hypertrophic cardiomyopathy	81405
ACTN4	ACTN4	Actinin, alpha 4	Focal segmental glomerulosclerosis	81406
ADRB2	ADRB2	Adrenergic beta-2 receptor surface	Drug metabolism	81401
AFF2	AFF2	AF4/FMR2 family, member 2 [FMR2]	Fragile X mental retardation 2 [FRAXE]	81171, 81172
AFG3L2	AFG3L2	AFG3 ATPase family gene 3-like 2 [S. cerevisiae]	Spinocerebellar ataxia	81406
AGL	AGL	Amylo-alpha-1, 6-glucosidase, 4-alpha-glucanotransferase	Glycogen storage disease type III	81407
AGTR1	AGTR1	Angiotensin II receptor, type 1	Essential hypertension	81400
AH1	AHI1	Abelson helper integration site 1	Joubert syndrome	81407
AIRE	AIRE	Autoimmune regulator	Autoimmune polyendocrinopathy syndrome type 1	81406
ALDH7A1	ALDH7A1	Aldehyde dehydrogenase 7 family, member A1	Pyridoxine-dependent epilepsy, epilepsy	81406, 81419
ALK	ALK	Anaplastic lymphoma receptor tyrosine kinase	Solid organ neoplasm or hematolymphoid neoplasm	81445, 81455
ANG	ANG	Angiogenin, ribonuclease, RNase A family, 5	Amyotrophic lateral sclerosis	81403
ANK2	ANK2	Ankyrin-2	Cardiac ion channelopathies	81413
ANKRD1	ANKRD1	Ankyrin repeat domain 1	Dilated cardiomyopathy	81405
ANO5	ANO5	Anoctamin 5	Limb-girdle muscular dystrophy	81406
ANOS1	ANOS1	Anosmin-1	Kallman syndrome 1	81406
	APC	Adenomatous polyposis coli	Familial adenomatosis polyposis [FAP], attenuated FAP, hereditary colon cancer disorders	81201, 81202, 81203, 81435
APOB	APOB	Apolipoprotein B	Familial hypercholesterolemia type B	81401, 81407
APOE	APOE	Apolipoprotein E	Hyperlipoproteinemia type III, cardiovascular disease, Alzheimer disease	81401
APP	APP	Amyloid beta [A4] precursor protein	Alzheimer disease	81406
APTX	APTX	Aprataxin	Ataxia with oculomotor apraxia 1	81405
AQP2	AQP2	Aquaporin 2 [collecting duct]	Nephrogenic diabetes insipidus	81404
AR	AR	Androgen receptor	Spinal and bulbar muscular atrophy, Kennedy disease, X chromosome inactivation, androgen insensitivity syndrome	81173, 81174, 81204
ARSA	ARSA	Arylsulfatase A	Arylsulfatase A deficiency, severe inherited conditions	81405, 81443
ARX	ARX	Aristaless related homeobox	X-linked lissencephaly with ambiguous genitalia, X-linked mental retardation, X-linked intellectual disability (XLID)	81403, 81404, 81470, 81471
	ASPA	Aspartoacylase	Canavan disease, Ashkenazi Jewish-associated disorders, severe inherited conditions	81200, 81412, 81443
ASPM	ASPM	Asp [abnormal spindle] homolog, microcephaly associated [Drosophila]	Primary microcephaly	81407

Separate Procedure   Unlisted Procedure   CCI Comp. Code   Non-specific Procedure

707

MOLECULAR PATHOLOGY GENE TABLE

Claim Designation	Abbreviated Gene Name	Full Gene Name	Commonly Associated Proteins/Disease	CPT Code(s)
ASS1	ASS1	Argininosuccinate synthase 1	Citrullinemia type I	81406
ASXL1	ASXL1	Additional sex combs like 1, transcriptional regulator	Myelodysplastic syndrome, myeloproliferative neoplasms, chronic myelomonocytic leukemia	81175, 81176
ATL1	ATL1	Atlastin GTPase 1	Spastic paraplegia	81406
ATM	ATM	Ataxia telangiectasia mutated	Ataxia telangiectasia	81408
ATN1	ATN1	Atrophin 1	Dentatorubral-pallidoluysian atrophy	81177
ATP1A2	ATP1A2	ATPase, Na+/K+ transporting, alpha 2 polypeptide	Familial hemiplegic migraine	81406
ATP7B	ATP7B	ATPase, Cu++ transporting, beta polypeptide	Wilson disease, severe inherited conditions	81406, 81443
ATRX	ATRX	Alpha thalassemia/mental retardation syndrome X-linked	X-linkned intellectual disability (XLID)	81470, 81471
ATXN1	ATXN1	Ataxin 1	Spinocerebellar ataxia	81178
ATXN2	ATXN2	Ataxin 2	Spinocerebellar ataxia	81179
ATXN3	ATXN3	Ataxin 3	Spinocerebellar ataxia, Machado-Joseph disease	81180
ATXN7	ATXN7	Ataxin 7	Spinocerebellar ataxia	81181
ATXN8OS	ATXN8OS	ATXN8 opposite strand [non-protein coding]	Spinocerebellar ataxia	81182
ATXN10	ATXN10	Ataxin 10	Spinocerebellar ataxia	81183
AVPR2	AVPR2	Arginine vasopressin receptor 2	Nephrogenic diabetes insipidus	81404
BBS1	BBS1	Bardet-Biedl syndrome 1	Bardet-Biedl syndrome	81406
BBS2	BBS2	Bardet-Biedl syndrome 2	Bardet-Biedl syndrome	81406
BBS10	BBS10	Bardet-Biedl syndrome 10	Bardet-Biedl syndrome	81404
BCKDHA	BCKDHA	Branched chain keto acid dehydrogenase E1, alpha polypeptide	Maple syrup urine disease, type 1A, severe inherited conditions	81400, 81405, 81443
BCKDHB	BCKDHB	Branched-chain keto acid dehydrogenase E1, beta polypeptide	Maple syrup urine disease, Maple syrup urine disease, type 1B, severe inherited conditions	81205, 81406, 81443
	BCR/ABL1	t(9;22)	Chronic myelogenous leukemia	81206, 81207, 81208
BCS1L	BCS1L	BCS1-like [S. cerevisiae]	Leigh syndrome, mitochondrial complex III deficiency, GRACILE syndrome, mitochondrial disorders	81405, 81440
BEST1	BEST1	Bestrophin 1	Vitelliform macular dystrophy	81406
	BLM	Bloom syndrome, RecQ helicase-like	Bloom syndrome, Ashkenazi Jewish-associated disorders, severe inherited conditions	81209, 81412, 81443
BMPR1A	BMPR1A	Bone morphogenetic protein receptor, type 1A	Hereditary colon cancer disorders	81435
BMPR2	BMPR2	Bone morphogenetic protein receptor, type II [serine/threonine kinase]	Heritable pulmonary arterial hypertension	81405, 81406
	BRAF	V-raf murine sarcoma viral oncogene homolog B1	Colon cancer	81210
BRAF	BRAF	B-Raf proto-oncogene, serine/threonine kinase	Noonan syndrome, Noonan spectrum disorders, solid organ neoplasm, hematolymphoid neoplasm or disorder	81406, 81442, 81445, 81450, 81455
	BRCA1	BRCA1, DNA repair associated	Hereditary breast and ovarian cancer, hereditary breast cancer-related disorders	81165, 81166, 81215, 81432, 81433
	BRCA2	BRCA2, DNA repair associated	Hereditary breast and ovarian cancer, hereditary breast cancer-related disorders	81167, 81216, 81217, 81432, 81433
	BRCA1 & BRCA2	BRCA1, DNA repair associated BRCA2, DNA repair associated	Hereditary breast and ovarian cancer	81162, 81163, 81164, 81212
BSCL2	BSCL2	Berardinelli-Seip congenital lipodystrophy 2 [seipin]	Berardinelli-Seip congenital lipodystrophy, hereditary peripheral neuropathies	81406, 81448
BTD	BTD	Biotinidase *	Biotinidase deficiency	81404
BTK	BTK	Bruton agammaglobulinemia tyrosine kinase	X-linked agammaglobulinemia, chronic lymphocytic leukemia	81406, 81233
C10ORF2	C10orf2	Chromosome 10 open reading frame 2	Mitochondrial DNA depletion syndrome, mitochondrial disorders	81404, 81440
C1P19Q	Chromosome 1p-/19q- deletion analysis	N/A	Glial tumors	81402

● New Code ▲ Revised Code + Add-On Code ⊘ Modifier -51 Exempt ★ Telemedicine

MOLECULAR PATHOLOGY GENE TABLE

Claim Designation	Abbreviated Gene Name	Full Gene Name	Commonly Associated Proteins/Disease	CPT Code(s)
CACNA1A	CACNA1A	Calcium channel, voltage-dependent, P/Q type, alpha 1A subunit	Spinocerebellar ataxia, epilepsy	81184, 81185, 81186, 81419
CACNB2	CACNB2	Calcium channel, voltage-dependent, beta 2 subunit	Brugada syndrome	81406
	CALR	Calreticulin	Myeloproliferative disorders	81219
CAPN3	CAPN3	Calpain 3	Limb-girdle muscular dystrophy [LGMD] type 2A, calpainopathy	81406
CASQ2	CASQ2	Calsequestrin 2 [cardiac muscle]	Catecholaminergic polymorphic ventricular tachycardia, cardiac ion channelopathies	81405, 81413
CASR	CASR	Calcium-sensing receptor	Hypocalcemia	81405
CAV3	CAV3	Caveolin 3	CAV3-related distal myopathy, limb-girdle muscular dystrophy type 1C, cardiac ion channelopathies	81404, 81413
CBFBMYH11	CBFB/MYH11	Inv(16)	Acute myeloid leukemia	81401
CBL	CBL	Cbl proto-oncogene, E3 ubiquitin protein ligase	Noonan spectrum disorders	81442
CBS	CBS	Cystathionine-beta-synthase	Homocystinuria, cystathionine beta-synthase deficiency	81401, 81406
CCND1/GH	CCND1/IGH	BCL1/IgH, t(11;14)	Mantle cell lymphoma	81401
CCR5	CCR5	Chemokine C-C motif receptor 5	HIV resistance	81400
CD40LG	CD40LG	CD40 ligand	X-linked hyper IgM syndrome	81404
CDH1	CDH1	Cadherin 1, type 1, E-Cadherin [epithelial]	Hereditary diffuse gastric cancer, herditary breast cancer-related disorders, hereditary colon cancer disorders	81406, 81432, 81435
CHD23	CDH23	Cadherin-related 23	Usher syndrome, type 1, hearing loss	81408, 81430
CDKL5	CDKL5	Cyclin-dependent kinase-like 5	Early infantile epileptic encephalopathy, X-linked intellectual disability (XLID), epilepsy	81405, 81406, 81419, 81470, 81471
CDKN2A	CDKN2A	Cyclin-dependent kinase inhibitor 2A	CDKN2A-related cutaneous malignant melanoma, solid organ neoplasm or hematolymphoid neoplasm	81404, 81445, 81455
	CEBPA	CCAAT/enhancer binding protein [C/EBP], alpha	Acute myeloid leukemia, hematolymphoid neoplasm or disorder, solid organ neoplasm	81218, 81450, 81455
CEL	CEL	Carboxyl ester lipase [bile salt-stimulated lipase]	Maturity-onset diabetes of the young [MODY]	81403
CEP290	CEP290	Centrosomal protein 290kDa	Joubert syndrome	81408
CFHARMS2	CFH/ARMS2	Complement factor H/age-related maculopathy susceptibility 2	Macular degeneration	81401
	CFTR	Cystic fibrosis transmembrane conductance regulator	Cystic fibrosis, Ashkenazi Jewish-associated disorders, severe inherited disorders	81220, 81221, 81222, 81223, 81224, 81412, 81443
Ch22Q13	Cytogenomic constitutional targeted microarray analysis of chromosome 22q13 by interrogation of genomic regins for copy number and single nucleotide polymorphism variants	N/A	N/A	81405
	CHD2	Chromodomain helicase DNA binding protein 2	Epilepsy	81419
CHD7	CHD7	Chromodomain helicase DNA binding protein 7	CHARGE syndrome	81407
	Chimerism engraftment analysis	N/A	Post-transplantation specimen (eg, hematopoietic stem cell)	81267, 81268
CHRNA4	CHRNA4	Cholinergic receptor, nicotinic, alpha 4	Nocturnal frontal lobe epilepsy	81405
CHRNB2	CHRNB2	Cholinergic receptor, nicotinic, beta 2 [neuronal]	Nocturnal frontal lobe epilepsy	81405
CHROM18Q	Chromosome 18q-		Colon cancer	81402
CLCN1	CLCN1	Chloride channel 1, skeletal muscle	Myotonia congenita	81406
CLCNKB	CLCNKB	Chloride channel, voltage-sensitive Kb	Bartter syndrome 3 and 4b	81406

Separate Procedure   Unlisted Procedure   CCI Comp. Code   Non-specific Procedure   **709**

MOLECULAR PATHOLOGY GENE TABLE

Claim Designation	Abbreviated Gene Name	Full Gene Name	Commonly Associated Proteins/Disease	CPT Code(s)
CLRN1	CLRN1	Clarin 1	Usher syndrome, type 3, hearing loss	81400, 81404, 81430
CNBP	CNBP	CCHC-type zinc finger, nucleic acid binding protein	Myotonic dystrophy type 2	81187
CNGA1	CNGA1	Cyclic nucleotide gated channel alpha 1	Hereditary retinal disorders	81434
CNTNAP2	CNTNAP2	Contactin associated protein-like 2	Pitt-Hopkins-like syndrome 1	81406
COL1A1	COL1A1	Collagen, type I, alpha 1	Osteogenesis imperfecta, type I	81408
COL1A1PDGFB	COL1A1/PDGFB	t(17;22)	Dermatofibrosarcoma protuberans	81402
COL1A2	COL1A2	Collagen, type I, alpha 2	Osteogenesis imperfecta, type I	81408
COL3A1	COL3A1	Collagen, type III, alpha 1	Aortic dysfunction or dilation	81410, 81411
COL4A1	COL4A1	Collagen, type IV, alpha 1	Brain small-vessel disease with hemorrhage	81408
COL4A3	COL4A3	Collagen, type IV, alpha 3 [Goodpasture antigen]	Alport syndrome	81408
COL4A4	COL4A4	Collagen, type IV, alpha 4	Alport syndrome	81407
COL4A5	COL4A5	Collagen, type IV, alpha 5	Alport syndrome	81407, 81408
COL6A1	COL6A1	Collagen, type VI, alpha 1	Collagen type VI-related disorders	81407
COL6A2	COL6A2	Collagen, type VI, alpha 2	Collagen type VI-related disorders	81406, 81407
COL6A3	COL6A3	Collagen, type VI, alpha 3	Collagen type VI-related disorders	81407
COQ2	COQ2	Coenzyme Q2, prolyprenyltransferase	Mitochondrial disorders	81440
COX10	COX10	COX10 homolog, cytochrome c oxidase assembly protein	Mitochondrial respiratory chain complex IV deficiency, mitochoncrial disorders	81405, 81440
COX15	COX15	COX15 homolog, cytochrome c oxidase assembly protein	Mitochondrial respiratory chain complex IV deficiency	81405
COX6B1	COX6B1	Cytochrome c oxidase subunit VIb polypeptide 1	Mitochondrial respiratory chain complex IV deficiency	81404
CPOX	CPOX	Coproporphyrinogen oxidase	Hereditary coproporphyria	81405
CPT1A	CPT1A	Carnitine palmitoyltransferase 1A [liver]	Carnitine palmitoyltransferase 1A [CPT1A] deficiency	81406
CPT2	CPT2	Carnitine palmitoyltransferase 2	Carnitine palmitoyltransferase II deficiency	81404
CRB1	CRB1	Crumbs homolog 1 [Drosophila]	Leber congenital amaurosis, hereditary retinal disorders	81406, 81434
CREBBP	CREBBP	CREB binding protein	Rubinstein-Taybi syndrome	81406, 81407
CRX	CRX	Cone-rod homeobox	Cone-rod dystrophy 2, Leber congenital amaurosis	81404
CSTB	CSTB	Cystatin B [stefin B]	Unverricht-Lundborg disease	81188, 81189, 81190
CTNNB1	CTNNB1	Catenin [cadherin- associated protein], beta 1, 88kDa	Desmoid tumors	81403
CTRC	CTRC	Chymotrypsin C	Hereditary pancreatitis	81405
CYP11B1	CYP11B1	Cytochrome P450, family 11, subfamily B, polypeptide 1	Congenital adrenal hyperplasia	81405
CYP17A1	CYP17A1	Cytochrome P450, family 17, subfamily A, polypeptide 1	Congenital adrenal hyperplasia	81405
CYP1B1	CYP1B1	Cytochrome P450, family 1, subfamily B, polypeptide 1	Primary congenital glaucoma	81404
CYP21A2	CYP21A2	Cytochrome P450, family 21, subfamily A, polypeptide 2	Congenital adrenal hyperplasia, 21-hydroxylase deficiency, steroid 21-hydroxylase isoform	81402, 81405
	CYP2C9	Cytochrome P450, family 2, subfamily C, polypeptide 9	Drug metabolism	81227
	CYP2C19	Cytochrome P450, family 2, subfamily C, polypeptide 19	Drug metabolism	81225
	CYP2D6	Cytochrome P450, family 2, subfamily D, polypeptide 6	Drug metabolism	81226
CYP3A4	CYP3A4	Cytochrome P450 family 3, subfamily A, member 4	Drug metabolism	81230
CYP3A5	CYP3A5	Cytochrome P450, family 3, subfamily A, member 5	Drug metabolism	81231

● New Code   ▲ Revised Code   ✛ Add-On Code   ⊘ Modifier -51 Exempt   ★ Telemedicine

MOLECULAR PATHOLOGY GENE TABLE

Claim Designation	Abbreviated Gene Name	Full Gene Name	Commonly Associated Proteins/Disease	CPT Code(s)
	Cytogenomic constitutional (genome-wide) microarray analysis	N/A	N/A	81228, 81229
	Cytogenomic neoplasia (genome-wide) microarray analysis	N/A	N/A	81277
DAZSRY	DAZ/SRY	Deleted in azoospermia and sex determining region Y	Male infertility	81403
DBT	DBT	Dihydrolipoamide branched chain transacylase E2	Maple syrup urine disease, type 2	81405, 81406
DCX	DCX	Doublecortin	X-linked lissencephaly	81405
DEKNUP214	DEK/NUP214	t(6;9)	Acute myeloid leukemia	81401
DES	DES	Desmin	Myofibrillar myopathy	81405
DFNB1	DFNB1	N/A	Hearing loss	81431
DFNB59	DFNB59	Deafness, autosomal recessive 59	Autosomal recessive nonsyndromic hearing impairment	81405
DGUOK	DGUOK	Deoxyguanosine kinase	Hepatocerebral mitochondrial DNA depletion syndrome, mitochondrial disorders	81405, 81440
DHCR7	DHCR7	7-dehydrocholesterol reductase	Smith-Lemli-Opitz syndrome, severe inherited disorders	81405, 81443
DLAT	DLAT	Dihydrolipoamide S-acetyltransferase	Pyruvate dehydrogenase E2 deficiency	81406
DLD	DLD	Dihydrolipoamide dehydrogenase	Maple syrup urine disease, type III	81406
	DMD	Dystrophin	Duchenne/Becker muscular dystrophy	81161
DMD	DMD	Dystrophin	Duchenne/Becker muscular dystrophy	81408
DMPK	DMPK	Dystrophia myotonica-protein kinase	Myotonic dystrophy, type 1	81234, 81239
DNMT3A	DNMT3A	DNA [cytosine-5-]- methyltransferase 3 alpha	Acute myeloid leukemia, hematolymphoid neoplasm or disorder, solid organ neoplasm	81403, 81450, 81455
DPYD	DPYD	Dihydropyrimidine dehydrogenase	5-fluorouracil/5-FU and capecitabine drug metabolism	81232
DSC2	DSC2	Desmocollin	Arrhythmogenic right ventricular dysplasia/ cardiomyopathy 11	81406
DSG2	DSG2	Desmoglein 2	Arrhythmogenic right ventricular dysplasia/ cardiomyopathy 10, hereditary cardiomyopathy	81406, 81439
DSP	DSP	Desmoplakin	Arrhythmogenic right ventricular dysplasia/ cardiomyopathy 8	81406
DYSF	DYSF	Dysferlin, limb girdle muscular dystrophy 2B [autosomal recessive]	Limb-girdle muscular dystrophy	81408
E2APBX1	E2A/PBX1	t(1;19)	Acute lymphocytic leukemia	81401
EFHC1	EFHC1	EF-hand domain [C-terminal] containing 1	Juvenile myoclonic epilepsy	81406
	EGFR	Epidermal growth factor receptor	Non-small cell lung cancer, solid organ neoplasm or hematolymphoid neoplasm	81235, 81445, 81455
EGR2	EGR2	Early growth response 2	Charcot-Marie-Tooth	81404
EIF2B2	EIF2B2	Eukaryotic translation initiation factor 2B, subunit 2 beta, 39kDa	Leukoencephalopathy with vanishing white matter	81405
EIF2B3	EIF2B3	Eukaryotic translation initiation factor 2B, subunit 3 gamma, 58kDa	Leukoencephalopathy with vanishing white matter	81406
EIF2B4	EIF2B4	Eukaryotic translation initiation factor 2B, subunit 4 delta, 67kDa	Leukoencephalopathy with vanishing white matter	81406
EIF2B5	EIF2B5	Eukaryotic translation initiation factor 2B, subunit 5 epsilon, 82kDa	Childhood ataxia with central nervous system hypomyelination/ vanishing white matter	81406
EMD	EMD	Emerin	Emery-Dreifuss muscular dystrophy	81404, 81405
EML4ALK	EML4/ALK	inv(2)	Non-small cell lung cancer	81401
ENG	ENG	Endoglin	Hereditary hemorrhagic telangiectasia, type 1	81405, 81406
EPCAM	EPCAM	Epithelial cell adhesion molecule	Lynch syndrome, hereditary colon cancer disorders	81403, 81436
EPM2A	EPM2A	Epilepsy, progressive myoclonus type 2A, Lafora disease [laforin]	Progressive myoclonus epilepsy	81404
ERBB2	ERBB2	V-Erb-B2 avian erythroblastic leukemia viral oncogene homolog 2	Solid organ neoplasm or hematolymphoid neoplasm	81445, 81455
ESR1PGR	ESR1/PGR	Receptor 1/progesterone receptor ratio	Breast cancer	81402

711

MOLECULAR PATHOLOGY GENE TABLE

Claim Designation	Abbreviated Gene Name	Full Gene Name	Commonly Associated Proteins/Disease	CPT Code(s)
ETV6RUNX1	ETV6/RUNX1	t(12;21)	acute lymphocytic Aeukemia	81401
EWSR1ATF1	EWSR1/ATF1	t(12;22)	Clear cell sarcoma	81401
EWSR1ERG	EWSR1/ERG	t(21;22)	Ewing sarcoma/ peripheral neuroectodermal tumor	81401
EWSR1FL1	EWSR1/FLI1	t(11;22)	Ewing sarcoma/ peripheral neuroectodermal tumor	81401
EWSR1WT1	EWSR1/WT1	t(11;22)	Desmoplastic small round cell tumor	81401
EYA1	EYA1	Eyes absent homolog 1 [Drosophila]	Bbranchio-oto-renal [BOR] spectrum disorders	81405, 81406
EYS	EYS	Eyes shut homolog (Drosophila)	Hereditary retinal disorders	81434
EZH2	EZH2	Enhancer of zeste polycomb repressive complex 2 subunit	Myelodysplastic syndrome, myeloproliferative neoplasms, diffuse large B-cell lymphoma	81236, 81237, 81450, 81455
	F2	Prothrombin, coagulation factor II	Hereditary hypercoagulability	81240
F2	F2	Prothrombin, coagulation factor II	Hereditary hypercoagulability	81400
	F5	Coagulation Factor V	Hereditary hypercoagulability	81241
F5	F5	Coagulation Factor V	Hereditary hypercoagulability	81400
F7	F7	Coagulation factor VII [serum prothrombin conversion accelerator]	Hereditary hypercoagulability	81400
F8	F8	Coagulation factor VIII	Hemophilia A	81403, 81406, 81407
F9	F9	Coagulation factor IX	Hemophilia B	81238
F11	F11	Coagulation factor XI	Coagulation disorder	81401
F12	F12	Coagulation factor XII [Hageman factor]	Angioedema, hereditary, type III; factor XII deficiency	81403
F13B	F13B	Coagulation factor XIII, B polypeptide	Hereditary hypercoagulability	81400
FAH	FAH	Fumarylacetoacetate hydrolase [fumarylaceto- acetase]	Tyrosinemia, type 1	81406
	FANCC	Fanconi anemia, complementation group C	Fanconi anemia, type C, Ashkenazi Jewish-associated disorders, severe inherited conditions	81242, 81412, 81443
FASTKD2	FASTKD2	FAST kinase domains 2	Mitochondrial respiratory chain complex IV deficiency	81406
FBN1	FBN1	Fibrillin 1	Marfan syndrome, aortic dysfunction or dilation	81408, 81410
FGB	FGB	Fibrinogen beta chain	Hereditary ischemic heart disease	81400
FGD1	FGD1	FYVE, RhoGEF and PH domain containing 1	X-linked intellectual disability (XLID)	81470, 81471
FGF23	FGF23	Fibroblast growth factor 23	Hypophosphatemic rickets	81404
FGFR1	FGFR1	Fibroblast growth factor receptor 1	Pfeiffer syndrome type 1, craniosynostosis	81400, 81405
FGFR2	FGFR2	Fibroblast growth factor receptor 2	Craniosynostosis, Apert syndrome, Crouzon syndrome	81404
FGFR3	FGFR3	Fibroblast growth factor receptor 3	Muenke syndrome	81400, 81401, 81403, 81404
FH	FH	Fumarate hydratase	Fumarate hydratase deficiency, hereditary leiomyomatosis with renal cell cancer	81405
FHL1	FHL1	Four and a half LIM domains 1	Emery-Dreifuss muscular dystrophy	81404
FIG4	FIG4	FIG4 homolog, SAC1 lipid phosphatase domain containing [S. cerevisiae]	Charcot-Marie-Tooth disease	81406
FIP1L1PDGFRA	FIP1L1/ PDGFRA	Del[4q12]	Imatinib-sensitive chronic eosinophilic leukemia	81401
FKRP	FKRP	Fukutin related protein	Congenital muscular dystrophy type 1C [MDC1C], limb-girdle muscular dystrophy [LGMD] type 2I	81404
FKTN	FKTN	Fukutin	Fukuyama congenital muscular dystrophy	81400, 81405
FLG	FLG	Filaggrin	Ichthyosis vulgaris	81401
	FLT3	FMS-related tyrosine kinase 3	Acute myeloid leukemia, hematolymphoid neoplasm or disorder, solid organ neoplasm	81245, 81426, 81450, 81455
	FMR1	Fragile X mental retardation 1	Fragile X mental retardation, X-linked intellectual disability (XLID)	81243, 81244, 81470, 81471
FOXG1	FOXG1	Forkhead box G1	Rett syndrome	81404
FOXO1PAX3	FOXO1/PAX3	t(12;13)	Ewing sarcoma/peripheral neuroectodermal tumor	81401
FOXO1PAX7	FOXO1/PAX7	t(2;13)	Ewing sarcoma/peripheral neuroectodermal tumor translocation analysis	81401
FSHMD1A	FSHMD1A	Facioscapulohumeral muscular dystrophy 1A	Facioscapulohumeral muscular dystrophy	81404

● New Code   ▲ Revised Code   ✛ Add-On Code   ⊘ Modifier -51 Exempt   ★ Telemedicine

MOLECULAR PATHOLOGY GENE TABLE

Claim Designation	Abbreviated Gene Name	Full Gene Name	Commonly Associated Proteins/Disease	CPT Code(s)
FTSJ1	FTSJ1	FtsJ RNA methyltransferase homolog 1 [E. coli]	X-linked mental retardation 9	81405, 81406
FUS	FUS	Fused in sarcoma	Amyotrophic lateral sclerosis	81406
FUSDDIT3	FUS/DDIT3	t(12;16)	Myxoid liposarcoma	81401
FXN	FXN	Frataxin	Friedreich ataxia	81284, 81285, 81286, 81289
G6PC	G6PC	Glucose-6-phosphatase, catalytic subunit	Glycogen storage disease, Type 1a, von Gierke disease, severe inherited conditions	81250, 81443
G6PD	G6PD	Glucose-6-phosphatase dehydrogenase	Hemolytic anemia, jaundice	81247, 81248, 81249
GAA	GAA	Glucosidase, alpha; acid	Glycogen storage disease type II [Pompe disease], severe inherited conditions	81406, 81443
GABRG2	GABRG2	Gamma-aminobutyric acid-[GABA] A receptor, gamma 2	Generalized epilepsy with febrile seizures, epilepsy	81405, 81419
GALC	GALC	Galactosyl- ceramidase	Krabbe disease	81401, 81406
GALT	GALT	Galactose-1- phosphate uridylyltransferase	Galactosemia, severe inherited conditions	81401, 81406, 81443
GARS	GARS	Glycyl-tRNA synthetase	Charcot-Marie-Tooth disease	81406
	GBA	Glucosidase, beta, acid	Gaucher disease, Ashkenazi Jewish-associated disorders, severe inherited conditions	81251, 81412, 81443
GBE1		1, 4-alpha-glucan branching enzyme 1	Severe inherited conditions	81443
GCDH	GCDH	Glutaryl-CoA dehydrogenase	Glutaricacidemia type 1	81406
GCH1	GCH1	GTP cyclohydrolase 1	Autosomal dominant dopa-responsive dystonia	81405
GCK	GCK	Glucokinase [hexokinase 4]	Maturity-onset diabetes of the young [MODY]	81406
GDAP1	GDAP1	Ganglioside-induced differentiation-associated protein 1	Charcot-Marie-Tooth disease	81405
GFAP	GFAP	Glial fibrillary acidic protein	Alexander disease	81405
GH1	GH1	Growth hormone 1	Growth hormone deficiency	81404
GHR	GHR	Growth hormone receptor	Laron syndrome	81405
GHRHR	GHRHR	Growth hormone releasing hormone receptor	Growth hormone deficiency	81405
GJB1	GJB1	Gap junction protein, beta 1	Charcot-Marie-Tooth X-linked, hereditary peripheral neuropathies	81403, 81448
	GJB2	Gap junction protein, beta 2, 26kDa, connexin 26	Nonsyndromic hearing loss	81252, 81253, 81430, 81431
	GJB6	Gap junction protein, beta 6, 30kDa, connexin 30	Nonsyndromic hearing loss	81254, 81431
GLA	GLA	Galactosidase, alpha	Fabry disease	81405
GLUD1	GLUD1	Glutamate dehydrogenase 1	Familial hyperinsulinism	81406
GNAQ	GNAQ	Guanine nucleotide- binding protein G[q] subunit alpha	Uveal melanoma	81403
GNE	GNE	Glucosamine [UDP-N-acetyl]-2-epimerase/N-acetylmanno samine kinase	Inclusion body myopathy 2 [IBM2], Nonaka myopathy	81400, 81406
GP1BB	GP1BB	Glycoprotein Ib [platelet], beta polypeptide	Bernard-Soulier syndrome type B	81404
GPR98	GPR98	G-protein couple receptor 98	Hearing loss	81430
	GRIN2A	Glutamate ionotropic receptor NMDA type subunit 2A	Epilepsy	81419
GRN	GRN	Granulin	Frontotemporal dementia	81406
H19	H19	Imprinted maternally expressed transcript [non-protein coding]	Beckwith-Wiedemann syndrome	81401
HADHA	HADHA	Hydroxyacyl-CoA dehydrogenase/3-ketoacyl-CoA thiolase/enoyl-CoA hydratase [trifunctional protein] alpha subunit	Long chain acyl-coenzyme A dehydrogenase deficiency	81406
HADHB	HADHB	Hydroxyacyl-CoA dehydrogenase/3-ketoacyl-CoA thiolase/enoyl-CoA hydratase [trifunctional protein], beta subunit	Trifunctional protein deficiency	81406
HBA1/HBA2	HBA1/HBA2	Alpha globin 1 and alpha globin 2	Alpha thalassemia, thalassemia, Hb Bart hyrdrops fetalis syndrme, HbH disease	81257, 81258, 81259, 81269

Separate Procedure	Unlisted Procedure	CCI Comp. Code	Non-specific Procedure	**713**

MOLECULAR PATHOLOGY GENE TABLE

Claim Designation	Abbreviated Gene Name	Full Gene Name	Commonly Associated Proteins/Disease	CPT Code(s)
HBB	HBB	Hemoglobin, subunit beta	Sickle cell anemia, beta thalassemia, hemoglobinopathy, severe inherited conditions	81361, 81362, 81363, 81364, 81443
HEA	HEA	Human erythrocyte antigen	Sickle cell disease, thalassemia, hemolytic transfusion reactions, hemolytic disease of fetus/newborn	81403
	HEXA	Hexosaminidase A [alpha polypeptide]	Tay-Sachs disease, Ashkenazi Jewish-associated disorders, severe inherited disorders	81255, 81406, 81412, 81443
	HFE	Hemochromatosis	Hereditary hemochromatosis	81256
	HLA	Human leukocyte antigene genes	Pretransplant and drug therapy testing	81370-81383
HLCS	HLCS	HLCS holocarboxylase synthetase	Holocarboxylase synthetase deficiency	81406
HMBS	HMBS	Hydroxymethylbilane synthetase	Acute intermittent porphyria	81406
HNF1A	HNF1A	HNF1 homeobox A	Maturity-onset diabetes of the young [MODY]	81405
HNF1B	HNF1B	HNF1 homeobox B	Maturity-onset diabetes of the young [MODY]	81404, 81405
HNF4A	HNF4A	Hepatocyte nuclear factor 4, alpha	Maturity-onset diabetes of the young [MODY]	81406
HPA1	Human platelet antigen 1 genotyping (HPA-1), ITGB3	Integrin, beta 3 [platelet glycoprotein IIIa], antigen CD61 [GPIIIa]	Neonatal alloimmune thrombocytopenia [NAIT], post-transfusion purpura	81105
HPA2	Human platelet antigen 2 genotyping (HPA-2), GP1BA	Glycoprotein Ib [platelet], alpha polypeptide [GPIba]	Neonatal alloimmune thrombocytopenia [NAIT], post-transfusion purpura	81106
HPA3	Human platelet antigen 3 genotyping (HPA-3), ITGA2B	Integrin, alpha 2b [platelet glycoprotein IIb of IIb/IIIa complex], antigen CD41 [GPIIb]	Neonatal alloimmune thrombocytopenia [NAIT], post-transfusion purpura	81107
HPA4	Human platelet antigen 4 genotyping (HPA-4), ITGB3	Integrin, beta 3 [platelet glycoprotein IIIa], antigen CD61 [GPIIIa]	Neonatal alloimmune thrombocytopenia [NAIT], post-transfusion purpura	81108
HPA5	Human platelet antigen 5 genotyping (HPA-5), ITGA2	Integrin, alpha 2 [CD49B, alpha 2 subunit of VLA-2 receptor] [GPIa]	Neonatal alloimmune thrombocytopenia [NAIT], post-transfusion purpura	81109
HPA6	Human platelet antigen 6 genotyping (HPA-6w), ITGB3	Integrin, beta 3 [platelet glycoprotein IIIa, antigen CD61] [GPIIIa]	Neonatal alloimmune thrombocytopenia [NAIT], post-transfusion purpura	81110
HPA9	Human platelet antigen 9 genotyping (HPA-9w), ITGA2B	Integrin, alpha 2b [platelet glycoprotein IIb of IIb/IIIa complex, antigen CD41] [GPIIb]	Neonatal alloimmune thrombocytopenia [NAIT], post-transfusion purpura	81111
HPA15	Human platelet antigen 15 genotyping (HPA-15), CD109	CD109 molecule	Neonatal alloimmune thrombocytopenia [NAIT], post-transfusion purpura	81112
HRAS	HRAS	v-Ha-ras Harvey rat sarcoma viral oncogene homolog	Costello syndrome, Noonan spectrum disorders	81403, 81404, 81442
HSD3B2	HSD3B2	Hydroxy-delta-5-steroid dehydrogenase, 3 beta- and steroid delta-isomerase 2	3-beta-hydroxysteroid dehydrogenase type II deficiency	81404
HSD11B2	HSD11B2	Hydroxysteroid [11-beta] dehydrogenase 2	Mineralocorticoid excess syndrome	81404
HSPB1	HSPB1	Heat shock 27kDa protein 1	Charcot-Marie-Tooth disease	81404
HTRA1	HTRA1	HtrA serine peptidase 1	Macular degeneration	81405
HTT	HTT	Huntingtin	Huntington disease	81271, 81274
HUWE1	HUWE1	HECT, UBA and WWE domain containing 1, E3 ubiquitin protein ligase	X-linked intellectual disability (XLID)	81470, 81471
IDH1	IDH1	Isocitrate dehydrogenase 1 [NADP+], soluble	Glioma, hematolymphoid neoplasm or disorder, solid organ neoplasm	81120, 81450, 81455
IDH2	IDH2	Isocitrate dehydrogenase 2 [NADP+], mitochondrial	Glioma, hematolymphoid neoplasm or disorder, solid organ neoplasm	81121, 81450, 81455
IDS	IDS	Iduronate 2-sulfatase	Mucopolysaccharidosis type II	81405
IDUA	IDUA	Iduronidase, alpha-L-	Mucopolysaccharidosis type I	81406

● New Code   ▲ Revised Code   + Add-On Code   ⊘ Modifier -51 Exempt   ★ Telemedicine

MOLECULAR PATHOLOGY GENE TABLE

Claim Designation	Abbreviated Gene Name	Full Gene Name	Commonly Associated Proteins/Disease	CPT Code(s)
IFNL3	IFNL3	Interferon, lambda 3	Drug response	81283
	IGH@	Immunoglobulin heavy chain locus	Leukemias and lymphomas, B-cell	81261, 81262, 81263
IGHBCL2	IGH@/BCL2	t(14;18)	Follicular lymphoma	81278, 81401
	IGK@	Immunoglobulin kappa light chain locus	Leukemia and lymphoma, B-cell	81264
	IKBKAP	Inhibitor of kappa light polypeptide gene enhancer in B-cells, kinase complex-associated protein	Familial dysautonomia, Ashkenazi Jewish-associated disorders, severe inherited disorders	81260, 81412, 81443
IL1RAPL	IL1RAPL	Interleukin 1 receptor accessory protein	X-linked intellectual disability (XLID)	81470, 81471
IL2RG	IL2RG	Interleukin 2 receptor, gamma	X-linked severe combined immunodeficiency	81405
INF2	INF2	Inverted formin, FH2 and WH2 domain containing	Focal segmental glomerulosclerosis	81406
INS	INS	Insulin	Diabetes mellitus	81404
ISPD	ISPD	Isoprenoid synthase domain containing	Muscle-eye-brain disease, Walker-Warburg syndrome	81405
ITPR1	ITPR1	Inositol 1,4,5-trisphosphate receptor, type 1	Spinocerebellar ataxia	81408
IVD	IVD	Isovaleryl-CoA dehydrogenase	Isovaleric acidemia	81400, 81406
JAG1	JAG1	Jagged 1	Alagille syndrome	81406, 81407
	JAK2	Janus kinase 2	Myeloproliferative disorder, hematolymphoid neoplasm or disorder, solid organ neoplasm	81270, 81279, 81450, 81455
JUP	JUP	Junction plakoglobin	Arrhythmogenic right ventricular dysplasia/ cardiomyopathy 11	81406
KCNC3	KCNC3	Potassium voltage-gated channel, Shaw-related subfamily, member 3	Spinocerebellar ataxia	81403
KCNE1	KCNE1	Potassium voltage-gated channel, subfamily E, member 1	Cardiac ion channelopathies	81413
KCNE2	KCNE2	Potassium voltage-gated channel, subfamily E, member 2	Cardiac ion channelopathies	81413
KCNH2	KCNH2	Potassium voltage- gated channel, subfamily H [eag-related], member 2	Short QT syndrome, long QT syndrome, cardiac ion channelopathies	81406, 81413, 81414
KCNJ1	KCNJ1	Potassium inwardly-rectifying channel, subfamily J, member 1	Bartter syndrome	81404
KCNJ2	KCNJ2	Potassium inwardly-rectifying channel, subfamily J, member 2	Andersen-Tawil syndrome, cardiac ion channelopathies	81403, 81413
KCNJ10	KCNJ10	Potassium inwardly-rectifying channel, subfamily J, member 10	SeSAME syndrome, EAST syndrome, sensorineural hearing loss	81404
KCNJ11	KCNJ11	Potassium inwardly-rectifying channel, subfamily J, member 11	Familial hyperinsulinism	81403
KCNQ1	KCNQ1	Potassium voltage-gated channel, KQT-like subfamily, member 1	Short QT syndrome, long QT syndrome, cardiac ion channelopathies	81406, 81413, 81414
KCNQ1OT1	KCNQ1OT1	KCNQ1 overlapping transcript 1 [non-protein coding]	Beckwith-Wiedemann syndrome	81401
KCNQ2	KCNQ2	Potassium voltage-gated channel, KQT-like subfamily, member 2	Epileptic encephalopathy, epilepsy	81406, 81419
KDM5C	KDM5C	Lysine [K]-specific demethylase 5C	X-linked mental retardation, X-linked intellectual disability (XLID)	81407, 81470, 81471
KIAA0196	KIAA0196	KIAA0196	Spastic paraplegia	81407
KIR	KIR	Killer cell immunoglobulin-like receptor	Hematopoietic stem cell transplantation	81403
	KIT	v-kit Hardy- Zuckerman 4 feline sarcoma viral oncogene homolog	Gstrointestinal stromal tumor, acute myeloid leukemia, melanoma, solid organ neoplasm, hematolymphoid neoplasm or disorder	81272, 81273, 81445, 81450, 81455
	KRAS	v-Ki-ras2 Kirsten rat sarcoma viral oncogene homolog	Carcinoma, Noonan syndrome	81275, 81276
KRAS	KRAS	Kirsten rat sarcoma viral oncogene homolog	Noonam syndrome, Noonam spectrum disorders, solid organ neoplasm, hematolymphoid neoplasm or disorder	81405, 81442, 81445, 81450, 81455
L1CAM	L1CAM	L1 cell adhesion molecule	MASA syndrome, X-linked hydrocephaly, X-linked intellectual disability (XLID)	81407, 81470, 81471
LAMA2	LAMA2	Laminin, alpha 2	Congenital muscular dystrophy	81408
LAMB2	LAMB2	Laminin, beta 2 [laminin S]	Pierson syndrome	81407
LAMP2	LAMP2	Lysosomal- associated membrane protein 2	Danon disease	81405
LCT	LCT	Lactase-phlorizin hydrolase	Lactose intolerance	81400

MOLECULAR PATHOLOGY GENE TABLE

Claim Designation	Abbreviated Gene Name	Full Gene Name	Commonly Associated Proteins/Disease	CPT Code(s)
LDB3	LDB3	LIM domain binding 3	Familial dilated cardiomyopathy, myofibrillar myopathy	81406
LDLR	LDLR	Low density lipoprotein receptor	Familial hypercholesterolemia	81405, 81406
LEPR	LEPR	Leptin receptor	Obesity with hypogonadism	81406
LHCGR	LHCGR	Luteinizing hormone/ choriogonadotropin receptor	Precocious male puberty	81406
LINC00518	LINC00518	Long intergenic non-protein coding RNA 518	Melanoma	81401
LITAF	LITAF	Lipopolysaccharide- induced TNF factor	Charcot-Marie-Tooth	81404
LMNA	LMNA	Lamin A/C	Emery-Dreifuss muscular dystrophy [EDMD1, 2 and 3] limb-girdle muscular dystrophy [LGMD] type 1B, dilated cardio-myopathy [CMD1A], familiar portal lipodystrophy [FPLD2]	81406
LRP5	LRP5	Low density lipoprotein receptor-related protein 5	Osteopetrosis	81406
LRRK2	LRRK2	Leucine-rich repeat kinase 2	Parkinson disease	81401, 81408
MAP2K1	MAP2K1	Mitogen-activated protein kinase 1	Cardiofaciocutaneous syndrome, Noonan spectrum disorders	81406, 81442
MAP2K2	MAP2K2	Mitogen-activated protein kinase 2	Cardiofaciocutaneous syndrome, Noonan spectrum disorders	81406, 81442
MAPT	MAPT	Microtubule- associated protein tau	Frontotemporal dementia	81406
MAX	MAX	MYC-associated factor X	Hereditary neuroendocrine tumor disorders	81437
MC4R	MC4R	Melanocortin 4 receptor	Obesity	81403
MCCC1	MCCC1	Methylcrotonyl-CoA carboxylase 1 [alpha]	3-methylcrotonyl-CoA carboxylase deficiency	81406
MCCC2	MCCC2	Methylcrotonyl-CoA carboxylase 2 [beta]	3-methylcrotonyl carboxylase deficiency	81406
	MCOLN1	Mucolipin 1	Mucolipidosis, type IV, Ashkenazi Jewish-associated disorders, severe inherited disorders	81290, 81412, 81443
	MECP2	Methyl CpG binding protein 2	Rett syndrome, X-linked intellectual disability (XLID), epilepsy	81302, 81303, 81304, 81419, 81470, 81471
MED12	MED12	Mediator complex subunit 12	FG syndrome type 1, Lujan syndrome, X-linked intellectual disability (XLID)	81401, 81470, 81471
MEFV	MEFV	Mediterranean fever	Familial Mediterranean fever	81402, 81404
MEG3DLK1	MEG3/DLK1	Maternally expressed 3 [non-protein coding]/delta-like 1 homolog [Drosophila]	Intrauterine growth retardation	81401
MEN1	MEN1	Multiple endocrine neoplasia I	Multiple endocrine neoplasia type 1, Wermer syndrome	81404, 81405
MET	MET	Met proto-oncogene	Solid organ neoplasm or hematolymphoid neoplasm	81445, 81455
MFN2	MFN2	Mitofusin 2	Charcot-Marie-Tooth disease, hereditary peripheral neuropathies	81406, 81448
	MGMT	0-6-methylguanine- DNA methyltransferase	Glioblastoma multiforme	81287
MICA	MICA	MHC class I polypeptide-related sequence A	Solid organ transplantation	81403
	Micro-satellite instability analysis	N/A	Hereditary nonpolyposis colorectal cancer, Lynch syndrome	81301
MID1	MID1	Midline 1	X-linked intellectual disability (XLID)	81470, 81471
	MLH1	mutL homolog 1, colon cancer, nonpolyposis type 2	Hereditary non-polyposis colorectal cancer, Lynch syndrome, hereditary breast cancer-related disorders, hereditary colon cancer disorders	81288, 81292, 81293, 81294, 81432, 81433, 81435, 81436
MLL	MLL	N/A	Hematolymphoid neoplasm or disorder, solid organ neoplasm	81450, 81455
MLLAFF1	MLL/AFF1	t(4;11)	Acute lymphoblastic leukemia	81401
MLLMLLT3	MLL/MLLT3	t(9;11)	Acute myeloid leukemia	81401
MMAA	MMAA	Methylmalonic aciduria [cobalamine deficiency] type A	MMAA-related methylmalonic acidemia	81405
MMB	MMAB	Methylmalonic aciduria [cobalamine deficiency] type B	MMAA-related methylmalonic acidemia	81405
MMACHC	MMACHC	Methylmalonic aciduria [cobalamin deficiency] cblC type, with homocystinuria	Methylmalonic acidemia and homocystinuria	81404
MPI	MPI	Mannose phosphate isomerase	Congenital disorder of glycosylation 1b	81405

● New Code   ▲ Revised Code   + Add-On Code   ⊘ Modifier -51 Exempt   ★ Telemedicine

MOLECULAR PATHOLOGY GENE TABLE

Claim Designation	Abbreviated Gene Name	Full Gene Name	Commonly Associated Proteins/Disease	CPT Code(s)
MPL	MPL	Myeloproliferative leukemia virus oncogene, thrombopoietin receptor, TPOR	Myeloproliferative disorder	81338, 81339
MPV17	MPV17	MpV17 mitochondrial inner membrane protein	Mitochondrial DNA depletion syndrome, mitochondrial disorders	81404, 81405, 81440
MPZ	MPZ	Myelin protein zero	Charcot-Marie-Tooth disease, hereditary peripheral neuropathies	81405, 81448
	MSH2	mutS homolog 2, colon cancer, nonpolyposis type 1	Hereditary non-polyposis colorectal cancer, Lynch syndrome, hereditary breast cancer-related disorders, hereditary colon cancer disorders	81295, 81296, 81297, 81432, 81433, 81435, 81436
	MSH6	mutS homolog 6 [E. coli]	Hereditary nonpolyposis colorectal cancer, Lynch syndrome, hereditary breast cancer-related disorders, hereditary colon cancer disorders	81298, 81299, 81300, 81432, 81435
MTATP6	MT-ATP6	Mitochondrially encoded ATP synthase 6	Neuropathy with ataxia and retinitis pigmentosa [NARP], Leigh syndrome	81401
	MTHFR	5,10-methylenetetrahydrofolate reductase	Hereditary hypercoagulability	81291
MTM1	MTM1	Myotubularin 1	X-linked centronuclear myopathy	81405, 81406
MTND4ND6	MT-ND4, MT-ND6	Mitochondrially encoded NADH dehydrogenase 4, mitochondrially encoded NADH dehydrogenase 6	Leber hereditary optic neuropathy [LHON]	81401
MTND5	MT-ND5	Mitochondrially encoded tRNA leucine 1 [UUA/G], mitochondrially encoded NADH dehydrogenase 5	Mitochondrial encephalopathy with lactic acidosis and stroke-like episodes [MELAS]	81401
MTRNR1	MT-RNR1	Mitochondrially encoded 12S RNA	Nonsyndromic hearing loss	81401, 81403, 81430
MTTK	MT-TK	Mitochondrially encoded tRNA lysine	Myoclonic epilepsy with ragged-red fibers [MERRF]	81401
MTTL1	MT-TL1	Mitochondrially encoded tRNA leucine 1 [UUA/G]	Diabetes and hearing loss	81401
MTTS1	MT-TS1	Mitochondrially encoded tRNA serine 1	Nonsyndromic hearing loss	81403
MTTS1RNR1	MT-TS1, MT-RNR1	Mitochondrially encoded tRNA serine 1 [UCN], mitochondrially encoded 12S RNA	Nonsyndromic sensori-neural deafness [including aminoglycoside-induced nonsyndromic deafness]	81401
MUT	MUT	Methylmalonyl CoA mutase	Methylmalonic acidemia	81406
MUTYH	MUTYH	mutY homolog [E. coli]	MYH-associated polyposis, hereditary colon cancer disorders	81401, 81406, 81435
MYBPC3	MYBPC3	Myosin binding protein C, cardiac	Familial hypertrophic cardiomyopathy, hereditary cardiomyopathy	81407, 81439
MYD88	MYD88	Myeloid differentiation primary response 88	Waldenstrom's macroglobulinemia, lymphoplasmacytic leukemia	81305
MYH6	MYH6	Myosin , heavy chain 6, cardiac muscle, alpha	Familial dilated cardiomyopathy	81407
MYH7	MYH7	Myosin, heavy chain 7, cardiac muscle, beta	Familial hypertrophic cardiomyopathy, Liang distal myopathy, hereditary cardiomyopathy	81407, 81439
MYH11	MYH11	Myosin, heavy chain 11, smooth muscle	Thoracic aortic aneurysms and aortic dissections, aortic dysfunction or dilation	81408, 81410, 81411
MYL2	MYL2	Myosin, light chain 2, regulatory, cardiac, slow	Familial hypertrophic cardiomyopathy	81405
MYL3	MYL3	Myosin, light chain 3, alkali, ventricular, skeletal, slow	Familial hypertrophic cardiomyopathy	81405
MYLK	MYLK	Myosin light chain kinase	Aortic dysfunction or dilation	81410
MYO7A	MYO7A	Myosin VIIA	Usher syndrome, type 1, hearing loss	81407, 81430
MYO15A	MYO15A	Myosin XVA	Hearing loss	81430
MYOT	MYOT	Myotilin	Limb-girdle muscular dystrophy	81405
NDP	NDP	Norrie disease [pseudoglioma]	Norrie disease	81403, 81404
NDUFA1	NDUFA1	NADH dehydrogenase [ubiquinone] 1 alpha subcomplex, 1, 7.5kDa	Leigh syndrome, mitochondrial complex I deficiency	81404
NDUFAF2	NDUFAF2	NADH dehydrogenase [ubiquinone] 1 alpha subcomplex, assembly factor 2	Leigh syndrome, mitochondrial complex I deficiency	81404
NDUFS1	NDUFS1	NADH dehydrogenase [ubiquinone] Fe-S protein 1, 75kDa [NADH-coenzyme Q reductase]	Leigh syndrome, mitochondrial complex I deficiency	81406

Separate Procedure   Unlisted Procedure   CCI Comp. Code   Non-specific Procedure

MOLECULAR PATHOLOGY GENE TABLE

Claim Designation	Abbreviated Gene Name	Full Gene Name	Commonly Associated Proteins/Disease	CPT Code(s)
NDUFS4	NDUFS4	NADH dehydrogenase [ubiquinone] Fe-S protein 4, 18kDa [NADH-coenzyme Q reductase]	Leigh syndrome, mitochondrial complex I deficiency	81404
NDUFS7	NDUFS7	NADH dehydrogenase [ubiquinone] Fe-S protein 7, 20kDa [NADH-coenzyme Q reductase]	Leigh syndrome, mitochondrial complex I deficiency	81405
NDUFS8	NDUFS8	NADH dehydrogenase [ubiquinone] Fe-S protein 8, 23kDa [NADH-coenzyme Q reductase]	Leigh syndrome, mitochondrial complex I deficiency	81405
NDUFV1	NDUFV1	NADH dehydrogenase [ubiquinone] flavoprotein 1, 51kDa	Leigh syndrome, mitochondrial complex I deficiency	81405
NEB	NEB	Nebulin	Nemaline myopathy 2	81400, 81408
NEFL	NEFL	Neurofilament, light polypeptide	Charcot-Marie-Tooth	81405
NF1	NF1	Neurofibromin 1	Neurofibromatosis, type 1	81408
NF2	NF2	Neurofibromin 2 [merlin]	Neurofibromatosis, type 2	81405, 81406
NHLRC1	NHLRC1	NHL repeat containing 1	Progressive myoclonus epilepsy	81403
NIPA1	NIPA1	Non-imprinted in Prader-Willi/ Angelman syndrome 1	Spastic paraplegia	81404
NLGN3	NLGN3	Neuroligin 3	Autism spectrum disorders	81405
NLGN4X	NLGN4X	Neuroligin 4, X-linked	Autism spectrum disorders	81404, 81405
NOD2	NOD2	Nucleotide-binding oligomerization domain containing 2	Crohn's disease, Blau syndrome	81401
NOS	Known familial variant NOS	N/A	N/A	81403
NOTCH1	NOTCH1	Notch 1	Aortic valve disease, hematolymphoid neoplasm or disorder, solid organ neoplasm	81407, 81450, 81455
NOTCH3	NOTCH3	Notch 3	Cerebral autosomal dominant arteriopathy with subcortical infarcts and leukoencephalopathy [CADASIL]	81406
NPC1	NPC1	Niemann-Pick disease, type C1	Niemann-Pick disease	81406
NPC2	NPC2	Niemann-Pick disease, type C2 [epididymal secretory protein E1]	Niemann-Pick disease type C2	81404
NPHP1	NPHP1	Nephronophthisis 1 [juvenile]	Joubert syndrome	81405, 81406
NPHS1	NPHS1	Nephrosis 1, congenital, Finnish type [nephrin]	Congenital Finnish nephrosis	81407
NPHS2	NPHS2	Nephrosis 2, idiopathic, steroid-resistant [podocin]	Steroid-resistant nephrotic syndrome	81405
	NPM1	Nucleophosmin	Acute myeloid leukemia, hematolymphoid neoplasm or disorder, solid organ neoplasm	81310, 81450, 81455
NPM1ALK	NPM1/ALK	t(2;5)	Anaplastic large cell lymphoma	81401
NR0B1	NR0B1	Nuclear receptor subfamily 0, group B, member 1	Congenital adrenal hypoplasia	81404
	NRAS	Neuroblastoma RAS viral [V-RAS] oncogene homolog	Colorectal carcinoma, Noonan spectrum disorders, solid organ neoplasm, hematolymphoid neoplasm or disorder	81311, 81442, 81445, 81450, 81455
NSD1	NSD1	Nuclear receptor binding SET domain protein 1	Sotos syndrome	81405, 81406
	NTRK	Neurotrophic-tropomyosin receptor tyrosine kinase 1, 2, and 3	Solid tumors	81194
	NTRK1	Neurotrophic receptor tyrosine kinase 1	Solid tumors	81191
	NTRK2	Neurotrophic receptor tyrosine kinase 2	Solid tumors	81192
	NTRK3	Neurotrophic receptor tyrosine kinase 3	Solid tumors	81193
	NUDT15	Nudix hydrolase 15	Drug metabolism	81306
OCRL	OCRL	Oculocerebrorenal syndrome of Lowe	X-linked intellectual disability (XLID)	81470, 81471
OPA1	OPA1	Optic atrophy 1	Optic atrophy, mitochondrial disorders	81406, 81407, 81440
OPTN	OPTN	Optineurin	Amyotrophic lateral sclerosis	81406
OTC	OTC	Ornithine carbamoyltransferase	Ornithine transcarbamylase deficiency	81405
OTOF	OTOF	Otoferlin	Hearing loss	81430
PABPN1	PABPN1	Poly[A] binding protein, nuclear 1	Oculopharyngeal muscular dystrophy	81312

● New Code   ▲ Revised Code   ✛ Add-On Code   ⊘ Modifier -51 Exempt   ★ Telemedicine

MOLECULAR PATHOLOGY GENE TABLE

Claim Designation	Abbreviated Gene Name	Full Gene Name	Commonly Associated Proteins/Disease	CPT Code(s)
PAFAH1B1	PAFAH1B1	Platelet-activating factor acetylhydrolase 1b, regulatory subunit 1 [45kDa]	Lissencephaly, Miller-Dieker syndrome	81405, 81406
PAH	PAH	Phenylalanine hydroxylase	Phenylketonuria, severe inherited disorders	81406, 81443
PALB2	PALB2	Partner and localizer of BRCA2	Breast and pancreatic cancer, hereditary breast cancer-related disorders	81307, 81308, 81432
PARK2	PARK2	Parkinson protein 2, E3 ubiquitin protein ligase [parkin]	Parkinson disease	81405, 81406
PAX2	PAX2	Paired box 2	Renal coloboma syndrome	81406
PAX8PPARG	PAX8/PPARG	t(2;3) (q13;p25)	Follicular thyroid carcinoma	81401
PC	PC	Pyruvate carboxylase	Pyruvate carboxylase deficiency	81406
	PCA3/KLK3	Prostate cancer antigen 3/kallikrein-related peptidase 3	Prostate cancer	81313
PCCA	PCCA	Propionyl CoA carboxylase, alpha polypeptide	Propionic acidemia, type 1	81405, 81406
PCCB	PCCB	Propionyl CoA carboxylase, beta polypeptide	Propionic acidemia	81406
PCDH15	PCDH15	Protocadherin-related 15	Usher syndrome type 1F, Usher syndrome type 1, hearing loss	81400, 81406, 81407, 81430
PCDH19	PCDH19	Protocadherin 19	Epileptic encephalopathy, epilepsy	81405, 81419
PCSK9	PCSK9	Proprotein convertase subtilisin/ kexin type 9	Familial hypercholesterolemia	81406
PDE6A	PDE6A	Phosphodiesterase 6A, CGMP-specific, rod, alpha	Hereditary retinal disorders	81434
PDE6B	PDE6B	Phosphodiesterase 6B, CGMP-specific, rod, beta	Hereditary retinal disorders	81434
	PDGFRA	Platelet-derived growth factor receptor alpha polypeptide	Gastrointestinal stromal tumor, solid organ neoplasm or hematolymphoid neoplasm	81314, 81445, 81455
	PDGFRB	Platelet-derived growth factor receptor beta polypeptide	Solid organ neoplasm or hematolymphoid neoplasm	81445, 81455
PDHA1	PDHA1	Pyruvate dehydrogenase [lipoamide] alpha 1	Lactic acidosis	81405, 81406
PDHB	PDHB	Pyruvate dehydrogenase [lipoamide] beta	Lactic acidosis	81405
PDHX	PDHX	Pyruvate dehydrogenase complex, component X	Lactic acidosis	81406
PDSS2	PDSS2	Decaprenyl diphosphate synthase subunit 2	Mitochondrial disorders	81440
PDX1	PDX1	Pancreatic and duodenal homeobox 1	Maturity-onset diabetes of the young [MODY]	81404
PGR	PGR	Progesterone receptor	Solid organ or hematolymphoid neoplasm	81445, 81455
PHEX	PHEX	Phosphate regulating endopeptidase homolog, X-linked	Hypophosphatemic rickets	81406
PHOX2B	PHOX2B	Paired-like homeobox 2b	Congenital central hypoventilation syndrome	81403, 81404
PIK3CA	PIK3CA	Phosphatidylinositol-4, 5-bisphosphate 3-kinase, catalytic subunit alpha	Colorectal cancer, solid organ neoplasm or hematolymphoid neoplasm	81309, 81445, 81455
PINK1	PINK1	PTEN induced putative kinase 1	Parkinson disease	81405
PKD1	PKD1	Polycystic kidney disease 1 [autosomal dominant]	Polycystic kidney disease	81407
PKD2	PKD2	Polycystic kidney disease 2 [autosomal dominant]	Polycystic kidney disease	81406
PKHD1	PKHD1	Polycystic kidney and hepatic disease 1	Autosomal recessive polycystic kidney disease	81408
PKLR	PKLR	Pyruvate kinase, liver and RBC	Pyruvate kinase deficiency	81405
PKP2	PKP2	Plakophilin 2	Arrhythmogenic right ventricular dysplasia/ cardiomyopathy 9, hereditary cardiomyopathy	81406, 81439
PLCE1	PLCE1	Phospholipase C, epsilon 1	Nephrotic syndrome type 3	81407
	PLCG2	Phospholipase C gamma 2	Chronic lymphocytic leukemia	81320
PLN	PLN	Phospholamban	Dilated cardiomyopathy, hypertrophic cardiomyopathy	81403
PLP1	PLP1	Proteolipid protein 1	Pelizaeus-Merzbacher disease, spastic paraplegia	81404, 81405
	PML/RARalpha	t(15;17) promyelocytic leukemia/retinoic acid receptor alpha	Promyelocytic leukemia	81315, 81316

| | Separate Procedure | | Unlisted Procedure | | CCI Comp. Code | | Non-specific Procedure | **719** |

MOLECULAR PATHOLOGY GENE TABLE

Claim Designation	Abbreviated Gene Name	Full Gene Name	Commonly Associated Proteins/Disease	CPT Code(s)
	PMP22	Peripheral myelin protein 22	Charcot-Marie-Tooth, hereditary neuropathy with liability to pressure palsies	81324, 81325, 81326
	PMS2	Postmeiotic segregation increased 2 [S. cerevisiae]	Hereditary non-polyposis colorectal cancer, Lynch syndrome	81317, 81318, 81319
PNKD	PNKD	Paroxysmal nonkinesigenic dyskinesia	Paroxysmal nonkinesigenic dyskinesia	81406
POLG	POLG	Polymerase [DNA directed], gamma	Alpers-Huttenlocher syndrome, autosomal dominant progressive external ophthalmoplegia, mitochondrial disorders, epilepsy	81406, 81419, 81440
POLG2	POLG2	Polymerase [DNA directed], gamma 2	Mitochondrial disorders	81440
POMGNT1	POMGNT1	Protein O-linked mannose beta1,2-N acetylglucosaminyltransferase	Muscle-eye-brain disease, Walker-Warburg syndrome	81406
POMT1	POMT1	Protein-O-mannosyltransferase 1	Limb-girdle muscular dystrophy [LGMD] type 2K, Walker-Warburg syndrome	81406
POMT2	POMT2	Protein-O-mannosyltransferase 2	Limb-girdle muscular dystrophy [LGMD] type 2N, Walker-Warburg syndrome	81406
POU1F1	POU1F1	POU class 1 homeobox 1	Combined pituitary hormone deficiency	81405
PPOX	PPOX	Protoporphyrinogen oxidase	Variegate porphyria	81406
PPP2R2B	PPP2R2B	Protein phosphatase 2, regulatory subunit B, beta	Spinocerebellar ataxia	81343
PQBP1	PQBP1	Polyglutamine binding protein 1	Renpenning syndrome	81404, 81405
PRAME	PRAME	Preferentially expressed antigen in melanoma	Melanoma	81401
PRKAG2	PRKAG2	Protein kinase, AMP-activated, gamma 2 non-catalytic subunit	Familial hypertrophic cardiomyopathy with Wolff-Parkinson-White syndrome, lethal congenital glycogen storage disease of heart	81406
PRKCG	PRKCG	Protein kinase C, gamma	Spinocerebellar ataxia, hyperkalemic periodic paralysis	81406
PRNP	PRNP	Prion protein	Genetic prion disease	81404
PROP1	PROP1	PROP paired-like homeobox 1	Combined pituitary hormone deficiency	81404
PRPF31	PRPF31	Pre-MRNA processing factor 31	Hereditary retinal disorders	81434
PRPH2	PRPH2	Peripherin 2 [retinal degeneration, slow]	Retinitis pigmentosa, hereditary retinal disorders	81404, 81434
	PRRT2	Proline rich transmembrane protein 2	Epilepsy	81419
PRSS1	PRSS1	Protease, serine, 1 [trypsin 1]	Hereditary pancreatitis	81401, 81404
PRX	PRX	Periaxin	Charcot-Marie-Tooth disease	81405
PSEN1	PSEN1	Presenilin 1	Alzheimer disease	81405
PSEN2	PSEN2	Presenilin 2 [Alzheimer disease 4]	Alzheimer disease	81406
	PTEN	Phosphatase and tensin homolog	Cowden syndrome, PTEN hamartoma tumor syndrome, hereditary breast cancer-related disorders, hereditary colon cancer disorders, solid organ neoplasm or hematolymphoid neoplasm	81321, 81322, 81323, 81432, 81435, 81445, 81455
PTPN11	PTPN11	Protein tyrosine phosphatase, non-receptor type 11	Noonan syndrome, LEOPARD syndrome, Noonan spectrum disorders	81406, 81442
PYGM	PYGM	Phosphorylase, glycogen, muscle	Glycogen storage disease type V, McArdle disease	81401, 81406
RAB7A	RAB7A	RAB7A, member RAS oncogene family	Charcot-Marie-Tooth disease	81405
RAF1	RAF1	v-raf-1 murine leukemia viral oncogene homolog 1	LEOPARD syndrome, Noonan spectrum disorder	81404, 81406, 81442
RAI1	RAI1	Retinoic acid induced 1	Smith-Magenis syndrome	81405
RDH12	RDH12	Retinol dehydrogenase 12 (All-Trans/9-Cis/11-Cis)	Hereditary retinal disorders	81434
REEP1	REEP1	Receptor accessory protein 1	Spastic paraplegia, hereditary peripheral neuropathies	81405, 81448
RET	RET	Ret proto-oncogene	Multiple endocrine neoplasia, type 2B and familial medullary thyroid carcinoma, Hirschsprung disease, solid organ neoplasm or hematolymphoid neoplasm	81404, 81405, 81406, 81445, 81455
RHDDA	RHD, deletion analysis	Rh blood group, D antigen	Hemolytic disease of fetus/newborn, Rh maternal/fetal compatibility	81403
RHDDAMB	RHD, deletion analysis, cell-free fetal DNA in maternal blood	Rh bood group D, antigen	Hemolytic disease of fetus/newborn, Rh maternal/fetal compatibility	81403
RHO	RHO	Rhodopsin	Retinitis pigmentosa, hereditary retinal disorders	81404, 81434

● New Code   ▲ Revised Code   ✛ Add-On Code   ⊘ Modifier -51 Exempt   ★ Telemedicine

MOLECULAR PATHOLOGY GENE TABLE

Claim Designation	Abbreviated Gene Name	Full Gene Name	Commonly Associated Proteins/Disease	CPT Code(s)
RIT1	RIT1	Ras-like without CAAX 1	Noonan spectrum disorders	81442
RP1	RP1	Retinitis pigmentosa 1	Retinitis pigmentosa, hereditary retinal disorders	81404, 81434
RP2	RP2	Retinitis pigmentosa 2	Hereditary retinal disorders	81434
RPE65	RPE65	Retinal pigment epithelium-specific protein 65kDa	Retinitis pigmentosa, Leber congenital amaurosis, hereditary retinal disorders	81406, 81434
RPGR	RPGR	Retinitis pigmentosa GTPase regulator	Hereditary retinal disorders	81434
RPS19	RPS19	Ribosomal protein S19	Diamond-Blackfan anemia	81405
RPS6KA3	RPS6KA3	Ribosomal protein S6 kinase, 90kDa, polypeptide3	X-linked intellectual disability (XLID)	81470, 81471
RRM2B	RRM2B	Ribonucleotide reductase M2 B [TP53 inducible]	Mitochondrial DNA depletion, mitochondrial disorders	81405, 81440
RUNX1	RUNX1	Runt related transcription factor 1	Acute myeloid leukemia, familial platelet disorder with associated myeloid malignancy	81334
RUNX1RUNX1T1	RUNX1/RUNX1T1	t(8;21)	Acute myeloid leukemia	81401
RYR1	RYR1	Ryanodine receptor 1, skeletal	Malignant hyperthermia	81406, 81408
RYR2	RYR2	Ryanodine receptor 2 [cardiac]	Catecholaminergic polymorphic ventricular tachycardia, arrhythmogenic right ventricular dysplasia, cardiac ion channelopathies	81408, 81413
scn1a	SCN1A	Sodium channel, voltage-gated, type 1, alpha subunit	Generalized epilepsy with febrile seizures, epilepsy	81407, 81419
SCN1B	SCN1B	Sodium channel, voltage-gated, type I, beta	Brugada syndrome, epilepsy	81404, 81419
	SCN2A	Sodium voltage-gated channel alpha subunit 2	Epilepsy	81419
SCN4A	SCN4A	Sodium channel, voltage-gated, type IV, alpha subunit	Hyperkalemic periodic paralysis	81406
	SCN8A	Sodium voltage-gated channel alpha subunit 8	Epilepsy	81419
SCN5A	SCN5A	Sodium channel, voltage-gated, type V, alpha subunit	Familial dilated cardiomyopathy, cardiac ion channelopathies	81407, 81413
SCNN1A	SCNN1A	Sodium channel, nonvoltage-gated 1 alpha	Pseudohypoaldo- steronism	81406
SCNN1B	SCNN1B	Sodium channel, nonvoltage-gated 1, beta	Liddle syndrome, pseudohypoaldo- steronism	81406
SCNN1G	SCNN1G	Sodium channel, nonvoltage-gated 1, gamma	Liddle syndrome, pseudohypoaldo- steronism	81406
SCO1	SCO1	SCO cytochrome oxidase deficient homolog 1	Mitochondrial respiratory chain complex IV deficiency, mitochondrial disorders	81405, 81440
SCO2	SCO2	SCO cytochrome oxidase deficient homolog 2 [SCO1L]	Mitochondrial respiratory chain complex IV deficiency, mitochondrial disorders	81404, 81440
SDHA	SDHA	Succinate dehydrogenase complex, subunit A, flavoprotein [Fp]	Leigh syndrome, mitochondrial complex II deficiency	81406
SDHB	SDHB	Succinate dehydrogenase complex, subunit B, iron sulfur	Hereditary paraganglioma, hereditary neuroendocrine tumor disorders	81405, 81437, 81438
SDHC	SDHC	Succinate dehydrogenase complex, subunit C, integral membrane protein, 15kDa	Hereditary paraganglioma- pheochromocytoma syndrome, hereditary neuroendocrine tumor disorders	81404, 81405, 81437, 81438
SDHD	SDHD	Succinate dehydrogenase complex, subunit D, integral membrane protein	Hereditary paraganglioma, hereditary neuroendocrine tumor disorders	81404, 81437, 81438
SEPT9	SEPT9	Septin 9	Colorectal cancer	81327
	SERPINA1	Serpin peptidase inhibitor, clade A, alpha-1 antiproteinase, antitrypsin, member 1	Alpha-1-antitrypsin deficiency	81332
SERPINE1	SERPINE1	Serpine peptidase inhibitor clade E, member 1, plasminogen activator inhibitor -1, PAI-1	Thrombophilia	81400
SETX	SETX	Senataxin	Ataxia	81406
	SF3B1	Splicing factor [3b] subunit B1	Myelodysplastic syndrome/acute myeloid leukemia	81347
SGCA	SGCA	Sarcoglycan, alpha [50kDa dystrophin-associated glycoprotein]	Limb-girdle muscular dystrophy	81405
SGCB	SGCB	Sarcoglycan, beta [43kDa dystrophin-associated glycoprotein]	Limb-girdle muscular dystrophy	81405
SGCD	SGCD	Sarcoglycan, delta [35kDa dystrophin-associated glycoprotein]	Limb-girdle muscular dystrophy	81405
SGCE	SGCE	Sarcoglycan, epsilon	Myoclonic dystonia	81405, 81406
SGCG	SGCG	Sarcoglycan, gamma [35kDa dystrophin-associated glycoprotein]	Limb-girdle muscular dystrophy	81404, 81405

| Separate Procedure | Unlisted Procedure | CCI Comp. Code | Non-specific Procedure | **721** |

MOLECULAR PATHOLOGY GENE TABLE

Claim Designation	Abbreviated Gene Name	Full Gene Name	Commonly Associated Proteins/Disease	CPT Code(s)
SH2D1A	SH2D1A	SH2 domain containing 1A	X-linked lymphoproliferative syndrome	81403, 81404
SH3TC2	SH3TC2	SH3 domain and tetratricopeptide repeats 2	Charcot-Marie-Tooth disease	81406
SHOC2	SHOC2	Soc-2 suppressor of clear homolog	Noonan-like syndrome with loose anagen hair, Noonan spectrum disorders	81400, 81405, 81442
	Short tandem repeat (STR)	N/A	Pretransplant recipient, donor germline testing, post-transplant recipient	81265, 81266
SHOX	SHOX	Short stature homeobox	Langer mesomelic dysplasia	81405
SIL1	SIL1	SIL1 homolog, endoplasmic reticulum chaperone [S. cerevisiae]	Ataxia	81405
SLC2A1	SLC2A1	Solute carrier family 2 [facilitated glucose transporter], member 1	Glucose transporter type 1 [GLUT 1] deficiency syndrome, epilepsy	81405, 81419
SLC2A10	SLC2A10	Solute carrier family 2 [facilitated glucose transporter], member 10	Aortic dysfunction or dilation	81410
SLC9A6	SLC9A6	Solute carrier family 9 [sodium/hydrogen exchanger], member 6	Christianson syndrome, epilepsy	81406, 81419
SLC12A1	SLC12A1	Solute carrier family 12 [sodium/potassium/chloride transporters], member 1	Bartter syndrome	81407
SLC12A3	SLC12A3	Solute carrier family 12 [sodium/chloride transporters], member 3	Gitelman syndrome	81407
SLC16A2	SLC16A2	Solute carrier family 16, member 2 [thyroid hormone transporter]	Specific thyroid hormone cell transporter deficiency, Allan-Herndon-Dudley syndrome, X-linked intellectual disability (XLID)	81404, 81405, 81470, 81471
SLC22A5	SLC22A5	Solute carrier family 22 [organic cation/carnitine transporter], member 5	Systemic primary carnitine deficiency	81405
SLC25A4	SLC25A4	Solute carrier family 25 [mitochondrial carrier; adenine nucleotide translocator], member 4	Progressive external ophthalmoplegia, mitochondrial disorders	81404, 81440
SLC25A20	SLC25A20	Solute carrier family 25 [carnitine/acylcarnitine translocase], member 20	Carnitine-acylcarnitine translocase deficiency	81404, 81405
SLC26A4	SLC26A4	Solute carrier family 26, member 4	Pendred syndrome, hearing loss	81406, 81430
SLC37A4	SLC37A4	Solute carrier family 37 [glucose-6-phosphate transporter], member 4	Glycogen storage disease type Ib	81406
SLCO1B1	SLCO1B1	Solute carrier organic anion transporter family, member 1B1	Adverse drug reaction	81328
SMAD3	SMAD3	SMAD family member 3	Aortic dysfunction or dilation	81410
SMAD4	SMAD4	SMAD family member 4	Hemorrhagic telangiectasia syndrome, juvenile polyposis, hereditary colon cancer disorders	81405, 81406, 81435, 81436
SMN1	SMN1	Survival of motor neuron 1, telomeric	Spinal muscular atrophy	81329, 81336, 81337
SMN1SMN2	SMN1/SMN2	Survival of motor neuron 1, telomeric/survival of motor neuron 2, centromeric	Spinal muscular atrophy	81329
	SMPD1	Sphingomyelin phospho-diesterase 1, acid lysosomal	Niemann-Pick disease, type A, Ashkenazi Jewish-associated disorders	81330, 81412
	SNRPN/ UBE3A	Small nuclear ribonucleoprotein polypeptide N and ubiquitin protein ligase E3A	Prader-Willi syndrome and/or Angelman syndrome	81331
SOD1	SOD1	Superoxide dismutase 1, soluble	Amyotrophic lateral sclerosis	81404
SOS1	SOS1	Son of sevenless homolog 1	Noonan syndrome, gingival fibromatosis, Noonan spectrum disorders	81406, 81442
SPAST	SPAST	Spastin	Spastic paraplegia, hereditary peripheral neuropathies	81405, 81406, 81448
SPG11	SPG11	Spastic paraplegia 11 [autosomal recessive]	Spastic paraplegia, hereditary peripheral neuropathies	81407, 81448
SPG7	SPG7	Spastic paraplegia 7 [pure and complicated autosomal recessive]	Spastic paraplegia	81405, 81406
SPINK1	SPINK1	Serine peptidase inhibitor, Kazal type 1	Hereditary pancreatitis	81404
SPRED1	SPRED1	Sprouty-related, EVH1 domain containing 1	Legius syndrome	81405
SPTBN2	SPTBN2	Spectrin, beta, non-erythrocytic 2	Spinocerebellar ataxia	81407

● New Code   ▲ Revised Code   ✛ Add-On Code   ⊘ Modifier -51 Exempt   ★ Telemedicine

MOLECULAR PATHOLOGY GENE TABLE

Claim Designation	Abbreviated Gene Name	Full Gene Name	Commonly Associated Proteins/Disease	CPT Code(s)
SPTLC1	SPTLC1	Serine palmitoyltransferase, long chain base subunit 1	Hereditary peripheral neuopathies	81448
	SRSF2	Serine and arginine-rich splicing factor 2	Myelodysplastic syndrome, acute myeloid leukemia	81348
SRY	SRY	Sex determining region Y	46,XX testicular disorder of sex development, gonadal dysgenesis	81400
SS18SSX1	SS18/SSX1	t(X;18)	Synovial sarcoma	81401
SS18SSX2	SS18/SSX2	t(X;18)	Synovial sarcoma	81401
STAT3	STAT3	Signal transducer and activator of transcription 3 [acute-phase response factor]	Autosomal dominant hyper-IgE syndrome	81405
STK11	STK11	Serine/threonine kinase 11	Peutz-Jeghers syndrome, hereditary breast cancer-related disordres, hereditary colon cancer disorders	81404, 81405, 81432, 81433, 81435, 81436
STRC	STRC	Stereocilin	Hearing loss	81431
STXBP1	STXBP1	Syntaxin binding protein 1	Epileptic encephalopathy, epilepsy	81406, 81419
SUCLA2	SUCLA2	Succinate-CoA ligase ADP-forming beta subunit	Mitochondrial disorders	81440
SUCLG1	SUCLG1	Succinate-CoA ligase alpha subunit	Mitochondrial disordres	81440
SURF1	SURF1	Surfeit 1	Mitochondrial respiratory chain complex IV deficiency	81405
	SYNGAP1	Synaptic Ras (GTPase activating protein 1	Epilepsy	81419
TACO1	TACO1	Translational activator of mitochondrial encoded cytochrome c oxidase I	Mitochondrial respiratory chain complex IV deficiency	81404
TARDBP	TARDBP	TAR DNA binding protein	Amyotrophic lateral sclerosis	81405
TAZ	TAZ	Tafazzin	Methylglutaconic aciduria type 2, Barth syndrome, mitochondrial disordres	81406, 81440
TBP	TBP	TATA box binding protein	Spinocerebellar ataxia	81344
TBX5	TBX5	T-box 5	Holt-Oram syndrome	81405
TCF4	TCF4	Transcription factor 4	Pitt-Hopkins syndrome, epilepsy	81405, 81406, 81419
	TERT	Telomerase reverse transcriptase	Thyroid carcinoma, glioblastoma multiforme	81345
	TGFBI	Transforming growth factor beta-induced	Corneal dystrophy	81333
TGFBR1	TGFBR1	Transforming growth factor, beta receptor 1	Marfan syndrome, aortic dysfunction or dilation	81405, 81410, 81411
TGFBR2	TGFBR2	Transforming growth factor, beta receptor 2	Marfan syndrome, aortic dysfunction or dilation	81405, 81410, 81411
TH	TH	Tyrosine hydroxylase	Segawa syndrome	81406
THAP1	THAP1	THAP domain containing, apoptosis associated protein 1	Torsion dystonia	81404
THRB	THRB	Thyroid hormone receptor, beta	Thyroid hormone resistance, thyroid hormone beta receptor deficiency	81405
TK2	TK2	Thymidine kinase 2, mitochondrial	Mitochondrial DNA depletion syndrome, mitochondrial disorders	81405, 81440
TMC1	TMC1	Transmembrane channel-like 1	Hearing loss	81430
TMEM43	TMEM43	Transmembrane protein 43	Arrhythmogenic right ventricular cardiomyopathy	81406
TMEM67	TMEM67	Transmembrane protein 67	Joubert syndrome	81407
TMEM127	TMEM127	Transmembrane protein 127	Hereditary neuroendocrine tumor disorders	81437
TMPRSS3	TMPRSS3	Transmembrane protease, serine 3	Hearing loss	81430
TNNC1	TNNC1	Troponin C type 1 [slow]	Hypertrophic cardiomyopathy or dilated cardiomyopathy	81405
TNNI3	TNNI3	Troponin I, type 3 [cardiac]	Familial hypertrophic cardiomyopathy	81405
TNNT2	TNNT2	Troponin T, type 2 [cardiac]	Familial hypertrophic cardiomyopathy	81406
TOR1A	TOR1A	Torsin family 1, member A [torsin A]	Early-onset primary dystonia [DYT1], torsion dystonia	81400, 81404
TP53	TP53	Tumor protein 53	Li-Fraumeni syndrome, hereditary breast cancer-related disorders	81351, 81352, 81353, 81432
TPM1	TPM1	Tropomyosin 1 [alpha]	Familial hypertrophic cardiomyopathy	81405
TPMT	TPMT	Thiopurine S-methyltransferase	Drug metabolism	81335
	TPP1	Tripeptidyl peptidase 1	Epilepsy	81419
	TRB@	T cell antigen receptor, beta	Leukemia and lymphoma	81340, 81341
TRD	TRD@	T cell antigen receptor, delta	Leukemia and lymphoma	81402

MOLECULAR PATHOLOGY GENE TABLE

Claim Designation	Abbreviated Gene Name	Full Gene Name	Commonly Associated Proteins/Disease	CPT Code(s)
	TRG@	T cell antigen receptor, gamma	Leukemia and lymphoma	81342
TRPC6	TRPC6	Transient receptor potential cation channel, subfamily C, member 6	Focal segmental glomerulosclerosis	81406
TSC1	TSC1	Tuberous sclerosis 1	Tuberous sclerosis, epilepsy	81405, 81406, 81419
TSC2	TSC2	Tuberous sclerosis 2	Tuberous sclerosis, epilepsy	81406, 81407, 81419
TTN	TTN	Titin	Hereditary cardiomyopathy	81439
TTPA	TTPA	Tocopherol [alpha] transfer protein	Ataxia	81404
TTR	TTR	Transthyretin	Familial transthyretin amyloidosis	81404
TWIST1	TWIST1	Twist homolog 1 [Drosophila]	Saethre-Chotzen syndrome	81403, 81404
TYMP	TYMP	Thymidine phosphorylase	Mitochondrial DNA depletion syndrome, mitochondrial disorders	81405, 81440
TYMS	TYMS	Thymidylate synthetase	5-fluorouracil/5-FU drug metabolism	81346
TYR	TYR	Tyrosinase [oculocutaneous albinism IA]	Oculocutaneous albinism IA	81404
	U2AF1	U2 small nuclear RNA auxiliary factor 1	Myelodysplastic syndrome, acute myeloid leukemia	81357
UBA1	UBA1	Ubiquitin-like modifier activating enzyme 1	Spinal muscular atrophy, X-linked	81403
UBE3A	UBE3A	Ubiquitin protein ligase E3A	Angelman syndrome	81406
UGT1A1	UGT1A1	UDP glucurono- syltransferase 1 family, polypeptide A1	Drug metabolism, Gilbert syndrome, Crigler-Najjar syndrome	81350, 81404
UMOD	UMOD	Uromodulin	Glomerulocystic kidney disease with hyperuricemia and isosthenuria	81406
UPD	Uniparental disomy	UPD	Russell-Silver syndrome, Prader-Willi/Angelman syndrome	81402
USH1C	USH1C	Usher syndrome 1C [autosomal recessive, severe]	Usher syndrome, type 1, hearing loss	81407, 81430
USH1G	USH1G	Usher syndrome 1G [autosomal recessive]	Usher syndrome, type 1, hearing loss	81404, 81430
USH2A	USH2A	Usher syndrome 2A [autosomal recessive, mild]	Usher syndrome, type 2, hearing loss, hereditary retinal disorders	81408, 81430, 81434
VHL	VHL	Von Hippel-Lindau tumor suppressor	Von Hippel-Lindau familial cancer syndrome, hereditary nueroendocrine tumor disorders	81403, 81404, 81437, 81438
	VKORC1	Vitamin K epoxide reductase complex, subunit 1	Warfarin metabolism	81355
VPS13B	VPS13B	Vacuolar protein sorting 13 homolog B [yeast]	Cohen syndrome	81407, 81408
VWF	VWF	Von Willebrand factor	Von Willebrand disease types 1, 1C, 2A, 2B, 2M, 2N, 3	81401, 81403, 81404 81405, 81406, 81408
WAS	WAS	Wiskott-Aldrich syndrome [eczema-thrombocytopenia]	Wiskott-Aldrich syndrome	81406
WDR62	WDR62	WD repeat domain 62	Primary autosomal recessive microcephaly	81407
WFS1	WFS1	Wolfram syndrome 1	Hearing loss	81430
WT1	WT1	Wilms tumor 1	Denys-Drash syndrome, familial Wilms tumor	81405
ZEB2	ZEB2	Zinc finger E-box binding homeobox 2	Mowat-Wilson syndrome, epilepsy	81404, 81405, 81419
ZNF41	ZNF41	Zinc finger protein 41	X-linked mental retardation 89	81404
	ZRSR2	Zinc finger CCCH type, RNA-binding motif and serine/arginine rich 2	Myelodysplastic syndrome, acute myeloid leukemia	81360

PATHOLOGY AND LABORATORY CODES

ORGAN OR DISEASE ORIENTED PANELS

CPT codes for organ or disease oriented panels were included in CPT due to the increased use of general screening programs by physicians, clinics, hospitals, and other health care facilities. Other codes in this section define profiles that combine laboratory tests together under a problem oriented classification. There is a list of specific laboratory tests under each of the panel CPT codes which define the components of each panel. However, each laboratory typically establishes its own profile and provides a listing of the components of that panel performed by the laboratory with test results.

● New Code   ▲ Revised Code   + Add-On Code   ⊘ Modifier -51 Exempt   ★ Telemedicine

The CPT coding system assigns CPT codes to organ or disease oriented panels consisting of a group of specified tests. If all tests of a CPT defined panel are performed, the provider may bill the panel code or the individual component test codes. The panel codes may be used when the tests are ordered as that panel or if the individual component tests of a panel are ordered separately. For example, if the individually ordered tests are cholesterol (CPT code 82465), triglycerides (CPT code 84478), and HDL cholesterol (CPT code 83718), the service could be billed as a lipid panel (CPT code 80061).

These panels were developed for coding purposes only and should not be interpreted as clinical parameters. The tests listed with each panel identify the defined components of that panel.

These panel components are not intended to limit the performance of other tests. If one performs tests in addition to those specifically indicated for a particular panel, those tests should be reported separately in addition to the panel code.

Do not report two or more panel codes that include any of the same constituent tests performed from the same patient collection. If a group of tests overlaps two or more panels, report the panel that incorporates the greater number of tests to fulfill the code definition and report the remaining tests using individual test codes (eg., do not report 80047 in conjunction with 80054).

80047 Basic metabolic panel (Calcium, ionized)

This panel must include the following:
Calcium, ionized (82330)
Carbon dioxide (82374)
Chloride (82435)
Creatinine (82565)
Glucose (82947)
Potassium (84132)
Sodium (84295)
Urea Nitrogen (BUN) (84520)

80048 Basic metabolic panel (Calcium, total)

This panel must include the following:
Calcium, total (82310)
Carbon dioxide (82374)
Chloride (82435)
Creatinine (82565)
Glucose (82947)
Potassium (84132)
Sodium (84295)
Urea Nitrogen (BUN) (84520)

80050 General health panel

This panel must include the following:
Comprehensive metabolic panel (80053)
Blood count, complete (CBC), automated and automated differential WBC count (85025 or 85027 and 85004)
OR
Blood count, complete (CBC), automated (85027) and appropriate manual differential WBC count (85007 or 85009)
Thyroid stimulating hormone (TSH) (84443)

80051 Electrolyte panel

This panel must include the following:
Carbon dioxide (82374)
Chloride (82435)
Potassium (84132)
Sodium (84295)

80053 Comprehensive metabolic panel

This panel must include the following:
Albumin (82040)
Bilirubin, total (82247)
Calcium, total (82310)

Carbon dioxide (bicarbonate) (82374)
Chloride (82435)
Creatinine (82565)
Glucose (82947)
Phosphatase, alkaline (84075)
Potassium (84132)
Protein, total (84155)
Sodium (84295)
Transferase, alanine amino (ALT) (SGPT) (84460)
Transferase, aspartate amino (AST) (SGOT) (84450)
Urea Nitrogen (BUN) (84520)

80055   Obstetric panel

This panel must include the following:
Blood count, complete (CBC), automated and automated differential WBC count (85025 or 85027 and 85004)
OR
Blood count, complete (CBC), automated (85027) and appropriate manual differential WBC count (85007 or 85009)
Hepatitis B surface antigen (HBsAg) (87340)
Antibody, rubella (86762)
Syphilis test, non-treponemal antibody; qualitative (eg, VDRL, RPR, ART) (86592)
Antibody screen, RBC, each serum technique (86850)
Blood typing, ABO (86900) AND
Blood typing, Rh (D) (86901)

(When syphilis screening is performed using a treponemal antibody approach [86780], do not use 80055. Use the individual codes for the tests performed in the obstetric panel)

80081   Obstetric panel (includes HIV testing)

This panel must include the following:
Blood count, complete (CBC), and automated differential WBC count (85025 or 85207 and 85004)
OR
Blood count, complete (CBC), automated (85027) and appropriate manual differential WBC count (85007 or 85009)
Hepatitis B surface antigen (HBsAg) (87340)
HIV-1 antigen(s), with HIV-1 and HIV-2 antibodies, single result (87389)
Antibody, rubella (86762)
Syphilis test, non-treponemal antibody; qualitative (eg, VDRL, RPR, ART) (86592)
Antibody screen, RBC, each serum technique (86850)
Blood typing, ABO (86900) AND
Blood typing, Rh (D) (86901)

(When syphilis screening is performed using a treponemal antibody approach [86780], do not use 80081. Use the individual codes for the tests performed in the obstetric panel)

80061   Lipid panel

This panel must include the following:
Cholesterol, serum, total (82465)
Lipoprotein, direct measurement, high density cholesterol (HDL cholesterol) (83718)
Triglycerides (84478)

80069   Renal function panel

This panel must include the following:
Albumin (82040)
Calcium, total (82310)
Carbon dioxide (bicarbonate) (82374)
Chloride (82435)
Creatinine (82565)
Glucose (82947)
Phosphorus inorganic (phosphate) (84100)
Potassium (84132)

Sodium (84295)
Urea nitrogen (BUN) (84520)

80074 Acute hepatitis panel

This panel must include the following:
Hepatitis A antibody (HAAb), IgM antibody (86709)
Hepatitis B core antibody (HbcAb), IgM antibody (86705)
Hepatitis B surface antigen (HbsAg) (87340)
Hepatitis C antibody (86803)

80076 Hepatic function panel

This panel must include the following:
Albumin (82040)
Bilirubin, total (82247)
Bilirubin, direct (82248)
Phosphatase, alkaline (84075)
Protein, total (84155)
Transferase, alanine amino (ALT) (SGPT) (84460)
Transferase, aspartate amino (AST) (SGOT) (84450)

80081 Code out of order. See page 726

DEFINITIONS AND ACRONYM CONVERSION LISTING	
Drug Testing Term/Acronym	**Definition**
6-MAM	Acronym for the heroin drug metabolite 6-monacetylmorphine
Acid	Descriptor for classifying drug/drug metabolite molecules based upon chemical ionization properties. Laboratory procedures for drug isolation and identification may include acid, base, or neutral groupings.
AM	A category of synthetic marijuana drugs discovered by and named after Alexandros Makriyannis at Northeastern Univ.
Analog	A structural derivative of a parent chemical compound that often differs from it by a single element.
Analyte	The substance or chemical constituent that is of interest in an analytical procedure.
Base	Descriptor for classifying drug/drug metabolite molecules based upon chemical ionization properties. Laboratory procedures for drug isolation and identification may include acid, base, or neutral groupings.
Card(s)	Multiplexed presumptive drug class(es) immunoassay product that is read by visual observation, including instrumented when performed
Cassette(s)	Multiplexed presumptive drug class immunoassay product(s) that is read by visual observation, including instrumented when performed
CEDIA	Acronym for Cloned-Enzyme-Donor-Immuno-Assay. CEDIA immunoassay is a competitive antibody binding procedure that utilizes enzyme donor fragment-labeled antigens (drugs) to compete for antigens (drugs) contained in the patient sample. Recombination of enzyme donor fragment and enzyme acceptor fragment produces a functional enzyme. CEDIA immunoassay enzyme activity is proportional to concentration of drug(s) detected.
Chromatograpy	An analytical technique used to separate components of a mixture. See thin layer chromatography, gas chromatography, and high performance chromatography.
Confirmatory	Term used to describe definitive identification/quantitation procedures that are secondary to presumptive screening methods.
DART	Acronym for Direct-Analysis-in-Real-Time. DART is an atmospheric pressure ionization method for mass spectrometry analysis.
Definitive Drug Procedure	A procedure that provides specific identification of individual drugs and drug metabolites.
DESI	Acronym for Desorption-ElectroSpray-Ionization. DESI is a combination of electrospray ionization and desorption ionization methods for mass spectrometry analysis.
Dipstick	A multiplexed presumptive drug class immunoassay product that is read by visual observation, including instrumented when performed.
Drug test cup	A multiplexed presumptive drug class immunoassay product that is read by visual observation, including instrumented when performed.
EDDP	Acronum for the methadone drug metabolite 2-ethylidene-1, 5-dimethyl-3, 3-diphenylpyrrolidine
EIA	Acronym for Enzyme-Immuno-Assay. Enzyme immunoassay is a competitive antibody binding procedure that utilizes enzyme-labeled antigens (drugs) to compete for antigens (drugs) contained in the patient sample. Enzyme immunoassay enzyme activity is proportional to concentration of drug(s) detected.
ELISA	Acronym for Enzyme-Linked Immunosorbent Assay. ELISA is a competitive binding immunoassay that is designed to measure antigens (drugs) or antibodies. ELISA immunoassay results are proportional to concentration of drug(s) detected.

DEFINITIONS AND ACRONYM CONVERSION LISTING

Drug Testing Term/Acronym	Definition
EMIT	Acronym for Enzyme-Multiplied-Immunoassay-Test. EMIT is a trade name for a type of enzyme immunoassay (EIA).
FPIA	Acronym for Fluorescence-Polarization-Immuno-Assay. FPIA is a competitive binding immunoassay that utilizes fluorexcein-labeled antigens (drugs) to compete for antigens (drugs) contained in the patient sample. The measure of polarized light emission is inversely proportional to the concentration of drug(s) detected.
Gas chromatography	Gas chromatography is a chromatography technique in which patient sample preparations are vaporized into a gas (mobile phase) which flows through a tubular column (containing a stational phase) and into a detector. The retention time of a drug on the column is determined by partitioning characteristics of the drug into the mobile and stationary phases. Chromatography column detectors may be non-specific (eg, flame ionization) or specific (eg, mass spectrometry). The combination of column retention time and specific detector response provides a definitive identification of the drug or drug metabolite.
GC	Acronym for gas chromatography.
GC-MS	Acronym for gas chromatography mass spectrometry.
GC-MS/MS	Acronym for gas chromatography mass spectrometry/mass spectrometry.
High performance liquid chromatography	High performance liquid chromatography is a chromatography technique in which patient sample preparations are injected into a liquid (mobile phase) which flows through a tubular column (containing a stationary phase) and into a detector. The retention time of a drug on the column is determined by partitioning characteristics of the drug into the mobile and stationary phases. Chromatography column detectors may be non-specific (eg, ultra-violet spectrophotometry) or specific (eg, mass spectrometry). The combination of column retention time and specific detector response provides a definitive identification of the drug or drug metabolite. High performance liquid chromatography is also called high pressure liquid chromatography.
HPLC	Acronym for high performance liquid chromatography
HU	A category of synthetic marijuana drugs discovered by and named after Raphael Mechoulam at Hebrew University.
IA	Acronym of immunoassay.
Immunoassay	Antigen-antibody binding procedures utilized to detect antigens (eg, drugs and/or drug metabolites) in patient samples. Immunoassay designs include competitive or non-competitive with various mechanisms for detection.
Isobaric	In mass spectrometry, ions with the same mass
Isomers	Compounds that have the same molecular formula but differ in structural formula
JWH	A category of synthetic marijuana drugs discovered by and named after John W. Huffman at Clemson University.
KIMS	Acronym for kinetic interaction of microparticles in solution. KIMS immunoassay is a competitive antibody binding procedure that utilizes microparticle-labeled antigens (drugs) to compete for antigens (drugs) contained in the patient sample. Microparticle immunoassay absorbance increase is inversely proportional to concentration of drug(s) detected.
LC-MS	Acronym for liquid chromatography mass spectrometry
LC-MS/MS	Acronym for liquid chromatography mass spectrometry/mass spectrometry
LDTD	Acronym for laser diode thermal desorption. LDTD is a combination of atmospheric pressure chemical ionization and laser diode thermal desorption methods for mass spectrometry analysis.
MALDI	Acronym for matrix assisted laser desorption/Ionization mass spectrometry. MALDI is a soft ionization technique that reduces molecular fragmentation.
MDA	Acronym for the drug 3,4-methylenedioxyamphetamine. MDA is also a drug metabolite of MDMA.
MDEA	Acronym for the drug 3,4-methylenedioxy-N-ethylamphetamine
MDMA	Acronym for the drug 3,4-methylenedioxy-N-methylamphetamine
MDPV	Acronym for the drug methylenedioxypyrovalerone
MS	Acronym for mass spectrometry. MS is an identification technique that measures the charge-to-mass ratio of charged particles. There are several types of mass spectrometry instruments, such as magnetic sectoring, time of flight, quadrapole mass filter, ion traps, and Fourier transformation. Mass spectrometry is used as part of the process to assign definitive identification of drugs and drug metabolites.
MS/MS	Acronym for mass spectrometry/mass spectrometry. MS/MS instruments combine multiple units of mass spectrometry filters into a single instrument. MS/MS is also called tandem mass spectrometry.
MS-TOF	Acronym for mass spectrometry time of flight. Time of flight is a mass spectrometry identification technique that utilizes ion velocity to determine the mass-to-charge ratio.
Multiplexed	Descriptor for a multiple component test device that simultaneously measures multiple analytes (drug classes) in a single analysis.
Neutral	Descriptor for classifying drug/drug metabolite molecules based upon chemical ionization properties. Laboratory procedures for drug isolation and identification may include acid, base, or neutral groupings.
ng/mL	Unit of measure for weight per volume calculated as nanograms per milliliter. The ng/mL unit of measure is equivalent to the ug/L unit of measure.
Optical observation	Optical observation refers to procedure results that are interpreted visually with or without instrumentation assistance.

● New Code ▲ Revised Code ✚ Add-On Code ⊘ Modifier -51 Exempt ★ Telemedicine

DEFINITIONS AND ACRONYM CONVERSION LISTING

Drug Testing Term/Acronym	Definition
Opiate	Medicinal category of narcotic alkaloid drugs that are natural products in the opium poppy plant Papaver somniferum. This immunoassay class of drugs typically includes detection of codeine, dihydrocodeine, hydrocodone, hydromorphone, and morphine.
Opioids	A category of medicinal synthetic or semi-synthetic narcotic alkaloid opioid receptor stimulating drugs including butorphanol, desomorphine, dextromethorphan, dextrorphan, levorphanol, meperidine, naloxone, naltrexone, normeperidine, and pentazocine.
Presumptive	Drug test results that indicate possible, but not definitive, presence of drugs and or drug metabolites.
QTOF	Acronym for Quadrapole-Time-Of-Flight mass spectrometry. QTOF is a hybrid mass spectrometry identification technique that combines ion velocity with tandem quadrapole mass spectrometry (MS or MS/MS) to determine the mass-to-charge ratio.
RCS	A category of synthetic marijuana drugs that are analogs of JHW compounds. See JWH
RIA	Acronym for radio-immuno-assay. Radioimmunoassay is a competitive antibody binding procedure that utilizes radioactive-labeled antigens (drugs) to compete for antigens (drugs) contained in the patient sample. The measure of radioactivity is inversely proportional to concentration of drug(s) detected.
Stereoisomers	Isomeric molecules that have the same molecular formula and sequence of bonded atoms (constitution), but that differ only in the three-dimensional orientations of their atoms in space.
Substance	A substance is a drug that does not have an established therapeutic use as distinguished from other analytes listed in the Chemistry section (82000-84999)
TDM	Acronym for Therapeutic Drug Monitoring
THC	Acronym for marijuana active drug ingredient tetrahydrocannabinol
Therapeutic Drug Monitoring	Analysis of blood (serum, plasma) drug concentration to monitor clinical response to therapy.
Time of Flight	A mass spectrometry technique that utilizes ion velocity to determine the mass-to-charge ratio.
TLC	Acronym for Thin Layer Chromatography
TOF	Acronym for Time Of Flight
ug/L	Unit of measure for mass per volume calculated as micrograms per liter. The ug/L unit of measure is equivalent to the ng/mL unit of measure.

DRUG ASSAY

Drug procedures are divided into three subsections: Therapeutic Drug Assay, Drug Assay, and Chemistry – with code selection dependent on the purpose and type of patient results obtained. Therapeutic Drug Assays are performed to monitor clinical response to a known, prescribed medication. The two major categories for drug testing in the drug assay subsection are:

1. **Presumptive drug class** procedures are used to identify possible use or non-use of a drug or drug class. A presumptive test may be followed by a definitive test in order to specifically identify drugs or metabolites.

2. **Definitive drug class** procedures are qualitative or quantitative tests to identify possible use or nonuse of a drug. These tests identify specific drugs and associated metabolites, if performed. A presumptive test is not required prior to a definitive drug test.

The material for drug class procedures may be any specimen type unless otherwise specified in the code descriptor (eg., urine, blood, oral fluid, meconium, hair). Procedures can be qualitative (eg., positive/negative or present/absent), semi quantitative, or quantitative (measured) depending on the purpose of the testing. Therapeutic drug assay (TDA) procedures are typically quantitative tests and the specimen type is whole blood, serum, plasma, and or cerebrospinal fluid.

When the same procedure(s) is performed on more than one specimen type (eg., blood and urine), the appropriate code is reported separately for each specimen type using modifier 59. Drugs or classes of drugs maybe commonly assayed first by a presumptive screening method followed by a definitive drug identification method. Presumptive methods include, but are not limited to, immunoassays (IA, EIA, ELISA, RIA, EMIT, FPIA, etc.), enzymatic methods (alcohol dehydrogenase, etc.), chromatographic methods without mass spectrometry (TLC, HPLC, GC, etc.), or mass spectrometry without adequate drug resolution by chromatography (MS-TOF, DART, DESI, LDTD, MALDI). LC-MS, LC-MS/MS, or mass spectrometry without adequate drug resolution by chromatography may also be used for presumptive testing if the chromatographic phase is not adequate to identify individual drugs and distinguish between structural isomers or isobaric compounds. All drug class immunoassays are considered presumptive, whether qualitative, semi-quantitative, or quantitative. Methods that cannot distinguish between structural isomers (such as morphine and hydromorephone or methamphetamine and phentermine) are also considered presumptive.

Definitive drug identification methods are able to identify individual drugs and distinguish between structural isomers but not necessarily stereoisomers. Definitive methods include, but are not limited to, gas chromatography with mass spectrometry (any

---

Separate Procedure	Unlisted Procedure	CCI Comp. Code	Non-specific Procedure	**729**

type, single or tandem) and liquid chromatography mass spectrometry (any type, single or tandem) and exclude immunoassays (eg., IA, EIA, ELISA, RIA, EMIT, FPIA), and enzymatic methods (eg., alcohol dehydrogenase).

For chromatography, each combination of stationary and mobile phase is to be counted as one procedure.

PRESUMPTIVE DRUG CLASS SCREENING

Drugs or classes of drugs may be commonly assayed first by a presumptive screening method followed by a definitive drug identification method. The methodology is considered when coding presumptive procedures. Each code (80305, 80306, 80307) represents all drugs and drug classes performed by the respective methodology per date of service. Each code also includes all sample validation procedures performed. Examples of sample validation procedures may include, but are not limited to, pH, specific gravity, and nitrite. The codes (80305, 80306, 80307) represent three different method categories:

1. Code 80305 is used to report procedures in which the results are read by direct optical observation. The results are visually read. Examples of these procedures are dipsticks, cups, cards, and cartridges. Report 80305 once, irrespective of the number of direct observation drug class procedures performed or results on any date of service.

2. Code 80306 is used to report procedures when an instrument is used to assist in determining the result of a direct optical observation methodology. Examples of these procedures are dipsticks, cards, and cartridges inserted into an instrument that determines the final result of an optical observation methodology. Report 80306 once, irrespective of the number of drug class procedures or results on any date of service.

3. Code 80307 is used to report any number of devices or procedures by instrumented chemistry analyzers. There are many different instrumented methodologies available to perform presumptive drug assays. Examples include immunoassay (eg, EIA, ELISA, EMIT, FPIA, IA, KIMS, RIA), chromatography (eg, GC, HPLC), and mass spectrometry, either with or without chromatography (eg, DART, DESI, GC-MS, GC-MS/MS, LC-MS, LC-MS/MS, LDTD, MALDI, TOF). Some of these methodologies may be used for definitive drug testing also, but, for the purpose of presumptive drug testing, the presumptive method is insufficient to provide definitive drug identification. Report 80307 once, irrespective of the number of drug class procedures or results on any date of service.

80305   Drug test(s), presumptive, any number of drug classes, any number of devices or procedures; capable of being read by direct optical observation only (eg, utilizing immunoassay [eg, dipsticks, cups, cards, or cartridges]), includes sample validation when performed, per date of service

80306   read by instrument assisted direct optical observation (eg, utilizing immunoassay [eg, dipsticks, cups, cards, or cartridges]), includes sample validation when performed, per date of service

80307   by instrument chemistry analyzers (eg, utilizing immunoassay [eg, EIA, ELISA, EMIT, FPIA, IA, KIMS, RIA]), chromatography (eg, GC, HPLC), and mass spectrometry either with or without chromatography, (eg, DART, DESI, GC-MS, GC-MS/MS, LC-MS, LC-MS/MS, LDTD, MALDI, TOF) includes sample validation when performed, per date of service

DEFINITIVE DRUG TESTING

Definitive drug identification methods are able to identify individual drugs and distinguish between structural isomers but not necessarily stereoisomers. Definitive methods include, but are not limited to, gas chromatography with mass spectrometry, any type, single or tandem and liquid chromatography mass spectrometry, any type, single or tandem, exclude immunoassays (eg., IA, EIA, ELISA, RIA, EMIT, FPIA), and enzymatic methods (e.g. alcohol dehydrogenase).

Use 80320-80377 to eport definitive drug class procedures. Definitive testing maybe qualitative, quantitative, or a combination of qualitative and quantitative for the same patient on the same date of service.

The Definitive Drug Classes Listing provides the drug classes, their associated CPT codes, and the drugs included in each class. Each category of a drug class, including metabolites if performed (except stereoisomers), is reported once per date of service. Metabolites not listed in the table may be reported using the code for the parent drug. Drug class metabolite(s) is not reported separately unless the metabolite(s) is listed as a separate category in Definitive Drug Classes Listing (e.g. heroin metabolite).

Drug classes may contain one or more codes based on the number of analytes. For example, an analysis in which five or more amphetamines and/or amphetamine metabolites would be reported with 80326. The code is based on the number of reported analytes and not the capacity of the analysis.

Definitive drug procedures that are not specified in 80320-80373 should be reported using the unlisted definitive procedure codes 80375, 80376, 80377, unless the specific analyte is listed in the Therapeutic Drug Assays (80143-80203) or Chemistry (82009-84830) sections.

See the Definitive Drug Classes Listing for a listing of the more common analytes within each drug class.

80320 Alcohols

(For alcohol [ethanol] by immunoassay and enzymatic methods, use 82077)

80321 Alcohol biomarkers; 1 or 2

80322   3 or more

80323 Alkaloids, not otherwise specified

80324 Amphetamines; 1 or 2

80325   3 or 4

80326   5 or more

80327 Anabolic steroids; 1 or 2

80328   3 or more

(For dihydrotestosterone analysis for endogenous hormone levels or therapeutic monitoring, use 82642)

80329 Analgesics, non-opiod; 1 or 2

80330   3-5

80331   6 or more

(For acetaminophen by immunoassay or enzymatic methods, use 80143)

(For salicylate by immunoassay or enzymatic methods, use 80179)

80332 Antidepressants, serotonergic class; 1 or 2

80333   3-5

80334   6 or more

80335 Antidepressants, tricyclic and other cyclicals; 1 or 2

80336   3-5

80337   6 or more

80338 Antidepressants, not otherwise specified

80339 Antiepileptics, not otherwsie specified; 1-3

80340   4-6

80341   7 or more

(To report definitive drug testing for antihistamines, see 80375, 80376, 80377)

(To report therapeutic drug assay for carbamazepine, see 80156, 80157, 80161)

80342 Antipsychotics, not otherwise specified; 1-3

80343   4-6

Separate Procedure   Unlisted Procedure   CCI Comp. Code   Non-specific Procedure   **731**

80344	7 or more
80345	Barbiturates
80346	Benzodiazepines; 1-12
80347	13 or more
80348	Buprenorphine
80349	Cannabinoids, natural
80350	Cannabinoids, synthetic; 1-3
80351	4-6
80352	7 or more
80353	Cocaine
80354	Fentanyl
80355	Gabapentin, non-blood

(For therapeutic drug assay, use 80171)

80356	Heroin metabolite
80357	Ketamine and norketamine
80358	Methadone
80359	Methylenedioxyamphetamines (MDA, MDEA, MDMA)
80360	Methylphenidate
80361	Opiates, 1 or more
80362	Opioids and opiate analogs; 1 or 2
80363	3 or 4
80364	5 or more
80365	Oxycodone
83992	Phencyclidine (PCP)

(Phenobarbital, use 80345)

80366	Pregabalin
80367	Propoxyphene
80368	Sedative hypnotics (non-benzodiazepines)
80369	Skeletal muscle relaxants; 1 or 2
80370	3 or more

● New Code ▲ Revised Code ＋ Add-On Code ⊘ Modifier -51 Exempt ★ Telemedicine

80371 Stimulants, synthetic

80372 Tapentadol

80373 Tramadol

80374 Stereoisomer (enantiomer) analysis; single drug class

(Use 80374 in conjunction with an index drug analysis when performed)

80375 Drug(s) or substance(s), definitive, qualitative or quantitative, not otherwise specified; 1-3

80376 4-6

80377 7 or more

(To report definitive drug testing for antihistamines, see 80375, 80376, 80377)

For Example:

To report amphetamine and methamphetamine using any number of definitive procedures, report 80324 once per facility per date of service.

To report codeine, hydrocodone, hydromorphone, morphine using any number of definitive procedures, report 80361 once per facility per date of service.

To report codeine, hydrocodone, hydromorphone, morphine, oxycodone, oxymorphone, naloxone, naltrexone performed using any number of definitive procedures, report 80361 x 1, 80362 x 1, and 80365 x 1 per facility per date of service.

DEFINITIVE DRUG CLASSES LISTING

Drugs and metabolites included in each definitive drug class are listed in the Definitive Drug Classes Listing table. This is not a comprehensive list. FDA classification of drugs not listed should be used where possible within the defined drug classes. Any metabolites that are not listed should be categorized with the parent drug. Drugs and metabolites not listed may be reported using codes from the Therapeutic Drug Assay (80143-80299) or Chemistry (82009-84999) sections.

DEFINITIVE DRUG CLASSES LISTING		
Codes	**Classes**	**Drugs**
80320	Alcohol(s)	Acetone, ethanol, ethchlorvynol, ethylene glycol, isopropanol, isopropyl alcohol, methanol
80321-80322	Alcohol Biomarker	Ethanol conjugates (ethyl glucuronid [ETG], ethyl sulfate [ETS], fatty acid ethyl esters, phosphatidylethanol)
80323	Alkaloids, not otherwise specified	7-Hydroxymitragynine, atropine, cotinine, lysergic acid diethylamoide
80324-80326	Amphetamines	Amphetamine, ephedrinelisdexamphetamine, methamphetamine, phentermihe, phenylpropanolamine, pseudoephedrine
80327-80328	Anabolic steroids	1-Androstenediol, 1-androstenedione, 1-testosterone, 4-hydroxy-testosterone, 6-oxo, 19-norandrostenedione, androstenedione, androstanolone, bolandiol, bolasterone, boldenone, boldione, calusterone, clostebol, danazol, dehydrochlormethyltestosterone, dihydrotestosterone, drostanolone, epiandrosterone, epitestosterone, fluoxymesterone, furazabol, mestanolone, mesterolone, methandienone, methandriol, methenolone, methydienolone, methyl-1-testosterone, methylnortestosterone, methyltestosterone, mibolerone, nandrolone, norbolethone, norclostebol, norethandrolone, norethindrone, oxabolone, oxandrolone, oxymesterone, oxymetholone, stanozolol, stenbolone, tibolone, trenbolone, zeranol
80329-80331	Analgesics, non-opioid	Acetaminophen, diclofenac ibuprofen, ketoprofen, naproxen, oxaprozin, salicylate
80332-80334	Antidepressants, serotonergic class	Citalopram, duloxetine, escitalopram, fluoxetine, fluvoxamine, paroxetine, sertraline
80335-80337	Antidepressants, tricyclic and other cyclicals	Amitriptyline, amoxapine, clomipramine, demexiptiline, desipramine, doxepin, imipramine, maprotiline, mirtazpine, nortriptyline, protriptyline

DEFINITIVE DRUG CLASSES LISTING

Codes	Classes	Drugs
80338	Antidepressants, not otherwise specified	Bupropion, desyenlafaxine, isocarboxazid, nefazodone, phenelzine, selegiline, tranylcypromine, trazodone, venlafaxine
80339-80341	Antiepileptics, not otherwise specified	Carbamazepine, clobazam, diamethadione, ethosuximide, ezogabine, lamotrigine, levetiracetam, methsuximide, oxcarbazepine, phenytoin, primidone, rufinamide, tiagabine, topiramate, trimethadione, valproic acid, zonisamide
80342-80344	Antipsychotics, not otherwise specified	Aripiprazole, chlorpromazine, clozapine, fluphenazine, haloperidol, loxapine, mesoridazine, molindone, olanzapine, paliperidone, perphenazine, phenothiazine, pimozide, prochlorperazine, quetiapine, risperidone, trifluoperazine, thiothixene, thoridazine, ziprasidone
80345	Barbiturates	Amobarbital, aprobarbital, butalbital, cyclobarbital, mephobarbital, pentobarbital, phenobarbital, secobarbital, talbutal, thiopental
80346, 80347	Benzodiazepines	Alprazolam, chlordiazepoxide, clonazepam, clorazepate, diazepam, estazolam, flunitrazepam, flurazepam, halazepamlorazepammidazolam, nitrazepam, nordazepam, oxazepam, prazepam, quazepam, temazepam
80348	Buprenorphine	Buprenorphine
80349	Cannabinoids, natural	Marijuana, dronabinol carboxy-THC
80350-80352	Cannabinoids, synth.	CP-47, 497, CP497 C8-homolog, JWH-018 and AM678, JWH-073, JWH-019, JWH-200, JWH-210, JWH-250, JWH-081, JWH-122, HWH-398, AM-2201, AM-694, SR-19 and RCS-4, SR-18 and RCS-8, JWH-203, UR-144, XLR-11, MAM-2201, AKB-48
80353	Cocaine	Benzoylecgonine, cocaethylene, cocaine, ecgonine methyl ester, norcocaine
80354	Fentanyls	Acetylfentanyl, alfentanil, fentanyl, remifentanil, sufentanil
80355	Gabapentin, non-blood	Gabapentin
80356	Heroin metabolite	6-acetylmorphine, acetylcodeine, diacetylmorphine
80368	Hypnotics, sedative (non-benzodiazepine)	See Sedative Hypnotics
80357	Ketamine and Norketamine	Ketamine, norketamine
80358	Methadone	Methadone and EDDP
80359	Methylenedioxy-amphetamines	MDA, MDEA, MDMA
80360	Methylphenidate	Methylphenidate, ritalinic acid
80357	Norketamine	See Ketamine
80368	Non-Benzodiazepine	See Hypnotics, sedative
80361	Opiates	Codeine, dihydrocodeine, hydrocodone, hydromorphone, morphine
80362-80364	Opiods and opiate analogs	Butorphanol, desomorphine, dextromethorphan, dextrorphan, levorphanol, meperidine, naloxone, naltrexone, normeperidine, pentazocine
80365	Oxycodone	Oxycodone, oxymorphone
83992	Phencyclidine	Phencyclidine
80366	Pregabalin	Pregabalin
80367	Propoxyphene	Norpropoxyphene, propoxyphene
80368	Sedative hypnotics (non-benzodiazepine)	Eszopiclone, zaleplon, zolpidem
80369, 80370	Skeletal muscle relaxants	Baclofen, carisoprodol, cyclobenzaprine, meprobamate, metaxalone, methocarbamol, orphenadrine, tizanidine
80371	Stimulants, synthetic	2C-B, 2C-E, 2C-I, 2C-H, 3TFMPP, 4-methylethcathinone, alpha-PVP, benzylpiperazine, bromodragonfly, cathinone, m-CPP, MDPBP, MDPPP, MDPV, mephedrone, methcathinone, methylone, phenethylamines, salvinorin, tryptamines
80372	Tapentadol	Tapentadol
80373	Tramadol	Tramadol

● New Code ▲ Revised Code + Add-On Code ⊘ Modifier -51 Exempt ★ Telemedicine

THERAPEUTIC DRUG ASSAYS

Therapeutic drug assays are performed to monitor levels of a known, prescribed, or over-the-counter medication.

The material for examination is whole blood, serum, plasma, or cerebrospinal fluid. Examination is quantitative. Coding is by parent drug; measured metabolites of the drug are included in the code, if performed..

● **80143** Acetaminophen

   (For definitive drug testing for acetaminophen, see 80329, 80330, 80331)

80145 Adalimumab

80150 Amikacin

● **80151** Amiodarone

80155 Caffeine

80156 Carbamazepine; total

80157   free

● **80161** -10, 11-epoxide

80158 Cyclosporine

80159 Clozapine

80161   This code is out of order. See page 735

80162 Digoxin; total

80163   free

80164   This code is out of order. See page 737

80165   This code is out of order. See page 737

80167   This code is out of order. See page 735

80168 Ethosuximide

80169 Everolimus

● **80167** Felbamate

● **80181** Flecainide

80171 Gabapentin, whole blood, serum, or plasma

80170 Gentamicin

80171   This code is out of order. See page 735

80173 Haloperidol

80230 Infliximab

● **80189** Itraconazole

	80235	Lacosamide
	80175	Lamotrigine
	80176	This code is out of order. See page 736
●	80193	Leflunomide
	80177	Levetiracetam
	80176	Lidocaine
	80178	Lithium
●	80204	Methotrexate
	80179	This code is out of order. See page736
	80180	Mycophenolate (mycophenolic acid)
	80181	This code is out of order. See page 735
	80183	Oxcarbazepine
	80184	Phenobarbital
	80185	Phenytoin; total
	80186	free
	80187	Posaconazole
	80188	Primidone
	80189	This code is out of order. See page 735
	80190	Procainamide;
	80192	with metabolites (eg, n-acetyl procainamide)
	80193	This code is out of order. See page 736
	80194	Quinidine
●	80210	Rufinamide
●	80179	Salicylate

(For definitive drug testing for salicylate, see 80329, 80330, 80331)

	80195	Sirolimus
	80197	Tacrolimus
	80198	Theophylline
	80199	Tiagabine
	80200	Tobramycin
	80201	Topiramate

● New Code   ▲ Revised Code   ✛ Add-On Code   ⊘ Modifier -51 Exempt   ★ Telemedicine

80164 Valproic acid (dipropylacetic acid); total

80165   free

80202 Vancomycin

80280 Vedolizumab

80285 Voriconazole

80203 Zonisamide

80204 This code is out of order. See page 736

80210 This code is out of order. See page 736

80230 This code is out of order. See page 735

80235 This code is out of order. See page 736

80280 This code is out of order. See page 737

80285 This code is out of order. See page 737

80299 Quantitation of therapeutic drug, not elsewhere specified

80305 This code is out of order. See Drug Assay, page 730

80306 This code is out of order. See Drug Assay, page 730

80307 This code is out of order. See Drug Assay, page 730

80320 This code is out of order. See Drug Assay, page 731

80321 This code is out of order. See Drug Assay, page 731

80322 This code is out of order. See Drug Assay, page 731

80323 This code is out of order. See Drug Assay, page 731

80324 This code is out of order. See Drug Assay, page 731

80325 This code is out of order. See Drug Assay, page 731

80326 This code is out of order. See Drug Assay, page 731

80327 This code is out of order. See Drug Assay, page 731

80328 This code is out of order. See Drug Assay, page 731

80329 This code is out of order. See Drug Assay, page 731

80330 This code is out of order. See Drug Assay, page 731

80331 This code is out of order. See Drug Assay, page 731

80332 This code is out of order. See Drug Assay, page 731

80333 This code is out of order. See Drug Assay, page 731

80334	This code is out of order. See Drug Assay, page 731
80335	This code is out of order. See Drug Assay, page 731
80336	This code is out of order. See Drug Assay, page 731
80337	This code is out of order. See Drug Assay, page 731
80338	This code is out of order. See Drug Assay, page 731
80339	This code is out of order. See Drug Assay, page 731
80340	This code is out of order. See Drug Assay, page 731
80341	This code is out of order. See Drug Assay, page 731
80342	This code is out of order. See Drug Assay, page 731
80343	This code is out of order. See Drug Assay, page 731
80344	This code is out of order. See Drug Assay, page 732
80345	This code is out of order. See Drug Assay, page 732
80346	This code is out of order. See Drug Assay, page 732
80347	This code is out of order. See Drug Assay, page 732
80348	This code is out of order. See Drug Assay, page 732
80349	This code is out of order. See Drug Assay, page 732
80350	This code is out of order. See Drug Assay, page 732
80351	This code is out of order. See Drug Assay, page 732
80352	This code is out of order. See Drug Assay, page 732
80353	This code is out of order. See Drug Assay, page 732
80354	This code is out of order. See Drug Assay, page 732
80355	This code is out of order. See Drug Assay, page 732
80356	This code is out of order. See Drug Assay, page 732
80357	This code is out of order. See Drug Assay, page 732
80358	This code is out of order. See Drug Assay, page 732
80359	This code is out of order. See Drug Assay, page 732
80360	This code is out of order. See Drug Assay, page 732
80361	This code is out of order. See Drug Assay, page 732
80362	This code is out of order. See Drug Assay, page 732
80363	This code is out of order. See Drug Assay, page 732
80364	This code is out of order. See Drug Assay, page 732

● New Code ▲ Revised Code + Add-On Code ⊘ Modifier -51 Exempt ★ Telemedicine

80365	This code is out of order. See Drug Assay, page 732
80366	This code is out of order. See Drug Assay, page 732
80367	This code is out of order. See Drug Assay, page 732
80368	This code is out of order. See Drug Assay, page 732
80369	This code is out of order. See Drug Assay, page 732
80370	This code is out of order. See Drug Assay, page 732
80371	This code is out of order. See Drug Assay, page 733
80372	This code is out of order. See Drug Assay, page 733
80373	This code is out of order. See Drug Assay, page 733
80374	This code is out of order. See Drug Assay, page 733
80375	This code is out of order. See Drug Assay, page 733
80376	This code is out of order. See Drug Assay, page 733
80377	This code is out of order. See Drug Assay, page 733

EVOCATIVE/SUPPRESSION TESTING

Evocative/suppression testing involves administration of agents to determine a patient's response to those agents. CPT codes 80400-80440 are to be used for reporting the laboratory components of the testing. When the test requires physician administration of the evocative/suppression agent, see codes 96390, 96361, 96372-96374, 96375. However, when physician attendance is not required, and the agent is administered by ancillary personnel, these codes are not to be separately reported.

In the inpatient setting, these codes are only reported if the physician performs the service personally. In the office setting, the service can be reported when performed by office personnel if the physician is directly supervising the service. While supplies necessary to perform the testing are included in the testing, the appropriate HCPCS J codes for the drugs can be separately reported for the diagnostic agents. Separate evaluation and management services are not to be reported, including prolonged services (in the case of prolonged infusions) unless a significant, separately identifiable service is provided and documented.

The following test panels involve the administration of evocative or suppressive agents, and the baseline and subsequent measurement of their effects on chemical constituents. These codes are to be used for the reporting of the laboratory component of the overall testing protocol. For the administration of the evocative or suppressive agents, see Hydration, Therapeutic, Prophylactic, Diagnostic Injections and Infusions, and Chemotherapy and Other Highly Complex drug or Highly Complex Biologic Agent Administration (eg, 96365, 96366, 96367, 96368, 96372, 96374, 96375, 96376). In the code descriptors where reference is made to a particular analyte (eg., Cortisol: 82533 x 2) the "x 2" refers to the number of times the test for that particular analyte is performed.

80400 ACTH stimulation panel; for adrenal insufficiency

This panel must include the following:
Cortisol (82533 x 2)

80402　　 for 21 hydroxylase deficiency

This panel must include the following:
Cortisol (82533 x 2)
17 hydroxyprogesterone (83498 x 2)

80406　　 for 3 beta-hydroxydehydrogenase deficiency

This panel must include the following:
Cortisol (82533 x 2)

17 hydroxypregnenolone (84143 x 2)

80408   Aldosterone suppression evaluation panel (eg, saline infusion)

This panel must include the following:
Aldosterone (82088 x 2)
Renin (84244 x 2)

80410   Calcitonin stimulation panel (eg, calcium, pentagastrin)

This panel must include the following:
Calcitonin (82308 x 3)

80412   Corticotropic releasing hormone (CRH) stimulation panel

This panel must include the following:
Cortisol (82533 x 6)
Adrenocorticotropic hormone (ACTH) (82024 x 6)

80414   Chorionic gonadotropin stimulation panel; testosterone response.

This panel must include the following:
Testosterone (84403 x 2 on 3 pooled blood samples)

▲ **80415**   estradiol response.

This panel must include the following:
Estradiol, total (82670 x 2 on 3 pooled blood samples)

80416   Renal vein renin stimulation panel (eg, captopril)

This panel must include the following:
Renin (84244 x 6)

80417   Peripheral vein renin stimulation panel (eg, captopril)

This panel must include the following:
Renin (84244 x 2)

80418   Combined rapid anterior pituitary evaluation panel

This panel must include the following:
Adrenocorticotropic hormone (ACTH) (82024 x 4)
Luteinizing hormone (LH) (83002 x 4)
Follicle stimulating hormone (FSH) (83001 x 4)
Prolactin (84146 x 4)
Human growth hormone (HGH)(83003 x 4)
Cortisol (82533 x 4)
Thyroid stimulating hormone (TSH) (84443 x 4)

80420   Dexamethasone suppression panel, 48 hour

This panel must include the following:
Free cortisol, urine (82530 x 2)
Cortisol (82533 x 2)
Volume measurement for timed collection (81050 x 2)

(For single dose dexamethasone, use 82533)

80422   Glucagon tolerance panel; for insulinoma

This panel must include the following:
Glucose (82947 x 3)
Insulin (83525 x 3)

80424 for pheochromocytoma.

This panel must include the following:
Catecholamines, fractionated (82384 x 2)

80426 Gonadotropin releasing hormone stimulation panel

This panel must include the following:
Follicle stimulating hormone (FSH) (83001 x 4)
Luteinizing hormone (LH)(83002 x 4)

80428 Growth hormone stimulation panel (eg, arginine infusion, l-dopa administration)

This panel must include the following:
Human growth hormone (HGH)(83003 x 4)

80430 Growth hormone suppression panel (glucose administration)

This panel must include the following:
Glucose (82947 x 3)
Human growth hormone (HGH)(83003 x 4)

80432 Insulin-induced C-peptide suppression panel

This panel must include the following:
Insulin (83525)
C-peptide (84681 x 5)
Glucose (82947 x 5)

80434 Insulin tolerance panel; for ACTH insufficiency

This panel must include the following:
Cortisol (82533 x 5)
Glucose (82947 x 5)

80435   for growth hormone deficiency

This panel must include the following:
Glucose (82947 x 5)
Human growth hormone (HGH) (83003 x 5)

80436 Metyrapone panel

This panel must include the following:
Cortisol (82533 x 2)
11 deoxycortisol (82634 x 2)

80438 Thyrotropin releasing hormone (TRH) stimulation panel; 1 hour

This panel must include the following:
Thyroid stimulating hormone (TSH) (84443 x 3)

80439   2 hour

This panel must include the following:
Thyroid stimulating hormone (TSH) (84443 x 4)

CONSULTATIONS (CLINICAL PATHOLOGY)

A clinical pathology consultation is a service, including a written report, rendered by the pathologist in response to a request from a physicia nor qualified health care professional in relation to a test result(s) requiring additional medical interpretive judgment. Reporting of a test result(s) without medical interpretive judgment is not considered a clinical pathology consultation.

80500 Clinical pathology consultation; limited, without review of patients history and medical records

80502 comprehensive, for a complex diagnostic problem, with review of patients history and medical records

(These codes may also be used for pharmacokinetic consultations)

(For consultations involving the examination and evaluation of the patient, see 99241-99275)

URINALYSIS

For specific analyses, see appropriate section.

81000 Urinalysis, by dip stick or tablet reagent for bilirubin, glucose, hemoglobin, ketones, leukocytes, nitrite, pH, protein, specific gravity,urobilinogen, any number of these constituents; non-automated, with microscopy

81001 automated, with microscopy

81002 non-automated, without microscopy

81003 automated, without microscopy

81005 Urinalysis; qualitative or semiquantitative, except immunoassays

(For non-immunoassay reagent strip urinalysis, see 81000, 81002)

(For immunoassay, qualitative or semiquantitative, use 83518)

(For microalbumin, see 82043, 82044)

81007 bacteriuria screen, except by culture or dipstick

(For culture, see 87086-87088)

(For dipstick, use 81000 or 81002)

81015 microscopic only

(For sperm evaluation for retrograde ejaculation, use 89331)

81020 2 or 3 glass test

81025 Urine pregnancy test, by visual color comparison methods

81050 Volume measurement for timed collection, each

81099 Unlisted urinalysis procedure

MOLECULAR PATHOLOGY

Molecular pathology procedures are medical laboratory procedures involving the analyses of nucleic acid (ie, DNA, RNA) to detect variants in genes that may be indicative of germline (eg, constitutional disorders) or somatic (eg, neoplasia) conditions, or to test for histocompatibility antigens (eg, HLA). Code selection is typically based on the specific gene(s) that is being analyzed. Genes are described using Human Genome Organization (HUGO) approved gene names and are italicized in the code descriptors. Gene names were taken from tables of the HUGO Gene Nomenclature Committee (HGNC) at the time the CPT codes were developed. For the most part, Human Genome Variation Society (HGVS) recommendations were followed for the names of specific molecular variants. The familiar name is used for some variants because defined criteria were not in place when the variant was first described or because HGVS recommendations were changed over time (eg, intronic variants, processed proteins). When the gene name is represented by an abbreviation, the abbreviation is listed first, followed by the full gene name italicized in parentheses (eg, "F5 [coagulation Factor V]"), except for the HLA series of codes. Proteins or diseases commonly associated with the genes are listed as examples in the code descriptors. The examples do not represent all conditions in which testing of the gene may be indicated

● New Code ▲ Revised Code ＋ Add-On Code ⊘ Modifier -51 Exempt ★ Telemedicine

Codes that describe tests to assess for the presence of gene variants use common gene variant names. Typically, all of the listed variants would be tested. However, these lists are not exclusive. If other variants are also tested in the analysis, they would be included in the procedure and not reported separately. Full gene sequencing should not be reported using codes that assess for the presence of gene variants unless specifically stated in the code descriptor.

The molecular pathology codes include all analytical services performed in the test (eg, cell lysis, nucleic acid stabilization, extraction, digestion, amplification, and detection). Any procedures required prior to cell lysis (eg, microdissection, codes 88380 and 88381) should be reported separately.

The results of the procedure may require interpretation by a physician or other qualified health care professional. When only the interpretation and report are performed, modifier 26 may be appended to the specific molecular pathology code.

All analyses are qualitative unless otherwise noted.

For microbial identification, see 87149-87153 and 87471-87801, and 87900-87904. For in situ hybridization analyses, see 88271-88275 and 88365-88368.

Molecular pathology procedures that are not specified in 81200-81383 should be reported using either the appropriate Tier 2 code (81400-81408) or the unlisted molecular pathology procedure code, 81479.

DEFINITIONS

For purposes of CPT reporting, the following definitions apply:

Abnormal allele: an alternative form of a gene that contains a disease-related variation from the normal sequence.

Breakpoint: the region at which a chromosome breaks during a translocation (defined elsewhere). These regions are often consistent for a given translocation.

Codon: a discrete unit of three nucleotides of a DNA or mRNA sequence that encodes a specific amino acid within, or signals the termination of, a polypeptide.

Common variants: variants (as defined elsewhere) that are associated with compromised gene function and are interrogated in a single round of laboratory testing (in a single, typically multiplex, assay format or using more than one assay to encompass all variants to be tested). These variants typically fit the definition of a "mutation," and are usually the predominant ones causing disease. Testing for additional uncommon variants may provide additional limited value in assessment of a patient. Often there are professional society recommendations or guidelines for which variants are most appropriate to test (eg, American College of Medical Genetics/American College of Obstetrics and Gynecology guidelines for variants used in population screening for cystic fibrosis).

Constitutional: synonymous with germline, often used in reference to the genetic code that is present at birth.

Copy number variants (CNVs): structural changes in the genome composed of large deletions or duplications. CNVs can be found in the germline, but can also occur in somatic cells. See also Duplication/Deletion (Dup/ Del).

Cytogenomic: chromosome analysis using molecular techniques.

DNA methylation: the process of adding methyl groups to a DNA sequence, specifically adenine and cytosine nucleotides, thereby affecting transcription of that sequence. DNA hyper-methylation in a gene promoter typically represses gene transcription. DNA methylation serves as a regulatory mechanism in numerous scenarios including development, chromosome inactivation, and carcinogenesis.

DNA methylation analysis: analytical protocols are designed to evaluate the degree of DNA methylation related to specific disease processes. This analysis has various applications, qualitative or quantitative, and could be gene specific or encompass global degrees of methylation. All assays employ specific maneuvers (eg, chemical, enzymatic) that allow for distinguishable evaluation of methylated and non-methylated sequences.

Duplication/Deletion (Dup/Del): terms that are usually used together with the "/" to refer to molecular testing, which assesses the dosage of a particular genomic region. The region tested is typically of modest to substantial size - from several dozen to several million or more nucleotides. Normal gene dosage is two copies per cell, except for the sex chromosomes (X and Y). Thus, zero or one copy represents a deletion, and three (or more) copies represent a duplication.

Dynamic mutation: polynucleotide (eg, trinucleotide) repeats that are in or associated with genes that can undergo disease-producing increases or decreases in the numbers of repeats within tissues and across generations.

Exome: DNA sequences within the human genome that code for proteins (coding regions).

Exon: typically, one of multiple nucleic acid sequences used to encode information for a gene product (polypeptide or protein). Exons are separated from each other by non-protein-coding sequences known as introns. Exons at the respective ends of a gene also contain nucleic acid sequence that does not code for the gene's protein product.

Gene: a nucleic acid sequence that typically contains information for coding a protein as well as for the regulated expression of that protein. Human genes usually contain multiple protein coding regions (exons) separated by non-protein coding regions (introns). See also exon, intron, and polypeptide.

Gene expression: the sequence of events that results in the production and assembly of a protein product corresponding to the information encoded in a specific gene. The process begins with the transcription of gene sequences to produce an mRNA intermediary, which is subsequently translated to produce a specific protein product.b

Genome: The total (nuclear) human genetic content.

Heteroplasmy: The copy number of a variant within a cell; it is expressed as a percent. It reflects the varied distribution and dosage of mutant mitochondria in tissues and organs (mitotic segregation).

Intron: a nucleic acid sequence found between exons in human genes. An intron contains essential sequences for its proper removal (by a process known as splicing) to join exons together and thus facilitate production of a functional protein from a gene. An intron is sometimes referred to as an intervening sequence (IVS).

Inversion: A defect in a chromosome in which a segment breaks and reinserts in the same place but in the opposite orientation.

Loss of heterozygosity (LOH, allelic imbalance): An event that can occur in dividing cells that are heterozygous for one or more alleles, in which a daughter cell becomes hemizygous or homozygous for the allele(s) through mitotic recombination, deletion, or other chromosomal event.

Microarray: surface(s) on which multiple specific nucleic acid sequences are attached in a known arrangement. Sometimes referred to as a 'gene chip'. Examples of uses of microarrays include evaluation of a patient specimen for gains or losses of DNA sequences (copy number variants, CNVs), identification of the presence of specific nucleotide sequence variants (also known as single nucleotide polymorphisms, SNPs), mRNA expression levels, or DNA sequence analysis.

Mitochondrial DNA (mtDNA): DNA located in the mitochondria, which are cytoplasmic organelles involved with energy production. MtDNA contains 37 genes coding for oxidative phosphorylation enzymes, transfer RNAs (tRNAs) and ribosomal RNAs (rRNAs).

Mutations: typically are variants associated with altered gene function that lead to functional deficits or disease (pathogenic).

Mutation scanning: a technique (eg, single strand conformation polymorphism, temperature gradient gel electrophoresis, etc.) typically employed on multiple PCR amplicons to indicate the presence of DNA sequence variants by differences in physical properties compared to normal. Variants are then further characterized by DNA sequence analysis only in amplicons which demonstrate differences.

Nuclear DNA: DNA located in the nucleus of a cell, generally packaged in chromosomes.

Polymorphisms: typically are variants that do not compromise gene function or produce disease (benign).

Polypeptide: a sequence of amino acids covalently linked in a specified order. Polypeptides alone or in combination with other polypeptide subunits are the building blocks of proteins.

Promoter: a region of DNA associated with a gene (on the same strand) which regulates gene expression. Promoter regions can affect gene transcription through the binding of specific transcription factors.

Short Tandem Repeat (STR): a region of DNA where a pattern of two or more nucleotides are repeated. The number of repeating segments can be used as genetic markers for human identity testing.

Single-nucleotide polymorphism (SNP): a DNA sequence variation existing at a significant frequency in the population, in which a single nucleotide (A, T, C, or G) differs between individuals and/or within an individual's paired chromosomes.

Somatic: synonymous with acquired, referring to genetic code alterations that develop after birth (eg, occurring in neoplastic cells).

Translocation: an abnormality resulting from the breakage of a chromosome and the relocation of a portion of that chromosome's DNA sequence to the same or another chromosome. Most common translocations involve a reciprocal exchange of DNA sequences between two differently numbered (ie, non-homologous) chromosomes, with or without a clinically significant loss of DNA.

Uniparental disomy (UPD): Abnormal inheritance of both members of a chromosome pair from one parent, with absence of the other parent's chromosome for the pair.

Variant: a nucleotide sequence difference from the "normal" (predominant) sequence for a given region. Variants are typically of two types: substitutions of one nucleotide for another, and deletions or insertions of nucleotides. Occasionally, variants reflect several nucleotide sequence changes in reasonably close proximity on the same chromosomal strand of DNA (a haplotype). These nucleotide sequence variants often result in amino acid changes in the protein made by the gene. The term variant does not itself carry a functional implication for those protein changes.

Variants in introns are typically described in one of two ways. The altered nucleotide(s) within a defined intervening sequence (eg, IVS3-2A>G) of a gene is listed with a "+" or "-" sign, which indicates the position relative to the first or last nucleotide of the intron. Or, the variant position is indicated relative to the last nucleotide of the preceding exon or first nucleotide of the following exon (eg, c.171+1G>A c.172-1G>T are single nucleotide changes at the first and last nucleotide of a given intron for a specific gene).

The majority of the variants described here are listed by the amino acid change using the single letter amino acid code for the original amino acid followed by the numerical position in the protein product and the amino acid substitution, eg, for ASPA E285A, Glutamic acid (E) at position 285 is replaced with an alanine (A). A few of the variants are described by the DNA change using the numerical position followed by the original nucleotide, a greater than sign (>) and the new nucleotide, eg, MTHFR. 677C>T.

A known familial variant is a specific mutation that has previously been identified within a patient's family.

TIER 1 MOLECULAR PATHOLOGY PROCEDURES

The following codes represent gene-specific and genomic procedures.

81105	This code is out of order. See page 752
81106	This code is out of order. See page 752
81107	This code is out of order. See page 752
81108	This code is out of order. See page 752
81109	This code is out of order. See page 752
81110	This code is out of order. See page 752
81111	This code is out of order. See page 753
81112	This code is out of order. See page 753
81120	This code is out of order. See page 753
81121	This code is out of order. See page 753
81161	This code is out of order. See page 750
81162	This code is out of order. See page 747
81163	This code is out of order. See page 748
81164	This code is out of order. See page 748

81165 This code is out of order. See page 748

81166 This code is out of order. See page 748

81167 This code is out of order. See page 748

81168 This code is out of order. See page 749

81170 *ABL1 (ABL proto-oncogene 1, non-receptor tyrosine kinase)* (eg, acquired imatinib tyrosine kinase inhibitor resistance), gene analysis, variants in the kinase domain

81171 *AFF2 (AF4/FMR2 family, member 2 [FMR2])* (eg, fragile X mental retardation 2 [FRAXE]) gene analysis; evaluation to detect abnormal (eg, expanded) alleles

81172 characterization of alleles (eg, expanded size and methylation status)

81173 This code is out of order. See page 746

81174 This code is out of order. See page 746

81201 *APC (adenomatous polyposis coli)* (eg, familial adenomatosis polyposis [FAP], attenuated FAP) gene analysis; full gene sequence

81202 known familiar variants

81203 duplication/deletion variants

81204 *AR (androgen receptor)* (eg, spinal and bulbar muscular atrophy, Kennedy disease, X chromosome inactivation) gene analysis; characterization of alleles (eg, expanded size or methylation status)

81173 full gene sequence

81174 known familial variant

81200 *ASPA (aspartoacylase)* (eg, Canavan disease) gene analysis, common variants (eg, E285A, Y231X)

81175 *ASXL1 (additional sex combs like 1, transcriptional regulator)* (eg, myelodysplastic syndrome, myeloproliferative neoplasms, chronic myelomonocytic leukemia), gene analysis; full gene sequence

81176 targeted sequence analysis (eg, exon 12)

81177 *ATN1 (atrophin 1)* (eg, dentatorubral-pallidoluysian atrophy) gene analysis, evaluation to detect abnormal (eg, expanded) alleles

81178 *ATXN1 (ataxin 1)* (eg, spinocerebellar ataxia) gene analysis, evaluation to detect abnormal (eg, expanded) alleles

81179 *ATXN2 (ataxin 2)* (eg, spinocerebellar ataxia) gene analysis, evaluation to detect abnormal (eg, expanded) alleles

81180 *ATXN3 (ataxin 3)* (eg, spinocerebellar ataxia, Machado-Joseph disease) gene analysis, evaluation to detect abnormal (eg, expanded) alleles

81181 *ATXN7 (ataxin 7)* (eg, spinocerebellar ataxia) gene analysis, evaluation to detect abnormal (eg, expanded) alleles

81182 *ATXN8OS (ATXN8 opposite strand [non-protein coding])* (eg, spinocerebellar ataxia) gene analysis, evaluation to detect abnormal (eg, expanded) alleles

81183 *ATXN10 (ataxin 10)* (eg, spinocerebellar ataxia) gene analysis, evaluation to detect abnormal (eg, expanded) alleles

● New Code ▲ Revised Code + Add-On Code ⊘ Modifier -51 Exempt ★ Telemedicine

81184   This code is out of order. See page 748

81185   This code is out of order. See page 748

81186   This code is out of order. See page 748

81187   This code is out of order. See page 749

81188   This code is out of order. See page 749

81189   This code is out of order. See page 749

81190   This code is out of order. See page 749

81191   This code is out of order. See page 755

81192   This code is out of order. See page 755

81193   This code is out of order. See page 755

81194   This code is out of order. See page 756

81200   This code is out of order. See page 746

81201   This code is out of order. See page 746

81202   This code is out of order. See page 746

81203   This code is out of order. See page 746

81204   This code is out of order. See page 746

81205   This code is out of order. See page 747

81206   This code is out of order. See page 747

81207   This code is out of order. See page 747

81208   This code is out of order. See page 747

81209   This code is out of order. See page 747

81210   This code is out of order. See page 747

81205   *BCKDHB (branched-chain keto acid dehydrogenase E1, beta polypeptide)* (eg, Maple syrup urine disease) gene analysis, common variants (eg, R183P, G278S, E422X)

81206   *BCR/ABL1 (t(9;22))* (eg, chronic myelogenous leukemia) translocation analysis; major breakpoint, qualitative or quantitative

81207   minor breakpoint, qualitative or quantitative

81208   other breakpoint, qualitative or quantitative

81209   *BLM (Bloom syndrome, RecQ helicase-like)* (eg, Bloom syndrome) gene analysis, 2281del6ins7 variant

81210   *BRAF (B-Raf proto-oncogene, serine/threonine kinase)* (eg, colon cancer), gene analysis, V600 variant(*s*)

81162   *BRCA1 (BRCA1, DNA repair associated)*, BRCA2 (BRCA2, DNA repair associated) (eg, hereditary breast and ovarian cancer) gene analysis; full sequence analysis and full duplication/deletion analysis (ie, detection of large gene rearrangements)

(Do not report 81162 in conjunction with 81163, 81164, 81165, 81166, 81167, 81216, 81217, 81432)

81163   full sequence analysis

81164   full duplication/deletion analysis (ie, detection of large gene rearrangements)

(To report BRCA1, BRCA2 full sequence analysis and full duplication/deletion analysis on the same date of service, use 81162)

(For analysis of common duplication/deletion variant(s) in BRCA1 [ie, exon 13 del 3.835kb, exon 13 dup 6kb, exon 14-20 del 26kb, exon 22 del 510bp, exon 8-9 del 7.1kb], use 81479)

(Do not report 81163 in conjunction with 81162, 81164, 81165, 81216, 81432)

(Do not report 81164 in conjunction with 81162, 81163, 81166, 81167, 81217)

81212   185delAG, 5385insC, 6174delT variants

(81211   deleted 2018 [2019 Edition]. To report, see 81162, 81163, 81164)

(81213   deleted 2018 [2019 Edition]. To report, see 81162, 81163, 81164)

(81214   deleted 2018 [2019 Edition]. To report, see 81165, 81166)

81165   *BRCA1 (BRCA1, DNA repair associated)* (eg, hereditary breast and ovarian cancer) gene analysis; full sequence analysis

81166   full duplication/deletion analysis (ie, detection of large gene rearrangements)

81215   known familial variant

(For analysis of common duplication/deletion variant(s) in BRCA1 [ie, exon 13 del 3.835kb, exon 13 dup 6kb, exon 14-20 del 26kb, exon 22 del 510bp, exon 8-9 del 7.1kb], use 81479)

(Do not report 81165 in conjunction with 81162, 81163, 81432)

(Do not report 81166 in conjunction with 81162, 81164)

81216   *BRCA2 (BRCA2, DNA repair associated)* (eg, hereditary breast and ovarian cancer) gene analysis; full sequence analysis

81167   full duplication/deletion analysis (ie, detection of large gene rearrangements)

81217   known familial variant

(Do not report 81216 in conjunction with 81162, 81163, 81432)

(Do not report 81167 in conjunction with 81162, 81164, 81217)

(Do not report 81217 in conjunction with 81162, 81164, 81167)

81233   *BTK (Bruton's tyrosine kinase)* (eg, chronic lymphocytic leukemia) gene analysis, common variants (eg, C481S, C481R, C481F)

81184   *CACNA1A (calcium voltage-gated channel subunit alpha1 A)* (eg, spinocerebellar ataxia) gene analysis; evaluation to detect abnormal (eg, expanded) alleles

81185   full gene sequence

81186   known familial variant

81219   *CALR (calreticulin)* (eg, myeloproliferative disorders), gene analysis, common variants in exon 9

● **81168** *CCND1/IGH (t(11;14))* (eg, mantle cell lymphoma) translocation analysis, major breakpoint, qualitative and quantitative, if performed

81218 *CEBPA (CCAAT/enhancer binding protein [C/EBP], alpha)* (eg, acute myeloid leukemia), gene analysis, full gene sequence

81219 This code is out of order. See page 748

81220 CFTR (cystic fibrosis transmembrane conductance regulator) (eg, cystic fibrosis) gene analysis; common variants (eg, ACMG/ACOG guidelines)

(When Intron 8 poly-T analysis is performed in conjunction with 81220 in a R117H positive patient, do not report 81224)

81221 known familial variants

81222 duplication/deletion variants

81223 full gene sequence

81224 intron 8 poly-T analysis (eg, male infertility)

81267 Chimerism (engraftment) analysis, post transplantation specimen (eg, hematopoietic stem cell), includes comparison to previously performed baseline analyses; without cell selection

81268 with cell selection (eg, CD3, CD33), each cell type

(If comparative STR analysis of recipient [using buccal swab or other germline tissue sample] and donor are performed after hematopoietic stem cell transplantation, report 81265, 81266 in conjunction with 81267, 81268 for chimerism testing)

81187 *CNBP (CCHC-type zinc finger nucleic acid binding protein)* (eg, myotonic dystrophy type 2) gene analysis, evaluation to detect abnormal (eg, expanded) alleles

81265 Comparative analysis using Short Tandem Repeat (STR) markers; patient and comparative specimen (eg, pre-transplant recipient and donor germline testing, post-transplant non-hematopoietic recipient germline [eg, buccal swab or other germline tissue sample] and donor testing, twin zygosity testing, or maternal cell contamination of fetal cells)

+ **81266** each additional specimen (eg, additional cord blood donor, additional fetal samples from different cultures, or additional zygosity in multiple birth pregnancies) (List separately in addition to code for primary procedure)

(Use 81266 in conjunction with 81265)

81188 *CSTB (cystatin B)* (eg, Unverricht-Lundborg disease) gene analysis; evaluation to detect abnormal (eg, expanded) alleles

81189 full gene sequence

81190 known familial variant(s)

81227 *CYP2C9 (cytochrome P450, family 2, subfamily C, polypeptide 9)* (eg, drug metabolism), gene analysis, common variants (eg, *2, *3, *5, *6)

81225 *CYP2C19 (cytochrome P450, family 2, subfamily C, polypeptide 19)* (eg, drug metabolism), gene analysis, common variants (eg, *2, *3, *4, *8, *17)

81226 *CYP2D6 (cytochrome P450, family 2, subfamily D, polypeptide 6)* (eg, drug metabolism), gene analysis, common variants (eg, *2, *3, *4, *5, *6, *9, *10, *17, *19, *29, *35, *41, *1XN, *2XN, *4XN)

81227 This code is out of order. See page 749

Separate Procedure   Unlisted Procedure   CCI Comp. Code   Non-specific Procedure   **749**

81230   *CYP3A4 (cytochrome P450 family 3 subfamily A member 4)* (eg, drug metabolism), gene analysis, common variant(s) (eg, *2, *22)

81231   *CYP3A5 (cytochrome P450 family 3 subfamily A member 5)* (eg, drug metabolism), gene analysis, common variants (eg, *2, *3, ·*4, *5, *6, *7)

81228   Cytogenomic constitutional (genome-wide) microarray analysis; interrogation of genomic regions for copy number variants (eg, Bacterial Artificial Chromosome [BAC] or oligo-based comparative genomic hybridization [CGH] microarray analysis)

81229   interrogation of genomic regions for copy number and single nucleotide polymorphism (SNP) variants for chromosomal abnormalities

(Do not report 81228 in conjunction with 81229)

(When performing cytogenomic constitutional microarray analysis that is not genome-wide [ie, regionally targeted], report the specific code for the targeted analysis if available [eg, 81405] or the unlisted molecular pathology code [81479])

(Do not report analyte-specific molecular pathology procedures separately in conjunction with 81228, 81229 when the specific analytes are included as part of the microarray analysis)

(Do not report 88271 when performing cytogenomic microarray analysis)

(For genomic sequencing procedures or other molecular multianalyte assays for copy number analysis using circulating cell-free fetal DNA in maternal blood, see 81420, 81422, 81479)

81277   Cytogenomic neoplasia (genome-wide) microarray analysis, interrogation of genomic regions for copy number and loss-of-heterozygosity variants for chromosomal abnormalities

(Do not report analyte-specific molecular pathology procedures separately when the specific analytes are included as part of the cytogenomic microarray analysis for neoplasia)

(Do not report 88271 when performing cytogenomic microarray analysis)

81230   This code is out of order. See page 750

81231   This code is out of order. See page 750

81161   *DMD (dystrophin)* (eg, Duchene/Becker muscular dystrophy) deletion analysis, and duplication analysis, if performed

81234   *DMPK (DM1 protein kinase)* (eg, myotonic dystrophy type 1) gene analysis; evaluation to detect abnormal (expanded) allele

81239   characterization of alleles (eg, expanded size)

81232   *DPYD (dihydropyrimidine dehydrogenase)* (eg, 5-fluorouracil/5-FU and capecitabine drug metabolism), gene analysis, common variant(s) (eg, *2A, *4, *5, *6)

81233   This code is out of order. See page 748

81234   This code is out of order. See page 750

81235   *EGFR (epidermal growth factor receptor)* (eg, non-small cell lunch cancer) gene analysis, common variants (eg, exon 19 LREA deletion, L858R, T790M, G719A, G719S, L861Q)

81236   *EZH2 (enhancer of zeste 2 polycomb repressive complex 2 subunit)* (eg, myelodysplastic syndrome, myeloproliferative neoplasms) gene analysis, full gene sequence

81237   *EZH2 (enhancer of zeste 2 polycomb repressive complex 2 subunit)* (eg, diffuse large B-cell lymphoma) gene analysis, common variant(s) (eg, codon 646)

81238   This code is out of order. See page 751

---

750   ● New Code   ▲ Revised Code   ✚ Add-On Code   ⊘ Modifier -51 Exempt   ★ Telemedicine

81239 This code is out of order. See page 750

81240 *F2 (prothrombin, coagulation factor II)* (eg, hereditary hypercoagulability) gene analysis, 20210G>A variant

81241 *F5 (coagulation Factor V)* (eg, hereditary hypercoagulability) gene analysis, Leiden variant

81238 *F9 (coagulation factor IX)* (eg, hemophilia B), full gene sequence

81242 *FANCC (Fanconi anemia, complementation group C)* (eg, Fanconi anemia, type C) gene analysis, common variant (eg, IVS4+4A>T)

81245 *FLT3 (fms-related tyrosine kinase 3)* (eg, acute myeloid leukemia), gene analysis; internal tandem duplication (ITD) variants (ie, exons 14, 15)

81246 tyrosine kinase domain (TKD) variants (eg., D835, I836)

81243 *FMR1 (Fragile X mental retardation 1)* (eg, fragile X mental retardation) gene analysis; evaluation to detect abnormal (eg, expanded) alleles

(For evaluation to detect and characterize abnormal alleles, see 81243, 81244)

(For evaluation to detect and characterize abnormal alleles using a single assay [eg, PCR], use 81243)

81244 characterization of alleles (eg, expanded size and promoter methylation status)

81245 This code is out of order. See page 751

81246 This code is out of order. See page 751

81284 *FXN (frataxin)* (eg, Friedreich ataxia) gene analysis; evaluation to detect abnormal (expanded) alleles

81285 characterization of alleles (eg, expanded size)

81286 full gene sequence

81289 known familial variant(s)

81250 *G6PC (glucose-6-phosphatase, catalytic subunit)* (eg, Glycogen storage disease, Type 1a, von Gierke disease) gene analysis, common variants (eg, R83C, Q347X)

81247 *G6PD (glucose-6-phosphate dehydrogenase)* (eg, hemolytic anemia, jaundice), gene analysis; common variant(s) (eg, A, A-)

81248 known familial variant(s)

81249 full gene sequence

81250 This code is out of order. See page 751

81251 *GBA (glucosidase, beta, acid)* (eg, Gaucher disease) gene analysis, common variants (eg, N370S, 84GG, L444P, IVS2+1G>A)

81252 *GJB2 (gap junction protein, beta 2, 26kDa; connexin 26)* (eg, nonsyndromic hearing loss) gene analysis; full gene sequence

81253 known familial variants

81254 *GJB6 (gap junction protein, beta 6, 30kDa, connexin 30)* (eg, nonsyndromic hearing loss) gene analysis, common variants (eg, 309kb [del(GJB6-D13S1830)] and 232kb [del(GJB6-D13S1854)])

Separate Procedure   Unlisted Procedure   CCI Comp. Code   Non-specific Procedure   **751**

81257   *HBA1/HBA2 (alpha globin 1 and alpha globin 2)* (eg, alpha thalassemia, Hb Bart hydrops fetalis syndrome, HbH disease), gene analysis; common deletions or variant (eg, Southeast Asian, Thai, Filipino, Mediterranean, alpha3.7, alpha4.2, alpha20.5, Constant Spring)

81258   known familial variant

81259   full gene sequence

81269   duplication/deletion variants

81361   *HBB (hemoglobin, subunit beta)* (eg, sickle cell anemia, beta thalassemia, hemoglobinopathy); common variant(s) (eg, HbS, HbC, HbE)

81362   known familial variant(s)

81363   duplication/deletion variant(s)

81364   full gene sequence

81255   *HEXA (hexosaminidase A [alpha polypeptide])* (eg, Tay-Sachs disease) gene analysis, common variants (eg, 1278insTATC, 1421+1G>C, G269S)

81256   *HFE (hemochromatosis)* (eg, hereditary hemochromatosis) gene analysis, common variants (eg, C282Y, H63D)

81257   This code is out of order. See page 752

81258   This code is out of order. See page 752

81259   This code is out of order. See page 752

81271   *HTT (huntingtin)* (eg, Huntington disease) gene analysis; evaluation to detect abnormal (eg, expanded) alleles

81274   characterization of alleles (eg, expanded size)

81105   *Human Platelet Antigen 1 genotyping (HPA-1), ITGB3(integrin, beta 3 [platelet glycoprotein IIIa], antigen CD61 [GPIIIa])* (eg, neonatal alloimmune thrombocytopenia [NAIT], post-transfusion purpura), gene analysis, common variant, HPA-1a/b (L33P)

81106   *Human Platelet Antigen 2 genotyping (HPA-2), GP1BA (glycoprotein Ib [platelet], alpha polypeptide [GPIba])* (eg, neonatal alloimmune thrombocytopenia [NAIT], posttransfusion purpura), gene analysis, common variant, HPA-2a/b (T145M)

81107   *Human Platelet Antigen 3 genotyping (HPA-3), ITGA2B (integrin, alpha 2b [platelet glycoprotein IIb of IIb/IIIa complex], antigen CD41 [GPIIb])* (eg, neonatal alloimmune thrombocytopenia [NAIT], post-transfusion purpura), gene analysis, common variant, HPA-3a/b (I843S)

81108   *Human Platelet Antigen 4 genotyping (HPA-4), ITGB3 (integrin, beta 3 [platelet glycoprotein IIIa], antigen CD61 [GPIIIa])* (eg, neonatal alloimmune thrombocytopenia [NAIT], post-transfusion purpura), gene analysis, common variant, HPA-4a/b (R143Q)

81109   *Human Platelet Antigen 5 genotyping (HPA-5), ITGA2 (integrin, alpha 2 [CD49B, alpha 2 subunit of VLA-2 receptor] [GPIa])* (eg, neonatal alloimmune thrombocytopenia [NAIT], post-transfusion purpura), gene analysis, common variant (eg, HPA-5a/b (K505E))

81110   *Human Platelet Antigen 6 genotyping (HPA-6w), ITGB3 (integrin, beta 3 [platelet glycoprotein IIIa, antigen CD61] [GPIIIa])* (eg, neonatal alloimmune thrombocytopenia [NAIT], post-transfusion purpura), gene analysis, common variant, HPA-6a/b (R489Q)

81111   *Human Platelet Antigen 9 genotyping (HPA-9w), ITGA2B (integrin, alpha 2b [platelet glycoprotein IIb of IIb/IIIa complex, antigen CD41] [GPIIb])* (eg, neonatal alloimmune thrombocytopenia [NAIT], post-transfusion purpura), gene analysis, common variant, HPA-9a/b (V837M)

81112   *Human Platelet Antigen 15 genotyping (HPA-15), CD109 (CD109 molecule)* (eg, neonatal alloimmune thrombocytopenia [NAIT], post-transfusion purpura), gene analysis, common variant, HPA-15a/b (S682Y)

81120   *IDH1 (isocitrate dehydrogenase 1 [NADP+], soluble)* (eg, glioma), common variants (eg, R132H, R132C)

81121   *IDH2 (isocitrate dehydrogenase 2 [NADP+], mitochondrial)* (eg, glioma), common variants (eg, R140W, R172M)

81283   *IFNL3 (interferon, lambda 3)* (eg, drug response), gene analysis, rs12979860 variant

81261   *IGH@ (Immunoglobulin heavy chain locus)* (eg, leukemias and lymphomas, B-cell), gene rearrangement analysis to detect abnormal clonal population(s); amplified methodology (eg, polymerase chain reaction)

81262   direct probe methodology (eg, Southern blot)

81263   *IGH@ (Immunoglobulin heavy chain locus)* (eg, leukemia and lymphoma, B-cell), variable region somatic mutation analysis

● **81278**   *IGH@/BCL2 (t(14;18))* (eg, follicular lymphoma) translocation analysis, major breakpoint region (MBR) and minor cluster region (mcr) breakpoints, qualitative or quantitative

81264   *IGK@ (Immunoglobulin kappa light chain locus)* (eg, leukemia and lymphoma, B-cell), gene rearrangement analysis, evaluation to detect abnormal clonal population(s)

(For immunoglobulin lambda gene [*IGL@*] rearrangement or immunoglobulin kappa deleting element, [*IGKDEL*] analysis, use 81479)

81260   *IKBKAP (inhibitor of kappa light polypeptide gene enhancer in B-cells, kinase complex-associated protein)* (eg, familial dysautonomia) gene analysis, common variants (eg, 2507+6T>C, R696P)

81261   This code is out of order. See page 752

81262   This code is out of order. See page 752

81263   This code is out of order. See page 752

81264   This code is out of order. See page 752

81265   This code is out of order. See page 749

81266   This code is out of order. See page 749

81267   This code is out of order. See page 749

81268   This code is out of order. See page 749

81269   This code is out of order. See page 752

81270   *JAK2 (Janus kinase 2)* (eg, myeloproliferative disorder) gene analysis, p.Val617Phe (V617F) variant

● **81279**   *JAK2 (Janus kinase 2)* (eg, myeloproliferative disorder) targeted sequence analysis (eg, exons 12 and 13)

81271   This code is out of order. See page 752

81272   *KIT (v-kit-Hardy-Zuckerman 4 feline sarcoma viral oncogene homolog)* (eg, gastrointestinal stromal tumor [GIST], acute myeloid leukemia, melanoma), gene analysis, targeted sequence analysis (eg, exons 8, 11, 13, 17, 18)

| ▉ Separate Procedure | ▉ Unlisted Procedure | ▉ CCI Comp. Code | ▉ Non-specific Procedure | **753** |

81273 *KIT (v-kit-Hardy-Zuckerman 4 feline sarcoma viral oncogene homolog)* (eg, mastocytosis), gene analysis, D816 variant(s)

81274 This code is out of order. See page 752

81275 *KRAS (Kirsten rat sarcoma viral oncogene homolog)* (eg, carcinoma) gene analysis, variants in exon 2 (eg, codons 12 and 13)

81276 additional variant(s) (eg, codon 61, codon 146)

81277 This code is out of order. See page 750

81278 This code is out of order. See page 753

81279 This code is out of order. See page 753

81283 This code is out of order. See page 753

81284 This code is out of order. See page 751

81285 This code is out of order. See page 751

81286 This code is out of order. See page 751

81287 This code is out of order. See page 754

81288 This code is out of order. See page 754

81289 This code is out of order. See page 751

81290 *MCOLN1 (mucolipin 1)* (eg, Mucolipidosis, type IV) gene analysis, common variants (eg, IVS3-2A>G, del6.4kb)

81302 *MECP2 (methyl CpG binding protein 2)* (eg, Rett syndrome) gene analysis; full sequence analysis

81303 known familial variant

81304 duplication/deletion variants

81287 MGMT (O-6-methylguanine-DNA methyltransferase) (eg, glioblastoma multiforme) promoter methylation analysis

81301 Microsatellite instability analysis (eg, hereditary non-polyposis colorectal cancer, Lynch syndrome) of markers for mismatch repair deficiency (eg, BAT25, BAT26), includes comparison of neoplastic and normal tissue, if performed

81292 *MLH1 (mutL homolog 1, colon cancer, nonpolyposis type 2)* (eg, hereditary non-polyposis colorectal cancer, Lynch syndrome) gene analysis; full sequence analysis

81288 promoter methylation analysis

81293 known familial variants

81294 duplication/deletion variants

● **81338** *MPL (MPL proto-oncogene, thrombopoietin receptor)* (eg, myeloproliferative disorder) gene analysis; common variants (eg, W515A, W515K, W515L, W515R)

● **81339** sequence analysis, exon 10

● New Code ▲ Revised Code ✦ Add-On Code ⊘ Modifier -51 Exempt ★ Telemedicine

81295 *MSH2 (mutS homolog 2, colon cancer, nonpolyposis type 1)* (eg, hereditary non-polyposis colorectal cancer, Lynch syndrome) gene analysis; full sequence analysis

81291 This code is out of order. See page 755

81292 This code is out of order. See page 754

81293 This code is out of order. See page 754

81294 This code is out of order. See page 754

81295 This code is out of order. See page 755

81296 known familial variants

81297 duplication/deletion variants

81298 *MSH6 (mutS homolog 6 [E. coli])* (eg, hereditary non-polyposis colorectal cancer, Lynch syndrome) gene analysis; full sequence analysis

81299 known familial variants

81300 duplication/deletion variants

81301 This code is out of order. See page 754

81302 This code is out of order. See page 754

81303 This code is out of order. See page 754

81304 This code is out of order. See page 754

81291 *MTHFR (5,10-methylenetetrahydrofolate reductase)* (eg, hereditary hypercoagulability) gene analysis, common variants (eg, 677T, 1298C)

81305 *MYD88 (myeloid differentiation primary response 88)* (eg, Waldenstrom's macroglobulinemia, lymphoplasmacytic leukemia) gene analysis, p.Leu265Pro (L265P) variant

81306 This code is out of order. See page 756

81307 This code is out of order. See page 756

81308 This code is out of order. See page 756

81309 This code is out of order. See page 756

81310 *NPM1 (nucleophosmin)* (eg, acute myeloid leukemia) gene analysis, exon 12 variants

81311 *NRAS (neuroblastoma RAS viral [v-ras] oncogene homolog)* (eg, colorectal carcinoma), gene analysis, variants in exon 2 (eg, codons 12 and 13) and exon 3 (eg, codon 61)

81312 This code is out of order. See page 756

● **81191** *NTRK1 (neurotrophic receptor tyrosine kinase 1)* (eg, solid tumors) translocation analysis

● **81192** *NTRK2 (neurotrophic receptor tyrosine kinase 2)* (eg, solid tumors) translocation analysis

● **81193** *NTRK3 (neurotrophic receptor tyrosine kinase 3)* (eg, solid tumors) translocation analysis

---

| | Separate Procedure | | Unlisted Procedure | | CCI Comp. Code | | Non-specific Procedure | **755** |

● **81194** *NTRK (neurotrophic-tropomyosin receptor tyrosine kinase 1, 2, and 3)* (eg, solid tumors) translocation analysis

(For translocation analysis NTRK1, NTRK2, and NTRK3 using a single assay, use 81194)

81306 *NUDT15 (nudix hydrolase 15)* (eg, drug metabolism) gene analysis, common variant(s) (eg, *2, *3, *4, *5, *6)

81312 *PABPN1 (poly[A] binding protein nuclear 1)* (eg, oculopharyngeal muscular dystrophy) gene analysis, evaluation to detect abnormal (eg, expanded) alleles

81307 PALB2 (partner and localizer of BRCA2) (eg, breast and pancreatic cancer) gene analysis; full gene sequence

81308 known familial variant

81313 *PCA3/KLK3 (prostate cancer antigen 3 [non-protein coding]/kallikrein-related peptidase 3 [prostate specific antigen])* ratio (eg, prostate cancer)

81314 *PDGFRA (platelet-derived growth factor receptor, alpha polypeptide)* (eg, gastrointestinal stromal tumor [GIST]), gene analysis, targeted sequence analysis (eg, exons 12,18)

81309 PIK3CA (phosphatidylinositol-4, 5-biphosphate 3-kinase, catalytic subunit alpha) (eg, colorectal and breast cancer) gene analysis, targeted sequence analysis (eg, exons 7, 9, 20)

81320 *PLCG2 (phospholipase C gamma 2)* (eg, chronic lymphocytic leukemia) gene analysis, common variants (eg, R665W, S707F, L845F)

81315 *PML/RAR-alpha, (t(15;17)),* (promyelocytic leukemia/retinoic acid receptor alpha) (eg, promyelocytic leukemia) translocation analysis; common breakpoints (eg, intron 3 and intron 6), qualitative or quantitative

81316 single breakpoint (eg, intron 3, intron 6 or exon 6), qualitative or quantitative

(For intron 3 and intron 6 [including exon 6 if performed] analysis, use 81315)

(If both intron 6 and exon 6 are analyzed, without intron 3, use one unit of 81316)

81324 *PMP22 (peripheral myelin protein 22)* (eg, Charcot-Marie-Tooth, hereditary neuropathy with liability to pressure palsies) gene analysis; duplication/deletion analysis

81325 full sequence analysis

81326 known familial variant

81317 *PMS2 (postmeiotic segregation increased 2 [S. cerevisiae])* (eg, hereditary non-polyposis colorectal cancer, Lynch syndrome) gene analysis; full sequence analysis

81318 known familial variants

81319 duplication/deletion variants

81320 This code is out of order. See page 756

81343 *PPP2R2B (protein phosphatase 2 regulatory subunit Bbeta)* (eg, spinocerebellar ataxia) gene analysis, evaluation to detect abnormal (eg, expanded) alleles

81321 *PTEN (phosphatase and tensin homolog)* (eg, Cowden syndrome, *PTEN* hamartoma tumor syndrome) gene analysis; full sequence analysis

81322 known familial variant

● New Code   ▲ Revised Code   ✛ Add-On Code   ⊘ Modifier -51 Exempt   ★ Telemedicine

81323   duplication/deletion variant

81324   This code is out of order. See page 756

81325   This code is out of order. See page 756

81326   This code is out of order. See page 756

81334   *RUNX1 (runt related transcription factor 1)* (eg, acute myeloid leukemia, familial platelet disorder with associated myeloid malignancy), gene analysis, targeted sequence analysis (eg, exons 3-8)

81327   *SEPT9 (Septin9)* (eg, colorectal cancer) promoter methylation analysis

81332   *SERPINA1 (serpin peptidase inhibitor, clade A, alpha-1 antiproteinase, antitrypsin, member 1)* (eg, alpha-1-antitrypsin deficiency), gene analysis, common variants (eg, *S and *Z)

● **81347**   *SF3B1 (splicing factor [3b] subunit B1)* (eg, myelodysplastic syndrome/acute myeloid leukemia) gene analysis, common variants (eg, A672T, E622D, L833F, R625C, R625L)

81328   *SLCO1B1 (solute carrier organic anion transporter family, member 1B1)* (eg, adverse drug reaction), gene analysis, common variant(s) (eg, *5)

81329   *SMN1 (survival of motor neuron 1, telomeric)* (eg, spinal muscular atrophy) gene analysis; dosage/deletion analysis (eg, carrier testing), includes SMN2 (survival of motor neuron 2, centromeric) analysis, if performed

81336   full gene sequence

81337   known familial sequence variant(s)

81330   *SMPD1(sphingomyelin phosphodiesterase 1, acid lysosomal)* (eg, Niemann-Pick disease, Type A) gene analysis, common variants (eg, R496L, L302P, fsP330)

81331   *SNRPN/UBE3A (small nuclear ribonucleoprotein polypeptide N and ubiquitin protein ligase E3A)* (eg, Prader-Willi syndrome and/or Angelman syndrome), methylation analysis

81332   This code is out of order. See page 757

● **81348**   *SRSF2 (serine and arginine-rich splicing factor 2)* (eg, myelodysplastic syndrome, acute myeloid leukemia) gene analysis, common variants (eg, P95H, P95L)

81344   *TBP (TATA box binding protein)* (eg, spinocerebellar ataxia) gene analysis, evaluation to detect abnormal eg, expanded) alleles

81345   *TERT (telomerase reverse transcriptase)* (eg, thyroid carcinoma, glioblastoma multiforme) gene analysis, targeted sequence analysis (eg, promoter region)

81333   *TGFBI (transforming growth factor beta-induced)* (eg, corneal dystrophy) gene analysis, common variants eg, R124H, R124C, R124L, R555W, R555Q)

81334   This code is out of order. See page 757

● **81351**   *TP53 (tumor protein 53)* (eg, Li-Fraumeni syndrome) gene analysis; full gene sequence

● **81352**   targeted sequence analysis (eg, 4 oncology)

● **81353**   known familial variant

81335   *TPMT (thiopurine S-methyltransferase)* (eg, drug metabolism), gene analysis, common variants (eg, *2, *3)

81336   This code is out of order. See page 757

■ Separate Procedure   ■ Unlisted Procedure   ■ CCI Comp. Code   ■ Non-specific Procedure   **757**

81337 This code is out of order. See page 757

81338 This code is out of order. See page 754

81339 This code is out of order. See page 754

81340 *TRB@ (T cell antigen receptor, beta)* (eg, leukemia and lymphoma), gene rearrangement analysis to detect abnormal clonal population(s); using amplification methodology (eg, polymerase chain reaction)

81341   using direct probe methodology (eg, Southern blot)

81342 *TRG@ (T cell antigen receptor, gamma)* (eg, leukemia and lymphoma), gene rearrangement analysis, evaluation to detect abnormal clonal population(s)

(For T cell antigen alpha [*TRA@*] gene rearrangement analysis, use 81479)

(For T cell antigen delta [*TRD@*] gene rearrangement analysis, report 81402)

81343 This code is out of order. See page 756

81344 This code is out of order. See page 757

81345 This code is out of order. See page 757

81346 TYMS (thymidylate synthetase) (eg, 5-fluorouracil/5-FU drug metabolism), gene analysis, common variant(s) (eg, tandem repeat variant)

81347 This code is out of order. See page 757

81348 This code is out of order. See page 757

● **81357** *U2AF1 (U2 small nuclear RNA auxiliary factor 1)* (eg, myelodysplastic syndrome, acute myeloid leukemia) gene analysis, common variants (eg, S34F, S34Y, Q157R, Q157P)

81350 UGT1A1 (UDP glucuronosyltransferase 1 family, polypeptide A1) (eg, drug metabolism, hereditary unconjugated hyperbilirubinemia [Gilbert syndrome]) gene analysis, common variants (eg, *28, *36, *37)

81351 This code is out of order. See page 757

81352 This code is out of order. See page 757

81353 This code is out of order. See page 757

81355 *VKORC1 (vitamin K epoxide reductase complex, subunit 1)* (eg, warfarin metabolism), gene analysis, common variant(s) (eg, -1639G>A, c.173+1000C>T)

81357 This code is out of order. See page 758

● **81360** *ZRSR2 (zinc finger CCCH-type, RNA binding motif and serine/arginine-rich 2)* (eg, myelodysplastic syndrome, acute myeloid leukemia) gene analysis, common variant(s) (eg, E65fs, E122fs, R448fs)

81361 This code is out of order. See page 746

81362 This code is out of order. See page 747

81363 This code is out of order. See page 747

81364 This code is out of order. See page 747

HUMAN LEUKOCYTE ANTIGEN (HLA) TYPING

Human Leukocyte Antigen (HLA) typing is performed to assess compatibility of recipients and potential donors as a part of solid organ and hematopoietic stem cell pre-transplant testing. HLA testing is also performed to identify HLA alleles and allele groups (antigen equivalents) associated with specific diseases and individualized responses to drug therapy (eg, HLA-B*27 and ankylosing spondylitis and HLA0B*57:01 and abacavir hypersensitivity). as well as other clinical uses. One of more HLA genes may be tested in specific clinical situations (eg, HLA-DQB1 for narcolepsy and HLA-A, -B, -C, -DRB1 and -DQB1 for kidney transplantation). Each HLA gene typically has multiple variant alleles or allele groups that can be identified by typing. For HLA result reporting, a low resolution HLA type is denoted by a two digit HLA name (eg, A*02) and intermediate resolution typing by a string of alleles or an NMDP (National Marrow Donor Program) code (eg, B*14:01/07N/08/12/14, B*39CKGN). Both low and intermediate resolution are considered low resolution for code assignment. High resolution typing resolves the common well defined (CWD) alleles and is usually denoted by at least 4 digits (eg, A*02:02, *03:01:01:01, A*26:01:01G, and C*03:04P), however, high resolution typing may include some ambiguities for rare alleles, which may be reported as a string of alleles or an NMDP code.

If additional testing is required to resolve ambiguous allele combinations for high resolution typing, this is included in the base HLA typing codes below. The gene names have been italicized similar to other molecular pathology codes.

(For HLA antigen typing by non-molecular pathology techniques, see 86812, 86813, 86816, 86817, 86821)

81370   HLA Class I and II typing, low resolution (eg, antigen equivalents); *HLA-A, -B, -C, -DRB1/3/4/5*, and *-DQB1*

81371   *HLA-A, -B,* and *-DRB1* (eg, verification typing)

(When HLA typing includes a determination of the presence or absence of the DRB3/4/5 genes, that service is included in the typing and is not separately reported)

81372   HLA Class I typing, low resolution (eg, antigen equivalents); complete (ie, *HLA-A, -B,* and *-C*)

(When performing both Class I and II low resolution HLA typing for *HLA-A, -B, -C, -DRB1/3/4/5*, and *-DQB1*, use 81370)

81373   one locus (eg, *HLA-A, -B,* or *-C*), each

(When performing a complete Class I [*HLA-A, -B* and *-C*] low resolution HLA typing, use 81372)

(When the presence or absence of a single antigen equivalent is reported using low resolution testing, use 81374)

81374   one antigen equivalent (eg, *B*27*), each

(When testing for presence or absence of more than 2 antigen equivalents at a locus, use 81373 for each locus tested)

81375   HLA Class II typing, low resolution (eg, antigen equivalents); *HLA-DRB1/3/4/5* and *-DQB1*

(When performing both Class I and II low resolution HLA typing for *HLA-A, -B, -C, -DRB1/3/4/5* and *-DQB1*, use 81370)

81376   one locus (eg, *HLA-DRB1, -DRB3/4/5, -DQB1, -DQA1, -DPB1,* or *-DPA1*), each

(When low resolution typing is performed for *HLA-DRG1/3/4/5* and *-DQB1*, use 81375)

(When HLA typing includes a determination of the presence or absence of the DRB3/4/5 genes, that service is included in the typing and is not separately reported. When low or intermediate resolution typing of any or all of the DRB3/4/5 genes is performed, treat as one locus)

81377   one antigen equivalent, each

(When testing for presence of absence of more than 2 antigen equivalents at a locus, use 81376 for each locus)

81378   HLA Class I and II typing, high resolution (ie, alleles or allele groups), *HLA-A, -B, -C,* and *-DRB1*

81379 HLA Class I typing, high resolution (ie, alleles or allele groups); complete (ie, *HLA-A, -B*, and *-C*)

81380 one locus (eg, *HLA-A, -B*, or *-C*), each

(When a complete Class I high resolution typing for *HLA-A, -B*, and *-C* is performed, use 81379)

(When the presence of absence of a single allele or allele group is reported using high resolution testing, use 81381)

81381 one allele or allele group (eg, *B*57:01P*), each

(When testing for the presence or absence of more than 2 alleles or allele groups at a locus, use 81380 for each locus)

81382 HLA Class II typing, high resolution (ie, alleles or allele groups); one locus (eg, *HLA-DRB1, -DRB3/4/5, -DQB1, -DQA1, -DPB1*, or *-DPA1*), each

(When only the presence or absence of a single allele or allele group is reported using high resolution testing, use 81383)

(When high resolution typing of any or all of the DRB3/4/5 genes is performed, treat as one locus)

81383 one allele or allele group (eg, *HLA-DQB1*06:02P*), each

(When testing for the presence or absence of more than 2 alleles or allele groups at a locus, use 81382 for each locus)

TIER 2 MOLECULAR PATHOLOGY PROCEDURES

The following molecular pathology procedures (Tier 2) codes are used to report procedures not listed in the Tier 1 molecular pathology codes (81200-81383). They represent medically useful procedures that are generally performed in lower volumes than Tier 1 procedures (eg, the incidence of the disease being tested is rare). They are arranged by level of technical resources and interpretive work by the physician or other qualified health care professional. The individual analyses listed under each code (ie, level of procedure) utilize the definitions and coding principles as described in the introduction preceding the Tier 1 molecular pathology codes. The parenthetical examples of methodologies presented near the beginning of each code provide general guidelines used to group procedures for a given level and are not all-inclusive.

Use the appropriate molecular pathology procedure level code that includes the specific analyte listed after the code descriptor. If the analyte tested is not listed under one of the Tier 2 codes or is not represented by a Tier 1 code, use the unlisted molecular pathology procedure code, 81479. See the Introduction section of the CPT code set for a complete list of the dates of release and implementation.b

81400 Molecular pathology procedure, Level 1 *(eg, identification of single germline variant [eg, SNP] by techniques such as restriction enzyme digestion or melt curve analysis)*

ACADM (acyl-CoA dehydrogenase, C-4 to C-12 straight chain, MCAD) (eg, medium chain acyl dehydrogenase deficiency), K304E variant

ACE (angiotensin converting enzyme) (eg, hereditary blood pressure regulation), insertion/deletion variant

AGTR1 (angiotensin II receptor, type 1) (eg, essential hypertension), 1166A>C variant

BCKDHA (branched chain keto acid dehydrogenase E1, alpha polypeptide) (eg, maple syrup urine disease, type 1A), Y438N variant

CCR5 (chemokine C-C motif receptor 5) (eg, HIV resistance), 32-bp deletion mutation/794 825del32 deletion

CLRN1 (clarin1) (eg, Usher syndrome, type3), N48K variant

F2 (coagulation factor 2) (eg, hereditary hypercoagulability), 1199G>A variant

F5 (coagulation factor V) (eg, hereditary hypercoagulability), HR2 variant

F7 (coagulation factor VII [serum prothrombin conversion accelerator]) (eg, hereditary hypercoagulability), R353Q variant

---

● New Code ▲ Revised Code ✛ Add-On Code ⊘ Modifier -51 Exempt ★ Telemedicine

F13B (coagulation factor XIII, B polypeptide) (eg, hereditary hypercoagulability), V34L variant

FGB (fibrinogen beta chain) (eg, hereditary ischemic heart disease), -455G>A variant

FGFR1 (fibroblast growth factor receptor 1) (eg, Pfeiffer syndrome type 1, craniosynostosis), P252R variant

FGFR3 (fibroblast growth factor receptor 3) (eg, Muenke syndrome), P250R variant

FKTN (fukutin) (eg, Fukuyama congenital muscular dystrophy), retrotransposon insertion variant

GNE (glucosamine [UDP-N-acetyl]-2-epimerase/ N-acetylmannosamine kinase) (eg, inclusion body myopathy 2 [IBM2], Nonaka myopathy), M727T variant

IVD (isovaleryl-CoA dehydrogenase) (eg, isovaleric acidemia), A282V variant

LCT (lactase-phlorizin hydrolase) (eg, lactose intolerance), 13910 C>T variant

NEB (nebulin) (eg, nemaline myopathy 2), exon 55 deletion variant

PCDH15 (protocadherin-related 15) (eg, Usher syndrome type 1F), R245X variant

SERPINE1 (serpine peptidase inhibitor clade E, member 1, plasminogen activator inhibitor -1, PAI-1) (eg, thrombophilia), 4G variant

SHOC2 (soc-2 suppressor of clear homolog) (eg, Noonan-like syndrome with loose anagen hair), S2G variant

SRY (sex determining region Y) (eg, 46,XX testicular disorder of sex development, gonadal dysgenesis), gene analysis

TOR1A (torsin family 1, member A [torsin A]) (eg, early-onset primary dystonia [DYT1]), 907_909delGAG (904_906delGAG) variant

▲ **81401**   Molecular pathology procedure, Level 2 (eg, 2-10 SNPs, 1 methylated variant, or 1 somatic variant [typically using nonsequencing target variant analysis], or detection of a dynamic mutation disorder/triplet repeat)

ABCC8 (ATP-binding cassette, sub-family C [CFTR/MRP], member 8) (eg, familial hyperinsulinism), common variants (eg, c.3898-9G>A [c.3992-9G>A], F1388del)

ABL1 (ABL proto-oncogene 1, non-receptor tyrosine kinase) (eg, acquired imatinib resistance), T315I variant

ACADM (acyl-CoA dehydrogenase, C-4 to C-12 straight chain, MCAD) (eg, medium chain acyl dehydrogenase deficiency), commons variants (eg, K304E, Y42H)

ADRB2 (adrenergic beta-2 receptor surface) (eg, drug metabolism), common variants (eg, G16R, Q27E)

APOB (apolipoprotein B) (eg, familial hypercholesterolemia type B), common variants (eg, R3500Q, R3500W)

APOE (apolipoprotein E) (eg, hyperlipoproteinemia type III, cardiovascular disease, Alzheimer disease), common variants (eg, *2, *3, *4)

CBFB/MYH11 (inv(16)) (eg, acute myeloid leukemia), qualitative, and quantitative, if performed

CBS (cystathionine-beta-synthase) (eg, homocystinuria, cystathionin beta-synthase deficiency), common variants (eg, I278T, G307S)

CFH/ARMS2 (complement factor H/age-related maculopathy susceptibility 2) (eg, macular degeneration), common variants (eg, Y402H [CFH], A69S [ARMS2])

DEK/NUP214 (t(6;9)) (eg, acute myeloid leukemia), translocation analsysis, qualitative, and quantitative, if performed

E2A/PBX1 (t(1;19)) (eg, acute lymphocytic leukemia), translocation analysis, qualitative and quantitative, if performed

EML4/ALK (inv(2)) (eg, non-small cell lunch cancer), translocation or inversion analysis

ETV6/RUNX1 (t(12;21)) (eg, acute lymphocytic leukemia), translocation analysis, qualitative, and quantitative if performed

EWSR1/ATF1 (t(12;22)) (eg, clear cell sarcoma), translocation analysis, qualitative, and quantitative, if performed

EWSR1/ERG (t(21;22)) (eg, Ewing sarcoma/peripheral neuroectodermal tumor), translocation analysis, qualitative, and quantitative, if performed

EWSR1/FLI1 (t(11;22)) (eg, Ewing sarcoma/peripheral neuroectodermal tumor), translocation analysis, qualitative, and quantitative, if performed

EWSR1/WT1 (t(11;22)) (eg, desmoplastic small round cell tumor), translocation analysis, qualitative, and quantitative, if performed

F11 (coagulation factor XI) (eg, coagulation disorder), common variants (eg, E117X [Type II], F283L [Type III], IVS14del14, and IVS14+1G>A [Type I])

FGFR3 (fibroblast growth factor receptor 3) (eg, achondroplasia), common variants (eg, 1138G>A, 1138G>C)

FIP1L1/PDGFRA (del[4q12]) (eg, imatinib-sensitive chronic eosinophilic leukemia), qualitative, and quantitative, if performed

FLG (filaggrin) (eg, icthyosis vulgaris), common variants (eg, R501X, 2282del4, R2447X, S3247X, 3702delG)

FOXO1/PAX3 (t(2;13)) (eg, alveolar rhabdomyosarcoma), translocation analysis, qualitative, and quantitative, if performed

FOXO1/PAX7 (t(1;13)) (eg, alveolar rhabdymyocarcoma), translocation analysis, qualitative, and quantitative, if performed

FUS/DDIT3 (t(12;16)) (eg, myxoid liposarcoma), translocation analysis, qualitative, and quantitative, if performed

GALC (galactosylceramidase) (eg, Krabbe disease), common variants (eg, c.857G>A, 30-kb deletion)

GALT (galactose-1-phosphate uridylyltransferase) (eg, galactosemia), common variants (eg, Q188R, S135L, K285N, T138M, L195P, Y209C, IVS2-2A>G, P171S, del5kb, N314D, L218L/N314D)

H19 (imprinted maternally expressed transcript [non-protein coding]) (eg, Beckwith-Wiedemann syndrome), methylation analysis

IGH@/BCL2 (t(14;18)) (eg, follicular lymphoma), translocation analysis; single breakpoint (eg, major breakpoint region [MBR] or minor cluster region [mcr]), qualitative or quantitative

(When both MBR and mcr breakpoints are performed, use 81278)

KCNQ1OT1 (KCNQ1 overlapping transcript 1 [non-protein coding]) (eg, Beckwith-Wiedemann syndrome), methylation analysis

LINC00518 (long intergenic non-protein coding RNA 518) (eg, melanoma), expression analysis

LRRK2 (leucine-rich repeat kinase 2) (eg, Parkinson disease), common variants (eg, R1441G, G2019S, I2020T)

MED12 (mediator complex subunit 12) (eg, FG syndrome type 1, Lujan syndrome), common variants (eg, R961W, N1007S)

MEG3/DLK1 (maternally expressed 3 [non-protein coding]/delta-like 1 homolog [Drosophila]) (eg, intrauterine growth retardation), methylation analysis

MLL/AFF1 (t(4;11)) (eg, acute lymphoblastic leukemia), translocation analysis, qualitative, and quantitative if performed

MLL/MLLT3 (t(9;11)) (eg, acute myeloid leukemia), translocation analysis, qualitative, and quantitative, if performed

MT-ATP6 (mitochondrially encoded ATP synthase 6) (eg, neuropathy with ataxia and retinitis pigmentosa [NARP], Leigh syndrome), common variants (eg, m.8993T>G, m.8993T>C)

MT-ND4, MT-ND6 (mitochondrially encoded NADH dehydrogenase 4, mitochondrially encoded NADH dehydrogenase 6) (eg, Leber hereditary optic neuropathy [LHON]), common variants (eg, m.11778G>A, M.3460G>A, m.14484T>C)

MT-ND5 (mitochondrially encoded tRNA leucine 1 [UUA/G], mitochondrially encoded NADH dehydrogenase 5) (eg, mitochondrial encephalopathy with lactic acidosis and stroke-like episodes [MELAS]), common variants (eg, m.3243A>G, m.3271T>C, m.3252A>G, m.13513G>A)

MT-RNR1 (mitochondrially encoded 12S RNA) (eg, nonsyndromic hearing loss), common variants (eg, m.1555A>G, m.1494C>T)

MT-TK (mitochondrially encoded tRNA lysine) (eg, myoclonic epilepsy with ragged-red fibers [MERRF]), common variants (eg, m.8344A>G, m.8356T>C)

MT-TL1 (mitochondrially encoded tRNA leucine 1 [UUA/G]) (eg, diabetes and hearing loss), common variants (eg, M3243A>G, M.14709T>C) MT-TL1,

MT-TS1, MT-RNR1 (mitochondrially encoded tRNA serine 1 [UCN], mitochondrially encoded 12S RNA) (eg, nonsyndromic sensorineural deafness [including aminoglycoside-induced nonsyndromic deafness]), common variants (eg, m.7445A>G, m.1555A>G)

MUTYH (mutY homolog [E.coli]) (eg, MYH-associated polyposis), common variants (eg, Y165C, G382D)

NOD2 (nucleotide-binding oligomerization domain containing 2) (eg, Crohn's disease, Blau syndrome), common variants (eg, SNP8, SNP 12, SNP 13)

NPM1/ALK (t(2;5)) (eg, anaplastic large cell lymphoma), transloation analysis

PAX8/PPARG (t(2;3) (q13;p25)) (eg, follicular thyroid carcinoma), translocation analysis

PRAME (preferentially expressed antigen in melanoma) (eg, melanoma), expression analysis

PRSS1 (protease, serine, 1 [trypsin1]) (eg, hereditary pancreatitis), common variants (eg, N29I, A16V, R122H)

PYGM (phosphorylase, glycogen, muscle) (eg, glycogen storage disease type V, McArdle disease), common variants (eg, R50X, G205S)

RUNX1/RUNX1T1 (t(8;21)) (eg, acute myeloid leukemia) translocation analysis, qualitative, and quantitative, if performed

SS18/SSX1 (t(X;18)) (eg, synovial sarcoma), translocation analysis, qualitative, and quantitative, if performed

SS18/SSX2 (t(X;18)) (eg, synovial sarcoma), translocation analysis, qualitative and quantitative if performed

VWF (von Willebrand factor) (eg, von Willebrand disease type 2N), common variants (eg, T791M, R816W, R854Q)

▲ **81402** Molecular pathology procedure, Level 3 (eg, >10 SNPs, 2-10 methylated variants, or 2-10 somatic variants [typically using non-sequencing target variant analysis], immunoglobulin and T-cell receptor gene rearrangements, duplication/deletion variants of 1 exon, loss of heterozygosity [LOH], uniparental disomy [UPD])

Chromosome 1p-/19q- (eg., glial tumors), deletion analysis

Chromosome 18q- (eg, D18S55, D18S58, D18S61, D18S64, and D18S69) (eg, colon cancer), allelic imbalance assessment (ie, loss of heterozygosity)

COL1A1/PDGFB (t(17;22)) (eg, dermatofibrosarcoma protuberans), translocation analysis, mutiple breakpoints, qualitative, and quantitative, if performed

CYP21A2 (cytochrome P450, family 21, subfamily A, polypeptide 2) (eg, congenital adrenal hyperplasia, 21-hydroxylase deficiency), common variants (eg, IVS2-13G, P30L, I172N, exon 6 mutation cluster [I235N, V236E, M238K], V281L, L307FfsX6, Q318X, R356W, P453S, G110VfsX21, 30-kb deletion variant)

ESR1/PGR (receptor 1/progesterone receptor) ratio (eg, breast cancer)

MEFV (Mediterranean fever) (eg, familial Mediterranean fever), common variants (eg, E148Q, P369S, F479L, M680I, I692del, M694V, M694I, K695R, V726A, A744S, R761H)

TRD@ (T cell antigen receptor, delta) (eg, leukemia and lymphoma), gene rearrangement analysis, evaluation to detect abnormal clonal population

Uniparental disomy (UPD) (eg, Russell-Silver syndrome, Prader-Willi/Angelman syndrome), short tandem repeat (STR) analysis

▲ **81403**   Molecular pathology procedure, Level 4 (eg, analysis of single exon by DNA sequence analysis, analysis of >10 amplicons using multiplex PCR in 2 or more independent reactions, mutation scanning or duplication/deletion variants of 2-5 exons)

ANG (angiogenin, ribonuclease, RNase A family, 5) (eg, amyotrophic lateral sclerosis), full gene sequence

ARX (aristaless-related homeobox) (eg, X-linked lissencephaly with ambiguous genitalia, X-linked mental retardation), duplication/deletion analysis

CEL (carboxyl ester lipase [bile salt-stimulated lipase]) (eg, maturity-onset diabetes of the young [MODY]), targeted sequence analysis of exon 11 (eg, c.1785delC, c.1686delT)

CTNNB1 (catenin [cadherin-associated protein], beta 1, 88kDa) (eg, desmoid tumors) targeted sequence analysis (ex, exon 3)

DAZ/SRY (deleted in azoospermia and sex determining region Y) (eg, male infertility), common deletions (eg, AZFa, AZFb, AZFc, AZFd)

DNMT3A (DNA [cytosine-5-]-methyltransferase 3 alpha) (eg, acute myeloid leukemia), targeted sequence analysis (eg, exon 23)

EPCAM (epithelial cell adhesion molecule) (eg, Lynch syndrome), duplication/deletion analysis

F8 (coagulation factor VIII) (eg, hemophilia A), inversion analysis, intron 1 and intron 22A

F12 (coagulation factor XII [Hageman factor]) (eg, angioedema, hereditary, type III, factor XII deficiency), targeted sequence analysis of exon 9

FGFR3 (fibroblast growth factor receptor 3) (eg, isolated craniosynostosis), targeted sequence analysis (ex, exon 7)

(For targeted sequence analysis of multiple FGFR3 exons, use 81404)

GJB1 (gap junction protein, beta 1) (eg, Charcot-Marie-Tooth X-linked), full gene sequence

GNAQ (guanine nucleotide-binding protein G[q] subunit alpha) (eg, uveal melanoma), common variants (eg, R183, Q209)

Human erythrocyte antigen gene analyses (eg., SLC14A1 [Kidd blood group], BCAM [Lutheran blood group], ICAM4 [Landsteiner-Wiener blood group], SLC4A1 [Diego blood group], AQP1 [Colton blood group], ERMAP [Scianna blood group], RHCE [Rh blood group, CcEe antigens], KEL [Kell blood group], DARC [Duffy blood group], GYPA, GYPB, GYPE [MNS blood group], ART4 {Dombrock blood group],) e(eg., sickle cell disease, thalassemia, hemolytic transfusion reactions, hemolytic disease of the fetus or newborn), common variants

HRAS (v-Ha-ras Harvey rat sarcoma viral oncogene homolog) (eg, Costello syndrome), exon 2 sequence

KCNC3 (potassium voltage-gated channel, Shaw-related subfamily, member 3) (eg, spinocerebellar ataxia), targeted sequence analysis (eg, exon 2)

KCNJ2 (potassium inwardly-rectifying channel, subfamily J, member 2) (eg, Andersen-Tawil syndrome), full gene sequence

KCNJ11 (potassium inwardly-rectifying channel, subfamily J, member 11) (eg, familial hyperinsulinism), full gene sequence

Killer cell immunoglobulin-like receptor (KIR) gene family (eg, hematopoietic stem cell transplantation), genotyping of KIR family genes

Known familial variant not otherwise specified, for gene listed in Tier 1 or Tier 2, or identified during a genomic sequencing procedure, DNA sequence analysis, each variant exon

---

(For a known familial variant that is considered a common variant, use specific common variant Tier 1 or Tier 2 code)

MC4R (melanocortin 4 receptor) (eg, obesity), full gene sequence

MICA (MHC class I polypeptide-related sequence A) (eg, solid organ transplantation), common varients (eg, *001, *002)

MT-RNR1 (mitochondrially encoded 12S RNA) (eg, nonsyndromic hearing loss), full gene sequence

MT-TS1 (mitochondrially encoded tRNA serine 1) (eg, nonsyndromic hearing loss), full gene sequence

NDP (Norrie disease [pseydoglioma]) (eg, Norrie disease), duplication/deletion analysis

NHLRC1 (NHL repeat containing 1) (eg, progressive myoclonus epilepsy), full gene sequence

PHOX2B (paired-like homeobox 2b) (eg, congenital central hypoventilation syndrome), duplication/deletion analysis

PLN (phospholamban) (eg, dilated cardiomyopathy, hypertrophic cardiomyopathy), full gene sequence

RHD (Rh blood group, D antigen) (eg., hemolytic disease of the fetus and newborn, Rh maternal/fetal compatibility), deletion analsysis (eg., exons 4, 5, and 7, pseudogene)

RHD (Rh blood group, D antigen) (eg., hemolytic disease of the fetus and newborn, Rh maternal/fetal compatibility), deletion analsysis (eg., exons 4, 5, and 7, pseudogene) performed on cell-free fetal DNA in maternal blood

(For human erythrocyte gene analysis of RHD, use a separate unit of 81403)

SH2D1A (SH2 domain containing 1A) (eg, X-linked ymphoproliferative syndrome), duplication/deletion analysis

TWIST1 (twist homolog 1 [Drosophila]) (eg, Saethre-Chotzen syndrome), duplication/deletion analysis

UBA1 (ubiquitin-like modifier activating enzyme 1) (eg, spinal muscular atrophy, X-linked), target sequence analysis (eg, exon 15)

VHL (von Hippel-Lindau tumor suppressor) (eg, von Hippel-Lindau familial cancer syndrome), deletion/duplication analysis

VWF (von Willebrand factor) (eg, von Willebrand disease types 2A, 2B, 2M), targeted sequence analysis (eg, exon 28)

▲ **81404**   Molecular pathology procedure, Level 5 (eg, analysis of 2-5 exons by DNA sequence analysis, mutation scanning or duplication/deletion variants of 6-10 exons, or characterization of a dynamic mutation disorder/triplet repeat by Southern blot analysis)

ACADS (acyl-CoA dehydrogenase, C-2 to C-3 short chain) (eg, short chain acyl-CoA dehydrogenase deficiency), targeted sequence analysis (eg, exons 5 and 6)

AQP2 (aquaporin 2 [collecting duct]) (eg, nephrogenic diabetes insipidus), full gene sequence

ARX (aristaless related homeobox) (eg, X-linked lissencephaly with ambiguous genitalia, X-linked mental retardation) full gene sequence

AVPR2 (arginine vasopressin receptor 2) (eg, nephrogenic diabetes insipidus), full gene sequence

BBS10 (Bardet-Biedl syndrome 10) (eg, Bardet-Biedl syndrome), full gene sequence

BTD (biotinidase) (eg, biotinidase deficiency), full gene sequence

C10orf2 (chromosome 10 open reading frame 2) (eg, mitochondrial DNA depletion syndrome), full gene sequence

CAV3 (caveolin 3) (eg, CAV3-related distal myopathy, limb-girdle muscular dystrophy type 1C), full gene sequence

CD4OLG (CD40 ligand) (eg, X-linked hyper IgM syndrome), full gene sequence

CDKN2A (cyclin-dependent kinase inhibitor 2A) (eg, CDKN2A-related cutaneous malignant melanoma, familiarl atypical mole-malignant melanoma syndrome), full gene sequence

CLRN1 (clarin 1) (eg, Usher syndrome, type 3), full gene sequence

COX6B1 (cytochrome c oxidase subunit VIb polypeptide 1) (eg, mitochondrial respiratory chain complex IV deficiency), full gene sequence

CPT2 (carnitine palmitoyltransferase 2) (eg, carnitine palmitoyltransferase II deficiency), full gene sequence

CRX (cone-rod homeobox) (eg, cone-rod dystrophy 2, Leber congenital amaurosis), full gene sequence

CYP1B1 (cytochrome P450, family 1, subfamily B, polypeptide 1) (eg, primary congenital glaucoma), full gene sequence

EGR2 (early growth response 2) (eg, Charcot-Marie-Tooth), full gene sequence

EMD (emerin) (eg, Emery-Dreifuss muscular dystrophy), duplication/deletion analysis

EPM2A (epilepsy, progressive myoclonus type 2A, Lafora disease [laforin]) (eg, progressive myoclonus epilepsy), full gene sequence

FGF23 (fibroblast growth factor 23) (eg, hypophosphatemic rickets), full gene sequence

FGFR2 (fibroblast growth factor receptor 2) (eg, craniosynostosis, Apert syndrome, Crouzon syndrome), targeted sequence analysis (eg, exons 8,10)

FGFR3 (fibroblast growth factor receptor 3) (eg, achondroplasia, hypochondroplasia), targeted sequence analysis (eg, exons 8, 11,12,13)

FHL1 (four and a half LIM domains 1) (eg, Emery-Dreifuss muscular dystrophy), full gene sequence

FKRP (Fukutin related protein) (eg, congenital muscular dystrophy type 1C [MDC1C], limb-girdle muscular dystrophy [LGMD] type 2I), full gene sequence

FOXG1 (forkhead box G1) (eg, Rett syndrome), full gene sequence

FSHMD1A (facioscapulohumeral muscular dystrophy 1A) (eg, facioscapulohumeral muscular dystrophy), evaluation to detect abnormal (eg, deleted) alleles

FSHMD1A (facioscapulohumeral muscular dystrophy 1A) (eg, facioscapulohumeral muscular dystrophy), characterization of haplotype(s) (ie, chromosome 4A and 4B haplotypes)

GH1 (growth hormone 1) (eg, growth hormone deficiency), full gene sequence

GP1BB (glycoprotein 1b [platelet], beta polypeptide) (eg, Bernard-Soulier syndrome type B), full gene sequence

(For common deletion variants of alpha globin 1 and alpha globin 2 genes, use 81257)

HNF1B (HNF1 homeobox B) (eg, maturity-onset diabetes of the young [MODY]), duplication/deletion analysis

HRAS (v-Ha-ras Harvey rat sarcoma viral oncogene homolog) (eg, Costello syndrome), full gene sequence

HSD3B2 (hydroxy-delta-5-steroid dehydrogenase, 3 beta- and steroid delta-isomerase 2) (eg, 3-beta-hydroxysteroid dehydrogenase type II deficiency), full gene sequence

HSD11B2 (hydroxysteroid [11-beta] dehydrogenase 2) (eg, mineralocorticoid excess syndrome), full gene sequence

HSPB1 (heat shock 27kDa protein 1) (eg, Charcot-Marie-Tooth disease), full gene sequence

INS (insulin) (eg, diabetes mellitus), full gene sequence

KCNJ1 (potassium inwardly-rectifying channel, subfamily J, member 1) (eg, Bartter syndrome), full gene sequence

KCNJ10 (potassium inwardly-rectifying channel, subfamily J, member 10) (eg, SeSAME syndrome, EAST syndrome, sensorineural hearing loss), full gene sequence

LITAF (lipopolysaccharide-induced TNF factor) (eg, Charcot-Marie-Tooth), full gene sequence

MEFV (Mediterranean fever) (eg, familial Mediterranean fever), full gene sequence

MEN1 (multiple endocrine neoplasia 1) (eg, multiple endocrine neoplasia type 1, Wermer syndrome), duplication/deletion analysis

MMACHC (methylmalonic aciduria [cobalamin deficiency] cblC type, with homocystinuria) (eg, methylmalonic acidemia and homocystinuria), full gene sequence

MPV17 (MpV17 mitochrondrial inner membrane protein) (eg., mitochondrial DNA depletion syndrome), duplication/deletion analysis

NDP (Norrie disease [pseudoglioma]) (eg, Norrie disease}, full gene sequence

NDUFA1 (NADH dehydrogenase [ubiquinone] 1 alpha subcomplex, 1, 7.5kDa) (eg, Leigh syndrome, mitochondrial complex 1 deficiency), full gene sequence

NDUFAF2 (NADH dehydrogenase [ubiquinone] 1 alpha subcomplex, assembly factor 2) (eg, Leigh syndrome, mitochondrial complex 1 deficiency), full gene sequence

NDUFS4 (NADH dehydrogenase [ubiquinone] Fe-S protein 4, 18kDa [NADH-coenzyme Q reductase]) (eg, Leigh syndrome, mitochondrial complex 1 deficiency), full gene sequence

NIPA1 (non-imprinted in Prader-Willi/Angelman syndrome 1) (eg, spastic paraplegia), full gene sequence

NLGN4X (neuroligin 4, X-linked) (eg, autism spectrum disorders), duplication/deletion analysis

NPC2 (Niemann-Pick disease, type C2 [epididymal secretory protein E1]) (eg, Niemann-Pick disease type C2), full gene sequence

NR0B1 (nuclear receptor subfamily 0, group B, member 1) (eg, congenital adrenal hypoplasia), full gene sequence

PDX1 (pancreatic and duodenal homeobox 1) (eg, maturity-onset diabetes of the young [MODY]), full gene sequence

PHOX2B (paired-like homeobox 2b) (eg, congenital central hypoventilation syndrome), full gene sequence

PLP1 (proteolipid protein 1) (eg, Pelizaeus-Merzbacher disease, spastic paraplegia), duplication/deletion analysis

PQBP1 (polyglutamine binding protein 1) (eg, Renpenning syndrome), duplication/deletion analysis

PRNP (prion protein) (eg, genetic prion disease), full gene sequence

PROP1 (PROP paired-like homeobox 1) (eg, combined pituitary hormone deficiency), full gene sequence

PRPH2 (peripherin 2[retinal degeneration, slow]) (eg, retinitis pigmentosa), full gene sequence

PRSS1 (protease, serine, 1[trypsin1]) (eg, hereditary pancreatitis), full gene sequence

RAF1 (v-raf-1 murine leukemia viral oncogene homolog 1) (eg, LEOPARD syndrome), targeted sequence analysis (eg, exons 7, 12, 14, 17)

RET (ret proto-oncogene) (eg, multiple endocrine neoplasia, type 2B and familial medullary thyroid carcinoma), common variants (eg, M918T, 2647_2648delinsTT, A883F)

RHO (rhodopsin) (eg, retinitis pigmentosa), full gene sequence

RP1 (retinitis pigmentosa 1) (eg, retinitis pigmentosa), full gene sequence

SCN!B (sodium channel, voltage-gated, type I, beta) (eg, Brugada syndrome), full gene sequence

SCO2 (SCO cytochrome oxidase deficient homolog 2 [SCO1L]) (eg, mitochondrial respiratory chain complex IV deficiency), full gene sequence

SDHC (succinate dehydrogenase complex, subunit C, integral membrane protein, 15kDa) (eg, hereditary paraganglioma-pheochromocytoma syndrome), duplication/deletion analysis

---

Separate Procedure   Unlisted Procedure   CCI Comp. Code   Non-specific Procedure   **767**

SDHD (succinate dehydrogenase complex, subunit D, integral membrane protein) (eg, hereditary paraganglioma), full gene sequence

SCGC (sarcoglycan, gamma [35kDa dystrophin-associated glycoprotein]) (eg, limb-girdle muscular dystrophy), duplication/deletion analysis

SH2D1A (SH2 domain containing 1A) (eg, X-linked lymphoproliferative syndrome), full gene sequence

SLC16A2 (solute carrier family 16, member 2 [thyroid hormone transporter]) (eg, specific thyroid hormone cell transporter deficiency, Allan-Herndon-Dudley syndrome), duplication/deletion analysis

SLC25A20 (solute carrier family 25 [carnitine/acylcarnitine translocase], member 20) (eg, carnitine-acylcarnitine translocase deficiency), duplication/deletion analysis

SLC25A4 (solute carrier family 25 [mitochondrial carrier; adenine nucleotide translocator], member 4) (eg, progressive external ophthalmoplegia), full gene sequence

SOD1 (superoxide dismutase 1, soluble) (eg, amyotrophic lateral sclerosis), full gene sequence

SPINK1 (serine peptidase inhibitor, Kazal type 1) (eg, hereditary pancreatitis), full gene sequence

STK11 (werine/threonine kinase 11) (eg, Peutz-Jeghers syndrome), duplication/deletion analysis

TACO1 (translational activator of mitochondrial encoded cytochrome c oxidase I) (eg, mitochondrial respiratory chain complex IV deficiency), full gene sequence

THAP1 (THAP domain continaing, apoptosis associated protein 1) (eg, torsion dystonia), full gene sequence

TOR1A (torsin family 1, member A [torsin A]) (eg, torsion dystonia), full gene sequence

TTPA (tocopherol [alpha] transfer protein) (eg, ataxia), full gene sequence

TTR (transthyretin) (eg, familial transthyretin amyloidosis), full gene sequence

TWIST1 (twist homolog 1 [Drosophila]) (eg, Saethre-Chotzen syndrome), full gene sequence

TYR (tyrosinase [oculocutaneous albinism IA]) (eg, oculocutaneous albinism IA), full gene sequence

UGT1A1 (UDP glucuronosyltransferase 1 family, polypeptide A1) (eg, hereditary unconjugated hyperbilirubinemia [Crigler-Najjar syndrome]) full gene sequence

USH1G (Usher syndrome 1G [autosomal recessive]) (eg, Usher syndrome type 1), full gene sequence

VHL (von Hippel-Lindau tumor suppressor) (eg, von Hippel-Lindau familial cancer syndrome), full gene sequence

VWF (von Willebrand factor) (eg, von Willebrand disease type 1C), targeted sequence analysis (eg, exons 26, 27, 37)

ZEB2 (zinc finger E-box binding homeobox 2) (eg, Mowat-Wilson syndrome), duplication/deletion analysis

ZNF41 (zinc finger protein 41) (eg, X-linked mental retardation 89), full gene sequence

▲ **81405** Molecular pathology procedure, Level 6 (eg, analysis of 6-10 exons by DNA sequence analysis, mutation scanning or duplication/deletion variants of 11-25 exons, regionally targeted cytogenomic array analysis)

ABCD1 (ATP-binding cassette, sub-family D [ALD], member 1) (eg, adrenoleukodystrophy), full gene sequence

ACADS (acyl-CoA dehydrogenase, C-2 to C-3 short chain) (eg, short chain acyl-CoA dehydrogenase deficiency) full gene sequence

ACTA2 (actin, alpha 2, smooth muscle, aorta) (eg, thoracic aortic aneurysms and aortic dissections), full gene sequence

ACTC1 (actin, alpha, cardiac muscle 1) (eg, familial hypertrophic cardiomyopathy), full gene sequence

ANKRD1 (ankyrin repeat domain 1) (eg, dilated cardiomyopathy), full gene sequence

APTX (aprataxin) (eg, ataxia with oculomotor apraxia 1), full gene sequence

● New Code   ▲ Revised Code   ✛ Add-On Code   ⊘ Modifier -51 Exempt   ★ Telemedicine

ARSA (arylsulfatase A) (eg, arylsulfatase A deficiency), full gene sequence

BCKDHA (branched chain keto acid dehydrogenase E1, alpha polypeptide) (eg, maple syrup urine disease, type 1A), full gene sequence

BCS1L (BCS1-like [S. cerevisiae]) (eg, Leigh syndrome, mitochondrial complex III deficiency, GRACILE syndrome), full gene sequence

BMPR2 (bone morphogenetic protein receptor, typye II [serine/threonine kinase]) (eg, heritable pulmonary arterial hypertension), duplication/deletioin analsyis

CASQ2 (calsequestrin 2 [cardiac muscle]) (eg, catecholaminergic polymorphic ventricular tachycardia), full gene sequence

CASR (calcium-sensing receptor) (eg, hypocalcemia), full gene sequence

CDKL5 (cyclin-dependent kinase-like 5) (eg, early infantile epileptic encephalopathy), duplication/deletion analysis

CHRNA4 (cholinergic receptor, nicotinic, alpha 4) (eg, nocturnal frontal lobe epilepsy), full gene sequence

CHRNB2 (cholinergic receptor, nicotinic, beta 2 [neuronal]) (eg, nocturnal frontal lobe epilepsy), full gene sequence

COX10 (COX10 homolog, cytochrome c oxidase assembly protein) (eg, mitochondrial respiratory chain complex IV deficiency), full gene sequence

COX15 (COX15 homolog, cytochrome c oxidase assembly protein) (eg, mitochondrial respiratory chain complex IV deficiency), full gene sequence

CPOX (coproporphyrinogen oxidase) (eg, hereditary coproporphyria), full gene sequence

CTRC (chymotrypsin C) (eg, hereditary pancreatitis), full gene sequence

CYP11B1 (cytochrome P450, family 11, subfamily B, polypeptide 1) (eg, congenital adrenal hyperplasia), full gene sequence

CYP17A1 (cytochrome P450, family 17, subfamily A, polypeptide 1) (eg, congenital adrenal hyperplasia), full gene sequence

CYP21A2 (cytochrome P450, family 21, subfamily A, polypeptide2) (eg, steroid 21-hydroxylase isoform, congenital adrenal hyperplasia), full gene sequence

Cytogenomic constitutional targeted microarray analysis of chromosome 22q13 by interrogation of genomic regions for copy number and single nucleotide polymorphism (SNP) variants for chromosomal abnormalities

(When performing genome-wide cystogenomic constitutional microarray analysis, see 81228, 81229)

(Do not report analyte-specific molecular pathology procedures separately when the specific analytes are included as part of the microarray analysis of chromosome 22q13)

(Do not report 88271 when performing cytogenomic microarray analysis)

DBT (dihydrolipoamide branched chain transacylase E2) (eg, maple syrup urine disease, type 2), duplication/deletion analysis

DCX (doublecortin) (eg, X-linked lissencephaly), full gene sequence

DES (desmin) (eg, myofibrillar myopathy), full gene sequence

DFNB59 (deafness, autosomal recessive 59) (eg, autosomal recessive nonsyndromic hearing impairment), full gene sequence

DGUOK (deoxyguanosine kinase) (eg, hepatocerebral mitochondrial DNA depletion syndrome), full gene sequence

DHCR7 (7-dehydrocholesterol reductase) (eg, Smith-Lemli-Opitz syndrome), full gene sequence

EIF2B2 (eukaryotic translation initiation factor 2B, subunit 2 beta, 39kDa) (eg, leukoencephalopathy with vanishing white matter), full gene sequence

---

Separate Procedure　　　Unlisted Procedure　　　CCI Comp. Code　　　Non-specific Procedure　　**769**

EMD (emerin) (eg, Emery-Dreifuss muscular dystrophy), full gene sequence

ENG (endoglin) (eg, hereditary hemorrhagic telangiectasia, type 1), duplication/deletion analysis

EYA1 (eyes absent homolog 1 [Drosophila]) (eg, branchio-oto- renal [BOR] spectrum disorders), duplication/deletion analysis

FGFR1 (fibrobast growth factor receptor 1) (eg, Kallmann syndrome 2), full gene sequence

FH (fumarate hydratase) (eg, fumarate hydratase deficiency, hereditary leiomyomatosis with renal cell cancer), full gene sequence

FKTN (fukutin) (eg, limb-girdle muscular dystrophy [LGMD] type 2M or 2L), full gene sequence

FTSJ1 (FtsJ RNA methyltransferase homolog 1 [E. coli]) (eg, X-linked mental retardation 9), duplication/deletion analysis

GABRG2 (gamma-aminobutyric acid [GABA] A receptor, gamma 2) (eg, generalized epilepsy with febrile seizures), full gene sequence

GCH1 (GTP cyclohydrolase 1) (eg, autosomal dominant dopa-responsive dystonia), full gene sequence

GDAP1 (ganglioside-induced differentiation-associated protein 1) (eg, Charcot-Marie-Tooth disease), full gene sequence

GFAP (glial fibrillary acidic protein) (eg, Alexander disease), full gene sequence

GHR (growth hormone receptor) (eg, Laron syndrome), full gene sequence

GHRHR (growth hormone releasing hormone receptor) (eg, growth hormone deficiency), full gene sequence

GLA (galactosidase, alpha) (eg, Fabry disease), full gene sequence

HNF1A (HNF1 homeobox A) (eg, maturity-onset diabetes of the young [MODY]), full gene sequence

HNF1B (HNF1 homeobox B) (eg, maturity-onset diabetes of the yound [MODY]), full gene sequence

HTRA1 (HtrA serine peptidase 1) (eg, macular degeneration), full gene sequence

IDS (iduronate 2-sulfatase) (eg, mucopolysacchridosis, type II), full gene sequence

IL2RG (interleukin 2 receptor, gamma) (eg, X-linked severe combined immunodeficiency), full gene sequence

ISPD (isoprenoid synthase domain containing) (eg, muscle-eye-brain disease, Walker-Warburg syndrome), full gene sequence

KRAS (Kirsten rat sarcoma viral oncogene homolog) (eg, Noonan syndrome), full gene sequence

LAMP2 (lysosomal-associated membrane protein 2) (eg, Danon disease), full gene sequence

LDLR (low density lipoprotein receptor) (eg, familial hypercholesterolemia), duplication/deletion analysis

MEN1 (multiple endocrine neoplasia 1) (eg, multiple endocrine neoplasia type 1, Wermer syndrome), full gene sequence

MMAA (methylmalonic aciduria [cobalamine deficiency] type A) (eg, MMAA-related methylmalonic acidemia), full gene sequence

MMAB (methylmalonic aciduria [cobalamine deficiency] type B) (eg, MMAB-related methylmalonic acidemia), full gene sequence

MPI (mannose phosphate isomerase) (eg, congenital disorder of slycosylation 1b), full gene sequence

MPV17 (MpV17 mitochòndrial inner membrane protein) (eg, mitochondrial DNA depletion syndrome), full gene sequence

MPZ (myelin protein zero) (eg, Charcot-Marie-Tooth), full gene sequence

MTM1 (myotubularin 1) (eg, X-linked centronuclear myopathy), duplication/deletion analysis

---

● New Code   ▲ Revised Code   ✚ Add-On Code   ⊘ Modifier -51 Exempt   ★ Telemedicine

MYL2 (myosin, light chain 2, regulatory, cardiac, slow) (eg, familial hypertrophic cardiomyopathy), full gene sequence

MYL3 (myosin, light chain 3, alkali, ventricular, skeletal, slow) (eg, familial hypertrophic cardiomyopathy), full gene sequence

MYOT (myotilin) (eg, limb-girdle muscular dystrophy), full gene sequence

NDUFS7 (NADH dehydrogenase [ubiquinone] Fe-S protein 7, 20kDa [NADH-coenzyme Q reductase]) (eg, Leigh syndrome, mitochondrial complex I deficiency), full gene sequence

NDUFS8 (NADH dehydrogenase [ubiquinone] Fe-S protein 8, 23kDa [NADH-coenzyme Q reductase]) (eg, Leigh syndrome, mitochondrial complex I deficiency), full gene sequence

NDUFV1 (NADH dehydrogenase [ubiquinone] flavoprotein 1, 51kDa) (eg, Leigh syndrome, mitochondrial complex I deficiency), full gene sequence

NEFL (neurofilament, light polypeptide) (eg, Charcot-Marie- Tooth), full gene sequence

NF2 (neurofibromin 2 [merlin]) (eg, neurofibromatosis, type 2), duplication/deletion analysis

NLGN3 (neuroligin 3) (eg, autism spectrum disorders), full gene sequence

NLGN4X (neuroligin 4, X-linked) (eg, autism spectrum disorders), full gene sequence

NPHP1 (nephronophthisis 1 [juvenile]) (eg, Joubert syndrome), deletion analysis, and duplication analysis if performed

NPHS2 (nephrosis 2, idiopathic, steroid-resistant [podocin]) (eg, steroid-resistant nephrotic syndrome), full gene sequence

NSD1 (nuclear receptor binding SET domain protein 1) (eg, Sotos syndrome), duplication/deletion analysis

OTC (ornithine carbamoyltransferase) (eg, ornithine transcarbamylase deficiency), full gene sequence

PAFAH1B1 (platelet-activating factor acetylhydrolase 1b, regulatory subunit 1 [45kDa]) (eg, lissencephaly, Miller-Dieker syndrome), duplication/deletion analysis

PARK2 (Parkinson protein 2, E3 ubiquitin protein ligase [parkin]) (eg, Parkinson disease), duplication/deletion anaysis

PCCA (propionyl CoA carboxylase, alpha polypeptide) (eg, propionic acidemia, type 1) duplication/deletion analysis

PCDH19 (protocadherin 19) (eg, epileptic encephalopathy), full gene sequence

PDHA1 (pyruvate dehydrogenase [lipoamide] alpha 1) (eg, lactic acidosis), duplication/deletion analysis

PDHB (pyruvate dehydrogenase [lipoamide] beta) (eg, lactic acidosis), full gene sequence

PINK1 (PTEN induced putative kinase 1) (eg, Parkinson disease), full gene sequence

PKLR (pyruvate kinase, liver and RBC) (eg, pyruvate kinase deficiency), full gene sequence

PLP1 (proteolipid protein 1) (eg, Pelizaeus-Merzbacher disease, spastic paraplegia), full gene sequence

POU1F1 (POU class 1 homeobox 1) (eg, combined pituitary hormone deficiency), full gene sequence

PRX (periaxin) (eg, Charcot-Marie-Tooth disease), full gene sequence

PQBP1 (polyglutamine binding protein 1) (eg, Renpenning syndrome), full gene sequence

PSEN1 (presenilin 1) (eg, Alzheimer disease), full gene sequence

RAB7A (RAB7A, member RAS oncogene family) (eg, Charcot-Marie-Toothe disease), full gene sequence

RAI1 (retinoic acid induced 1) (eg, Smith-Magenis syndrome), full gene sequence

REEP1 (receptor accessory protein 1) (eg, spastic paraplegia), full gene sequence

RET (ret proto-oncogene) (eg, multiple endocrine neoplasia, type 2A and familial medullary thyroid carcinoma), targeted sequence analysis (eg, exons 10, 11, 13-16)

RPS19 (ribosomal protein S19) (eg, Diamond-Blackfan anemia), full gene sequence

RRM2B (ribonucleotide reductase M2 B[TP53 inducible]) (eg, mitochondrial DNA depletion), full gene sequence

SCO1 (SCO cytochrome oxidase deficient homolog 1) (eg, mitochondrial respiratory chain complex IV deficiency), full gene sequence

SDHB (succinate dehydrogenase complex, subunit B, iron sulfur) (eg, hereditary paraganglioma), full gene sequence

SDHC (succinate dehydrogenase complex, submit C, integral membrane protein, 15kDa) (eg, hereditary paraganglioma-pheochromocytoma syndrome), full gene sequence

SGCA (sarcoglycan, alpha [50kDa dystrophin-associated glycoprotein]) (eg, limb-girdle muscular dystrophy), full gene sequence

SGCB (sarcoglycan, beta [43kDa dystrophin-associated glycoprotein]) (eg, limb-girdle muscular dystrophy), full gene sequence

SGCD (sarcoglycanm delta [35kDa dystrophin-associated glycoprotein]) (eg, limb-girdle muscular dystrophy), full gene sequence

SGCE (sarcoglycan, epsilon) (eg, myoclonic dystonia), duplication/deletion analysis

SGCG (sarcoglycan, gamma [35kDa dystrophin-associated glycoprotein]) (eg, limb-girdle muscular dystrophy), full gene sequence

SHOC2 (soc-2 suppressor of clear homolog) (eg, Noonan-like syndrome with loose anagen hair), full gene sequence

SHOX (short stature homeobox) (eg, Langer mesomelic dysplasia), full gene sequence

SIL1 (SIL 1 homolog, endoplasmic reticulum chaperone [S. cerevisiae]) (eg, ataxia), full gene sequence

SLC2A1 (solute carrier family 2 [facilitated glucose transporter], member 1) (eg, glucose transporter type 1 [GLUT 1] deficiency syndrome), full gene sequence

SLC16A2 (solute carrier family 16, member 2 [thyroid hormone transporter]) (eg, specific thyroid hormone cell transporter deficiency, Allan-Herndon-Dudley syndrome), full gene sequence

SLC22A5 (solute carrier family 22 [organic cation/carnitine transporter], member 5) (eg, systemic primary carnitine deficiency),, full gene sequence

SLC25A20 (solute carrier family 25 [carnitine/acylcarnitine translocase], member 20) (eg, carnitine-acylcarnitine translocase deficiency), full gene sequence

SMAD4 (SMAD family member 4) (eg, hemorrhagic telangiectasia syndrome, juvenile polyposis), duplication/deletion analsysi

SPAST (spastin) (eg, spastic paraplegia), duplication/deletion analsysis

SPG7 (spastic paraplegia 7 [pure and complicated autosomal recessive]) (eg, spastic paraplegia), duplication/deletion analysis

SPRED1 (sprouty-related, EVH1 domain containing 1) (eg, Legius syndrome), full gene sequence

STAT3 (signal transducer and activator of transcription 3 [acute-phase response factor]) (eg, autosomal dominant hyper-Ig-E syndrome), targeted sequence analysis (eg, exons 12, 13, 14, 16, 17, 20, 21)

STK11 (serine/threonine kinase 11) (eg, Peutz-Jeghers syndrome), full gene sequence

SURF1 (surfeit 1) (eg, mitochondrial respiratory chain complex IV deficiency), full gene sequence

TARDBP (TAR DNA binding protein) (eg, amyotrophic lateral sclerosis), full gene sequence

TBX5 (T-box 5) (eg, Holt-Oram syndrome), full gene sequence

TCF4 (transcription factor 4) (eg, Pitt-Hopkins syndrome), duplication/deletion analysis

TGFBR1 (transforming growth factor, beta receptor 1) (eg, Marfan syndrome), full gene sequence

---

● New Code   ▲ Revised Code   + Add-On Code   ⊘ Modifier -51 Exempt   ★ Telemedicine

TGFBR2 (transforming growth factor, beta receptor 2) (eg, Marfan syndrome), full gene sequence

THRB (thyroid hormone receptor, beta) (eg, thyroid hormone resistance, thyroid hormone beta receptor deficiency), full gene sequence or targeted sequence analysis of >5 exons

TK2 (thymidine kinase 2, mitochondrial) (eg, mitochondrial DNA depletion syndrome), full gene sequence

TNNC1 (troponin C type 1 [slow]) (eg, hypertrophic cardiomyopathy or dilated cardiomyopathy), full gene sequence

TNNI3 (troponin I, type 3 [cardiac]) (eg, familial hypertrophic cardiomyopathy), full gene sequence

TPM1 (tropomyosin 1 [alpha]) (eg, familial hypertrophic cardiomyopathy), full gene sequence

TSC1 (tuberous sclerosis 1) (eg, tuberous sclerosis), duplication/ deletion analysis

TYMP (thymidine phosphorylase) (eg, mitochondrial DNA depletion syndrome), full gene sequence

VWF (von Willebrand factor) (eg, von Willebrand disease type 2N), targeted sequence analysis (eg, exons 18-20, 23-25)

WT1 (Wilms tumor 1) (eg, Denys-Drash syndrome, familial Wilms tumor), full gene sequence

ZEB2 (zinc finger E-box binding homeobox 2) (eg, Mowat-Wilson syndrome), full gene sequence

81406　　Molecular pathology procedure, Level 7 (eg, analysis of 11-25 exons by DNA sequence analysis, mutation scanning or duplication/deletion variants of 26-50 exons)

ACADVL (acyl-CoA dehydrogenase, very long chain) (eg, very long chain acyl-coenzyme A dehydrogenase deficiency), full gene sequence

ACTN4 (actinin, alpha 4) (eg, focal segmental glomerulosclerosis), full gene sequence

AFG3L2 (AFG3 ATPase family gene 3-like 2 [S. cerevisiae]) (eg, spinocerebellar ataxia), full gene sequence

AIRE (autoimmune regulator) (eg, autoimmune polyendocrinopathy syndrome type 1), full gene sequence

ALDH7A1 (aldehyde dehydrogenase 7 family, member A1) (eg, pyridoxine-dependent epilepsy), full gene sequence

ANO5 (anoctamin 5) (eg, limb-girdle muscular dystrophy), full gene sequence

ANOS1 (anosmin-1) (eg, Kallmann syndrome 1), full gene sequence

APP (amyloid beta [A4] precursor protein) (eg, Alzheimer disease), full gene sequence

ASS1 (argininosuccinate synthase 1) (eg, citrullinemia type I), full gene sequence

ATL1 (atlastin GTPase 1) (eg, spastic paraplegia), full gene sequence

ATP1A2 (ATPase, Na+/K+ transporting, alpha 2 polypeptide) (eg, familial hemiplegic migraine), full gene sequence

ATP7B (ATPase, Cu++ transporting, beta polypeptide) (eg, Wilson disease), full gene sequence

BBS1 (Bardet-Biedl syndrome 1) (eg, Bardet-Biedl syndrome), full gene sequence

BBS2 (Bardet-Biedl syndrome 2) (eg, Bardet-Biedl syndrome), full gene sequence

BCKDHB (branched-chain keto acid dehydrogenase E1, beta polypeptide) (eg, maple syrup urine disease, type 1B), full gene sequence

BEST1 (bestrophin 1) (eg, vitelliform macular dystrophy), full gene sequence

BMPR2 (bone morphogenetic protein receptor, type II [serine/threonine kinase]) (eg, heritable pulmonary arterial hypertension), full gene sequence

BRAF (B-raf proto-oncogene, serine/threonine kinase) (eg, Noonan syndrome), full gene sequence

BSCL2 (Berardinelli-Seip congenital lipodystrophy 2 [seipin]) (eg, Berardinelli-Seip congenital lipodystrophy), full gene sequence

---

Separate Procedure　　　　Unlisted Procedure　　　　CCI Comp. Code　　　　Non-specific Procedure　　**773**

BTK (Bruton agammaglobulinemia tyrosine kinase) (eg, X-linked agammaglobulinemia), full gene sequence

CACNB2 (calcium channel, voltage-dependent beta 2 subunit) (eg, Brugada syndrome), full gene sequence

CAPN3 (Calpain 3) (eg, limb-girdle muscular dystrophy [LGMD] type 2A, calpainopathy), full gene sequence

CBS (cystathionine-beta-synthase) (eg, homocystinuria, cystathionine beta-synthase deficiency), full gene sequence

CDH1 (cadherin 1, type 1, E-cadherin [epithelial]) (eg, hereditary diffuse gastric cancer), full gene sequence

CDKL5 (cyclin-dependent kinase-like 5) (eg, early infantile epileptic encephalopathy), full gene sequence

CLCN1 (chloride channel 1, skeletal muscle) (eg, myotonia congenita), full gene sequence

CLCNKB (chlorid channel, voltage-sensitive Kb) (eg, Bartter syndrome 3 and 4b), full gene sequence

CNTNAP2 (contactin-associated protein-like 2) (eg, Pitt-Hopkins-like syndrome 1), full gene sequence

COL6A2 (collagen, type VI, alpha 2) (eg, collagen type VI-related disorders), duplication/deletion analysis

CPT1A (carnitine palmitoyltransferase 1A [liver]) (eg, carnitine palmitoyltransferase 1A[CPT1A] deficiency), full gene sequence

CRB1 (crumbs homolog 1 [Drosophila]) (eg, Leber congenital amaurosis), full gene sequence

CREBBP (CREB binding protein) (eg, Rubinstein-Taybi syndrome), duplication/deletion analisys

DBT (dihydrolipoamide branched chain transacylase E2) (eg, maple syrup urine disease, type 2), full gene sequence

DLAT (dihydrolipoamide S-acetyltransferase) (eg, pyruvate dehydrogenase E2 deficiency), full gene sequence

DLD (dihydrolipoamide dehydrogenase) (eg, maple syrup urine disease, type III), full gene sequence

DSC2 (desmocollin) (eg, arrhythmogenic right ventricular dysplasia/cardiomyopathy 11), full gene sequence

DSG2 (dismoglein 2) (eg, arrhythmogenic right ventricular dysplasia/cardiomyopathy 10), full gene sequence

DSP (desmoplakin) (eg, arrhythmogenic right ventricular dysplasia/cadiomyopathy 8), full gene sequence

EFHC1 (EG-hand domain [C-terminal] containing 1) (eg, juvenile myoclonic epilepsy), full gene sequence

EIF2B3 (eukaryotic translation initiation factor 2B, subunit 3 gamma, 58kDa) (eg, leukoencephalopathy with vanishing white matter), full gene sequence

EIF2B4 (eukaryotic translation initiation factor 2B, subunit 4 delta, 67kDa) (eg, leukoencephalopathy with vanishing white matter), full gene sequence

EIF2B5 (eukaryotic translation initiation factor 2B, subunit 5 epsilon, 82kDa) (eg, childhood ataxia with central nervous system hypomyelination/vanishing white matter), full gene sequence

ENG (endoglin) (eg, hereditary hemorrhagic telangiectasia, type 1), full gene sequence

EYA1 (eyes absent homolog 1 [Drosophila]) (eg, branchio-otorenal [BOR] spectrum disorders), full gene sequence

F8 (coagulation factor VIII) (eg, hemophilia A), duplication/ deletion analysis

FAH (fumarylacetoacetate hydrolase [fumarylacetoacetase]) (eg, tyrosinemia, type 1), full gene sequence

FASTKD2 (FAST kinase domains2) (eg, mitochrondrial respiratory chain complex IV deficiency), full gene sequence

FIG4 (FIG4 homolog, SAC1 lipid phosphatase domain containing [S. cerevisiae]) (eg, Charcot-Marie-Tooth disease), full gene sequence

FTSJ1 (FtsJ RNA methyltransferase homolog 1 [E. coli]) (eg, X-linked mental retardation 9), full gene sequence

FUS (fused in sarcoma) (eg, amyotrophic lateral sclerosis), full gene sequence

GAA (glucosidase, alpha; acid) (eg, glycogen storage disease type II [Pompe disease]), full gene sequence

GALC (galactosylceramidase) (eg, Krabbe disease), full gene sequence

GALT (galactose-1-phosphate uridylyltransferase) (eg, galactosemia), full gene sequence

GARS (glycyl-tRNA synthetase) (eg, Charcot-Marie-Tooth disease), full gene sequence

GCDH (glutaryl-CoA dehydrogenase) (eg, glutaricacidemia type 1), full gene sequence

GCK (glucokinase [hexokinase 4]) (eg, maturity-onset diabetes of the young [MODY]), full gene sequence

GLUD1 (glutamate dehydrogenase 1) (eg, familial hyperinsulinism), full gene sequence

GNE (glucosamine [UDP-N-acetyl]-2-epimerase/N- acetylmannosamine kinase) (eg, inclusion body myopathy 2 [EBM2], Nonaka myopathy), full gene sequence

GRN (granulin) (eg, frontotemporal dementia), full gene sequence

HADHA (hydroxyacyl-CoA dehydrogenase/3-ketoacyl-CoA thiolase/enoyl-CoA hydratase [trifunctional protein] alpha subunit) (eg, long chain acyl-coenzyme A dehydrogenase deficiency), full gene sequence

HADHB (hydroxyacyl-CoA dehydrogenase/3-ketoacyl-CoA thiolase/enoyl-CoA hydratase [trifunctional protein], beta subunit) (eg, trifunctional protein deficiency), full gene sequence

HEXA (hexosaminidase A, alpha polypeptide) (eg, Tay-Sachs disease), full gene sequence

HLCS (HLCS holocarboxylase synthetase) (eg, holocarboxylase synthetase deficiency), full gene sequence

HMBS (hydroxymethylbilane synthase) (eg, acute intermittent porphyria), full gene sequence

HNF4A (hepatocyte nuclear factor 4, alpha) (eg, maturity-onset diabetes of the young [MODY]), full gene sequence

IDUA (iduronidase, alpha-L-) (eg, mucopolysaccharidosis type I), full gene sequence

INF2 (inverted formin, FH2 and WH2 domain containing) (eg, focal segmental glomerulosclerosis), full gene sequence

IVD (isovaleryl-CoA dehydrogenase) (eg, isovaleric acidemia), full gene sequence

JAG1 (jagged 1) (eg, Alagille syndrome), duplication/deletion analysis

JUP (junction plakoglobin) (eg, arrhythmogenic right ventricular dysplasia/cardiomyopathy 11), full gene sequence

KCNH2 (potassium voltage-gated channel, subfamily H [eag-related], member 2) (eg, short QT syndrome, long QT syndrome), full gene sequence

KCNQ1 (potassium voltage-gated channel, KQT-like subfamily, member 1) (eg, short QT syndrome, long QT syndrome), full gene sequence

KCNQ2 (potassium voltage-gated channel, KQT-like subfamily, member 2) (eg, epileptic encephalopathy), full gene sequence

LDB3 (LIM domain binding 3) (eg, familial dilated cardiomyopathy, myofibrillar myopathy), full gene sequence

LDLR (low density lipoprotein receptor) (eg, familial hypercholesterolemia), full gene sequence

LEPR (leptin receptor) (eg, obesity with hypogonadism), full gene sequence

LHCGR (luteinizing hormone/choriogonadotropin receptor) (eg, precocious male puberty), full gene sequence

LMNA (lamin A/C) (eg, Emery-Dreifuss muscular dystrophy [EDMD1, 2 and 3] limb-girdle muscular dystrophy [LGMD] type 1B, dilated cardiomyopathy [CMD1A], familial partial lipodystrophy [FPLD2]), full gene sequence

LRP5 (low density lipoprotein receptor-related protein 5) (eg, osteopetrosis), full gene sequence

MAP2K1 (mitogen-activated protein kinase 1) (eg, cardiofaciocutaneous syndrome), full gene sequence

MAP2K2 (mitogen-activated protein kinase 2) (eg, cardiofaciocutaneous syndrome), full gene sequence

MAPT (microtubule-associated protein tau) (eg, frontotemporal dementia), full gene sequence

MCCC1 (methylcrotonoyl-CoA carboxylase 1 [alpha]) (eg, 3-methylcrotonyl-CoA-carboxylase deficiency), full gene sequence

MCCC2 (methylcrotonoyl-CoA carboxylase 2 [beta]) (eg, 3-methylcrotonyl carboxylase deficiency), full gene sequence

MFN2 (mitofusin 1) (eg, Charcot-Marie-Tooth disease), full gene sequence

MTM1 (myotubularin 1) (eg, X-linked centronuclear myopathy), full gene sequence

MUT 9methylmalonyl CoA mutase) (eg, methylmalonic acidemia), full gene sequence

MUTYH (mutY homolog [E. coli]) (eg, MYH-associated polyposis), full gene sequence

NDUFS1 (NADH dehydrogenase [ubiquinone] Fe-S protein 1, 75kDa [NADH-coenzyme Q reductase]) (eg, Leigh syndrome, mitochondrial complex I deficiency), full gene sequence

NF2 (neurofibromin 2 [merlin]) (eg, neurofibromatosis, type 2), full gene sequence

NOTCH3 (notch 3) (eg, cerebral autosomal dominant arteriopathy with subcortical infarcts and leukoencephalopathy [CADASIL]), targeted sequence analysis (eg, exons 1-23)

NPC1 (Niemann-Pick disease, type C1) (eg, Niemann-Pick disease), full gene sequence

NPHP1 (nephronophthisis 1 [juvenile]) (eg, Joubert syndrome), full gene sequence

NSD1 (nuclear receptor binding SET domain protein 1) (eg, Sotos syndrome), full gene sequence

OPA1 (optic atrophy 1) (eg, optic atrophy), duplication/deletion analysis

OPTN (optineurin) (eg, amyotrophic lateral sclerosis), full gene sequence

PAFAH1B1 (platelet-activating factor acetylhydrolase 1b, regulatory subunit 1 [45kDa]) (eg, lissencephaly, Miller-Dieker syndrome), full gene sequence

PAH (phenylalanine hydroxylase) (eg, phenylketonuria), full gene sequence

PARK2 (Parkinson protein 2, E3 ubiquitin protein ligase [parkin]) (eg, Parkinson disease), full gene sequence

PAX2 (paired box 2) (eg, renal coloboma syndrome), full gene sequence

PC (pyruvate carboxylase) (eg, pyruvate carboxylase deficiency), full gene sequence

PCCA (propionyl CoA-carboxylase, alpha polypeptide) (eg, propionic acidemia, type 1), full gene sequence

PCCB (propionyl CoA carboxylase, beta polypeptide) (eg, propionic acidemia), full gene sequence

PCDH15 (protocadherin-related 15) (eg, Usher syndrome type 1F), duplication/deletion analysis

PCSK9 (proprotein convertase subtilisin/kexin type 9) (eg, familial hypercholesterolemia), full gene sequence

PDHA1 (pyruvate dehydrogenase [lipoamide] alpha 1) (eg, lactic acidosis), full gene sequence

PDHX (pyruvate dehydrogenase complex, component X) (eg, lactic acidosis), full gene sequence

PHEX (phosphate-regulating endopeptidase homolog, X-linked) (eg, hypophosphatemic rickets), full gene sequence

---

● New Code   ▲ Revised Code   + Add-On Code   ⊘ Modifier -51 Exempt   ★ Telemedicine

PKD2 (polycystic kidney disease 2 [autosomal dominant]) (eg, polycystic kidney disease), full gene sequence

PKP2 (plakophilin 2) (eg, arrhythmogenic right ventricular dysplasia/cardiomyopathy 9), full gene sequence

PNKD (eg, paroxysmal nonkinesigenic dyskinesia) (eg, paroxysmal nonkinesigenic dyskinesia), full gene sequence

POLG (polymerase [DNA directed], gamma) (eg, Alpers-Huttenlocher syndrome, autosomal dominant progressive external ophthalmoplegia), full gene sequence

POMGNT1 (protein O-linked mannose beta1,2-N acetylglucosaminyltransferase) (eg, muscle-eye-brain disease, Walker-Warburg syndrome), full gene sequence

POMT1 (protein-O-mannosyltransferase 1) (eg, limb-girdle muscular dystrophy [LGMD] type 2K, Walker-Warburg syndrome), full gene sequence

POMT2 (protein-O-mannosyltransferase 2) (eg, limb-girdle muscular dystrophy [LGMD] type 2N, Walker-Warburg syndrome), full gene sequence

PPOX (protoporphyrinogen oxidase) (eg, variegate porphyria), full gene sequence

PRKAG2 (protein kinase, AMP-activated, gamma 2 non-catalytic subunit) (eg, familial hypertrophic cardiomyopathy with Wolff-Parkinson-White syndrome, lethal congenital glycogen storage disease of heart), full gene sequence

PRKCG (protein kinase C, gamma) (eg, spinocerebellar ataxia), full gene sequence

PSEN2 (presenilin 2 [Alzheimer disease 4]) (eg, Alzheimer disease), full gene sequence

PTPN11 (protein tyrosine phosphatase, non-receptor type 11) (eg, Noonan syndrome, LEOPARD syndrome), full gene sequence

PYGM (phosphorylase, glycogen, muscle) (eg, glycogen storage disease type V, McArdle disease), full gene sequence

RAF1 (v-raf-1 murine leukemia viral oncogene homolog 1) (eg, LEOPARD syndrome), full gene sequence

RET (ret proto-oncogene) (eg, Hirschsprung disease), full gene sequence

RPE65 (retinal pigment epithelium-specific protein 65kDa) (eg, retinitis pigmentosa, Leber congenital amaurosis), full gene sequence

RYR1 (ryanodine receptor 1, skeletal) (eg, malignant hyperthermia), targeted sequence analysis of exons with functionally-confirmed mutations

SCN4A (sodium channel, voltage-gated, type IV, alpha subunit) (eg, hyperkalemic periodic paralysis), full gene sequence

SCNN1A (sodium channel, nonvoltage-gated 1 alpha) (eg, pseudohypoaldosteronism), full gene sequence

SCNN1B (sodium channel, nonvoltage-gated 2, beta) (eg, Liddle syndrome, pseudohypoaldosteronism), full gene sequence

SCNN1G (sodium channel, nonvoltage-gated 1, gamma) (eg, Liddle syndrome, pseudohypoaldosteronism), full gene sequence

SDHA (succinate dehydrogenase complex, subunit A, flavoprotein [Fp]) (eg, Leigh syndrome, mitochondrial complex II deficiency), full gene sequence

SETX (senataxin) (eg, ataxia), full gene sequence

SGCE (sarcoglycan, epsilon) (eg, myoclonic dystonia), full gene sequence

SH3TC2 (SH3 domain and tetratricopeptide repeats 2) (eg, Charcot-Marie-Tooth disease), full gene sequence

SLC9A6 (solute carrier family 9 [sodium/hydrogen exchanger], member 6) (eg, Christianson syndrome), full gene sequence

SLC26A4 (solute carrier family 26, member 4) (eg, Pendred syndrome), full gene sequence

SLC37A4 (solute carrier family 37 [glucose-6-phosphate transporter], member 4) (eg, glycogen storage disease type Ib), full gene sequence

SMAD4 (SMAD family member 4) (eg, hemorrhagic telangiectasia syndrome, juvenile polyposis), full gene sequence

SOS1 (son of sevenless homolog 1) (eg, Noonan syndrome, gingival fibromatosis), full gene sequence

SPAST (spastin) (eg, spastic paraplegia), full gene sequence

SPG7 (spastic paraplegia 7 [pure and complicated autosomal recessive]) (eg, spastic paraplegia), full gene sequence

STXBP1 (syntaxin-binding protein 1) (eg, epileptic encephalopathy), full gene sequence

TAZ (tafazzin) (eg, methylglutaconic aciduria type 2, Barth syndrome), full gene sequence

TCF4 (transcription factor 4) (eg, Pitt-Hopkins syndrome), full gene sequence

TH (tyrosine hydroxylase) (eg, Segawa syndrome), full gene sequence

TMEM43 (transmembrane protein 43) (eg, arrhythmogenic right ventricular cardiomyopathy), full gene sequence

TNNT2 (troponin T, type 2 [cardiac]) (eg, familial hypertrophic cardiomyopathy), full gene sequence

TRPC6 (transient receptor potential cation channel, subfamily C, member 6) (eg, focal segmental glomerulosclerosis), full gene sequence

TSC1 (tuberous sclerosis 1) (eg, tuberous sclerosis), full gene sequence

TSC2 (tuberous sclerosis 2) (eg, tuberous sclerosis), duplication/deletion analysis

UBE3A (ubiquitin protein ligase E3A) (eg, Angelman syndrome), full gene sequence

UMOD (uromodulin) (eg, glomerulocystic kidney disease with hyperuricemia and isosthenuria), full gene sequence

VWF (von Willebrand factor) (von Willebrand disease type 2A), extended targeted sequence analysis (eg, exons 11-16, 24-26, 51, 52)

WAS (Wiskott-Aldrich syndrome [eczema-thrombocytopenia]) (eg, Wiskott-Aldrich syndrome), full gene sequence

81407 Molecular pathology procedure, Level 8 (eg, analysis of 26-50 exons by DNA sequence analysis, mutation scanning or duplication/deletion variants of >50 exons, sequence analysis of multiple genes on one platform)

ABCC8 (ATP-binding cassette, sub-family C [CFTR/MRP], member 8) (eg, familial hyperinsulinism), full gene sequence

AGL (amylo-alpha-1, 6-glucosidase, 4-alpha-glucanotransferase) (eg, glycogen storage disease type III), full gene sequence

AHI1 (Abelson helper integration site 1) (eg, Joubert syndrome), full gene sequence

APOB (apolipoprotein B) (eg, familial hypercholesterolemia type B) full gene sequence

ASPM (asp [abnormal spindle] homolog, microcephaly associated [Drosophila]) (eg, primary microcephaly), full gene sequence

CHD7 (chromodomain helicase DNA binding protein 7) (eg, CHARGE syndrome), full gene sequence

COL4A4 (collagen, type IV, alpha 4) (eg, Alport syndrome), full gene sequence

COL4A5 (collagen, type IV, alpha 5) (eg, Alport syndrome), duplication/deletion analysis

COL6A1 (collagen, type VI, alpha 1) (eg, collagen type VI-related disorders), full gene sequence

COL6A2 (collagen, type VI, alpha 2) (eg, collagen type VI-related disorders), full gene sequence

---

● New Code ▲ Revised Code + Add-On Code ⊘ Modifier -51 Exempt ★ Telemedicine

COL6A3 (collagen, type VI, alpha 3) (eg, collagen type VI-related disorders), full gene sequence

CREBBP (CREB binding protein) (eg, Rubinstein-Taybi syndrome), full gene sequence

F8 (coagulation factor VIII) (eg, hemophilia A), full gene sequence

JAG1 (jagged 1) (eg, Alagille syndrome), full gene sequence

KDM5C (lysine [K]-specific demethylase 5C) (eg, X-linked mental retardation), full gene sequence

KIAA0196 (KIAA0196) (eg, spastic paraplegia), full gene sequence

L1CAM (L1 cell adhesion molecule) (eg, MASA syndrome, X-linked hydrocephaly), full gene sequence

LAMB2 (laminin, beta 2 [laminin S]) (eg, Pierson syndrome), full gene sequence

MYBPC3 (myosin binding protein C, cardiac) (eg, familial hypertrophic cardiomyopathy), full gene sequence

MYH6 (myosin, heavy chain 6, cardiac muscle, alpha) (eg, familial dilated cardiomyopathy), full gene sequence

MYH7 (myosin, heavy chain 7, cardiac muscle, beta) (eg, familial hypertrophic cardiomyopathy, Liang distal myopathy), full gene sequence

MYO7A (myosin VIIA) (eg, Usher syndrome, type 1), full gene sequence

NOTCH1 (notch 1) (eg, aortic valve disease), full gene sequence

NPHS1 (nephrosis 1, congenital, Finnish type [nephrin]) (eg, congenital Finnish nephrosis), full gene sequence

OPA1 (optic atrophy 1) (eg, optic atrophy), full gene sequence

PCDH15 (protocadherin-related 15) (eg, Usher syndrome, type 1), full gene sequence

PKD1 (polycystic kidney disease 1 [autosomal dominant]) (eg, polycystic kidney disease), full gene sequence

PLCE1 (phospholipase C, epsilon 1) (eg, nephrotic syndrome type 3), full gene sequence

SCN1A (sodium channel, voltage-gated, type 1, alpha subunit) (eg, generalized epilepsy with febrile seizures), full gene sequence

SCN5A (sodium channel, voltage-gated, type V, alpha subunit) (eg, familial dilated cardiomyopathy), full gene sequence

SLC12A1 (solute carrier family 12 [sodium/potassium/chloride transporters], member 1) (eg, Bartter syndrome), full gene sequence

SLC12A3 (solute carrier family 12 [sodium/chloride transporters], member 3) (eg, Gitelman syndrome), full gene sequence

SPG11 (spastic paraplegia 11 [autosomal recessive]) (eg, spastic paraplegia), full gene sequence

SPTBN2 (spectrin, beta, non-erythrocytic 2) (eg, spinocerebellar ataxia), full gene sequence

TMEM67 (transmembrane protein 67) (eg, Joubert syndrome), full gene sequence

TSC2 (tuberous sclerosis 2) (eg, tuberous sclerosis), full gene sequence

USH1C (Usher syndrome 1C [autosomal recessive, severe]) (eg, Usher syndrome, type 1), full gene sequence

VPS13B (vacuolar protein sorting 13 homolog B [yeast]) (eg, Cohen syndrome), duplication/deletion analysis

WDR62 (WD repeat domain 62) (eg, primary autosomal recessive microcephaly), full gene sequence

81408   Molecular pathology procedure, Level 9 (eg, analysis of >50 exons in a single gene by DNA sequence analysis)

ABCA4 (ATP-binding cassette, sub-family A [ABC1], member 4) (eg, Stargardt disease, age-related macular degeneration), full gene sequence

ATM (ataxia telangiectasia mutated) (eg, ataxia telangiectasia), full gene sequence

CDH23 (cadherin-related 23) (eg, Usher syndrome, type 1), full gene sequence

CEP290 (centrosomal protein 290kDa) (eg, Joubert syndrome), full gene sequence

COL1A1 (collagen, type I, alpha 1) (eg, osteogenesis imperfecta, type I), full gene sequence

COL1A2 (collagen, type I, alpha 2) (eg, osteogenesis imperfecta, type I), full gene sequence

COL4A1 (collagen, type IV, alpha 1) (eg, brain small-vessel disease with hemorrhage), full gene sequence

COL4A3 (collagen, type IV, alpha 3 [Goodpasture antigen]) (eg, Alport syndrome), full gene sequence

COL4A5 (collagen, type IV, alpha 5) (eg, Alport syndrome), full gene sequence

DMD (dystrophin) (eg, Duchenne/Becker muscular dystrophy), full gene sequence

DYSF (dysferlin, limb girdle muscular dystrophy 2B [autosomal recessive]) (eg, limb-girdle muscular dystrophy), full gene sequence

FBN1 (fibrillin 1) (eg, Marfan syndrome), full gene sequence

ITPR1 (inositol 1, 4, 5-trisphosphate receptor, type 1) (eg, spinocerebellar ataxia), full gene sequence

LAMA2 (laminin, alpha 2) (eg, congenital muscular dystrophy), full gene sequence

LRRK2 (leucine-rich repeat kinase 2) (eg, Parkinson disease), full gene sequence

MYH11 (myosin, heavy chain 11, smooth muscle) (eg, thoracic aortic aneurysms and aortic dissections), full gene sequence

NEB (nebulin) (eg, nemaline myopathy 2), full gene sequence

NF1 (neurofibromin 1) (eg, neurofibromatosis, type 1), full gene sequence

PKHD1 (polycystic kidney and hepatic disease 1) (eg, autosomal recessive polycystic kidney disease), full gene sequence

RYR1 (ryanodine receptor 1, skeletal) (eg, malignant hyperthermia), full gene sequence

RYR2 (ryanodine receptor 2 [cardiac]) (eg, catecholaminergic polymorphic ventricular tachycardia, arrhythmogenic right ventricular dysplasia), full gene sequence or targeted sequence analysis of > 50 exons

USH2A (Usher syndrome 2A [autosomal recessive, mild]) (eg, Usher syndrome, type 2), full gene sequence

VPS13B (vacuolar protein sorting 13 homolog B [yeast]) (eg, Cohen syndrome), full gene sequence

VWF (von Willebrand factor) (eg, von Willebrand disease types 1 and 3), full gene sequence

81479   Unlisted molecular pathology procedure

GENOMIC SEQUENCING PROCEDURES AND OTHER MOLECULAR MULTIANALYTE ASSAYS

Genomic sequencing procedures (GSPs) and other molecular multianalyte assays GSPs are DNA or RNA sequence analysis methods that simultaneously assay multiple genes or genetic regions relevant to a clinical situation. They may target specific combinations of genes or genetic material, or assay the exome or genome. The technology used for genomic sequencing is commonly referred to as next generation sequencing (NGS) or massively parallel sequencing (MPS). GSPs are performed on nucleic acids from germline or neoplastic samples. Examples of applications include aneuploidy analysis of cell-free circulating fetal DNA, gene panels for somatic alterations in neoplasms, and sequence analysis of the exome or genome to determine the cause of developmental delay. The exome and genome procedures are designed to evaluate the genetic material in totality or near totality. Although commonly used to identify sequence (base) changes, they can also be used to identify copy number, structural changes, and abnormal zygosity patterns. Another unique feature of GSPs is the ability to "re-query" or re-evaluate the sequence data (eg, complex phenotype such as developmental delay is reassessed when new genetic knowledge is attained, or for a separate unrelated clinical indication). The analyses listed below represent groups of genes that are often performed by GSPs; however, the analyses may also be performed by other molecular techniques (polymerase chain reaction [PCR] methods and microarrays). These codes should be used when the components of the descriptor(s) are fulfilled regardless of the technique used to provide the analysis, unless specifically noted in the code descriptor. When a GSP assay includes gene(s) that is listed in more than one code descriptor, the code for the most specific test for the primary disorder sought should be reported, rather than reporting multiple codes for the same gene(s). When all of the components of the descriptor are not performed, use individual Tier 1 codes, Tier 2 codes, or 81479 (Unlisted molecular pathology procedure).

The assays in this section represent discrete genetic values, properties, or characteristics in which the measurement or analysis of each analyte is potentially of independent medical significance or useful in medical management. In contrast to multianalyte assays with algorithmic analyses (MAAAs), the assays in this section do not represent algorithmically combined results to obtain a risk score or other value, which in itself represents a new and distinct medical property that is of independent medical significance relevant to the individual, component test results.

(For cytogenetic MicroArray analyses, see 81228, 81229, 81405, 81406)

81410 Aortic dysfunction or dilation (eg, Marfan syndrome, Loeys Dietz syndrome, Ehler Danlos syndrome type IV, arterial tortuosity syndrome); genomic sequence analysis panel, must include sequencing of at least 9 genes, including *FBN1, TGFBR1, TGFBR2, COL3A1, MYH11, ACTA2, SLC2A10, SMAD3,* and *MYLK*

81411 duplication/deletion analysis panel, must include analyses for *TGFBR1, TGFBR2, MYH11,* and *COL3A1*

81412 Ashkenazi Jewish associated disorders (eg, Bloom syndrome, Canavan disease, cystic fibrosis, familial dysautonomia, Fanconi anemia group C, Gaucher disease, Tay-Sachs disease), genomic sequence analysis panel, must include sequencing of at least 9 genes, including *ASPA, BLM, CFTR, FANCC,GBA, HEXA, IKBKAP, MCOLN1,* and *SMPD1*

81413 Cardiac ion channelopathies (eg, Brugada syndrome, long QT syndrome, short QT syndrome, catecholaminergic polymorphic ventricular tachycardia); genomic sequence analysis panel, must include sequencing of at least 10 genes, including *ANK2, CASQ2, CAV3, KCNE1, KCNE2, KCNH2, KCNJ2, KCNQ1, RYR2,* and *SCN5A*

81414 duplication/deletion gene analysis panel, must include analysis of at least 2 genes, including KCNH2 and KCNQ1

(For genomic sequencing panel testing for cardiomyopathies, use 81439)

(Do not report 81413, 81414 in conjunction with 81439 when performed on the same date of service)

● **81419** Epilepsy genomic sequence analysis panel, must include analyses for *ALDH7A1, CACNA1A, CDKL5, CHD2, GABRG2, GRIN2A, KCNQ2, MECP2, PCDH19, POLG, PRRT2, SCN1A, SCN1B, SCN2A, SCN8A, SLC2A1, SLC9A6, STXBP1, SYNGAP1, TCF4, TPP1, TSC1, TSC2,* and *ZEB2*

81415 Exome (eg, unexplained constitutional or heritable disorder or syndrome); sequence analysis

+ **81416** sequence analysis, each comparator exome (eg, parents, siblings) (List separately in addition to code for primary procedure)

(Use 81416 in conjunction with 81415)

81417 re-evaluation of previously obtained exome sequence (eg, updated knowledge or unrelated condition/syndrome)

(Do not report 81417 for incidental findings)

(For exome-wide copy number assessment by microarray, see 81228, 81229)

81419 This code is out of order. See page 781

81420 Fetal chromosomal aneuploidy (eg, trisomy 21, monosomy X) genomic sequence analysis panel, circulating cell-free fetal DNA in maternal blood, must include analysis of chromosomes 13, 18, and 21

(Do not report 81228, 81229, 88271 when performing genomic sequencing procedures or other molecular multianalyte assays for copy number analysis)

81422 Fetal chromosomal microdeletion(s) genomic sequence analysis (eg, DiGeorge syndrome, Cri-du-chat syndrome), circulating cell-free fetal DNA in maternal blood

(Do not report 81228, 81229, 88271 when performing genomic sequencing procedures or other molecular multianalyte assays for copy number analysis)

81443 Genetic testing for severe inherited conditions (eg, cystic fibrosis, Ashkenazi Jewish-associated disorders [eg, Bloom syndrome, Canavan disease, Fanconi anemia type C, mucolipidosis type VI, Gaucher disease, Tay-Sachs disease], beta hemoglobinopathies, phenylketonuria, galactosemia), genomic sequence analysis panel, must include sequencing of at least 15 genes (eg, ACADM, ARSA, ASPA, ATP7B, BCKDHA, BCKDHB, BLM, CFTR, DHCR7, FANCC, G6PC, GAA, GALT, GBA, GBE1, HBB, HEXA, IKBKAP, MCOLN1, PAH)

(If spinal muscular atrophy testing is performed separately, use 81401)

(If testing is performed only for Ashkenazi Jewishassociated disorders, use 81412)

(If FMR1 [expanded allele] testing is performed separately, use 81243)

(If hemoglobin A testing is performed separately, use 81257)

(Do not report 81443 in conjunction with 81412)

81425 Genome (eg, unexplained constitutional or heritable disorder or syndrome); sequence analysis

+ 81426 sequence analysis, each comparator genome (eg, parents, siblings) (List separately in addition to code for primary procedure)

(Use 81426 in conjunction with 81425)

81427 re-evaluation of previously obtained genome sequence (eg, updated knowledge or unrelated condition/syndrome)

(Do not report 81427 for incidental findings)

(For genome-wide copy number assessment by microarray, see 81228, 81229)

81430 Hearing loss (eg, nonsyndromic hearing loss, Usher syndrome, Pendred syndrome); genomic sequence analysis panel, must include sequencing of at least 60 genes, including *CDH23, CLRN1, GJB2, GPR98, MTRNR1, MYO7A, MYO15A, PCDH15, OTOF, SLC26A4, TMC1, TMPRSS3, USH1C, USH1G, USH2A, and WFS1*

81431 duplication/deletion analysis panel, must include copy number analyses for *STRC* and *DFNB1* deletions in *GJB2* and *GJB6* genes

81432 Hereditary breast cancer-related disorders (eg, hereditary breast cancer, hereditary ovarian cancer, hereditary endometrial cancer); genomic sequence analysis panel, must include sequencing of at least 10 genes, always including *BRCA1, BRCA2, CDH1, MLH1, MSH2, MSH6, PALB2, PTEN, STK11, and TP53*

81433 duplication/deletion analysis panel, must include analyses for *BRCA1, BRCA2, MLH1, MSH2, and STK11*

81434 Hereditary retinal disorders (eg, retinitis pigmentosa, Leber congenital amaurosis, cone-rod dystrophy), genomic sequence analysis panel, must include sequencing of at least 15 genes, including *ABCA4, CNGA1, CRB1, EYS, PDE6A, PDE6B, PRPF31, PRPH2, RDH12, RHO, RP1, RP2, RPE65, RPGR, and USH2A*

81435 Hereditary colon cancer disorders (eg, Lynch syndrome, PTEN hamartoma syndrome, Cowden syndrome, familial adenomatosis polyposis); genomic sequence analysis panel, must include sequencing of at least 10 genes, including *APC, BMPR1A, CDH1, MLH1, MSH2, MSH6, MUTYH, PTEN, SMAD4, and STK11*

81436 duplication/deletion analysis panel, must include analysis of at least 5 genes, including *MLH1, MSH2, EPCAM, SMAD4, and STK11*

● New Code ▲ Revised Code + Add-On Code ⊘ Modifier -51 Exempt ★ Telemedicine

81437 Hereditary neuroendocrine tumor disorders (eg, medullary thyroid carcinoma, parathyroid carcinoma, malignant pheochromocytoma or paraganglioma); genomic sequence analysis panel, must include sequencing of at least 6 genes, including *MAX, SDHB, SDHC, SDHD, TMEM127,* and *VHL*

81438 Hereditary neuroendocrine tumor disorders (eg, medullary thyroid carcinoma, parathyroid carcinoma, malignant pheochromocytoma or paraganglioma); duplication/deletion analysis panel, must include analyses for *SDHB, SDHC, SDHD,* and *VHL*

81448 Hereditary peripheral neuropathies (eg, Charcot-Marie- Tooth, spastic paraplegia), genomic sequence analysis panel, must include sequencing of at least 5 peripheral neuropathy-related genes (eg, *BSCL2, GJB1, MFN2, MPZ, REEP1, SPAST, SPG11, SPTLC1*)

81439 Hereditary cardiomyopathy (eg, hypertrophic cardiomyopathy, dilated cardiomyopathy, arrhythmogenic right ventricular cardiomyopathy), genomic sequence analysis panel, must include sequencing of at least 5 cardiomyopathy-related genes (eg, *DSG2, MYBPC3, MYH7, PKP2, TTN*)

(Do not report 81439 in conjunction with 81413, 81414 when performed on the same date of service)

(For genomic sequencing panel testing for cardiac ion channelopathies, see 81413, 81414)

81440 Nuclear encoded mitochondrial genes (eg, neurologic or myopathic phenotypes), genomic sequence panel, must include analysis of at least 100 genes, including *BCS1L, C10orf2, COQ2, COX10, DGUOK, MPV, OPA1, PDSS2, POLG, POLG2, RRM2B, SCO1, SCO2, SLC25A4, SUCLA2, SUCLG1, TAZ, TK2,* and *TYMP*

81442 Noonan spectrum disorders (eg, Noonan syndrome, cardio-facio-cutaneous syndrome, Costello syndrome, LEOPARD syndrome, Noonan-like syndrome), genomic sequence analysis panel, must include sequencing of at least 12 genes, including *BRAF, CBL, HRAS, KRAS, MAP2K1, MAP2K2, NRAS, PTPN11, RAF1, RIT1, SHOC2,* and *SOS1*

81443 This code is out of order. See page 782

81445 Targeted genomic sequence analysis panel, solid organ neoplasm, DNA analysis, and RNA analysis when performed, 5-50 genes (eg, *ALK, BRAF, CDKN2A, EGFR, ERBB2, KIT, KRAS, NRAS, MET, PDGFRA, PDGFRB, PGR, PIK3CA, PTEN, RET*), interrogation for sequence variants and copy number variants or rearrangements, if performed

(For copy number assessment by microarray, use 81406)

81448 This code is out of order. See page 783

81450 Targeted genomic sequence analysis panel, hematolymphoid neoplasm or disorder, DNA analysis, and RNA analysis when performed, 5-50 genes (eg, *BRAF, CEBPA, DNMT3A, EZH2, FLT3, IDH1, IDH2, JAK2, KRAS, KIT, MLL, NRAS, NPM1, NOTCH1*), interrogation for sequence variants, and copy number variants or rearrangements, or isoform expression or mRNA expression levels, if performed

(For copy number assessment by microarray, use 81406)

81455 Targeted genomic sequence analysis panel, solid organ or hematolymphoid neoplasm, DNA analysis, and RNA analysis when performed, 51 or greater genes (eg, *ALK, BRAF, CDKN2A, CEBPA, DNMT3A, EGFR, ERBB2, EZH2, FLT3, IDH1, IDH2, JAK2, KIT, KRAS, MLL, NPM1, NRAS, MET, NOTCH1, PDGFRA, PDGFRB, PGR, PIK3CA, PTEN, RET*), interrogation for sequence variants and copy number variants or rearrangements, if performed

(For copy number assessment by microarray, use 81406)

81460 Whole mitochondrial genome (eg, Leigh syndrome, mitochondrial encephalomyopathy, lactic acidosis, and stroke-like episodes [MELAS], myoclonic epilepsy with ragged-red fibers [MERFF], neuropathy, ataxia, and retinitis pigmentosa [NARP], leber hereditary optic neuropathy [LHON]), genomic sequence, must include sequence analysis of entire mitochondrial genome with heteroplasmy detection

81465 Whole mitochondrial genome large deletion analysis panel (eg, Kearns-Sayre syndrome, chronic progressive external ophthalmoplegia), including heteroplasmy detection, if performed

---

Separate Procedure   Unlisted Procedure   CCI Comp. Code   Non-specific Procedure   **783**

81470 X-linked intellectual disability (XLID) (eg, syndromic and non-syndromic XLID); genomic sequence analysis panel, must include sequencing of at least 60 genes, including *ARX, ATRX, CDKL5, FGD1, FMR1, HUWE1, IL1RAPL, KDM5C, L1CAM, MECP2, MED12, MID1, OCRL, RPS6KA3,* and *SLC16A2*

81471 duplication/deletion gene analysis, must include analysis of at least 60 genes, including *ARX, ATRX, CDKL5, FGD1, FMR1, HUWE1, IL1RAPL, KDM5C, l1CAM, MECP2, MED12, MID1, OCRL, RPS6KA3,* and *SLC16a2*

81479 This code is out of order. See 780

MULTIANALYTE ASSAYS WITH ALGORITHMIC ANALYSES

Multianalyte Assays with Algorithmic Analyses (MAAAs) are procedures that utilize multiple results derived from panels of analyses of various types, including molecular pathology assays, fluorescent in situ hybridization assays and non-nucleic acid based assays (eg, proteins, polypeptides, lipids, carbohydrates). Algorithmic analysis using the results of these assays as well as other patient information (if used) is then performed, and typically reported as a numeric score(s) or as a probability. MAAAs are typically unique to a single clinical laboratory or manufacturer. The results of individual component procedure(s) that are inputs to the MAAAs may be provided on the associated laboratory report; however these assays are not separately reported using additional codes.

The format for the code descriptors of MAAAs usually include (in order):

Disease type (eg, oncology, autoimmune, tissue rejection),

Material(s) analyzed (eg, DNA, RNA, protein, antibody),

Number of markers (eg, number of genes, number of proteins),

Methodology(ies) (eg, microarray, real-time [RT]-PCR, in situ hybridization [ISH], enzyme linked immunosorbent assays [ELISA],

Number of functional domains (if indicated),

Specimen type (eg, blood, fresh tissue, formalin-fixed paraffin embedded),

Algorithm result type (eg, prognostic, diagnostic),

Report (eg, probability index, risk score)

In contrast to GSPs and other molecular multianalyte assays, the assays in this section represent alorithmically combined results of analyses of multiple analytes to obtain a risk score or other value which in itself represents a new and distinct medical property that is of independent medical significance relative to the individual component test results in clinical context in which the assay is performed.

MAAAs, including those that do not have a Category I code, may be found in Appendix O. MAAAs that do not have a Category I code are identified in Appendix O by a four-digit number followed by the letter "M." The Category 1 MAAA codes that are included in this subsection are also included in Appendix O. All MAAA codes are listed in Appendix O along with the procedure's proprietary name. In order to report a MAAA code, the analysis performed must fulfill the code descriptor AND, if proprietary, must be the test represented by the proprietary name listed in Appendix O.

When a specific MAAA procedure is not listed below or in Appendix O, the procedure must be reported using the Category 1 MAAA unlisted code (81599).

These codes encompass all analytical services required (eg, cell lysis, nucleic acid stabilization, extraction, digestion, amplification, hybridization, adn detection) in addition to the algorithmic analysis itself. Procedures that are required prior to cell lysis (eg, microdissection, codes 88380 and 88381) should be reported separately.

81490 Autoimmune (rheumatoid arthritis), analysis of 12 biomarkers using immunoassays, utilizing serum, prognostic algorithm reported as a disease activity score

(Do not report 81490 in conjunction with 86140)

● New Code ▲ Revised Code ✚ Add-On Code ⊘ Modifier -51 Exempt ★ Telemedicine

81595 Cardiology (heart transplant), mRNA, gene expression profiling by real-time quantitative PCR of 20 genes (11 content and 9 housekeeping), utilizing subfraction of peripheral blood, algorithm reported as a rejection risk score

81493 Coronary artery disease, mRNA, gene expression profiling by real-time RT-PCR of 23 genes, utilizing whole peripheral blood, algorithm reported as a risk score

81500 This code is out of order. See page 786

81503 This code is out of order. See page 786

81504 This code is out of order. See page 787

81506 Endocrinology (type 2 diabetes), biochemical assays of seven analytes (glucose, HbA1c, insulin, hs-CRP, adoponectin, ferritin, interleukin 2-receptor alpha), utilizing serum or plasma, algorithm reporting a risk score

(Do not report 81506 in conjunction with constituent components [ie, 82728, 82947, 83036, 83525, 86141], 84999 [for adopectin], and 83520 [for interleukin 2-receptor alpha])

81507 Fetal aneuploidy (trisomy 21, 18, and 13) DNA sequence analysis of selected regions using maternal plasma, algorithm reported as a risk score for each trisomy

(Do not report 81228, 81229, 88271 when performing genomic sequencing procedures or other molecular multianalyte assays for copy number analysis)

81508 Fetal congenital abnormalities, biochemical assays of two proteins (PAPP-A, hCG [any form]), utilizing maternal serum, algorithm reported as a risk score

(Do not report 81508 in conjunction with 84163, 84702)

81509 Fetal congenital abnormalities, biochemical assays of three proteins (PAPP-A, hCG [any form], DIA), utilizing maternal serum, algorithm reported as a risk score

(Do not report 81509 in conjunction with 84163, 84702, 86336)

81510 Fetal congenital abnormalities, biochemical assays of three analytes (AFP, uE3, hCG [any form]), utilizing maternal serum, algorithm reported as a risk score

(Do note report 81510 in conjunction with 82105, 82677, 84702)

81511 Fetal congenital abnormalities, biochemical assays of four analytes (AFP, uE3, hCG [any form], DIA) utilizing maternal serum, algorithm reported as a risk score (may include additional results from previous biochemical testing)

(Do not report 81511 in conjunction with 82105, 82677, 84702,. 86336)

81512 Fetal congenital abnormalities, biochemical assays of five analytes (AFP, uE3, total hCG, hyperglycosylated hCG, DIA) utilizing maternal serum, algorithm reported as a risk score

(Do not report 81512 in conjunction with 82105, 82677, 84702, 86336)

● **81513** Infectious disease, bacterial vaginosis, quantitative realtime amplification of RNA markers for Atopobium vaginae, Gardnerella vaginalis, and Lactobacillus species, utilizing vaginal-fluid specimens, algorithm reported as a positive or negative result for bacterial vaginosis

● **81514** Infectious disease, bacterial vaginosis and vaginitis, quantitative real-time amplification of DNA markers for Gardnerella vaginalis, Atopobium vaginae, Megasphaera type 1, Bacterial Vaginosis Associated Bacteria-2 (BVAB- 2), and Lactobacillus species (L. crispatus and L. jensenii), utilizing vaginal-fluid specimens, algorithm reported as a positive or negative for high likelihood of bacterial vaginosis, includes separate detection of Trichomonas vaginalis and/or Candida species (C. albicans, C. tropicalis, C. parapsilosis, C. dubliniensis), Candida glabrata, Candida krusei, when reported

(Do not report 81514 in conjunction with 87480, 87481, 87482, 87510, 87511, 87512, 87660, 87661)

Separate Procedure   Unlisted Procedure   CCI Comp. Code   Non-specific Procedure   **785**

81596 Infectious disease, chronic hepatitis C virus (HCV) infection, six biochemical assays (ALT, A2-macroglobulin, apolipoprotein A-1, total bilirubin, GGT, and haptoglobin) utilizing serum, prognostic algorithm reported as scores for fibrosis and necroinflammatory activity in liver

81518 Oncology (breast), mRNA, gene expression profiling by real-time RT-PCR of 11 genes (7 content and 4 housekeeping), utilizing formalin-fixed paraffinembedded tissue, algorithms reported as percentage risk for metastatic recurrence and likelihood of benefit from extended endocrine therapy

81522 Oncology (breast), mRNA, gene expression profiling by RT-PCR of 12 genes (8 content and 4 housekeeping), utilizing formalin-fixed paraffin-embedded tissue, algorithm reported as recurrence risk score

81519 Oncology (breast), mRNA, gene expression profiling by real-time RT-PCR of 21 genes, utilizing formalin-fixed paraffin embedded tissue, algorithm reported as recurrence score

81520 Oncology (breast), mRNA gene expression profiling by hybrid capture of 58 genes (50 content and 8 housekeeping), utilizing formalin-fixed paraffinembedded tissue, algorithm reported as a recurrence risk score

81521 Oncology (breast), mRNA, microarray gene expression profiling of 70 content genes and 465 housekeeping genes, utilizing fresh frozen or formalin-fixed paraffinembedded tissue, algorithm reported as index related to risk of distant metastasis

81522 This code is out of order. See page 786

81525 Oncology (colon), mRNA, gene expression profiling by real-time RT-PCR of 12 genes (7 content and 5 housekeeping), utilizing formalin-fixed paraffin-embedded tissue, algorithm reported as a recurrence score

81528 Oncology (colorectal) screening, quantitative real-time target and signal amplification of 10 DNA markers (KRAS mutations, promoter methylation of NDRG4 and BMP3) and fecal hemoglobin, utilizing stool, algorithm reported as a positive or negative result

(Do not report 81528 in conjunction with 81275, 82274)

● **81529** Oncology (cutaneous melanoma), mRNA, gene expression profiling by real-time RT-PCR of 31 genes (28 content and 3 housekeeping), utilizing formalin-fixed paraffinembedded tissue, algorithm reported as recurrence risk, including likelihood of sentinel lymph node metastasis

81535 Oncology (gynecologic), live tumor cell culture and chemotherapeutic response by DAPI stain and morphology, predictive algorithm reported as a drug response score; first single drug or drug combination

+ **81536** each additional single drug or drug combination (List separately in addition to code for primary procedure)

(Use 81536 in conjunction with 81535)

81538 Oncology (lung), mass spectrometric 8-protein signature, including amyloid A, utilizing serum, prognostic and predictive algorithm reported as good versus poor overall survival

81500 Oncology (ovarian), biochemical assays of two proteins (CA-125 adn HE4), utilizing serum, with menopausal status, algorithm reported as a risk score

(Do note report 81500 in conjunction with 86304, 86305)

81503 Oncology (ovarian), biochemical assays of five proteins (CA-125, apolipoprotein A1, beta-2 microglobulin, transferrin, and pre-albumin), utilizing serum, algorithm reported as a risk score

(Do not report 81503 in conjunction with 82172, 82232, 84134, 84466, 86304)

81539 Oncology (high-grade prostate cancer), biochemical assay of four proteins (Total PSA, Free PSA, Intact PSA, and human kallikrein-2 [hK2]), utilizing plasma or serum, prognostic algorithm reported as a probability score

● New Code   ▲ Revised Code   + Add-On Code   ⊘ Modifier -51 Exempt   ★ Telemedicine

81540   This code is out of order. See page 787

81541   Oncology (prostate), mRNA gene expression profiling by real-time RT-PCR of 46 genes (31 content and 15 housekeeping), utilizing formalin-fixed paraffinembedded tissue, algorithm reported as a diseasespecific mortality risk score

81542   Oncology (prostate), mRNA, microarray gene expression profiling of 22 content genes, utilizing formalin-fixed paraffin-embedded tissue, algorithm reported as metastasis risk score

(**81545**   deleted 2020 [2021 Edition])

81546   This code is out of order. See page 787

81551   Oncology (prostate), promoter methylation profiling by real-time PCR of 3 genes (GSTP1, APC, RASSF1), utilizing formalin-fixed paraffin-embedded tissue, algorithm reported as a likelihood of prostate cancer detection on repeat biopsy

● **81546**   Oncology (thyroid), mRNA, gene expression analysis of 10,196 genes, utilizing fine needle aspirate, algorithm reported as a categorical result (eg, benign or suspicious)

81504   Oncology (tissue of origin), microarray gene expression profiling of > 2000 genes, utilizing formalin-fixed paraffin-embedded tissue, algorithm reported as tissue similarity scores

81540   Oncology (tumor of unknown origin), mRNA, gene expression profiling by real-time RT-PCR of 92 genes (87 content and 5 housekeeping) to classify tumor into main cancer type and subtype, utilizing formalin-fixed paraffin-embedded tissue, algorithm reported as a probability of a predicted main cancer type and subtype

81552   Oncology (uveal melanoma), mRNA, gene expression profiling by real-time RT-PCR of 15 genes (12 content and 3 housekeeping), utilizing fine needle aspirate or formalin-fixed paraffin-embedded tissue, algorithm reported as risk of metastasis

● **81554**   Pulmonary disease (idiopathic pulmonary fibrosis [IPF]), mRNA, gene expression analysis of 190 genes, utilizing transbronchial biopsies, diagnostic algorithm reported as categorical result (eg, positive or negative for high probability of usual interstitial pneumonia [UIP])

81595   This code is out of order. See page 785

81596   This code is out of order. See page 786

81599   Unlisted multianalyte assay with algorithmic analysis

   (Do not report 81599 for multianalyte assays with algorithmic analyses listed in Appendix O)

CHEMISTRY

The material for examination may be from any source unless otherwise specified in the code descriptor. When an analyte is measured in multiple specimens from different sources, or in specimens that are obtained at different times, the analyte is reported separately for each source and for each specimen. The examination is quantitative unless specified. To report an organ or disease oriented panel, see codes 80048-80076.

When a code describes a method where measurement of multiple analytes may require one or several procedures, each procedure is coded separately (eg., 82491-82492, 82541-82544). For example, if two analytes are measured using column chromatography using a single stationary or mobile phase, use 82492. If the same two analytes are measured using different stationary or mobile phase conditions, 82491 would be used twice. If a total of four analytes are measured where two analytes are measured with a single stationary and mobile phase, and the other two analytes are measured using a different stationary and mobile phase, use 82492 twice. If a total of three analytes are measured where two analytes are measured using a single stationary or mobile phase condition, and the third analyte is measured separately using a different stationary or mobile phase procedure, use 82492 once for the two analytes measured under the same condition, and use 82491 once for the third analyte measured separately.

Clinical information or mathematically calculated values, which are not specifically requested by the ordering physician and are derived from the results of other ordered or performed laboratory tests, are considered part of the ordered test procedure(s) and therefore are not separately reportable service(s).

When the requested analyte result is derived using a calculation that requires values from nonrequested laboratory analyses, only the requested analyte code should be reported.

When the calculated analyte determination requires values derived from other requested and nonrequested laboratory analyses, the requested analyte codes (including those calculated) should be reported.

An exception to the above is when an analyte (eg, urinary creatinine) is performed to compensate for variations in urine concentration (eg, microalbumin, thromboxane metabolites) in random urine samples; the appropriate CPT code is reported for both the ordered analyte and the additional required analyte. When the calculated result(s) represent an algorithmically derived numeric score or probability, see the appropriate multianalyte assay with algorithmic analyses (MAAA) code or the MAAA unlisted code (81599).

82009 Ketone body(s) (eg, acetone, acetoacetic acid, beta-hydroxybutyrate); qualitative

82010   quantitative

82013 Acetylcholinesterase

     (For gastric acid analysis, use 82930)

     (Acid phosphatase, see 84060-84066)

82016 Acylcarnitines; qualitative, each specimen

82017   quantitative, each specimen

     (For carnitine, use 82379)

82024 Adrenocorticotropic hormone (ACTH)

82030 Adenosine, 5-monophosphate, cyclic (cyclic AMP)

82040 Albumin; serum, plasma or whole blood

82042 This code is out of order. See page 788

82043   urine (eg, microalbumin), quantitative

82044   urine (eg, microalbumin), semiquantitative (eg, reagent strip assay)

     (For prealbumin, use 84134)

82045   ischemia modified

82042   other source, quantitative, each specimen

     (For total protein, see 84155, 84156, 84157, 84160)

▲ **82075** Alcohol (ethanol); breath

● **82077**   any specimen except urine and breath, immunoassay (eg, IA, EIA, ELISA, RIA, EMIT, FPIA) and enzymatic methods (eg, alcohol dehydrogenase)

     (For definitive drug testing for alcohol [ethanol], use 80320)

82085 Aldolase

82088 Aldosterone

(Alkaline phosphatase, see 84075, 84080)

(Alphaketoglutarate, see 82009, 82010)

(Alpha tocopherol (Vitamin E), use 84446)

82103 Alpha-1-antitrypsin; total

82104 phenotype

82105 Alpha-fetoprotein; serum

82106 amniotic fluid

82107 AFP-L3 fraction isoform and total AFP (including ratio)

82108 Aluminum

82120 Amines, vaginal fluid, qualitative

(For combined pH and amines test for vaginitis, use 82120 and 83986)

82127 Amino acids; single, qualitative, each specimen

82128 multiple, qualitative, each specimen

82131 single, quantitative, each specimen

82135 Aminolevulinic acid, delta (ALA)

82136 Amino acids, 2 to 5 amino acids, quantitative, each specimen

82139 Amino acids, 6 or more amino acids, quantitative, each specimen

82140 Ammonia

82143 Amniotic fluid scan (spectrophotometric)

(For L/S ratio, use 83661)

(Amobarbital, use 80345)

82150 Amylase

82154 Androstanediol glucuronide

82157 Androstenedione

82160 Androsterone

82163 Angiotensin II

82164 Angiotensin I - converting enzyme (ACE)

(Antidiuretic hormone (ADH), use 84588)

(Antimony, use 83015)

(Antitrypsin, alph-1-, see 82103, 82104)

82172 Apolipoprotein, each

Separate Procedure   Unlisted Procedure   CCI Comp. Code   Non-specific Procedure   **789**

82175   Arsenic

(For heavy metal screening, use 83015)

82180   Ascorbic acid (Vitamin C), blood

(Aspirin, see acetylsalicylic acid, 80329, 80330, 80331)

(For salicylate by immunoassay or enzymatic methods, use 80179)

(Atherogenic index, blood, ultracentrifugation, quantitative, use 83717)

82190   Atomic absorption spectroscopy, each analyte

82232   Beta-2 microglobulin

(Bicarbonate, use 82374)

82239   Bile acids; total

82240   cholylglycine

(For bile pigments, urine, see 81000-81005)

82247   Bilirubin; total

82248   direct

82252   feces, qualitative

82261   Biotinidase, each specimen

82270   Blood, occult, by peroxidase activity (eg, guaiac), qualitative; feces, consecutive collected specimens with single determination, for colorectal neoplasm screening (ie, patient was provided three cards or single triple card for consecutive collection)

82271   other sources

82272   Blood, occult, by peroxidase activity (eg, guaiac), qualitative, feces, 1-3 simultaneous determinations, performed for other than colorectal neoplasm screening

(Blood urea nitrogen (BUN), see 84520, 84525)

82274   Blood, occult, by fecal hemoglobin determination by immunoassay, qualitative, feces, 1-3 simultaneous determinations

82286   Bradykinin

82300   Cadmium

82306   Vitamin D; 25 hydroxy, includes fraction(s), if performed

82652   1, 25-dihydroxy, includes fraction(s), if performed

82308   Calcitonin

82310   Calcium; total

82330   ionized

82331   after calcium infusion test

   ● New Code   ▲ Revised Code   + Add-On Code   ⊘ Modifier -51 Exempt   ★ Telemedicine

82340	urine quantitative, timed specimen
82355	Calculus; qualitative analysis
82360	quantitative analysis, chemical
82365	infrared spectroscopy
82370	x-ray diffraction

(Carbamates, see individual listings)

82373	Carbohydrate deficient transferrin
82374	Carbon dioxide (bicarbonate)

(See also 82803)

82375	Carboxyhemoglobin; quantitative
82376	qualitative

(For transcutaneous measurement of carboxyhemoglobin, use 88740)

82378	Carcinoembryonic antigen (CEA)
82379	Carnitine (total and free), quantitative, each specimen

(For acylcarnitine, see 82016, 82017)

82380	Carotene
82382	Catecholamines; total urine
82383	blood
82384	fractionated

(For urine metabolites, see 83835, 84585)

82387	Cathepsin-D
82390	Ceruloplasmin
82397	Chemiluminescent assay
82415	Chloramphenicol
82435	Chloride; blood
82436	urine
82438	other source

(For sweat collection by iontophoresis, use 89230)

82441	Chlorinated hydrocarbons, screen

(Chlorpromazine, use 84022)

(Cholecalciferol [Vitamin D], use 82306)

82465   Cholesterol, serum or whole blood, total

       (For high density lipoprotein (HDL), use 83718)

82480   Cholinesterase; serum

82482   RBC

82485   Chondroitin B sulfate, quantitative

       (Chorionic gonadotropin, see gonadotropin, 84702, 84703)

82495   Chromium

82507   Citrate

       (Cocaine, qualitative analysis, use 80353)

       (Codeine, qualitative analysis, see 80361)

       (Complement, see 86160-86162)

82523   Collagen cross links, any method

82525   Copper

       (Coproporphyrin, see 84119, 84120)

       (Corticosteroids, use 83491)

82528   Corticosterone

82530   Cortisol; free

82533   total

       (C-peptide, use 84681)

82540   Creatine

82542   Column chromatography, includes mass spectrometry, if performed (eg, HPLC, LC, LC/MS, LC/MS-MS, GC, GC/MS-MS, GC/MS, HPLC/MS), non-drug analyte(s) not elsewhere specified, qualitative or quantitative, each specimen

       (Do not report more than one unit of 82542 for each specimen)

       (For column chromatography/mass spectrometry of drugs or substances, see 80305, 80306, 80307, 80320-80377, or specific analyte code[s] in Chemistry section)

82550   Creatine kinase (CK), (CPK); total

82552   isoenzymes

82553   MB fraction only

82554   isoforms

82565   Creatinine; blood

82570   other source

82575   clearance

   ● New Code   ▲ Revised Code   ✛ Add-On Code   ⦵ Modifier -51 Exempt   ★ Telemedicine

82585   Cryofibrinogen

82595   Cryoglobulin, qualitative or semi-quantitative (eg,cryocrit)

(For quantitative, cryoglobulin, see 82784, 82785)

(Crystals, pyrophosphate vs. urate, use 89060)

82600   Cyanide

82607   Cyanocobalamin (Vitamin B-12);

82608   unsaturated binding capacity

(Cyclic AMP, use 82030)

(Cyclosporine, use 80158)

82610   Cystatin C

82615   Cystine and homocystine, urine, qualitative

82626   Dehydroepiandrosterone (DHEA)

(Do not report 82626 in conjunction with 80327, 80328 to identify anabolic steroid testing for testosterone)

82627   Dehydroepiandrosterone-sulfate (DHEA-S)

(Delta-aminolevulinic acid (ALA), use 82135)

82633   Desoxycorticosterone, 11-

82634   Deoxycortisol, 11-

(Dexamethasone suppression test, use 80420)

(Diastase, urine, use 82150)

82638   Dibucaine number

(Dichloroethane, use 82441)

(Dichloromethane, use 82441)

(Diethylether, use 84600)

82642   Dihydrotestosterone (DHT)

(For dihydrotestosterone analysis for anabolic drug testing, see 80327, 80328)

(Dipropylacetic acid, use 80164)

(Dopamine, see 82382-82384)

(Duodenal contents, see individual enzymes; for intubation and collection, see 43756, 43757)

82652   This code is out of order. See page 790

82656   Elastase, pancreatic (EL-1), fecal, qualitative or semi-quantitative

82657   Enzyme activity in blood cells, cultured cells, or tissue, not elsewhere specified; nonradioactive substrate, each specimen

82658   radioactive substrate, each specimen

    Separate Procedure   Unlisted Procedure   CCI Comp. Code   Non-specific Procedure   **793**

82664 Electrophoretic technique, not elsewhere specified

(Endocrine receptor assays, see 84233-84235

82668 Erythropoietin

▲ **82670** Estradiol; total

● **82681** free, direct measurement (eg, equilibrium dialysis)

82671 Estrogens; fractionated

82672 total

(Estrogen receptor assay, use 84233)

82677 Estriol

82679 Estrone

(For definitive drug testing for alcohol [ethanol], use 80320)

(For alcohol [ethanol] by immunoassay or enzymatic methods, use 82077)

82681 This code is out of order. See page 794

82693 Ethylene glycol

82696 Etiocholanolone

(For fractionation of ketosteroids, use 83593)

82705 Fat or lipids, feces; qualitative

82710 quantitative

82715 Fat differential, feces, quantitative

82725 Fatty acids, nonesterified

82726 Very long chain fatty acids

(For long-chain (C20-22) omega-3 fatty acids in red blood cell (RBC) membranes, use Category III code 0111T)

82728 Ferritin

(Fetal hemoglobin, see hemoglobin 83030, 83033, and 85460)

(Fetoprotein, alpha-1, see 82105, 82106)

82731 Fetal fibronectin, cervicovaginal secretions, semi-quantitative

82735 Fluoride

(Foam stability test, use 83662)

82746 Folic acid; serum

82747 RBC

(Follicle stimulating hormone (FSH), use 83001)

● New Code ▲ Revised Code ✛ Add-On Code ⊘ Modifier -51 Exempt ★ Telemedicine

82757 Fructose, semen

(Fructosamine, use 82985)

(Fructose, TLC screen, use 84375)

82759 Galactokinase, RBC

82760 Galactose

82775 Galactose-1-phosphate uridyl transferase; quantitative

82776 screen

82777 Galectin-3

82784 Gammaglobulin (immunoglobulin); IgA, IgD, IgG, IgM, each

82785 IgE

(For allergen specific IgE, see 86003, 86005)

82787 immunoglobulin subclasses (eg, IgG1, 2, 3, or 4), each

(Gamma-glutamyltransferase (GGT), use 82977)

82800 Gases, blood, pH only

82803 Gases, blood, any combination of pH, pCO_2, pO_2, CO_2, HCO_3 (including calculated O_2 saturation);

(Use 82803 for two or more of the above listed analytes)

82805 with O_2 saturation, by direct measurement, except pulse oximetry

82810 Gases, blood, O_2 saturation only, by direct measurement, except pulse oximetry

(For pulse oximetry, use 94760)

82820 Hemoglobin-oxygen affinity (pO_2 for 50% hemoglobin saturation with oxygen)

(For gastric acid analysis, use 82930)

82930 Gastric acid analysis, includes pH if performed, each specimen

82938 Gastrin after secretin stimulation

82941 Gastrin

(Gentamicin, use 80170)

(GGT, use 82977)

(For a qualitative column chromatography procedure [eg, gas liquid chromatography], use the appropriate specific analyte code, if available, or 82542)

82943 Glucagon

82945 Glucose, body fluid, other than blood

82946 Glucagon tolerance test

82947 Glucose; quantitative, blood, (except reagent strip)

82948	blood, reagent strip
82950	post glucose dose (includes glucose)
82951	tolerance test (GTT), 3 specimens (includes glucose)
+ 82952	tolerance test, each additional beyond 3 specimens (List separately in addition to code for primary procedure)

(Use 82952 in conjunction with 82951)

(For insulin tolerance test, see 80434, 80435)

(For leucine tolerance test, use 80428)

(For semiquantitative urine glucose, see 81000, 81002, 81005, 81099)

82955	Glucose-6-phosphate dehydrogenase (G6PD); quantitative
82960	screen

(For glucose tolerance test with medication, use 96374 in addition)

82962	Glucose, blood by glucose monitoring device(s) cleared by the FDA specifically for home use
82963	Glucosidase, beta
82965	Glutamate dehydrogenase
82977	Glutamyltransferase, gamma (GGT)
82978	Glutathione
82979	Glutathione reductase, RBC

(Glycohemoglobin, use 83036)

82985	Glycated protein

(Gonadotropin, chorionic, see 84702, 84703)

83001	Gonadotropin; follicle stimulating hormone (FSH)
83002	luteinizing hormone (LH)

(For luteinizing releasing factor (LRH), use 83727)

83003	Growth hormone, human (HGH) (somatotropin)

(For antibody to human growth hormone, use 86277)

83006	Growth stimulation expressed gene 2 (ST2, Interleukin 1 receptor like1)
83009	Helicobacter pylori, blood test analysis for urease activity, non-radioactive isotope (eg, C-13)

(For H. pylori, breath test analysis for urease activity, see 83013, 83014)

83010	Haptoglobin; quantitative
83012	phenotypes
83013	Helicobacter pylori; breath test analysis for urease activity, non-radioactive isotope (eg, C-13)

● New Code   ▲ Revised Code   + Add-On Code   ⊘ Modifier -51 Exempt   ★ Telemedicine

83014   drug administration

(For H. pylori, stool, use 87338. For H. pylori, liquid scintillation counter, see 78267, 78268. For H. pylori immunoassay, use 87339)

(For H. pylori, blood test analysis for urease activity, use 83009)

83015 Heavy metal (eg, arsenic, barium, beryllium, bismuth, antimony, mercury); qualitative, any number of analytes

83018   quantitative, each, not elsewhere specified

(Use an analyte-specific heavy metal quantitative code, instead of 83018, when available)

83020 Hemoglobin fractionation and quantitation; electrophoresis (eg, A2, S, C, and/or F)

83021   chromotography (eg, A2, S, C,and/or F)

(For glycosylated [A1c] hemoglobin analysis, by electrophoresis or chromatography, in the absence of an identified hemoglobin variant, use 83036)

83026 Hemoglobin; by copper sulfate method, non-automated

83030   F (fetal), chemical

83033   F (fetal), qualitative

83036   glycosylated (A1C)

(For glycosylated [A1C] hemoglobin analysis, by electrophoresis or chromatography, in the setting of an identified hemoglobin variant, use 83020, 83021)

(For fecal hemoglobin detection by immunoassay, use 82274)

83037   glycosylated (A1C) by device cleared by FDA for home use

83045   methemoglobin, qualitative

83050   methemoglobin, quantitative

(For transcutaneous quantitative methemoglobin determination, use 88741)

83051   plasma

83060   sulfhemoglobin, quantitative

83065   thermolabile

83068   unstable, screen

83069   urine

83070 Hemosiderin; qualitative

(HIAA, use 83497)

(For a qualitative column chromatography procedure [eg, high performance liquid chromatography], use the appropriate specific analyte code, if available, or 82542)

83080 b-Hexosaminidase, each assay

83088 Histamine

| Separate Procedure | Unlisted Procedure | CCI Comp. Code | Non-specific Procedure | **797** |

(Hollander test, see 43754, 43755)

83090 Homocystine

83150 Homovanillic acid (HVA)

(Hormones, see individual alphabetic listings in Chemistry section)

(For hydrogen/methane breath test, use 91065)

83491 Hydroxycorticosteroids, 17- (17-OHCS)

(For cortisol, see 82530, 82533. For deoxycortisol, use 82634)

83497 Hydroxyindolacetic acid, 5-(HIAA)

(For urine qualitative test, use 81005)

(5-Hydroxytryptamine, use 84260)

83498 Hydroxyprogesterone, 17-d

83500 Hydroxyproline; free

83505   total

83516 Immunoassay for analyte other than infectious agent antibody or infectious agent antigen; qualitative or semiquantitative, multiple step method

83518   qualitative or semiquantitative, single step method (eg, reagent strip)

83519   quantitative, by radioimmunoassay (eg, RIA)

83520   quantitative, not otherwise specified

(For immunoassays for antibodies to infectious agent antigens, see analyte and method specific codes in the Immunology section)

(For immunoassay of tumor antigen not elsewhere specified, use 86316)

(Immunoglobulins, see 82784, 82785)

83525 Insulin; total

(For proinsulin, use 84206)

83527   free

83528 Intrinsic factor

(For intrinsic factor antibodies, use 86340)

83540 Iron

83550 Iron binding capacity

83570 Isocitric dehydrogenase (IDH)

(Isonicotinic acid hydrazide, INH, see code for specific method)

(Isopropyl alcohol, use 80320)

83582 Ketogenic steroids, fractionation

● New Code   ▲ Revised Code   ✛ Add-On Code   ⊘ Modifier -51 Exempt   ★ Telemedicine

(Ketone bodies, for serum, see 82009, 82010; for urine, see 81000-81003)

83586 Ketosteroids, 17- (17-KS); total

83593   fractionation

83605 Lactate (lactic acid)

83615 Lactate dehydrogenase (LD), (LDH);

83625   isoenzymes, separation and quantitation

83630 Lactoferrin, fecal; qualitative

83631   quantitative

83632 Lactogen, human placental (HPL) human chorionic somatomammotropin

83633 Lactose, urine; qualitative

(For tolerance, see 82951, 82952)

(For breath hydrogen/methane test for lactase deficiency, use 91065)

83655 Lead

83661 Fetal lung maturity assessment; lecithin-sphingomyelin ratio (L/S ratio)

83662   foam stability test

83663   fluorescence polarization

83664   lamellar body density

(For phosphatidylglycerol, use 84081)

83670 Leucine aminopeptidase (LAP)

83690 Lipase

83695 Lipoprotein (a)

83698 Lipoprotein-associated phospholipase A_2, (Lp-PLA_2)

(For secretory type II phospholipase A2 [sPLA2-IIA], use 0423T)

83700 Lipoprotein, blood; electrophoretic separation and quantitation

83701   high resolution fractionation and quantitation of lipoproteins including lipoprotein subclasses when performed (eg, electrophoresis, ultracentrifugation)

83704   quantitation of lipoprotein particle number(s) (eg, by nuclear magnetic resonance spectroscopy), includes lipoprotein particle subclass(es), when performed

83718 Lipoprotein, direct measurement; high density cholesterol (HDL cholesterol)

83719   VLDL cholesterol

83721   LDL cholesterol

83722   small dense LDL cholesterol

Separate Procedure   Unlisted Procedure   CCI Comp. Code   Non-specific Procedure   **799**

(For fractionation by high resolution electrophoresis or ultracentrifugation, use 83701)

(For lipoprotein particle numbers and subclasses analysis by nuclear magnetic resonance spectroscopy, use 83695)

83727 Luteinizing releasing factor (LRH)

(Luteinizing hormone (LH), use 83002)

(Macroglobulins, alpha-2, use 86329)

83735 Magnesium

83775 Malate dehydrogenase

(Maltose tolerance, see 82951, 82952)

(Mammotropin, use 84146)

83785 Manganese

83789 Mass spectrometry and tandem mass spectrometry (eg, MS, MS/MS, MALDI, MS-TOF, QTOF), non-drug analyte(s) not elsewhere specified, qualitative or quantitative, each specimen

(Do not report more than one unit of 83789 for each specimen)

(For column chromatography/mass spectrometry of drugs or substances, see 80305, 80306, 80307, 80320-80377, or specific analyte code[s] in the Chemistry section)

83825 Mercury, quantitative

(Mercury screen, use 83015)

83835 Metanephrines

(For catecholamines, see 82382-82384)

(Methamphetamine, see 80324, 80325, 80326)

(Methane breath test, use 91065)

83857 Methemalbumin

(Methemoglobin, see hemoglobin 83045, 83050)

(Methyl alcohol, use 80320)

(Microalbumin, see 82043 for quantitative, see 82044 for semiquantitative)

83861 Microfluidic analysis utilizing an integrated collection and analysis device, tear osmolarity

(Microglobulin, beta-2, use 82232)

(For microfluidic tear osmolarity of both eyes, report 83861 twice)

83864 Mucopolysaccharides, acid; quantitative

83872 Mucin, synovial fluid (Ropes test)

83873 Myelin basic protein, cerebrospinal fluid

(For oligoclonal bands, use 83916)

83874 Myoglobin

83876 Myeloperoxidase (MPO)

● New Code   ▲ Revised Code   ✚ Add-On Code   ⊘ Modifier -51 Exempt   ★ Telemedicine

83880   Natriuretic peptide

83883   Nephelometry, each analyte not elsewhere specified

83885   Nickel

83915   Nucleotidase 5-

83916   Oligoclonal immune (oligoclonal bands)

83918   Organic acids; total, quantitative, each specimen

83919   qualitative, each specimen

83921   Organic acid, single; quantitative

83930   Osmolality; blood

83935   urine

(For tear osmolarity using microfluidic analysis, use 83861)

83937   Osteocalcin (bone g1a protein)

83945   Oxalate

83950   Oncoprotein; HER-2/neu

(For tissue, see 88342, 88365)

83951   des-gamma-carboxy-prothrombin (DCP)

83970   Parathormone (parathyroid hormone)

(Pesticide, quantitative, see code for specific method. For screen for chlorinated hydrocarbons, use 82441)

83986   pH; body fluid, not otherwise specified

83987   exhaled breath condensate

(For blood pH, see 82800, 82803)

(Phenobarbital, use 80345)

83992   This code is out of order. See page 732

83993   Calprotectin, fecal

84030   Phenylalanine (PKU), blood

(Phenylalanine-tyrosine ratio, see 84030, 84510)

84035   Phenylketones, qualitative

84060   Phosphatase, acid; total

(**84061**   deleted 2017 [2018 edition])

84066   prostatic

84075   Phosphatase, alkaline;

Separate Procedure   Unlisted Procedure   CCI Comp. Code   Non-specific Procedure   **801**

84078   heat stable (total not included)

84080   isoenzymes

84081   Phosphatidylglycerol

(Phosphates inorganic, use 84100)

(Phosphates, organic, see code for specific method. For cholinesterase, see 82480, 82482)

84085   Phosphogluconate, 6-, dehydrogenase, RBC

84087   Phosphohexose isomerase

84100   Phosphorus inorganic (phosphate);

84105   urine

(Pituitary gonadotropins, see 83001-83002)

(PKU, see 84030, 84035)

84106   Porphobilinogen, urine; qualitative

84110   quantitative

84112   Evaluation of cervicovaginal fluid for specific amniotic fluid protein(s) (eg, placental alpha microglobulin-1 [PAMG-1], placental protein 12 [PP12], alpha-fetoprotein), qualitative, each specimen

84119   Porphyrins, urine; qualitative

84120   quantitation and fractionation

84126   Porphyrins, feces; quantitative

(Porphyrin precursors, see 82135, 84106, 84110)

(For protoporphyrin, RBC, see 84202, 84203)

84132   Potassium; serum, plasma or whole blood

84133   urine

84134   Prealbumin

(For microalbumin, see 82043, 82044)

84135   Pregnanediol

84138   Pregnanetriol

84140   Pregnenolone

84143   17-hydroxypregnenolone

84144   Progesterone

(Progesterone receptor assay, use 84234)

(For proinsulin, use 84206)

84145   Procalcitonin (PCT)

● New Code   ▲ Revised Code   ✚ Add-On Code   ⊘ Modifier -51 Exempt   ★ Telemedicine

84146 Prolactin

84150 Prostaglandin, each

84152 Prostate specific antigen (PSA); complexed (direct measurement)

84153   total

84154   free

84155 Protein, total, except by refractometry; serum, plasma or whole blood

84156   urine

84157   other source (eg, synovial fluid, cerebrospinal fluid)

84160 Protein, total, by refractometry, any source

(For urine total protein by dipstick method, use 81000-81003)

84163 Pregnancy-associated plasma protein-A (PAPP-A)

84165 Protein; electrophoretic fractionation and quantitation, serum

84166   electrophoretic fractionation and quantitation, other fluids with concentration (eg, urine, CSF)

84181   Western Blot, with interpretation and report, blood or other body fluid

84182   Western Blot, with interpretation and report, blood or other body fluid, immunological probe for band identification, each

(For Western Blot tissue analysis, use 88371)

84202 Protoporphyrin, RBC; quantitative

84203   screen

84206 Proinsulin

(Pseudocholinesterase, use 82480)

84207 Pyridoxal phosphate (Vitamin B-6)

84210 Pyruvate

84220 Pyruvate kinase

84228 Quinine

84233 Receptor assay; estrogen

84234   progesterone

84235   endocrine, other than estrogen or progesterone (specify hormone)

84238   non-endocrine (specify receptor)

84244 Renin

84252 Riboflavin (Vitamin B-2)

Separate Procedure   Unlisted Procedure   CCI Comp. Code   Non-specific Procedure   **803**

(Salicylates, see 80329, 80330, 80331)

(For salicylate by immunoassay or enzymatic methods, use 80179)

(Secretin test, see 99070, 43756, 43757 and appropriate analyses)

84255 Selenium

84260 Serotonin

(For urine metabolites (HIAA), use 83497)

84270 Sex hormone binding globulin (SHBG)

84275 Sialic acid

(Sickle hemoglobin, use 85660)

84285 Silica

84295 Sodium; serum, plasma or whole blood

84300   urine

84302   other source

(Somatomammotropin, use 83632)

(Somatotropin, use 83003)

84305 Somatomedin

84307 Somatostatin

84311 Spectrophotometry, analyte not elsewhere specified

84315 Specific gravity (except urine)

(For specific gravity, urine, see 81000-81003)

(Stone analysis, see 82355-82370)

(For suppression of growth stimulation expressed gene 2 [ST2] testing, use 83006)

84375 Sugars, chromatographic, TLC or paper chromatography

84376 Sugars (mono, di, and oligosaccharides); single qualitative, each specimen

84377   multiple qualitative, each specimen

84378   single quantitative, each specimen

84379   multiple quantitative, each specimen

84392 Sulfate, urine

(Sulfhemoglobin, use hemoglobin, 83060)

(T-3, see 84479-84481)

(T-4, see 84436-84439)

84402 Testosterone; free

84403	total

84410   bioavailable, direct measurement (eg, differential precipitation)

(Do not report 84402, 84403 in conjunction with 80327, 80328 to identify anabolic steroid testing for testosterone)

84425   Thiamine (Vitamin B-1)

84430   Thiocyanate

84431   Thromboxane metabolite(s), including thromboxane if performed, urine

(For concurrent urine creatinine determination, use 84431 in conjunction with 82470)

84432   Thyroglobulin

(Thyroglobulin, antibody, use 86800)

(Thyrotropin releasing hormone (TRH) test, see 80438, 80439)

84436   Thyroxine; total

84437   requiring elution (eg, neonatal)

84439   free

84442   Thyroxine binding globulin (TBG)

84443   Thyroid stimulating hormone (TSH)

84445   Thyroid stimulating immune globulins (TSI)

(Tobramycin, use 80200)

84446   Tocopherol alpha (Vitamin E)

84449   Transcortin (cortisol binding globulin)

84450   Transferase; aspartate amino (AST) (SGOT)

84460   alanine amino (ALT) (SGPT)

84466   Transferrin

(Iron binding capacity, use 83550)

84478   Triglycerides

84479   Thyroid hormone (T3 or T4) uptake or thyroid hormone binding ratio (THBR)

84480   Triiodothyronine T3; total (TT-3)

84481   free

84482   reverse

84484   Troponin, quantitative

(For Troponin, qualitative assay, use 84512)

84485   Trypsin; duodenal fluid

84488	feces, qualitative
84490	feces, quantitative, 24-hour collection
84510	Tyrosine

(Urate crystal identification, use 89060)

84512	Troponin, qualitative

(For Troponin, quantitative assay, use 84484)

84520	Urea nitrogen; quantitative
84525	semiquantitative (eg, reagent strip test)
84540	Urea nitrogen, urine
84545	Urea nitrogen, clearance
84550	Uric acid; blood
84560	other source
84577	Urobilinogen, feces, quantitative
84578	Urobilinogen, urine; qualitative
84580	quantitative, timed specimen
84583	semiquantitative

(Uroporphyrins, use 84120)

(Valproic acid (dipropylacetic acid), ues 80164)

84585	Vanillylmandelic acid (VMA), urine
84586	Vasoactive intestinal peptide (VIP)
84588	Vasopressin (antidiuretic hormone, ADH)
84590	Vitamin A

(Vitamin B-1, use 84425)

(Vitamin B-2, use 84252)

(Vitamin B-6, use 84207)

(Vitamin B-12, use 82607)

(Vitamin B-12, absorption (Schilling), see 78270, 78271)

(Vitamin C, use 82180)

(Vitamin D, see 82306, 82652)

(Vitamin E, use 84446)

84591	Vitamin, not otherwise specified
84597	Vitamin K

● New Code ▲ Revised Code + Add-On Code ⊘ Modifier -51 Exempt ★ Telemedicine

(VMA, use 84585)

84600   Volatiles (eg, acetic anhydride, diethylether)

(For carbon tetrachloride, dichloroethane, dichloromethane, use 82441)

(For isopropyl alcohol and methanol, use 80320)

(Volume, blood, RISA or Cr-51, see 78110, 78111)

84620   Xylose absorption test, blood and/or urine

(For administration, use 99070)

84630   Zinc

84681   C-peptide

84702   Gonadotropin, chorionic (hCG); quantitative

84703   qualitative

(For urine pregnancy test by visual color comparison, use 81025)

84704   free beta chain

84830   Ovulation tests, by visual color comparison methods for human luteinizing hormone

84999   Unlisted chemistry procedure

(For definitive testing of a drug, not otherwise specified, see 80299, 80375, 80376, 80377)

HEMATOLOGY AND COAGULATION

(For blood banking procedures, see Transfusion Medicine)

(Agglutinins, see Immunology)

(Antiplasmin, use 85410)

(Antithrombin III, see 85300, 85301)

85002   Bleeding time

85004   Blood count; automated differential WBC count

85007   blood smear, microscopic examination with manual differential WBC count

85008   blood smear, microscopic examination without manual differential WBC count

(For other fluids (eg, CSF), see 89050, 89051)

85009   manual differential WBC count, buffy coat

(Eosinophils, nasal smear, use 89190)

85013   spun microhematocrit

85014   hematocrit (Hct)

85018   hemoglobin (Hgb)

(For other hemoglobin determination, see 83020-83069)

(For immunoassay, hemoglobin, fecal, use 82274)

(For transcutaneous hemoglobin measurement, use 88738)

85025 complete (CBC), automated (Hgb, Hct, RBC, WBC and platelet count) and automated differential WBC count

85027 complete (CBC), automated (Hgb, Hct, RBC, WBC and platelet count)

85032 manual cell count (erythrocyte, leukocyte, or platelet) each

85041 red blood cell (RBC), automated

(Do not report code 85041 in conjunction with 85025 or 85027)

85044 reticulocyte, manual

85045 reticulocyte, automated

85046 reticulocytes, automated, including 1 or more cellular parameters (eg, reticulocyte hemoglobin content [CHr], immature reticulocyte fraction [IRF], reticulocyte volume [mrv], RNA content), direct measurement

85048 leukocyte (WBC), automated

85049 platelet, automated

85055 Reticulated platelet assay

85060 Blood smear, peripheral, interpretation by physician with written report

85097 Bone marrow, smear interpretation

(For special stains, see 85540, 88312, 88313)

(For bone biopsy, see 20220, 20225, 20240, 20245, 20250, 20251)

85130 Chromogenic substrate assay

(Circulating anti-coagulant screen (mixing studies), see 85611, 85732)

85170 Clot retraction

85175 Clot lysis time, whole blood dilution

(Clotting factor I (fibrinogen), see 85384, 85385)

85210 Clotting; factor II, prothrombin, specific

(See also 85610-85613)

85220 factor V (AcG or proaccelerin), labile factor

85230 factor VII (proconvertin, stable factor)

85240 factor VIII (AHG), 1 stage

85244 factor VIII related antigen

85245 factor VIII, VW factor, ristocetin cofactor

85246 factor VIII, VW factor antigen

● New Code ▲ Revised Code ＋ Add-On Code ⊘ Modifier -51 Exempt ★ Telemedicine

85247	factor VIII, von Willebrands factor, multimetric analysis	
85250	factor IX (PTC or Christmas)	
85260	factor X (Stuart-Prower)	
85270	factor XI (PTA)	
85280	factor XII (Hageman)	
85290	factor XIII (fibrin stabilizing)	
85291	factor XIII (fibrin stabilizing), screen solubility	
85292	prekallikrein assay (Fletcher factor assay)	
85293	high molecular weight kininogen assay (Fitzgerald factor assay)	
85300	Clotting inhibitors or anticoagulants; antithrombin III, activity	
85301	antithrombin III, antigen assay	
85302	protein C, antigen	
85303	protein C, activity	
85305	protein S, total	
85306	protein S, free	
85307	Activated Protein C (APC) resistance assay	
85335	Factor inhibitor test	
85337	Thrombomodulin	

(For mixing studies for inhibitors, use 85732)

85345	Coagulation time; Lee and White	
85347	activated	
85348	other methods	

(Differential count, see 85007 et seq)

(Duke bleeding time, use 85002)

(Eosinophils, nasal smear, use 89190)

85360 Euglobulin lysis

(Fetal hemoglobin, see 83030, 83033, 85460)

85362 Fibrin(ogen) degradation (split) products (FDP)(FSP); agglutination slide, semiquantitative

(Immunoelectrophoresis, use 86320)

85366	paracoagulation	
85370	quantitative	

85378 Fibrin degradation products, D-dimer; qualitative or semiquantitative

85379 quantitative

(For ultrasensitive and standard sensitivity quantitative D-dimer, use 85379)

85380 ultrasensitive (eg., for evaluation for venous thromboembolism), qualitative or semiquantitative

85384 Fibrinogen; activity

85385 antigen

85390 Fibrinolysins or coagulopathy screen, interpretation and report

85396 Coagulation/fibrinolysis assay, whole blood (eg, viscoelastic clot assessment), including use of any pharmacologic additive(s), as indicated, including interpretation and written report, per day

85397 Coagulation and fibrinolysis, functional activity, not otherwise specified (eg, adamts-13), each analyte

85400 Fibrinolytic factors and inhibitors; plasmin

85410 alpha-2 antiplasmin

85415 plasminogen activator

85420 plasminogen, except antigenic assay

85421 plasminogen, antigenic assay

(Fragility, red blood cell, see 85547, 85555-85557)

85441 Heinz bodies; direct

85445 induced, acetyl phenylhydrazine

(Hematocrit (PCV), see 85014)

(Hemoglobin, see 83020-83068, 85018-85027)

85460 Hemoglobin or RBCs, fetal, for fetomaternal hemorrhage; differential lysis (Kleihauer-Betke)

(See also 83030, 83033)

(Hemolysins, see 86940, 86941)

85461 rosette

85475 Hemolysin, acid

(See also 86940, 86941)

85520 Heparin assay

85525 Heparin neutralization

85530 Heparin-protamine tolerance test

85536 Iron stain, peripheral blood

(For iron stains on bone marrow or other tissues with physician evaluation, use 88313)

85540 Leukocyte alkaline phosphatase with count

● New Code   ▲ Revised Code   ✚ Add-On Code   ⊘ Modifier -51 Exempt   ★ Telemedicine

85547 Mechanical fragility, RBC

85549 Muramidase

(Nitroblue tetrazolium dye test, use 86384)

85555 Osmotic fragility, RBC; unincubated

85557   incubated

(Packed cell volume, use 85013)

(Partial thromboplastin time, see 85730, 85732)

(Parasites, blood (eg, malaria smears), use 87207)

(Plasmin, use 85400)

(Plasminogen, use 85420)

(Plasminogen activator, use 85415)

85576 Platelet; aggregation (in vitro), each agent

(For thromboxane metabolite[s], including thromboxane, if performed, measurement[s] in urine, use 84431)

85597 Phospholipid neutralization; platelet

85598   hexagonal phospholipid

85610 Prothrombin time;

85611   substitution, plasma fractions, each

85612 Russell viper venom time (includes venom); undiluted

85613   diluted

(Red blood cell count, see 85025, 85027, 85041)

85635 Reptilase test

(Reticulocyte count, see 85044, 85045)

85651 Sedimentation rate, erythrocyte; non-automated

85652   automated

85660 Sickling of RBC, reduction

(Hemoglobin electrophoresis, use 83020)

(Smears (eg, for parasites, malaria), use 87207)

85670 Thrombin time; plasma

85675   titer

85705 Thromboplastin inhibition, tissue

(For individual clotting factors, see 85245-85247)

85730 Thromboplastin time, partial (PTT); plasma or whole blood

---

85732	substitution, plasma fractions, each
85810	Viscosity

(von Willebrand factor assay, see 85245-85247)

(WBC count, see 85025-85031, 85048, 89050)

85999	Unlisted hematology and coagulation procedure

IMMUNOLOGY

(Acetylcholine receptor antibody, see 83519, 86255, 86256)

(Actinomyces, antibodies to, use 86602)

(Adrenal cortex antibodies, see 86255, 86256)

86000	Agglutinins, febrile (eg, Brucella, Francisella, Murine typhus, Q fever, Rocky Mountain spotted fever, scrub typhus), each antigen

(For antibodies to infectious agents, see 86602-86804)

86001	Allergen specific IgG quantitative or semiquantitative, each allergen

(Agglutinins and autohemolysins, see 86940, 86941)

86003	Allergen specific IgE; quantitative or semiquantitative, crude allergen extract, each

(For total quantitative IgE, use 82785)

86005	qualitative, multiallergen screen (eg, disk, sponge, card)
86008	quantitative or semiquantitative, recombinant or purified component, each

(For total qualitative IgE, use 83518)

(Alpha-1 antitrypsin, see 82103, 82104)

(Alpha-1 feto-protein, see 82105, 82106)

(Anti-AChR (acetylcholine receptor) antibody titer, see 86255, 86256)

(Anticardiolipin antibody, use 86147)

(Anti-DNA, use 86225)

(Anti-deoxyribonuclease titer, use 86215)

86021	Antibody identification; leukocyte antibodies
86022	platelet antibodies
86023	platelet associated immunoglobulin assay
86038	Antinuclear antibodies (ANA);
86039	titer

(Antistreptococcal antibody, ie, anti-DNAse, use 86215)

(Antistreptokinase titer, use 86590)

86060	Antistreptolysin 0; titer

(For antibodies to infectious agents, see 86602-86804)

86063   screen

(For antibodies to infectious agents, see 86602-86804)

(Blastomyces, antibodies to, use 86612)

86077   Blood bank physician services; difficult cross match and/or evaluation of irregular antibody(s), interpretation and written report

86078   investigation of transfusion reaction including suspicion of transmissible disease, interpretation and written report

86079   authorization for deviation from standard blood banking procedures (eg, use of outdated blood, transfusion of Rh incompatible units), with written report

(Brucella, antibodies to, use 86622)

(Candida, antibodies to, use 86628. For skin testing, use 86485)

86140   C-reactive protein;

(Candidiasis, use 86628)

86141   high sensitivity (hsCRP)

86146   Beta 2 Glycoprotein 1 antibody, each

86147   Cardiolipin (phospholipid) antibody, each Ig class

86152   Cell enumeration using immunologic selection and identification in fluid specimen (eg, circulating tumor cells in blood);

(For physician interpretation and report, use 86153. For cell enumeration with interpretation and report, use 86152 and 86153)

86153   physician interpretation and report, when required

(For cell enumeration, use 86152. For cell enumeration with interpretation and report, use 86152 and 86153)

(For flow cytometric immunophenotyping, see 88184-88189)

(For flow cytometric quantitation, see 86355, 86356, 86357, 86359, 86360, 86361, 86367)

86148   Anti-phosphatidylserine (phospholipid) antibody

(To report antiprothrombin (phospholipid cofactor) antibody, use 86849)

86152   Code out of order. See page 813

86153   Code out of order. See page 813

86155   Chemotaxis assay, specify method

(Clostridium difficile toxin, use 87230)

(Coccidioides, antibodies, to, see 86635. For skin testing, use 86490)

86156   Cold agglutinin; screen

86157   titer

86160   Complement; antigen, each component

| Separate Procedure | Unlisted Procedure | CCI Comp. Code | Non-specific Procedure | **813** |

86161	functional activity, each component
86162	total hemolytic (CH50)
86171	Complement fixation tests, each antigen

(Coombs test, see 86880-86886)

(**86185** deleted 2017 [2018 edition])

86200 Cyclic citrullinated peptide (CCP), antibody

86215 Deoxyribonuclease, antibody

86225 Deoxyribonucleic acid (DNA) antibody; native or double stranded

(Echinococcus, antibodies to, see code for specific method)

(For HIV antibody tests, see 86701-86703)

86226 single stranded

(Anti D.S., DNA, IFA, eg, using C.Lucilae, see 86255 and 86256)

86235 Extractable nuclear antigen, antibody to, any method (eg, nRNP, SS-A, SS-B, Sm, RNP, Sc170, J01), each antibody

(**86243** deleted 2017 [2018 edition])

86255 Fluorescent noninfectious agent antibody; screen, each antibody

86256 titer, each antibody

(Fluorescent technique for antigen identification in tissue, use 88346; for indirect fluorescence, see 88346, 88350)

(FTA, use 86780)

(Gel (agar) diffusion tests, use 86331)

86277 Growth hormone, human (HGH), antibody

86280 Hemagglutination inhibition test (HAI)

(For rubella, use 86762)

(For antibodies to infectious agents, see 86602-86804)

86294 Immunoassay for tumor antigen, qualitative or semiquantitative (eg, bladder tumor antigen)

(for qualitative NMP22 protein, use 86386)

86300 Immunoassay for tumor antigen, quantitative; CA 15-3 (27.29)

86301 CA 19-9

86304 CA 125

(For measurement of serum HER-2/neu oncoprotein, see 83950)

(For hepatitis delta agent, antibody, use 86692)

86305 Human epididymis protein 4 (HE4)

● New Code ▲ Revised Code ✛ Add-On Code ⊘ Modifier -51 Exempt ★ Telemedicine

86308   Heterophile antibodies; screening

(For antibodies to infectious agents, see 86602-86804)

86309   titer

(For antibodies to infectious agents, see 86602-86804)

86310   titers after absorption with beef cells and guinea pig kidney

(Histoplasma, antibodies to, use 86698. For skin testing, use 86510)

(For antibodies to infectious agents, see 86602-86804)

(Human growth hormone antibody, use 86277)

86316   Immunoassay for tumor antigen, other antigen, quantitative (eg, CA 50, 72-4, 549), each

86317   Immunoassay for infectious agent antibody, quantitative, not otherwise specified

(For immunoassay techniques for antigens, see 83516, 83518, 83519, 83520, 87301-87450, 87810-87899)

(For particle agglutination procedures, use 86403)

▲ **86318**   Immunoassay for infectious agent antibody(ies), qualitative or semiquantitative, single-step method (eg, reagent strip);

● **86328**   severe acute respiratory syndrome coronavirus 2 (SARS-CoV-2) (Coronavirus disease [COVID-19])

(For severe acute respiratory syndrome coronavirus 2 [SARS-CoV-2] [Coronavirus disease {COVID-19}] antibody testing using multiple-step method, use 86769)

86320   Immunoelectrophoresis; serum

86325   other fluids (eg, urine, cerebrospinal fluid) with concentration

86327   crossed (2-dimensional assay)

86328   This code is out of order. See page 815

86329   Immunodiffusion; not elsewhere specified

86331   gel diffusion, qualitative (Ouchterlony), each antigen or antibody

86332   Immune complex assay

86334   Immunofixation electrophoresis; serum

86335   other fluids with concentration (eg, urine, CSF)

86336   Inhibin A

86337   Insulin antibodies

86340   Intrinsic factor antibodies

(Leptospira, antibodies to, use 86720)

(Leukoagglutinins, use 86021)

86341   Islet cell antibody

86343   Leukocyte histamine release test (LHR)

86344 Leukocyte phagocytosis

86352 Cellular function assay involving stimulation (eg, mitogen or antigen) and detection of biomarker (eg, ATP)

86353 Lymphocyte transformation, mitogen (phytomitogen) or antigen induced blastogenesis

(Malaria antibodies, use 86750)

(For cellular function assay involving stimulation and detection of biomarker, use 86352)

86355 B cells, total count

86356 Mononuclear cell antigen, quantitive (eg, flow cytometry), not otherwise specified, each antigen

(Do not report 88187-88189 for interpretation of 86355, 86356, 86357, 86359, 86360, 86361, 86367)

86357 Natural killer (NK) cells, total count

86359 T cells; total count

86360   absolute CD4 and CD8 count, including ratio

86361   absolute CD4 count

86367 Stem cells (ie, CD34), total count

(For flow cytometric immunophenotyping for the assessment of potential hematolymphoid neoplasia, see 88184-88189)

86376 Microsomal antibodies (eg, thyroid or liver-kidney), each

(86378 deleted 2017 [2018 edition])

86382 Neutralization test, viral

86384 Nitroblue tetrazolium dye test (NTD)

86386 Nuclear Matrix Protein 22 (NMP22), qualitative

(Ouchterlony diffusion, use 86331)

(Platelet antibodies, see 86022, 86023)

86403 Particle agglutination; screen, each antibody

86406   titer, each antibody

(Pregnancy test, see 84702, 84703)

(Rapid plasma reagin test (RPR), see 86592, 86593)

86430 Rheumatoid factor; qualitative

86431   quantitative

(Serologic test for syphilis, see 86592, 86593)

86480 Tuberculosis test, cell mediated immunity antigen response measurement; gamma interferon

86481   enumeration of gamma interferon-producing T-cells in cell suspension

86485 Skin test; candida

● New Code   ▲ Revised Code   + Add-On Code   ⊘ Modifier -51 Exempt   ★ Telemedicine

(For antibody, candida, use 86628)

86486   unlisted antigen, each

86490   coccidioidomycosis

86510   histoplasmosis

(For histoplasma, antibody, use 86698)

86580   tuberculosis, intradermal

(For tuberculosis test, cell mediated immunity measurement of gamma interferon antigen response, use 86480)

(For skin tests for allergy, see 95012-95199)

(Smooth muscle antibody, see 86255, 86256)

(Sporothrix, antibodies to, see code for specific method)

86590   Streptokinase, antibody

(For antibodies to infectious agents, see 86602-86804)

(Streptolysin O antibody, see antistreptolysin O, 86060, 86063)

86592   Syphilis test, non-treponemal antibody; qualitative (eg, VDRL, RPR, ART)

(For antibodies to infectious agents, see 86602-86804)

86593   quantitative

(For antibodies to infectious agents, see 86602-86804)

(Tetanus antibody, use 86774)

(Thyroglobulin antibody, use 86800)

(Thyroglobulin, use 84432)

(Thyroid microsomal antibody, use 86376)

(For toxoplasma antibody, see 86777-86778)

The following codes (86602-86804) are qualitative or semiquantitative immunoassays performed by multiplestep methods for the detection of antibodies to infectious agents. For immunoassays by single-step method (eg, reagent strips), see codes 86318, 86328. Procedures for the identification of antibodies should be coded as precisely as possible. For example, an antibody to a virus could be coded with increasing specificity for virus, family, genus, species, or type. In some cases, further precision may be added to codes by specifying the class of immunoglobulin being detected. When multiple tests are done to detect antibodies to organisms classified more precisely than the specificity allowed by available codes, it is appropriate to code each as a separate service. For example, a test for antibody to an enterovirus is coded as 86658. Coxsackie viruses are enteroviruses, but there are no codes for the individual species of enterovirus. If assays are performed for antibodies to coxsackie A and B species, each assay should be separately coded. Similarly, if multiple assays are performed for antibodies of different immunoglobulin classes, each assay should be coded separately. When a coding option exists for reporting IgM specific antibodies (eg, 86632), the corresponding nonspecific code (eg, 86631) may be reported for performance of either an antibody analysis not specific for a particular immunoglobulin class or for an IgG analysis.

(For the detection of antibodies other than those to infectious agents, see specific antibody [eg, 86021, 86022, 86023, 86376, 86800, 86850-86870] or specific method [eg, 83516, 86255, 86256])

(For infectious agent/antigen detection, see 87260-87899)

86602   Antibody; actinomyces

86603   adenovirus

86606	Aspergillus
86609	bacterium, not elsewhere specified
86611	Bartonella
86612	Blastomyces
86615	Bordetella
86617	Borrelia burgdorferi (Lyme disease) confirmatory test (eg, Western blot or immunoblot)
86618	Borrelia burgdorferi (Lyme disease)
86619	Borrelia (relapsing fever)
86622	Brucella
86625	Campylobacter
86628	Candida

(For skin test, candida, use 86485)

86631	Chlamydia
86632	Chlamydia, IgM

(For chlamydia antigen, see 87270, 87320. For fluorescent antibody technique, see 86255, 86256)

86635	Coccidioides

(For severe acute respiratory syndrome coronavirus 2 [SARS-CoV-2] [Coronavirus disease {COVID-19}] antibody testing, see 86328, 86769)

86638	Coxiella Brunetii (Q fever)
86641	Cryptococcus
86644	cytomegalovirus (CMV)
86645	cytomegalovirus (CMV), IgM
86648	Diphtheria
86651	encephalitis, California (La Crosse)
86652	encephalitis, Eastern equine
86653	encephalitis, St. Louis
86654	encephalitis, Western equine
86658	enterovirus (eg, coxsackie, echo, polio)

(Trichinella, antibodies to, use 86784)

(Trypanosoma, antibodies to, see code for specific method)

(Tuberculosis, use 86580 for skin testing)

(Viral antibodies, see code for specific method)

● New Code   ▲ Revised Code   ✛ Add-On Code   ⊘ Modifier -51 Exempt   ★ Telemedicine

86663	Epstein-Barr (EB) virus, early antigen (EA)
86664	Epstein-Barr (EB) virus, nuclear antigen (EBNA)
86665	Epstein-Barr (EB) virus, viral capsid (VCA)
86666	Ehrlichia
86668	Francisella Tularensis
86671	fungus, not elsewhere specified
86674	Giardia Lamblia
86677	Helicobacter Pylori
86682	helminth, not elsewhere specified
86684	Hemophilus influenza
86687	HTLV-I
86688	HTLV-II
86689	HTLV or HIV antibody, confirmatory test (eg, Western Blot)
86692	hepatitis, delta agent

(For hepatitis delta agent, antigen, use 87380)

86694	herpes simplex, non-specific type test
86695	herpes simplex, type 1
86696	herpes simplex, type 2
86698	histoplasma
86701	HIV-1
86702	HIV-2
86703	HIV-1 and HIV-2, single result

(For HIV-1 antigen(s) with HIV-1 and HIV-2 antibodies, single result, use 87389)

(When HIV immunoassay [HIV testing 86701-86703 or 87389] is performed using a kit or transportable instrument that wholly or in part consists of a single use, disposable analytical chamber, the service may be identified by adding modifier 92 to the usual code)

(For HIV-1 antigen, use 87390)

(For HIV-2 antigen, use 87391)

(For confirmatory test for HIV antibody (eg, Western Blot), use 86689)

86704	Hepatitis B core antibody (HBcAb); total
86705	IgM antibody
86706	Hepatitis B surface antibody (HBsAb)

86707	Hepatitis Be antibody (HBeAb)
86708	Hepatitis A antibody (HAAb)
86709	Hepatitis A antibody (HAAb), IgM antibody
86710	Antibody; influenza virus
86711	JC (John Cunningham) virus
86713	Legionella
86717	Leishmania
86720	Leptospira
86723	Listeria monocytogenes
86727	lymphocytic choriomeningitis
(86729	deleted 2017 [2018 edition])
86732	mucormycosis
86735	mumps
86738	Mycoplasma
86741	Neisseria meningitidis
86744	Nocardia
86747	parvovirus
86750	Plasmodium (malaria)
86753	protozoa, not elsewhere specified
86756	respiratory syncytial virus
86757	Rickettsia
86759	rotavirus
86762	rubella
86765	rubeola
86768	Salmonella
● 86769	severe acute respiratory syndrome coronavirus 2 (SARS-CoV-2) (Coronavirus disease [COVID-19])

(For severe acute respiratory syndrome coronavirus 2 [SARS-CoV-2] [Coronavirus disease {COVID-19}] antibody testing using single-step method, use 86328)

86771	Shigella
86774	tetanus
86777	Toxoplasma

86778	Toxoplasma, IgM
86780	Treponema pallidum

(For syphilis testing by non-treponemal antibody analysis, see 86592-86593)

86784	Trichinella
86787	varicella-zoster
86788	West Nile virus, IgM
86789	West Nile virus
86790	virus, not elsewhere specified
86793	Yersinia
86794	Zika virus, IgM
86800	Thyroglobulin antibody

(For thyroglobulin, use 84432)

86803	Hepatitis C antibody;
86804	confirmatory test (eg, immunoblot)

TISSUE TYPING

86805	Lymphocytotoxicity assay, visual crossmatch; with titration
86806	without titration
86807	Serum screening for cytotoxic percent reactive antibody (PRA); standard method
86808	quick method
86812	HLA typing; A, B, or C (eg, A10, B7, B27), single antigen
86813	A, B, or C, multiple antigens
86816	DR/DQ, single antigen
86817	DR/DQ, multiple antigens
86821	lymphocyte culture, mixed (MLC)
(86822	deleted 2017 [2018 edition])
86825	Human leukocyte antigen (HLA) crossmatch, non cytotoxic (eg, using flow cytometry); first serum sample or dilution
+ 86826	each additional serum sample or sample dilution (List separately in addition to primary procedure)

(Use 86826 in conjunction with 86825)

(Do not report 86825, 86826 in conjunction with 86355, 86359, 88184-88189 for antibody surface markers integral to crossmatch testing)

(For autologous HLA crossmatch, see 86825, 86826)

(For lymphocytotoxicity visual crossmatch, see 86805, 86806)

86828   Antibody to human leukocyte antigens (HLA), solid phase assays (eg, microspheres or beads, ELISA, flow cytometry); qualitative assessment of the presence of absence of antibody(ies) to HLA Class I and Class II HLA antigens

86829   qualitative assessment of the presence or absence of antibody(ies) to HLA Class I or Class II HLA antigens

(If solid phase testing is performed to assess presence or absence of antibody to both HLA classes, use 86828)

86830   antibody identification by qualitative panel using complete HLA phenotypes, HLA Class I

86831   antibody identification by qualitative panel using complete HLA phenotypes, HLA Class II

86832   high definition qualitative panel for identification of antibody sepcificities (eg, individual antigen per bead methodology), HLA Class I

86833   high definition qualitative panel for identification of antibody specificities (eg, individual antigen per bead methodology), HLA Class II

(If solid phase testing is performed to test for HLA Class I or II antibody after treatment [eg, to remove IgM antibodies or other interfering substances], report 86828-86833 once for each panel with the untreated serum and once for each panel with the treated serum)

86834   semi-quantitative panel (eg, titer), HLA Class I

86835   semi-quantiative panel (eg, titer), HLA Class II

86849   Unlisted immunology procedure

TRANSFUSION MEDICINE

(For apheresis, see 36511-36512)

(For therapeutic phlebotomy, use 99195)

86850   Antibody screen, RBC, each serum technique

86860   Antibody elution (RBC), each elution

86870   Antibody identification, RBC antibodies, each panel for each serum technique

86880   Antihuman globulin test (Coombs test); direct, each antiserum

86885   indirect, qualitative, each reagent red cell

86886   indirect, each antibody titer

(For indirect antihuman globulin [Coombs] test for RBC antibody screening, use 86850)

(For indirect·antihuman globulin [Coombs] test for RBC antibody identification using reagent red cell panels, use 86870)

86890   Autologous blood or component, collection processing and storage; predeposited

86891   intra-or postoperative salvage

86900   Blood typing, serologic; ABO

86901   Rh (D)

86902   antigen testing of donor blood using reagent serum, each antigen test

(If multiple blood units are tested for the same antigen, 86902 should be reported once for each antigen for each unit tested.)

86904   antigen screening for compatible unit using patient serum, per unit screened

86905   RBC antigens, other than ABO or Rh (D), each

86906   Rh phenotyping, complete

(For human erythrocyte antigen typing by molecular pathology techniques, use 81403)

86910   Blood typing, for paternity testing, per individual; ABO, Rh and MN

86911   each additional antigen system

86920   Compatibility test each unit; immediate spin technique

86921   incubation technique

86922   antiglobulin technique

86923   electronic

(Do not use 86923 in conjunction with 86920-86922 for same unit crossmatch)

86927   Fresh frozen plasma, thawing, each unit

86930   Frozen blood, each unit; freezing (includes preparation)

86931   thawing

86932   freezing (includes preparation) and thawing

86940   Hemolysins and agglutinins; auto, screen, each

86941   incubated

86945   Irradiation of blood product, each unit

86950   Leukocyte transfusion

(For allogenic lymphocyte infusion, use 38242)

(For leukapheresis, use 36511)

86960   Volume reduction of blood or blood product (eg, red blood cells or platelets), each unit

86965   Pooling of platelets or other blood products

(For harvesting, preparation, and injection[s] of platelet rich plasma, use 0232T)

(For harvesting, preparation, and injection[s] of autologous white blood cell/autologous protein solution, use 0481T)

86970   Pretreatment of RBCs for use in RBC antibody detection, identification, and/or compatibility testing; incubation with chemical agents or drugs, each

86971   incubation with enzymes, each

Separate Procedure   Unlisted Procedure   CCI Comp. Code   Non-specific Procedure   **823**

86972   by density gradient separation

86975   Pretreatment of serum for use in RBC antibody identification; incubation with drugs, each

86976   by dilution

86977   incubation with inhibitors, each

86978   by differential red cell absorption using patient RBCs or RBCs of known phenotype, each absorption

86985   Splitting of blood or blood products, each unit

86999   Unlisted transfusion medicine procedure

MICROBIOLOGY

Includes bacteriology, mycology, parasitology, and virology.

Presumptive identification of microorganisms is defined as identification by colony morphology, growth on selective media, Gram stains, or up to three tests (eg., catalase, oxidase, indole, urease). Definitive identification of microorganisms is defined as an identification to the genus or species level that requires additional tests (eg., biochemical panels, slide cultures). If additional studies involve molecular probes, nucleic acid sequencing, chromatography, or immunologic techniques, these should be separately coded using 87140-87158, in addition to definitive identification codes. The molecular diagnostic codes (eg., 81200-81408) are not to be used in combination with or instead of the procedures represented by 87140-87158. For multiple specimens/sites, used modifier 59. For repeat laboratory tests performed on the same day, use modifier 91.

87003   Animal inoculation, small animal, with observation and dissection

87015   Concentration (any type), for infectious agents

     (Do not report 87015 in conjunction with 87177)

87040   Culture, bacterial; blood, aerobic, with isolation and presumptive identification of isolates (includes anaerobic culture, if appropriate)

87045   stool, aerobic, with isolation and preliminary examination (eg, KIA, LIA), Salmonella and Shigella species

87046   stool, aerobic, additional pathogens, isolation and presumptive identification of isolates, each plate

87070   any other source except urine, blood or stool, aerobic, with isolation and presumptive identification of isolates

     (For urine, use 87088)

87071   quantitative, aerobic with isolation and presumptive identification of isolates, any source except urine, blood or stool

     (For urine, use 87088)

87073   quantitative, anaerobic with isolation and presumptive identification of isolates, any source except urine, blood or stool

     (For definitive identification of isolates, use 87076 or 87077. for typing of isolates see 87140-87158)

87075   any source, except blood, anaerobic with isolation and presumptive identification of isolates

87076   anaerobic isolate, additional methods required for definitive identification, each isolate

87077   aerobic isolate, additional methods required for definitive identification, each isolate

---

824   ● New Code   ▲ Revised Code   + Add-On Code   ⊘ Modifier -51 Exempt   ★ Telemedicine

87081 Culture, presumptive, pathogenic organisms, screening only;

87084   with colony estimation from density chart

87086 Culture, bacterial; quantitative colony count, urine

87088   with isolation and presumptive identification of each isolate, urine

87101 Culture, fungi (mold or yeast) isolation, with presumptive identification of isolates; skin, hair, or nail

87102   other source (except blood)

87103   blood

87106 Culture, fungi, definitive identification, each organism; yeast

87107   mold

87109 Culture, mycoplasma, any source

87110 Culture, chlamydia, any source

(For immunofluorescence staining of shell vials, use 87140)

87116 Culture, tubercle or other acid-fast bacilli (eg, TB, AFB, mycobacteria) any source, with isolation and presumptive identification of isolates

(For concentration, use 87015)

87118 Culture, mycobacterial, definitive identification, each isolate

87140 Culture, typing; immunofluorescent method, each antiserum

87143   gas liquid chromatography (GLC) or high pressure liquid chromotography (HPLC) method

87147   immunologic method, other than immunofluorescence (eg, agglutination grouping), per antiserum

87149   identification by nucleic acid (DNA or RNA) probe, direct probe technique, per culture or isolate, each organism probed

(Do not report 87149 in conjunction with 81200-81408)

87150   identification by nucleic acid (DNA or RNA) probe, amplified probe technique, per culture or isolate, each organism probed

(Do not report 87150 in conjunction with 81200-81408)

87152   identification by pulse field gel typing

(Do not report 87152 in conjunction with 81200-81408)

87153   identification by nucleic acid sequencing method, each isolate (eg, sequencing of the 16S rRNA gene)

87158   other methods

87164 Dark field examination, any source (eg, penile, vaginal, oral, skin); includes specimen collection

87166   without collection

87168 Macroscopic examination; arthropod

87169   parasite

87172   Pinworm exam (eg, cellophane tape prep)

87176   Homogenization, tissue, for culture

87177   Ova and parasites, direct smears, concentration and identification

(Do not report 87177 in conjunction with 87015)

(For direct smears from a primary source, use 87207)

(For coccidia or microsporidia exam, use 87207)

(For complex special stain (trichrome, iron hematoxylin), use 87209)

(For nucleic acid probes in cytologic material, use 88365)

87181   Susceptibility studies, antimicrobial agent; agar diffusion method, per agent (eg, antibiotic gradient strip)

87184   disk method, per plate (12 or fewer disks)

87185   enzyme detection (eg, beta lactamase), per enzyme

87186   microdilution or agar dilution (minimum inhibitory concentration [MIC] or breakpoint), each multi-antimicrobial, per plate

+ **87187**   microdilution or agar dilution, minimum lethal concentration (MLC), each plate ((List separately in addition to code for primary procedure)

(Use 87187 in conjunction with 87186 or 87188)

87188   macrobroth dilution method, each agent

87190   mycobacteria, proportion method, each agent

(For other mycobacterial susceptibility studies, see 87181, 87184, 87186, or 87188)

87197   Serum bactericidal titer (Schlicter test)

87205   Smear, primary source with interpretation; Gram or Giemsa stain for bacteria, fungi, or cell types

87206   fluorescent and/or acid fast stain for bacteria, fungi, or cell types

87207   special stain for inclusion bodies or parasites (eg, malaria, coccidia, microsporidia, trypanosomes, herpes viruses)

(For direct smears with concentration and identification, use 87177)

(For thick smear preparation, use 87015)

(For fat, meat, fibers, nasal eosinophils, and starch, see miscellaneous section)

87209   complex special stain (eg, trichrome, iron hemotoxylin) for ova and parasites

87210   wet mount for infectious agents (eg, saline, India ink, KOH preps)

(For KOH examination of skin, hair or nails, see 87220)

87220   Tissue examination by KOH slide of samples from skin, hair, or nails for fungi or ectoparasite ova or mites (eg, scabies)

87230   Toxin or antitoxin assay, tissue culture (eg, Clostridium difficile toxin)

87250 Virus isolation; inoculation of embryonated eggs, or small animal, includes observation and dissection

87252 tissue culture inoculation, observation, and presumptive identification by cytopathic effect

87253 tissue culture, additional studies or definitive identification (eg, hemabsorption, neutralization, immunofluorescence stain) each isolate

(Electron microscopy, use 88348)

(Inclusion bodies in tissue sections, see 88304-88309; in smears, see 87207-87210; in fluids, use 88106)

87254 centrifuge enhanced (shell vial) technique, includes identification with immunofluorescence stain, each virus

(Report 87254 in addition to 87252 as appropriate)

87255 including identification by non-immunologic method, other than by cytopathic effect (eg., virus specific enzymatic activity)

These codes are intended for primary source only. For similar studies on culture material, refer to codes 87140-87158. Infectious agents by antigen detection, immunofluorescence microscopy, or nucleic acid probe techniques should be reported as precisely as possible. The molecular pathology procedures codes (81161, 81200-81408) are not to be used in combination with or instead of the procedures represented by 87471-87801. The most specific code possible should be reported. If there is no specific agent code, the general methodology code (eg, 87299, 87449, 87450, 87797, 87798, 87799, 87899) should be used. For identification of antibodies to many of the listed infectious agents, see 86602-86804. When separate results are reported for different species or strain of organisms, each result should be coded separately. Use modifier 59 when separate results are reported for different species or strains that are described by the same code.

87260 Infectious agent antigen detection by immunofluorescent technique; adenovirus

87265 Bordetella pertussis/parapertussis

87267 Enterovirus, direct fluorescent antibody (DFA)

87269 giardia

87270 Chlamydia trachomatis

87271 Cytomegalovirus, direct fluorescent antibody (DFA)

87272 cryptosporidium

87273 Herpes simplex virus type 2

87274 Herpes simplex virus 1

87275 Influenza B virus

87276 influenza A virus

(**87277** deleted 2017 [2018 edition])

87278 Legionella pneumophila

87279 Parainfluenza virus, each type

87280 respiratory syncytial virus

87281 Pneumocystis carinii

87283 Rubeola

87285	Treponema pallidum
87290	Varicella zoster virus
87299	not otherwise specified, each organism
87300	Infectious agent antigen detection by immunofluorescent technique, polyvalent for multiple organisms, each polyvalent antiserum

(For physican evaluation of infectious disease agents by immunofluorescence, use 88346)

87301	Infectious agent antigen detection by immunoassay technique, (eg, enzyme immunoassay [EIA], enzyme-linked immunosorbent assay [ELISA], immunochemiluminometric assay [IMCA]) qualitative or semiquantitative, multiple-step method; adenovirus enteric types 40/41
87305	Aspergillus
87320	Chlamydia trachomatis
87324	Clostridium difficile toxin(s)
87327	Cryptococcus neoformans

(For Cryptococcus latex agglutination, use 86403)

87328	cryptosporidium
87329	giardia
87332	cytomegalovirus
87335	Escherichia coli 0157

(For giardia antigen, use 87329)

87336	Entamoeba histolytica dispar group
87337	Entamoeba histolytica group
87338	Helicobacter pylori, stool
87339	Helicobacter pylori

(For H. pylori, stool, use 87338. For H. pylori, breath and blood by mass spectrometry, see 83013, 83014. For H. pylori, liquid scintillation counter, see 78267, 78268)

87340	hepatitis B surface antigen (HBsAg)
87341	hepatitis B surface antigen (HBsAg) neutralization
87350	hepatitis Be antigen (HBeAg)
87380	hepatitis, delta agent
87385	Histoplasma capsulatum
87389	HIV-1 antigen(s), with HIV-1 and HIV-2 antibodies, single result
87390	HIV-1
87391	HIV-2

● New Code ▲ Revised Code + Add-On Code ⊘ Modifier -51 Exempt ★ Telemedicine

87400   Influenza, A or B, each

87420   respiratory syncytial virus

87425   rotavirus

87427   Shiga-like toxin

87430   Streptococcus, group A

87449   Infectious agent antigen detection by immunoassay technique, (eg, enzyme immunoassay [EIA], enzyme-linked immunosorbent assay [ELISA], immunochemiluminometric assay [IMCA]), qualitative or semiquantitative; multiple-step method, not otherwise specified, each organism

(**87450**   deleted December 31, 2020)

87451   multiple step method, polyvalent for multiple organisms, each polyvalent antiserum

(**87470**   deleted 2017 [2018 edition])

87471   Infectious agent detection by nucleic acid (DNA or RNA); Bartonella henselae and Bartonella quintana, amplified probe technique

87472   Bartonella henselae and Bartonella quintana, quantification

87475   Borrelia burgdorferi, direct probe technique

87476   Borrelia burgdorferi, amplified probe technique

(**87477**   deleted 2017 [2018 edition])

87480   Candida species, direct probe technique

87481   Candida species, amplified probe technique

87482   Candida species, quantification

87483   Central nervous system pathogen (eg, Neisseria meningitidis, Streptococcus pneumoniae, Listeria, Haemophilus influenzae, E. coli, Streptococcus agalactiae, enterovirus, human parechovirus, herpes simplex virus type 1 and 2, human herpesvirus 6, cytomegalovirus, varicella zoster virus, Cryptococcus), includes multiplex reverse transcription, when performed, and multiplex amplified probe technique, multiple types or subtypes, 12-25 targets

87485   Chlamydia pneumoniae, direct probe technique

87486   Chlamydia pneumoniae, amplified probe technique

87487   Chlamydia pneumoniae, quantification

87490   Chlamydia trachomatis, direct probe technique

87491   Chlamydia trachomatis, amplified probe technique

87492   Chlamydia trachomatis, quantification

87493   Clostridium difficile, toxin gene(s), amplified probe technique

87495   cytomegalovirus, direct probe technique

87496	cytomegalovirus, amplified probe technique
87497	cytomegalovirus, quantification
87498	enterovirus, amplified probe technique, includes reverse transcription when performed
87500	vancomycin resistance (eg, enterococcus species van A, van B), amplified probe technique
87501	influenza virus, includes reverse transcription, when performed, and amplified probe technique, each type or subtype
87502	influenza virus, for multiple types or sub-types, includes multiplex reverse transcription, when performed, and multiplex amplified probe technique, first 2 types or sub-types
+ 87503	influenza virus, for multiple types or sub-types, includes multiplex reverse transcription, when performed, and multiplex amplified probe technique, each additional influenza virus type or sub-type beyond 2 (List separately in addition to code for primary procedure)

(Use 87503 in conjunction with 87502)

87505	gastrointestinal pathogen (eg, Clostridium difficile, E. coli, Salmonella, Shigella, norovirus, Giardia), includes multiplex reverse transcription, when performed, and multiplex amplified probe technique, multiple types or subtypes, 3-5 targets
87506	gastrointestinal pathogen (eg, Clostridium difficile, E.coli, Salmonella, Shigella, norovirus, Giardia), includes multiplex reverse transcription, when performed, and multiplex amplified probe technique, multiple types or subtypes, 6-11 targets
87507	gastrointestinal pathogen (eg, Clostridium difficile, E. coli, Salmonella, Shigella, norovirus, Giardia), includes multiplex reverse transcription, when performed, and multiplex amplified probe technique, multiple types or subtypes, 12-25 targets
87510	Gardnerella vaginalis, direct probe technique
87511	Gardnerella vaginalis, amplified probe technique
87512	Gardnerella vaginalis, quantification
(87515	deleted 2017 [2018 edition])
87516	hepatitis B virus, amplified probe technique
87517	hepatitis B virus, quantification
87520	hepatitis C, direct probe technique
87521	hepatitis C, amplified probe technique, includes reverse transcription when performed
87522	hepatitis C, quantification, includes reverse transcription when performed
87525	hepatitis G, direct probe technique
87526	hepatitis G, amplified probe technique
87527	hepatitis G, quantification
87528	Herpes simplex virus, direct probe technique
87529	Herpes simplex virus, amplified probe technique

● New Code   ▲ Revised Code   + Add-On Code   ⊘ Modifier -51 Exempt   ★ Telemedicine

87530	Herpes simplex virus, quantification
87531	Herpes virus-6, direct probe technique
87532	Herpes virus-6, amplified probe technique
87533	Herpes virus-6, quantification
87534	HIV-1, direct probe technique
87535	HIV-1, amplified probe technique, includes reverse transcription when performed
87536	HIV-1, quantification, includes reverse transcription when performed
87537	HIV-2, direct probe technique
87538	HIV-2, amplified probe technique, includes reverse transcription when performed
87539	HIV-2, quantification, includes reverse transcription when performed
87623	Human Papillomavirus (HPV), low-risk types (eg., 6, 11, 42, 43, 44)
87624	Human Papillomavirus (HPV), high-risk types (eg., 16, 18, 31, 33, 35, 39, 45, 51, 56, 58, 59, 68)

(When both low-risk and high-risk HPV types are performed in a single assay, use only 87624)

| 87625 | Human Papillomavirus (HPV), types 16 and 18 only, includes type 45, if performed |

(For Human Papillomavirus [HPV] detection of five or greater separately reported high-risk HPV types [ie, genotyping], use 0500T)

87540	Legionella pneumophila, direct probe technique
87541	Legionella pneumophila, amplified probe technique
87542	Legionella pneumophila, quantification
87550	Mycobacteria species, direct probe technique
87551	Mycobacteria species, amplified probe technique
87552	Mycobacteria species, quantification
87555	Mycobacteria tuberculosis, direct probe technique
87556	Mycobacteria tuberculosis, amplified probe technique
87557	Mycobacteria tuberculosis, quantification
87560	Mycobacteria avium-intracellulare, direct probe technique
87561	Mycobacteria avium-intracellulare, amplified probe technique
87562	Mycobacteria avium-intracellulare, quantification
87563	Mycoplasma genitalium, amplified probe technique
87580	Mycoplasma pneumoniae, direct probe technique

87581	Mycoplasma pneumoniae, amplified probe technique
87582	Mycoplasma pneumoniae, quantification
87590	Neisseria gonorrhoeae, direct probe technique
87591	Neisseria gonorrhoeae, amplified probe technique
87592	Neisseria gonorrhoeae, quantification
87623	This code is out of order. See page 831
87624	This code is out of order. See page 831
87625	This code is out of order. See page 831

87631   respiratory virus (eg, adenovirus, influenza virus, coronavirus, metapneumovirus, parainfluenza virus, respiratory syncytial virus, rhinovirus), includes multiplex reverse transcription, when performed, and multiplex amplified probe technique, multiple types or subtypes, 3-5 targets

87632   respiratory virus (eg, adenovirus, influenza virus, coronavirus, metapneumovirus, parainfluenza virus, respiratory syncytial virus, rhinovirus), includes multiplex reverse transcription, when performed, and multiplex amplified probe technique, multiple types or subtypes, 6-11 targets

87633   respiratory virus (eg, adenovirus, influenza virus, coronavirus, metapneumovirus, parainfluenza virus, respiratory syncytial virus, rhinovirus), includes multiplex reverse transcription, when performed, and multiplex amplified probe technique, multiple types or subtypes, 12-25 targets

(Use 87631-87633 for nucleic acid assays which detect multiple respiratory viruses in a multiplex reaction [ie, single procedure with multiple results])

(For assays that are used to type or subtype influenza viruses only, see 87501-87503)

(For assays that include influenza viruses with additional respiratory viruses, see 87631-87633)

(For detection of multiple infectious agents not otherwise specified which report a single result, see 87800, 87801)

87634   respiratory syncytial virus, amplified probe technique

(For assays that include respiratory syncytial virus with additional respiratory viruses, see 87631, 87632, 87633)

● 87635   severe acute respiratory syndrome coronavirus 2 (SARS-CoV-2) (Coronavirus disease [COVID-19]), amplified probe technique

● 87636   severe acute respiratory syndrome coronavirus 2 (SARS-CoV-2) (Coronavirus disease [COVID-19]) and influenza virus types A and B, multiplex amplified probe technique

● 87637   severe acute respiratory syndrome coronavirus 2 (SARS-CoV-2) (Coronavirus disease [COVID-19]), influenza virus types A and B, and respiratory syncytial virus, multiplex, amplified probe technique

87640   Staphylococcus aureus, amplified probe technique

87641   Staphylococcus aureus, methicillin resistant, amplified probe technique

(For assays that detect methicillin resistance and identify Staphylococcus aureus using a single nucleic acid sequenc, use 87641)

87650   Streptococcus, group A, direct probe technique

87651   Streptococcus, group A, amplified probe technique

● New Code   ▲ Revised Code   + Add-On Code   ⊘ Modifier -51 Exempt   ★ Telemedicine

87652	Streptococcus, group A, quantification
87653	Streptococcus, group B, amplified probe technique
87660	Trichomonas vaginalis, direct probe technique
87661	Trichomonas vaginalis, amplified probe technique
87662	Zika virus, amplified probe technique
87797	Infectious agent detection by nucleic acid (DNA or RNA), not otherwise specified; direct probe technique, each organism
87798	amplified probe technique, each organism
87799	quantification, each organism
87800	Infectious agent detection by nucleic acid (DNA or RNA), multiple organisms; direct probe(s) technique
87801	amplified probe(s) technique

(For each specific organism nucleic acid detection from a primary source, see 87471-87660. For detection of specific infectious agents not otherwise specified, see 87797, 87798, or 87799 1 time for each agent)

(For detection of multiple infectious agents not otherwise specified which report a single result, see 87800, 87801)

(Do not use 87801 for nucleic acid assays that detect multiple respiratory viruses in a multiplex reaction [ie, single procedure with multiple results], see 87631-87633)

87802	Infectious agent antigen detection by immunoassay with direct optical observation; Streptococcus, group B
87803	Clostridium difficile toxin A
87806	HIV-1 antigen(s), with HIV-1 and HIV-2 antibodies
87804	Influenza
87806	This code is out of order. See page 833
87807	respiratory syncytial virus
87808	Trichomonas vaginalis
87809	adenovirus
87810	Chlamydia trachomatis
● 87811	severe acute respiratory syndrome coronavirus 2 (SARS-CoV-2) (Coronavirus disease [COVID-19])
87850	Neisseria gonorrhoeae
87880	Streptococcus, group A
87899	not otherwise specified
87900	Infectious agent drug susceptibility phenotype prediction using regularly updated genotypic bioinformatics
87910	Infectious agent genotype analysis by nucleic acid (DNA or RNA); cytomegalovirus

(For infectious agent drug susceptibility phenotype prediction for HIV-1, use 87900)

| Separate Procedure | Unlisted Procedure | CCI Comp. Code | Non-specific Procedure | **833** |

(For Human Papillomavirus [HPV] for high-risk types (ie, genotyping), of five or greater separately reported HPV types, use 0500T)

87901 HIV-1, reverse transciptase and protease regions

87906 HIV-1, other region (eg, integrase, fusion)

(For infectious agent drug susceptibility phenotype prediction for HIV-1, use 87900)

87912 Hepatitis B virus

87902 Hepatitis C virus

87903 Infectious agent phenotype analysis by nucleic acid (DNA or RNA) with drug resistance tissue culture analysis, HIV 1; first through 10 drugs tested

+ 87904 each additional drug tested (List separately in addition to code for primary procedure)

(Use 87904 in conjunction with code 87903)

87905 Infectious agent enzymatic activity other than virus (eg, sialidase activity in vaginal fluid)

(For virus isolation including identification by non-immunologic method, other than by cytopathic effect, use 87255)

87906 This code is out of order. See page 834

87910 This code is out of order. See page 833

87912 This code is out of order. See page 834

87999 Unlisted microbiology procedure

ANATOMIC PATHOLOGY

POSTMORTEM EXAMINATION

Procedures 88000 through 88099 represent physician services only. Use modifier 90 for outside laboratory services.

88000 Necropsy (autopsy), gross examination only; without CNS

88005 with brain

88007 with brain and spinal cord

88012 infant with brain

88014 stillborn or newborn with brain

88016 macerated stillborn

88020 Necropsy (autopsy), gross and microscopic; without CNS

88025 with brain

88027 with brain and spinal cord

88028 infant with brain

88029 stillborn or newborn with brain

● New Code ▲ Revised Code + Add-On Code ⊘ Modifier -51 Exempt ★ Telemedicine

88036	Necropsy (autopsy), limited, gross and/or microscopic; regional
88037	single organ
88040	Necropsy (autopsy); forensic examination
88045	coroner's call
88099	Unlisted necropsy (autopsy) procedure

CYTOPATHOLOGY

When cytopathology codes are reported, the appropriate CPT code to bill is that which describes, to the highest level of specificity, what services were rendered. Accordingly, for a given specimen, only one code from a group of related codes describing a group of services that could be performed on a specimen with the same end result (e.g. 88104-88112, 88142- 88143, 88150-88154, 88164-88167, etc.) is to be reported.

If multiple services (i.e., separate specimens from different anatomic sites) are reported, modifier -59 should be used to indicate that different levels of service were provided for different specimens from different anatomic sites. This should be reflected in the cytopathologic reports. A cytopathology preparation from a fluid, washing, or brushing is to be reported using one code from the range of CPT codes 88104-88112. It is inappropriate to additionally use CPT codes 88160-88162 because the smears are included in the codes referable to fluids (or washings or brushings) and 88160-88162 references any other source which would exclude fluids, washings, or brushings.

88104	Cytopathology, fluids, washings or brushings, except cervical or vaginal; smears with interpretation
88106	simple filter method with interpretation

(Do not report 88106 in conjunction with 88104)

(For nongynecological selective cellular enhancement including filter transfer techniques, use 88112)

88108	Cytopathology, concentration technique, smears and interpretation (eg, Saccomanno technique)

(For cervical or vaginal smears, see 88150-88155)
(For gastric intubation with lavage, see 43754, 43755)

(For x-ray localization, use 74340)

88112	Cytopathology, selective cellular enhancement technique with interpretation (eg, liquid based slide preparation method), except cervical or vaginal

(Do not report 88112 with 88108)

88120	Cytopathology, in situ hybridization (eg, fish), urinary tract specimen with morphometric analysis, 3-5 molecular probes, each specimen; manual
88121	using computer-assisted technology

(For morphometric in situ hybridization on cytologic specimens other than urinary tract, see 88367, 88368)

(For more than 5 probes, use 88399)

88125	Cytopathology, forensic (eg, sperm)
88130	Sex chromatin identification; Barr bodies
88140	peripheral blood smear, polymorphonuclear drumsticks

(For Guard stain, use 88313)

Codes 88141-88155, 88164-88167, 88174-88175 are used to report cervical or vaginal screening by various methods and to report physician interpretation services. Use codes 88150, 88152, 88153 to report conventional Pap smears that are examined using non-Bethesda reporting. Use codes 88164-88167 to report conventional Pap smears that are examined using the Bethesda System of reporting. Use codes 88142-88143 to report liquidbased specimens processed as thin-layer preparations that are examined using any system of reporting (Bethesda or non-Bethesda). Use codes 88174-88175 to report automated screening of liquid-based specimens that are examined using any system of reporting (Bethesda or non-Bethesda).Within each of these three code families choose the one code that describes the screening method(s) used. Codes 88141 and 88155 should be reported in addition to the screening code chosen when the additional services are provided. Manual rescreening requires a complete visual reassessment of the entire slide initially screened by either an automated or manual process. Manual review represents an assessment of selected cells or regions of a slide identified by initial automated review.

88141 Cytopathology, cervical or vaginal (any reporting system), requiring interpretation by physician

(Use 88141 in conjunction with 88142, 88143, 88147, 88148, 88150, 88152, 88153, 88164-88167, 88174-88175)

88142 Cytopathology, cervical or vaginal (any reporting system), collected in preservative fluid, automated thin layer preparation; manual screening under physician supervision

88143 with manual screening and rescreening under physician supervision

(For automated screening of automated thin layer preparation, see 88174, 88175)

88147 Cytopathology smears, cervical or vaginal; screening by automated system under physician supervision

88148 screening by automated system with manual rescreening under physician supervision

88150 Cytopathology, slides, cervical or vaginal; manual screening under physician supervision

88152 with manual screening and computer-assisted rescreening under physician supervision

88153 with manual screening and rescreening under physician supervision

(**88154** deleted 2017 [2018 edition])

+ **88155** Cytopathology, slides, cervical or vaginal, definitive hormonal evaluation (eg, maturation index, karyopyknotic index, estrogenic index) (List separately in addition to code[s] for other technical and interpretation services)

(Use 88155 in conjunction with 88142, 88143, 88147, 88148, 88150, 88152, 88153, 88164-88167, 88174-88175)

88160 Cytopathology, smears, any other source; screening and interpretation

88161 preparation, screening and interpretation

88162 extended study involving over 5 slides and/or multiple stains

(For aerosol collection of sputum, use 89350)

(For special stains, see 88312-88314)

88164 Cytopathology, slides, cervical or vaginal (the Bethesda System); manual screening under physician supervision

88165 with manual screening and rescreening under physician supervision

88166 with manual screening and computer-assisted rescreening under physician supervision

88167 with manual screening and computer-assisted rescreening using cell selection and review under physician supervision

---

● New Code   ▲ Revised Code   + Add-On Code   ⊘ Modifier -51 Exempt   ★ Telemedicine

(For collection of specimen via fine needle aspiration biopsy, see 10004, 10005, 10006, 10007, 10008, 10009, 10010, 10011, 10012, 10021)

88172 Cytopathology, evaluation of fine needle aspirate; immediate cytohistologic study to determine adequacy for diagnosis, first evaluation episode, each site

(The evaluation episode represents a complete set of cytologic material submitted for evaluation and is independent of the number of needle passes or slides prepared. A separate evaluation episode occurs if the proceduralist provider obtains additional material from the same site, based on the prior immediate adequacy assessment, or a separate lesion is aspirated.)

88173 interpretation and report

(Report one unit of 88173 for the interpretation and report from each anatomic site, regardless of the number of passes or evaluation episodes performed during the aspiration procedure)

(For fine needle aspirate biopsy, see 10004, 10005, 10006, 10007, 10008, 10009, 10010, 10011, 10012, 10021)

(Do not report 88172, 88173 in conjunction with 88333 and 88334 for the same specimen)

+ 88177 immediate cytohistologic study to determine adequacy for diagnosis, each separate additional evaluation episode, same site (List separately in addition to code for primary procedure)

(When repeat immediate evaluation episode(s) is required on subsequent cytologic material from the same site, eg, following determination the prior sampling that was not adequate for diagnosis, use 1 unit of 88177 for each additional evaluation episode)

(Use 88177 in conjunction with 88172)

88174 Cytopathology, cervical or vaginal (any reporting system), collected in preservative fluid, automated thin layer preparation; screening by automated system, under physician supervision

88175 with screening by automated system and manual rescreening or review, under physician supervision

(For manual screening, see 88142, 88143)

88177 This code is out of order. See page 837

88182 Flow cytometry; cell cycle or DNA analysis

(For DNA ploidy analysis by morphometric techniques, use 88358)

88184 Flow cytometry, cell surface, cytoplasmic, or nuclear marker, technical component only; first marker

+ 88185 each additional marker (List separately in addition to code for first marker)

(Report 88185 in conjunction with 88184)

88187 Flow cytometry, interpretation; 2 to 8 markers

88188 9 to 15 markers

88189 16 or more markers

(Do not report 88187-88189 for interpretation of 86355, 86356, 86357, 86359, 86360, 86361, 86367)

(For assessment of circulating antibodies by flow cytometric techniques, see analyte and method-specific codes in the Chemistry section [83516-83520] or Immunology section [86000-86849])

(For cell enumeration using immunologic selection and identification in fluid specimen [eg, circulating tumor cells in blood], see 0279T, 0280T)

88199 Unlisted cytopathology procedure

(For electron microscopy, see 88348)

CYTOGENETIC STUDIES

Molecular pathology procedures should be reported using the appropriate code from Tier 1 (81161, 81200-81383), Tier 2 (81400-81408), Genomic Sequencing Procedures and Other Molecular Multianalyte Assays (81410-81471), or Multianalyte Assays wit Algorithmic Analyses (81500-81512) sections. If no specific code exists, one of the unlisted codes (81479 or 81599) should be used.

(For acetylcholinesterase, use 82013)

(For alpha-fetoprotein, serum or amniotic fluid, see 82105, 82106)

(For laser microdissection of cells from tissue sample, see 88380)

88230	Tissue culture for non-neoplastic disorders; lymphocyte
88233	skin or other solid tissue biopsy
88235	amniotic fluid or chorionic villus cells
88237	Tissue culture for neoplastic disorders; bone marrow, blood cells
88239	solid tumor
88240	Cryopreservation, freezing and storage of cells, each cell line

(For therapeutic cryopreservation and storage, use 38207)

88241	Thawing and expansion of frozen cells, each aliquot

(For therapeutic thawing of previous harvest, use 38208)

88245	Chromosome analysis for breakage syndromes; baseline Sister Chromatid Exchange (SCE), 20-25 cells
88248	baseline breakage, score 50-100 cells, count 20 cells, 2 karyotypes (eg, for ataxia telangiectasia, Fanconi anemia, fragile X)
88249	score 100 cells, clastogen stress (eg, diepoxybutane, mitomycin C, ionizing radiation, UV radiation)
88261	Chromosome analysis; count 5 cells, 1 karyotype, with banding
88262	count 15-20 cells, 2 karyotypes, with banding
88263	count 45 cells for mosaicism, 2 karyotypes, with banding
88264	analyze 20-25 cells
88267	Chromosome analysis, amniotic fluid or chorionic villus, count 15 cells, 1 karyotype, with banding
88269	Chromosome analysis, in situ for amniotic fluid cells, count cells from 6-12 colonies, 1 karyotype, with banding
88271	Molecular cytogenetics; DNA probe, each (eg, FISH)

(For cytogenomic microarray analysis, see 81228, 81229, 81405, 81406, 81479)

(For genomic sequencing procedures or other molecular multianalyte assays for copy number analysis using circulating cell-free fetal DNA in maternal blood, see 81420, 81422, 81479)

88272	chromosomal in situ hybridization, analyze 3-5 cells (eg, for derivatives and markers)

● New Code   ▲ Revised Code   ＋ Add-On Code   ⊘ Modifier -51 Exempt   ★ Telemedicine

88273	chromosomal in situ hybridization, analyze 10-30 cells (eg, for microdeletions)
88274	interphase in situ hybridization, analyze 25-99 cells
88275	interphase in situ hybridization, analyze 100-300 cells
88280	Chromosome analysis; additional karyotypes, each study
88283	additional specialized banding technique (eg, NOR, C-banding)
88285	additional cells counted, each study
88289	additional high resolution study
88291	Cytogenetics and molecular cytogenetics, interpretation and report
88299	Unlisted cytogenetic study

SURGICAL PATHOLOGY

Services 88300 through 88309 include accession, examination, and reporting. They do not include the services designated in codes 88311 through 88365 and 88399, which are coded in addition when provided.

The unit of service for codes 88300 through 88309 is the specimen.

A specimen is defined as tissue or tissues that is (are) submitted for individual and separate attention, requiring individual examination and pathologic diagnosis. Two or more such specimens from the same patient (eg., separately identified endoscopic biopsies, skin lesions), are each appropriately assigned an individual code reflective of its proper level of service.

Service code 88300 is used for any specimen that in the opinion of the examining pathologist can be accurately diagnosed without microscopic examination. Service code 88302 is used when gross and microscopic examination is performed on a specimen to confirm identification and the absence of disease. Service codes 88304 through 88309 describe all other specimens requiring gross and microscopic examination, and represent additional ascending levels of physician work. Levels 88302 through 88309 are specifically defined by the assigned specimens.

Any unlisted specimen should be assigned to the code which most closely reflects the physician work involved when compared to other specimens assigned to that code.

(Do not report 88302-88309 on the same specimen as part of Mohs surgery)

88300	Level I - Surgical pathology, gross examination only
88302	Level II - Surgical pathology, gross and microscopic examination

Appendix, Incidental
Fallopian Tube, Sterilization
Fingers/Toes, Amputation, Traumatic
Foreskin, Newborn
Hernia Sac, Any Location
Hydrocele Sac
Nerve
Skin, Plastic Repair
Sympathetic Ganglion
Testis, Castration
Vaginal Mucosa, Incidental
Vas Deferens, Sterilization

88304 Level III - Surgical pathology, gross and microscopic examination

Abortion, Induced
Abscess
Aneurysm - Arterial/Ventricular
Anus, Tag
Appendix, Other than Incidental
Artery, Atheromatous Plaque
Bartholin's Gland Cyst
Bone Fragment(s), Other than Pathologic Fracture
Bursa/Synovial Cyst
Carpal Tunnel Tissue
Cartilage, Shavings
Cholesteatoma
Colon, Colostomy Stoma
Conjunctiva - Biopsy/Pterygium
Cornea
Diverticulum - Esophagus/Small Intestine
Dupuytren's Contracture Tissue
Femoral Head, Other than Fracture
Fissue/Fistula
Foreskin, Other than Newborn
Gallbladder
Ganglion Cyst
Hematoma
Hemorrhoids
Hydatid of Morgagni
Intervertebral Disc
Joint, Loose Body
Meniscus
Mucocele, Salivary
Neuroma - Morton's/Traumatic
Pilonidal Cyst/Sinus
Polyps, Inflammatory - Nasal/Sinusoidal
Skin - Cyst/Tag/Debridement
Soft Tissue, Debridement
Soft Tissue, Lipoma
Spermatocele
Tendon/Tendon Sheath
Testicular Appendage
Thrombus or Embolus
Tonsil and/or Adenoids
Varicocele
Vas Deferens, Other than Sterilizaton
Vein, Varicosity

88305 Level IV - Surgical pathology, gross and microscopic examination

Abortion - Spontaneous/Missed
Artery, Biopsy
Bone Marrow, Biopsy
Bone Exostosis
Brain/Meninges, Other than for Tumor Resection
Breast Biopsy, Not Requiring Microscopic Evaluation of Surgical Margins
Breast, Reduction Mammoplasty
Bronchus, Biopsy
Cell Block, Any Source
Cervix, Biopsy
Colon, Biopsy
Duodenum, Biopsy
Endocervix, Curettings/Biopsy
Endometrium, Currettings/Biopsy
Esophagus, Biopsy
Extremity, Amputation, Traumatic
Fallopian Tube, Biopsy

● New Code   ▲ Revised Code   + Add-On Code   ⊘ Modifier -51 Exempt   ★ Telemedicine

Fallopian Tube, Ectopic Pregnancy
Femoral Head, Fracture
Fingers/Toes, Amputation, Non-Traumatic
Gingiva/Oral Mucosa, Biopsy
Heart Valve
Joint, Resection
Kidney, Biopsy
Larynx, Biopsy
Leiomyoma(s), Uterine Myomectomy - without Uterus
Lip, Biopsy/Wedge Resection
Lung, Transbronchial Biopsy
Lymph Node, Biopsy
Muscle, Biopsy
Nasal Mucosa, Biopsy
Nasopharynx/Oropharynx, Biopsy
Nerve, Biopsy
Odontogenic/Dental Cyst
Omentum, Biopsy
Ovary with or without Tube, Non-neoplastic
Ovary, Biopsy/Wedge Resection
Parathyroid Gland
Peritoneum, Biopsy
Pituitary Tumor
Placenta, Other than Third Trimester
Pleura/Pericardium - Biopsy/Tissue
Polyp, Cervical/Endometrial
Polyp, Colorectal
Polyp, Stomach/Small Intestine
Prostate, Needle Biopsy
Prostate, TUR
Salivary Gland, Biopsy
Sinus, Paranasal Biopsy
Skin, Other than Cyst/Tag/Debridement/Plastic Repair
Small Intestine, Biopsy
Soft Tissue, Other than Tumor/Mass/Lipoma/Debridement
Spleen
Stomach, Biopsy
Synovium
Testis, Other than Tumor/Biopsy/Castration
Thyroglossal Duct/Brachial Cleft Cyst
Tongue, Biopsy
Tonsil, Biopsy
Trachea, Biopsy
Ureter, Biopsy
Urethra, Biopsy
Urinary Bladder, Biopsy
Uterus, with or without Tubes and Ovaries, for Prolapse
Vagina, Biopsy
Vulva/Labia, Biopsy

88307   Level V - Surgical pathology, gross and microscopic examination

Adrenal, Resection
Bone - Biopsy/Curettings
Bone Fragment(s), Pathologic Fracture
Brain, Biopsy
Brain/Meninges, Tumor Resection
Breast, Excision of Lesion, Requiring Microscopic Evaluation of Surgical Margins
Breast, Mastectomy - Partial/Simple
Cervix, Conization
Colon, Segmental Resection, Other than for Tumor
Extremity, Amputation, Non-traumatic
Eye, Enucleation
Kidney, Partial/Total Nephrectomy
Larynx, Partial/Total Resection

Liver, Biopsy - Needle/Wedge
Lung, Wedge Biopsy
Lymph Nodes, Regional Resection
Mediastinum, Mass
Myocardium, Biopsy
Odontogenic Tumor
Ovary with or without Tube, Neoplastic
Pancreas, Biopsy
Placenta, Third Trimester
Prostate, Except Radical Resection
Salivary Gland
Sentinel Lymph Node
Small Intestine, Resection, Other Than for Tumor
Soft Tissue Mass (except Lipoma) - Biopsy/Simple Excision
Stomach - Subtotal/Total Resection, Other than for Tumor
Testis, Biopsy
Thymus, Biopsy
Thyroid, Total/Lobe
Ureter, Resection
Urinary Bladder, TUR
Uterus, with or without Tubes and Ovaries, Other than Neoplastic/Prolapse

88309   Level VI - Surgical pathology, gross and microscopic examination

Bone Resection
Breast, Mastectomy - with Regional Lymph Nodes
Colon, Segmental Resection for Tumor
Colon, Total Resection
Esophagus, Partial/Total Resection
Extremity, Disarticulation
Fetus, with Dissection
Larynx, Partial/Total Resection - with Regional Lymph Nodes
Lung - Total/Lobe/Segment Resection
Pancreas, Total/Subtotal Resection
Prostate, Radical Resection
Small Intestine, Resection for Tumor
Soft Tissue Tumor, Extensive Resection
Stomach - Subtotal/Total Resection for Tumor
Testis, Tumor
Tongue/Tonsil - Resection for Tumor
Urinary Bladder, Partial/Total Resection
Uterus, with or without Tubes and Ovaries, Neoplastic
Vulva, Total/Subtotal Resection

(For fine needle aspiration biopsy, see 10004, 10005, 10006, 10007, 10008, 10009, 10010, 10011, 10012, 10021)

(For evaluation of fine needle aspirate, see 88172-88173)

(Do not report 88302-88309 on the same specimen as part of Mohs surgery)

+ 88311   Decalcification procedure (List separately in addition to code for surgical pathology examination)

88312   Special stain including interpretation and report; Group I for microorganisms (eg, acid fast, methenamine silver)

(Report one unit of 88312 for each special stain, on each surgical pathology block, cytologic specimen, or hematologic smear)

88313   Group II, all other, (eg, iron, trichrome), except stain for microorganisms, stains for enzyme constituents, or immunocytochemistry and immunohistochemistry

(Report one unit of 88313 for each special stain, on each surgical pathology block, cytologic specimen, or hematologic smear)

(For immunocytochemistry and immunohistochemistry, use 88342)

   ● New Code   ▲ Revised Code   + Add-On Code   ⊘ Modifier -51 Exempt   ★ Telemedicine

+ 88314   histochemical stain on frozen tissue block (List separately in addition to code for primary procedure)

(Use 88314 in conjunction with 17311-17315, 88302-88309, 88331, 88332)

(Do not report 88314 with 17311-17315 for routine frozen section stain [eg., hematoxylin and eosin, toluidine blue], performed during Mohs surgery. When a nonroutine histochemical stain on frozen tissue during Mohs surgery is utilized, report 88314 with modifier 59)

(Report one unit of 88314 for each special stain on each frozen surgical pathology block)

(For a special stain performed on frozen tissue section material to identify enzyme constituents, use 88319)

(For determinative histochemistry to identify chemical components, use 88313)

88319   Group III, for enzyme constituents

(For each stain on each surgical pathology block, cytologic specimen, or hematologic smear, use one unit of 88319)

(For detection of enzyme constituents by immunohistochemical or immunocytochemical technique, see 88342)

88321   Consultation and report on referred slides prepared elsewhere

88323   Consultation and report on referred material requiring preparation of slides

88325   Consultation, comprehensive, with review of records and specimens, with report on referred material

88329   Pathology consultation during surgery;

88331   first tissue block, with frozen section(s), single specimen

+ 88332   each additional tissue block with frozen section(s) (List separately in addition to code for primary procedure)

(Use 88332 in conjunction with 88331)

88333   cytologic examination (eg, touch prep, squash prep), initial site

+ 88334   cytologic examination (eg, touch prep, squash prep), each additional site (List separately in addition to code for primary procedure)

(Use 88334 in conjunction with 88331, 88333)

(For intraoperative consultation on a specimen requiring both frozen section and cytologic evaluation, use 88331 and 88334)

(For percutaneous needle biopsy requiring intraprocedural cytologic examination, use 88333)

(Do not report 88333 and 88334 for non-intraoperative cytologic examination, see 88160-88162)

(Do not report 88333 and 88334 for intraprocedural cytologic evaluation of fine needle aspirate, see 88172).

88341   This code is out of order. See page 843

88342   Immunohistochemistry or immunocytochemistry, per specimen; initial single antibody stain procedure

(For quantitative or semiquantitative immunohistochemistry, see 88360, 88361)

+ 88341   each additional single antibody stain procedure (List separately in addition to code for primary procedure)

(Use 88341 in conjunction with 88342)

(For multiplex antibody stain procedure, use 88344)

88344   each multiplex antibody stain procedure

(Do not use more than one unit of 88341, 88342, or 88344 for the same separately identifiable antibody per specimen)

(Do not report 88341, 88342, 88344 in conjunction with 88360, 88361 unless each procedure is for a different antibody)

(When multiple separately identifiable antibodies are applied to the same specimen [ie, multiplex antibody stain procedure], use one unit of 88344)

(When multiple antibodies are applied to the same slide that are not separately identifiable [eg, antibody cocktails], use 88342, unless an additional separately identiable antibody is also used, then use 88344)

88346   Immunofluorescence, per specimen; initial single antibody stain procedure

+ **88350**   each additional single antibody stain procedure (List separately in addition to code for primary procedure)

(Report 88350 in conjunction with 88346)

(Do not report 88346 and 88350 for fluorescent in situ hybridization studies, see 88364, 88365, 88366, 88367, 88368, 88369, 88373, 88374, and 88377)

(Do not report 88346 and 88350 for multiplex immunofluorescence analysis, use 88399)

88348   Electron microscopy; diagnostic

88350   This code is out of order. See page 844

88355   Morphometric analysis; skeletal muscle

88356   nerve

88358   tumor (eg, DNA ploidy)

(Do not report 88358 with 88313 unless each procedure is for a different special stain)

88360   Morphometric analysis, tumor immunohistochemistry (eg, Her-2/neu, estrogen receptor/progesterone receptor), quantitative or semiquantitative, per specimen, each single antibody stain procedure; manual

88361   using computer-assisted technology

(Do not report 88360, 88361 in conjunction with 88341, 88342, or 88344 unless each procedure is for a different antibody)

(Morphometric analysis of a multiplex antibody stain should be reported with one unit of 88360 or 88361, per specimen)

(For morphometric analysis using in situ hyvridization techniques, see 88367, 88368)

(When semi-thin plastic-embedded sections are performed in conjunction with morphometric analysis, only the morphometric analysis should be coded; if performed as an independent procedure, see codes 88300-88309 for surgical pathology)

88362   Nerve teasing preparations

88363   Examination and selection of retrieved archival (ie, previously diagnosed) tissue(s) for molecular analysis (eg, Kras mutational analysis)

88364   This code is out of order. See page 844

88365   In situ hybridization (eg, FISH), per specimen; initial single probe stain procedure

+ **88364**   each additional single probe stain procedure (List separately in addition to code for primary procedure)

(Use 88364 in conjunction with 88365)

88366 each multiplex probe stain procedure

(Do not report 88365, 88366 in conjunction with 88367, 88368, 88374, 88377 for the same probe)

88367 Morphometric analysis, in situ hybridization, (quantitative or semi-quantitative), using computer-assisted technology, per specimen; initial single probe stain procedure

+ 88373 each additional single probe stain procedure (List separately in addition to code for primary procedure)

(Use 88373 in conjunction with 88367)

88374 each multiplex probe stain procedure

(Do not report 88367, 88374 in conjunction with 88365, 88366, 88368, 88377 for the same probe)

88368 Morphometric analysis, in situ hybridization (quantitative or semi-quantitative), manual, per specimen; initial single probe stain procedure

+ 88369 each additional single probe stain procedure (List separately in addition to code for primary procedure)

(Use 88369 in conjunction with 88368)

88377 each multiplex probe stain procedure

(Do not report 88368 or 88377 in conjunction with 88365, 88366, 88367, 88374 for the same probe)

(For morphometric in situ hybridization evaluation of urinary tract cytologic specimens, see 88120, 88121)

88371 Protein analysis of tissue by Western Blot, with interpretation and report;

88372 immunological probe for band identification, each

88373 This code is out of order. See page 845

88374 This code is out of order. See page 845

88375 Optical endomicroscopic image(s), interpretation and report, real-time or referred, each endoscopic session

(Do not report 88375 in conjunction with 43206, 43252, 0397T)

88377 This code is out of order. See page 845

88380 Microdissection (ie, sample preparation of microscopically identified target); laser capture

88381 manual

(Do not report 88380 in conjunction with 88381)

88387 Macroscopic examination, dissection, and preparation of tissue for non microscopic analytical studies (eg, nucleic acid based molecular studies); each tissue preparation (eg, a single lymph node)

(Do not report 88387 for tissue preparation for microbiologic cultures or flow cytometric studies)

(Do not report 88387 in conjunction with 88388, 88329-88334)

+ 88388 in conjunction with a touch imprint, intraoperative consultation, or frozen section, each tissue preparation (eg, a single lymph node) (List separately in addition to code for primary procedure)

(Use 88388 in conjunction with 88329-88334)

(Do not report 88387 or 88388 for tissue preparation for microbiologic cultures or flow cytometric studies)

88399   Unlisted surgical pathology procedure

IN VIVO (eg, TRANSCUTANEOUS) LABORATORY PROCEDURES

(For all in vivo measurements not specifically listed, use 88749)

(For wavelength fluorescent spectroscopy of advanced glycation end products [skin], use 88749)

(For transcutaneous oxyhemoglobin measurement in a lower extremity wound by near infrared spectroscopy, use 0493T)

88720   Bilirubin, total, transcutaneous

(For transdermal oxygen saturation, see 94760-94762)

88738   Hemoglobin (Hgb), quantitative, transcutaneous

(For in vitro hemoglobin measurement, use 85018)

88740   Hemoglobin, quantitative, transcutaneous, per day; carboxyhemoglobin

(For in vitro carboxyhemoglobin measurement, use 82375)

88741   methemoglobin

(For in vitro quantitative methemoglobin determination, use 83050)

88749   Unlisted in vivo (eg, transcutaneous) laboratory service

OTHER PROCEDURES

89049   Caffeine halothane contracture test (CHCT) for malignant hyperthermia susceptibility, including interpretation and report

89050   Cell count, miscellaneous body fluids (eg, cerebrospinal fluid, joint fluid), except blood;

89051   with differential count

89055   Leukocyte assessment, fecal, qualitative or semiquantitative

89060   Crystal identification by light microscopy with or without polarizing lens analysis, tissue or any body fluid (except urine)

(Do not report 89060 for crystal identification on paraffin-embedded tissue)

89125   Fat stain, feces, urine, or respiratory secretions

89160   Meat fibers, feces

89190   Nasal smear for eosinophils

(Occult blood, feces, use 82270)

(Paternity tests, use 86910)

89220   Sputum, obtaining specimen, aerosol induced technique (separate procedure)

89230   Sweat collection by iontophoresis

89240   Unlisted miscellaneous pathology test

● New Code   ▲ Revised Code   ✚ Add-On Code   ⊘ Modifier -51 Exempt   ★ Telemedicine

REPRODUCTIVE MEDICINE PROCEDURES

89250 Culture of oocyte(s)/embryo(s), less than 4 days;

89251   with co-culture of oocyte(s)/embryo(s)

       (For extended culture of oocyte(s)/embryo(s), see 89272)

89253 Assisted embryo hatching, microtechniques (any method)

89254 Oocyte identification from follicular fluid

89255 Preparation of embryo for transfer (any method)

89257 Sperm identification from aspiration (other than seminal fluid)

       (For semen analysis, see 89300-89320)

       (For sperm identification from testis tissue, use 89264)

89258 Cryopreservation; embryo(s)

89259   sperm

       (For cryopreservation of reproductive tissue, testicular, use 89335)

89260 Sperm isolation; simple prep (eg, sperm wash and swim-up) for insemination or diagnosis with semen analysis

89261   complex prep (eg, Percoll gradient, albumin gradient) for insemination or diagnosis with semen analysis

       (For semen analysis without sperm wash or swim-up, use 89320)

89264 Sperm identification from testis tissue, fresh or cryopreserved

       (For biopsy of testis, see 54500, 54505)

       (For sperm identification from aspiration, use 89257)

       (For semen analysis, see 89300-89320)

89268 Insemination of oocytes

89272 Extended culture of oocyte(s)/embryo(s), 4-7 days

89280 Assisted oocyte fertiliation, microtechnique; less than or equal to 10 oocytes

89281   greater than 10 oocytes

89290 Biopsy, oocyte polar body or embryo blastomere, microtechnique (for pre-implantation genetic diagnosis); less than or equal to 5 embryos

89291   greater than 5 embryos

89300 Semen analysis; presence and/or motility of sperm including Huhner test (post coital)

89310   motility and count (not including Huhner test)

89320   volume, count, motility, and differential

       (Skin tests, see 86485-86580 and 95012-95199)

Separate Procedure   Unlisted Procedure   CCI Comp. Code   Non-specific Procedure   **847**

| 89321 | sperm presence and motility of sperm, if performed |

(To report Hyaluronan binding assay [HBA], use 89398)

| 89322 | volume, count, motility, and differential using strict morphologic criteria (eg, Kruger) |

| 89325 | Sperm antibodies |

(For medicolegal identification of sperm, use 88125)

| 89329 | Sperm evaluation; hamster penetration test |

| 89330 | cervical mucus penetration test, with or without spinnbarkeit test |

| 89331 | Sperm evaluation, for retrograde ejaculation, urine (sperm concentration, motility, and morphology, as indicated) |

(For semen analysis on concurrent semen specimen, see 89300-89322 in conjunction with 89331)

(For detection of sperm in urine, use 81015)

| 89335 | Cryopreservation, reproductive tissue, testicular |

(For cryopreservation of embryo[s], use 89258. For cryopreservation of sperm, use 89259; for mature oocytes, use 89337)

| 89337 | Cryopreservation, mature oocyte(s) |

| 89342 | Storage, (per year); embryo(s) |

| 89343 | sperm/semen |

| 89344 | reproductive tissue, testicular/ovarian |

| 89346 | oocyte(s) |

| 89352 | Thawing of cryopreserved; embryo(s) |

| 89353 | sperm/semen, each aliquot |

| 89354 | reproductive tissue, testicular/ovarian |

| 89356 | oocytes, each aliquot |

| 89398 | Unlisted reproductive medicine laboratory procedure |

PROPRIETARY LABORATORY ANALYSES

Proprietary laboratory analyses (PLA) codes describe proprietary clinical laboratory analyses and can be provided either by a single ("sole-source") laboratory or licensed or marketed to multiple providing laboratories (eg, cleared or approved by the Food and Drug Administration [FDA]).

This subsection includes advanced diagnostic laboratory tests (ADLTs) and clinical diagnostic laboratory tests (CDLTs) as defined under the Protecting Access to Medicare Act (PAMA) of 2014. These analyses may include a range of medical laboratory tests including, but not limited to, multianalyte assays with algorithmic analyses (MAAA) and genomic sequencing procedures (GSP). The descriptor nomenclature follows, where possible, existing code conventions (eg, MAAA, GSP).

Unless specifically noted, even though the Proprietary Laboratory Analyses section of the code set is located at the end of the Pathology and Laboratory section of the code set, a PLA code does not fulfill Category I code criteria. PLA codes are not required to fulfill the Category I criteria. The standards for inclusion in the PLA section are:

1.The test must be commercially available in the United States for use on human specimens and

2.The clinical laboratory or manufacturer that offers the test must request the code.

For similar laboratory analyses that fulfill Category I criteria, see codes listed in the numeric 80000 series.

When a PLA code is available to report a given proprietary laboratory service, that PLA code takes precedence. The service should not e reported with any other CPT code(s) and other CPT code(s) should not be used to report services that may be reported with that specific PLA code. These codes encompass allanalytical services required for the analysis (eg, cell lysis, nucleic acid stabilization, extraction, digestion, amplification, hybridization adn detection). For molecular analyses, additional procedures that are required prior to cell lysis (eg, microdissection [codes 88380 and 88381]) may be reported separately.

Codes in this subsection are released on a quarterly basis to expedite dissemination for reporting. PLA codes will be published electronically on the AMA CPT website (ama-assn.org/cpt-pla-codes), distributed via CPT data files on a quarterly basis, and, at a minimum, made available in print annually in the CPT codebook. See the Introduction section of the CPT code set for a complete list of the dates of release and implementation.

If a proprietary test has already been accepted for a Category I code and a code has not been published, subsequent application for a PLA code will take precedence. The code will only be placed in the PLA section.

The accuracy of a PLA code is to be maintained by the original applicant, or the current owner of the test kit or laboratory performing the proprietary test.

A new PLA code is required when:

1. Additional nucleic acid (DNA or RNA) and/or protein analysis(es) are added to the current PLA test, or

2. The name of the PLA test has changed in association with changes in test performance or test characteristics.

The addition or modification of the therapeutic applications of the test require submission of a code change application, but it may not require a new code number.

0001U Red blood cell antigen typing, DNA, human erythrocyte antigen gene analysis of 35 antigens from 11 blood groups, utilizing whole blood, common RBC alleles reported

0002U Oncology (colorectal), quantitative assessment of three urine metabolites (ascorbic acid, succinic acid and carnitine) by liquid chromatography with tandem mass spectrometry (LC-MS/MS) using multiple reaction monitoring acquisition, algorithm reported as likelihood of adenomatous polyps

0003U Oncology (ovarian) biochemical assays of five proteins (apolipoprotein A-1, CA 125 II, follicle stimulating hormone, human epididymis protein 4, transferrin), utilizing serum, algorithm reported as a likelihood score

(0004U deleted 2018 [2019 Edition])

0005U Oncology (prostate) gene expression profile by real-time RT-PCR of 3 genes (ERG, PCA3, and SPDEF), urine, algorithm reported as risk score

(0006U deleted 2020 [2021 Edition])

0007U Drug test(s), presumptive, with definitive confirmation of positive results, any number of drug classes, urine, includes specimen verification including DNA authentication in comparison to buccal DNA, per date of service

(For additional PLA code with identical clinical descriptor, see 0020U. See Appendix O to determine appropriate code assignment)

0008U Helicobacter pylori detection and antibiotic resistance, DNA, 16S and 23S rRNA, gyrA, pbp1, rdxA and rpoB, next generation sequencing, formalin-fixed paraffin-embedded or fresh tissue or fecal sample, predictive, reported as positive or negative for resistance to clarithromycin, fluoroquinolones, metronidazole, amoxicillin, tetracycline, and rifabutin

---

0009U Oncology (breast cancer), ERBB2 (HER2) copy number by FISH, tumor cells from formalin-fixed paraffin-embedded tissue isolated using image-based dielectrophoresis (DEP) sorting, reported as ERBB2 gene amplified or nonamplified

0010U Infectious disease (bacterial), strain typing by whole genome sequencing, phylogenetic-based report of strain relatedness, per submitted isolate

0011U Prescription drug monitoring, evaluation of drugs present by LC-MS/MS, using oral fluid, reported as a comparison to an estimated steady-state range, per date of service including all drug compounds and metabolites

0012U Germline disorders, gene rearrangement detection by whole genome next-generation sequencing, DNA, whole blood, report of specific gene rearrangement(s)

0013U Oncology (solid organ neoplasia), gene rearrangement detection by whole genome next-generation sequencing, DNA, fresh or frozen tissue or cells, report of specific gene rearrangement(s)

0014U Hematology (hematolymphoid neoplasia), gene rearrangement detection by whole genome nextgeneration sequencing, DNA, whole blood or bone marrow, report of specific gene rearrangement(s)

(0015U deleted 2018 [2019 Edition])

0016U Oncology (hematolymphoid neoplasia), RNA, BCR/ABL1 major and minor breakpoint fusion transcripts, quantitative PCR amplification, blood or bone marrow, report of fusion not detected or detected with quantitation

0017U Oncology (hematolymphoid neoplasia), JAK2 mutation, DNA, PCR amplification of exons 12-14 and sequence analysis, blood or bone marrow, report of JAK2 mutation not detected or detected

0018U Oncology (thyroid), microRNA profiling by RT-PCR of 10 microRNA sequences, utilizing fine needle aspirate, algorithm reported as a positive or negative result for moderate to high risk of malignancy

0019U Oncology, RNA, gene expression by whole transcriptome sequencing, formalin-fixed paraffin-embedded tissue or fresh frozen tissue, predictive algorithm reported as potential targets for therapeutic agents

(0020U deleted 2019 [2020 Edition])

0021U Oncology (prostate), detection of 8 autoantibodies (ARF 6, NKX3-1, 5'-UTR-BMI1, CEP 164, 3'-UTR-Ropporin, Desmocollin, AURKAIP-1, CSNK2A2), multiplexed immunoassay and flow cytometry serum, algorithm reported as risk score

0022U Targeted genomic sequence analysis panel, non-small cell lung neoplasia, DNA and RNA analysis, 23 genes, interrogation for sequence variants and rearrangements, reported as presence/absence of variants and associated therapy(ies) to consider

0023U Oncology (acute myelogenous leukemia), DNA, genotyping of internal tandem duplication, p.D835, p.I836, using mononuclear cells, reported as detection or non-detection of FLT3 mutation and indication for or against the use of midostaurin

0024U Glycosylated acute phase proteins (GlycA), nuclear magnetic resonance spectroscopy, quantitative

0025U Tenofovir, by liquid chromatography with tandem mass spectrometry (LC-MS/MS), urine, quantitative

0026U Oncology (thyroid), DNA and mRNA of 112 genes, nextgeneration sequencing, fine needle aspirate of thyroid nodule, algorithmic analysis reported as a categorical result ("Positive, high probability of malignancy" or "Negative, low probability of malignancy")

0027U JAK2 (Janus kinase 2) (eg, myeloproliferative disorder) gene analysis, targeted sequence analysis exons 12-15

(0028U deleted 2019 [2020 Edition]

● New Code ▲ Revised Code + Add-On Code ⊘ Modifier -51 Exempt ★ Telemedicine

0029U Drug metabolism (adverse drug reactions and drug response), targeted sequence analysis (ie, CYP1A2, CYP2C19, CYP2C9, CYP2D6, CYP3A4, CYP3A5, CYP4F2, SLCO1B1, VKORC1 and rs12777823)

0030U Drug metabolism (warfarin drug response), targeted sequence analysis (ie, CYP2C9, CYP4F2, VKORC1, rs12777823)

0031U CYP1A2 (cytochrome P450 family 1, subfamily A, member 2) (eg, drug metabolism) gene analysis, common variants (ie, *1F, *1K, *6, *7)

0032U COMT (catechol-O-methyltransferase) (eg, drug metabolism) gene analysis, c.472G>A (rs4680) variant

0033U HTR2A (5-hydroxytryptamine receptor 2A), HTR2C (5-hydroxytryptamine receptor 2C) (eg, citalopram metabolism) gene analysis, common variants (ie, HTR2A rs7997012 [c.614-2211T>C], HTR2C rs3813929 [c.-759C>T] and rs1414334 [c.551-3008C>G])

0034U TPMT (thiopurine S-methyltransferase), NUDT15 (nudix hydroxylase 15) (eg, thiopurine metabolism) gene analysis, common variants (ie, TPMT *2, *3A, *3B, *3C, *4, *5, *6, *8, *12; NUDT15 *3, *4, *5)

0035U Neurology (prion disease), cerebrospinal fluid, detection of prion protein by quaking-induced conformational conversion, qualitative

0036U Exome (ie, somatic mutations), paired formalin-fixed paraffin-embedded tumor tissue and normal specimen, sequence analyses

0037U Targeted genomic sequence analysis, solid organ neoplasm, DNA analysis of 324 genes, interrogation for sequence variants, gene copy number amplifications, gene rearrangements, microsatellite instability and tumor mutational burden

0038U Vitamin D, 25 hydroxy D2 and D3, by LC-MS/MS, serum microsample, quantitative

0039U Deoxyribonucleic acid (DNA) antibody, double stranded, high avidity

0040U BCR/ABL1 (t(9;22)) (eg, chronic myelogenous leukemia) translocation analysis, major breakpoint, quantitative

0041U Borrelia burgdorferi, antibody detection of 5 recombinant protein groups, by immunoblot, IgM

0042U Borrelia burgdorferi, antibody detection of 12 recombinant protein groups, by immunoblot, IgG

0043U Tick-borne relapsing fever Borrelia group, antibody detection to 4 recombinant protein groups, by immunoblot, IgM

0044U Tick-borne relapsing fever Borrelia group, antibody detection to 4 recombinant protein groups, by immunoblot, IgG

0045U Oncology (breast ductal carcinoma in situ), mRNA, gene expression profiling by real-time RT-PCR of 12 genes (7 content and 5 housekeeping), utilizing formalin-fixed paraffin-embedded tissue, algorithm reported as recurrence score

0046U FLT3 (fms-related tyrosine kinase 3) (eg, acute myeloid leukemia) internal tandem duplication (ITD) variants, quantitative

0047U Oncology (prostate), mRNA, gene expression profiling by real-time RT-PCR of 17 genes (12 content and 5 housekeeping), utilizing formalin-fixed paraffinembedded tissue, algorithm reported as a risk score

0048U Oncology (solid organ neoplasia), DNA, targeted sequencing of protein-coding exons of 468 cancerassociated genes, including interrogation for somatic mutations and microsatellite instability, matched with normal specimens, utilizing formalin-fixed paraffinembedded tumor tissue, report of clinically significant mutation(s)

0049U NPM1 (nucleophosmin) (eg, acute myeloid leukemia) gene analysis, quantitative

---

0050U Targeted genomic sequence analysis panel, acute myelogenous leukemia, DNA analysis, 194 genes, interrogation for sequence variants, copy number variants or rearrangements

0051U Prescription drug monitoring, evaluation of drugs present by LC-MS/MS, urine, 31 drug panel, reported as quantitative results, detected or not detected, per date of service

0052U Lipoprotein, blood, high resolution fractionation and quantitation of lipoproteins, including all five major lipoprotein classes and subclasses of HDL, LDL, and VLDL by vertical auto profile ultracentrifugation

0053U Oncology (prostate cancer), FISH analysis of 4 genes (ASAP1, HDAC9, CHD1 and PTEN), needle biopsy specimen, algorithm reported as probability of higher tumor grade

0054U Prescription drug monitoring, 14 or more classes of drugs and substances, definitive tandem mass pectrometry with chromatography, capillary blood, quantitative report with therapeutic and toxic ranges, including steady-state range for the prescribed dose when detected, per date of service

0055U Cardiology (heart transplant), cell-free DNA, PCR assay of 96 DNA target sequences (94 single nucleotide polymorphism targets and two control targets), plasma

0056U Hematology (acute myelogenous leukemia), DNA, whole genome next-generation sequencing to detect gene rearrangement(s), blood or bone marrow, report of specific gene rearrangement(s)

(0057U deleted 2019 [2020 Edition]

0058U Oncology (Merkel cell carcinoma), detection of antibodies to the Merkel cell polyoma virus oncoprotein (small T antigen), serum, quantitative

0059U Oncology (Merkel cell carcinoma), detection of antibodies to the Merkel cell polyoma virus capsid protein (VP1), serum, reported as positive or negative

0060U Twin zygosity, genomic-targeted sequence anlysis of chromosome 2, using circulating cell-free fetal DNA in maternal blood

0061U Transcutaneous measurement of five biomarkers (tissue oxygenation [StO2], oxyhemoglobin [ctHbO2], deoxyhemoglobin [ctHbR], papillary and reticular dermal hemoglobin concentrations [ctHb1 and ctHb2]), using spatial frequency domain imaging (SFDI) and multispectral analysis

0062U Autoimmune (systemic lupus erythematosus), IgG and IgM analysis of 80 biomarkers, utilizing serum, algorithm reported with a risk score

0063U Neurology (autism), 32 amines by LC-MS/MS, using plasma, algorithm reported as metabolic signature associated with autism spectrum disorder

0064U Antibody, Treponema pallidum, total and rapid plasma reagin (RPR), immunoassay, qualitative

0065U Syphilis test, non-treponemal antibody, immunoassay, qualitative (RPR)

0066U Placental alpha-micro globulin-1 (PAMG-1), immunoassay with direct optical observation, cervico-vaginal fluid, each specimen

0067U Oncology (breast), immunohistochemistry, protein expression profiling of 4 biomarkers (matrix metalloproteinase-1 [MMP-1], carcinoembryonic antigenrelated cell adhesion molecule 6 [CEACAM6], hyaluronoglucosaminidase [HYAL1], highly expressed in cancer protein [HEC1]), formalin-fixed paraffin-embedded precancerous breast tissue, algorithm reported as carcinoma risk score

0068U Candida species panel (C. albicans, C. glabrata, C. parapsilosis, C. kruseii, C. tropicalis, and C. auris), amplified probe technique with qualitative report of the presence or absence of each species

0069U Oncology (colorectal), microRNA, RT-PCR expression profiling of miR-31-3p, formalin-fixed paraffin-embedded tissue, algorithm reported as an expression score

---

● New Code ▲ Revised Code ✛ Add-On Code ⊘ Modifier -51 Exempt ★ Telemedicine

0070U   CYP2D6 (cytochrome P450, family 2, subfamily D, polypeptide 6) (eg, drug metabolism) gene analysis, common and select rare variants (ie, *2, *3, *4, *4N, *5, *6, *7, *8, *9, *10, *11, *12, *13, *14A, *14B, *15, *17, *29, *35, *36, *41, *57, *61, *63, *68, *83, *xN)

+ 0071U   CYP2D6 (cytochrome P450, family 2, subfamily D, polypeptide 6) (eg, drug metabolism) gene analysis, full gene sequence (List separately in addition to code for primary procedure)

(Use 0071U in conjunction with 0070U)

+ 0072U   CYP2D6 (cytochrome P450, family 2, subfamily D, polypeptide 6) (eg, drug metabolism) gene analysis, targeted sequence analysis (ie, CYP2D6-2D7 hybrid gene) (List separately in addition to code for primary procedure)

(Use 0072U in conjunction with 0070U)

+ 0073U   CYP2D6 (cytochrome P450, family 2, subfamily D, polypeptide 6) (eg, drug metabolism) gene analysis, targeted sequence analysis (ie, CYP2D7-2D6 hybrid gene) (List separately in addition to code for primary procedure)

(Use 0073U in conjunction with 0070U)

+ 0074U   CYP2D6 (cytochrome P450, family 2, subfamily D, polypeptide 6) (eg, drug metabolism) gene analysis, targeted sequence analysis (ie, non-duplicated gene when duplication/multiplication is trans) (List separately in addition to code for primary procedure)

(Use 0074U in conjunction with 0070U)

+ 0075U   CYP2D6 (cytochrome P450, family 2, subfamily D, polypeptide 6) (eg, drug metabolism) gene analysis, targeted sequence analysis (ie, 5' gene duplication/multiplication) (List separately in addition to code for primary procedure)

(Use 0075U in conjunction with 0070U)

+ 0076U   CYP2D6 (cytochrome P450, family 2, subfamily D, polypeptide 6) (eg, drug metabolism) gene analysis, targeted sequence analysis (ie, 3' gene duplication/multiplication) (List separately in addition to code for primary procedure)

(Use 0076U in conjunction with 0070U)

0077U   Immunoglobulin paraprotein (M-protein), qualitative, immunoprecipitation and mass spectrometry, blood or urine, including isotype

0078U   Pain management (opioid-use disorder) genotyping panel, 16 common variants (ie, ABCB1, COMT, DAT1, DBH, DOR, DRD1, DRD2, DRD4, GABA, GAL, HTR2A, HTTLPR, MTHFR, MUOR, OPRK1, OPRM1), buccal swab or other germline tissue sample, algorithm reported as positive or negative risk of opioid-use disorder

0079U   Comparative DNA analysis using multiple selected single-nucleotide polymorphisms (SNPs), urine and buccal DNA, for specimen identity verification

0080U   Oncology (lung), mass spectrometric analysis of galectin- 3-binding protein and scavenger receptor cysteine-rich type 1 protein M130, with five clinical risk factors (age, smoking status, nodule diameter, nodule-spiculation status and nodule location), utilizing plasma, algorithm reported as a categorical probability of malignancy

(0081U has been deleted. To report, use 81552)

0082U   Drug test(s), definitive, 90 or more drugs or substances, definitive chromatography with mass spectrometry, and presumptive, any number of drug classes, by instrument chemistry analyzer (utilizing immunoassay), urine, report of presence or absence of each drug, drug metabolite or substance with description and severity of significant interactions per date of service

0083U   Oncology, response to chemotherapy drugs using motility contrast tomography, fresh or frozen tissue, reported as likelihood of sensitivity or resistance to drugs or drug combinations

---

0084U   Red blood cell antigen typing, DNA, genotyping of 10 blood groups with phenotype prediction of 37 red blood cell antigens

(0085U   deleted 2020 [2021 Edition])

0086U   Infectious disease (bacterial and fungal), organism identification, blood culture, using rRNA FISH, 6 or more organism targets, reported as positive or negative with phenotypic minimum inhibitory concentration (MIC)-based antimicrobial susceptibility

0087U   Cardiology (heart transplant), mRNA gene expression profiling by microarray of 1283 genes, transplant biopsy tissue, allograft rejection and injury algorithm reported as a probability score

0088U   Transplantation medicine (kidney allograft rejection), microarray gene expression profiling of 1494 genes, utilizing transplant biopsy tissue, algorithm reported as a probability score for rejection

0089U   Oncology (melanoma), gene expression profiling by RTqPCR, PRAME and LINC00518, superficial collection using adhesive patch(es)

0090U   Oncology (cutaneous melanoma), mRNA gene expression profiling by RT-PCR of 23 genes (14 content and 9 housekeeping), utilizing formalin-fixed paraffin-embedded tissue, algorithm reported as a categorical result (ie, benign, indeterminate, malignant)

0091U   Oncology (colorectal) screening, cell enumeration of circulating tumor cells, utilizing whole blood, algorithm, for the presence of adenoma or cancer, reported as a positive or negative result

0092U   Oncology (lung), three protein biomarkers, immunoassay using magnetic nanosensor technology, plasma, algorithm reported as risk score for likelihood of malignancy

0093U   Prescription drug monitoring, evaluation of 65 common drugs by LC-MS/MS, urine, each drug reported detected or not detected

0094U   Genome (eg, unexplained constitutional or heritable disorder or syndrome), rapid sequence analysis

0095U   Inflammation (eosinophilic esophagitis), ELISA analysis of eotaxin-3 (CCL26 [C-C motif chemokine ligand 26]) and major basic protein (PRG2 [proteoglycan 2, pro eosinophil major basic protein]), specimen obtained by swallowed nylon string, algorithm reported as predictive probability index for active eosinophilic esophagitis

0096U   Human papillomavirus (HPV), high-risk types (ie, 16, 18, 31, 33, 35, 39, 45, 51, 52, 56, 58, 59, 66, 68), male urine

0097U   Gastrointestinal pathogen, multiplex reverse transcription and multiplex amplified probe technique, multiple types or subtypes, 22 targets (Campylobacter [C. jejuni/C. coli/C. upsaliensis], Clostridium difficile [C. difficile] toxin A/B, Plesiomonas shigelloides, Salmonella, Vibrio [V. parahaemolyticus/V. vulnificus/V. cholerae], including specific identification of Vibrio cholerae, Yersinia enterocolitica, Enteroaggregative Escherichia coli [EAEC], Enteropathogenic Escherichia coli [EPEC], Enterotoxigenic Escherichia coli [ETEC] lt/st, Shiga-like toxin-producing Escherichia coli [STEC] stx1/stx2 [including specific identification of the E. coli O157 serogroup within STEC], Shigella/Enteroinvasive Escherichia coli [EIEC], Cryptosporidium, Cyclospora cayetanensis, Entamoeba histolytica, Giardia lamblia [also known as G. intestinalis and G. duodenalis], adenovirus F 40/41, astrovirus, norovirus GI/GII, rotavirus A, sapovirus [Genogroups I, II, IV, and V])

0098U   Respiratory pathogen, multiplex reverse transcription and multiplex amplified probe technique, multiple types or subtypes, 14 targets (adenovirus, coronavirus, human metapneumovirus, influenza A, influenza A subtype H1, influenza A subtype H3, influenza A subtype H1-2009, influenza B, parainfluenza virus, human rhinovirus/ enterovirus, respiratory syncytial virus, Bordetella pertussis, Chlamydophila pneumoniae, Mycoplasma pneumoniae)

0099U   Respiratory pathogen, multiplex reverse transcription and multiplex amplified probe technique, multiple types or subtypes, 20 targets (adenovirus, coronavirus 229E, coronavirus HKU1, coronavirus, coronavirus OC43, human metapneumovirus, influenza A, influenza A subtype, influenza A subtype H3, influenza A subtype H1-2009, influenza, parainfluenza virus, parainfluenza virus 2, parainfluenza virus 3, parainfluenza virus 4, human rhinovirus/enterovirus, respiratory syncytial virus, Bordetella pertussis, Chlamydophila pneumonia, Mycoplasma pneumoniae)

0100U Respiratory pathogen, multiplex reverse transcription and multiplex amplified probe technique, multiple types or subtypes, 21 targets (adenovirus, coronavirus 229E, coronavirus HKU1, coronavirus NL63, coronavirus OC43, human metapneumovirus, human rhinovirus/enterovirus, influenza A, including subtypes H1, H1-2009, and H3, influenza B, parainfluenza virus 1, parainfluenza virus 2, parainfluenza virus 3, parainfluenza virus 4, respiratory syncytial virus, Bordetella parapertussis [IS1001], Bordetella pertussis [ptxP], Chlamydia pneumoniae, Mycoplasma pneumoniae)

0101U Hereditary colon cancer disorders (eg, Lynch syndrome, PTEN hamartoma syndrome, Cowden syndrome, familial adenomatosis polyposis), genomic sequence analysis panel utilizing a combination of NGS, Sanger, MLPA, and array CGH, with mRNA analytics to resolve variants of unknown significance when indicated (15 genes [sequencing and deletion/duplication], EPCAM and GREM1 [deletion/duplication only])

0102U Hereditary breast cancer-related disorders (eg, hereditary breast cancer, hereditary ovarian cancer, hereditary endometrial cancer), genomic sequence analysis panel utilizing a combination of NGS, Sanger, MLPA, and array CGH, with mRNA analytics to resolve variants of unknown significance when indicated (17 genes [sequencing and deletion/duplication])

0103U Hereditary ovarian cancer (eg, hereditary ovarian cancer, hereditary endometrial cancer), genomic sequence analysis panel utilizing a combination of NGS, Sanger, MLPA, and array CGH, with mRNA analytics to resolve variants of unknown significance when indicated (24 genes [sequencing and deletion/duplication], EPCAM [deletion/duplication only])

(0104U has been deleted)

0105U Nephrology (chronic kidney disease), multiplex electrochemiluminescent immunoassay (ECLIA) of tumor necrosis factor receptor 1A, receptor superfamily 2 (TNFR1, TNFR2), and kidney injury molecule-1 (KIM-1) combined with longitudinal clinical data, including APOL1 genotype if available, and plasma (isolated fresh or frozen), algorithm reported as probability score for rapid kidney function decline (RKFD)

0106U Gastric emptying, serial collection of 7 timed breath specimens, non-radioisotope carbon-13 (13C) spirulina substrate, analysis of each specimen by gas isotope ratio mass spectrometry, reported as rate of 13CO2 excretion

0107U Clostridium difficile toxin(s) antigen detection by immunoassay technique, stool, qualitative, multiplestep method

0108U Gastroenterology (Barrett's esophagus), whole slide- digital imaging, including morphometric analysis, computer-assisted quantitative immunolabeling of 9 protein biomarkers (p16, AMACR, p53, CD68, COX-2, CD45RO, HIF1a, HER-2, K20) and morphology, formalinfixed paraffin-embedded tissue, algorithm reported as risk of progression to high-grade dysplasia or cancer

0109U Infectious disease (Aspergillus species), real-time PCR for detection of DNA from 4 species (A. fumigatus, A. terreus, A. niger, and A. flavus), blood, lavage fluid, or tissue, qualitative reporting of presence or absence of each species

0110U Prescription drug monitoring, one or more oral oncology drug(s) and substances, definitive tandem mass spectrometry with chromatography, serum or plasma from capillary blood or venous blood, quantitative report with steady-state range for the prescribed drug(s) when detected

0111U Oncology (colon cancer), targeted KRAS (codons 12, 13, and 61) and NRAS (codons 12, 13, and 61) gene analysis, utilizing formalin-fixed paraffin-embedded tissue

0112U Infectious agent detection and identification, targeted sequence analysis (16S and 18S rRNA genes) with drugresistance gene

0113U Oncology (prostate), measurement of PCA3 and TMPRSS2-ERG in urine and PSA in serum following prostatic massage, by RNA amplification and fluorescence-based detection, algorithm reported as risk score

0114U Gastroenterology (Barrett's esophagus), VIM and CCNA1 methylation analysis, esophageal cells, algorithm reported as likelihood for Barrett's esophagus

---

Separate Procedure   Unlisted Procedure   CCI Comp. Code   Non-specific Procedure   **855**

0115U Respiratory infectious agent detection by nucleic acid (DNA and RNA), 18 viral types and subtypes and 2 bacterial targets, amplified probe technique, including multiplex reverse transcription for RNA targets, each analyte reported as detected or not detected

0116U Prescription drug monitoring, enzyme immunoassay of 35 or more drugs confirmed with LC-MS/MS, oral fluid, algorithm results reported as a patient-compliance measurement with risk of drug to drug interactions for prescribed medications

0117U Pain management, analysis of 11 endogenous analytes (methylmalonic acid, xanthurenic acid, homocysteine, pyroglutamic acid, vanilmandelate, 5-hydroxyindoleacetic acid, hydroxymethylglutarate, ethylmalonate, 3-hydroxypropyl mercapturic acid (3-HPMA), quinolinic acid, kynurenic acid), LC-MS/MS, urine, algorithm reported as a pain-index score with likelihood of atypical biochemical function associated with pain

0118U Transplantation medicine, quantification of donor-derived cell-free DNA using whole genome next-generation sequencing, plasma, reported as percentage of donorderived cell-free DNA in the total cell-free DNA

0119U Cardiology, ceramides by liquid chromatography-tandem mass spectrometry, plasma, quantitative report with risk score for major cardiovascular events

0120U Oncology (B-cell lymphoma classification), mRNA, gene expression profiling by fluorescent probe hybridization of 58 genes (45 content and 13 housekeeping genes), formalin-fixed paraffin-embedded tissue, algorithm reported as likelihood for primary mediastinal B-cell lymphoma (PMBCL) and diffuse large B-cell lymphoma (DLBCL) with cell of origin subtyping in the latter

0121U Sickle cell disease, microfluidic flow adhesion (VCAM-1), whole blood

0122U Sickle cell disease, microfluidic flow adhesion (P-Selectin), whole blood

0123U Mechanical fragility, RBC, shear stress and spectral analysis profiling

(**0124U** deleted 2020 [2021 Edition])

(**0125U** deleted 2020 [2021 Edition])

(**0126U** deleted 2020 [2021 Edition])

(**0127U** deleted 2020 [2021 Edition])

(**0128U** deleted 2020 [2021 Edition])

0129U Hereditary breast cancer-related disorders (eg, hereditary breast cancer, hereditary ovarian cancer, hereditary endometrial cancer), genomic sequence analysis and deletion/duplication analysis panel (ATM, BRCA1, BRCA2, CDH1, CHEK2, PALB2, PTEN, and TP53)

+ **0130U** Hereditary colon cancer disorders (eg, Lynch syndrome, PTEN hamartoma syndrome, Cowden syndrome, familial adenomatosis polyposis), targeted mRNA sequence analysis panel (APC, CDH1, CHEK2, MLH1, MSH2, MSH6, MUTYH, PMS2, PTEN, and TP53) (List separately in addition to code for primary procedure)

(Use 0130U in conjunction with 81435, 0101U)

+ **0131U** Hereditary breast cancer-related disorders (eg, hereditary breast cancer, hereditary ovarian cancer, hereditary endometrial cancer), targeted mRNA sequence analysis panel (13 genes) (List separately in addition to code for primary procedure)

(Use 0131U in conjunction with 81162, 81432, 0102U)

+ **0132U** Hereditary ovarian cancer-related disorders (eg, hereditary breast cancer, hereditary ovarian cancer, hereditary endometrial cancer), targeted mRNA sequence analysis panel (17 genes) (List separately in addition to code for primary procedure)

(Use 0132U in conjunction with 81162, 81432, 0103U)

+ **0133U**   Hereditary prostate cancer-related disorders, targeted mRNA sequence analysis panel (11 genes) (List separately in addition to code for primary procedure)

(Use 0133U in conjunction with 81162)

+ **0134U**   Hereditary pan cancer (eg, hereditary breast and ovarian cancer, hereditary endometrial cancer, hereditary colorectal cancer), targeted mRNA sequence analysis panel (18 genes) (List separately in addition to code for primary procedure)

(Use 0134U in conjunction with 81162, 81432, 81435)

+ **0135U**   Hereditary gynecological cancer (eg, hereditary breast and ovarian cancer, hereditary endometrial cancer, hereditary colorectal cancer), targeted mRNA sequence analysis panel (12 genes) (List separately in addition to code for primary procedure)

(Use 0135U in conjunction with 81162)

+ **0136U**   ATM (ataxia telangiectasia mutated) (eg, ataxia telangiectasia) mRNA sequence analysis (List separately in addition to code for primary procedure)

(Use 0136U in conjunction with 81408)

+ **0137U**   PALB2 (partner and localizer of BRCA2) (eg, breast and pancreatic cancer) mRNA sequence analysis (List separately in addition to code for primary procedure)

(Use 0137U in conjunction with 81307)

+ **0138U**   BRCA1 (BRCA1, DNA repair associated), BRCA2 (BRCA2, DNA repair associated) (eg, hereditary breast and ovarian cancer) mRNA sequence analysis (List separately in addition to code for primary procedure)

(Use 0138U in conjunction with 81162)

● **0139U**   Neurology (autism spectrum disorder [ASD]), quantitative measurements of 6 central carbon metabolites (ie, a-ketoglutarate, alanine, lactate, phenylalanine, pyruvate, and succinate), LC-MS/MS, plasma, algorithmic analysis with result reported as negative or positive (with metabolic subtypes of ASD)

● **0140U**   Infectious disease (fungi), fungal pathogen identification, DNA (15 fungal targets), blood culture, amplified probe technique, each target reported as detected or not detected

● **0141U**   Infectious disease (bacteria and fungi), gram-positive organism identification and drug resistance element detection, DNA (20 gram-positive bacterial targets, 4 resistance genes, 1 pan gram-negative bacterial target, 1 pan Candida target), blood culture, amplified probe technique, each target reported as detected or not detected

● **0142U**   Infectious disease (bacteria and fungi), gram-negative bacterial identification and drug resistance element detection, DNA (21 gram-negative bacterial targets, 6 resistance genes, 1 pan gram-positive bacterial target, 1 pan Candida target), amplified probe technique, each target reported as detected or not detected

● **0143U**   Drug assay, definitive, 120 or more drugs or metabolites, urine, quantitative liquid chromatography with tandem mass spectrometry (LC-MS/MS) using multiple reaction monitoring (MRM), with drug or metabolite description, comments including sample validation, per date of service *Duplicate PLA Test*

(For additional PLA code with identical clinical descriptor, see 0150U. See Appendix O to determine appropriate code assignment)

● **0144U**   Drug assay, definitive, 160 or more drugs or metabolites, urine, quantitative liquid chromatography with tandem mass spectrometry (LC-MS/MS) using multiple reaction monitoring (MRM), with drug or metabolite description, comments including sample validation, per date of service

● **0145U**   Drug assay, definitive, 65 or more drugs or metabolites, urine, quantitative liquid chromatography with tandem mass spectrometry (LC-MS/MS) using multiple reaction monitoring (MRM), with drug or metabolite description, comments including sample validation, per date of service

● **0146U** Drug assay, definitive, 80 or more drugs or metabolites, urine, by quantitative liquid chromatography with tandem mass spectrometry (LC-MS/MS) using multiple reaction monitoring (MRM), with drug or metabolite description, comments including sample validation, per date of service

● **0147U** Drug assay, definitive, 85 or more drugs or metabolites, urine, quantitative liquid chromatography with tandem mass spectrometry (LC-MS/MS) using multiple reaction monitoring (MRM), with drug or metabolite description, comments including sample validation, per date of service

● **0148U** Drug assay, definitive, 100 or more drugs or metabolites, urine, quantitative liquid chromatography with tandem mass spectrometry (LC-MS/MS) using multiple reaction monitoring (MRM), with drug or metabolite description, comments including sample validation, per date of service

● **0149U** Drug assay, definitive, 60 or more drugs or metabolites, urine, quantitative liquid chromatography with tandem mass spectrometry (LC-MS/MS) using multiple reaction monitoring (MRM), with drug or metabolite description, comments including sample validation, per date of service

● **0150U** Drug assay, definitive, 120 or more drugs or metabolites, urine, quantitative liquid chromatography with tandem mass spectrometry (LC-MS/MS) using multiple reaction monitoring (MRM), with drug or metabolite description, comments including sample validation, per date of service ***Duplicate PLA Test***

(For additional PLA code with identical clinical descriptor, see 0143U. See Appendix O to determine appropriate code assignment)

● **0151U** Infectious disease (bacterial or viral respiratory tract infection), pathogen specific nucleic acid (DNA or RNA), 33 targets, real-time semi-quantitative PCR, bronchoalveolar lavage, sputum, or endotracheal aspirate, detection of 33 organismal and antibiotic resistance genes with limited semi-quantitative results 3 CPT Changes: An Insider's View 2021

● **0152U** Infectious disease (bacteria, fungi, parasites, and DNA viruses), DNA, PCR and next-generation sequencing, plasma, detection of >1,000 potential microbial organisms for significant positive pathogens

● **0153U** Oncology (breast), mRNA, gene expression profiling by next-generation sequencing of 101 genes, utilizing formalin-fixed paraffin-embedded tissue, algorithm reported as a triple negative breast cancer clinical subtype(s) with information on immune cell involvement

● **0154U** Oncology (urothelial cancer), RNA, analysis by real-time RT-PCR of the FGFR3 (fibroblast growth factor receptor 3) gene analysis (ie, p.R248C [c.742C>T], p.S249C [c.746C>G], p.G370C [c.1108G>T], p.Y373C [c.1118A>G], FGFR3-TACC3v1, and FGFR3-TACC3v3), utilizing formalinfixed paraffin-embedded urothelial cancer tumor tissue, reported as FGFR gene alteration status

● **0155U** Oncology (breast cancer), DNA, PIK3CA (phosphatidylinositol-4,5-bisphosphate 3-kinase, catalytic subunit alpha) (eg, breast cancer) gene analysis (ie, p. C420R, p.E542K, p.E545A, p.E545D [g.1635G>T only], p. E545G, p.E545K, p.Q546E, p.Q546R, p.H1047L, p.H1047R, p.H1047Y), utilizing formalin-fixed paraffin-embedded breast tumor tissue, reported as PIK3CA gene mutation status

● **0156U** Copy number (eg, intellectual disability, dysmorphology), sequence analysis

●+**0157U** APC (APC regulator of WNT signaling pathway) (eg, familial adenomatosis polyposis [FAP]) mRNA sequence analysis (List separately in addition to code for primary procedure)

(Use 0157U in conjunction with 81201)

●+**0158U** MLH1 (mutL homolog 1) (eg, hereditary non-polyposis colorectal cancer, Lynch syndrome) mRNA sequence analysis (List separately in addition to code for primary procedure)

(Use 0158U in conjunction with 81292)

●+**0159U** MSH2 (mutS homolog 2) (eg, hereditary colon cancer, Lynch syndrome) mRNA sequence analysis (List separately in addition to code for primary procedure)

(Use 0159U in conjunction with 81295)

●+**0160U** MSH6 (mutS homolog 6) (eg, hereditary colon cancer, Lynch syndrome) mRNA sequence analysis (List separately in addition to code for primary procedure)

(Use 0160U in conjunction with 81298)

● New Code   ▲ Revised Code   + Add-On Code   ⊘ Modifier -51 Exempt   ★ Telemedicine

●+**0161U**   PMS2 (PMS1 homolog 2, mismatch repair system component) (eg, hereditary non-polyposis colorectal cancer, Lynch syndrome) mRNA sequence analysis (List separately in addition to code for primary procedure)

(Use 0161U in conjunction with 81317)

●+**0162U**   Hereditary colon cancer (Lynch syndrome), targeted mRNA sequence analysis panel (MLH1, MSH2, MSH6, PMS2) (List separately in addition to code for primary procedure)

(Use 0162U in conjunction with 81292, 81295, 81298, 81317, 81435)

● **0163U**   Oncology (colorectal) screening, biochemical enzymelinked immunosorbent assay (ELISA) of 3 plasma or serum proteins (teratocarcinoma derived growth factor-1 [TDGF-1, Cripto-1], carcinoembryonic antigen [CEA], extracellular matrix protein [ECM]), with demographic data (age, gender, CRC-screening compliance) using a proprietary algorithm and reported as likelihood of CRC or advanced adenomas

● **0164U**   Gastroenterology (irritable bowel syndrome [IBS]), immunoassay for anti-CdtB and anti-vinculin antibodies, utilizing plasma, algorithm for elevated or not elevated qualitative results

● **0165U**   Peanut allergen-specific quantitative assessment of multiple epitopes using enzyme-linked immunosorbent assay (ELISA), blood, individual epitope results and probability of peanut allergy

● **0166U**   Liver disease, 10 biochemical assays (a2-macroglobulin, haptoglobin, apolipoprotein A1, bilirubin, GGT, ALT, AST, triglycerides, cholesterol, fasting glucose) and biometric and demographic data, utilizing serum, algorithm reported as scores for fibrosis, necroinflammatory activity, and steatosis with a summary interpretation

● **0167U**   Gonadotropin, chorionic (hCG), immunoassay with direct optical observation, blood

● **0168U**   Fetal aneuploidy (trisomy 21, 18, and 13) DNA sequence analysis of selected regions using maternal plasma without fetal fraction cutoff, algorithm reported as a risk score for each trisomy

● **0169U**   NUDT15 (nudix hydrolase 15) and TPMT (thiopurine S-methyltransferase) (eg, drug metabolism) gene analysis, common variants

● **0170U**   Neurology (autism spectrum disorder [ASD]), RNA, nextgeneration sequencing, saliva, algorithmic analysis, and results reported as predictive probability of ASD diagnosis

● **0171U**   Targeted genomic sequence analysis panel, acute myeloid leukemia, myelodysplastic syndrome, and myeloproliferative neoplasms, DNA analysis, 23 genes, interrogation for sequence variants, rearrangements and minimal residual disease, reported as presence/absence

● **0172U**   Oncology (solid tumor as indicated by the label), somatic mutation analysis of BRCA1 (BRCA1, DNA repair associated), BRCA2 (BRCA2, DNA repair associated) and analysis of homologous recombination deficiency pathways, DNA, formalin-fixed paraffin-embedded tissue, algorithm quantifying tumor genomic instability score

● **0173U**   Psychiatry (ie, depression, anxiety), genomic analysis panel, includes variant analysis of 14 genes

● **0174U**   Oncology (solid tumor), mass spectrometric 30 protein targets, formalin-fixed paraffin-embedded tissue, prognostic and predictive algorithm reported as likely, unlikely, or uncertain benefit of 39 chemotherapy and targeted therapeutic oncology agents

● **0175U**   Psychiatry (eg, depression, anxiety), genomic analysis panel, variant analysis of 15 genes

● **0176U**   Cytolethal distending toxin B (CdtB) and vinculin IgG antibodies by immunoassay (ie, ELISA)

● **0177U**   Oncology (breast cancer), DNA, PIK3CA (phosphatidylinositol-4,5-bisphosphate 3-kinase catalytic subunit alpha) gene analysis of 11 gene variants utilizing plasma, reported as PIK3CA gene mutation status

● **0178U**   Peanut allergen-specific quantitative assessment of multiple epitopes using enzyme-linked immunosorbent assay (ELISA), blood, report of minimum eliciting exposure for a clinical reaction

● **0179U**   Oncology (non-small cell lung cancer), cell-free DNA, targeted sequence analysis of 23 genes (single nucleotide variations, insertions and deletions, fusions without prior knowledge of partner/breakpoint, copy number variations), with report of significant mutation(s)

Separate Procedure   Unlisted Procedure   CCI Comp. Code   Non-specific Procedure   **859**

- **0180U** Red cell antigen (ABO blood group) genotyping (ABO), gene analysis Sanger/chain termination/conventional sequencing, ABO (ABO, alpha 1-3-N-acetylgalactosaminyltransferase and alpha 1-3-galactosyltransferase) gene, including subtyping, 7 exons

- **0181U** Red cell antigen (Colton blood group) genotyping (CO), gene analysis, AQP1 (aquaporin 1 [Colton blood group]) exon 1

- **0182U** Red cell antigen (Cromer blood group) genotyping (CROM), gene analysis, CD55 (CD55 molecule [Cromer blood group]) exons 1-10

- **0183U** Red cell antigen (Diego blood group) genotyping (DI), gene analysis, SLC4A1 (solute carrier family 4 member 1 [Diego blood group]) exon 19

- **0184U** Red cell antigen (Dombrock blood group) genotyping (DO), gene analysis, ART4 (ADP-ribosyltransferase 4 [Dombrock blood group]) exon 2

- **0185U** Red cell antigen (H blood group) genotyping (FUT1), gene analysis, FUT1 (fucosyltransferase 1 [H blood group]) exon 4

- **0186U** Red cell antigen (H blood group) genotyping (FUT2), gene analysis, FUT2 (fucosyltransferase 2) exon 2

- **0187U** Red cell antigen (Duffy blood group) genotyping (FY), gene analysis, ACKR1 (atypical chemokine receptor 1 [Duffy blood group]) exons 1-2

- **0188U** Red cell antigen (Gerbich blood group) genotyping (GE), gene analysis, GYPC (glycophorin C [Gerbich blood group]) exons 1-4

- **0189U** Red cell antigen (MNS blood group) genotyping (GYPA), gene analysis, GYPA (glycophorin A [MNS blood group]) introns 1, 5, exon 2

- **0190U** Red cell antigen (MNS blood group) genotyping (GYPB), gene analysis, GYPB (glycophorin B [MNS blood group]) introns 1, 5, pseudoexon 3

- **0191U** Red cell antigen (Indian blood group) genotyping (IN), gene analysis, CD44 (CD44 molecule [Indian blood group]) exons 2, 3, 6

- **0192U** Red cell antigen (Kidd blood group) genotyping (JK), gene analysis, SLC14A1 (solute carrier family 14 member 1 [Kidd blood group]) gene promoter, exon 9

- **0193U** Red cell antigen (JR blood group) genotyping (JR), gene analysis, ABCG2 (ATP binding cassette subfamily G member 2 [Junior blood group]) exons 2-26

- **0194U** Red cell antigen (Kell blood group) genotyping (KEL), gene analysis, KEL (Kell metallo-endopeptidase [Kell blood group]) exon 8

- **0195U** KLF1 (Kruppel-like factor 1), targeted sequencing (ie, exon 13)

- **0196U** Red cell antigen (Lutheran blood group) genotyping (LU), gene analysis, BCAM (basal cell adhesion molecule [Lutheran blood group]) exon 3

- **0197U** Red cell antigen (Landsteiner-Wiener blood group) genotyping (LW), gene analysis, ICAM4 (intercellular adhesion molecule 4 [Landsteiner-Wiener blood group]) exon 1

- **0198U** Red cell antigen (RH blood group) genotyping (RHD and RHCE), gene analysis Sanger/chain termination/conventional sequencing, RHD (Rh blood group D antigen) exons 1-10 and RHCE (Rh blood group CcEe antigens) exon 5

- **0199U** Red cell antigen (Scianna blood group) genotyping (SC), gene analysis, ERMAP (erythroblast membrane associated protein [Scianna blood group]) exons 4, 12

- **0200U** Red cell antigen (Kx blood group) genotyping (XK), gene analysis, XK (X-linked Kx blood group) exons 1-3

- **0201U** Red cell antigen (Yt blood group) genotyping (YT), gene analysis, ACHE (acetylcholinesterase [Cartwright blood group]) exon 2

● New Code   ▲ Revised Code   + Add-On Code   ⊘ Modifier -51 Exempt   ★ Telemedicine

● **0202U** Infectious disease (bacterial or viral respiratory tract infection), pathogen-specific nucleic acid (DNA or RNA), 22 targets including severe acute respiratory syndrome coronavirus 2 (SARS-CoV-2), qualitative RT-PCR, nasopharyngeal swab, each pathogen reported as detected or not detected

● **0203U** Autoimmune (inflammatory bowel disease), mRNA, gene expression profiling by quantitative RT-PCR, 17 genes (15 target and 2 reference genes), whole blood, reported as a continuous risk score and classification of inflammatory bowel disease aggressiveness

● **0204U** Oncology (thyroid), mRNA, gene expression analysis of 593 genes (including BRAF, RAS, RET, PAX8, and NTRK) for sequence variants and rearrangements, utilizing fine needle aspirate, reported as detected or not detected

● **0205U** Ophthalmology (age-related macular degeneration), analysis of 3 gene variants (2 CFH gene, 1 ARMS2 gene), using PCR and MALDI-TOF, buccal swab, reported as positive or negative for neovascular age-related maculardegeneration risk associated with zinc supplements

● **0206U** Neurology (Alzheimer disease); cell aggregation using morphometric imaging and protein kinase C-epsilon (PKCe) concentration in response to amylospheroid treatment by ELISA, cultured skin fibroblasts, each reported as positive or negative for Alzheimer disease

●+**0207U** quantitative imaging of phosphorylated ERK1 and ERK2 in response to bradykinin treatment by in situ immunofluorescence, using cultured skin fibroblasts, reported as a probability index for Alzheimer disease (List separately in addition to code for primary procedure)

(Use 0207U in conjunction with 0206U)

● **0208U** Oncology (medullary thyroid carcinoma), mRNA, gene expression analysis of 108 genes, utilizing fine needle aspirate, algorithm reported as positive or negative for medullary thyroid carcinoma

● **0209U** Cytogenomic constitutional (genome-wide) analysis, interrogation of genomic regions for copy number, structural changes and areas of homozygosity for chromosomal abnormalities

● **0210U** Syphilis test, non-treponemal antibody, immunoassay, quantitative (RPR)

● **0211U** Oncology (pan-tumor), DNA and RNA by next-generation sequencing, utilizing formalin-fixed paraffin-embedded tissue, interpretative report for single nucleotide variants, copy number alterations, tumor mutational burden, and microsatellite instability, with therapy association

● **0212U** Rare diseases (constitutional/heritable disorders), whole genome and mitochondrial DNA sequence analysis, including small sequence changes, deletions, duplications, short tandem repeat gene expansions, and variants in non-uniquely mappable regions, blood or saliva, identification and categorization of genetic variants, proband

(Do not report 0212U in conjunction with 81425)

● **0213U** Rare diseases (constitutional/heritable disorders), whole genome and mitochondrial DNA sequence analysis, including small sequence changes, deletions, duplications, short tandem repeat gene expansions, and variants in non-uniquely mappable regions, blood or saliva, identification and categorization of genetic variants, each comparator genome (eg, parent, sibling)

(Do not report 0213U in conjunction with 81426)

● **0214U** Rare diseases (constitutional/heritable disorders), whole exome and mitochondrial DNA sequence analysis, including small sequence changes, deletions, duplications, short tandem repeat gene expansions, and variants in non-uniquely mappable regions, blood or saliva, identification and categorization of genetic variants, proband

(Do not report 0214U in conjunction with 81415)

● **0215U** Rare diseases (constitutional/heritable disorders), whole exome and mitochondrial DNA sequence analysis, including small sequence changes, deletions, duplications, short tandem repeat gene expansions, and variants in non-uniquely mappable regions, blood or saliva, identification and categorization of genetic variants, each comparator exome (eg, parent, sibling)

(Do not report 0215U in conjunction with 81416)

Separate Procedure   Unlisted Procedure   CCI Comp. Code   Non-specific Procedure   **861**

● **0216U** Neurology (inherited ataxias), genomic DNA sequence analysis of 12 common genes including small sequence changes, deletions, duplications, short tandem repeat gene expansions, and variants in non-uniquely mappable regions, blood or saliva, identification and categorization of genetic variants

● **0217U** Neurology (inherited ataxias), genomic DNA sequence analysis of 51 genes including small sequence changes, deletions, duplications, short tandem repeat gene expansions, and variants in non-uniquely mappable regions, blood or saliva, identification and categorization of genetic variants

● **0218U** Neurology (muscular dystrophy), DMD gene sequence analysis, including small sequence changes, deletions, duplications, and variants in non-uniquely mappable regions, blood or saliva, identification and characterization of genetic variants

● **0219U** Infectious agent (human immunodeficiency virus), targeted viral next-generation sequence analysis (ie, protease [PR], reverse transcriptase [RT], integrase [INT]), algorithm reported as prediction of antiviral drug susceptibility

● **0220U** Oncology (breast cancer), image analysis with artificial intelligence assessment of 12 histologic and immunohistochemical features, reported as a recurrence score

● **0221U** Red cell antigen (ABO blood group) genotyping (ABO), gene analysis, next-generation sequencing, ABO (ABO, alpha 1-3-N-acetylgalactosaminyltransferase and alpha 1-3-galactosyltransferase) gene

● **0222U** Red cell antigen (RH blood group) genotyping (RHD and RHCE), gene analysis, next-generation sequencing, RH proximal promoter, exons 1-10, portions of introns 2-3

● **0223U** Infectious disease (bacterial or viral respiratory tract infection), pathogen-specific nucleic acid (DNA or RNA), 22 targets including severe acute respiratory syndrome coronavirus 2 (SARS-CoV-2), qualitative RT-PCR, nasopharyngeal swab, each pathogen reported as detected or not detected

● **0224U** Antibody, severe acute respiratory syndrome coronavirus 2 (SARS-CoV-2) (Coronarvirus disease [COVID-19]), inlcudes titer(s), when performed

● **0225U** Infectious disease (bacterial or viral respiratory tract infection) pathogen-specific DNA and RNA, 21 targets, including severe acute respiratory syndrome coronavirus 2 (SARS-CoV-2), amplified probe technique, including multiple reverse transcription for RNA targets, each analyte reported as detected or not detected

● **0226U** Surrogate viral neutralization test (sVNT), severe acute respiratory syndrome coronavirus 2 (SARS-CoV-2) (Coronavirus disease [COVID-19]), ELISA, plasma, serum

● **0240U** Infectious disease (viral respiratory tract infection), pathogen-specific RNA, 3 targets (severe acute respiratory syndrome coronavirus 2 [SARS-CoV-2], influenza A, influenza B), upper respiratory specimen, each pathogen reported as detected or not detected

● **0241U** Infectious disease (viral respiratory tract infection), pathogen-specific RNA, 4 targets (severe acute respiratory syndrome coronavirus 2 [SARS-CoV-2], influenza A, influenza B, respiratory syncytial virus [RSV]), upper respiratory specimen, each pathogen reported as detected or not detected

---

● New Code   ▲ Revised Code   ✛ Add-On Code   ⊘ Modifier -51 Exempt   ★ Telemedicine

MEDICINE SECTION OVERVIEW

The sixth section of the CPT coding system is the medicine section, which includes codes for immunizations, therapeutic or diagnostic injections, psychiatric services, dialysis, ophthalmology services, specialty specific diagnostic services, chemotherapy administration, physical medicine and rehabilitation services, osteopathic and chiropractic services. Within each subsection, the CPT codes are arranged by the type of service provided.

SEPARATE PROCEDURES

Some procedures or services listed in the CPT coding system that are usually provided as an integral component of another total service or procedure are identified by the inclusion of the term (separate procedure). Codes designated as (separate procedure) should not be reported in addition to the code for the total procedure or service of which it is considered an integral component.

However, when a procedure or service designated as a (separate procedure) is provided independently or is considered to be unrelated or distinct from other procedures/services provided at the same time, the CPT code may be reported by itself. If the (separate procedure) is provided in addition to other procedures or services, the modifier -59 should be added to the (separate procedure) code to indicate that it is a distinct, independent procedure.

UNLISTED SERVICE OR PROCEDURE

A medicine service or procedure may be provided that is not listed in the CPT codebook. When reporting such service(s), the appropriate "Unlisted Procedure" code should be used to indicate the service, identifying it by "Special Report" as discussed below. The "Unlisted Procedures" and accompanying code forMedicine is as follows:

90399	Unlisted immune globulin
90749	Unlisted vaccine/toxoid
90899	Unlisted psychiatric service or procedure
90999	Unlisted dialysis procedure, inpatient or outpatient
91299	Unlisted diagnostic gastroenterology procedure
92499	Unlisted ophthalmological service or procedure
92700	Unlisted otorhinolaryngological service or procedure
93799	Unlisted cardiovascular service or procedure
93998	Unlisted noninvasive vascular diagnostic study
94799	Unlisted pulmonary service or procedure
95199	Unlisted allergy/clinical immunologic service or procedure
95999	Unlisted neurological or neuromuscular diagnostic procedure
96379	Unlisted therapeutic, prophylactic, or diagnostic intravenous or intra-arterial injection or infusion
96549	Unlisted chemotherapy procedure
96999	Unlisted special dermatological service or procedure
97039	Unlisted modality (specify type and time if constant attendance)
97139	Unlisted therapeutic procedure (specify)

MED 90000

97799   Unlisted physical medicine/rehabilitation service or procedure

99199   Unlisted special service, procedure or report

99600   Unlisted home visit service or procedure

SPECIAL REPORT

A service that is rarely provided, unusual, variable, or new may require a special report. Pertinent information should include an adequate definition or description of the nature, extent, and need for the procedure and the time, effort, and equipment necessary to provide the service.

SUPPLIES AND MATERIALS

Supplies and materials provided (eg, sterile trays, drugs) over and above those usually included with the office visit or anesthesia services rendered may be listed separately. Drugs, tray supplies, and materials provided should be listed and identified with 99070 or the appropriate supply code. For Medicare claims, HCPCS Level II codes should be used to report supplies and materials.

MEDICINE SUBSECTIONS

The MEDICINE section of CPT is divided into the following subsections:

Immune Globulins, Serums or Recombinant Products	90281-90399
Immunization Administration for Vaccines/Toxoids	90460-90474
Vaccines, Toxoids	90476-90749
Psychiatry	90785-90899
Biofeedback	90901-90913
Dialysis	90935-90999
Gastroenterology	91010-91299
Ophthalmology	92002-92499
Special Otorhinolaryngologic Services	92502-92700
Cardiovascular	92920-93799
Noninvasive Vascular Diagnostic Studies	93880-93998
Pulmonary	94002-94799
Allergy and Clinical Immunology	95004-95199
Endocrinology	95249-95251
Neurology and Neuromuscular Procedures	95700-96020
Medical Genetics and Genetic Counseling Services	96040
Adaptive Behavior Services	97151-97158
Central Nervous System Assessments/Tests	96105-96146
Health Behavior Assessment and Intervention	96156-96171
Hydration, Therapeutic, Prophylactic, Diagnostic Injections and Infusions, and Chemotherapy	96360-96549
Photodynamic Therapy	96567-96574
Special Dermatological Procedures	96900-96999
Physical Medicine and Rehabilitation	97161-97799
Medical Nutrition Therapy	97802-97804
Acupuncture	97810-97814
Osteopathic Manipulative Treatment	98925-98929
Chiropractic Manipulative Tretment	98940-98943
Education and Training for Patient Self-Management	98960-98962
Non-Face-to-Face Non-Physician Services	98966-98972
Special Services, Procedures and Reports	99000-99082
Qualifying Circumstances for Anesthesia	99100-99140
Moderate (Conscious) Sedation	99151-99157
Other Services and Procedures	99170-99199
Home Health Procedures/Services	99500-99602
Medication Therapy Management	99605-99607

Most of the subsections have special needs or instructions unique to that section which should be reviewed carefully before reporting.

● New Code   ▲ Revised Code   ✚ Add-On Code   ⊘ Modifier -51 Exempt   ★ Telemedicine

MEDICINE SERVICES MODIFIERS

MEDICINE services and procedures may be modified under certain circumstances. When applicable, the modifying circumstance is identified by the addition of the appropriate modifier code. The following modifiers are frequently used with MEDICINE services.

-22 Unusual services

-26 Professional component

-51 Multiple procedures

This modifier may be used to report multiple medical procedures performed at the same session, as well as a combination of medical and surgical procedures.

-52 Reduced services

-76 Repeat procedure by same physician

-77 Repeat procedure by another physician

-90 Reference (outside) laboratory

-99 Multiple modifiers

This page intentionally left blank

● New Code ▲ Revised Code + Add-On Code ⊘ Modifier -51 Exempt ★ Telemedicine

MEDICINE CODES

IMMUNE GLOBULINS, SERUM OR RECOMBINANT PRODUCTS

Codes 90281-90399 identify the serum globulins, extracted from human blood; or recombinant immune globulin products created in a laboratory through genetic modification of human and/or animal proteins. Both are reported in addition to the administration codes 96365, 96366, 96367, 96368, 96369, 96370, 96371, 96372, 96374, 96375, as appropriate. Modifier 51 should not be reported with this section of products codes when performed with another procedure. The serum or recombinant globulin products listed here include broadspectrum anti-infective immune globulins, antitoxins, various isoantibodies, and monoclonal antibodies. See the Introduction section of the CPT code set for a complete list of the dates of release and implementation.b

90281	Immune globulin (Ig), human, for intramuscular use	
90283	Immune globulin (IgIV), human, for intravenous use	
90284	Immune globulin (SCIg), human, for use in subcutaneous infusions, 100 mg, each	
90287	Botulinum antitoxin, equine, any route	
90288	Botulism immune globulin, human, for intravenous use	
90291	Cytomegalovirus immune globulin (CMV-IgIV), human, for intravenous use	
90296	Diphtheria antitoxin, equine, any route	
90371	Hepatitis B immune globulin (HBIg), human, for intramuscular use	
90375	Rabies immune globulin (RIg), human, for intramuscular and/or subcutaneous use	
90376	Rabies immune globulin, heat-treated (RIg-HT), human, for intramuscular and/or subcutaneous use	
● **90377**	Rabies immune globulin, heat- and solvent/detergenttreated (RIg-HT S/D), human, for intramuscular and/or subcutaneous use	
90378	Respiratory syncytial virus monoclonal antibody, recombinant, for intramuscular use, 50 mg, each	
90384	Rho(D) immune globulin (RhIg), human, full-dose, for intramuscular use	
90385	Rho(D) immune globulin (RhIg), human, mini-dose, for intramuscular use	
90386	Rho(D) immune globulin (RhIgIV), human, for intravenous use	
90389	Tetanus immune globulin (TIg), human, for intramuscular use	
90393	Vaccinia immune globulin, human, for intramuscular use	
90396	Varicella-zoster immune globulin, human, for intramuscular use	
90399	Unlisted immune globulin	

IMMUNIZATION ADMINISTRATION FOR VACCINES/TOXOIDS

Immunization is the administration of a vaccine or toxoid to stimulate the immune system to provide protection against disease. Immunizations are usually given in conjunction with an evaluation and management service. When an immunization is the only service performed, a minimal evaluation and management service code may be listed in addition to the injection code.

Coding Rules

1. *When an immunization is the only service provided, evaluation and management service code 99211, Minimal service, may be reported in addition to the immunization.*

2. *Immunization administration CPT codes must be reported in addition to the vaccine and toxoid CPT codes.*

3. *Supplies or equipment used to inject the vaccine or toxoid are not reported separately.*

Report vaccine immunization administration codes 90460, 90461, 90471-90474 in addition to the vaccine and toxoid code(s) 90476-90749.

Report codes 90460 and 90461 only when the physician or qualified health care professional provides face-to-face counseling of the patient/family during the administration of a vaccine. For immunization administration of any vaccine that is not accompanied by face-to-face physician or qualified health care professional counseling to the patient/family, or for administration of vaccines to patients over 18 years of age, report codes 90471-90474.

If a significant separately identifiable evaluation and management service (eg, new or established patient office or other outpatient services [99202-99215], office or other outpatient consultations [99241-99245], emergency department services [99281-99285], preventive medicine services [99381-99429]) is performed, the appropriate E/M service code should be reported in addition to the vaccine and toxoid administration codes.

A component refers to all antigen in a vaccine that prevent disease(s) caused by one organism (90460 and 90461). Multi-valent antigens or multiple serotypes of antigens against a single organism are considered a single component of vaccines. Combination vaccines are those vaccines that contain multiple vaccine components. Conjugates or adjuvants contained in vaccines are not considered to be component parts of the vaccine as defined above.

IMMUNIZATION ADMINISTRATION

> (For allergy testing, see 95004 et seq)
>
> (For skin testing of bacterial, viral, fungal extracts, see 86485-86580)
>
> (For therapeutic or diagnostic injections, see 96372-96379)

90460 Immunization administration through 18 years of age via any route of administration, with counseling by physician or other qualified health care professional; first or only component of each vaccine or toxoid administered

+ **90461** each additional vaccine or toxoid component administered (List separately in addition to code for primary procedure)

> (Use 90460 for each vaccine administered. For vaccines with multiple components [combination vaccines], report 90460 in conjunction with 90461 for each additional component in a given vaccine)

90471 Immunization administration (includes percutaneous, intradermal, subcutaneous, or intramuscular injections); 1 vaccine (single or combination vaccine/toxoid)

> (Do not report 90471 in conjunction with 90473)

+ **90472** each additional vaccine (single or combination vaccine/toxoid) (List separately in addition to code for primary procedure)

> (Use 90472 in conjunction with 90460, 90471, 90473)
>
> (For immune globulins, see 90281-90399. For administration of immune globulins, see 96365, 96366, 96367, 96368, 96369, 96370, 96371, 96374)
>
> (For intravesical administration of BCG vaccine, use 51720, and see 90586)

90473 Immunization administration by intranasal or oral route; 1 vaccine (single or combination vaccine/toxoid)

> (Do not report 90473 in conjunction with 90471)

+ 90474   each additional vaccine (single or combination vaccine/toxoid) (List separately in addition to code for primary procedure)

(Use 90474 in conjunction with 90460, 90471, 90473)

VACCINES, TOXOIDS

Codes 90476-90749 identify the vaccine product **only**. To report the administration of a vaccine/toxoid, the vaccine/toxoid product codes 90476-90749 must be used in addition to an immunization administration code(s) 90460, 90461, 90471, 90472, 90473, 90474. Modifier -51 should not be reported with vaccine/toxoid codes 90476-90479, when reported in conjunction with administratino codes 90460, 90461, 90471-90474.

If a significant separately identifiable E/M service (eg., office or other outpatient services, preventive medicine services) is performed, the appropriate E/M service code should be reported in addition to the vaccine and toxoid administration codes.

To meet the reporting requirements of immunization registries, vaccine distribution programs, and reporting systems (eg., Vaccine Adverse Event Reporting System) the exact vaccine product administered needs to be reported. Multiple codes for a particular vaccine are provided in the CPT codebook when the schedule (number of doses or timing) differs for two or more products of the same vaccine type (eg., hepatitis A, Hib) or the vaccine product is available in more than one chemical formulation, dosage, or route of administration.

The "when administered to" age descriptions included in CPT vaccine codes are not intended to identify a product's licensed age indication. The term "preservative free" includes use for vaccines that contain no preservative and vaccines that contain trace amounts of preservative agents that are not present in a sufficient concentration for the purpose of preserving the final vaccine formulation. The absence of a designation regarding a preservative does not necessarily indicate the presence or absence of preservative in the vaccine. Refer to the product's prescribing information (PI) for the licensed age indication before administering vaccine to a patient.

Separate codes are available for combination vaccines (eg., DTP-Hib, DTaP-Hib, HepB-Hib). It is inappropriate to code each component of a combination vaccine separately. If a specific vaccine code is not available, the unlisted procedure code should be reported, until a new code becomes available.

(For immune globulins, see 90281-90399. For administration of immune globulins, see 96365-96375)

90476   Adenovirus vaccine, type 4, live, for oral use

90477   Adenovirus vaccine, type 7, live, for oral use

90581   Anthrax vaccine, for subcutaneous or intramuscular use

90585   Bacillus Calmette-Guerin vaccine (BCG) for tuberculosis, live, for percutaneous use

90586   Bacillus Calmette-Guerin vaccine (BCG) for bladder cancer, live, for intravesical use

90587   Dengue vaccine, quadrivalent, live, 3 dose schedule, for subcutaneous use

90619   This code is out of order .See page 872

90620   This code is out of order .See page 872

90621   This code is out of order. See page 872

90625   This code is out of order. See page 872

90630   This code is out of order. See page 870

90632   Hepatitis A vaccine (HepA), adult dosage, for intramuscular use

90633   Hepatitis A vaccine (HepA), pediatric/adolescent dosage-2 dose schedule, for intramuscular use

90634 Hepatitis A vaccine (HepA), pediatric/adolescent dosage-3 dose schedule, for intramuscular use

90636 Hepatitis A and hepatitis B vaccine (HepA-HepB), adult dosage, for intramuscular use

90644 This code is out of order. See page 872

90647 Hemophilus influenza tybe b vaccine (Hib), PRP-OMP conjugate 3 dose schedule, for intramuscular use

90648 Hemophilus influenza type b vaccine (Hib), PRP-T conjugate, 4 dose schedule, for intramuscular use

90649 Human Papillomavirus (HPV) vaccine, types 6, 11, 16, 18, quadrivalent (4vHPV), 3 dose schedule, for intramuscular use

90650 Human Papillomavirus (HPV) vaccine, types 16, 18, bivalent (2vHPV), 3 dose schedule, for intramuscular use

90651 Human Papillomavirus vaccine types 6, 11, 16, 18, 31, 33, 45, 52, 58, nonavalent (9vHPV), 2 or 3 dose schedule, for intramuscular use

90653 Influenza vaccine, inactivated (IIV), subunit, adjuvanted, for intramuscular use

90654 Influenza virus vaccine, trivalent (IIV3), split virus, preservative-free, for intradermal use

90630 Influenza virus vaccine, quadrivalent (IIV4), split virus, preservative free, for intradermal use

90655 Influenza virus vaccine, trivalent (IIV3), split virus, preservative free, 0.25 mL dosage, for intramuscular use

90656 Influenza virus vaccine, trivalent (IIV3), split virus, preservative free, 0.5 mL dosage, for intramuscular use

90657 Influenza virus vaccine, trivalent (IIV3), split virus, 0.25 mL dosage, for intramuscular use

90658 Influenza virus vaccine, trivalent (IIV3), split virus, 0.5 mL dosage, for intramuscular use

90660 Influenza virus vaccine, trivalent, live (LAIV3), for intranasal use

90672 Influenza virus vaccine, quadrivalent, live (LAIV4), for intranasal use

90661 Influenza virus vaccine, trivalent (ccIIV3), derived from cell cultures, subunit, preservative and antibiotic free, 0.5 mL dosage, for intramuscular use

90674 Influenza virus vaccine, quadrivalent (ccIIV4), derived from cell cultures, subunit, preservative and antibiotic free, 0.5 mL dosage, for intramuscular use

90756 Influenza virus vaccine, quadrivalent (ccIIV4), derived from cell cultures, subunit, antibiotic free, 0.5 mL dosage, for intramuscular use

90673 Influenza virus vaccine, trivalent (RIV3), derived from recombinant DNA, hemagglutinin (HA) protein only, preservative and antibiotic free, for intramuscular use

90662 Influenza virus vaccine (IIV), split virus, preservative free, enhanced immunogenicity via increased antigen content, for intramuscular use

90664 Influenza virus vaccine, live (LAIV), pandemic formulation, for intranasal use

90666 Influenza virus vaccine (IIV), pandemic formulation, split virus, preservative free, for intramuscular use

(FDA approval pending)

90667 Influenza virus vaccine (IIV), pandemic formulation, split virus, adjuvanted, for intramuscular use

---

● New Code ▲ Revised Code + Add-On Code ⊘ Modifier -51 Exempt ★ Telemedicine

(FDA approval pending)

90668 Influenza virus vaccine (IIV), pandemic formulation, split virus, for intramuscular use

(FDA approval pending)

90670 Pneumococcal conjugate vaccine, 13 valent (PCV13), for intramuscular use

90672 This code is out of order. See page 870

90673 This code is out of order. See page 870

90674 This code is out of order. See page 870

90675 Rabies vaccine, for intramuscular use

90676 Rabies vaccine, for intradermal use

90680 Rotavirus vaccine, pentavalent (RV5), 3 dose schedule, live, for oral use

90681 Rotavirus vaccine, human, attenuated (RV1), 2 dose schedule, live, for oral use

90682 Influenza virus vaccine, quadrivalent (RIV4), derived from recombinant DNA, hemagglutinin (HA) protein only, preservative and antibiotic free, for intramuscular use

90685 Influenza virus vaccine, quadrivalent (IIV4), split virus, preservative free, 0.25 mL dosage, for intramuscular use

90686 Influenza virus vaccine, quadrivalent (IIV4), split virus, preservative free, 0.5 mL dosage, for intramuscular use

90687 Influenza virus vaccine, quadrivalent (IIV4), split virus, 0.25 mL dosage, for intramuscular use

90688 Influenza virus vaccine, quadrivalent (IIV4), split virus, 0.5 mL dosage, for intramuscular use

90689 Influenza virus vaccine, quadrivalent (IIV4), inactivated, adjuvanted, preservative free, 0.25 mL dosage, for intramuscular use

90694 Influenza virus vaccine, quadrivalent (aIIV4), inactivated, adjuvanted, preservative free, 0.5 mL dosage, for intramuscular use

90690 Typhoid vaccine, live, oral

90691 Typhoid vaccine, Vi capsular polysaccharide (ViCPs), for intramuscular use

90694 This code is out of order. See page 871

90696 Diphtheria, tetanus toxoids, acellular pertussis vaccine and inactivated poliovirus vaccine (DTaP-IPV), when administered to children 4 through 6 years of age, for intramuscular use

90697 Diphtheria, tetanus toxoids, acellular pertussis vaccine, inactivated poliovirus vaccine, Haemophilus influenzae type b PRP-OMP conjugate vaccine, and hepatitis B vaccine (DTaP-IPV-Hib-HepB), for intramuscular use

90698 Diphtheria, tetanus toxoids, acellular pertussis vaccine, Haemophilus influenza type b, and inactivated poliovirus vaccine (DTaP-IPV/Hib), for intramuscular use

90700 Diphtheria, tetanus toxoids, and acellular pertussis vaccine (DTaP), when administered to individuals younger than 7 years, for intramuscular use

90702 Diphtheria and tetanus toxoids adsorbed (DT), when administered to individuals younger than 7 years, for intramuscular use

90707 Measles, mumps and rubella virus vaccine (MMR), live, for subcutaneous use

90710 Measles, mumps, rubella, and varicella vaccine (MMRV), live, for subcutaneous use

90713 Poliovirus vaccine, inactivated, (IPV), for subcutaneous or intramuscular use

90714 Tetanus and diphtheria toxoids adsorbed (Td), preservative free, when administered to individuals 7 years or older, for intramuscular use

90715 Tetanus, diphtheria toxoids and acellular pertussis vaccine (Tdap), when administered to individuals 7 years or older, for intramuscular use

90716 Varicella virus vaccine (VAR), live, for subcutaneous use

90717 Yellow fever vaccine, live, for subcutaneous use

90723 Diphtheria, tetanus toxoids, acellular pertussis vaccine, hepatitis B, and inactivated poliovirus vaccine (DTaP-HepB-IPV), for intramuscular use

90625 Cholera vaccine, live, adult dosage, 1 dose schedule, for oral use

90732 Pneumococcal polysaccharide vaccine, 23-valent (PPSV23), adult or immunosuppressed patient dosage, when administered to individuals 2 years or older, for subcutaneous or intramuscular use

90644 Meningococcal conjugate vaccine, serogroups C & Y and Haemophilus influenzae type b vaccine (Hib-MenCY), 4 dose schedule, when administered to children 6 weeks-18 months of age, for intramuscular use

90733 Meningococcal polysaccharide vaccine, serogroups A, C, Y, W-135, quadrivalent (MPSV4), for subcutaneous use

90734 Meningococcal conjugate vaccine, serogroups A, C, W, Y, quadrivalent, diphtheria toxoid carrier (MenACWY-D) or CRM197 carrier (MenACWY-CRM), for intramuscular use

90619 Meningococcal conjugate vaccine, serogroups A, C, W, Y, quadrivalent, tetanus toxoid carrier (MenACWY-TT), for intramuscular use

90620 Meningococcal recombinant protein and outer membrane vesicle vaccine, serogroup B (MenB-4C), 2 dose schedule, for intramuscular use

90621 Meningococcal recombinant lipoprotein vaccine, serogroup B (MenB-FHbp), 2 or 3 dose schedule, for intramuscular use

90736 Zoster (shingles) vaccine (HZV), live, for subcutaneous injection

90750 Zoster (shingles) vaccine (HZV), recombinant, subunit, adjuvanted, for intramuscular use

90738 Japanese encephalitis virus vaccine, inactivated, for intramuscular use

90739 Hepatitis B vaccine (HepB), adult dosage, 2 dose schedule, for intramuscular use

90740 Hepatitis B vaccine (HepB), dialysis or immunosuppressed patient dosage, 3 dose schedule, for intramuscular use

90743 Hepatitis B vaccine (HepB), adolescent, 2 dose schedule, for intramuscular use

90744 Hepatitis B vaccine (HepB), pediatric/adolescent dosage, 3 dose schedule, for intramuscular use

● New Code ▲ Revised Code ✛ Add-On Code ⃠ Modifier -51 Exempt ★ Telemedicine

90746 Hepatitis B vaccine (HepB), adult dosage, 3 dose schedule, for intramuscular use

90747 Hepatitis B vaccine (HepB), dialysis or immunosuppressed patient dosage, 4 dose schedule, for intramuscular use

90748 Hepatitis B and Haemophilus influenza type b vaccine (Hib-HepB), for intramuscular use

90749 Unlisted vaccine/toxoid

90750 This code is out of order. See page 872

90756 This code is out of order. See page 870

PSYCHIATRY

Psychiatry services include diagnostic services, psychotherapy, and other services to an individual, family, or group. Patient condition, characteristics, or situational factors may require services described as being with interactive complexity. Services may be provided to a patient in crisis. Services are provided in all settings of care and psychiatry services codes are reported without regard to setting. Services may be provided by a physician or other qualified health care professional. Some psychiatry services may be reported with evaluation and management services (99202-99255, 99281-99285, 99304-99337, 99341-99350) or other services when performed. Evaluation and management services (99202-99285, 99304-99337, 99341-99350) may be reported for treatment of psychiatric conditions, rather than using psychiatry services codes, when appropriate.

Hospital care in treating a psychiatric inpatient or partial hospitalization may be initial or subsequent in nature (see 99221-99233).

Some patients receive hospital evaluation and management services only and others receive evaluation and management services and other procedures. If other procedures such as electroconvulsive therapy or psychotherapy are rendered in addition to hospital evaluation and management services, these should be listed separately (ie., hospital care services [99221-99223, 99231-99233] plus electroconvulsive therapy [90870] or when psychotherapy is done, with appropriate code(s) defining psychotherapy services.

Consultation for psychiatric evaluation of a patient includes examination of a patient and exchange of information with the primary physician and other informants, such as nurses or family members, and preparation of a report. These services may be reported usin consultation codes.

> (Do not report 90785-90899 in conjunction with 90839, 90840, 97151, 97152, 97153, 97154, 97155, 97156, 97157, 97158, 0362T, 0373T)

INTERACTIVE COMPLEXITY

Code 90785 is an add-on code for interactive complexity to be reported in conjunction with codes for diagnostic psychiatric evaluation (90791, 90792), psychotherapy (90832, 90834, 90837), psychotherapy when performed with an evaluation and management service (90833, 90836, 90838, 99202-99255, 99304-99337, 99341-99350), and group psychotherapy (90853).

Interactive complexity refers to specific communication factors that complicate the delivery of a psychiatric procedure. Common factors include more difficult communication with discordant or emotional family members and engagement of young and verbally undeveloped or impaired patients. Typical patients are those who have third parties, such as parents, guardians, other family members, interpreters, language translators, agencies, court officers, or schools involved in their psychiatric care.

Psychiatric procedures may be reported "with interactive complexity" when at least one of the following is present:

1. The need to manage maladaptive communication (related to, eg, high anxiety, high reactivity, repeated questions, or disagreement) among participants that complicates delivery of care.

2. Caregiver emotions or behavior that interferes with the caregiver's understanding and ability to assist in the implementation of the treatment plan.

3. Evidence or disclosure of a sentinel event and mandated report to third party (eg, abuse or neglect with report to state agency) with initiation of discussion of the sentinel event and/or report with patient and other visit participants.

4. Use of play equipment, other physical devices, interpreter or translator to communicate with the patient to overcome barriers to therapeutic or diagnostic interaction between the physician or other qualified health care professional and a patient who:

* is not fluent in the same language as the physician or other qualified health care professional, or

* has not developed or has lost either the expressive language communication skills to explain his/her symptoms and response to treatment, or the receptive communication skills to understand the physician or other qualified health care professional if he/she were to use typical language for communication.

When provided in conjunction with the psychotherapy services (90832-90838), the amount of time spent by a physician or other qualified health care professional providing interactive complexity services should be reflected in the timed service code for psychotherapy (90832, 90834, 90837) or the psychotherapy add-on code performed with an evaluation and management service (90833, 90836, 90838) and must relate to the psychotherapy service only. Interactive complexity is not a factor for evaluation and management services selection (99202-99255, 99281-99285, 99304-99337, 99341-99350), except as it directly affects key components as defined in the Evaluation and Management Services Guidelines (ie, history, examination, and medical decision making).

+ 90785 Interactive complexity (List separately in addition to the code for primary procedure)

> (Use 90785 in conjunction with codes for diagnostic psychiatric evaluation [90791, 90792], psychotherapy [90832, 90834, 90837], psychotherapy when performed with an evaluation and management service [90833, 90836, 90838, 99202-99255, 99304-99337, 99341-99350], and group psychotherapy [90853])

> (Do not report 90785 in conjunction with 90839, 90840, 0364T, 0365T, 0366T, 0367T, 0373T, 0374T)

> (Do not report 90785 in conjunction with 90839, 90840, 97151, 97152, 97153, 97154, 97155, 97156, 97157, 97158, 0362T, 0373T)

PSYCHIATRIC DIAGNOSTIC PROCEDURES

Psychiatric diagnostic evaluation is an integrated biopsychosocial assessment, including history, mental status and recommendations. The evaluation may include communication with family or other sources and review and ordering of diagnostic services.

Psychiatric diagnostic evaluation with medical services is an integrated biopsychosocial and medical assessment, including history, mental status, other physical examination elements as indicated, and recommendations. The evaluation may include communication with family or other sources, prescription of medications, and review and ordering of laboratory or other diagnostic studies.

In certain circumstances one or more other informants (family members, guardians, or significant others) may be seen in lieu of the patient. Codes 90791, 90792 may be reported more than once for the patient when separate diagnostic evaluations are conducted with the patient and other informants. Report services as being provided to the patient and not the informant or other party in such circumstances. Codes 90791, 90792 may be reported once per day and not on the same day as an evaluation and management service performed by the same individual for the same patient.

The psychiatric diagnostic evaluation may include interactive complexity services when factors exist that complicate the delivery of the psychiatric procedure. These services should be reported with add-on code 90785 used in conjunction with the diagnostic psychiatric evaluation codes 90791, 90792.

Codes 90791, 90792 are used for the diagnostic assessment(s) or reassessment(s) if required, and do not include psychotherapeutic services. Psychotherapy services, including for crisis, may not be reported on the same day.

> (Do not report 90791-90899 in conjunction with 90839, 90840, 97151, 97152, 97153, 97154, 97155, 97156, 97157, 97158, 0362T, 0373T)

★ 90791 Psychiatric diagnostic evaluation

★ 90792 Psychiatric diagnostic evaluation with medical services

> (Do not report 90791 or 90792 in conjunction with 99202-99337, 99341-99350, 99366-99368, 99401-99443, 97151, 97152, 97153, 97154, 97155, 97156, 97157, 97158, 0362T, 0373T)

> (Use 90785 in conjunction with 90791, 90792 when the diagnostic evaluation includes interactive complxity services)

PSYCHOTHERAPY

Psychotherapy is the treatment of menal illness and behavioral disturbances in which the physician or other qualified health care professional, through definitive therapeutic communication, attempts to alleviate the emotional disturbances, reverse or change maladaptive patterns of behavior, and encourage personality growth and development.

The psychotherapy service codes 90832-90838 include ongoing assessment and adjustment of psychotherapeutic interventions, and may include involvement of informants in the treatment process.

Codes 90832, 90833, 90834, 90836, 90837, 90838 describe psychotherapy for the individual patient, although times are for face-to-face services with patient and may include informant(s). The patient must be present for all or a majority of the service.

See codes 90846, 90847 when utilizing family psychotherapy techniques, such as focusing on family dynamics. Do not report 90846, 90847 for family psychotherapy services less than 26 minutes. Codes 90832, 90833, 90834, 90836, 90837, 90838 may be reported on the same day as codes 90846, 90847, when the services are separate and distinct.

In reporting, choose the code closest to the actual time (ie, 16-37 minutes for 90832 and 90833, 38-52 minutes for 90834 and 90836, and 53 or more minutes for 90837 and 90838). Do not report psychotherapy of less than 16 minutes duration. (See instructions for the usage of time in the Introduction of the CPT code set.)

Psychotherapy provided to a patient in a crisis state is reported with codes 90839 and 90840 and cannot be reported in addition to the psychotherapy codes 90832-90838. For psychotherapy for crisis, see "Other Psychotherapy."

Code 90785 is an add-on code to report interactive complexity services when provided in conjunction with the psychotherapy codes 90832-90838. For family psychotherapy, see 90846, 90847. The amount of time spent by a physician or other qualified health care professional providing interactive complexity services should be reflected in the timed service code for psychotherapy (90832, 90834, 90837) or the psychotherapy add-on code performed with an evaluation and management service (90833, 90836, 90838)

Some psychiatric patients receive a medical evaluation and management (E/M) service on the same day as the psychotherapy service by the same physician or other qualified health care professional. To report both E/M and psychotherapy, the two services must be significant and separately identifiable. These services are reported by using codes specific for psychotherapy when performed with evaluation and managment services (90833, 90836, 90838) as add-on codes to the evaluation and management service.

Medical symptoms and disorders inform treatment choices of psychotherapeutic interventions, and data from therapeutic communications are used to evaluate the presence, type, and severity of medical symptoms and disorders. For the purposes of reporting, the medical and psychotherapeutic components of the service may be separately identified as follows:

1. The type and level of E/M service is selected first based upon the key components of history, examination and medical decision making

2. Time associated with activities used to meet criteria for the E/M service is not included in the time used for reporting the psychotherapy service (ie, time spent on history, examination and medical decision making **when used for the E/M service** is not psychotherapy time). Time may not be used as the basis of E/M code selection and Prolonged Services may not be reported when psychotherapy with E/M (90833, 90836, 90838) are reported.

3. A separate diagnosis is not required for the reportin of E/M and psychotherapy on the same date of service.

★ **90832** Psychotherapy, 30 minutes with patient

★+**90833** Psychotherapy, 30 minutes with patient when performed with an evaluation and management service (List separately in addition to the code for primary procedure)

    (Use 90833 in conjunction with 99202-99255, 99304- 99337, 99341-99350)

★ **90834** Psychotherapy, 45 minutes with patient

★+**90836** Psychotherapy, 45 minutes with patient when performed with an evaluation and management service (List separately in addition to the code for primary procedure)

    (Use 90836 in conjunction with 99202-99255, 99304- 99337, 99341-99350)

    Separate Procedure   Unlisted Procedure   CCI Comp. Code   Non-specific Procedure   **875**

★ **90837**   Psychotherapy, 60 minutes with patient

> (Use the appropriate prolonged service code [99354, 99355, 99356, 99357] for psychotherapy services not performed with an E/M service of 90 minutes or longer face-to-face with the patient)

★+**90838**   Psychotherapy, 60 minutes with patientn when performed with an evaluation and management service (List separately in addition to the code for primary procedure)

> (Use 90838 in conjunction with 99202-99255, 99304- 99337, 99341-99350)

> (Use 90785 in conjunction with 90832, 90833, 90834, 90836, 90837, 90838 when psychotherapy includes interactive complexity services)

PSYCHOTHERAPY FOR CRISIS

Psychotherapy for crisis is an urgent assessment and history of a crisis state, a mental status exam, and a disposition. The treatment includes psychotherapy, mobilization of resources to defuse the crisis and restore safety, and implementation of psychotherapeutic interventions to minimize the potential for psychological trauma. The presenting problem is typically life threatening or complex and requires immediate attention to a patient in high distress.

Codes 90839, 90840 are used to report the total duration of time face-to-face with the patient and/or family spent by the physician or other qualified health care professional providing psychotherapy for crisis, even if the time spent on that date is not continuous. For any given period of time spent providing psychotherapy for crisis state, the physician or other qualified health care professional must devote his or her full attention to the patient and, therefore, cannot provide services to any other patients during the same time period. The patient must be present for all or some of the service. Do not report with 90791 or 90792.

Code 90839 is used to report the first 30-74 minutes of psychotherapy for crisis on a given date. It should be used only once per date if the time spent by the physician or other qualified health care professional is not continuous on that date. Psychotherapy for crisis of less than 30 minutes total duration on a given date should be reported with 90832 or 90833 (when provided with evaluation and management services). Code 90840 is used to report additional block(s) of time, up to 30 minutes each beyond the first 74 minutes.

90839   Psychotherapy for crisis; first 60 minutes

+ **90840**   each additional 30 minutes (List separately in addition to code for primary service)

> (Use 90840 in conjunction with 90839)

> (Do not report 90839, 90840 in conjunction with 90791, 90792, psychotherapy codes 90832-90838 or other psychiatric services, or 90785-90899)

OTHER PSYCHOTHERAPY

★ **90845**   Psychoanalysis

★ **90846**   Family psychotherapy (without the patient present), 50 minutes

★ **90847**   Family psychotherapy (conjoint psychotherapy) (with patient present), 50 minutes

> (Do not report 90846, 90847 for family psychotherapy services less than 26 minutes)

> (Do not report 90846, 90847 in conjunction with 97151, 97152, 97153, 97154, 97155, 97156, 97157, 97158, 0362T, 0373T)

> (For family psychotherapy services (90847) of 80 minutes or more, see the appropriate prolonged services code (99354, 99355, 99356, 99357))

90849   Multiple-family group psychotherapy

90853   Group psychotherapy (other than of a multiple-family group)

> (Use 90853 in conjunction with 90785 for the specified patient when group psychotherapy includes interactive complexity)

(Do not report 90853 in conjunction with 97151, 97152, 97153, 97154, 97155, 97156, 97157, 97158, 0362T, 0373T)

OTHER PSYCHIATRIC SERVICES OR PROCEDURES

(For electronic analysis with programming, when performed, of vagal nerve neurostimulators, see 95970, 95976, 95977)

★+90863   Pharmacologic management, including prescription and review of medication, when performed with psythotherapy services (List separately in addition to the code for primary procedure)

(Use 90863 in conjunction with 90832, 90834, 90837)

(For pharmacologic management with psychotherapy services performed by a physician or other qualified health care professional who may report evaluation and management codes, use the appropriate evaluation and management codes 99202-99255, 99281-99285, 99304-99337, 99341-99350 and the appropriate psychotherapy with evaluation and management service 90833, 90836, 90838)

(Do not count time spent on providing pharmacologic management services in the time used for selection of the psychotherapy service)

90865   Narcosynthesis for psychiatric diagnostic and therapeutic purposes (eg, sodium amobarbital (Amytal) interview)

90867   Therapeutic repetitive transcranial magnetic stimulation (TMS) treatment; initial, including cortical mapping, motor threshold determination, delivery and management

(Report only once per course of treatment)

(Do not report 90867 in conjunction with 90868, 90869, 95860-95870, 95928, 95929, 95939)

90868   subsequent delivery and management, per session

90869   subsequent motor threshold re-determination with delivery and management

(Do not report 90869 in conjunction with 90867, 90868, 95860-95870, 95928, 95929, 95939)

(If a significant, separately identifiableevaluation and management, medication management, or psychotherapy service is performed, the appropriate E/M or psychotherapy code may be reported in addition to 90867-90869. Evaluation and management activities directly related to cortical mapping, motor threshold determination, delivery and management of TMS are not separately reported)

90870   Electroconvulsive therapy (includes necessary monitoring)

90875   Individual psychophysiological therapy incorporating biofeedback training by any modality (face-to-face with the patient), with psychotherapy (eg, insight oriented, behavior modifying or supportive psychotherapy); 30 minutes

90876   45 minutes

90880   Hypnotherapy

90882   Environmental intervention for medical management purposes on a psychiatric patients behalf with agencies, employers, or institutions

90885   Psychiatric evaluation of hospital records, other psychiatric reports, psychometric and/or projective tests, and other accumulated data for medical diagnostic purposes

90887   Interpretation or explanation of results of psychiatric, other medical examinations and procedures, or other accumulated data to family or other responsible persons, or advising them how to assist patient

(Do not report 90887 in conjunction with 97151, 97152, 97153, 97154, 97155, 97156, 97157, 97158, 0362T, 0373T)

Separate Procedure   Unlisted Procedure   CCI Comp. Code   Non-specific Procedure   **877**

90889   Preparation of report of patient's psychiatric status, history, treatment, or progress (other than for legal or consultative purposes) for other individuals, agencies, or insurance carriers

90899   Unlisted psychiatric service or procedure

BIOFEEDBACK

Biofeedback is the process of detecting information about a patient's biological functions, eg. heart rate, breathing rate, skin temperature, and amount of muscle tension, picked up by surface electrodes (sensors) and electronically amplified to provide feedback, usually in the form of an audio-tone and/or visual read-out to the patient. Biofeedback training uses the information that has been monitored from the sensors attached to a muscle on the skin's surface, or to the skin only for thermal or other readings. With the help of a trained clinician, the patient can learn how to make voluntary changes in those biological functions and bring them under control.

Biofeedback services involve the use of electromyographic techniques to detect and record muscle activity. The CPT codes 95860-95872 (EMG) should not be reported with biofeedback services based on the use of electromyography during a biofeedback session. If an EMG is performed as a separate medically necessary service for diagnosis or follow-up of organic muscle dysfunction, the appropriate EMG codes (e.g. CPT codes 95860-95872) may be reported.

Modifier -59 should be added to indicate that the service performed was a separately identifiable diagnostic service. Reporting only an objective electromyographic response to biofeedback is not sufficient to bill the codes referable to diagnostic EMG.

(For psychophysiological therapy incorporating biofeedback training, see 90875, 90876)

90901   Biofeedback training by any modality

(90911   deleted 2019 [2020 Edition]. To report, see 90912, 90913)

90912   Biofeedback training, perineal muscles, anorectal or urethral sphincter, including EMG and/or mamometry, when performed; initial 15 minutes of one-on-one physician or other qualified health care professional contact with the patient

+ 90913   each additional 15 minutes of one-on-one physician or other qualified health care professional contact with the patient (List separately in addition to to code for primary procedure)

(Use 90913 in conjunction with 90912)

(For testing of rectal sensation, tone and compliance, use 91120)

(For incontinence treatment by pulsed magnetic neuromodulation, use 53899)

DIALYSIS

(For therapeutic apheresis for white blood cells, red blood cells, platelets and plasma pheresis, see 36511, 36512, 36513, 36514)

(For therapeutic apheresis extracorporeal adsorption procedures, use 36516)

(90918   deleted 2009 edition. To report ESRD-related services for patients younger than 2 years of age, see 90951-90953, 90963, 90967)

(90919   deleted 2009 edition. To report ESRD-related services for patients between 2 and 11 years of age, see 90954-90956, 90964, 90968)

(90920   deleted 2009 edition. To report ESRD-related services for patients between 12 and 19 years of age, see 90957-90959, 90965, 90969)

(90921   deleted 2009 edition. To report ESRD-related services for patients 20 years of age and older, see 90960-90962, 90966, 90970)

(90922   deleted 2009 edition. To report ESRD-related services for patients younger than 2 years of age, see 90951-90953, 90963, 90967)

(**90923**   deleted 2009 edition. To report ESRD-related services for patients between 2 and 11 years of age, see 90954-90956, 90964, 90968)

(**90924**   deleted 2009 edition. To report ESRD-related services for patients between 12 and 19 years of age, see 90957-90959, 90965, 90969)

(**90925**   deleted 2009 edition. To report ESRD-related services for patients 20 years of age and older, see 90960-90962, 90966, 90970)

HEMODIALYSIS

Codes 90935, 90937 are reported to describe the hemodialysis procedure with all evaluation and management services related to the patient's renal disease on the day of the hemodialysis procedure. These codes are used for inpatient end-stage renal disease (ESRD) and non-ESRD procedures or for outpatient non-ESRD dialysis services. Code 90935 is reported if only one evaluation of the patient is required related to that hemodialysis procedure. Code 90937 is reported when patient re-evaluation(s) is required during a hemodialysis procedure. Use modifier 25 with evaluation and management codes including new or established patient office or other outpatient services (99202-99215), office or other outpatient consultations (99241-99245), observation care (99217-99220, 99224-99226), observation or inpatient care including admission and discharge (99234-99236), initial hospital care (99221-99226, 99231-99239), new or established patient emergency department services (99281-99285), critical care services (99291, 99292), inpatient neonatal intensive care services and pediatric and neonatal critical care services (99466-99480), nursing facility services (99304-99318), domiciliary, rest home services, or custodial care (99324-99337), and home services (99341-99350), for separately identifiable services unrelated to the dialysis procedure or renal failure which cannot be rendered during the dialysis session.

> (For home visit hemodialysis services performed by a non-physician health care professional, use 99512)
>
> (For cannula declotting, see 36831, 36833, 36860, 36861)
>
> (For declotting of implanted vascular access device or catheter by thrombolytic agent, use 36593)
>
> (For collection of blood specimen from a partially or completely implantable venous access device, use 36591)
>
> (For prolonged attendance by a physician or other qualified health care professional, see 99354-99360)

90935   Hemodialysis procedure with single evaluation by a physician or other qualified health care professional

90937   Hemodialysis procedure requiring repeated evaluation(s) with or without substantial revision of dialysis prescription

90940   Hemodialysis access flow study to determine blood flow in grafts and arteriovenous fistulae by an indicator method

> (For duplex scan of hemodialysis access, use 93990)

MISCELLANEOUS DIALYSIS PROCEDURES

Codes 90945, 90947 describe dialysis procedures other than hemodialysis (eg, peritoneal dialysis, hemofiltration or continuous renal replacement therapies), and all evaluation and management services related to the patient's renal disease on the day of the procedure. Code 90945 is reported if only one evaluation of the patient is required related to that procedure. Code 90947 is reported when patient re-evaluation(s) is required during a procedure. Use modifier 25 with evaluation and management codes including office or other outpatient services (99202-99215), office or other outpatient consultations (99241-99245), observation care (99217-99220, 99224-99226), observation or inpatient care including admission and discharge (99234-99239), hospital care (99221-99226, 99231-99239), new or established patient emergency department services (99281-99285), critical care services (99291, 99292), inpatient neonatal intensive care services and pediatric and neonatal critical care services (99466-99480), nursing facility services (99304-99318), domiciliary, rest home, or custodial care services (99324-99337), and home services (99341-99350) for separately identifiable services unrelated to the procedure or the renal failure which cannot be rendered during the dialysis session.

> (For percutaneous insertion of intraperitoneal tunneled catheter, use 49418. For open insertion of tunneled intraperitoneal catheter, use 49421.)
>
> (For prolonged attendance by a physician or other qualified heatlh care professional, see 99354-99360)

90945 Dialysis procedure other than hemodialysis (eg, peritoneal dialysis, hemofiltration or other continuous renal replacement therapies), with single evaluation by a physician or other qualified health care professional

(For home infusion of peritoneal dialysis, use 99559)

90947 Dialysis procedure other than hemodialysis (eg, peritoneal dialysis, hemofiltration, or other continuous renal replacement therapies) requiring repeated evaluation by a physician or other qualified health care professional, with or without substantial revision of dialysis prescription

END-STAGE RENAL DISEASE SERVICES

Codes 90951-90962 are reported **once** per month to distinguish age-specific services related to the patient's end-stage renal disease (ESRD) performed in an outpatient setting with three levels of service based on the number of face-to-face visits. ESRD-related services by a physician or other qualified health care professional include establishment of a dialyzing cycle, outpatient evaluation and management of the dialysis visits, telephone calls, and patient management during the dialysis provided during a full month. In circumstances in which the patient has had a complete assessment visit during the month and services are provided over a period of less than a month, 90951-90962 may be used according to the number of visits performed.

Codes 90963-90966 are reported once per month for a full month of service to distinguish age-specific services for end-stage renal disease (ESRD) services for home dialysis patients.

For ESRD and non-ESRD dialysis services performed in an inpatient setting, and for non-ESRD dialysis services performed in an outpatient setting, see 90935-90937 and 90945-90947.

Evaluation and Management services unrelated to ESRD services that cannot be performed during the dialysis session may be reported separately.

Codes 90967-90970 are reported to distinguish age-specific services for end-stage renal disease (ESRD) services for less than a full month of service, per day, for services provided under the following circumstances: transient patients, partial month where there was one or more face-to-face visits without the complete assessment, the patient was hospitalized before a complete assessment was furnished, dialysis was stopped due to recovery or death, or the patient received a kidney transplant. For reporting purposes, each month is considered 30 days.

(Do not report 90951-90970 during the same month in conjunction with 99439, 99487, 99489, 99490, 99491)

★ **90951** End-stage renal disease (ESRD) related services monthly, for patients younger than 2 years of age to include monitoring for the adequacy of nutrition, assessment of growth and development, and counseling of parents; with 4 or more face-to-face visits by a physician or other qualified health care professional, per month

★ **90952** with 2-3 face-to-face visits by a physician or other qualified health care professional, per month

90953 with 1 face-to-face visit by a physician or other qualified health care professional per month

★ **90954** End-stage renal disease (ESRD) related services monthly, for patients 2-11 years of age to include monitoring for the adequacy of nutrition, assessment of growth and development, and counseling of parents; with 4 or more face-to-face visits by a physician or other qualified health care professional per month

★ **90955** with 2-3 face-to-face visits by a physician or other qualified health care professional per month

90956 with 1 face-to-face visits by a physician or other qualified health care professional per month

★ **90957** End-stage renal disease (ESRD) related services monthly, for patients 12-19 years of age to include monitoring for the adequacy of nutrition, assessment of growth and development, and counseling of parents; with 4 or more face-to-face visits by a physician or other qualified health care professional per month

★ **90958** with 2-3 face-to-face visits by a physician or other qualified health care professional per month

90959 with 1 face-to-face visit by a physician or other qualified health care professional per month

● New Code ▲ Revised Code ✛ Add-On Code ⊘ Modifier -51 Exempt ★ Telemedicine

★ **90960** End-stage renal disease (ESRD) related services monthly, for patients 20 years of age and older; with 4 or more face-to-face visits by a physician or other qualified health care professional per month

★ **90961** with 2-3 face-to-face visits by a physician or other qualified health care professional per month

90962 with 1 face-to-face visit by a physician or other qualified health care professional per month

90963 End-stage renal disease (ESRD) related services for home dialysis per full month, for patients younger than 2 years of age to include monitoring for the adequacy of nutrition, assessment of growth and development, and counseling of parents

90964 End-stage renal disease (ESRD) related services for home dialysis per full month, for patients 2-11 years of age to include monitoring for the adequacy of nutrition, assessment of growth and development, and counseling of parents

90965 End-stage renal disease (ESRD) related services for home dialysis per full month, for patients 12-19 years of age to include monitoring for the adequacy of nutrition, assessment of growth and development, and counseling of parents

90966 End-stage renal disease (ESRD) related services for home dialysis per full month, for patients 20 years of age and older

90967 End-stage renal disease (ESRD) related services for dialysis less than a full month of service, per day; for patients younger than 2 years of age

90968 for patients 2-11 years of age

90969 for patients 12-19 years of age

90970 for patients 20 years of age and older

OTHER DIALYSIS PROCEDURES

90989 Dialysis training, patient, including helper where applicable, any mode, completed course

90993 Dialysis training, patient, including helper where applicable, any mode, course not completed, per training session

90997 Hemoperfusion (eg, with activated charcoal or resin)

90999 Unlisted dialysis procedure, inpatient or outpatient

GASTROENTEROLOGY

91010 Esophageal motility (manometric study of the esophagus and/or gastroesophageal junction) study with interpretation and report;

+ **91013** with stimulation or perfusion (eg, stimulant, acid or alkali perfusion) (List separately in addition to code for primary procedure)

(Use 91013 in conjunction with 91010)

(Do not report 91013 more than once per session)

(To report esophageal motility studies with high resolution esophageal pressure topography, use 91299)

91020 Gastric motility (manometric) studies

91022 Duodenal motility (manometric) study

(If gastrointestinal endoscopy is performed, use 43235)

Separate Procedure   Unlisted Procedure   CCI Comp. Code   Non-specific Procedure   **881**

(If fluoroscopy is performed, use 76000)

(If gastric motility study is performed, use 91020)

(Do not report 91020, 91022 in conjunction with 91112)

91030 Esophagus, acid perfusion (Bernstein) test for esophagitis

91034 Esophagus, gastroesophageal reflux test; with nasal catheter pH electrode(s) placement, recording, analysis and interpretation

91035 with mucosal attached telemetry pH electrode placement, recording, analysis and interpretation

91037 Esophageal function test, gastroesophageal reflux test with nasal catheter intraluminal impedance electrode(s) placement, recording, analysis and interpretation;

91038 prolonged (greater than 1 hour, up to 24 hours)

91040 Esophageal balloon distension provocation study, diagnostic, with provocation when performed

(Do not report 91040 more than once per session)

91065 Breath hydrogen or methane test (eg, for detection of lactase deficiency, fructose intolerance, bacterial overgrowth, or oro-cecal gastrointestinal transit)

(Report 91065 once for each administered challenge)

(For H. pylori breath test analysis, use 83013 for non-radioactive (C-13) isotope or 78268 for radioactive (C-14) isotope)

(To report placement of an esophageal tamponade tube for management of variceal bleeding, use 43460. To report placement of a long intestinal Miller-Abbott tube, use 44500)

(For abdominal paracentesis, see 49082, 49083, 49084; with instillation of medication, see 96440, 96446)

(For peritoneoscopy, use 49320; with biopsy, use 49321)

(For splenoportography, see 38200, 75810)

91110 Gastrointestinal tract imaging, intraluminal (eg, capsule endoscopy), esophagus through ileum, with interpretation and report

(Do not report 91110 in conjunction with 91111, 0355T)

(Visualization of the colon is not reported separately)

(Append modifier -52 if the ileum is not visualized)

91111 Gastrointestinal tract imaging, intraluminal (eg, capsule endoscopy), esophagus with interpretation and report

(Do not report 91111 in conjunction with 91110, 0355T)

(For measurement of gastrointestinal tract transit times or pressure using wireless capsule, use 91112)

91112 Gastrointestinal transit and pressure measurement, stomach through colon, wireless capsule, with interpretation and report

(Do not report 91112 in conjunction with 83986, 91020, 91022, 91117)

91117 Colon motility (manometric) study, minimum 6 hours continuous recording (including provocation tests, eg, meal, intracolonic balloon distension, pharmacologic agents, if performed), with interpretation and report

(For wireless capsule pressure measurements, use 91112)

(Do not report 91117 in conjunction with 91120, 91122)

● New Code   ▲ Revised Code   + Add-On Code   ⊘ Modifier -51 Exempt   ★ Telemedicine

91120 Rectal sensation, tone, and compliance test (ie, response to graded balloon distention)

(For biofeedback training, see 90912, 90913)

(For anorectal manometry, use 91122)

91122 Anorectal manometry

(Do not report 91120, 91122 in conjunction with 91117)

GASTRIC PHYSIOLOGY

91132 Electrogastrography, diagnostic, transcutaneous;

91133   with provocative testing

OTHER PROCEDURES

91200 Liver elastography, mechanically induced shear wave (eg, vibration), without imaging, with interpretation and report

(Do not report 91200 in conjunction with 76981, 76982, 76983)

91299 Unlisted diagnostic gastroenterology procedure

OPHTHALMOLOGY

(For surgical procedures, see Surgery, Eye and Ocular Adnexa, 65091 et seq)

Ophthalmology is the study and treatment of diseases of the eye. Ophthalmological diagnostic and treatment services are reported using CPT Medicine codes 92002-92499.

Coding Rules

1. *Minimal, brief and limited office services, and hospital, home, extended care, emergency department and consultations are reported using appropriate evaluation and management service codes.*

2. *Surgical procedures on the eye(s) are reported using CPT codes from the Eye and Ocular Adnexa subsection of the SURGERY section of CPT.*

3. *To report intermediate ophthalmological services, the following must be performed and documented: a) evaluation of new or existing condition, b) complications of new diagnostic or management problems (not necessarily related to the primary diagnosis), c) history, d) general medical observation e) external ocular and adnexal examination, f) other diagnostic procedures as indicated, and g) may include the use of mydriasis. Intermediate ophthalmological services do not usually include determination of refractive state but may in an established patient under continuing active treatment.*

4. *To report comprehensive ophthalmological services the following must be performed and documented: a) reported as a single service but may be performed at more than one session, b) history, c) general medical observation, d) external and ophthalmoscopic examination, e) gross visual fields, f) basic sensorimotor examination, g. may include, as indicated; biomicroscopy, examination with cycloplegia or mydriasis and tonometry, h) always includes initiation of diagnostic and treatment programs.*

5. *For both intermediate and comprehensive ophthalmological services, service components, such as slip lamp examination, keratomy, ophthalmoscopy, retinoscopy, tonometry and motor evaluation are not reported separately.*

For procedures requiring intravenous injection of dye or other diagnostic agent, insertion of an intravenous catheter and dye injection are necessary to accomplish the procedure and are included in the procedure. Accordingly, HCPCS/CPT codes 36000 (introduction of a needle or catheter), 36410 (venipuncture), G0345-G0350 (90760-90768 in 2006)(IV infusion), and G0353-G0354 (90774-90775 in 2006)(IV injection)as well as selective vascular catheterization codes are not to be separately reported with services requiring intravenous injection (e.g. CPT codes 92230, 92235, 92240, 92287, for angioscopy and angiography).

Fundus photography (CPT code 92250) and scanning ophthalmic computerized diagnostic imaging (CPT code 92135) are generally mutually exclusive of one another in that a provider would use one technique or the other to evaluate fundal disease. However, there are a limited number of clinical conditions where both techniques are medically reasonable and necessary on the ipsilateral eye. In these situations, both CPT codes may be reported appending modifier -59 to CPT code 92250.

GENERAL OPHTHALMOLOGICAL SERVICES

General ophthalmological services (e.g. CPT codes 92002-92014) describe components of the ophthalmologic examination. When evaluation and management codes are reported, these general ophthalmological service codes (e.g. CPT codes 92002-92014) are not to be reported; the same services would be represented by both series of codes.

NEW PATIENT

(For distinguishing between new and established patients, see E/M guidelines)

92002   Ophthalmological services: medical examination and evaluation with initiation of diagnostic and treatment program; intermediate, new patient

(Do not report 92002 in conjunction with 99173, 99174, 99177, 0469T)

92004   comprehensive, new patient, 1 or more visits

(Do not report 92004 in conjunction with 99173, 99174, 99177, 0469T)

ESTABLISHED PATIENT

(For distinguishing between new and established patients, see E/M guidelines)

92012   Ophthalmological services: medical examination and evaluation, with initiation or continuation of diagnostic and treatment program; intermediate, established patient

(Do not report 92012 in conjunction with 99173, 99174, 99177, 0469T)

92014   comprehensive, established patient, 1 or more visits

(Do not report 92014 in conjunction with 99173, 99174, 99177, 0469T)

(For surgical procedures, see Surgery, Eye and Ocular Adnexa, 65091 et seq)

SPECIAL OPHTHALMOLOGICAL SERVICES

Special ophthalmological services are defined as a level of service in which a special evaluation of part of the visual system is made which goes beyond the services usually included under general ophthalmological services, or in which special treatment is given. Fluorescein angioscopy, quantitative visual field examination, or extended color vision examination should be specifically reported as special ophthalmological services.

Special ophthalmologic services represent specific services not described as part of a general or routine ophthalmological examination. Special ophthalmological services are recognized as significant, separately identifiable services.

92015   Determination of refractive state

(Do not report 92015 in conjunction with 99173, 99174, 99177)

(For instrument-based ocular screening, use 99174, 99177)

92018   Ophthalmological examination and evaluation, under general anesthesia, with or without manipulation of globe for passive range of motion or other manipulation to facilitate diagnostic examination; complete

92019   limited

92020   Gonioscopy (separate procedure)

(Do not report 92020 in conjunction with 0621T, 0622T)

(For gonioscopy under general anesthesia, use 92018)

● New Code   ▲ Revised Code   ✚ Add-On Code   ⊘ Modifier -51 Exempt   ★ Telemedicine

92025 Computerized corneal topography, unilateral or bilateral, with interpretation and report

(Do not report 92025 in conjunction with 65710-65771)

(92025 is not used for manual keratoscopy, which is part of a single system of E/M or ophthalmological service)

92060 Sensorimotor examination with multiple measurements of ocular deviation (eg, restrictive or paretic muscle with diplopia) with interpretation and report (separate procedure)

92065 Orthoptic and/or pleoptic training, with continuing medical direction and evaluation

92071 Fitting of contact lens for treatment of ocular surface disease

(Do not report 92071 in conjunction with 92072)

(Report supply of lens separately with 99070 or appropriate supply codes)

92072 Fitting of contact lens for management of keratoconus, initial fitting

(For subsequent fittings, report using E/M services or General Ophthalmological services)

(Do not report 92072 in conjunction with 92071)

(Report supply of lens separately with 99070 or appropriate supply code)

92081 Visual field examination, unilateral or bilateral, with interpretation and report; limited examination (eg, tangent screen, Autoplot, arc perimeter, or single stimulus level automated test, such as Octopus 3 or 7 equivalent)

92082 intermediate examination (eg, at least 2 isopters on Goldmann perimeter, or semiquantitative, automated suprathreshold screening program, Humphrey suprathreshold automatic diagnostic test, Octopus program 33)

92083 extended examination (eg, Goldmann visual fields with at least 3 isopters plotted and static determination within the central 30 degrees, or quantitative, automated threshold perimetry, Octopus programs G-1, 32 or 42, Humphrey visual field analyzer full threshold programs 30-2, 24-2, or 30/60-2)

(Gross visual field testing (eg, confrontation testing) is a part of general ophthalmological services and is not reported separately)

(For visual field assessment by patient activated data transmission to a remote surveillance center, see 0378T, 0379T)

92100 Serial tonometry (separate procedure) with multiple measurements of intraocular pressure over an extended time period with interpretation and report, same day (eg, diurnal curve or medical treatment of acute elevation of intraocular pressure)

(For monitoring of intraocular pressure for 24 hours or longer, use 0329T)

(Ocular blood flow measurements are reported with 0198T. Single-episode tonomemtry is a component of general ophthalmological service or E/M service)

92132 Scanning computerized ophthalmic diagnostic imaging, anterior segment, with interpretation and report, unilateral or bilateral

(For spectral microscopy and endothelial cell analysis, use 92286)

(For tear film imaging, use 0330T)

92133 Scanning computerized ophthalmic diagnostic imaging, posterior segment, with interpretation and report, unilateral or bilateral; optic nerve

92134 retina

(Do not report 92133 and 92134 at the same patient encounter)

(For scanning computerized ophthalmic diagnostic imaging of the optic nerve and retina, see 92133, 92134)

92136 Ophthalmic biometry by partial coherence interferometry with intraocular lens power calculation

(For tear film imaging, use 0330T)

92145 Corneal hysteresis determination, by air impulse stimulation, unilateral or bilateral, with interpretation and report

OPHTHALMOSCOPY

Routine ophthalmoscopy is part of general and special ophthalmologic services whenever indicated. It is a non-itemized service and is not reported separately.

92201 Ophthalmoscopy, extended; with retinal drawing and scleral depression of peripheral retinal disease (eg, for retinal tear, retinal detachment, retinal tumor) with interpretation and report, unilateral or bilateral

92202 with drawing of optic nerve or macula (eg, for glaucoma, macular pathology, tumor) with interpretation and report, unilateral or bilateral

(Do not report 92201, 92202 in conjunction with 92250)

(**92225** deleted 2019 [2020 Edition]. To report, see 99202, 99202)

(**92226** deleted 2019 [2020 Edition]. To report, see 99202, 99202)

▲★**92227** Imaging of retina for detection or monitoring of disease; with remote clinical staff review and report, unilateral or bilateral

(Do not report 92227 in conjunction with 92133, 92134, 92228, 92229, 92250)

▲★**92228** with remote physician or other qualified health care professional interpretation and report, unilateral or bilateral

(Do not report 92228 in conjunction with 92133, 92134, 92227, 92229, 92250)

● **92229** point-of-care automated analysis and report, unilateral or bilateral

(Do not report 92229 in conjunction with 92133, 92134, 92227, 92228, 92250)

92230 Fluorescein angioscopy with interpretation and report

92235 Fluorescein angiography (includes multiframe imaging) with interpretation and report, unilateral or bilateral

(When fluorescein and indocyanine-green angiography are performed at the same patient encounter, use 92242)

92240 Indocyanine-green angiography (includes multiframe imaging) with interpretation and report, unilateral or bilateral

(When indocyanine-green and fluorescein angiography are performed at the same patient encounter, use 92242)

92242 Fluorescein angiography and indocyanine-green angiography (includes multiframe imaging) performed at the same patient encounter with interpretation and report, unilateral or bilateral

(To report fluorescein angiography and indocyaninegreen angiography not performed at the same patient encounter, see 92235, 92240)

92250 Fundus photography with interpretation and report

● New Code ▲ Revised Code ✛ Add-On Code ⊘ Modifier -51 Exempt ★ Telemedicine

92260 Ophthalmodynamometry

(For opthalmoscopy under general anesthesia, use 92018)

OTHER SPECIALIZED SERVICES

For prescription, fitting, and/or medical supervision of ocular prosthetic (artificial eye) adaptation by a physician, see evaluation and management services including office or other outpatient services (99202-99215), office or other outpatient consultations (99241-99245), or general ophthalmological service codes 92002-92014.

Electroretinography (ERG) is used to evaluate function of the retina and optic nerve of the eye, including photoreceptors and ganglion cells. A number of techniques are used which target different areas of the eye, including full field (flash and flicker) (92273) for a global response of photoreceptors of the retina, multifocal (92274) for photoreceptors in multiple separate locations in the retina including the macula, and pattern (0509T) for retinal ganglion cells. Multiple additional terms and techniques are used to describe various types of ERG. If the technique used is not specifically named in the code descriptors for 92273, 92274, or 0509T, use the unlisted procedure code 92499.

92265 Needle oculoelectromyography, 1 or more extraocular muscles, one or both eyes, with interpretation and report

92270 Electro-oculography with interpretation and report

(For vestibular function tests with recording, see 92537, 92538, 92540, 92541, 92542, 92544, 92545, 92546, 92547, 92548)

(Do not report 92270 in conjunction with 92537, 92538, 92540, 92541, 92542, 92544, 92545, 92546, 92547, 92548, 92549)

(To report saccadic eye movement testing with recording, use 92700)

92273 Electroretinography (ERG), with interpretation and report; full field (ie, ffERG, flash ERG, Ganzfeld ERG)

92274 multifocal (mfERG)

(For pattern ERG, use 0509T)

(**92275** deleted 2018 [2019 Edition]. To report electroretinography, see 92273, 92274, 0509T)

(For electronystagmography for vestibular function studies, see 92541 et seq)

(For ophthalmic echography (diagnostic ultrasound), see 76511-76529)

92283 Color vision examination, extended, eg, anomaloscope or equivalent

(Color vision testing with pseudoisochromatic plates (such as HRR or Ishihara) is not reported separately. It is included in the appropriate general or ophthalmological service, or 99172)

92284 Dark adaptation examination with interpretation and report

92285 External ocular photography with interpretation and report for documentation of medical progress (eg, close-up photography, slit lamp photography, goniophotography, stereo-photography)

(For tear film imaging, use 0330T)

(For meibomian gland imaging, use 0507T)

92286 Anterior segment imaging with interpretation and report; with specular microscopy and endothelial cell analysis

92287 with fluorescein angiography

CONTACT LENS SERVICES

Follow-up of successfully fitted extended wear lenses is reported as part of a general ophthalmological service (92012 et seq).

The supply of contact lenses may be reported as part of the service of fitting. It may also be reported separately by using the appropriate supply codes.

> (For therapeutic or surgical use of contact lens, see 68340, 92071, 92072)

92310 Prescription of optical and physical characteristics of and fitting of contact lens, with medical supervision of adaptation; corneal lens, both eyes, except for aphakia

> (For prescription and fitting of one eye, add modifier -52)

92311 corneal lens for aphakia, 1 eye

92312 corneal lens for aphakia, both eyes

92313 corneoscleral lens

92314 Prescription of optical and physical characteristics of contact lens, with medical supervision of adaptation and direction of fitting by independent technician; corneal lens, both eyes except for aphakia

> (For prescription and fitting of one eye, add modifier -52)

92315 corneal lens for aphakia, 1 eye

92316 corneal lens for aphakia, both eyes

92317 corneoscleral lens

92325 Modification of contact lens (separate procedure), with medical supervision of adaptation

92326 Replacement of contact lens

> (For prescription, fitting, and/or medical supervision of ocular prosthetic adaptation by a physician, see Evaluation and Management services or General Ophthalmological service codes 92002-92014)

SPECTACLE SERVICES (INCLUDING PROSTHESIS FOR APHAKIA)

Prescription of lenses, when required, is included in 92015, Determination of refractive state. It includes specification of lens type (monofocal, bifocal, other), lens power, axis, prism, absorptive factor, impact resistance, and other factors.

When provided, fitting of spectacles is a separate service and is reported as indicated by 92340-92371.

Fitting includes measurement of anatomical facial characteristics, the writing of laboratory specifications, and the final adjustment of the spectacles to the visual axes and anatomical topography. Presence of the physician or other qualified health care professional is not required.

Supply of materials is a separate service component; it is not part of the service of fitting spectacles.

92340 Fitting of spectacles, except for aphakia; monofocal

92341 bifocal

92342 multifocal, other than bifocal

92352 Fitting of spectacle prosthesis for aphakia; monofocal

92353 multifocal

92354 Fitting of spectacle mounted low vision aid; single element system

---

● New Code   ▲ Revised Code   + Add-On Code   ⊘ Modifier -51 Exempt   ★ Telemedicine

92355	telescopic or other compound lens system
92358	Prosthesis service for aphakia, temporary (disposable or loan, including materials)
92370	Repair and refitting spectacles; except for aphakia
92371	spectacle prosthesis for aphakia

OTHER PROCEDURES

92499	Unlisted ophthalmological service or procedure

SPECIAL OTORHINOLARYNGOLOGIC SERVICES

Otorhinolaryngology is the study and treatment of diseases of the head and neck, including the ears, nose and throat.

Diagnostic or treatment procedures that are reported as evaluation and management services (eg, otoscopy, anterior rhinoscopy, tuning fork test, removal of non-impacted cerumen) are not reported separately.

Special otorhinolaryngologic services are those diagnostic and treatment services not included in an evaluation and management service, including office or other outpatient services (99202-99215) or office or other outpatient consultations (99241-99245).

Codes 92507, 92508, 92520, 92521, 92522, 92523, 92524, and 92526 are used to report evaluation and treatment of speech sound production, receptive language, and expressive language abilities, voice and resonance production, speech fluency, and swallowing. Evaluations may include examination of speech sound production, articulatory movements of oral musculature, oral-pharyngeal swallowing function, qualitative analysis of voice and resonance, and measures of frequency, type, and duration of stuttering. Evaluations may also include the patient's ability to understand the meaning and intent of written and verbal expressions, as well as the appropriate formulation and utterance of expressive thought. In contrast, 92626 and 92627 are reported for an evaluation of auditory rehabilitation status determining the patient's ability to use residual hearing in order to identify the acoustic characteristics of sounds associated with speech communication.

(For laryngoscopy with stroboscopy, use 31579)

92502	Otolaryngologic examination under general anesthesia
92504	Binocular microscopy (separate diagnostic procedure)
92507	Treatment of speech, language, voice, communication, and/or auditory processing disorder; individual

(Do not report 92507 in conjunction with 97153, 97155)

92508	group, two or more individuals

(Do not report 92508 in conjunction with 97154, 97158)

(For auditory rehabilitation, prelingual hearing loss, use 92630)

(For auditory rehabilitation, postlingual hearing loss, use 92633)

(For cochlear implant programming, see 92601-92604)

92511	Nasopharyngoscopy with endoscope (separate procedure)

(Do not report 92511 in conjunction with 31575, 43197, 43198)

(For nasopharyngoscopy, surgical, with dilation of eustachian tube, see 69705, 69706)

92512	Nasal function studies (eg, rhinomanometry)
92516	Facial nerve function studies (eg, electroneuronography)
92517	This code is out of order. See page 891

| | Separate Procedure | | Unlisted Procedure | | CCI Comp. Code | | Non-specific Procedure | **889** |

92518   This code is out of order. See page 891

92519   This code is out of order. See page 891

92520   Laryngeal function studies (ie, aerodynamic testing and acoustic testing)

       (For performance of a single test, use modifier 52)

       (To report flexible fiberoptic laryngeal evaluation of swallowing and laryngeal sensory testing, see 92611-92617)

       (To report other testing of laryngeal function (eg, electroglottography), use 92700)

92521   Evaluation of speech fluency (eg, stuttering, cluttering)

92522   Evaluation of speech sound production (eg, articulation, phonological process, apraxia, dysarthria);

92523   with evaluation of language comprehension and expression (eg, receptive and expressive language)

92524   Behavioral and qualitative analysis of voice and resonance

92526   Treatment of swallowing dysfunction and/or oral function for feeding

VESTIBULAR FUNCTION TESTS, WITHOUT ELECTRICAL RECORDING

92531   Spontaneous nystagmus, including gaze

92532   Positional nystagmus test

       (Do not report 92531, 92532 with evaluation and management services including office or other outpatient services [99202-99215], observation care [99218-99220, 99224-99226], observation or inpatient care including admission and discharge [99234-99236], hospital care [99221-99223, 99231-99233], office or other outpatient consultations [99241-99245], nursing facility services [99304-99318], and domiciliary, rest home, or custodial care services [99324-99337])

92533   Caloric vestibular test, each irrigation (binaural, bithermal stimulation constitutes 4 tests)

92534   Optokinetic nystagmus test

VESTIBULAR FUNCTION TESTS, WITH RECORDING (eg, ENG)

92537   Caloric vestibular test with recording, bilateral; bithermal (ie, one warm and one cool irrigation in each ear for a total of four irrigations)

       (Do not report 92537 in conjunction with 92270, 92538)

       (For three irrigations, use modifier 52)

       (For monothermal caloric vestibular testing, use 92538)

92538   monothermal (ie, one irrigation in each ear for a total of two irrigations)

       (Do not report 92538 in conjunction with 92270, 92537)

       (For one irrigation, use modifier 52)

       (For bilateral, bithermal caloric vestibular testing, use 92537)

92540   Basic vestibular evaluation, includes spontaneous nystagmus test with eccentric gaze fixation nystagmus, with recording, positional nystagmus test, minimum of 4 positions, with recording, optokinetic nystagmus test, bidirectional foveal and peripheral stimulation, with recording, and oscillating tracking test, with recording

       (Do not report 92540 in conjunction with 92270, 92541, 92542, 92544, 92545)

92541   Spontaneous nystagmus test, including gaze and fixation nystagmus, with recording

(Do not report 92541 in conjunction with 92270, 92540 or the set of 92542, 92544, and 92545)

92542   Positional nystagmus test, minimum of 4 positions, with recording

(Do not report 92542 in conjunction with 92270, 92540 or the set of 92541, 92544, and 92545)

92544   Optokinetic nystagmus test, bidirectional, foveal or peripheral stimulation, with recording

(Do not report 92544 in conjunction with 92270, 92540 or the set of 92541, 92542, and 92545)

92545   Oscillating tracking test, with recording

(Do not report 92545 in conjunction with 92270, 92540 or the set of 92541, 92542, and 92544)

92546   Sinusoidal vertical axis rotational testing

(Do not report 92546 in conjunction with 92270)

+ **92547**   Use of vertical electrodes (List separately in addition to code for primary procedure)

(Use 92547 in conjunction with codes 92540-92546)

(For unlisted vestibular tests, use 92700)

(Do not report 92547 in conjunction with 92270)

92548   Computerized dynamic posturography sensory organization test (CDP-SOT), 6 conditions (ie, eyes open, eyes closed, visual sway, platform sway, eyes closed platform sway, platform and visual sway), including interpretation and report;

92549   with motor control test (MCT) and adaptation test (ADT)

(Do not report 92548, 92549 in conjunction with 92270)

● **92517**   Vestibular evoked myogenic potential (VEMP) testing, with interpretation and report; cervical (cVEMP)

(Do not report 92517 in conjunction with 92270, 92518, 92519)

● **92518**   ocular (oVEMP)

(Do not report 92518 in conjunction with 92270, 92517, 92519)

● **92519**   cervical (cVEMP) and ocular (oVEMP)

(Do not report 92519 in conjunction with 92270, 92517, 92518)

AUDIOLOGIC FUNCTION TESTS

The audiometric tests listed below require the use of calibrated electronic equipment, recording of results and a report with interpretation. Hearing tests (such as whispered voice, tuning fork) that are otorhinolaryngologic E/M services are not reported separately. All services include testing of both ears. Use modifier 52 if a test is applied to one ear instead of two ears. All codes (except 92559) apply to testing of individuals. For testing of groups, use 92559 and specify test(s) used.

(For evaluation of speech, language and/or hearing problems through observation and assessment of performance, see 92521, 92522, 92523, 92524)

92550   Tympanometry and reflex threshold measurements

(Do not report 92550 in conjunction with 92567, 92568)

92551   Screening test, pure tone, air only

92552   Pure tone audiometry (threshold); air only

92553		air and bone
92555	Speech audiometry threshold;	
92556		with speech recognition
92557	Comprehensive audiometry threshold evaluation and speech recognition (92553 and 92556 combined)	

(For hearing aid evaluation and selection, see 92590-92595)

(For automated audiometry, see 0208T-0212T)

92558 Code out of order. See page 893

92559 Audiometric testing of groups

92560 Bekesy audiometry; screening

92561 diagnostic

92562 Loudness balance test, alternate binaural or monaural

92563 Tone decay test

92564 Short increment sensitivity index (SISI)

92565 Stenger test, pure tone

92567 Tympanometry (impedance testing)

92568 Acoustic reflex testing; threshold

92570 Acoustic immittance testing, includes tympanometry (impedance testing), acoustic reflex threshold testing, and acoustic reflex decay testing

(Do not report 92570 in conjunction with 92567, 92568)

92571 Filtered speech test

92572 Staggered spondaic word test

92575 Sensorineural acuity level test

92576 Synthetic sentence identification test

92577 Stenger test, speech

92579 Visual reinforcement audiometry (VRA)

92582 Conditioning play audiometry

92583 Select picture audiometry

92584 Electrocochleography

(**92585** deleted 2020 [2021 Edition]. To report, see 92652, 92653)

(**92586** deleted 2020 [2021 Edition]. To report, see 92650, 92651)

● **92650** Auditory evoked potentials; screening of auditory potential with broadband stimuli, automated analysis

---

● New Code ▲ Revised Code + Add-On Code ⊘ Modifier -51 Exempt ★ Telemedicine

● **92651**   for hearing status determination, broadband stimuli, with interpretation and report

● **92652**   for threshold estimation at multiple frequencies, with interpretation and report

(Do not report 92652 in conjunction with 92651)

● **92653**   neurodiagnostic, with interpretation and report

92558 Evoked otoacoustic emissions, screening (qualitative measurement of distortion product or transient evoked otoacoustic emissions), automated analysis

92587 Distortion product evoked otoacoustic emissions; limited evaluation (to confirm the presence or absence of hearing disorder, 3-6 frequencies) or transient evoked otoacoustic emissions, with interpretation and report

92588   comprehensive diagnostic evaluation (quantitative analysis of outer hair cell function by cochlear mapping, minimum of 12 frequencies), with interpretation and report

(For central auditory function evaluation, see 92620, 92621)

92590 Hearing aid examination and selection; monaural

92591   binaural

92592 Hearing aid check; monaural

92593   binaural

92594 Electroacoustic evaluation for hearing aid; monaural

92595   binaural

92596 Ear protector attenuation measurements

92597 This code is out of order. See page 893

EVALUATIVE AND THERAPEUTIC SERVICES

Codes 92601 and 92603 describe post-operative analysis and fitting of previously placed external devices, connection to the cochlear implant, and programming of the stimulator. Codes 92602 and 92604 describe subsequent sessions for measurements and adjustments of the external transmitter and re-programming of the internal stimulator.

(For placement of cochlear implant, use 69930)

92601 Diagnostic analysis of cochlear implant, patient under 7 years of age; with programming

92602   subsequent reprogramming

(Do not report 92602 in addition to 92601)

(For aural rehabilitation services following cochlear implant, including evaluation of rehabilitation status, see 92626-92627, 92630-92633)

92603 Diagnostic analysis of cochlear implant, age 7 years or older; with programming

92604   subsequent reprogramming

(Do not report 92604 in addition to 92603)

92597 Evaluation for use and/or fitting of voice prosthetic device to supplement oral speech

(To report augmentative and alternative communication device services, see 92605, 92607, 92608, 92618)

92605 Evaluation for prescription of non-speech-generating augmentative and alternative communication device, face-to-face with the patient; first hour

(To report evaluation for use and/or fitting of voice prosthetic device, use 92597)

+ 92618 each additional 30 minutes (List separately in addition to code for primary procedure)

(Use 92618 in conjunction with 92605)

92606 Therapeutic service(s) for the use of non-speech-generating device, including programming and modification

92607 Evaluation for prescription for speech-generating augmentative and alternative communication device, face-to-face with the patient; first hour

(To report evaluation for use and/or fitting of voice prosthetic device, use 92597)

(For evaluation for prescription of a non-speech-generating device, use 92605)

+ 92608 each additional 30 minutes (List separately in addition to code for primary procedure)

(Use 92608 in conjunction with 92607)

92609 Therapeutic services for the use of speech-generating device, including programming and modification

(For therapeutic service(s) for the use of a non-speech-generating device, use 92606)

92610 Evaluation of oral and pharyngeal swallowing function

(For motion fluoroscopic evaluation of swallowing function, use 92611)

(For flexible endoscopic examination, use 92612-92617)

92611 Motion fluoroscopic evaluation of swallowing function by cine or video recording

(For radiological supervision and interpretation, use 74230)

(For evaluation of oral and pharyngeal swallowing function, use 92610)

(For flexible diagnostic laryngoscopy, use 31575.)

92612 Flexible endoscopic evaluation of swallowing by cine or video recording;

(If flexible or endoscopic evaluation of swallowing is performed without cine or video recording, use 92700)

(Do not report 92612 in conjunction with 31575)

92613 interpretation and report only

(To report an evaluation of oral and pharyngeal swallowing function, use 92610)

(To report motion fluoroscopic evaluation of swallowing function, use 92611)

92614 Flexible endoscopic evaluation, laryngeal sensory testing by cine or video recording;

(If flexible endoscopic evaluation of swallowing is performed without cine or video recording, use 92700)

(Do not report 92614 in conjunction with 31575)

92615 interpretation and report only

92616 Flexible endoscopic evaluation of swallowing and laryngeal sensory testing by cine or video recording;

(If flexible endoscopic evaluation of swallowing is performed without cine or video recording, use 92700)

(Do not report 92616 in conjunction with 31575)

---

894 ● New Code ▲ Revised Code ✛ Add-On Code ⊘ Modifier -51 Exempt ★ Telemedicine

92617	interpretation and report only
92618	Code out of order. See page 894
92620	Evaluation of central auditory function, with report; initial 60 minutes
+ 92621	each additional 15 minutes (List separately in addition to code for primary procedure)

(Use 92621 in conjunction with 92620)

(Do not report 92620, 92621 in conjunction with 92521, 92522, 92523, 92524)

92625	Assessment of tinnitus (includes pitch, loudness matching, and masking)

(Do not report 92625 in conjunction with 92562)

(For unilateral assessment, use modifier 52)

92626	Evaluation of auditory function for surgically implanted device(s) candidacy or postoperative status of a surgically implanted device(s); first hour
+ 92627	each additional 15 minutes (List separately in addition to code for primary procedure)

(Use 92627 in conjunction with 92626)

(When reporting 92626, 92627, use the face-to-face time with the patient or family)

(Do not report 92626, 92627 in conjunction with 92590, 92591, 92592, 92593, 92594, 92595 for hearing aid evaluation, fitting, follow-up, or selection)

92630	Auditory rehabilitation; pre-lingual hearing loss
92633	post-lingual hearing loss

SPECIAL DIAGNOSTIC PROCEDURES

92640	Diagnostic analysis with programming of auditory brainstem implant, per hour

(Report nonprogramming services separately [eg., cardiac monitoring])

92650	This code is out of order. See page 892
92651	This code is out of order. See page 893
92652	This code is out of order. See page 893
92653	This code is out of order. See page 893

OTHER PROCEDURES

92700	Unlisted otorhinolaryngological service or procedure

CARDIOVASCULAR

Cardiovascular services refers to the study and treatment of diseases of the heart and vascular (arteries and veins) system. Cardiovascular services CPT codes are used to report therapeutic services such as cardiopulmonary resuscitation (CPR), cardioversion and percutaneous transluminal coronary angioplasty (PTCA) and diagnostic procedures such as electrocardiography, echocardiography and cardiac catheterization.

Cardiovascular medicine services include non-invasive and invasive diagnostic testing (including intracardiac testing) as well as therapeutic services (e.g. electrophysiological procedures).

When cardiopulmonary resuscitation is performed without other evaluation and management services (e.g. a physician responds to a "code blue" and directs cardiopulmonary resuscitation with the patient's attending physician then resuming the care of the patient after the patient has been revived), only the CPT code 92950 for CPR should be reported. Levels of critical care services and prolonged management services are determined by time; when CPT code 92950 is reported, the time required to perform CPR is not included in critical care or other timed evaluation and management services.

In keeping with the policies outlined previously, procedures routinely performed as part of a comprehensive service are included in the comprehensive service and not separately reported. A number of therapeutic and diagnostic cardiovascular procedures (e.g. CPT codes 92950-92998, 93501-93545, 93600-93624, 93640- 93652) routinely utilize intravenous or intra-arterial vascular access, routinely require electrocardiographic monitoring, and frequently require agents administered by injection or infusion techniques; accordingly, separate codes for routine access, monitoring, injection or infusion services are not to be reported.

Fluoroscopic guidance procedures are integral to invasive intravascular procedures and are included in those services. In unique circumstances, where these services are performed, not as an integral part of the procedure, the appropriate code can be separately reported with modifier -59. When supervision and interpretation codes are identified in the CPT code book for a given procedure, these can be separately reported.

Cardiac output measurement (e.g. CPT codes 93561-93562) is routinely performed during cardiac catheterization procedures per CPT definition and, therefore, CPT codes 93561-93562 are not to be reported with cardiac catheterization codes.

THERAPEUTIC SERVICES AND PROCEDURES

92920   This code is out of order. See page 899

92921   This code is out of order. See page 899

92924   This code is out of order. See page 899

92925   This code is out of order. See page 899

92928   This code is out of order. See page 899

92929   This code is out of order. See page 899

92933   This code is out of order. See page 899

92934   This code is out of order. See page 899

92937   This code is out of order. See page 899

92938   This code is out of order. See page 899

92941   This code is out of order. See page 899

92943   This code is out of order. See page 900

92944   This code is out of order. See page 900

OTHER THERAPEUTIC SERVICES AND PROCEDURES

92950   Cardiopulmonary resuscitation (eg, in cardiac arrest)

(See also critical care services, 99291, 99292)

92953   Temporary transcutaneous pacing

(For direction of ambulance or rescue personnel outside the hospital by a physician or other qualified health care professional, use 99288)

92960   Cardioversion, elective, electrical conversion of arrhythmia; external

92961   internal (separate procedure)

(Do not report 92961 in conjunction with 93282-93284, 93287, 93289, 93295, 93296, 93618-93624, 93631, 93640-93642, 93650, 93653-93657, 93662)

92970 Cardioassist-method of circulatory assist; internal

92971 external

(For balloon atrial septostomy, use 33741)

(For placement of catheters for use in circulatory assist devices such as intra-aortic balloon pump, use 33970)

92973 This code is out of order. See page 900

92974 This code is out of order. See page 900

92975 This code is out of order. See page 900

92977 This code is out of order. See page 900

92978 This code is out of order. See page 900

92979 This code is out of order. See page 900

92986 Percutaneous balloon valvuloplasty; aortic valve

92987 mitral valve

92990 pulmonary valve

(**92992** deleted 2020 [2021 Edition]. For atrial septectomy or septostomy, transvenous method, balloon or blade, use 33741)

(**92993** deleted 2020 [2021 Edition]. For atrial septectomy or septostomy, transvenous method, balloon or blade, use 33741)

92997 Percutaneous transluminal pulmonary artery balloon angioplasty; single vessel

+ **92998** each additional vessel (List separately in addition to code for primary procedure)

(Use 92998 in conjunction with code 92997)

CORONARY THERAPEUTIC SERVICES AND PROCEDURES

Codes 92920-92944 describe percutaneous revascularization services performed for occlusive disease of the coronary vessels (major coronary arteries, coronary artery branches, or coronary artery bypass grafts). These percutaneous coronary intervention (PCI) codes are built on progressive hierarchies with more intensive services inclusive of lesser intensive services. These PCI codes all include the work of accessing and selectively catheterizing the vessel, traversing the lesion, radiological supervision and interpretation directly related to the intervention(s) performed, closure of the arteriotomy when performed through the access sheath, and imaging performed to document completion of the intervention in addition to the intervention(s) performed. These codes include angioplasty (eg, balloon, cutting balloon, wired balloons, cryoplasty), atherectomy (eg, directional, rotational, laser), and stenting (eg, balloon expandable, self-expanding, bare metal, drug eluting, covered). Each code in this family includes balloon angioplasty, when performed. Diagnostic coronary angiography may be reported separately under specific circumstances.

Diagnostic coronary angiography codes (93454-93461) and injection procedure codes (93563-93564) should not be used with percutaneous coronary revascularization services (92920-92944) to report:

1. Contrast injections, angiography, roadmapping, and/or fluoroscopic guidance for the coronary intervention,

2. Vessel measurement for the coronary intervention, or

3. Post-coronary angioplasty/stent/atherectomy angiography, as this work is captured in the percutaneous coronary revascularization services codes (92920-92944).

Diagnostic angiography performed at the time of a coronary interventional procedure may be separately reportable if:

1. No prior catheter-based coronary angiography study is available, and a full diagnostic study is performed, and a decision to intervene is based on the diagnostic angiography, OR

2. A prior study is available, but as documented in the medical record:

   a. The patient's condition with respect to the clinical indication has changed since the prior study, OR

   b. There is inadequate visualization of the anatomy and/or pathology, OR

   c. There is a clinical change during the procedure that requires a new evaluation outside the target area of intervention.

Diagnostic coronary angiography performed at a separate session from an interventional procedure is separately reportable.

Major coronary arteries: The major coronary arteries are the left main, left anterior descending, left circumflex, right, and ramus intermediate arteries. All PCI procedures performed in all segments (proximal, mid, distal) of a single major coronary artery through the native coronary circulation are reported with one code. When one segment of a major coronary artery is treated through the native circulation and treatment of another segment of the same artery requires access through a coronary artery bypass graft, the intervention through the bypass graft is reported separately.

Coronary artery branches: Up to two coronary artery branches of the left anterior descending (diagonals), left circumflex (marginals), and right (posterior descending, posterolaterals) coronary arteries are recognized. The left main and ramus intermedius coronary arteries do not have recognized branches for reporting purposes. All PCI(s) performed in any segment (proximal, mid, distal) of a coronary of artery branch is reported with one code. PCI is reported for up to two branches of a major coronary artery. Additional PCI in a third branch of the same major coronary artery is not separately reportable.

Coronary artery bypass grafts: Each coronary artery bypass graft represents a coronary vessel. A sequential bypass graft with more than one distal anastomosis represents only one graft. A branching bypass graft (eg, Y graft) represents a coronary vessel for the main graft, and each branch off the main graft constitutes an additional coronary vessel. PCI performed on major coronary arteries or coronary artery branches by access through a bypass graft is reported using the bypass graft PCI codes. All bypass graft PCI codes include the use of coronary artery embolic protection devices when performed.

Only one base code from this family may be reported for revascularization of a major coronary artery and its recognized branches. Only one base code should be reported for revascularization of a coronary artery bypass graft, its subtended coronary artery, and recognized branches of the subtended coronary artery. If one segment of a major coronary artery and its recognized branches is treated through the native circulation, and treatment of another segment of the same vessel requires access through a coronary artery bypass graft, an additional base code is reported to describe the intervention performed through the bypass graft. The PCI base codes are 92920, 92924, 92928, 92933, 92937, 92941, and 92943. The PCI base code that includes the most intensive service provided for the target vessel should be reported. The hierarchy of these services is built on an intensity of service ranked from highest to lowest as 92943 = 92941 = 92933 > 92924 > 92937 = 92928 > 92920.

PCI performed during the same session in additional recognized branches of the target vessel should be reported using the applicable add-on code(s). The add-on codes are 92921, 92925, 92929, 92934, 92938, and 92944 and follow the same principle in regard to reporting the most intensive service provided. The intensity of service is ranked from highest to lowest as 92944 = 92938 > 92934 > 92925 > 92929 > 92921.

PCI performed during the same session in additional major coronary or in additional coronary artery bypass grafts should be reported using the applicable additional base code(s). PCI performed during the same session in additional coronary artery branches should be reported using the applicable additional add-on code(s).

If a single lesion extends from one target vessel (major coronary artery, coronary artery bypass graft, or coronary artery branch) into another target vessel, but can be revascularized with a single intervention bridging the two vessels, this PCI should be reported with a single code despite treating more than one vessel. For example, if a left main coronary lesion extends into the proximal left circumflex coronary artery and a single stent is placed to treat the entire lesion, this PCI should be reported as a single vessel stent (92928). In this example, a code for additional vessel treatment (92929) would not be additionally reported.

When bifurcation lesions are treated, PCI is reported for both vessels treated. For example, when a bifurcation lesion involving the left anterior descending artery and the first diagonal artery is treated by stenting both vessels, 92928 and 92929 are both reported.

Target vessel PCI for acute myocardial infarction is inclusive of all balloon angioplasty, atherectomy, stenting, manual aspiration thrombectomy, distal protection, and intracoronary rheolytic agent administration performed. Mechanical thrombectomy is reported separately.

● New Code   ▲ Revised Code   + Add-On Code   ⊘ Modifier -51 Exempt   ★ Telemedicine

Chronic total occlusion of a coronary vessel is present when there is no antegrade flow through the true lumen, accompanied by suggestive angiographic and clinical criteria (eg, antegrade "bridging" collaterals present, calcification at the occlusion site, no current presentation with ST elevation or Q wave acute myocardial infarction attributable to the occluded target lesion). Current presentation with ST elevation or Q wave acute myocardial infarction attributable to the occluded target lesion, subtotal occlusion, and occlusion with dye staining at the site consistent with fresh thrombus are not considered chronic total occlusion.

Codes 92973 (percutaneous transluminal coronary thrombectomy, mechanical), 92974 (coronary brachytherapy), 92978 and 92979 (intravascular ultrasound/optical coherence tomography), and 93571 and 93572 (intravascular Doppler velocity and/or pressure [fractional flow reserve (FFR) or coronary flow reserve (CFR)]) are add-on codes for reporting procedures performed in addition to coronary and bypass graft diagnostic and interventional services, unless included in the base code. Non-mechanical, aspiration thrombectomy is not reported with 92973, and is included in the PCI code for acute myocardial infarction (92941), when performed

> (To report transcatheter placement of radiation delivery device for coronary intravascular brachytherapy, use 92974)
>
> (For intravascular radioelement application, see 77770, 77771, 77772)
>
> (For nonsurgical septal reduction therapy [eg, alcohol ablation], use 93799)

92920 Percutaneous transluminal coronary angioplasty; single major coronary artery or branch

+ **92921** each additional branch of a major coronary artery (List separately in addition to code for primary procedure)

> (Use 92921 in conjunction with 92920, 92924, 92928, 92933, 92937, 92941, 92943)

92924 Percutaneous transluminal coronary atherectomy, with coronary angioplasty when performed; single major coronary artery or branch

+ **92925** each additional branch of a major coronary artery (List separately in addition to code for primary procedure)

> (Use 92925 in conjunction with 92924, 92928, 92933, 92937, 92941, 92943)

92928 Percutaneous transcatheter placement of intracoronary stent(s), with coronary angioplasty when performed; single majore coronary artery or branch

+ **92929** each additional branch of a major coronary artery (List separately in addition to code for primary procedure)

> (Use 92929 in conjunction with 92928, 92933, 92937, 92941, 92943)

92933 Percutaneous transluminal coronary atherectomy, with intracoronary stent, with coronary angioplasty when performed; single major coronary artery or branch

+ **92934** each additional branch of a major coronary artery (List separately in addition to code for primary procedure)

> (Use 92934 in conjunction with 92933, 92937, 92941, 92943)

92937 Percutaneous transluminal revascularization of or through coronary artery bypass graft (internal mammary, free arterial, venous), any combination of intracoronary stent, atherectomy and angioplasty, including distal protection when performed; single vessel

+ **92938** each additional branch subtended by the bypass graft (List separately in addition to code for primary procedure)

> (Use 92938 in conjunction with 92937)

92941 Percutaneous transluminal revascularization of acute total/subtotal occlusion during acute myocardial infarction, coronary artery or coronary artery bypass graft, any combination of intracoronary stent, atherectomy and angioplasty, including aspiration thrombectomy when performed; single vessel

> (For additional vessels treated, see 92920-92938, 92943, 92944)

Separate Procedure	Unlisted Procedure	CCI Comp. Code	Non-specific Procedure

899

92943 Percutaneous transluminal revascularization of chronic total occlusion, coronary artery, coronary artery branch, or coronary artery bypass graft, any combination of intracoronary stent, atherectomy and angioplasty; single vessel

+ 92944 each additional coronary artery, coronary artery branch, or bypass graft (List separately in addition to code for primary procedure)

(Use 92944 in conjunction with 92924, 92928, 92933, 92937, 92941, 92943)

(To report transcatheter placement of radiation delivery device for coronary intravascular brachytherapy, use 92974)

(For intravascular radioelement application, see 77770, 77771, 77772)

+ 92973 Percutaneous transluminal coronary thrombectomy, mechanical (List separately in addition to code for primary procedure)

(Use 92973 in conjunction with codes 92920, 92924, 92928, 92933, 92937, 92941, 92943, 92975, 93454-93461, 93563, 93564)

(Do not report 92973 for aspiration thrombectomy)

+ 92974 Transcatheter placement of radiation delivery device for subsequent coronary intravascular brachytherapy (List separately in addition to code for primary procedure)

(Use 92974 in conjunction with 92920, 92924, 92928, 92933, 92937, 92941, 92943, 93454-93461)

(For intravascular radioelement application, see 77770, 77771, 77772)

92975 Thrombolysis, coronary; by intracoronary infusion, including selective coronary angiography

92977 by intravenous infusion

(For thrombolysis of vessels other than coronary, see 37211-37214)

(For cerebral thrombolysis, use 37195)

+ 92978 Endoluminal imaging of coronary vessel or graft using intravascular ultrasound (IVUS) or optical coherence tomography (OCT) during diagnostic evaluation and/or therapeutic intervention including imaging supervision, interpretation and report; initial vessel (List separately in addition to code for primary procedure)

(Report 92978 once per session)

(Use 92978 in conjunction with 92975, 92920, 92924, 92928, 92933, 92937, 92941, 92943, 93454-93461, 93563, 93564)

+ 92979 each additional vessel (List separately in addition to code for primary procedure)

(Report 92979 once per additional vessel)

(Use 92979 in conjunction with code 92978)

(Intravascular ultrasound and optical coherence tomography services include all transducer manipulations and repositioning within the specific vessel being examined, both before and after therapeutic intervention [eg, stent placement])

CARDIOGRAPHY

Routine monitoring of EKG rhythm and review of daily hemodynamics, including cardiac outputs, is a part of critical care evaluation and management. Separate billing for review of EKG rhythm strips and cardiac output measurements (e.g. CPT codes 93040-93042, 93561, 93562) and critical care services is inappropriate.

An exception to this may include a sudden change in patient status associated with a change in cardiac rhythm requiring a return to the ICU or telephonic transmission to review a rhythm strip. If reported separately, time included for this service is not included in the critical care time calculated for the critical care service.

● New Code   ▲ Revised Code   + Add-On Code   ⊘ Modifier -51 Exempt   ★ Telemedicine

Codes 93040-93042 are appropriate when an order for the test is triggered by an event, the rhythm strip is used to help diagnose the presence or absence of an arrhythmia, and a report is generated.

> (For echocardiography, see 93303-93350)

> (For acoustic cardiography services, use 93799)

93000 Electrocardiogram, routine ECG with at least 12 leads; with interpretation and report

93005 tracing only, without interpretation and report

93010 interpretation and report only

> (For ECG monitoring, see 99354-99360)

> (Do not report 93000, 93005, 93010 in conjunction with 0525T, 0526T, 0527T, 0528T, 0529T, 0530T, 0531T, 0532T)

93015 Cardiovascular stress test using maximal or submaximal treadmill or bicycle exercise, continuous electrocardiographic monitoring, and/or pharmacological stress; with supervision, with interpretation and report

93016 supervision only, without interpretation and report

93017 tracing only, without interpretation and report

93018 interpretation and report only

93024 Ergonovine provocation test

93025 Microvolt T-wave alternans for assessment of ventricular arrhythmias

93040 Rhythm ECG, 1 to 3 leads; with interpretation and report

93041 tracing only without interpretation and report

93042 interpretation and report only

93050 Arterial pressure waveform analysis for assessment of central arterial pressures, includes obtaining waveform(s), digitization and application of nonlinear mathematical transformations to determine central arterial pressures and augmentation index, with interpretation and report, upper extremity artery, non-invasive

> (Do not report 93050 in conjunction with diagnostic or interventional intra-arterial procedures)

CARDIOVASCULAR MONITORING SERVICES

Cardiovascular monitoring services are diagnostic medical procedures using in-person and remote technology to assess cardiovascular rhythm (ECG) data. Holter monitors (93224-93227) include up to 48 hours of continuous recording. Mobile cardiac telemetry monitors (93228, 93229) have the capability of transmitting a tracing at any time, always have internal ECG analysis algorithms designed to detect major arrhythmias, and transmit to an attended surveillance center. Event monitors (93268-93272) record segments of ECGs with recording initiation triggered either by patient activation or by an internal automatic, preprogrammed detection algorithm (or both) and transmit the recorded electrocardiographic data when requested (but cannot transmit immediately based upon the patient or algorithmic activation rhythm) and require attended surveillance. Long-term continuous recorders (93241, 93242, 93243, 93244, 93245, 93246, 93247, 93248) continuously record and store for greater than 48 hours and up to 7 days or for greater than 7 days up to 15 days.

Attended surveillance: is the immediate availability of a remote technician to respond to rhythm or device alert transmissions from a patient, either from an implanted or wearable monitoring or therapy device, as they are generated and transmitted to the remote surveillance location or center.

Electrocardiographic rhythm derived elements: elements derived from recordings of the electrical activation of the heart including, but not limited to heart thythm, rate, ST analysis, heart rate variability, T-wave alternans.

Long-term continuous recorders: Continuously record the electrocardiographic rhythm from a device applied to the patient. The electrocardiographic rhythm recording data collected is analyzed and annotated with frequency, duration, and symptomatic rhythm correlations. The processing center technician reviews the data and notifies the physician or other qualified health care professional depending on the prescribed criteria. An initial findings report is generated for physician review and final interpretation.

Mobile cardiovascular telemetry (MCT): continuously records the electrocardiographic rhythm from external electrodes placed on the patient's body. Segments of the ECG data are automatically (without patient intervention) transmitted to a remote surveillance location by cellular or landline telephone signal. The segments of the rhythm, selected for transmission, are triggered automatically (MCT device algorithm) by rapid and slow heart rates or by the patient during a symptomatic episode. There is continuous realtime data analysis by preprogrammed algorithms in the device and attended surveillance of the transmitted rhythm segments by a surveillance center technician to evaluate any arrhythmias and to determine signal quality. The surveillance center technician reviews the data and notifies the physician or other qualified health care professional depending on the prescribed criteria.

ECG rhythm derived elements are distinct from physiologic data, even when the same device is capable of producing both. Implantable cardiovascular physiologic monitor device services are always separately reported from implantable cardioverter-defibrillator (ICD) service.

93224 External electrocardiographic recording up to 48 hours by continuous rhythm recording and storage; includes recording, scanning analysis with report, review and interpretation

93225 recording (includes connection, recording, and disconnection)

93226 scanning analysis with report

93227 review and interpretation by a physician or other qualified health care professional

(For less than 12 hours of continuous recording, use modifier 52)

(For greater than 48 hours of monitoring, see 93241, 93242, 93243, 93244, 93245, 93246, 93247, 93248)

● **93241** External electrocardiographic recording for more than 48 hours up to 7 days by continuous rhythm recording and storage; includes recording, scanning analysis with report, review and interpretation

● **93242** recording (includes connection and initial recording)

● **93243** scanning analysis with report

● **93244** review and interpretation

(Do not report 93241, 93242, 93243, 93244 in conjunction with 93224, 93225, 93226, 93227, 93228, 93229, 93245, 93246, 93247, 93248, 93268, 93270, 93271, 93272, 99091, 99453, 99454, 0497T, 0498T, for the same monitoring period)

● **93245** External electrocardiographic recording for more than 7 days up to 15 days by continuous rhythm recording and storage; includes recording, scanning analysis with report, review and interpretation

● **93246** recording (includes connection and initial recording)

● **93247** scanning analysis with report

● **93248** review and interpretation

(Do not report 93245, 93246, 93247, 93248 in conjunction with 93224, 93225, 93226, 93227, 93228, 93229, 93241, 93242, 93243, 93244, 93268, 93270, 93271, 93272, 99091, 99453, 99454, 0497T, 0498T, for the same monitoring period)

★ **93228** External mobile cardiovascular telemetry with electrocardiographic recording, concurrent computerized real time data analysis and greater than 24 hours of accessible ECG data storage (retrievable with query) with ECG triggered and patient selected events transmitted to a remote attended surveillance center for up to 30 days; review and interpretation with report by a physician or other qualified health care professional

(Report 93228 only once per 30 days)

(Do not report 93228 in conjunction with 93224, 93227)

★ **93229** technical support for connection and patient instructions for use, attended surveillance, analysis and transmission of daily and emergent data reports as prescribed by a physician or other qualified health care professional

(Report 93229 only once per 30 days)

(Do not report 93229 in conjunction with 93224, 93226)

(For external cardiovascular monitors that do not perform automatic ECG triggered transmissions to an attended surveillance center, see 93224-93227, 932268-93272)

93241 This code is out of order. See page 902

93242 This code is out of order. See page 902

93243 This code is out of order. See page 902

93244 This code is out of order. See page 902

93245 This code is out of order. See page 902

93246 This code is out of order. See page 902

93247 This code is out of order. See page 902

93248 This code is out of order. See page 902

93260 This code is out of order. See page 907

93261 This code is out of order. See page 908

93264 This code is out of order. See page 906

★ **93268** External patient and, when performed, auto activated electrocardiographic rhythm derived event recording with symptom-related memory loop with remote download capability up to 30 days, 24-hour attended monitoring; includes transmission, review and interpretation by a physician or other qualified health care professional

★ **93270** recording (includes connection, recording, and disconnection)

★ **93271** transmission download and analysis

★ **93272** review and interpretation by a physician or other qualified health care professional

(For subcutaneous cardiac rhythm monitoring, see 33285, 93285, 93291, 93298)

93278 Signal-averaged electrocardiography (SAECG), with or without ECG

(For interpretation and report only, use 93278 with modifier -26)

(For unlisted cardiographic procedure, use 93799)

IMPLANTABLE, INSERTABLE, AND WEARABLE CARDIAC DEVICE EVALUATIONS

Cardiac device evaluation services are diagnostic medical procedures using in-person and remote technology to assess device therapy and cardiovascular physiologic data. Codes 93260, 93261, 93279-93298 describe this technology and technical/professional and service center practice. Codes 93260, 93261, 93279- 93292 are reported per procedure. Codes 93293, 93294, 93295, 93296 are reported no more than once every 90 days. Do not report 93293, 93294, 93295, 93296, if the monitoring period is less than 30 days. Codes 93297, 93298 are reported no more than once up to every 30 days, per patient. Do not report 93297, 93298, if the monitoring period is less than 10 days. Do not report 93264 if the monitoring period is less than 30 days. Code 93264 is reported no more than once up to every 30 days, per patient.

A service center may report 93296 during a period in which a physician or other qualified health care professional performs an in-person interrogation device evaluation. The same individual may not report an in-person and remote interrogation of the same device during the same period. Report only remote services when an in-person interrogation device evaluation is performed during a period of remote interrogation device evaluation. A period is established by the initiation of the remote monitoring or the 91st day of a pacemaker or implantable defibrillator monitoring or the 31st day of monitoring a subcutaneous cardiac rhythm monitor or implantable cardiovascular physiologic monitor, and extends for the subsequent 90 or 30 days respectively, for which remote monitoring is occurring. Programming device evaluations and in-person interrogation device evaluations may not be reported on the same date by the same individual. Programming device evaluations and remote interrogation device evaluations may both be reported during the remote interrogation device evaluation period.

For monitoring by wearable devices, see 93224-93272.

ECG rhythm derived elements are distinct from physiologic data, even when the same device is capable of producing both. Implantable cardiovascular physiologic monitor services are always separately reported from implantable defibrillator services. When cardiac rhythm data are derived from an implantable defibrillator or pacemaker, do not report subcutaneous cardiac rhythm monitor services with pacemaker or implantable defibrillator services.

Do not report 93268-93272 when performing 93260, 93261, 93279-93289, 93291-93296, or 93298. Do not report 93040, 93041, 93042 when performing 93260, 93261, 93279-93289, 93291-93296, or 93298.

The pacemaker and implantable defibrillator interrogation device evaluations, peri-procedural device evaluations and programming, and programming device evaluations may not be reported in conjunction with pacemaker or implantable defibrillator device and/or lead insertion or revision services by the same individual.

The following definitions and instructions apply to codes 93260, 93261, 93279-93298:

Attended surveillance: the immediate availability of a remote technician to respond to rhythm or device alert transmissions from a patient, either from an implanted, inserted, or wearable monitoring or therapy device, as they are generated and transmitted to the remote surveillance location or center.

Device, leadless: a leadless cardiac pacemaker system thatincludes a pulse generator with built-in battery and electrode for implantation into the cardiac chamber via a transcatheter approach.

Device, single lead: a pacemaker or implantable defibrillator with pacing and sensing function in only one chamber of the heart or a subcutaneous electrode..

Device, dual lead: a pacemaker or implantable defibrillator with pacing and sensing function in only two chambers of the heart.

Device, multiple lead: a pacemaker or implantable defibrillator with pacing and sensing function in three or more chambers of the heart.

Electrocardiographic rhythm derived elements: elements derived from recordings of the electrical activation of the heart including, but not limited to heart rhythm, rate, ST analysis, heart rate variability, T-wave alternans.

Implantable cardiovascular physiologic monitor: an implantable cardiovascular device used to assist the physician or other qualified health care professional in the management of non-rhythm related cardiac conditions such as heart failure. The device collects longitudinal physiologic cardiovascular data elements from one or more internal sensors (such as right ventricular pressure, pulmonary artery pressure, left atrial pressure, or an index of lung water) and/or external sensors (such as blood pressure or body weight) for patient assessment and management. The data are stored and transmitted by either local telemetry or remotely to an Internet-based file server or surveillance technician. The function of the implantable cardiovascular physiologic monitor may be an additional function of an implantable cardiac device (eg, implantable defibrillator) or a function of a stand-alone device. When implantable cardiovascular physiologic monitor functionality is included in an implantable defibrillator device or pacemaker, the implantable cardiovascular physiologic monitor data and the implantable defibrillator or pacemaker,

● New Code   ▲ Revised Code   ✛ Add-On Code   ⊘ Modifier -51 Exempt   ★ Telemedicine

heart rhythm data such as sensing, pacing, and tachycardia detection therapy are distinct and, therefore, the monitoring processes are distinct.

Implantable defibrillator: two general categories of implantable defibrillators exist: transvenous mplantable pacing cardioverter-defibrillator (ICD) and subcutaneous implantable defibrillator (SICD). An implantable pacing cardioverter-defibrillator device provides high-energy and low-energy stimulation to one or more chambers of the heart to terminate rapid heart rhythms called tachycardia or fibrillation. Implantable pacing cardioverterdefibrillators also have pacemaker functions to treat slow heart rhythms called bradycardia. In addition to the tachycardia and bradycardia functions, the implantable pacing cardioverter-defibrillator may or may not include the functionality of an implantable cardiovascular physiologic monitor or a subcutaneous cardiac rhythm monitor. The subcutaneous implantable defibrillator uses a single subcutaneous electrode to treat ventricular tachyarrhythmias. Subcutaneous implantable defibrillators differ from transvenous implantable pacing cardioverter-defibrillators in that subcutaneous implantable defibrillators do not provide antitachycardia pacing or chronic pacing. For subcutaneous implantable defibrillator device evaluation, see 93260, 93261.

Interrogation device evaluation: an evaluation of an implantable device such as a cardiac pacemaker, implantable defibrillator, implantable cardiovascular physiologic monitor, or subcutaneous cardiac rhythm monitor. Using an office, hospital, or emergency room instrument or via a remote interrogation system, stored and measured information about the lead(s) when present, sensor(s) when present, battery and the implanted device function, as well as data collected about the patient's heart rhythm and heart rate is retrieved. The retrieved information is evaluated to determine the current programming of the device and to evaluate certain aspects of the device function such as battery voltage, lead impedance, tachycardia detection settings, and rhythm treatment settings.

The components that must be evaluated for the various types of implantable or insertable cardiac devices are listed below. (The required components for both remote and in-person interrogations are the same.)

  Pacemaker: Programmed parameters, with or without lead(s), battery, capture and sensing function and heart rhythm.

  Implantable defibrillator: Programmed parameters, lead(s), battery, capture and sensing function, presence or absence of therapy for ventricular tachyarrhythmias and underlying heart rhythms.

  Implantable cardiovascular physiologic monitor: programmed parameters and analysis of at least one recorded physiologic cardiovascular data element from either internal or external sensors.

  Subcutaneous cardiac rhythm monitor: programmed parameters and the heart rate and rhythm during recorded episodes from both patient initiated and device algorithm detected events, when present.

Interrogation device evaluation (remote): a procedure performed for patients with pacemakers, implantable defibrillators, or subcutaneous cardiac rhythm monitors using data obtained remotely. All device functions, including the programmed parameters, lead(s), battery, capture and sensing function, presence or absence of therapy for ventricular tachyarrhythmias (for implantable defibrillators) and underlying heart rhythm are evaluated.

The components that must be evaluated for the various types of implantable or insertable cardiac devices are listed below. (The required components for both remote and in person interrogations are the same.)

  Pacemaker: programmed parameters, with or without lead(s), battery, capture and sensing function, and heart rhythm.

  Implantable defibrillator: Programmed parameters, lead(s), battery, capture and sensing function, presence or absence of therapy for ventricular tachyarrhythmias and underlying heart rhythms.

  Implantable cardiovascular physiologic monitor: programmed parameters and analysis of at least one recorded physiologic cardiovascular data element from either internal or external sensors.

  Subcutaneous cardiac rhythm monitor: programmed parameters and the heart rate and rhythm during recorded episodes from both patient-initiated and device algorithm detected events, when present.

Pacemaker: an implantable device that provides low energy localized stimulation to one or more chambers of the heart to initiate contraction in that chamber. Two general categories of pacemakers exist: (1) pacemakers with a subcutaneous generator plus transvenous/epicardial lead(s); and (2) leadless pacemakers. A leadless pacemaker does not require a subcutaneous pocket for the generator. It combines a miniaturized generator with an integrated electrode for implantation in a heart chamber via a transcatheter approach.

Peri-procedural device evaluation and programming: an evaluation of an implantable device system (either a pacemaker or implantable defibrillator) to adjust the device to settings appropriate for the patient prior to a surgery, procedure, or test. The device system data are interrogated to evaluate the lead(s) when present, sensor(s), and battery in addition to review of stored information, including patient and system measurements. The device is programmed to settings appropriate for the surgery, procedure, or test, as required. A second evaluation and programming are performed after the surgery, procedure, or test to provide settings appropriate to the post procedural situation, as required. If one performs both the pre- and post-evaluation and programming service, the appropriate code, either 93286 or 93287, would be reported two times. If one performs the pre-surgical service and a separate individual performs the post-surgical service, each reports either 93286 or 93287 only one time.

Physiologic cardiovascular data elements: data elements from one or more internal sensors (such as right ventricular pressure, left atrial pressure, or an index of lung water) and/or external sensors (such as blood pressure or body weight) for patient assessment and management. It does not include ECG rhythm derived data elements.

Programming device evaluations (in person): a procedure performed for patients with a pacemaker, implantable defibrillator, or subcutaneous cardiac rhythm monitor. All device functions, including the battery, programmable settings and lead(s), when present, are evaluated. To assess capture thresholds, iterative adjustments (eg, progressive changes in pacing output of a pacing lead) of the programmable parameters are conducted. The iterative adjustments provide information that permits the operator to assess and select the most appropriate final program parameters to provide for consistent delivery of the appropriate therapy and to verify the function of the device. The final program parameters may or may not change after evaluation.

The programming device evaluation includes all of the components of the interrogation device evaluation (remote) or the interrogation device evaluation (in person), and it includes the selection of patient specific programmed parameters depending on the type of device.

The components that must be evaluated for the various types of programming device evaluations are listed below. (See also required interrogation device evaluation [remote and in person] components above.)

> **Pacemaker:** programmed parameters, lead(s) when present, battery, capture and sensing function, and heart rhythm. Often, but not always, the sensor rate response, lower and upper heart rates, AV intervals, pacing voltage and pulse duration, sensing value, and diagnostics will be adjusted during a programming evaluation.

> **Implantable defibrillator:** Programmed parameters, lead(s), battery, capture and sensing function, presence or absence of therapy for ventricular tachyarrhythmias and underlying heart rhythms. Often, but not always, the sensor rate response, lower and upper heart rates, AV intervals, pacing voltage and pulse duration, sensing value, and diagnostics will be adjusted during a programming evaluation. In addition, ventricular tachycardia detection and therapies are sometimes altered depending on the interrogated data, patient's rhythm, symptoms, and condition.

> **Subcutaneous cardiac rhythm monitor:** programmed parameters and the heart rhythm during recorded episodes from both patient initiated and device algorithm detected events. Often, but not always, the tachycardia and bradycardia detection criteria will be adjusted during a programming evaluation.

Subcutaneous cardiac rhythm monitor: an implantable or insertable device that continuously records the electrocardiographic rhythm triggered automatically by rapid, irregular, and/or slow heart rates or by the patient during a symptomatic episode. The cardiac rhythm monitor function may be the only function of the device or it may be part of a pacemaker or implantable defibrillator device. The data are stored and transmitted by either local telemetry or remotely to an Internet-based file server or surveillance technician. Extraction of data and compilation or report for physician or qualified health care professional interpretation is usually performed in the office setting.

Transtelephonic rhythm strip pacemaker evaluation: service of transmission of an electrocardiographic rhythm strip over the telephone by the patient using a transmitter and recorded by a receiving location using a receiver/recorder (also commonly known as transtelephonic pacemaker monitoring). The electrocardiographic rhythm strip is recorded both with and without a magnet applied over the pacemaker. The rhythm strip is evaluated for heart rate and rhythm, atrial and ventricular capture (if observed) and atrial and ventricular sensing (if observed). In addition, the battery status of the pacemaker is determined by measurement of the paced rate on the electrocardiographic rhythm strip recorded with the magnet applied. For remote monitoring of an implantable wireless pulmonary artery pressure sensor, use 93264.

Implantable wireless pulmonary artery sensor: an implantable cardiovascular device used to assist the physician or other qualified health care professional in monitoring heart failure. The device collects longitudinal physiologic cardiovascular data elements from an internal sensor located in the pulmonary artery. The data are transmitted and stored remotely to an Internet-based file server

93264 Remote monitoring of a wireless pulmonary artery pressure sensor for up to 30 days, including at least weekly downloads of pulmonary artery pressure recordings, interpretation(s), trend analysis, and report(s) by a physician or other qualified health care professional

(Report 93264 only once per 30 days)

● New Code   ▲ Revised Code   ✛ Add-On Code   ⊘ Modifier -51 Exempt   ★ Telemedicine

(Do not report 93264 if download[s], interpretation[s], trend analysis, and report[s] do not occur at least weekly during the 30-day time period)

(Do not report 93264 if review does not occur at least weekly during the 30-day time period)

(Do not report 93264 if monitoring period is less than 30 days)

93279 Programming device evaluation (in person) with iterative adjustment of the implantable device to test the function of the device and select optimal permanent programmed values with analysis, review and report by a physician or other qualified health care professional; single lead pacemaker system or leadless pacemaker system in one cardiac chamber

(Do not report 93279 in conjunction with 93286, 93288)

93280   dual lead pacemaker system

(Do not report 93280 in conjunction with 93286, 93288)

93281   multiple lead pacemaker system

(Do not report 93281 in conjunction with 93286, 93288)

93282   single lead transvenous implantable defibrillator system

(Do not report 93282 in conjunction with 93260, 93287, 93289, 93745)

93283   dual lead transvenous implantable defibrillator system

(Do not report 93283 in conjunction with 93287, 93289)

93284   multiple lead transvenous implantable defibrillator system

(Do not report 93284 in conjunction with 93287, 93289)

93260   implantable subcutaneous lead defibrillator system

(Do not report 93260 in conjunction with 93261, 93282, 93287)

(Do not report 93260 in conjunction with pulse generator and lead insertion or repositioning codes 33240, 33241, 33262, 33270, 33271, 33272, 33273)

93285   subcutaneous cardiac rhythm monitor system

(Do not report 93285 in conjunction with 33285, 93279-93284, 93291)

93286 Peri-procedural device evaluation (in person) and programming of device system parameters before or after a surgery, procedure, or test with analysis, review and report by a physician or other qualified health care professional; single, dual, or multiple lead pacemaker system, or leadless pacemaker system

(Report 93286 once before and once after surgery, procedure, or test, when device evaluation and programming is performed before and after surgery, procedure, or test)

(Do not report 93286 in conjunction with 93279-93281, 93288, 0408T, 0409T, 0410T, 0411T, 0414T, 0415T)

93287   single, dual, or multiple lead implantable defibrillator system

(Report 93287 once before and once after surgery, procedure, or test, when device evaluation and programming is performed before and after surgery, procedure, or test)

(Do not report 93287 in conjunction with 93260, 93261, 93282, 93283, 93284, 93289, 0408T, 0409T, 0410T, 0411T, 0414T, 0415T)

93288 Interrogation device evaluation (in person) with analysis, review and report by a physician or other qualified health care professional, includes connection, recording and disconnection per patient encounter; single, dual, or multiple lead pacemaker system, or leadless pacemaker system

(Do not report 93288 in conjunction with 93279-93281, 93286, 93294, 93296)

93289 single, dual, or multiple lead transvenous implantable defibrillator system, including analysis of heart rhythm derived data elements

(For monitoring physiologic cardiovascular data elements derived froman implantable defibrillator, use 93290)

(Do not report 93289 in conjunction with 93261, 93282, 93283, 93284, 93287, 93295, 93296)

93261 implantable subcutaneous lead defibrillator system

(Do not report 93261 in conjunction with 93260, 93287, 93289)

(Do not report 93261 in conjunction with pulse generator and lead insertion or repositioning codes 33240, 33241, 33262, 33270, 33271, 33272, 33273)

93290 implantable cardiovascular physiologic monitor system, including analysis of 1 or more recorded physiologic cardiovascular data elements from all internal and external sensors

(For heart rhythm derived data elements, use 93289)

(Do not report 93290 in conjunction with 93297)

93291 subcutaneous cardiac rhythm monitor system, including heart rhythm derived data analysis

(Do not report 93291 in conjunction with 33285, 93288-93290, 93298)

93292 wearable defibrillator system

(Do not report 93292 in conjunction with 93745)

93293 Transtelephonic rhythm strip pacemaker evaluation(s) single, dual, or multiple lead pacemaker system, includes recording with and without magnet application with analysis, review and report(s) by a physician or other qualified health care professional, up to 90 days

(Do not report 93293 in conjunction with 93294)

(For in person evaluation, see 93040, 93041, 93042)

(Report 93293 only once per 90 days)

93294 Interrogation device evaluation(s) (remote), up to 90 days; single, dual, or multiple lead pacemaker system, or leadless pacemaker system with interim analysis, review(s) and report(s) by a physician or other qualified health care professional

(Do not report 93294 in conjunction with 93288, 93293)

(Report 93294 only once per 90 days)

93295 single, dual, or multiple lead implantable defibrillator system with interim analysis, review(s) and report(s) by a physician or other qualified health care professional

(For remote monitoring of physiologic cardiovascular data elements derived from an ICD, use 93297)

(Do not report 93295 in conjunction with 93289)

(Report 93295 only once per 90 days)

(For remote interrogation device evaluation[s] of implantable cardioverter-defibrillator with substernal lead, see 0578T, 0579T)

93296 single, dual, or multiple lead pacemaker system, leadless pacemaker system, or implantable defibrillator system, remote data acquisition(s), receipt of transmissions and technician review, technical support and distribution of results

(Do not report 93296 in conjunction with 93288, 93289)

● New Code ▲ Revised Code ✚ Add-On Code ⊘ Modifier -51 Exempt ★ Telemedicine

(Report 93296 only once per 90 days)

(For remote interrogation device evaluation[s] of implantable cardioverter-defibrillator with substernal lead, see 0578T, 0579T)

93297 Interrogation device evaluation(s), (remote) up to 30 days; implantable cardiovascular physiologic monitor system, including analysis of 1 or more recorded physiologic cardiovascular data elements from all internal and external sensors, analysis, review(s) and report(s) by a physician or other qualified health care professional

(For heart rhythm derived data elements, use 93295)

(Do not report 93297 in conjunction with 93264, 93290, 93298, 99091, 99454)

(Report 93297 only once per 30 days)

★ **93298** subcutaneous cardiac rhythm monitor system, including analysis of recorded heart rhythm data, analysis, review(s) and report(s) by a physician or other qualified health care professional

(Do not report 93298 in conjunction with 33285, 93291, 93297, 99091, 99454)

(Report 93298 only once per 30 days)

(**93299** deleted 2019 [2020 Edition]. To report, see 93297, 93298)

(For remote monitoring of an implantable wireless pulmonary artery pressure sensor, use 93264)

ECHOCARDIOGRAPHY

An echocardiogram is an ultrasound of the heart. Using standard ultrasound techniques, two-dimensional slices of the heart can be imaged. The latest ultrasound systems employ 3D real-time imaging. The standard echocardiogram is also known as a transthoracic echocardiogram, or TTE. In this case, the echocardiography transducer (or probe) is placed on the chest wall (or thorax) of the subject, and images are taken through the chest wall. This is a non-invasive, highly accurate and quick assessment of the overall health of the heart.

Another method to perform an echocardiogram is to insert a specialized scope containing an echocardiography transducer (TOE probe) into the patient's esophagus and record pictures from there. This is known as a transesophageal echocardiogram, or TEE. The advantages of TEE over TTE are clearer images, since the transducer is closer to the heart. Some structures are better imaged with the TEE. These structures include the aorta, the pulmonary artery, the valves of the heart, and the left and right atria. While TTE can be performed easily and without pain for the patient, TEE may require light sedation and a local anesthetic lubricant for the esophagus. Unlike the TTE, the TEE is considered an invasive procedure.

In addition to creating two-dimensional pictures of the cardiovascular system, the echocardiogram can also produce accurate assessment of the direction of blood flow and the velocity of blood and cardiac tissue at any arbitrary point using Doppler ultrasound. This allows assessment of cardiac valve areas and function, any abnormal communications between the left and right side of the heart, any leaking of blood through the valves (valvular regurgitation), and calculation of the cardiac output as well as the ejection fraction.

Echocardiography includes obtaining ultrasonic signals from the heart and great vessels, with real time image and/or Doppler ultrasonic signal documentation, with interpretation and report. When interpretation is performed separately, use modifier 26.

A complete transthoracic echocardiogram without spectral or color flow Doppler (93307) is a comprehensive procedure that includes 2-dimensional and, when performed, selected M-mode examination of: the left and right atria; left and right ventricles; the aortic, mitral, and tricuspid valves; the pericardium; and adjacent portions of the aorta. Multiple views are required to obtain a complete functional and anatomic evaluation, and appropriate measurements are obtained and recorded. Despite significant effort, identification and measurement of some structures may not always be possible. In such instances, the reason that an element could not be visualized must be documented. Additional structures that may be visualized (eg., pulmonary veins, pulmonary artery, pulmonic valve, inferior vena cava) would be included as part of the service.

A complete transthoracic echocardiogram with spectral and color flow Doppler (93306) is a comprehensive procedure that includes spectral Doppler and color flow Doppler in addition to the 2-dimensional and selected M-mode examinations, when performed. Spectral Doppler (93320, 93321) and color flow Doppler (93325) provide information regarding intracardiac blood flow and hemodynamics.

A follow-up or limited echocardiographic study (93308) is an examination that does not evaluate or document the attempt to evaluate all the structures that comprise the complete echocardiographic exam. This is typically limited to, or performed in follow-up of a focused clinical concern.

When a stress echocardiogram is performed with a complete cardiovascular stress test (continuous electrocardiographic monitoring, supervision, interpretation and report by a physician or other qualified health care professional), use 93351. When only the professional components of a complete stress test and a stress echocardiogram are provided (eg, in a facility setting) by the same physician, use 93351 with modifier 26. When all professional services of a stress test are not performed by the same physician performing the stress echocardiogram, use 93350 in conjunction with the appropriate codes (93016-93018) for the components of the cardiovascular stress test that are provided.

When left ventricular endocardial borders cannot be adequately identified by standard echocardiographic imaging, echocardiographic contrast may be infused intravenously both at rest and with stress to achieve that purpose. Code 93352 is used to report the administration of echocardiographic contrast agent in conjunction with the stress echocardiography codes (93350 or 93351). Supply of contrast agent and/or drugs used for pharmacological stress is reported separately in addition to the procedure code.

Code 93355 is used to report transesophageal echocardiography (TEE) services during transcatheter intracardiac therapies. Code 93355 is reported once per interventin and only by an individual who is not performing the interventional procedure. Code 93355 includes the work of passing the endoscopic ultrasound transducer through the mouth into the esophagus, when performed by the individual performing the TEE, diagnostic transesophageal echocardiography adn ongoing manipulation of the transducer to guide sizing and/or placement of implants, determination of adequacy of the intervention, and assessment for potential complications. Real-time image acquisition, measurements, and interpretation of image(s), documentation of completion of the intervention, and final written report are included in this code.

A range of intracardiac therapies may be performed with TEE guidance. Code 93355 describes TEE during advanced transcatheter structural heart procedures (eg., transcatheter aortic valve replacement [TAVE], left atrial appendage closure [LAA], or percutaneous mitral valve repair).

See 93313 for separate reporting of the probe insertion by a physician other than the physician performing the TEE.

Report of an echocardiographic study, whether complete or limited, includes an interpretation of all obtained information, documentation of all clinically relevant findings including quantitative measurements obtained, plus a description of any recognized abnormalities. Pertinent images, videotape, and/or digital data are archived for permanent storage and are available for subsequent review. Use of echocardiography not meeting these criteria is not separately reportable.

Use of ultrasound, without thorough evaluation of organ(s) or anatomic region, image documentation and final, written report, is not separately reportable.

(For fetal echocardiography, see 76825-76828)

93303 Transthoracic echocardiography for congenital cardiac anomalies; complete

93304 follow-up or limited study

93306 Echocardiography, transthoracic, real-time with image documentation (2D), includes M-mode recording, when performed, complete, with spectral doppler echocardiography, and with color flow doppler echocardiography

(For transthoracic echocardiography without spectral and color Doppler, use 93307)

93307 Echocardiography, transthoracic, real-time with image documentation (2D) includes M-mode recording, when performed, complete, without spectral or color Doppler echocardiography

(Do not report 93307 in conjunction with 93320, 93321, 93325)

93308 Echocardiography, transthoracic, real-time with image documentation (2D), includes M-mode recording, when performed, follow-up or limited study

93312 Echocardiography, transesophageal, real-time with image documentation (2D) (with or without M-mode recording); including probe placement, image acquisition, interpretation and report

(Do not report 93312 in conjunction with 93355)

● New Code   ▲ Revised Code   + Add-On Code   ⊘ Modifier -51 Exempt   ★ Telemedicine

93313   placement of transesophageal probe only

(The same individual may not report 93313 in conjunction with 93355)

93314   image acquisition, interpretation and report only

(Do not report 93314 in conjunction with 93355)

93315   Transesophageal echocardiography for congenital cardiac anomalies; including probe placement, image acquisition, interpretation and report

(Do not report 93315 in conjunction with 93355)

93316   placement of transesophageal probe only

(Do not report 93316 in conjunction with 93355)

93317   image acquisition, interpretation and report only

(Do not report 93317 in conjunction with 93355)

93318   Echocardiography, transesophageal (TEE) for monitoring purposes, including probe placement, real time 2-dimensional image acquisition and interpretation leading to ongoing (continuous) assessment of (dynamically changing) cardiac pumping function and to therapeutic measures on an immediate time basis

(Do not report 93318 in conjunction with 93355)

+ **93320**   Doppler echocardiography, pulsed wave and/or continuous wave with spectral display (List separately in addition to codes for echocardiographic imaging); complete

(Use 93320 in conjunction with 93303, 93304, 93312, 93314, 93315, 93317, 93350, 93351)

(Do not report 93320 in conjunction with 93355)

+ **93321**   follow-up or limited study (List separately in addition to codes for echocardiographic imaging)

(Use 93321 in conjunction with 93303, 93304, 93308, 93312, 93314, 93315, 93317, 93350, 93351)

(Do not report 93321 in conjunction with 93355)

+ **93325**   Doppler echocardiography color flow velocity mapping (List separately in addition to codes for echocardiography)

(Use 93325 in conjunction with 76825, 76826, 76827, 76828, 93303, 93304, 93308, 93312, 93314, 93315, 93317, 93350, 93351)

(Do not report 93325 in conjunction with 93355)

93350   Echocardiography, transthoracic, real-time with image documentation (2D), includes M-mode recording, when performed, during rest and cardiovascular stress test using treadmill, bicycle exercise and/or pharmacologically induced stress, with interpretation and report

(Stress testing codes 93016-93018 should be reported, when appropriate, in conjunction with 93350 to capture the cardiovascular stress portion of the study)

(Do not report 93350 in conjunction with 93015)

93351   including performance of continuous electrocardiographic monitoring, with supervision by a physician or other qualified health care professional

(Do not report 93351 in conjunction with 93015-93018, 93350. Do not report 93351-26 in conjunction with 93016, 93018, 93350-26))

+ **93356**   Myocardial strain imaging using speckle tracking-derived assessment of myocardial mechanics (List separately in addition to codes for echocardiography imaging)

(Use 93356 in conjunction with 93303, 93304, 93306, 93307, 93308, 93350, 93351)

(Report 93356 once per session)

+ **93352** Use of echocardiographic contrast agent during stress echocardiography (list separately in addition to code for primary procedure)

(Do not report 93352 more than once per stress echocardiogram)

(Use 93352 in conjunction with 93350, 93351)

93355 Echocardiography, transesophageal (TEE) for guidance of a transcatheter intracardiac or great vessel(s) structural intervention(s) (eg,TAVR, transcathether pulmonary valve replacement, mitral valve repair, paravalvular regurgitation repair, left atrial appendage occlusion/closure, ventricular septal defect closure) (peri-and intra-procedural), real-time image acquisition and documentation, guidance with quantitative measurements, probe manipulation, interpretation, and report, including diagnostic transesophageal echocardiography and, when performed, administration of ultrasound contrast, Doppler, color flow, and 3D

(To report placement of transesophageal probe by separate physician, use 93313)

(Do not report 93355 in conjunction with 76376, 76377, 93312, 93313, 93314, 93315, 93316, 93317, 93318, 93320, 93321, 93325)

93356 This code is out of order. See page 911

CARDIAC CATHETERIZATION

A coronary catheterization is a minimally invasive procedure to access the coronary circulation and blood filled chambers of the heart using a catheter. It is performed for both diagnostic and interventional (treatment) purposes.

Specifically, coronary catheterization is a visually interpreted test performed to recognize occlusion, stenosis, restenosis, thrombosis or aneurysmal enlargement of the coronary artery lumens, heart chamber size, heart muscle contraction performance and some aspects of heart valve function. Important internal heart and lung blood pressures, not measurable from outside the body, can be accurately measured during the test. The relevant problems that the test deals with most commonly occur as a result of advanced atherosclerosis, atheroma activity within the wall of the coronary arteries. Less frequently, other issues, valvular, heart muscle or arrhythmia issues are the primary focus of the test.

Coronary artery luminal narrowing reduces the flow reserve for oxygenated blood to the heart, typically producing intermittent angina if very advanced; luminal occlusion usually produces a heart attack. However, it has been increasingly recognized, since the late 1980s, that coronary catheterization does not allow the recognition of the presence or absence of coronary atherosclerosis itself, only significant luminal changes which have occurred as a result of end stage complications of the atherosclerotic process. See IVUS and atheroma for a better understanding of this issue.

Coronary catheterization is performed in a cardiac catheterization lab, usually located within a hospital.

Catheterization to treat luminal disease

By changing the diagnostic catheter to a guiding catheter, physicians can also pass a variety of instruments through the catheter and into the artery to a lesion site. The most commonly used are guide wires and the balloon dilation catheters.

By injecting radiocontrast agent through a tiny passage extending down the balloon catheter and into the balloon, the balloon is progressively expanded. The hydraulic pressures are chosen and applied by the physician, according to how the balloon within the stenosis responds. The radiocontrast filled balloon is watched under fluoroscopy (it typically assumes a "dog bone" shape imposed on the outside of the balloon by the stenosis as the balloon is expanded), as it opens. As much hydraulic brute force is applied as judged needed and visualized to be effective to make the stenosis of the artery lumen visibly enlarge.

Additionally, several other devices can be advanced into the artery via a guiding catheter. These include laser catheters, stent catheters, IVUS catheters, Doppler catheter, pressure or temperature measurement catheter and various clot and grinding or removal devices. Most of these devices have turned out to be niche devices, only useful in a small percentage of situations or for research.

Stents, specially manufactured expandable stainless steel mesh tubes, mounted on a balloon catheter, are the most commonly used device beyond the balloon catheter. When the stent/balloon device is positioned within the stenosis, the balloon is inflated which, in turn, expands the stent and the artery. The balloon is removed and the stent remains in place, supporting the inner artery walls in the more open, dilated position.

There are two code families for cardiac catheterization: one for congenital heart disease, and one for all other conditions. Anomalous coronary arteries, patent foramen ovale, mitral valve prolapse, and bicuspid aortic valve are to be reported with 93451-93464, 93566-93568.

Right heart catheterization includes catheter placement in one or more right-sided cardiac chamber(s) or structures (ie, the right atrium, right ventricle, pulmonary artery, pulmonary wedge), obtaining blood samples for measurement of blood gases, and cardiac output measurements (Fick or other method), when performed. Left heart catheterization involves catheter placement in a left-sided (systemic) cardiac chamber(s) (left ventricle or left atrium) and includes left ventricular injection(s) when performed. Do not report code 93503 in conjunction with other diagnostic cardiac catheterization codes. When right heart catheterization is performed in conjunction with other cardiac catheterization services, report 93453, 93456, 93457, 93460 or 93461. For placement of a flow directed catheter (eg, Swan-Ganz) performed for hemodynamic monitoring purposes not in conjunction with other catheterization services, use 93503. Right heart catheterization does not include right ventricular or right atrial angiography (93566). When left heart catheterization if performed using either transapical puncture of the left ventricle or transeptal puncture of an intact septum, report 93462 in conjunction with 93452, 93453, 93458-93461, 93653, 93654. Catheter placement(s) in coronary artery(ies) involves selective engagement of the origins of the native coronary artery(ies) for the purpose of coronary angiography. Catheter placement(s) in bypass graft(s) (venous, internal mammary, free arterial graft[s]) involve selective engagement of the origins of the graft(s) for the purpose of bypass angiography. It is typically performed only in conjunction with coronary angiography of native vessels.

The cardiac catheterization codes (93452-93462), other than those for congenital heart disease, include contrast injection(s), imaging supervision, interpretation, and report for imaging typically performed. Codes for left heart catheterization (93452, 93453, 93458-93461) other than those for congenital heart disease, include intraprocedural injection(s) for left ventricular/left atrial angiography, imaging supervision, and interpretation, when performed. Codes for coronary catheter placement(s) (93454-93461), other than those for congenital heart disease, include intraprocedural injection(s) for coronary angiography, imaging supervision, and interpretation. Codes for catheter placement(s) in bypass graft(s) (93455, 93457, 93459, 93461) other than those for congenital heart disease, include intraprocedural injection(s) for bypass graft angiography, imaging supervision, and interpretation. Do not report 93563-93565 in conjunction with 93452-93461.

For cardiac catheterization for congenital cardiac anomalies, see 93530-93533. When contrast injection(s) are performed in conjunction with cardiac catheterization for congenital anomalies, see 93563-93568.

Cardiac catheterization (93451-93461) includes all roadmapping angiography in order to place the catheters, including any injections and imaging supervision, interpretation, and report. It does not include contrast injection(s) and imaging supervision, interpretation, and report for imaging that is separately identified by specific procedure code(s). For right ventricular or right atrial angiography performed in conjunction with cardiac catheterization for congenital or noncongenital heart disease (93451-93461, 93530-93533), use 93566. For aortography, use 93567. For pulmonary angiography, use 93568. For angiography of noncoronary arteries and veins, performed as a distinct service, use appropriate codes from the Radiology section and the Vascular Injection Procedures section.

When cardiac catheterization is combined with pharmacologic agent administration with the specific purpose of repeating hemodynamic measurements to evaluate hemodynamic response, use 93463 in conjunction with 93451-93453 and 93456-93461. Do not report 93463 for intracoronary administration of pharmacologic agents during percutaneous coronary interventional procedures, during intracoronary assessment of coronary pressure, flow or resistance, or during intracoronary imaging procedures. Do not report 93463 in conjunction with 92920-92944, 92975, 92977.

When cardiac catheterization is combined with exercise (eg, walking or arm or leg ergometry protocol) with the specific purpose of repeating hemodynamic measurements to evaluate hemodynamic response, report 93464 in conjunction with 93451-93453, 93456-93461, and 93530-93533.

Contrast injection to image the access site(s) for the specific purpose of placing a closure device is inherent to the catheterization procedure and not separately reportable. Closure device placement at the vascular access site is inherent to the catheterization procedure and not separately reportable.

Modifier 51 should not be appended to 93451, 93456, 93503.

Please see the cardiac catheterization table, located following 93572.

93451 Right heart catheterization including measurement(s) of oxygen saturation and cardiac output, when performed

(Do not report 93451 in conjunction with 33289, 93453, 93456, 93457, 93460, 93461, 0613T, 0632T)

(Do not report 93451 in conjunction with 33418, 0345T, 0483T, 0484T, 0544T, 0545T for diagnostic right heart catheterization procedures intrinsic to the valve repair or annulus reconstruction procedure)

93452 Left heart catheterization including intraprocedural injection(s) for left ventriculography, imaging supervision and interpretation, when performed

(Do not report 93452 in conjunction with 33418, 0345T, 0483T, 0484T, 0544T, 0545T for diagnostic left heart catheterization procedures intrinsic to the valve repair or annulus reconstruction procedure)

93453 Combined right and left heart catheterization including intraprocedural injection(s) for left ventriculography, imaging supervision and interpretation, when performed

(Do not report 93453 in conjunction with 93451, 93452, 93456-93461, 0408T, 0409T, 0410T, 0411T, 0414T, 0415T)

(Do not report 93453 in conjunction with 33418, 0345T, 0483T, 0484T, 0544T, 0545T for diagnostic left and right heart catheterization procedures intrinsic to the valve repair or annulus reconstruction procedure)

93454 Catheter placement in coronary artery(s) for coronary angiography, including intraprocedural injection(s) for coronary angiography, imaging supervision and interpretation

(Do not report 93454 in conjunction with 33418, 0345T, 0483T, 0484T, 0544T, 0545T for coronary angiography intrinsic to the valve repair or annulus reconstruction procedure)

93455 with catheter placement(s) in bypass graft(s) (internal mammary, free arterial venous grafts) including intraprocedural injection(s) for bypass graft angiography

(Do not report 93455 in conjunction with 33418, 0345T, 0483T, 0484T, 0544T, 0545T for coronary angiography intrinsic to the valve repair or annulus reconstruction procedure)

93456 with right heart catheterization

(Do not report 93456 in conjunction with 33418, 0345T, 0483T, 0484T, 0544T, 0545T for diagnostic coronary angiography or right heart catheterization procedures intrinsic to the valve repair or annulus reconstruction procedure)

93457 with catheter placement(s) in bypass graft(s) (internal mammary, free arterial, venous grafts) including intraprocedural injection(s) for bypass graft angiography and right heart catheterization

(Do not report 93457 in conjunction with 33418, 0345T, 0483T, 0484T, 0544T, 0545T for diagnostic coronary angiography or right heart catheterization procedures intrinsic to the valve repair or annulus reconstruction procedure)

93458 with left heart catheterization including intraprocedural injection(s) for left ventriculography, when performed

(Do not report 93458 in conjunction with 33418, 0345T, 0483T, 0484T, 0544T, 0545T for diagnostic coronary angiography or left heart catheterization procedures intrinsic to the valve repair or annulus reconstruction procedure)

(Do not report 93458 in conjunction with 0408T, 0409T, 0410T, 0411T, 0414T, 0415T)

93459 with left heart catheterization including intraprocedural injection(s) for left ventriculography, when performed, catheter placement(s) in bypass graft(s) (internal mammary, free arterial, venous grafts) with bypass graft angiography

(Do not report 93459 in conjunction with 33418, 0345T, 0483T, 0484T, 0544T, 0545T for diagnostic coronary angiography or left heart catheterization procedures intrinsic to the valve repair or annulus reconstruction procedure)

(Do not report 93459 in conjunction with 0408T, 0409T, 0410T, 0411T, 0414T, 0415T)

93460 with right and left heart catheterization including intraprocedural injection(s) for left ventriculography, when performed

(Do not report 93460 in conjunction with 33418, 0345T, 0483T, 0484T, 0544T, 0545T for diagnostic coronary angiography or left and right heart catheterization procedures intrinsic to the valve repair or annulus reconstruction procedure)

(Do not report 93460 in conjunction with 0408T, 0409T, 0410T, 0411T, 0414T, 0415T)

93461 with right and left heart catheterization including intraprocedural injection(s) for left ventriculography, when performed, catheter placement(s) in bypass graft(s) (internal mammary, free arterial, venous grafts) with bypass graft angiography

(Do not report 93461 in conjunction with 33418, 0345T, 0483T, 0484T, 0544T, 0545T for diagnostic coronary angiography or left and right heart catheterization procedures intrinsic to the valve repair or annulus reconstruction procedure)

(Do not report 93461 in conjunction with 0408T, 0409T, 0410T, 0411T, 0414T, 0415T)

+ **93462** Left heart catheterization by transseptal puncture through intact septum or by transapical puncture (List separately in addition to code for primary procedure)

(Use 93462 in conjunction with 33477, 93452, 93453, 93458, 93459, 93460, 93461, 93582, 93653, 93654)

(Use 93462 in conjunction with 93590, 93591 for transapical puncture performed for left heart catheterization and percutaneous transcatheter closure of paravalvular leak)

(Do not report 93462 in conjunction with 93590 for transeptal puncture through intact septum performed for left heart catheterization and percutaneous transcatheter closure of paravalvular leak)

(Do not report 93462 in conjunction with 93656)

(Do not report 93462 in conjunction with 0345T, 0544T unless transapical puncture is performed)

+ **93463** Pharmacologic agent administration (eg, inhaled nitric oxide, intravenous infusion of nitroprusside, dobutamine, milrinone, or other agent) including assessing hemodynamic measurements before, during, after and repeat pharmacologic agent administration, when performed (List separately in addition to code for primary procedure)

(Use 93463 in conjunction with 33477, 93451-93453, 93456-93461, 93530, 93531, 93532, 93533, 93580, 93581)

(Report 93463 only once per catheterization procedure)

(Do not report 93463 for pharmacologic agent administration in conjunction with coronary interventional procedure codes 92920-92944, 92975, 92977)

+ **93464** Physiologic exercise study (eg, bicycle or arm ergometry) including assessing hemodynamic measurements before and after (List separately in addition to code for primary procedure)

(Use 93464 in conjunction with 33477, 93451-93453, 93456-93461, 93530-93533)

(Report 93464 only once per catheterization procedure)

(For pharmacologic agent administration, use 93463)

(For bundle of His recording, use 93600)

93503 Insertion and placement of flow directed catheter (eg, Swan-Ganz) for monitoring purposes

(Do not report 93503 in conjunction with 0632T)

(For subsequent monitoring, see 99356-99357)

93505 Endomyocardial biopsy

93530 Right heart catheterization, for congenital cardiac anomalies

93531 Combined right heart catheterization and retrograde left heart catheterization, for congenital cardiac anomalies

---

Table of Catheterization Codes

CPT Code	Catheter Placement Type				Add-On Procedures (Can be reported separately)					
	RHC	LHC	Coronary Artery Placement	Bypass Graft(s)	With Transseptal or Transapical Puncture 93462	With Pharmacological Study 93463	With Exercise Study 93464	Injection Procedure for Selective Rt Ventricular or Rt Atrial Angiography 93566	Injection Procedure for Supravalvular Aortography 93567	Injection Procedure for Pulmonary Angiography 93568
93451	•					•	•	•		•
93452		•			•	•	•		•	
93453	•	•			•	•	•	•	•	•
93454			•						•	
93455			•	•					•	
93456	•		•			•	•	•	•	•
93457	•		•	•		•	•	•	•	•
93458		•	•		•	•	•		•	
93459		•	•	•	•	•	•		•	
93460	•	•	•		•	•	•	•	•	•
93461	•	•	•	•	•	•	•	•	•	•

93532 Combined right heart catheterization and transseptal left heart catheterization through intact septum with or without retrograde left heart catheterization, for congenital cardiac anomalies

93533 Combined right heart catheterization and transseptal left heart catheterization through existing septal opening, with or without retrograde left heart catheterization, for congenital cardiac anomalies

INJECTION PROCEDURES

All injection codes include radiological supervision, interpretation, and report. Cardiac catheterization codes (93452-93461), other than those for congenital heart disease, include contrast injection(s) for imaging typically performed during these procedures (see Cardiac Catheterization above.) Do not report 93563-93565 in conjunction with 93452-93461. When injection procedures for right ventricular, right atrial, aortic, or pulmonary angiography are performed in conjunction with cardiac catheterization, these services are reported separately (93566-93568). When right ventricular or right atrial angiography is performed at the time of heart catheterization, use 93566 with the appropriate catheterization code ((93451, 93453, 93456, 93457, 93460, or 93461). Use 93567 when supravalvular ascending aortography is performed at the t ime of heart catheterization. Use 93568 with the appropriate right heart catheterization code when pulmonary angiography is preformed. Separately reported injection procedures do not include introduction of catheters but do include repositioning of catheters when necessary and use of automatic power injectors, when performed.

When contrast injection(s) are performed in conjunction with cardiac catheterization for congenital cardiac anomalies (93530-93533), see 93563-93568. Injection procedure codes 93563-93568 include imaging supervision, interpretation, and report.

Injection procedures 93563-93568 represent separate identifiable services and may be coded in conjunction with one another when appropriate. The technical details of angiography, supervision of imaging and processing, interpretation, and report are included.

93561 Indicator dilution studies such as dye or thermodilution, including arterial and/or venous catheterization; with cardiac output measurement (separate procedure)

93562 subsequent measurement of cardiac output

(Do not report 93561, 93562 in conjunction with 93451-93462, 93582)

(For radioisotope method of cardiac output, see 78472, 78473 or 78481)

+ **93563** Injection procedure during cardiac catheterization including imaging supervision, interpretation, and report; for selective coronary angiography during congenital heart catheterization (List separately in addition to code for primary procedure)

+ **93564** for selective opacification of aortocoronary venous or arterial bypass graft(s) (eg, aortocoronary saphenous vein, free radial artery, or free mammary artery graft) to one or more coronary arteries and in situ arterial conduits (eg, internal mammary), whether native or used for bypass to one or more

● New Code   ▲ Revised Code   + Add-On Code   ⊘ Modifier -51 Exempt   ★ Telemedicine

coronary arteries during congenital heart catheterization, when performed (List separately in addition to code for primary procedure)

(Do not report 93563, 93564 in conjunction with 33418, 0345T, 0483T, 0484T, 0544T, 0545T for coronary angiography intrinsic to the valve repair or annulus reconstruction procedure)

+ **93565**   for selective left ventricular or left atrial angiography (List separately in addition to code for primary procedure)

(Do not report 93563-93565 in conjunction with 93452-93461)

(Use 93563-93565 in conjunction with 93530-93533)

+ **93566**   for selective right ventricular or right atrial angiography (List separately in addition to code for primary procedure)

(Use 93566 in conjunction with 93451, 93453, 93456, 93457, 93460, 93461, 93530-93533)

(Do not report 93566 in conjunction with 33274 for right ventriculography performed during leadless pacemaker insertion)

(Do not report 93566 in conjunction with 0545T for right ventricular or right atrial angiography procedures intrinsic to the annulus reconstruction procedure)

+ **93567**   for supravalvular aortography (List separately in addition to code for primary procedure)

(Use 93567 in conjunction with 93451-93461, 93530-93533)

(For non-supravalvular thoracic aortography or abdominal aortography performed at the time of cardiac catheterization, use the appropriate radiological supervision and interpretation codes [36221, 75600-75630])

+ **93568**   for pulmonary angiography (List separately in addition to code for primary procedure)

(Use 93568 in conjunction with 93451, 93453, 93456, 93457, 93460, 93461, 93530-93533)

(Do not report 93568 in conjunction with 0632T)

+ **93571**   Intravascular Doppler velocity and/or pressure derived coronary flow reserve measurement (coronary vessel or graft) during coronary angiography including pharmacologically induced stress; initial vessel (List separately in addition to code for primary procedure)

(Use 93571 in conjunction with 92920, 92924, 92928, 92933, 92937, 92941, 92943, 92975, 93454-93461, 93563, 93564)

(Do not report 93571 in conjunction with 0523T)

+ **93572**   each additional vessel (List separately in addition to code for primary procedure)

(Use 93572 in conjunction with 93571)

(Intravascular distal coronary blood flow velocity measurements include all Doppler transducer manipulations and repositioning within the specific vessel being examined, during coronary angiography or therapeutic intervention (eg, angioplasty))

(For unlisted cardiac catheterization procedure, use 93799)

(Do not report 93572 in conjunction with 0523T)

REPAIR OF SEPTAL HEART DEFECT

93580   Percutaneous transcatheter closure of congenital interatrial communication (i.e., fontan fenestration, atrial septal defect) with implant

(Percutaneous transcatheter closure of atrial septal defect includes a right heart catheterization procedure. Code 93580 includes injection of contrast for atrial and ventricular angiograms. Codes 93451-93453, 93455-93461, 93530-93533, 93564-93566 should not be reported separately in addition to code 93580)

93581   Percutaneous transcatheter closure of a congenital ventricular septal defect with implant

---

| | Separate Procedure | | Unlisted Procedure | | CCI Comp. Code | | Non-specific Procedure | **917** |

(Percutaneous transcatheter closure of ventricular septal defect includes a right heart catheterization procedure. Code 93581 includes injection of contrast for atrial and ventricular angiograms. Codes 93451-93453, 93455-93461, 93530-93533, 93564-93566 should not be reported separately in addition to 93581)

(For echocardiographic services performed in addition to 93580, 93581, see 93303-93317 as appropriate)

93582   Percutaneous transcatheter closure of patent ductus arteriosus

(93582 includes congenital right and left heart catheterization, catheter placement in the aorta, and aortic arch angiography, when performed)

(Do not report 93582 in conjunction with 36013, 36014, 36200, 75600, 75605, 93451-93461, 93530, 93531, 93532, 93533, 93567)

(For other cardiac angiographic procedures performed at the time of transcatheter PDA closure, see 93563, 93564, 93565, 93566, 93568 as appropriate)

(For left heart catheterization by transseptal puncture through intact septum or by transapical puncture performed at the time of transcatheter PDA closure, use 93462)

(For repair of patent ductus arteriosus by ligation, see 33820, 33822, 33824)

(For intracardiac echocardiographic services performed at the time of transcatheter PDA closure, use 93662. Other echocardiographic services provided by a separate individual are reported using the appropriate echocardiography service codes, 93315, 93316, 93317)

93583   Percutaneous transcatheter septal reduction therapy (eg, alcohol septal ablation) including temporary pacemaker insertion when performed

(93583 includes insertion of temporary pacemaker, when performed, and left heart catheterization)

(Do not report 93583 in conjunction with 33210, 93452, 93453, 93458, 93459, 93460, 93461, 93531, 93532, 93533, 93565)

(93583 includes left anterior descending coronary angiography for the purpose of roadmapping to guide the intervention. Do not report 93454, 93455, 93456, 93457, 93458, 93459, 93460, 93461, 93563 for coronary angiography performed during alcohol septal ablation for the purpose of roadmapping, guidance of the intervention, vessel measurement, and completion angiography)

(Diagnostic cardiac catheterization procedures may be separately reportable when no prior catheter-based diagnostic study of the treatment zone is available, the prior diagnostic study is inadequate, or the patient's condition with respect to the clinical indication has changed since the prior study or during the intervention. Use the appropriate codes from 93451, 93454, 93455, 93456, 93457, 93530, 93563, 93564, 93566, 93567, 93568)

(Do not report 93583 in conjunction with 33210, 33211)

(Do not report 93463 for the injection of alcohol for this procedure)

(For intracardiac echocardiographic services performed at the time of alcohol septal ablation, use 93662)

(Other echocardiographic services provided by a separate physician are reported using the appropriate echocardiography services codes, 93312, 93313, 93314, 93315, 93316, 93317)

(For surgical ventriculomyotomy [–mectomy] for idiopathic hypertrophic subaortic stenosis, use 33416)

Transcatheter Closure of Paravalvular Leak

Codes 93590, 93591, 93592 are used to report transcatheter closure of paravalvular leak (PVL). Codes 93590 and 93591 include, when performed, percutaneous access, placing the access sheath(s), advancing the delivery system to the paravalvular leak, positioning the closure device, repositioning the closure device as needed, and deploying the device.

Codes 93590 and 93591 include, when performed, fluoroscopy (76000), angiography, radiological supervision and interpretation services performed to guide the PVL closure (eg, guiding the device placement and documenting completion of the intervention).

● New Code   ▲ Revised Code   ＋ Add-On Code   ⊘ Modifier -51 Exempt   ★ Telemedicine

Code 93590 includes transseptal puncture, and left heart catheterization/left ventriculography (93452, 93453, 93458, 93459, 93460, 93461, 93531, 93532, 93533, 93565), when performed. Transapical left heart catheterization (93462) may be reported separately, when performed.

Code 93591 includes, when performed, supravalvular aortography (93567), left heart catheterization/left ventriculography (93452, 93453, 93458, 93459, 93460, 93461, 93531, 93532, 93533, 93565). Transapical left heart catheterization (93462) may be reported separately, when performed.

Diagnostic right heart catheterization codes (93451, 93456, 93457, 93530) and diagnostic coronary angiography codes (93454, 93455, 93456, 93457, 93563, 93564) may be reported with 93590, 93591, representing separate and distinct services from PVL closure, if:

1. No prior study is available and a full diagnostic study is performed, or

2. A prior study is available, but as documented in the medical record:

a. there is inadequate visualization of the anatomy and/or pathology, or

b. the patient's condition with respect to the clinical indication has changed since the prior study, or

c. there is a clinical change during the procedure that requires new evaluation.

Other cardiac catheterization services may be reported separately, when performed for diagnostic purposes not intrinsic to PVL closure.

For same session/same day diagnostic cardiac catheterization services, report the appropriate diagnostic cardiac catheterization code(s) appended with modifier 59 indicating separate and distinct procedural service from PVL closure.

93590   Percutaneous transcatheter closure of paravalvular leak; initial occlusion device, mitral valve

      (Do not report 93590 in conjunction with 93462 for transseptal puncture)

      (For transapical puncture performed in conjunction with 93590, use 93462)

93591   initial occlusion device, aortic valve

      (For transseptal or transapical puncture performed in conjunction with 93591, use 93462)

+ 93592   each additional occlusion device (List separately in addition to code for primary procedure)

      (Use 93592 in conjunction with 93590, 93591)

INTRACARDIAC ELECTROPHYSIOLOGICAL PROCEDURES/STUDIES

Intracardiac electrophysiology study (EPS) involves placing wire electrodes within the heart to determine the characteristics of heart arrhythmias. Before performing EPS, which is invasive, the cardiologist will try to identify a suspected arrhythmia using other, less invasive tests like ambulatory cardiac monitoring. If the abnormal rhythm is not detected by these other methods and symptoms suggest an arrhythmia, EPS may be recommended. Additional reasons that EPS may be considered include:

- *To find the location of a known arrhythmia and determine the best therapy*

- *To assess the severity of the arrhythmia and determine if the patient is at risk for future cardiac events, especially sudden cardiac death*

- *To evaluate the effectiveness of medication in controlling an arrhythmia*

- *To determine if the focus (the place where the arrhythmia is coming from) should be ablated*

- *To evaluate the need for a permanent pacemaker or an implantable cardioverter-defibrillator (ICD)*

During EPS, the cardiologist inserts a catheter through a small incision in a groin vein after cleansing the site and numbing it with a local anesthetic. This catheter is equipped with an electrode connected to electrocardiographic monitors. The catheter is then carefully threaded into the heart using an x-ray imaging technique called fluoroscopy to guide the insertion. Electrodes are placed in the heart to measure electrical activity along the heart's conduction system and within heart muscle cells themselves.

Separate Procedure	Unlisted Procedure	CCI Comp. Code	Non-specific Procedure

919

Normal electrical activity is signaled from the heart's natural pacemaker known as the sinoatrial (SA) node. It then travels through the atria, the atrioventricular (AV) node, and the ventricles. Abnormal electrical activity can occur anywhere along this conduction system, including in the muscle cells of either the atria or ventricles. The electrodes inserted during EPS will map the type of arrhythmia the patient has and where the problem arises in the heart.

If ablation is thought to be the appropriate therapy, it is performed at the time of EPS.

Definitions

Arrhythmia Induction: In most electrophysiologic studies, an attempt is made to induce arrhythmia(s) from single or multiple sites within the heart. Arrhythmia induction may be achieved by multiple techniques, eg. by performing pacing at different rates or programmed stimulation (introduction of critically timed electrical impulses). Because arrhythmia induction occurs via the same catheter(s) inserted for the electrophysiologic study(ies), catheter insertion and temporary pacemaker codes are not additionally reported. Codes 93600-93603, 93610-93612 and 93618 are used to describe unusual situations where there may be recording, pacing or an attempt at arrhythmia induction from only one site in the heart. Code 93619 describes only evaluation of the sinus node, atrioventricular node, and His-Purkinje conduction system, without arrhythmia induction. Codes 93620-93624, 93640-93642, 93653, 93654 and 93656 all include recording, pacing and attempted arrhythmia induction from one or more site(s) in the heart.

Mapping: When a tachycardia is induced, the site of tachycardia origination or its electrical path through the heart is often defined by mapping. Mapping creates a multidimensional depiction of a tachycardia by recording multiple electrograms obtained sequentially or simultaneously from multiple catheter sites in the heart. Depending upon the technique, certain types of mapping catheters may be repositioned from point-to-point within the heart, allowing sequential recording from the various sites to construct maps. Other types of mapping catheters allow mapping without a point-to-point technique by allowing simultaneous recording from many electrodes on the same catheter and computer-assisted three-dimensional reconstruction of the tachycardia activation sequence.

Mapping is a distinct procedure performed in addition to a diagnostic electrophysiologic study or ablation procedure and may be separately reported using 93609 or 93613. Do not report standard mapping (93609) in addition to 3-dimensional mapping (93613).

Ablation: Once the part of the heart involved in the tachycardia is localized, the tachycardia may be treated by ablation (the delivery of a radiofrequency or cryo-energy to the area to selectively destroy cardiac tissue). Ablation procedures (93653-93657) are performed at the same session as electrophysiology studies and therefore represent a combined code description. When reporting ablation therapy codes (93653-93657), the single site electrophysiology studies (93600-93603, 93610, 93612, 93618) and the comprehensive electrophysiology studies (93619, 93620) may not be reported separately. Code 93622 may be reported separately with 93653 and 93656. Code 93623 may be reported separately with 93653, 93654, and 93656. However, 93621 for left atrial pacing and recording from coronary sinus or left atrium should not be reported in conjunction with 93656 as this procedure is a component of 93656. Codes 93653 and 93654 include right ventricular pacing and recording and His bundle recording when clinically indicated. When performance of one or more components is not possible or indicated, document the reason for not performing. Code 93656 includes each of left atrial pacing/recording, right ventricular pacing/recording, and His bundle recording when clinically indicated. When performance of one or more components is not possible or indicated, document the reason for not performing.

The differences in the techniques involved for ablation of supraventricular arrhythmias, ventricular arrhythmias, and atrial fibrillation are reflected within the descriptions for 93653-93657. Code 93653 is a primary code for catheter ablation for treatment of supraventricular tachycardia caused by dual atrioventricular nodal pathways, accessory atrioventricular connections, or other atrial foci. Code 93654 describes catheter ablation for treatment of ventricular tachycardia or focus of ventricular ectopy. Code 93656 is a primary code for reporting treatment of atrial fibrillation by ablation to achieve complete pulmonary vein electrical isolation. Codes 93653, 93654 and 93656 are distinct primary procedure codes and may not be reported together.

Codes 93655 and 93657 are add-on codes listed in addition to the primary ablation code to report ablation of sites distinct from the primary ablation site. After ablation of the primary target site, post-ablation electrophysiologic evaluation is performed as part of those ablation services (93653, 93654, 93656) and additional mechanisms of tachycardia may be identified. For example, if the primary tachycardia ablated was atrioventricular nodal reentrant tachycardia and during post-ablation testing an atrial tachycardia, atrial flutter, or accessory pathway with orthodromic reentry tachycardia was identified, this would be considered a separate mechanism of tachycardia. Pacing maneuvers are performed to define the mechanism(s) of the new tachycardia(s). Catheter ablation of this distinct mechanism of tachycardia is then performed at the newly discovered atrial or ventricular origin. Appropriate post-ablation attempts at re-induction and observation are again performed. Code 93655 is listed in conjunction with 93653 when repeat ablation is for treatment of an additional supraventricular tachycardia mechanism and with 93654 when the repeat ablation is for treatment of an additional ventricular tachycardia mechanism. Code 93655 may be reported with 93656 when an additional non-atrial fibrillation tachycardia is separately diagnosed after pulmonary vein isolation. Code 93657 is

● New Code   ▲ Revised Code   + Add-On Code   ⊘ Modifier -51 Exempt   ★ Telemedicine

reported in conjunction with 93656 when successful pulmonary vein isolation is achieved, attempts at re-induction of atrial fibrillation identify an additional left or right atrial focus for atrial fibrillation, and further ablation of this new focus is performed.

In certain circumstances, depending on the chamber of origin, a catheter or catheters may be maneuvered into the left ventricle to facilitate arrhythmia diagnosis. This may be accomplished via a retrograde aortic approach by means of the arterial access or through a transseptal puncutre. For ablation treatment of supraventricular tachycardia (93653) and ventricular tachycardia (93654), the left heart catheterization by transseptal puncture through intact septum (93462) may be reported separately as an add-on code. However, for ablation treatment of atrial fibrillation (93656), the transseptal puncture (93462) is a standard component of the procedure and may not be reported separately. Do not report 93462 in conjunction with 93656.

Modifier 51 should not be appended to 93600-93603, 93610, 93612, 93615-93618.

⊘ **93600**   Bundle of His recording

(Do not report 93600 in conjunction with 93619, 93620, 93653, 93654, 93656)

⊘ **93602**   Intra-atrial recording

(Do not report 93602 in conjunction with 93619, 93620, 93653, 93654, 93656)

⊘ **93603**   Right ventricular recording

(Do not report 93603 in conjunction with 93619, 93620, 93653, 93654, 93656)

+ **93609**   Intraventricular and/or intra-atrial mapping of tachycardia site(s) with catheter manipulation to record from multiple sites to identify origin of tachycardia (List separately in addition to code for primary procedure)

(Use 93609 in conjunction with 93620, 93653, 93656)

(Do not report 93609 in conjunction with 93613, 93654)

⊘ **93610**   Intra-atrial pacing

(Do not report 93610 in conjunction with 93619, 93620, 93653, 93654, 93656)

⊘ **93612**   Intraventricular pacing

(Do not report 93612 in conjunction with 93619, 93620, 93621, 93622, 93653, 93654, 93656)

+ **93613**   Intracardiac electrophysiologic 3-dimensional mapping (List separately in addition to code for primary procedure)

(Use 93613 in conjunction with 93620, 93653, 93656)

(Do not report 93613 in addition to 93609, 93654)

⊘ **93615**   Esophageal recording of atrial electrogram with or without ventricular electrogram(s);

⊘ **93616**   with pacing

⊘ **93618**   Induction of arrhythmia by electrical pacing

(Do not report 93618 in conjunction with 93619, 93620, 93621, 93622, 93653, 93654, 93656)

(For intracardiac phonocardiogram, use 93799)

93619   Comprehensive electrophysiologic evaluation with right atrial pacing and recording, right ventricular pacing and recording, His bundle recording, including insertion and repositioning of multiple electrode catheters without induction or attempted induction of arrhythmia

(Do not report 93619 in conjunction with 93600, 93602, 93603, 93610, 93612, 93618, 93620, 93621, 93622, 93653, 93654, 93655, 93656, 93657)

93620   Comprehensive electrophysiologic evaluation including insertion and repositioning of multiple electrode catheters with induction or attempted induction of arrhythmia; with right atrial pacing and recording, right ventricular pacing and recording, His bundle recording

(Do not report 93620 in conjunction with 93600, 93602, 93603, 93610, 93612, 93618, 93619, 93653, 93654, 93655, 93656, 93657)

+ 93621   with left atrial pacing and recording from coronary sinus or left atrium (List separately in addition to code for primary procedure)

(Use 93621 in conjunction with 93620, 93653, 93654)

(Do not report 93621 in conjunction with 93656)

+ 93622   with left ventricular pacing and recording (List separately in addition to code for primary procedure)

(Use 93622 in conjunction with 93620, 93653, 93654)

(Do not report 93622 in conjunction with 93654)

+ 93623 Programmed stimulation and pacing after intravenous drug infusion (List separately in addition to code for primary procedure)

(Use 93623 in conjunction with 93610, 93612, 93619, 93620, 93653, 93654, 93656)

(Do not report 93623 more than once per day)

93624 Electrophysiologic follow-up study with pacing and recording to test effectiveness of therapy, including induction or attempted induction of arrhythmia

93631 Intra-operative epicardial and endocardial pacing and mapping to localize the site of tachycardia or zone of slow conduction for surgical correction

(For operative ablation of an arrhythmogenic focus or pathway by a separate individual, see 33250-33261)

93640 Electrophysiologic evaluation of single or dual chamber pacing cardioverter-defibrillator leads including defibrillation threshold evaluation (induction of arrhythmia, evaluation of sensing and pacing for arrhythmia termination) at time of initial implantation or replacement;

93641   with testing of single or dual chamber pacing cardioverter-defibrillator pulse generator

(For subsequent or periodic electronic analysis and/or reprogramming of single or dual chamber pacing cardioverter-defibrillators, see 93282, 93283, 93289, 93292, 93295, 93642)

93642 Electrophysiologic evaluation of single or dual chamber transvenous pacing defibrillator (includes defibrillation threshold evaluation, induction of arrhythmia, evaluation of sensing and pacing for arrhythmia termination, and programming or reprogramming of sensing or therapeutic parameters)

93644 Electrophysiologic evaluation of subcutaneous implantable defibrillator (includes defibrillation threshold evaluation, induction of arrhythmia, evaluation of sensing for arrhythmia termination, and programming or reprogramming of sensing or therapeutic parameters)

(Do not report 93644 in conjunction with 33270 at the time of subcutaneous implantable defibrillator device insertion)

(For subsequent electrophysiologic evaluation of a subcutaneous implantable defibrillator device, see 93260, 93261)

(For electrophysiological evaluation of subcutaneous implantable defibrillator system, with substernal electrode, use 0577T)

93650 Intracardiac catheter ablation of atrioventricular node function, atrioventricular conduction for creation of complete heart block, with or without temporary pacemaker placement

93653 Comprehensive electrophysiologic evaluation including insertion and repositioning of multiple electrode catheters with induction or attempted induction of an arrhythmia with right atrial pacing and recording, right ventricular pacing and recording (when necessary), and His recording (when necessary) with intracardiac catheter ablation of arrhythmogenic focus; with treatment of supraventricular tachycardia by ablation of fast or slow atrioventricular pathway, accessory atrioventricular connection, cavo-tricuspid isthmus or other single atrial focus or source of atrial re-entry.

(Do not report 93653 in conjunction with 93600-93603, 93610, 93612, 93618-93620, 93642, 93654, 93656)

93654   with treatment of ventricular tachycardia or focus of ventricular ectopy including intracardiac electrophysiologic 3D mapping, when performed, and left ventricular pacing and recording, when performed

(Do not report 93654 in conjunction with 93279-93284, 93286-93289, 93600-93603, 93609, 93610, 93612, 93613, 93618-93620, 93622, 93642, 93653, 93656)

+ 93655   Intracardiac catheter ablation of a discrete mechanism of arrhythmia which is distinct from the primary ablated mechanism, including repeat diagnostic maneuvers, to treat a spontaneous or induced arrhythmia (List separately in addition to code for primary procedure)

(Use 93655 in conjunction with 93653, 93654, 93656)

93656   Comprehensive electrophysiologic evaluation including transseptal catheterizations, insertion and repositioning of multiple electrode catheters with induction or attempted induction of an arrhythmia including left or right atrial pacing/recording when necessary, right ventricular pacing/recording when necessary, and His bundle recording when necessary with intracardiac catheter ablation of atrial fibrillation by pulmonary vein isolation

(Do not report 93656 in conjunction with 93279-93284, 93286-93289, 93462, 93600, 93602, 93603, 93610, 93612, 93618, 93619, 93620, 93621, 93653, 93654)

+ 93657   Additional linear or focal intracardiac catheter ablation of the left or right atrium for treatment of atrial fibrillation remaining after completion of pulmonary vein isolation (List separately in addition to code for primary procedure)

(Use 93657 in conjunction with 93656)

93660   Evaluation of cardiovascular function with tilt table evaluation, with continuous ECG monitoring and intermittent blood pressure monitoring, with or without pharmacological intervention

(For testing of autonomic nervous system function, see 95921, 95924, 95943)

+ 93662   Intracardiac echocardiography during therapeutic/diagnostic intervention, including imaging supervision and interpretation (List separately in addition to code for primary procedure)

(Use 93662 in conjunction with 92987, 93453, 93460-93462, 93532, 93580, 93581, 93620, 93621, 93622, 93653, 93654, 93656 as appropriate)

(Do not report 93662 in conjunction with 92961, 0569T, 0570T, 0613T)

PERIPHERAL ARTERIAL DISEASE REHABILITATION

Peripheral arterial disease (PAD) rehabilitative physical exercise consists of a series of sessions, lasting 45-60 minutes per session, involving use of either a motorized treadmill or a track to permit each patient to achieve symptom-limited claudication. Each session is supervised by an exercise physiologist or nurse. The supervising provider monitors the individual patient's claudication threshold and other cardiovascular limitations for adjustment of workload. During this supervised rehabilitation program, the development of new arrhythmias, symptoms that might suggest angina or the continued inability of the patient to progress to an adequate level of exercise may require review and examination of the patient by a physician or other qualified health care professional. These services would be separately reported with an appropriate level E/M service code including office or other outpatient services (99202- 99215), initial hospital care (99221-99223), subsequent hospital care (99231-99233), critical care services (99291-99292).

93668   Peripheral arterial disease (PAD) rehabilitation, per session

NONINVASIVE PHYSIOLOGIC STUDIES AND PROCEDURES

(For arterial cannulization and recording of direct arterial pressure, use 36620)

(For radiographic injection procedures, see 36000-36299)

(For vascular cannulization for hemodialysis, see 36800-36821)

(For chemotherapy for malignant disease, see 96409-96549)

(For penile plethysmography, use 54240)

93701 Bioimpedance-derived physiologic cardiovascular analysis

(For bioelectrical impedance analysis whole body composition, use 0358T. For left ventricular filling pressure indirect measurement by computerized calibration of the arterial waveform response to Valsalva, use 93799)

93702 Bioimpedance spectroscopy (BIS), extracellular fluid analysis for lymphedema assessment(s)

(For bioelectrical impedance analysis whole body composition, use 0358T)

(For bioimpedance-derived physiological cardiovascular analysis, use 93701)

93724 Electronic analysis of antitachycardia pacemaker system (includes electrocardiographic recording, programming of device, induction and termination of tachycardia via implanted pacemaker, and interpretation of recordings)

93740 Temperature gradient studies

93745 Initial set-up and programming by a physician or other qualified health care professional of wearable cardioverter-defibrillator includes initial programming of system, establishing baseline electronic ECG, transmission of data to data repository, patient instruction in wearing system and patient reporting of problems or events

(Do not report 93745 in conjunction with 93282, 93292)

93750 Interrogation of ventricular assist device (VAD), in person, with physician or other qualified health care professional analysis of device parameters (eg, drivelines, alarms, power surges), review of device function (eg, flow and volume status, septum status, recovery), with programming, if performed, and report

(Do not report 93750 in conjunction with 33975, 33976, 33979, 33981-33983)

(93760, 93762 have been deleted)

93770 Determination of venous pressure

(For central venous cannulization see 36555-36556, 36500)

93784 Ambulatory blood pressure monitoring, utilizing reportgenerating software, automated, worn continuously for 24 hours or longer; including recording, scanning analysis, interpretation and report

93786 recording only

93788 scanning analysis with report

93790 review with interpretation and report

(For self measured blood pressure monitoring, see 99473, 99474)

HOME AND OUTPATIENT INTERNATIONAL NORMALIZED RATIO (INR) MONITORING SERVICES

Home and outpatient international normalized ratio (INR) monitoring services describe the management of warfarin therapy, including ordering, review, and interpretation of new INR test result(s), patient instructions, and dosage adjustments as needed.

If a significantly, separately identifiable evaluation and management (E/M) service is performed on the same day as 93792, the appropriate E/M service may be reported using modifier 25.

Do not report 93793 on the same day as an E/M service.

● New Code ▲ Revised Code + Add-On Code ⊘ Modifier -51 Exempt ★ Telemedicine

Do not report 93792, 93793 in conjunction with 98966, 98967, 98968, 98970, 98971, 98972, 99421, 99422, 99423, 99441, 99442, 99443, when telephone or online digital evaluation and management services address home and outpatient INR monitoring.

Do not count time spent in 93792, 93793 in the time of 99439, 99487, 99489, 99490, 99491, when reported in the same calendar month.

93792 Patient/caregiver training for initiation of home international normalized ratio (INR) monitoring under the direction of a physician or other qualified health care professional, face-to-face, including use and care of the INR monitor, obtaining blood sample, instructions for reporting home INR test results, and documentation of patient's/caregiver's ability to perform testing and report results

(For provision of test materials and equipment for home INR monitoring, see 99070 or the appropriate supply code)

93793 Anticoagulant management for a patient taking warfarin, must include review and interpretation of a new home, office, or lab international normalized ratio (INR) test result, patient instructions, dosage adjustment (as needed), and scheduling of additional test(s), when performed

(Do not report 93793 in conjunction with 99202, 99203, 99204, 99205, 99211, 99212, 99213, 99214, 99215, 99241, 99242, 99243, 99244, 99245)

(Report 93793 no more than once per day, regardless of the number of tests reviewed)

OTHER PROCEDURES

93797 Physician or other qualified health care professional services for outpatient cardiac rehabilitation; without continuous ECG monitoring (per session)

93798 with continuous ECG monitoring (per session)

93799 Unlisted cardiovascular service or procedure

NON-INVASIVE VASCULAR DIAGNOSTIC STUDIES

Vascular studies refers to diagnostic procedures performed to determine blood flow and/or the condition of arteries and/or veins. Vascular studies include patient care required to perform the studies, supervision of the studies and interpretation of the study results with copies for patient records of hard copy output with analysis of all data, including bi-directional vascular flow or imaging when provided.

The use of a simple hand-held or other Doppler device that does not produce hard copy output, or that produces a record that does not permit analysis of bi-directional vascular flow, is considered to be part of the physical examination of the vascular system and is not reported separately. To report unilateral non-invasive diagnostic studies, add modifier -52 to the basic code.

Coding Rules

1. *Non-invasive vascular studies are usually performed in addition to evaluation and management service, such as a consultation or visit, and should be reported separately in addition to the evaluation and management service.*

2. *All of the non-invasive vascular services fall under the Medicare Purchased Diagnostic Services guidelines; therefore, reporting should be as instructed by your local Medicare carrier.*

The use of a simple hand-held or other Doppler device that does not produce hard copy output, or that produces a record that does not permit analysis of bidirectional vascular flow, is considered to be part of the physical examination of the vascular system and is not separately reported. The Ankle-Brachial Index (or ABI) is reportable with 93922 or 93923 as logn as simultaneous Doppler recording and analysis of bidirectional blood flow, volume plethysmography, or transcutaneous oxygen tension measurements are also performed.

Duplex scan (eg., 93880, 93882) describes an ultrasonic scanning procedure for characterizing the pattern and direction of blood flow in arteries or veins with the production of real-time images integrating B-mode two-dimensional vascular structure, Doppler spectral analysis and color flow Doppler imaging.

Physiologic studies: Noninvasive physiologic studies are performed using equipment separate and distinct from the duplex ultrasound imager. Codes 93922, 93923, 93924 describe the evaluation of non-imaging physiologic recordings of pressures with Doppler analysis of bi-directional blood flow, plethysmography, and/or oxygen tension measurements appropriate for the anatomic area studied.

CEREBROVASCULAR ARTERIAL STUDIES

A complete transcranial Doppler (TCD) study (93886) includes ultrasound evaluation of the right and left anterior circulation territories and the posterior circulation territory (to include vertebral arteries and basilar artery). In a limited TCD study (93888) there is ultrasound evaluation of two or fewer of these territories. For TCD, ultrasound evaluation is a reasonable and concerted attempt to identify arterial signals through an acoustic window.

Code 93895 includes the acquisition and storage of images of the common carotid arteries, carotid bulbs, and internal carotid arteries bilaterally with quantification of intima media thickness (common carotid artery mean and maximal values) and determination of presence of atherosclerotic plaque.

93880 Duplex scan of extracranial arteries; complete bilateral study

(Do not report 93880 in conjunction with 93895)

93882 unilateral or limited study

(Do not report 93882 in conjunction with 93895)

(To report common carotid intima-media thickness (IMT) study for evaluation of atherosclerotic burden or coronary heart disease risk factor assessment, use Category III code 0126T)

93886 Transcranial Doppler study of the intracranial arteries; complete study

93888 limited study

93890 vasoreactivity study

93892 emboli detection without intravenous microbubble injection

93893 emboli detection with intravenous microbubble injection

93895 Quantitative carotid intima media thickness and carotid atheroma evaluation, bilateral

(Do not report 93895 in conjunction with 93880, 93882)

(Do not report 93890-93893 in conjunction with 93888)

EXTREMITY ARTERIAL STUDIES (INCLUDING DIGITS)

93922 Limited bilateral non-invasive physiologic studies of upper or lower extremity arteries, (eg, for lower extremity: ankle/brachial indices at distal posterior tibial and anterior tibial/dorsalis pedis arteries plus bidirectional, Doppler waveform recording and analysis at 1-2 levels, or ankle/brachial indices at distal posterior tibial and anterior tibial/dorsalis pedis arteries plus volume plethysmography at 1-2 levels, or ankle/brachial indices at distal posterior tibial and anterior tibial/dorsalis pedis arteries with transcutaneous oxygen tension measurements at 1-2 levels)

(When only 1 arm or leg is available for study, report 93922 with modifier 52 for a unilateal study when recording 1-2 levels. Report 93922 when recording 3 or more levels or performing provocative functional maneuvers.)

(Report 93922 only once in the upper extremity(s) and/or once in the lower extremity(s). When both the upper and lower extremities are evaluated in the same setting, 93922 may be reported twice by adding modifier 59 to the second procedure)

(For transcutaneous oxyhemoglobin measurement in a lower extremity wound by near infrared spectroscopy, use 0493T)

(For transcutaneous visible light hyperspectral imaging measurement of oxyhemoglobin, deoxyhemoglobin, and tissue oxygenation, use 0631T)

93923 Complete bilateral non-invasive physiologic studies of upper or lower extremity arteries, 3 or more levels (eg, for lower extremity: ankle/brachial indices at distal posterior tibial and anterior tibial/dorsalis pedis arteries plus segmental blood pressure measurements with bidirectional Doppler waveform recording and analysis, at 3 or more levels, or ankle/brachial indices at distal posterior tibial and anterior tibial/dorsalis pedis arteries plus segmental volume plethysmography at 3 or more levels, or ankle/brachial indices at distal posterior tibial and anterior tibial/dorsalis pedis arteries plus segmental transcutaneous oxygen tension measurements at 3 or more levels), or single level study—with provocative functional maneuvers (eg, measurements with postural provocative tests or measurements with reactive hyperemia)

(When only 1 arm or leg is available for study, report 93922 for a unilateral study when recording 3 or more levels or when performing provocative functional maneuvers.)

(Report 93923 only once in the upper extremity(s) and/or once in the lower extremity(s). When both the upper and lower extremities are evaluated in the same setting, 93923 may be reported twice by adding modifier 59 to the second procedure.)

(For transcutaneous visible light hyperspectral imaging measurement of oxyhemoglobin, deoxyhemoglobin, and tissue oxygenation, use 0631T)

93924 Non-invasive physiologic studies of lower extremity arteries, at rest and following treadmill stress testing, (ie, bidirectional Doppler waveform or volume plethysmography recording and analysis at rest with ankle/brachial indices immediately after and at timed intervals following performance of a standardized protocol on a motorized treadmill plus recording of time of onset of claudication or other symptoms, maximal walking time, and time to recovery) complete bilateral study

(Do not report 93924 in conjunction with 93922, 93923)

93925 Duplex scan of lower extremity arteries or arterial bypass grafts; complete bilateral study

(Do not report 93925 in conjunction with 93985 for the same extremities)

93926 unilateral or limited study

(Do not report 93926 in conjunction with 93986 for the same extremity)

93930 Duplex scan of upper extremity arteries or arterial bypass grafts; complete bilateral study

(Do not report 93930 in conjunction with 93985, 93986 for the same extremity[ies])

93931 unilateral or limited study

(Do not report 93931 in conjunction with 93985, 93986 for the same extremity)

EXTREMITY VENOUS STUDIES (INCLUDING DIGITS)

93970 Duplex scan of extremity veins including responses to compression and other maneuvers; complete bilateral study

(Do not report 93970 in conjunction with 93985, 93986 for the same extremity[ies])

93971 unilateral or limited study

(Do not report 93970, 93971 in conjunction with 364745, 36476, 36478, 36479)

(Do not report 93971 in conjunction with 93985, 93986 for the same extremity)

VISCERAL AND PENILE VASCULAR STUDIES

93975 Duplex scan of arterial inflow and venous outflow of abdominal, pelvic, scrotal contents and/or retroperitoneal organs; complete study

93976 limited study

93978   Duplex scan of aorta, inferior vena cava, iliac vasculature, or bypass grafts; complete study

93979   unilateral or limited study

   (For ultrasound screening study for abdominal aortic aneurysm [AAA], real time with image documentation, use 76706)

93980   Duplex scan of arterial inflow and venous outflow of penile vessels; complete study

93981   follow-up or limited study

(**93982**   deleted 2017 [2018 edition])

EXTREMITY ARTERIAL-VENOUS STUDIES

A complete extremity duplex scan (93985, 93986) includes evaluation of both arterial inflow and venous outflow for preoperative vessel assessment prior to creation of hemodialysis access. If only an arterial extremity duplex scan is performed, see 93925, 93926, 93930, 93931. If only a venous extremity duplex scan is performed, see 93970, 93971. If a physiologic arterial evaluation of extremities is performed, see 93922, 93923, 93924.

93985   Duplex scan of arterial inflow and venous outflow for preoperative vessel assessment prior to creation of hemodialysis access; complete bilateral study

   (Do not report 93985 in conjunction with 93925, 93930, 93970 for the same extremity[ies])

   (Do not report 93985 in conjunction with 93990 for the same extremity)

93986   complete unilateral study

   (Do not report 93986 in conjunction with 93926, 93931, 93971, 93990 for the same extremity)

93990   Duplex scan of hemodialysis access (including arterial inflow, body of access and venous outflow)

   (For measurement of hemodialysis access flow using indicator dilution methods, use 90940)

OTHER NONINVASIVE VASCULAR DIAGNOSTIC STUDIES

93998   Unlisted noninvasive vascular diagnostic study

PULMONARY

Pulmonary disease is concerned with diseases of the lungs and airways. The Pulmonologist diagnoses and treats pneumonia, cancer, pleurisy, asthma, occupational diseases, bronchitis, sleep disorders, emphysema, and other complex disorders of the lungs. Pulmonologists test lung functions in many ways, endoscope the bronchial airways and prescribe and monitor mechanical assistance to ventilation. Many pulmonary disease physicians are also expert in critical care.

Pulmonary services refer to diagnostic procedures performed to determine air flow, blood gases, and the condition of the lungs and respiratory system. Pulmonary services include the laboratory procedure(s), interpretation, and physician's services (except surgical and anesthesia services) unless otherwise stated. It is common for pulmonologists to provide interpretation services only, under contract to medical facilities.

CPT coding for pulmonary function tests includes both comprehensive and component codes to accommodate variation among pulmonary function laboratories. As a result of these code combinations, several issues are addressed in this policy section.

Alternate methods of reporting data obtained during a spirometry or other pulmonary function session cannot be separately reported. Specifically, the flow volume loop is an alternative method of calculating a standard spirometric parameter. The CPT code 94375 is included in standard spirometry (rest and exercise) studies.

When a physician who is in attendance for a pulmonary function study, obtains a limited history, and performs a limited examination referable specifically to the pulmonary function testing, separately coding for an evaluation and management service is not appropriate. If a significant, separately identifiable service is performed unrelated to the technical performance of the pulmonary function test, an evaluation and management service may be reported.

● New Code   ▲ Revised Code   ✚ Add-On Code   ⊘ Modifier -51 Exempt   ★ Telemedicine

When multiple spirometric determinations are necessary (e.g. CPT code 94070) to complete the service described in the CPT code, only one unit of service is reported.

Complex pulmonary stress testing (e.g. CPT code 94621) is a comprehensive stress test with a number of component tests separately defined in the CPT code book. It is inappropriate to separately code venous access, EKG monitoring, spirometric parameters performed before, during and after exercise, oximetry, O2 consumption, CO2 production, rebreathing cardiac output calculations, etc., when performed as part of a complex pulmonary stress test. It is also inappropriate to bill for a cardiac stress test and the component codes used to perform a simple pulmonary stress test (CPT code 94620), when a complex pulmonary stress test is performed. If using a standard exercise protocol, serial electrocardiograms are obtained, and a separate report describing a cardiac stress test (professional component) is included in the medical record, the professional components for both a cardiac and pulmonary stress test may be reported. Modifier -59 should be reported with the secondary procedure. Both tests must satisfy the requirement for medical necessity. (Since a complex pulmonary stress test includes electrocardiographic recordings, the technical components for both the cardiac stress test and the pulmonary stress test should not be reported separately.)

VENTILATOR MANAGEMENT

94002 Ventilation assist and management, initiation of pressure or volume preset ventilators for assisted or controlled breathing; hospital inpatient/observation, initial day

94003   hospital inpatient/observation, each subsequent day

94004   nursing facility, per day

(Do not report 94002-94004 in conjunction with evaluation and management services 99202-99499)

94005 Home ventilator management care plan oversight of a patient (patient not present) in home, domiciliary or rest home (eg, assisted living) requiring review of status, review of laboratories and other studies and revision of orders and respiratory care plan (as appropriate),within a calendar month, 30 min. or more

(Do not report 94005 in conjunction with 99339-99340, 99374-99378)

(Ventilator management care plan oversight is reported separately from home or domiciliary, rest home [eg., assisted living] services. A physician or other qualified health care professional may report 94005, when performed, including when a different Individual reports 99339, 99340, 99374-99378 for the same 30 days)

PULMONARY DIAGNOSTIC TESTING AND THERAPIES

Codes 94010-94799 include laboratory procedure(s) and interpretation of test results. If a separate identifiable evaluation and management service is performed, the appropriate E/M service code including new or established patient office or other outpatient services (99202-99215), office or other outpatient consultations (99241-99245), emergency department services (99281-99285), nursing facility services (99304-99318), domiciliary, rest home, or custodial care services (99324-99337), and home services (99341-99350) may be reported in addition to 94010-94799.

Spirometry (94010) measures expiratory airflow and volumes and forms the basis of most pulmonary function testing. When spirometry is performed before and after administration of a bronchodilator, report 94060. Measurement of vital capacity (94150) is a component of spirometry and is only reported when performed alone. The flow-volume loop (94375) is used to identify patterns of inspiratory and/or expiratory obstruction in central or peripheral airways. Spirometry (94010, 94060) includes maximal breathing capacity (94200) and flow-volume loop (94375), when performed.

Measurement of lung volumes may be performed using plethysmography, helium dilution or nitrogen washout. Plethysmography (94726) is utilized to determine total lung capacity, residual volume, functional residual capacity, and airway resistance. Nitrogen washout or helium dilution (94727) may be used to measure lung volumes, distribution of ventilation and closing volume. Oscillometry (94728) assesses airway resistance and may be reported in addition to gas dilution techniques. Spirometry (94010, 94060) and bronchial provocation (94070) are not included in 94726 and 94727 and maybe reported separately.

Diffusing capacity (94729) is most commonly performed in conjunction with lung volumes or spirometry and is an add-on code to 94726-94728, 94010, 94060, 94070, and 94375.

Pulmonary function tests (94011-94013) are reported for measurements in infants and young children though 2 years of age.

| | Separate Procedure | | Unlisted Procedure | | CCI Comp. Code | | Non-specific Procedure | **929** |

Pulmonary function testing measurements are reported as actual values and as a percent of predicted values by age, gender, height and race.

Chest wall manipulation for the mobilization of secretions and improvement in lung function can be performed using manual (94667, 94668) or mechanical (94669) methods. Manual techniiques include cupping, percussing, and use of a hand-held vibration device. A mechanical technique is the application of an external vest or wrap that delivers mechanical oscillation.

94010 Spirometry, including graphic record, total and timed vital capacity, expiratory flow rate measurement(s), with or without maximal voluntary ventilation

(Do not report 94010 in conjunction with 94150, 94200, 94375, 94728)

94011 Measurement of spirometric forced expiratory flows in an infant or child through 2 years of age

94012 Measurement of spirometric forced expiratory flows, before and after bronchodilator, in an infant or child through 2 years of age

94013 Measurement of lung volumes (ie, functional residual capacity [FRC], forced vital capacity [FVC], and expiratory reserve volume [ERV]) in an infant or child through 2 years of age

94014 Patient-initiated spirometric recording per 30-day period of time; includes reinforced education, transmission of spirometric tracing, data capture, analysis of transmitted data, periodic recalibration, and review and interpretation by a physician or other qualified health care professional

94015 recording (includes hook-up, reinforced education, data transmission, data capture, trend analysis, and periodic recalibration)

94016 review and interpretation only by a physician or other qualified health care professional

94060 Bronchodilation responsiveness, spirometry as in 94010, pre- and post-bronchodilator administration

(Do not report 94060 in conjunction with 94150, 94200, 94375, 94640, 94728)

(Report bronchodilator supply separately with 99070 or appropriate supply code)

(For exercise test for bronchospasm with pre- and postspirometry, see 94617, 94619)

94070 Bronchospasm provocation evaluation, multiple spirometric determinations as in 94010, with administered agents (eg, antigen(s), cold air, methacholine)

(Do not report 94070 in conjunction with 94640)

(Report antigen(s) administration separately with 99070 or appropriate supply code)

94150 Vital capacity, total (separate procedure)

(Do not report 94150 in conjunction with 94010, 94060, 94728. To report thoracic gas volumes, see 94726, 94727)

94200 Maximum breathing capacity, maximal voluntary ventilation

(Do not report 94200 in conjunction with 94010, 94060)

(**94250** deleted 2020 [2021 Edition])

94375 Respiratory flow volume loop

(Do not report 94375 in conjunction with 94010, 94060)

(**94400** deleted 2020 [2021 Edition])

94450 Breathing response to hypoxia (hypoxia response curve)

(For high altitude simulation test (HAST), see 94452, 94453)

● New Code ▲ Revised Code ✚ Add-On Code ⊘ Modifier -51 Exempt ★ Telemedicine

94452 High altitude simulation test (HAST), with interpretation and report by a physician or other qualified health care professional;

(For obtaining arterial blood gases, use 36600)

(Do not report 94452 in conjunction with 94453, 94760, 94761)

94453 with supplemental oxygen titration

(For obtaining arterial blood gases, use 36600)

(Do not report 94453 in conjunction with 94452, 94760, 94761)

⊘ **94610** Intrapulmonary surfactant administration by a physician or other qualified health care professional through endotracheal tube

(Do not report 94610 in conjunction with 99468-99472)

(For endotracheal intubation, use 31500)

(Report 94610 once per dosing episode)

▲ **94617** Exercise test for bronchospasm, including pre- and postspirometry and pulse oximetry; with electrocardiographic recording(s)

● **94619** without electrocardiographic recording(s)

94618 Pulmonary stress testing (eg, 6-minute walk test), including measurement of heart rate, oximetry, and oxygen titration, when performed

94619 This code is out of order. See page 931

(**94620** deleted 2017 [2018 edition]. To report pulmonary stress testing, use 94618)

94621 Cardiopulmonary exercise testing, including measurements of minute ventilation, CO2 production, O2 uptake, and electrocardiographic recordings

(Do not report 94617, 94619, 94621 in conjunction with 93000, 93005, 93010, 93040, 93041, 93042 for ECG monitoring performed during the same session)

(Do not report 94617, 94619, 94621 in conjunction with 93015, 93016, 93017, 93018)

(Do not report 94621 in conjunction with 94680, 94681, 94690)

(Do not report 94617, 94618, 94619, 94621 in conjunction with 94760, 94761)

94640 Pressurized or nonpressurized inhalation treatment for acute airway obstruction for therapeutic purposes and/or for diagnostic purposes such as sputum induction with an aerosol generator, nebulizer, metered dose inhaler or intermittent positive pressure breathing (IPPB) device

(Do not report 94640 in conjunction with 94060, 94070)

(For more than one inhalation treatment performed on the same date, append modifier -76)

(For continuous inhalation treatment of 1 hour or more, see 94644, 94645)

94642 Aerosol inhalation of pentamidine for pneumocystis carinii pneumonia treatment or prophylaxis

94644 Continuous inhalation treatment with aerosol medication for acute airway obstruction; first hour

(For services of less than 1 hour, use 94640)

+ **94645** each additional hour (List separately in addition to code for primary procedure)

(Use 94645 in conjunction with 94644)

94660 Continuous positive airway pressure ventilation (CPAP), initiation and management

94662 Continuous negative pressure ventilation (CNP), initiation and management

94664 Demonstration and/or evaluation of patient utilization of an aerosol generator, nebulizer, metered dose inhaler or IPPB device

(94664 can be reported one time only per day of service)

94667 Manipulation chest wall, such as cupping, percussing, and vibration to facilitate lung function; initial demonstration and/or evaluation

94668 subsequent

94669 Mechanical chest wall oscillation to facilitate lung function, per session

94680 Oxygen uptake, expired gas analysis; rest and exercise, direct, simple

94681 including CO_2 output, percentage oxygen extracted

94690 rest, indirect (separate procedure)

(For single arterial puncture, use 36600)

(Do not report 94680, 94681, 94690 in conjunction with 94621)

94726 Plethysmography for determination of lung volumes and, when performed, airway resistance

(Do not report 94726 in conjunction with 94727, 94728)

94727 Gas dilution or washout for determination of lung volumes and, when performed, distribution of ventilation and closing volumes

(Do not report 94727 in conjunction with 94726)

94728 Airway resistance by oscillometry

(Do not report 94728 in conjunction with 94010, 94060, 94070, 94375, 94726)

+ **94729** Diffusing capacity (eg, carbon monoxide, membrane) (List separately in addition to code for primary procedure)

(Report 94729 in conjunction with 94010, 94060, 94070, 94375, 94726-94728)

(**94750** deleted 2020 [2021 Edition]) ·

94760 Noninvasive ear or pulse oximetry for oxygen saturation; single determination

(For blood gases, see 82803-82810)

94761 multiple determinations (eg, during exercise)

(Do not report 94760, 94761 in conjunction with 94617, 94618, 94619, 94621)

94762 by continuous overnight monitoring (separate procedure)

(For other in vivo laboratory procedures, see 88720-88741)

(**94770** deleted 2020 [2021 Edition])

94772 Circadian respiratory pattern recording (pediatric pneumogram), 12 to 24 hour continuous recording, infant

(Separate procedure codes for electromyograms, EEG, ECG, and recordings of respiration are excluded when 94772 is reported)

● New Code   ▲ Revised Code   ✛ Add-On Code   ⊘ Modifier -51 Exempt   ★ Telemedicine

94774   Pediatric home apnea monitoring event recording including respiratory rate, pattern and heart rate per 30-day period of time; includes monitor attachment, download of data, review, interpretation, and preparation of a report by a physician or other qualified health care professional

     (Do not report 94774 in conjunction with 94775-94777 during the same reporting period)

94775   monitor attachment only (includes hook-up, initiation of recording and disconnection)

94776   monitoring, download of information, receipt of transmission(s) and analyses by computer only

94777   review, interpretation and preparation of report only by a physician or other qualified health care professional

     (When oxygen saturation monitoring is used in addition to heart rate and respiratory monitoring, it is not reported separately)

     (Do not report 94774-94777 in conjunction with 93224-93272)

     (Do not report apnea recording device separately)

     (For sleep study, see 95805-95811)

94780   Car seat/bed testing for airway integrity, for infants through 12 months of age, with continual clinical staff observation and continuous recording of pulse oximetry, heart rate and respiratory rate, with interpretation and report; 60 minutes

     (Do not report 94780 for less than 60 minutes)

     (Do not report 94780 in conjunction with 93040-93042, 94760, 94761, 99468-99472, 99477-99480)

+ 94781   each additional full 30 minutes (List separately in addition to code for primary procedure)

     (Use 94781 in conjunction with 94780)

94799   Unlisted pulmonary service or procedure

ALLERGY AND CLINICAL IMMUNOLOGY

Allergy and Immunology refers to diagnostic services performed to determine a patient's sensitivity to specific substances, the treatment of patients with allergens by the administration or allergenic extracts, and/or medical conference services.

The CPT coding system divides allergy and clinical immunology into testing and immunotherapy. Immunotherapy is divided into codes that include preparation of the antigen when it is administered at the same session and when it is prepared but delivered for immunotherapy by a different physician. Several specific issues are identified regarding allergy testing and immunotherapy.

If percutaneous or intracutaneous (intradermal)single test (CPT codes 95004 or 95024) and "sequential and incremental" tests (CPT codes 95010, 95015, or 95027) are performed on the same date of service, both the "sequential and incremental" test and single test codes may be reported if the tests are for different allergens or different dilutions of the same allergen. The unit of service to report is the number of separate tests. Do not report both a single test and a sequential and incremental test for the same dilution of an allergen. For example, if the single test for an antigen is positive and the provider proceeds to sequential and incremental tests with three additional different dilutions of the same antigen, the provider may report one unit of service for the single test code and three units of service for the sequential and incremental test code.

When photo patch tests (e.g. CPT code 95052) are performed (same antigen/same session) with patch or application tests, only the photo patch testing should be reported. Additionally, if photo testing is performed including application or patch testing, the code for photo patch testing (CPT code 95052) is to be reported, not CPT code 95044 (patch or application tests) and CPT code 95056 (photo tests).

Evaluation and management codes reported with allergy testing or allergy immunotherapy are appropriate only if a significant, separately identifiable service is administered. Obtaining informed consent, is included in the immunotherapy. If E & M services are reported, medical documentation of the separately identifiable service should be in the medical record.

     Separate Procedure   Unlisted Procedure   CCI Comp. Code   Non-specific Procedure   **933**

Allergy testing is not performed on the same day as allergy immunotherapy in standard medical practice. These codes should, therefore, not be reported together. Additionally, the testing becomes an integral part to rapid desensitization kits (CPT code 95180) and would therefore not be reported separately.

Do not report evaluation and management (E/M) services for test interpretation and report. If a significant separately identifiable E/M service is performed, the appropriate E/M service code, which may include new or established patient office or other outpatient services (99202-99215), hospital observation services (99217-99220, 99224-99226), hospital care (99221-99223, 99231-99233), consultations (99241-99255), emergency department services (99281-99285), nursing facility services (99304-99318), domiciliary, rest home, or custodial care services (99324-99337), home services (99341-99350), or preventive medicine services (99381-99429), should be reported using modifier 25.

ALLERGY TESTING

(For allergy laboratory tests, see 86000-86999)

(For administration of medications [eg, epinephrine, steroidal agents, antihistamines] for therapy for severe or intractable allergic reaction, use 96372)

95004 Percutaneous tests (scratch, puncture, prick) with allergenic extracts, immediate type reaction, including test interpretation and report, specify number of tests

95012 Nitric oxide expired gas determination

95017 Allergy testing, any combination of percutaneous (scratch, puncture, prick) and intracutaneous (intradermal), sequential and incremental, with venoms, immediate type reaction, including test interpretation and report, specify number of tests

95018 Allergy testing, any combination of percutaneous (scratch, puncture, prick) and intracutaneous (intradermal), sequential and incremental, with drugs or biologicals, immediate type reaction, including test interpretation and report, specify number of tests

95024 Intracutaneous (intradermal) tests with allergenic extracts, immediate type reaction, including test interpretation and report, specify number of tests

95027 Intracutaneous (intradermal) tests, sequential and incremental, with allergenic extracts for airborne allergens, immediate type reaction, including test interpretation and report, specify number of tests

95028 Intracutaneous (intradermal) tests with allergenic extracts, delayed type reaction, including reading, specify number of tests

95044 Patch or application test(s) (specify number of tests)

95052 Photo patch test(s) (specify number of tests)

95056 Photo tests

95060 Ophthalmic mucous membrane tests

95065 Direct nasal mucous membrane test

▲ **95070** Inhalation bronchial challenge testing (not including necessary pulmonary function tests), with histamine, methacholine, or similar compounds

(For pulmonary function tests, see 94060, 94070)

(**95071** deleted 2020 [2021 Edition])

INGESTION CHALLENGE TESTING

Codes 95076 and 95079 re used to report ingestion challenge testing. Report 95076 for initial 120 minutes of testing time (ie, not physician face-to-face time). Report 95079 for each additional 60 minutes of testing time (ie, not physician face-to-face time). For

● New Code ▲ Revised Code ✚ Add-On Code ⊘ Modifier -51 Exempt ★ Telemedicine

total testing time less than 61 minutes (eg, positive challenge resulting in cessation of testing), report and evaluation and management service, if appropriate. Patient assessment/monitoring activities for allergic reactin (eg, blood pressure testing, peak flow meter testing) are not separately reported. Intervention therapy (eg, injection of steroid or epinephrine) may be reported separately as appropriate.

For purposes of reporting testing times, if an E/M service is required, then testing time ends.

95076   Ingestion challenge test (sequential and incremental ingestion of test items, eg. food, drug or other substance); initial 120 minutes of testing

+ 95079   each additional 60 minutes of testing (List separately in addition to code for primary procedure

     (Use 95079 in conjunction with 95076)

ALLERGEN IMMUNOTHERAPY

Allergen immunotherapy CPT codes include the professional services necessary for allergen immunotherapy. Evaluation and management service codes may be reported in addition to allergen immunotherapy if other identifiable services are provided at the same time.

Codes 95115-95199 include the professional services necessary for allergen immunotherapy. Office visit codes may be used in addition to allergen immunotherapy if other identifiable services are provided at that time.

95115   Professional services for allergen immunotherapy not including provision of allergenic extracts; single injection

95117   2 or more injections

95120   Professional services for allergen immunotherapy in the office or institution of the prescribing physician or other qualified health care professional, including provision of allergenic extract; single injection

95125   2 or more injections

95130   single stinging insect venom

95131   2 stinging insect venoms

95132   3 stinging insect venoms

95133   4 stinging insect venoms

95134   5 stinging insect venoms

95144   Professional services for the supervision of preparation and provision of antigens for allergen immunotherapy; single dose vials(s) (specify number of vials)

     (A single dose vial contains a single dose of antigen administered in one injection)

95145   Professional services for the supervision of preparation and provision of antigens for allergen immunotherapy (specify number of doses); single stinging insect venom

95146   2 single stinging insect venoms

95147   3 single stinging insect venoms

95148   4 single stinging insect venoms

95149   5 single stinging insect venoms

95165   Professional services for the supervision of preparation and provision of antigens for allergen immunotherapy; single or multiple antigens (specify number of doses)

Separate Procedure	Unlisted Procedure	CCI Comp. Code	Non-specific Procedure

935

95170   whole body extract of biting insect or other arthropod (specify number of doses)

(For allergy immunotherapy reporting, a dose is the amount of antigen(s) administered in a single injection from a multiple dose vial)

95180   Rapid desensitization procedure, each hour (eg, insulin, penicillin, equine serum)

95199   Unlisted allergy/clinical immunologic service or procedure

(For skin testing of bacterial, viral, fungal extracts, see 86485-86580, 95028)

(For special reports on allergy patients, use 99080)

(For testing procedures such as radioallergosorbent testing (RAST), rat mast cell technique (RMCT), mast cell degranulation test (MCDT), lymphocytic transformation test (LTT), leukocyte histamine release (LHR), migration inhibitory factor test (MIF), transfer factor test (TFT), nitroblue tetrazolium dye test (NTD), see Immunology section in Pathology or use 95199)

ENDOCRINOLOGY

Codes 95249 and 95250 are used to report the service for subcutaneous interstitial sensor placement, hook-up of the sensor to the transmitter, calibration of continuous glucose monitoring (CGM) device, patient training on CGM device functions and management, removal of the interstitial sensor, and the print-out of captured data recordings. For the CGM device owned by the physician's or other qualified health care professional's office, use 95250 for the data capture occurring over a minimum period of 72 hours.

Code 95249 may be reported only once during the time that a patient owns a given data receiver, including the initial episode of data collection.

Code 95249 may not be reported for subsequent episodes of data collection, unless the patient obtains a new and/or different model of data receiver. Obtaining a new sensor and/or transmitter without a change in receiver may not be reported with 95249.

Code 95249 may not be reported unless the patient brings the data receiver in to the physician's or other qualified health care professional's office with the entire initial data collection procedure conducted in the physician's or other qualified health care professional's office.

95249   This code is out of order. See page 936

95250   Ambulatory continuous glucose monitoring of interstitial tissue fluid via a subcutaneous sensor for a minimum of 72 hours; physician or other qualified health care professional (office) provided equipment, sensor placement, hook-up, calibration of monitor, patient training, removal of sensor, and printout of recording

(Do not report 95250 more than once per month)

(Do not report 95250 in conjunction with 99091, 0446T)

95249   patient-provided equipment, sensor placement, hookup, calibration of monitor, patient training, and printout of recording

(Do not report 95249 more than once for the duration that the patient owns the data receiver)

(Do not report 95249 in conjunction with 99091, 0446T)

95251   analysis, interpretation and report

(Do not report 95251 more than once per month)

(Do not report 95251 in conjunction with 99091)

NEUROLOGY AND NEUROMUSCULAR PROCEDURES

Neurology refers to the study and treatment of the nervous system. Neurology services are usually performed in conjunction with a medical consultation. The consultation should be reported separately using the appropriate evaluation and management consultation code.

Neurologic services are typically consultative, and any of the levels of consultation (99241-99255) may be appropriate.

The EEG, autonomic function, evoked potential, reflex tests, EMG, NCV, and MEG services (95812-95829 and 95860-95967) include recording, interpretation by a physician, and report. For interpretation only, use modifier 26. For EMG guidance, see 95873, 95874.

The CPT coding system defines codes for neuromuscular diagnostic or therapeutic services not requiring surgical procedures. Sleep testing, nerve and muscle testing and electroencephalographic procedures are included. The CPT code book guidelines regarding sleep testing are very precise and should be reviewed carefully before billing for these services.

Sleep testing differs from polysomnography in that the latter requires the presence of sleep staging. Sleep staging includes a qualitative and quantitative assessment of sleep as determined by standard sleep scoring techniques. Accordingly, at the same session, a "sleep study" and "polysomnography" are not reported together.

Polysomnography requires at least one central and usually several other EEG electrodes. EEG procurement for polysomnography (sleep staging) differs greatly from that required for diagnostic EEG testing (i.e. speed of paper, number of channels, etc.). Accordingly, EEG testing is not to be reported with polysomnography unless performed separately; the EEG tests, if rendered with a separate report, are to be reported with modifier -59, indicating that this represents a different session from the sleep study.

Continuous electroencephalographic monitoring services (CPT codes 95950- 95962) represent different services than those provided during sleep testing; accordingly these codes are only to be reported when a separately identifiable service is performed and documented. Additionally, billing standard EEG services would only be appropriate if a significant, separately identifiable service is provided. These codes are to be reported with modifier -59 to indicate that a different service is clearly documented.

When nerve testing (EMG, nerve conduction velocity, etc.) is performed to assess the level of paralysis during anesthesia or during mechanical ventilation, the series of CPT codes 95851-95937 are not to be separately reported; these codes reflect significant, separately identifiable diagnostic services requiring a formal report in the medical record. Additionally, electrical stimulation used to identify or locate nerves as part of a procedure involving treatment of a cranial or peripheral nerve (e.g. nerve block, nerve destruction, neuroplasty, transection, excision, repair, etc.) is part of the primary procedure.

Intraoperative neurophysiology testing (CPT code 95920) should not be reported by the physician performing an operative procedure since it is included in the global package. However, when performed by a different physician during the procedure, it is separately reportable by the second physician. The physician performing an operative procedure should not bill other 90000 neurophysiology testing codes for intraoperative neurophysiology testing since they are also included in the global package.

The NCCI edit with column one CPT code 95903 (Motor nerve conduction studies with F-wave study, each nerve) and column two CPT code 95900 (Motor nerve conduction studies without F-wave study, each nerve) is often bypassed by utilizing modifier -59. Use of modifier -59 with the column two CPT code 95900 of this NCCI edit is only appropriate if the two procedures are performed on different nerves or in separate patient encounters.

Neurologic services are typically consultative, and any of the levels of consultation (99241-99255) may be appropriate. In addition, services and skills outlined under Evaluation and Management levels of service appropriate to neurologic illnesses should be reported similarly.

The electroencephalogram (EEG), video electroencephalogram (VEEG), autonomic function, evoked potential, reflex tests, electromyography (EMG), nerve conduction velocity (NCV), and magnetoencephalography (MEG) services (95700-95726, 95812-95829, and 95860-95967) include recording, interpretation, and report by a physician or other qualified health care professional. For interpretation only, use modifier 26 with 95812-95829, 95860-95967. For interpretation only for long-term EEG services, report 95717, 95718, 95719, 95720, 95721, 95722, 95723, 95724, 95725, 95726.

Codes 95700-95726 and 95812-95822 use EEG/VEEG recording time as a basis for code use. Recording time is when the recording is underway and diagnostic EEG data is being collected. Recording time excludes set up and take down time. If diagnostic EEG recording is disrupted, recording time stops until diagnostic EEG recording is resumed. Codes 95961-95962 use physician or other qualified health care professional attendance time as a basis for code use.

(Do not report codes 95860-95875 in addition to 96000-96004)

SLEEP MEDICINE TESTING

Polysomnography includes sleep staging that is refined to include a 1-4 lead electroencephalogram (EEG), an electro-oculogram (EOG), and a submental electromyogram (EMG). For a study to be reported as polysomnography, sleep must be recorded and staged. Additional parameters of sleep include:

Electrocardiogram (ECG)

airflow

ventilation and respiratory effort

gas exchange by oximetry, transcutaneous monitoring, or end tidal gas analysis

extremity muscle activity, motor activity-movement

extended EEG monitoring

penile tumescence

gastroesophageal reflux

continuous blood pressure monitoring

snoring

body positions, etc.

For a study to be reported as a polysomnogram:

studies must be performed for 6 hours

sleep must be recorded and staged

an attendant must be present throughout the course of the study

Diagnostic testing is covered when a patient has the symptoms or complaints of one of the following conditions:

Narcolepsy - Narcolepsy is a neurologic disorder of unknown etiology characterized predominantly by abnormalities of REM, some abnormalities of NREM sleep and the presence of excessive daytime sleepiness often with involuntary daytime sleep episodes (e.g., while driving, in the middle of a meal, amnesiac episodes).

Sleep Apnea - Sleep Apnea is defined as a cessation of airflow for at least 10 seconds. These cessations of breathing may be due to either an occlusion of the airway (obstructive sleep apnea), absence of respiratory effort (central sleep apnea), or a combination of these factors (mixed sleep apnea).

Parasomnias - Parasomnias are a group of behavioral disorders during sleep that are associated with brief or partial arousals but not with marked sleep disruption or impaired daytime alertness. The presenting complaint is usually related to the behavior itself.

All sleep services (95800-95811) include recording, interpretation and report. (Report with modifier 52 if less than 6 hours of recording for 95800, 95801 and 95806, 95807, 95810, 95811; if less than 7 hours of recording for 95782, 95783, or if less than 4 nap opportunities are recorded for 95805).

> (Report with modifier 52 if less than 6 hours of recording or in other cases of reduced services as appropriate)
>
> (For unattended sleep study, use 95806)

95700   This code is out of order. See page 950

95705   This code is out of order. See page 951

95706   This code is out of order. See page 951

95707	This code is out of order. See page 951
95708	This code is out of order. See page 951
95709	This code is out of order. See page 951
95710	This code is out of order. See page 951
95711	This code is out of order. See page 951
95712	This code is out of order. See page 951
95713	This code is out of order. See page 951
95714	This code is out of order. See page 951
95715	This code is out of order. See page 951
95716	This code is out of order. See page 951
95717	This code is out of order. See page 951
95718	This code is out of order. See page 951
95719	This code is out of order. See page 951
95720	This code is out of order. See page 951
95721	This code is out of order. See page 952
95722	This code is out of order. See page 952
95723	This code is out of order. See page 952
95724	This code is out of order. See page 952
95725	This code is out of order. See page 952
95726	This code is out of order. See page 952
95782	This code is out of order. See page 940
95783	This code is out of order. See page 940
95800	This code is out of order. See page 940
95801	This code is out of order. See page 940

95803 Actigraphy testing, recording, analysis, interpretation, and report (minimum of 72 hours to 14 consecutive days of recording)

(Do not report 95803 more than once in any 14 day period)

(Do not report 95803 in conjunction with 95806-95811)

95805 Multiple sleep latency or maintenance of wakefulness testing, recording, analysis and interpretation of physiological measurements of sleep during multiple trials to assess sleepiness

95806 Sleep study, unattended, simultaneous recording of heart rate, oxygen saturation, respiratory airflow and respiratory effort (eg, thoracoabdominal movement)

(Do not report 95806 in conjunction with 93041-93227, 93228, 93229, 93268-93272, 95800, 95801)

(For unattended sleep study that measures heart rate, oxygen saturation, respiratory analysis, and sleep time, use 95800)

(For unattended sleep study that measures a minimum heart rate, oxygen saturation, and respiratory analysis, use 95801)

95800 Sleep study, unattended, simultaneous recording; heart rate, oxygen saturation, respiratory analysis (eg, by airflow or peripheral arterial tone), and sleep time

(Do not report 95800 in conjunction with 93041-93227, 93228, 93229, 93268-93272, 95803, 95806, 95801)

(For unattended sleep study that measures a minimum of heart rate, oxygen saturation, and respiratory analysis, use 95801)

95801 minimum of heart rate, oxygen saturation, and respiratory analysis (eg, by airflow or peripheral arterial tone)

(Do not report 95801 in conjunction with 93041-93227, 93228, 93229, 93268-93272, 95806, 95800)

(For unattended sleep study that measures heart rate, oxygen saturation, respiratory analysis, and sleep time, use 95800)

95807 Sleep study, simultaneous recording of ventilation, respiratory effort, ECG or heart rate, and oxygen saturation, attended by a technologist

95808 Polysomnography; any age, sleep staging with 1-3 additional parameters of sleep, attended by a technologist

95810 age 6 years or older, sleep staging with 4 or more additional parameters of sleep, attended by a technologist

95811 age 6 years or older, sleep staging with 4 or more additional parameters of sleep, with initiation of continuous positive airway pressure therapy or bilevel ventilation, attended by a technologist

95782 younger than 6 years, sleep staging with 4 or more additional parameters of sleep, attended by a technolgist

95783 younger than 6 years, sleep staging with 4 or more additional parameters of sleep, with initiation of continuous positive airway pressure therapy or bi-level ventilation, attended by a technologist

ROUTINE ELECTROENCEPHALOGRAPHY (EEG)

EEG codes 95812-95822 include hyperventilation and/or photic stimulation when appropriate. Routine EEG codes 95816-95822 include 20 to 40 minutes of recording. Extended EEG codes 95812-95813 include reporting times longer than 40 minutes.

95812 Electroencephalogram (EEG) extended monitoring; 41-60 minutes

(Do not report 95812 in conjunction with 95700-95726)

95813 61-119 minutes

(Do not report 95813 in conjunction with 95700-95726)

(For long-term EEG services [2 hours or more], see 95700-95726)

95816 Electroencephalogram (EEG) including recording awake and drowsy

(Do not report 95816 in conjunction with 95700-95726)

95819 including recording awake and asleep

(Do not report 95819 in conjunction with 95700-95726)

● New Code ▲ Revised Code ＋ Add-On Code ⊘ Modifier -51 Exempt ★ Telemedicine

95822   recording in coma or sleep only

(Do not report 95822 in conjunction with 95700-95726)

95824   cerebral death evaluation only

(**95827**   deleted 2019 [2020 Edition]. To report all night EEG recording, see 95705, 95706, 95707, 95711, 95712, 95713, 95717, 95718)

(For long-term EEG monitoring, see 95700-95726)

(For EEG during nonintracranial surgery, use 95955)

(For Wada test, use 95958)

95829   This code is out of order. See page 941

95830   Insertion by physician or other qualified health care professional of sphenoidal electrodes for electroencephalographic (EEG) recording

ELECTROCORTICOGRAPHY

Electrocorticography (ECoG) is the recording of EEG from electrodes directly on or in the brain.

Code 95829 describes intraoperative recordings of ECoG from electrode arrays implanted in or placed directly on the brain exposed during surgery. Code 95829 includes review and interpretation during surgery.

Code 95836 describes recording of ECoG from electrodes chronically implanted on or in the brain. Chronically implanted electrodes allow for intracranial recordings to continue after the patient has been discharged from the hospital. Code 95836 includes unattended ECoG recording with storage for later review and interpretation during a single 30-day period. Code 95836 may be reported only once for each 30-day period. The dates encompassed by the 30-day period must be documented in the report.

For report of programming for a brain neurostimulator pulse generator/transmitter during the ECoG (95836) 30-day period, see 95983, 95984.

95829   Electrocorticogram at surgery (separate procedure)

95836   Electrocorticogram from an implanted brain neurostimulator pulse generator/transmitter, including recording, with interpretation and written report, up to 30 days

(Report 95836 only once per 30 days)

(Do not report 95836 in conjunction with 95957)

(For programming a brain neurostimulator pulse generator/transmitter when performed in conjunction with ECoG [95836], see 95983, 95984)

RANGE OF MOTION TESTING

(**95831**   deleted 2019 [2020 Edition]. To report manual muscle testing, see Physical Medicine and Rehabilitation services 97161-97172)

(**95832**   deleted 2019 [2020 Edition]. To report manual muscle testing, see Physical Medicine and Rehabilitation services 97161-97172)

(**95833**   deleted 2019 [2020 Edition]. To report manual muscle testing, see Physical Medicine and Rehabilitation services 97161-97172)

(**95834**   deleted 2019 [2020 Edition]. To report manual muscle testing, see Physical Medicine and Rehabilitation services 97161-97172)

95836   This code is out of order. See page 941

95851	Range of motion measurements and report (separate procedure); each extremity (excluding hand) or each trunk section (spine)

95852	hand, with or without comparison with normal side

95857	Cholinesterase inhibitor challenge test for myasthenia gravis

ELECTROMYOGRAPHY

Needle electromyographic (EMG) procedures include the interpretation of electrical waveforms measured by equipment that produces both visible and audible components of electrical signals recorded from the muscle(s) studied by the needle electrode.

Use 95870 or 95885 when four or fewer muscles are tested in an extremity. Use 95860-95864 or 95886 when five or more muscles are tested in an extremity.

Use EMG codes (95860-95864 and 95867-95870) when no nerve conduction studies (95907-95913) are performed on that day. Use 95885, 95886 and 95887 for EMG services when nerve conduction studies (95907-95913) are performed in conjunction with EMG on the same day.

Report either 95885 or 95886 once per extremity. Codes 95885 and 95886 can be reported together up to a combined total of four units of service per patient when all four extremities are tested.

Report 95887 once per anatomic site (ie, cervical paraspinal muscle[s], thoracic paraspinal muscle[s], lumbar paraspinal muscle[s], chest wall muscle[s], and abdominal wall muscle[s]). Use 95887 for a unilateral study of the cranial nerve innervated muscles (excluding extra-ocular and larynx); when performed bilaterally, 95887 may be reported twice.

Use 95887 when a study of the cervical paraspinal muscle(s) or the lumbar paraspinal muscle(s) is performed with no corresponding limb study (95885 or 95886) on the same day.

(For needle electromyography of anal or urethral sphincter, use 51785)

(For non-needle electromyography of anal or urethral sphincter, use 51784)

(For needle electromyography of larynx, use 95865)

(For needle electromyography of hemidiaphram, use 95866)

(For needle electromyography of extra-ocular muscles, use 92265)

95860	Needle electromyography; 1 extremity with or without related paraspinal areas

95861	2 extremities with or without related paraspinal areas

(For dynamic electromyography performed during motion analysis studies, see 96002-96003)

95863	3 extremities with or without related paraspinal areas

95864	4 extremities with or without related paraspinal areas

95865	larynx

(Do not report modifier 50 in conjunction with 95865)

(For unilateral procedure, report modifier 52 in conjunction with 95865)

95866	hemidiaphragm

95867	cranial nerve supplied muscle(s), unilateral

95868	cranial nerve supplied muscles, bilateral

95869	thoracic paraspinal muscles (excluding T1 or T12

● New Code ▲ Revised Code + Add-On Code ⊘ Modifier -51 Exempt ★ Telemedicine

95870   limited study of muscles in 1 extremity or non-limb (axial) muscles (unilateral or bilateral), other than thoracic paraspinal, cranial nerve supplied muscles, or sphincters

(To report a complete study of the extremities, see 95860-95864)

(For anal or urethral sphincter, detrusor, urethra, perineum musculature, see 51785-51792)

(For eye muscles, use 92265)

95872   Needle electromyography using single fiber electrode, with quantitative measurement of jitter, blocking and/or fiber density, any/all sites of each muscle studied

+ 95885   Needle electromyography, each extremity, with related paraspinal areas, when performed, done with nerve conduction, amplitude and latency/velocity study; limited (List separately in addition to code for primary procedure)

+ 95886   complete, five or muscles studied, innervated by three or more nerves or four or more spinal levels (List separately in addition to code for primary procedure)

(Use 95885, 95886 in conjunction with 95907-95913)

(Do not report 95885, 95886 in conjunction with 95860-95864, 95870, 95905)

+ 95887   Needle electromyography, non-extremity (cranial nerve supplied or axial) muscle(s) done with nerve conduction, amplitude and latency/velocity study (List separately in addition to code for primary procedure)

(Use 95887 in conjunction with 95907-95913)

(Do not report 95887 in conjunction with 95867-95870, 95905)

ISCHEMIC MUSCLE TESTING AND GUIDANCE FOR CHEMODENERVATION

+ 95873   Electrical stimulation for guidance in conjunction with chemodenervation (List separately in addition to code for primary procedure)

(Do not report 95873 in conjunction with 64451, 64617, 64625, 95860-95870, 95874)

+ 95874   Needle electromyography for guidance in conjunction with chemodenervation (List separately in addition to code for primary procedure)

(Use 95873, 95874 in conjunction with 64612, 64615, 64616, 64642, 64643, 64644, 64645, 64646, 64647)

(Do not report more than one guidance code for each corresponding chemodenervation code)

(Do not report 95874 in conjunction with 64451, 64617, 64625, 95860-95870, 95873)

95875   Ischemic limb exercise test with serial specimen(s) acquisition for muscle(s) metabolite(s)

95885   Code out of order. See page 943

95886   Code out of order. See page 943

95887   Code out of order. See page 943

NERVE CONDUCTION TESTS

Codes 95907-95913 describe nerve conduction tests when performed with individually placed stimulating, recording, and ground electrodes.

For the purposes of coding, a single conduction study is defined as a sensory conduction test, a motor conduction test with or without a F wave test, or an H-reflex test. Each type of study (sensory, motor with or without F wave, or H-reflex) for each nerve includes all orthodromic and antidromic impulses associated with that nerve and constitutes a distinct study when determining the number of studies in each grouping (eg. 1-2 or 3-4 nerve conduction studies). Each type of nerve conduction study is counted only once when multiple sites on the same nerve are stimulated or recorded. The numbers of these separate tests should be added to determine which code to use. Use 95885-95887 in conjunction with 95907-95913 when performing eletromyography with nerve conduction studies.

Code 95905 describes nerve conduction tests when performed with preconfigured electrodes customized to a specific anatomic site.

⊘ **95905** Motor and/or sensory nerve conduction, using preconfigured electrode array(s), amplitude and latency/velocity study, each limb, includes F wave study when performed, with interpretation and report

(Report 95905 only once per limb studied)

(Do not report 95905 in conjunction with 95885, 95886, 95907-95913)

95907 Nerve conduction studies; 1-2 studies

95908 3-4 studies

95909 5-6 studies

95910 7-8 studies

95911 9-10 studies

95912 11-12 studies

95913 13 or more studies

INTRAOPERATIVE NEUROPHYSIOLOGY

Codes 95940, 95941 describe ongoing neurophysiologic monitoring, testing, and data interpretation distinct from performance of specific type(s) of baseline neurophysiologic study(s) performed during surgical procedures. When the service is performed by a surgeon or anesthesiologist, the professional services are included in the surgeon's or anesthesiologist's primary service code(s) for the procedure and are not reported separately. Do not report these codes for automated monitoring devices that do not require continuous attendance by a professional qualified to interpret the testing and monitoring.

Recording and testing are performed either personally or by a technologist who is physically present with the patient during the service. Supervision is performed either in the operating room or by real time connection outside the operating room. The monitoring professional must be solely dedicated to performing the intraoperative neurophysiologic monitoring and must be available to intervene at all times during the service as necessary, for the reported time period(s). For any given period of time spent providing these services, the service takes full attention and therefore other clinical activities beyond providing and interpreting of monitoring cannot be provided during the same period.

Throughout the monitoring, there must be provisions for continuous and immediate communication directly with the operating room team in the surgical suite. One or more simultaneous cases may be reported (95941). When monitoring more than one procedure, there must be the immediate ability to transfer patient monitoring to another monitoring professional during the surgical procedure should that individual's exclusive attention be required for another procedure. Report 95941 for all remote or non-one-on-one monitoring time connected to each case regardless of overlap with other cases.

Codes 95940, 95941 include only the ongoing neurophysiologic monitoring time distinct from performance of specific type(s) of baseline neurophysiologic study(ies) or other services such as intraoperative functional cortical or subcortical mapping. Codes 95940 and 95941 are reported based upon the time spent monitoring only, and not the number of baseline tests performed or parameters monitored. The time spent performing or interpreting the baseline neurophysiologic study(ies) should not be counted as intraoperative monitoring, but represents separately reportable procedures. When reporting 95940 and 95941, the same neurophysiologic study(ies) performed at baseline should be reported not more than once per operative session. Baseline study reporting is based upon the total unique studies performed. For example, if during the course of baseline testing and one-on-one monitoring, two separate nerves have motor testing performed in conjunction with limited single extremity EMG, then 95885 and 95907 would be reported in addition to 95940. Time spent monitoring (95940, 95941) excludes time to set up, record, and interpret the baseline studies, and to remove electrodes at the end of the procedure. To report time spent waiting on standby for a case to start, use 99360. For procedures that last beyond midnight, report services using the day on which the monitoring began and using the total time monitored.

Code 95940 is reported per 15 minutes of service. Code 95940 requires reporting only the portion of time the monitoring professional was physically present in the operating room providing one-on-one patient monitoring, and no other cases may be monitored at the same time. Time spent in the operating room is cumulative. To dtermine units of service of 95940, use the total minutes monitoring in the operating room one-on-one. Monitoring may begin prior to incision (eg, when positioning on the table is a time of risk). Report continuous intraoperative neurophysiologic monitoring in the operating room (95940) in addition to the services related to monitoring from outside the operating room (95941).

Code 95941 should be used once per hour even if multiple methods of neurophysiologic monitoring are used during the time. Code 95941 requires the monitoring of neurophysiological data that is collected from the operating room continuously on-line in real time via a secure data link. When reporting 95941, real-time ability must be available through sufficient data bandwidth transfer rates to view and interrogate the neurophysiologic data contemporaneously.

Report 95941 for all cases in which there was no physical presence by the monitoring professional in the operating room during the monitoring time or when monitoring more than one case in an operating room. It is also used to report the time of monitoring physically performed outside of the operating room in those cases where monitoring occurred both within and outside the operating room. Do not report 95941 if monitoring lasts 30 minutes or less.

Intraoperative neurophysiology monitoring codes 95940 and 95941 are each used to report the total duration of respective time spent providing each service, even if that time is not in a single continuous block.

+ **95940**   Continuous intraoperative neurophysiology monitoring in the operating room, one on one monitoring requiring personal attendance, each 15 minutes (List separately in addition to code for primary procedure)

        (Use 95940 in conjunction with the study performed, 92653, 95822, 95860-95870, 95907-95913, 95925, 95926, 95927, 95928, 95929, 95930-95937, 95938, 95939)

+ **95941**   Continuous intraoperative neurophysiology monitoring, from outside the operating room (remote or nearby) or for monitoring of more than one case while in the operating room, per hour (List separately in addition to code for primary procedure)

        (Use 95941 in conjunction with the study performed, 92653, 95822, 95860-95870, 95907-95913, 95925, 95926, 95927, 95928, 95929, 95930-95937, 95938, 95939)

        (For time spent waiting on standby before monitoring, use 99360)

        (For electrocorticography, use 95829)

        (For intraoperative EEG during nonintracranial surgery, use 95955)

        (For intraoperative functional cortical or subcortical mapping, see 95961-95962)

        (For intraoperative neurostimulator programming, see 95971, 95972, 95976, 95977, 95983, 95984)

AUTONOMIC FUNCTION TESTS

The purpose of autonomic nervous sytem function testing is to determine the presence of autonomic dysfunction, the site of autonomic dysfunction, and the various autonomic subsystems that may be disordered.

Code 95921 should be reported only when electrocardiographic monitoring of heart rate derived from the time elapsing between two consecutive R waves in the electrocardiogram, or the R-R interval, is displayed on a monitor and stored for subsequent analysis of waveforms. Testing is typically performed in the prone position. A tilt table may be used, but is not required equipment for testing of the parasympathetic function. At least two of the following components need to be included in testing:

1.   Heart rate response to deep breathing derived from a visual quantitative analysis of recording with subject breathing at a rate of 5-6 breaths per minute

2.   Valsalva ratio determined by dividing the maximum heart rate by the lowest heart rate. The initial heart rate responses to sustained oral pressure (blowing into a tube with an open glottis) consist of tachycardia followed by a bradycardia at 15-45 seconds after the Valsalva pressure has been released. A minimum of two Valsalva maneuvers are to be performed. The initial cardioacceleration is an exercise reflex while the subsequent tachycardia and bradycardia are baroreflex-mediated.

3.   A 30:15 ratio (R-R interval at beat 30)/(R-R interval at beat 15) used as an index of cardiovascular function.

Code 95922 should be reported only when all of the following components are included in testing:

1. Continuous recording of beat-to-beat BP and heart rate. The heart rate needs to be derived from an electrocardiogram (ECG) unit such that an accurate quantitative graphical measurement of the R-R interval is obtained.

2. A period of supine rest of at least 20 minutes prior to testing.

3. The performance and recording of beat-to-beat blood pressure and heart rate during a minimum of two (2) Valsalva maneuvers.

4. The performance of passive head-up tilt with continuous recording of beat-to-beat blood pressure and heart rate for a minimum of five minutes, followed by passive tilt-back to the supine position. This must be performed using a tilt table.

Code 95924 should be reported only when both the parasympathetic function and the adrenergic function are tested together with the use of a tilt table.

(To report autonomic function testing that does not include beat-to-beat recording or for testing without use of a tilt table, use 95943)

95921 Testing of autonomic nervous system function; cardiovagal innervation (parasympathetic function), including 2 or more of the following: heart rate response to deep breathing with recorded R-R interval, Valsalva ratio, and 30:15 ratio

95922 vasomotor adrenergic innervation (sympathetic adrenergic function), including beat-to-beat blood pressure and R-R interval changes during Valsalva maneuver and at least 5 minutes of passive tilt

(Do not report 95922 in conjunction with 95921)

95923 sudomotor, including 1 or more of the following: quantitative sudomotor axon reflex test (QSART), silastic sweat imprint, thermoregulatory sweat test, and changes in sympathetic skin potential

95924 combined parasympathetic and sympathetic adrenergic function testing with at least 5 minutes of passive tilt

(Do not report 95924 in conjunction with 95921 or 95922)

95943 Simultaneous, independent, quantitative measures of both parasympathetic function and sympathetic function, based on time-frequency analysis of heart rate variability concurrent with time-frequency analysis of continuous respiratory activity, with mean heart rate and blood pressure measures, during rest, paced (deep) breathing, Valsalva maneuvers, and head-up postural change

(Do not report 95943 in conjunction with 93040, 95921, 95922, 95924)

EVOKED POTENTIALS AND REFLEX TESTS

95925 Short-latency somatosensory evoked potential study, stimulation of any/all peripheral nerves or skin sites, recording from the central nervous system; in upper limbs

(Do not report 95925 in conjunction with 95926)

95926 in lower limbs

(Do not report 95926 in conjunction with 95925)

95938 in upper and lower limbs

(Do not report 95938 in conjunction with 95925, 95926)

95927 in the trunk or head

(To report a unilateral study, use modifier -52)

(For auditory evoked potentials, use 92653)

95928 Central motor evoked potential study (transcranial motor stimulation); upper limbs

---

● New Code   ▲ Revised Code   + Add-On Code   ⊘ Modifier -51 Exempt   ★ Telemedicine

(Do not report 95928 in conjunction with 95929)

95929   lower limbs

(Do not report 95929 in conjunction with 95928)

95939   in upper and lower limbs

(Do not report 95939 in conjunction with 95928, 95929)

95930   Visual evoked potential (VEP) checkerboard or flash testing, central nervous system except glaucoma, with interpretation and report

(For visual evoked potential testing for glaucoma, use 0464T)

(For screening of visual acuity using automated visual evoked potential devices, use 0333T)

95933   Orbicularis oculi (blink) reflex, by electrodiagnostic testing

95937   Neuromuscular junction testing (repetitive stimulation, paired stimuli), each nerve, any 1 method

95938   Code out of order, See page 946

95939   Code out of order. See page 947

95940   Code out of order. See page 945

95941   Code out of order. See page 945

95943   Code out of order. See page 946

SPECIAL EEG TESTS

Codes 95961 and 95962 use physician or other qualified health care professional time as a basis for unit of service. Report 95961 for the first hour of attendance. Use modifier 52 with 95961 for 30 minutes or less. Report 95962 for each additional hour of attendance. Codes 95961, 95962 may be reported with 95700-95726 when functional cortical or subcortical mapping is performed with long-term EEG monitoring.

Codes 95700-95726 describe long-term continuous recording services for electroencephalography (EEG), which are performed to differentiate seizures from other abnormalities, determine type or location of seizures, monitor treatment of seizures and status epilepticus, establish if the patient is a candidate for epilepsy surgery, and/or screen for adverse change in critically ill patients.

The set of codes that describe long-term continuous recording EEG services (95700-95726) is divided into two major groups: (1) technical services, and (2) professional services. Codes 95700-95726 may be reported for any site of service. The technical component of the services is reported with 95700-95716. The professional component of the services is reported with 95717, 95718, 95719, 95720, 95721, 95722, 95723, 95724, 95725, 95726. Diagnostic EEG recording time of less than 2 hours (ie, 1 minute, up to 1 hour and 59 minutes) is not reported separately as a long-term EEG service.

Long-term continuous recording EEG services (95700-95726) are different than routine EEGs (95812, 95813, 95816, 95819, 95822). Routine EEGs capture brainwave activity within a short duration of testing, defined as less than 2 hours. Long-term continuous recording EEGs capture brain-wave activity for durations of time equal to or greater than 2 hours. The length of recording is based on a number of factors, including the clinical indication for the test and the frequency of seizures.

Use of automated spike and seizure detection and trending software is included in 95700-95726, when performed. Do not report 95957 for use of automated software.

Definitions

<u>EEG technologist</u>: An individual who is qualified by education, training, licensure/certification/regulation (when applicable) in seizure recognition. An EEG technologist(s) performs EEG setup, takedown when performed, patient education, technical description, maintenance, and seizure recognition when within his or her scope of practice and as allowed by law, regulation, and facility policy (when applicable).

Unmonitored: Services that have no real-time monitoring by an EEG technologist(s) during the continuous recording. If the criteria for intermittent or continuous monitoring are not met, then the study is an unmonitored study.

Intermittent monitoring (remote or on-site): Requires an EEG technologist(s) to perform and document realtime review of data at least every 2 hours during the entire recording period to assure the integrity and quality of the recording (ie, EEG, VEEG), identify the need for maintenance, and, when necessary, notify the physician or other qualified health care professional of clinical issues. For intermittent monitoring, a single EEG technologist may monitor a maximum of 12 patients concurrently. If the number of intermittently monitored patients exceeds 12, then all of the studies are reported as unmonitored.

Continuous real-time monitoring (may be provided remotely): Requires all elements of intermittent monitoring. In addition, the EEG technologist(s) performs and documents real-time concurrent monitoring of the EEG data and video (when performed) during the entire recording period. The EEG technologist(s) identifies when events occur and notifies, as instructed, the physician or other qualified health care professional. For continuous monitoring, a single EEG technologist may monitor a maximum of four patients concurrently. If the number of concurrently monitored patients exceeds four, then all of the studies are reported as either unmonitored or intermittent studies. If there is a break in the real-time monitoring of the EEG recording, the study is an intermittent study.

Technical description: The EEG technologist(s)'s written documentation of the reviewed EEG/VEEG data, including technical interventions. The technical description is based on the EEG technologist(s)'s review of data and includes the following required elements: uploading and/or transferring EEG/VEEG data from EEG equipment to a server or storage device; reviewing raw EEG/VEEG data and events and automated detection, as well as patient activations; and annotating, editing, and archiving EEG/VEEG data for review by the physician or other qualified health care professional. For unmonitored services, the EEG technologist(s) annotates the recording for review by the physician or other qualified health care professional and creates a single summary.

Maintenance of long-term EEG equipment: Performed by the EEG technologist(s) and involves ensuring the integrity and quality of the recording(s) (eg, camera position, electrode placement, and impedances).

Setup: Performed in person by the EEG technologist(s) and includes preparing supplies and equipment and securing electrodes using the 10/20 system. Code 95700 is reported only once per recording period on the date the setup was performed. "In person" means that the EEG technologist(s) must be physically present with the patient.

Technical Component Services

Code 95700 describes any long-term continuous EEG/VEEG recording, setup, takedown when performed, and patient/caregiver education by the EEG technologist(s). To report 95700, the setup must include a minimum of eight channels of EEG. Services with fewer than eight channels may be reported using 95999. Eight to 15 channels are typically used for neonates and when electrodes cannot be placed on certain regions of the scalp that are sterile. Twenty or more channels are typically used for children and adults. If setup is performed by someone who does not meet the definition of an EEG technologist(s), report 95999.

Codes 95705-95716 describe monitoring, maintenance, review of data, and creating a summary technical description. These codes are divided into four groups based on duration and whether video is utilized. Key elements in determining the appropriate technical code (95705-95716) for long-term EEG continuous recording are: (1) whether diagnostic video recording is captured in conjunction and simultaneously with the EEG service, which is referred to as video EEG (VEEG), and (2) technologist monitoring for the study (ie, unmonitored, intermittently monitored, or continuously monitored). Codes 95711, 95712, 95713, 95714, 95715, 95716 are reported if diagnostic video of the patient is recorded a minimum of 80% of the time of the entire long-term VEEG service, concurrent with diagnostic EEG recording (ie, the entire study is reported as an EEG without video if concurrent diagnostic video occurs less than 80% of the entire study). Diagnostic EEG recording is an essential component of all long-term EEG services. If diagnostic EEG recording stops, timing stops until the diagnostic EEG is resumed.

Codes 95705, 95706, 95707, 95711, 95712, 95713 are reported when total diagnostic recording time is between 2 and 12 hours, or to capture the final increment of a multiple-day service when the final increment extends 2 to 12 hours beyond the time reported by the appropriate greater-than-12-hour-up-to-26-hour code(s) (95708, 95709, 95710, 95714, 95715, 95716). A maximum of one 2-12 hour code may be reported for an entire longterm EEG service. For example, if the testing lasts 48 hours, but diagnostic recording occurs only in the initial 11 hours and the final 11 hours of the testing period, a single greater-than-12-hour-up-to-26-hour technical code is reported, rather than two 2-12 hour codes for the 48-hour service (see the Long-Term EEG Monitoring Table).

Professional Component Services

Codes 95717, 95718, 95719, 95720, 95721, 95722, 95723, 95724, 95725, 95726 describe the professional services performed by a physician or other qualified health care professional for reviewing, analyzing, interpreting, and reporting the results of the

---

● New Code ▲ Revised Code + Add-On Code ⊘ Modifier -51 Exempt ★ Telemedicine

Long-Term EEG Monitoring Table					
	Professoinal Services		Technical Services		
Duration of Long-Term EEG/VEE\G Recording	With report each 24 hours	With report at conclusion of entire recording period	Unmonitored	Intermittent	Continuous
Less than 120 minutes (w/video or w/o video)	Not reported separately	See 95812/95813	Not reported separately	Not reported separately	Not reported separately
2 to 12 hours (w/o video)	95717 x 1		95705 x 1	95706 x 1	95707 x 1
2 to 12 hours (w/video)	95718 x 1		95711 x 1	95712 x 1	95713 x 1
12 hours and 1 minute to 26 hours (w/o video)	95719 x 1		95708 x 1	95709 x 1	95710 x 1
12 hours and 1 minute to 26 hours (w/video)	95720 x 1		95714 x 1	95715 x 1	95716 x 1
26 hours and 1 minute to 36 hours (w/o video)	95719 x 1 and 95717 x 1		95708 x 1 and 95705 x 1	95709 x 1 and 95706 x 1	95710 x 1 and 95707 x 1
26 hours and 1 minute to 36 hours (wvideo)	95720 x 1 and 95718 x 1		95714 x 1 and 95711 x 1	95715 x 1 and 95712 x 1	95716 x 1 and 95713 x 1
36 hours and 1 minute to 50 hours (w/o video)	95719 x 2	95721 x 1	95708 x 2	95709 x 2	95710 x 2
36 hours and 1 minute to 50 hours (w/video)	95720 x 2	95722 x 1	95714 x 2	95715 x 2	95716 x 2
50 hours and 1 minute to 60 hours (w/o video)	95719 x 2 and 95717 x 1	95721 x 1	95708 x 1 and 95705 x 1	95709 x 2 and 95706 x 1	95710 x 2 and 95707 x 1
50 hours and 1 minute to 60 hours (w/video)	95720 x 2 and 95718 x 1	95722 x 1	95714 x 2 and 95711 x 1	95715 x 2 and 95712 x 1	95716 x 2 and 95713 x 1
60 hours and 1 minute to 74 hours (w/o video)	95719 x 3	95723 x 1	95708 x 3	95709 x 3	95710 x 3
60 hours and 1 minute to 74 hours (w/video)	95720 x 3	95724 x 1	95714 x 3	95715 x 3	95716 x 3
74 hours and 1 minute to 84 hours (w/o video)	95719 x 3 and 95717 x 1	95723 x 1	95708 x 3 and 95705 x 1	95709 x 3 and 95706 x 1	95710 x 3 and 95707 x 1
74 hours and 1 minute to 84 hours (w/video)	95720 x 3 and 95718 x 1	95724 x 1	95714 x 3 and 95711 x 1	95715 x 3 and 95712 x 1	95716 x 3 and 95713 x 1
84 hours and 1 minute to 98 hours (w/o video)	95719 x 4	95725 x 1	95708 x 4	95709 x 4	95710 x 4
84 hours and 1 minute to 98 hours (w/video)	95720 x 4	95726 x 1	95714 x 4	95715 x 4	95716 x 4

continuous recording EEG/VEEG with recommendations based on the findings of the studies. These codes do not include E/M services, which may be reported separately.

Codes 95719, 95720 are used for greater than 12 hours (ie, 12 hours and 1 minute) up to 26 hours of recording. Code selection for professional interpretation for longterm EEG is based on: (1) length of the recording being interpreted, and (2) when the physician or other qualified health care professional reports are generated (ie, whether diagnostic interpretations and reports are made daily during the study, or whether the entire professional interpretation is performed after the entire study is completed). Codes 95717, 95718, 95719, 95720 are reported when: (1) daily professional reports are generated during the long-term recording, even if the entire study extends over multiple days or (2) the time of recording for the entire study is between 2 hours and 36 hours. Codes 95717, 95718 are reported once for each 2-12 hour recording and reported a maximum of once for an entire long-term EEG service. Codes 95719, 95720 are reported once for each greater-than-12-hours-up-to-26-hours recording period. Studies lasting 26 to 36 hours or longer are reported using building blocks and reported using one or more of the greater-than-12-hours-up-to-26- hour code with one 2-12 hour code. The recorded data are reviewed, interpreted, and reported daily by the physician or other qualified health care professional, and summary reports are made for the entire multiple-day study. The summary reports are included in each code (95717, 95718, 95719, 95720, 95721, 95722, 95723, 95724, 95725, 95726) and not reported separately (see the Long-Term EEG Monitoring Table).

For 95721, 95722, 95723, 95724, 95725, 95726, the entire professional interpretation (including retrospective daily reports and a summary report) is made after the entire study is recorded and downloaded at the completion of the study. When the entire professional interpretation is provided for a multiple-day study that is greater than 36 hours, 95721, 95722, 95723, 95724, 95725, 95726 are used to report the entire professional service with the appropriate code determined by the span of diagnostic recording

	Separate Procedure		Unlisted Procedure		CCI Comp. Code		Non-specific Procedure

time, as defined by the codes. A single code (95721, 95722, 95723, 95724, 95725, 95726) is reported for the multiple-day study. For example, a long-Term EEG recording that spans three days with a total of 50 hours of VEEG recording would be reported with 95722. Sixty hours and one minute of diagnostic VEEG recording is reported with 95724 (see the Long-Term EEG Monitoring Table)

(**95950** deleted 2019 [2020 Edition]. To report, see 95700-95726. See Long-Term EEG Monitoring Table for guidance)

(**95951** deleted 2019 [2020 Edition]. To report, see 95700-95726. See Long-Term EEG Monitoring Table for guidance)

(**95953** deleted 2019 [2020 Edition]. To report, see 95700-95726. See Long-Term EEG Monitoring Table for guidance)

95954 Pharmacological or physical activation requiring physician or other qualified health care professional attendance during EEG recording of activation phase (eg, thiopental activation test)

95955 Electroencephalogram (EEG) during nonintracranial surgery (eg, carotid surgery)

(**95956** deleted 2019 [2020 Edition]. To report, see 95700-95726. See Long-Term EEG Monitoring Table for guidance)

95957 Digital analysis of electroencephalogram (EEG) (eg, for epileptic spike analysis)

(Do not report 95957 for use of automated software. For use of automated spike and seizure detection and trending software when performed with long-term EEG, see 95700-95726)

95958 Wada activation test for hemispheric function, including electroencephalographic (EEG) monitoring

95961 Functional cortical and subcortical mapping by stimulation and/or recording of electrodes on brain surface, or of depth electrodes, to provoke seizures or identify vital brain structures; initial hour of attendance by a physician or other qualified health care professional

+ **95962** each additional hour of attendance by a physician or other qualified health care professional (List separately in addition to code for primary procedure)

(Use 95962 in conjunction with code 95961)

95965 Magnetoencephalography (MEG), recording and analysis; for spontaneous brain magnetic activity (eg, epileptic cerebral cortex localization)

95966 for evoked magnetic fields, single modality (eg, sensory, motor, language, or visual cortex localization)

+ **95967** for evoked magnetic fields, each additional modality (eg, sensory, motor, language, or visual cortex localization) (List separately in addition to code for primary procedure)

(Use 95967 in conjunction with code 95966)

(For electroencephalography performed in addition to magnetoencephalography, see 95812-95824)

(For somatosensory evoked potentials, auditory evoked potentials, and visual evoked potentials performed in addition to magnetic evoked field responses, see 92653, 95925, 95926, and/or 95930)

(For computerized tomography performed in addition to magnetoencephalography, see 70450-70470, 70496)

(For magnetic resonance imaging performed in addition to magnetoencephalography, see 70551-70553)

LONG-TERM EEG SETUP

95700 Electroencephalogram (EEG) continuous recording, with video when performed, setup, patient education, and takedown when performed, administered in person by EEG technologist, minimum of 8 channels

(95700 should be reported once per recording period)

● New Code ▲ Revised Code + Add-On Code ⊘ Modifier -51 Exempt ★ Telemedicine

(For EEG using patient-placed electrode sets, use 95999)

(For setup performed by non-EEG technologist or remotely supervised by an EEG technologist, use 95999)

MONITORING

95705 Electroencephalogram (EEG), without video, review of data, technical description by EEG technologist, 2-12 hours; unmonitored

95706 with intermittent monitoring and maintenance

95707 with continuous, real-time monitoring and maintenance

95708 Electroencephalogram (EEG), without video, review ofdata, technical description by EEG technologist, eachincrement of 12-26 hours; unmonitored

95709 with intermittent monitoring and maintenance

95710 with continuous, real-time monitoring andmaintenance

95711 Electroencephalogram with video (VEEG), review of data, technical description by EEG technologist, 2-12 hours; unmonitored

95712 with intermittent monitoring and maintenance

95713 with continuous, real-time monitoring and maintenance

95714 Electroencephalogram with video (VEEG), review of data, technical description by EEG technologist, each increment of 12-26 hours; unmonitored

95715 with intermittent monitoring and maintenance

95716 with continuous, real-time monitoring and maintenance

(95705, 95706, 95707, 95711, 95712, 95713 may be reported a maximum of once for an entire longer-term EEG service to capture either the entire time of service or the final 2-12 hour increment of a service extending beyond 26 hours)

95717 Electroencephalogram (EEG), continuous recording, physician or other qualified health care professional review of recorded events, analysis of spike and seizure detection, interpretation and report, 2-12 hours of EEG recording; without video

95718 with video (VEEG)

(For recording greater than 12 hours, see 95719, 95720, 95721, 95722, 95723, 95724, 95725, 95726)

(95717, 95718 may be reported a maximum of once for an entire long-term EEG service to capture either the entire time of service or the final 2-12 hour increment of a service extending beyond 24 hours)

95719 Electroencephalogram (EEG), continuous recording, physician or other qualified health care professional review of recorded events, analysis of spike and seizure detection, each increment of greater than 12 hours, up to 26 hours of EEG recording, interpretation and report after each 24-hour period; without video

95720 with video (VEEG)

(95719, 95720 may be reported only once for a recording period greater than 12 hours up to 26 hours. For multiple-day studies, 95719, 95720 may be reported after each 24-hour period during the extended recording period. 95719, 95720 describe reporting for a 26-hour recording period, whether done as a single report or as multiple reports during the same time)

(95717, 95718 may be reported in conjunction with 95719, 95720 for studies lasting greater than 26 hours)

(Do not report 95717, 95718, 95719, 95720 for professional interpretation of long-term EEG studies when the recording is greater than 36 hours and the entire professional report is retroactively generated, even if separate daily reports are rendered after the completion of recording)

(When the entire study includes recording greater than 36 hours, and the professional interpretation is performed after the entire recording is completed, see 95721, 95722, 95723, 95724, 95725, 95726)

95721 Electroencephalogram (EEG), continuous recording, physician or other qualified health care professional review of recorded events, analysis of spike and seizure detection, interpretation, and summary report, complete study; greater than 36 hours, up to 60 hours of EEG recording, without video

95722   greater than 36 hours, up to 60 hours of EEG recording, with video (VEEG)

95723   greater than 60 hours, up to 84 hours of EEG recording, without video

95724   greater than 60 hours, up to 84 hours of EEG recording, with video (VEEG)

95725   greater than 84 hours of EEG recording, without video

95726   greater than 84 hours of EEG recording, with video (VEEG)

(When the entire study includes recording greater than 36 hours, and the professional interpretation is performed after the entire recording is completed, see 95721, 95722, 95723, 95724, 95725, 95726)

(Do not report 95721, 95722, 95723, 95724, 95725, 95726 in conjunction with 95717, 95718, 95719, 95720)

NEUROSTIMULATORS, ANALYSIS-PROGRAMMING

Electronic analysis of an implanted neurostimulator pulse generator/transmitter involves documenting settings and electrode impedances of the system parameters prior to programming. Programming involves adjusting the system parameter(s) to address clinical signs and patient symptoms. Parameters available for programming can vary between systems and may need to be adjusted multiple times during a single programming session. The iterative adjustments to parameters provide information that is required for the physician or other qualified health care professional to assess and select the most appropriate final program parameters to provide for consistent delivery of appropriate therapy. The values of the final program parameters may differ from the starting values after the programming session.

Examples of parameters include: contact group(s), interleaving, amplitude, pulse width, frequency (Hz), on/off cycling, burst, magnet mode, dose lockout, patient-selectable parameters, responsive neurostimulation, detection algorithms, closed-loop parameters, and passive parameters. Not all parameters are available for programming in every neurostimulator pulse generator/transmitter.

For coding purposes, a neurostimulator system is considered implanted when the electrode array(s) is inserted into the target area for either permanent or trial placement.

There are several types of implantable neurostimulator pulse generator/transmitters and they are differentiated by the nervous system region that is stimulated. A brain neurostimulator may stimulate either brain surface regions (cortical stimulation) or deep brain structures (deep brain stimulation). A brain neurostimulation system consists of array(s) that targets one or more of these regions.

A cranial nerve neurostimulator targets the fibers of the cranial nerves or their branches and divisions. There are 12 pairs of cranial nerves (see nerve anatomy figure on page 706). Each cranial nerve has its origin in the brain and passes through one or more foramina in the skull to innervate extracranial structures. A cranial nerve neurostimulator stimulates the nerve fibers of either the extracranial or intracranial portion(s) of one or more cranial nerve(s) (eg, vagus nerve, trigeminal nerve).

A spinal cord or peripheral nerve neurostimulator targets nerve(s) that originate in the spinal cord and exit the spine through neural foramina and gives rise to peripheral nerves. The peripheral nervous system consists of the nerves and ganglia outside of the brain and spinal cord. Peripheral nerves may give rise to independent branches or branches that combine with other peripheral nerves in neural plexuses (ie, brachial plexus, lumbosacral plexus). Under the lumbosacral plexus, the sacral nerves (specifically S2, S3, S4) are located in the lower back just above the tailbone. Neurostimulation of the sacral nerves affect pelvic floor muscles and urinary organs (eg, bladder, urinary sphincter).

● New Code   ▲ Revised Code   ✛ Add-On Code   ⦰ Modifier -51 Exempt   ★ Telemedicine

Physician or Other Qualified Health Care Professional Face-to-Face Time for Brain Neurostimulator Analysis w/ Programming	Code(s)
Less than 8 minutes	Not reported
8 - 22 minutes	95983 x 1
23 - 37 minutes	95983 x 1 + 95986 x 1
38 - 52 minutes	95983 x 1 + 95984 x 2
53 - 67 minutes	95983 x 1 + 95984 x 3
68 minutes or longer	add units of 95984

Cranial nerve, spinal cord, peripheral nerve, and sacral nerve neurostimulator analysis with programming (95971, 95972, 95976, 95977) are reported based on the number of parameters adjusted during a programming session. Brain neurostimulator analysis with programming (95983, 95984) is reported based on physician or other qualified health care professional face-to-face time.

Code 95970 describes electronic analysis of the implanted brain, cranial nerve, spinal cord, peripheral nerve, or sacral nerve neurostimulator pulse generator/transmitter without programming. Electronic analysis is inherent to implantation codes 43647, 43648, 43881, 43882, 61850, 61860, 61863, 61864, 61867, 61868, 61880, 61885, 61886, 61888, 63650, 63655, 63661, 63662, 63663, 63664, 63685, 63688, 64553, 64555, 64561, 64566, 64568, 64569, 64570, 64575, 64580, 64581, 64585, 64590, 64595, and is not separately reportable at the same operative session.

Codes 95971, 95972, 95976, 95977 describe electronic analysis with simple or complex programming of the implanted neurostimulator pulse generator/transmitter. Simple programming of a neurostimulator pulse generator/transmitter includes adjustment of one to three parameter(s). Complex programming includes adjustment of more than three parameters. For purposes of counting the number of parameters being programmed, a single parameter that is adjusted two or more times during a programming session counts as one parameter.

Code 95971 describes electronic analysis with simple programming of an implanted spinal cord or peripheral nerve (eg, sacral nerve) neurostimulator pulse generator/transmitter.

Code 95972 describes electronic analysis with complex programming of an implanted spinal cord or peripheral nerve (eg, sacral nerve) neurostimulator pulse generator/transmitter.

Code 95976 describes electronic analysis with simple programming of an implanted cranial nerve neurostimulator pulse generator/transmitter.

Code 95977 describes electronic analysis with complex programming of an implanted cranial nerve neurostimulator pulse generator/transmitter.

Codes 95983, 95984 describe electronic analysis with programming of an implanted brain neurostimulator pulse generator/transmitter. Code 95983 is reported for the first 15 minutes of physician or other qualified health care professional face-to-face time for analysis and programming. Code 95984 is reported for each additional 15 minutes. A unit of service is attained when the mid-point is passed. Physician or other qualified health care professional face-to-face time of less than eight minutes is not separately reportable.

Code 95980 describes intraoperative electronic analysis of an implanted gastric neurostimulator pulse generator system, with programming; code 95981 describes subsequent analysis of the device; code 95982 describes subsequent analysis and reprogramming. For electronic analysis and reprogramming of gastric neurostimulator, lesser curvature, see 95980-95982.

Codes 95971, 95972, 95976, 95977, 95983, 95984 are reported when programming a neurostimulator is performed by a physician or other qualified health care professional. Programming may be performed in the operating room, postoperative care unit, inpatient, and/or outpatient setting. Programming a neurostimulator in the operating room is not inherent in the service represented by the implantation code and may be reported by either the implanting surgeon or other qualified health care professional, when performed.

Test stimulations are typically performed during an implantation procedure (43647, 43648, 43881, 43882, 61850, 61860, 61863, 61864, 61867, 61868, 61880, 61885, 61886, 61888, 63650, 63655, 63661, 63662, 63663, 63664, 63685, 63688, 64553, 64555, 64561, 64566, 64568, 64569, 64570, 64575, 64580, 64581, 64585, 64590, 64595) to confirm correct target site placement of the electrode array(s) and/or to confirm the functional status of the system. Test stimulation is not considered electronic analysis or programming of the neurostimulator system (test stimulation is included in the service described by the implantation code) and should not be reported with 95970, 95971, 95972, 95980, 95981, 95982, 95983, 95984. Electronic analysis of a device (95970) is not reported separately at the time of implantation.

(For insertion of neurostimulator pulse generator, see 61885, 61886, 63685, 64568, 64590)

(For revision or removal of neurostimulator pulse generator or receiver, see 61888, 63688, 64569, 64570, 64595)

(For implantation of neurostimulator electrodes, see 43647, 43881, 61850-61868, 63650, 63655, 64553-64581. For revision or removal of neurostimulator electrodes, see 43648, 43882, 61880, 63661, 63662, 63663, 63664, 64569, 64570, 64585)

(For analysis and programming of implanted integrated neurostimulation system, posterior tibial nerve, see 0589T, 0590T)

95970 Electronic analysis of implanted neurostimulator pulse generator/transmitter (eg, contact group[s], interleaving, amplitude, pulse width, frequency [Hz], on/off cycling, burst, magnet mode, dose lockout, patient selectable parameters, responsive neurostimulation, detection algorithms, closed loop parameters, and passive parameters) by physician or other qualified health care professional; with brain, cranial nerve, spinal cord, peripheral nerve, or sacral nerve, neurostimulator pulse generator/transmitter, without programming

(Do not report 95970 in conjunction with 43647, 43648, 43881, 43882, 61850, 61860, 61863, 61864, 61867, 61868, 61880, 61885, 61886, 61888, 63650, 63655, 63661, 63662, 63663, 63664, 63685, 63688, 64553, 64555, 64561, 64566, 64568, 64569, 64570, 64575, 64580, 64581, 64585, 64590, 64595, during the same operative session)

(Do not report 95970 in conjunction with 95971, 95972, 95976, 95977, 95983, 95984)

95971 with simple spinal cord or peripheral nerve (eg, sacral nerve) neurostimulator pulse generator/transmitter programming by physician or other qualified health care professional

(Do not report 95971 in conjunction with 95972)

95972 with complex spinal cord or peripheral nerve (eg, sacral nerve) neurostimulator pulse generator/transmitter programming by physician or other qualified health care professional

(For percutaneous implantation or replacement of integrated neurostimulation system, posterior tibial nerve, use 0587T)

(95974 deleted 2018 [2019 Edition]. To report, see 95976, 95977)

(95975 deleted 2018 [2019 Edition]. To report, see 95976, 95977)

95976 with simple cranial nerve neurostimulator pulse generator/transmitter programming by physician or other qualified health care professional

(Do not report 95976 in conjunction with 95977)

95977 with complex cranial nerve neurostimulator pulse generator/transmitter programming by physician or other qualified health care professional

95983 with brain neurostimulator pulse generator/transmitter programming, first 15 minutes face-to-face time with physician or other qualified health care professional

+ 95984 with brain neurostimulator pulse generator/transmitter programming, each additional 15 minutes face-to-face time with physician or other qualified health care professional (List separately in addition to code for primary procedure)

(Use 95984 in conjunction with 95983)

(Do not report 95970, 95971, 95972, 95976, 95977, 95983, 95984 in conjunction with 0587T, 0588T, 0589T, 0590T)

(For percutaneous implantation or replacement of integrated neurostimulation system, posterior tibial nerve, use 0587T)

(95978 deleted 2018 [2019 Edition]. To report, see 95983, 95984)

(95979 deleted 2018 [2019 Edition]. To report, see 95983, 95984)

---

954 ● New Code ▲ Revised Code + Add-On Code ⊘ Modifier -51 Exempt ★ Telemedicine

95980 Electronic analysis of implanted neurostimulator pulse generator system (eg, rate, pulse amplitude and duration, configuration of wave form, battery status, electrode selectability, output modulation, cycling, impedance and patient measurement(s) gastric neurostimulator pulse generator/transmitter; intraoperative, with programming

95981 subsequent, without reprogramming

95982 subsequent, with reprogramming

(For intraoperative or subsequent analysis, with programming, when performed, of vagus nerve trunk stimulator used for blocking therapy [morbid obesity], see 0312T, 0317T)

95983 This code is out of order. See page 954

95984 This code is out of order. See page 954

OTHER PROCEDURES

95990 Refilling and maintenance of implantable pump or reservoir for drug delivery, spinal (intrathecal, epidural) or brain (intraventricular), includes electronic analysis of pump, when performed;

95991 requiring skill of a physician or other qualified health care professional

(Do not report 95990, 95991 in conjunction with 62367-62370. For analysis and/or reprogramming of implantable infusion pump, see 62367-62370)

(For refill and maintenance of implanted infusion pump or reservoir for systemic drug therapy [eg, chemotherapy] use 96522)

95992 Canalith repositioning procedure(s) (eg, Epley maneuver, Semont maneuver), per day

(Do not report 95992 in conjunction with 92531, 92532)

95999 Unlisted neurological or neuromuscular diagnostic procedure

MOTION ANALYSIS

Codes 96000-96004 describe services performed as part of a major therapeutic or diagnostic decision making process. Motion analysis is performed in a dedicated motion analysis laboratory (ie., facility capable of performing videotaping from the front, back and both sides, computerized 3D kinematics, 3D kinetics, and dynamic electromyography). Code 96000 may include 3D kinetics and stride characteristics. Codes 96002-96003 describe dynamic electromyography.

Code 96004 should only be reported once regardless of the number of studies reviewed/interpreted.

(For performance of needle electromyography procedures, see 95860-95870, 95872, 95885-95887)

(For gait training, use 97116)

96000 Comprehensive computer-based motion analysis by video-taping and 3-D kinematics;

96001 with dynamic plantar pressure measurements during walking

96002 Dynamic surface electromyography, during walking or other functional activities, 1-12 muscles

96003 Dynamic fine wire electromyography, during walking or other functional activities, 1 muscle

(Do not report 96002, 96003 in conjunction with 95860-95866, 95869-95872, 95885-95887)

96004 Review and interpretation by physician or other qualified health care professional of comprehensive computer-based motion analysis, dynamic plantar pressure measurements, dynamic surface electromyography during walking or other functional activities, and dynamic fine wire electromyography, with written report

| Separate Procedure | Unlisted Procedure | CCI Comp. Code | Non-specific Procedure | **955** |

FUNCTIONAL BRAIN MAPPING

Code 96020 includes selection and administration of testing of language, memory, cognition, movement, sensation, and other neurological functions when conducted in association with functional neuroimaging, monitoring of performance of this testing, and determination of validity of neurofunctional testing relative to separately interpreted functional magnetic resonance images.

96020   Neurofunctional testing selection and administration during noninvasive imaging functional brain mapping, with test administered entirely by a physician or other qualified health care professional (ie, psychologist), with review of test results and report

(For functional magnetic resonance imaging [fMRI], brain, use 70555)

(Do not report 96020 in conjunction with 96112, 96113, 96116, 96121, 96130, 96131, 96132, 96133)

(Do not report 96020 in conjunction with 70554)

(Evaluation and Management services codes should not be reported on the same day as 96020)

MEDICAL GENETICS AND GENETIC COUNSELING SERVICES

These sevices are provided by trained genetic counselors and may include obtaining a structured family genetic history, pedigree construction, analysis for genetic risk assessment, and counseling of the patient and family. These activities may be provided during one or more sessions and may include review of medical data and family information, face-to-face interviews, and counseling services.

Code 96040 is reported for each 30-minute increment of face-to-face time. Do not report 96040 for 15 minutes or less of face-to-face time. Report 96040 once for 16 to 30 minutes of face-to-face time.

★ **96040**   Medical genetics and genetic counseling services, each 30 minutes face-to-face with patient/family

(For genetic counseling and education provided to an individual by a physician or other qualified health care professional who may report E/M services, see the appropriate E/M codes)

(For genetic counseling and education provided to a group by a physician or other qualified health care professional, use 99078)

(For education regarding genetic risks by a nonphysician to a group, see 98961, 98962)

(For genetic counseling and/or risk factor reduction intervention provided to patient(s) without symptoms or established disease, by a physician or other qualified health care professional who may report evaluation and management services, see 99401-99412)

ADAPTIVE BEHAVIOR SERVICES

Adaptive behavior services address deficient adaptive behaviors (eg, impaired social, communication, or selfcare skills), maladaptive behaviors (eg, repetitive and stereotypic behaviors, behaviors that risk physical harm to the patient, others, and/or property), or other impaired functioning secondary to deficient adaptive or maladaptive behaviors, including, but not limited to, instruction-following, verbal and nonverbal communication, imitation, play and leisure, social interactions, self-care, daily living, and personal safety.

Definitions

Functional behavior assessment: comprises descriptive assessment procedures designed to identify environmental events that occur just before and just after occurrences of potential target behaviors and that may influence those behaviors. That information may be gathered by interviewing the patient's caregivers; having caregivers complete checklists, rating scales, or questionnaires; and/or observing and recording occurrences of target behaviors and environmental events in everyday situations.

Functional analysis: an assessment procedure for evaluating the separate effects of each of several environmental events on a potential target behavior by systematically presenting and withdrawing each event to a patient multiple times and observing and measuring occurrences of the behavior in response to those events. Graphed data are analyzed visually to determine which events produced relatively high and low occurrences of the behavior.

Standardized instruments and procedures: include, but not limited to, behavior checklists, rating scales, and adaptive skill assessment instruments that comprise a fixed set of items and are administered and scored in a uniform way with all patients (eg,

Pervasive Developmental Disabilities Behavior Inventory, Brigance Inventory of Early Development, Vineland Adaptive Behavior Scales).

Nonstandardized instruments and procedures: include, but not limited to, curriculum-referenced assessments, stimulus preference-assessment procedures, and other procedures for assessing behaviors and associated environmental events that are specific to the individual patient and behaviors.

ADAPTIVE BEHAVIOR ASSESSMENTS

Behavior identification assessment (97151) is conducted by the physician or other qualified health care professional and may include analysis of pertinent past data (including medical diagnosis), a detailed behavioral history, patient observation, administration of standardized and/or nonstandardized instruments and procedures, functional behavior assessment, functional analysis, and/or guardian/caregiver interview to identify and describe deficient adaptive behaviors, maladaptive behaviors, and other impaired functioning secondary to deficient adaptive or maladaptive behaviors. Code 97151 includes the physician's or other qualified health care professional's scoring of assessments, interpretation of results, discussion of findings and recommendations with the primary guardian(s)/caregiver(s), preparation of report, and development of plan of care, which may include behavior identification supporting assessment (97152) or behavior identification-supporting assessment with four required components (0362T).

Behavior identification supporting assessment (97152) is administered by a technician under the direction of a physician or other qualified health care professional. The physician or other qualified health care professional may or may not be on site during the face-to-face assessment process. Code 97152 includes the physician's or other qualified health care professional's interpretation of results and may include functional behavior assessment, functional analysis, and other structured observations and/or standardized and/or nonstandardized instruments and procedures to determine levels of adaptive and maladaptive behavior.

Codes 97152, 0362T may be reported separately with 97151 based on the time that the patient is face-to-face with one or more technician(s). Only count the time of one technician when two or more are present.

For behavior identification-supporting assessment with four required components, use 0362T.

Guide to Selection of Codes 97152 and 0362T		
	97152	0362T
Physician or other qualified health care professional required to be on site		X
Physician or other qualified health care professional not required to be on site	X	
Number of technicians	1	2 or more
Deficient adaptive behavior(s), maladaptive behavior(s), or other impaired functioning secondary to deficient adaptive or maladaptive behaviors	X	
Destructive behavior(s)		X
May include functional behavior assessment		X
May include functional analysis	X	X
Environment customized to patient and behavior		X

97151 **Behavior identification assessment**, administered by a physician or other qualified health care professional, each 15 minutes of the physician's or other qualified health care professional's time face-to-face with patient and/or guardian(s)/caregiver(s) administering assessments and discussing findings and recommendations, and non-face-to-face analyzing past data, scoring/interpreting the assessment, and preparing the report/treatment plan

97152 **Behavior identification-supporting assessment,** administered by one technician under the direction of a physician or other qualified health care professional, face-to-face with the patient, each 15 minutes

(97151, 97152, 0362T may be repeated on the same or different days until the behavior identification assessment [97151] and, if necessary, supporting assessment[s] [97152, 0362T], is complete)

(For psychiatric diagnostic evaluation, see 90791, 90792)

(For speech evaluations, see 92521, 92522, 92523, 92524)

(For occupational therapy evaluation, see 97165, 97166, 97167, 97168)

(For medical team conference, see 99366, 99367, 99368)

(For health and behavior assessment/intervention, see 96156, 96158, 96159, 96164, 96165, 96167, 96168, 96170, 96171)

(For neurobehavioral status examination, see 96116, 96121)

(For neuropsychological testing, see 96132, 96133, 96136, 96137, 96138, 96139, 96146)

ADAPTIVE BEHAVIOR TREATMENT

Adaptive behavior treatment codes 97153, 97154, 97155, 97156, 97157, 97158, 0373T describe services that address specific treatment targets and goals based on results of previous assessments (see 97151, 97152, 0362T), and include ongoing assessment and adjustment of treatment protocols, targets, and goals.

Adaptive behavior treatment by protocol (97153) and **group adaptive behavior treatment by protocol** (97154) are administered by a technician under the direction of a physician or other qualified health care professional, utilizing a treatment protocol designed in advance by the physician or other qualified health care professional, who may or may not provide direction during the treatment. Code 97153 describes face-to-face services with one patient and code 97154 describes face-to-face services with two or more patients. Do not report 97154 if the group has more than eight patients.

Adaptive behavior treatment with protocol modification (97155) is administered by a physician or other qualified health care professional face-to-face with a single patient. The physician or other qualified health care professional resolves one or more problems with the protocol and may simultaneously direct a technician in administering the modified protocol while the patient is present. Physician or other qualified health care professional direction to the technician without the patient present is not reported separately.

Family adaptive behavior treatment guidance and **multiple-family group adaptive behavior treatment guidance** (97156, 97157) are administered by a physician or other qualified health care professional face-to-face with guardian(s)/caregiver(s) and involve identifying potential treatment targets and training guardian(s)/caregiver(s) of one patient (97156) or multiple patients (97157) to implement treatment protocols designed to address deficient adaptive or maladaptive behaviors. Services described by 97156 may be performed with or without the patient present. Services described by 97157 are performed without the patient present. Do not report 97157 if the group has more than eight patients' guardian(s)/caregiver(s).

Group adaptive behavior treatment with protocol modification (97158) is administered by a physician or other qualified health care professional face-to-face with multiple patients. The physician or other qualified health care professional monitors the needs of individual patients and adjusts the treatment techniques during the group sessions, as needed. In contrast to group adaptive behavior treatment by protocol (97154), protocol adjustments are made in real time rather than for a subsequent service. Do not report 97158 if the group has more than eight patients.

For adaptive behavior treatment with protocol modification with four required components, use 0373T.

97153 Adaptive behavior treatment by protocol, administered by technician under the direction of a physician or other qualified health care professional, face-to-face with one patient, each 15 minutes

(Do not report 97153 in conjunction with 90785-90899, 92507, 96105-96171, 97129)

97154 Group adaptive behavior treatment by protocol, administered by technician under the direction of a physician or other qualified health care professional, face-to-face with two or more patients, each 15 minutes

(Do not report 97154 if the group has more than 8 patients)

(Do not report 97154 in conjunction with 90785-90899, 92508, 96105-96171, 97150)

97155 Adaptive behavior treatment with protocol modification, administered by physician or other qualified health care professional, which may include simultaneous direction of technician, face-to-face with one patient, each 15 minutes

(Do not report 97155 in conjunction with 90785-90899, 92507, 96105-96171, 97129)

97156 Family adaptive behavior treatment guidance, administered by physician or other qualified health care professional (with or without the patient present), face-to-face with guardian(s)/caregiver(s), each 15 minutes

● New Code   ▲ Revised Code   ✛ Add-On Code   ⊘ Modifier -51 Exempt   ★ Telemedicine

Guide to Selection of Codes 97153, 97155, and 0373T			
	97153	**97155**	**0373T**
By protocol	X		
With protocol modification		X	X
Physician or other qualified health care professional face-to-face with patient		X	
Physician or other qualified health care professional required to be on site			X
Physician or other qualified health care professional not required to be on site	X		
Number of technicians	1	0 - 1	2 or more
Deficient adaptive behavior(s), maladaptive behavior(s), or other impaired functioning secondary to deficient adaptive or maladaptive behavior(s)	X	X	
Destructive behavior(s)		X	X
Environment customized to patient and behavior			X

(Do not report 97156 in conjunction with 90785-90899, 96105-96171)

97157 Multiple-family group adaptive behavior treatment guidance, administered by physician or other qualified health care professional (without the patient present), face-to-face with multiple sets of guardians/caregivers, each 15 minutes

(Do not report 97157 if the group has more than 8 families)

(Do not report 97156, 97157 in conjunction with 90785- 90899, 96105-96171)

97158 Group adaptive behavior treatment with protocol modification, administered by physician or other qualified health care professional, face-to-face with multiple patients, each 15 minutes

(Do not report 97158 if the group has more than 8 patients)

(Do not report 97158 in conjunction with 90785-90899, 96105-96171, 92508, 97150)

CENTRAL NERVOUS SYSTEM ASSESSMENTS/TESTS (eg, NEURO-COGNITIVE, MENTAL STATUS, SPEECH TESTING)

The following codes are used to report the services provided during testing of the central nervous system functions. The central nervous system assessments include, but are not limited to, memory, language, visual motor responses, and abstract reasoning/problem-solving abilities. It is accomplished by the combination of several types of testing procedures. Testing procedures include assessment of aphasia and cognitive performance testing, developmental screening and behavioral assessments and testing, and psychological/neuropsychological testing. The administration of these tests will generate material that will be formulated into a report or an automated result.

(For development of cognitive skills, see 97129, 97533)

(For dementia screens, [eg, Folstein Mini-Mental State Examination, by a physician or other qualified health care professional], see Evaluation and Management services codes)

(Do not report assessment of aphasia and cognitive performance testing services [96105, 96125], developmental/behavioral screening and testing services [96110, 96112, 96113, 96127], and psychological/neuropsychological testing services [96116, 96121, 96130, 96131, 96132, 96133, 96136, 96137, 96138, 96139, 96146] in conjunction with 97151, 97152, 97153, 97154, 97155, 97156, 97157, 97158, 0362T, 0373T)

Definitions: Codes in this family (96105-96146) describe a number of services that are defined below:

Cognitive performance testing: assesses the patient's ability to complete specific functional tasks applicable to the patient's environment in order to identify or quantify specific cognitive deficits. The results are used to determine impairments and develop therapeutic goals and objectives.

Interactive feedback: used to convey the implications of psychological or neuropsychological test findings and diagnostic formulation. Based on patient-specific cognitive and emotional strengths and weaknesses, interactive feedback may include promoting adherence to medical and/or psychological treatment plans; educating and engaging the patient about his or her condition to maximize patient collaboration in their care; addressing safety issues; facilitating psychological coping; coordinating care; and engaging the patient in planning given the expected course of illness or condition, when performed.

Central Nervous System Assessments/Tests (eg, Neuro-Cognitive, Mental Status, Speech Testing) Tables

Assessment of Aphasia and Cognitive Performance Testing

Code	Unit	Cognitive Services		Test Administration/Scoring		Interpretation and Report or Automated Result	
		Evaluation	Interactive Feedback	Physician or Qual. Health Care Prof.	Technician	Physician or Qual. Health Care Prof.	Automated Result
96105	Per hour	X		X		X	
96125	Per hour	X		X		X	

Developmental/Behavioral Screening and Testing

Code	Unit	Cognitive Services		Test Administration/Scoring		Interpretation and Report or Automated Result	
		Evaluation	Interactive Feedback	Physician or Qual. Health Care Prof.	Technician	Physician or Qual. Health Care Prof.	Automated Result
96110	Per instrument				X		
96112	Per hour	X		X		X	
+96113	Per hour (add-on)	X		X		X	
96127	Per instrument				X		

Psychological/Neuropsychological Testing

Code	Unit	Cognitive Services		Test Administration/Scoring		Interpretation and Report or Automated Result	
		Evaluation	Interactive Feedback	Physician or Qual. Health Care Prof.	Technician	Physician or Qual. Health Care Prof.	Automated Result

Neurobehavioral Status Examinations

Code	Unit	Evaluation	Interactive Feedback	Physician or Qual. Health Care Prof.	Technician	Physician or Qual. Health Care Prof.	Automated Result
96116	Per hour	X		X		X	
+96121	Per hour (add-on)	X		X		X	

Testing Evaluation Services

Code	Unit	Evaluation	Interactive Feedback	Physician or Qual. Health Care Prof.	Technician	Physician or Qual. Health Care Prof.	Automated Result
96130	Per hour	X	X	Not included in code	Not included in code	X	
+96131	Per hour (add-on)	X	X	Not included in code	Not included in code	X	
96132	Per hour	X	X	Not included in code	Not included in code	X	
+96133	Per hour (add-on)	X	X	Not included in code	Not included in code	X	

Test Administration and Scoring

Code	Unit	Evaluation	Interactive Feedback	Physician or Qual. Health Care Prof.	Technician	Physician or Qual. Health Care Prof.	Automated Result
96136	Per 30 min.	Not included in code	Not included in code	X		Not included in code	Not included in code
+96137	Per 30 min. (add-on)	Not included in code	Not included in code	X		Not included in code	Not included in code
96138	Per 30 min.	Not included in code	Not included in code		X	Not included in code	Not included in code
+96139	Per 30 min. (add-on)	Not included in code	Not included in code		X	Not included in code	Not included in code

Automated Testing and Result

Code	Unit	Evaluation	Interactive Feedback	Physician or Qual. Health Care Prof.	Technician	Physician or Qual. Health Care Prof.	Automated Result
96146	Automated report(s)	Not included in code	Not included in code				X

Interpretation and report: performed by a physician or other qualified health care professional. In some circumstances, a result is generated through the use of a computer, tablet computer, or other device(s).

Neurobehavioral status examination: a clinical assessment of cognitive functions and behavior, and may include an interview with the patient, other informant(s), and/or staff, as well as integration of prior history and other sources of clinical data with clinical decision making, further assessment and/or treatment planning and report. Evaluation domains may include acquired knowledge, attention, language, memory, planning and problem solving, and visual spatial abilities.

Neuropsychological testing evaluation services: typically include integration of patient data with other sources of clinical data, interpretation, clinical decision making, and treatment planning and report. It may include interactive feedback to the patient, family member(s) or caregiver(s), when performed. Evaluation domains for neuropsychological evaluation may include

● New Code   ▲ Revised Code   ✛ Add-On Code   ⊘ Modifier -51 Exempt   ★ Telemedicine

intellectual function, attention, executive function, language and communication, memory, visual-spatial function, sensorimotor function, emotional and personality features, and adaptive behavior.

Psychological testing evaluation services: typically include integration of patient data with other sources of clinical data, interpretation, clinical decision making, and treatment planning and report. It may include interactive feedback to the patient, family member(s) or caregiver(s), when performed. Evaluation domains for psychological evaluation may include emotional and interpersonal functioning, intellectual function, thought processes, personality, and psychopathology.

Standardized instruments: used in the performance of these services. Standardized instruments are validated tests that are administered and scored in a consistent or "standard" manner consistent with their validation.

Testing: administered by a physician, other qualified health care professional, and technician, or completed by the patient. The mode of completion can be manual (eg, paper and pencil) or via automated means.

Assessment of aphasia and cognitive performance testing, which includes interpretation and report, are described by 96105, 96125.

Developmental screening services are described by 96110. Developmental/behavioral testing services, which include interpretation and report, are described by 96112, 96113.

Neurobehavioral status examination, which includes interpretation and report, is described by 96116, 96121.

Psychological and neuropsychological test evaluation services, which include integration of patient data, interpretation of test results and clinical data, treatment planning and report, and interactive feedback, are described by 96130, 96131, 96132, 96133.

Testing and administration services (96136, 96137) are performed by a physician or other qualified health care professional. For 96136, 96137, do not include time for evaluation services (eg, integration of patient data or interpretation of test results). This time is included with psychological and neuropsychological test evaluation services (96130, 96131, 96132, 96133). Testing and administration services (96138, 96139) are performed by a technician. The tests selected, test administration and method of testing and scoring are the same, regardless whether the testing is performed by a physician, other qualified health care professional, or a technician, for 96136, 96137, 96138, 96139. Automated testing and result code 96146 describes testing performed by a single automated instrument with an automated result.

Some of these services are typically performed together. For example, psychological/neuropsychological testing evaluation services (96130, 96131, 96132, 96133) may be reported with psychological/neuropsychological test administration and scoring services (96136, 96137, 96138, 96139).

A requirement of testing services (96105, 96125, 96112, 96113, 96130, 96131, 96132, 96133, 96146) is that there is an interpretation and report when performed by a qualified health care professional, or a result when generated by automation. These services follow standard CPT time definitions (ie, a minimum of 16 minutes for 30 minutes codes and 31 minutes for 1-hour codes must be provided to report any per hour code). The time reported in 96116, 96121, 96130, 96131, 96132, 96133, 96125 is the face-to-face time with the patient and the time spent integrating and interpreting data.

Report the total time at the completion of the entire episode of evaluation.

(**96101**   deleted 2018 [2019 Edition])

(**96102**   deleted 2018 [2019 Edition])

(**96103**   deleted 2018 [2019 Edition])

> (To report psychological testing evaluation and administration and scoring services, see 96130, 96131, 96136, 96137, 96138, 96139, 96146)

> (To report psychological test administration using a single automated instrument, use 96146)

ASSESSMENT OF APHASIA AND COGNITIVE PERFORMANCE TESTING

96105   Assessment of aphasia (includes assessment of expressive and receptive speech and language function, language comprehension, speech production ability, reading, spelling, writing, eg, by Boston Diagnostic Aphasia Examination) with interpretation and report, per hour

---

| | Separate Procedure | | Unlisted Procedure | | CCI Comp. Code | | Non-specific Procedure | **961** |

96125 Standardized cognitive performance testing (eg, Ross Information Processing Assessment) per hour of a qualified health care professional's time, both face-to-face time administering tests to the patient and time interpreting these test results and preparing the report

(To report neuropsychological testing evaluation and administration and scoring services, see 96132, 96133, 96136, 96137, 96138, 96139, 96146)

DEVELOPMENTAL/BEHAVIORAL SCREENING AND TESTING

96110 Developmental screening (eg., developmental milestone survey, speech and language delay screen), with scoring adn documentation, per standardized instrument

(For an emotional/behavioral assessment, use 96127)

(96111 deleted 2018 [2019 Edition])

(To report developmental testing, see 96112, 96113)

96112 Developmental test administration (including assessment of fine and/or gross motor, language, cognitive level, social, memory and/or executive functions by standardized developmental instruments when performed), by physician or other qualified health care professional, with interpretation and report; first hour

+ 96113 each additional 30 minutes (List separately in addition to code for primary procedure)

96127 Brief emotional/behavioral assessment (eg, depression inventory, attention-deficit/hyperactivity disorder [adhd] scale), with scoring and documentation, per standardized instrument

(For developmental screening, use 96110)

PSYCHOLOGICAL/NEUROPSYCHOLOGICAL TESTING

NEUROBEHAVIORAL STATUS EXAMINATION

★ **96116** Neurobehavioral status examination (clinical assessment of thinking, reasoning and judgment, [eg, acquired knowledge, attention, language, memory, planning and problem solving, and visual spatial abilities]), by physician or other qualified health care professional, both face-to-face time with the patient and time interpreting test results and preparing the report; first hour

(96118 deleted 2018 [2019 Edition])

(96119 deleted 2018 [2019 Edition])

(96120 deleted 2018 [2019 Edition])

(To report neuropsychological testing evaluation and administration and scoring services, see 96132, 96133, 96136, 96137, 96138, 96139, 96146)

(To report neuropsychological test administration using a single automated instrument, use 96146)

+ 96121 each additional hour (List separately in addition to code for primary procedure)

(Use 96121 in conjunction with 96116)

96125 This code is out of order. See page 962

96127 This code is out of order. See page 962

TESTING EVALUATION SERVICES

96130 Psychological testing evaluation services by physician or other qualified health care professional, including integration of patient data, interpretation of standardized test results and clinical data, clinical decision making, treatment planning and report, and interactive feedback to the patient, family member(s) or caregiver(s), when performed; first hour

● New Code ▲ Revised Code + Add-On Code ⊘ Modifier -51 Exempt ★ Telemedicine

+ **96131**   each additional hour (List separately in addition to code for primary procedure)

96132   Neuropsychological testing evaluation services by physician or other qualified health care professional, including integration of patient data, interpretation of standardized test results and clinical data, clinical decision making, treatment planning and report, and interactive feedback to the patient, family member(s) or caregiver(s), when performed; first hour

+ **96133**   each additional hour (List separately in addition to code for primary procedure)

TEST ADMINISTRATION AND SCORING

96136   Psychological or neuropsychological test administration and scoring by physician or other qualified health care professional, two or more tests, any method; first 30 minutes

+ **96137**   each additional 30 minutes (List separately in addition to code for primary procedure)

(96136, 96137 may be reported in conjunction with 96130, 96131, 96132, 96133 on the same or different days)

96138   Psychological or neuropsychological test administration and scoring by technician, two or more tests, any method; first 30 minutes

+ **96139**   each additional 30 minutes (List separately in addition to code for primary procedure)

(96138, 96139 may be reported in conjunction with 96130, 96131, 96132, 96133 on the same or different days)

(For 96136, 96137, 96138, 96139, do not include time for evaluation services [eg, integration of patient data or interpretation of test results]. This time is included in 96130, 96131, 96132, 96133)

AUTOMATED TESTING AND RESULT

96146   Psychological or neuropsychological test administration, with single automated, standardized instrument via electronic platform, with automated result only

(If test is administered by physician, other qualified health care professional, or technician, do not report 96146. To report, see 96127, 96136, 96137, 96138, 96139)

HEALTH BEHAVIOR ASSESSMENT AND INTERVENTION

Health behavior assessment and intervention services are used to identify and address the psychological, behavioral, emotional, cognitive, and interpersonal factors important to the assessment, treatment, or management of physical health problems.

The patient's primary diagnosis is physical in nature and the focus of the assessment and intervention is on factors complicating medical conditions and treatments. These codes describe assessments and interventions to improve the patient's health and well-being utilizing psychological and/or psychosocial interventions designed to ameliorate specific disease-related problems.

Health behavior assessment: includes evaluation of the patient's responses to disease, illness or injury, outlook, coping strategies, motivation, and adherence to medical treatment. Assessment is conducted through healthfocused clinical interviews, observation, and clinical decision making.

Health behavior intervention: includes promotion of functional improvement, minimizing psychological and/ or psychosocial barriers to recovery, and management of and improved coping with medical conditions. These services emphasize active patient/family engagement and involvement. These interventions may be provided individually, to a group (two or more patients), and/or to the family, with or without the patient present.

Codes 96156, 96158, 96159, 96164, 96165, 96167, 96168, 96170, 96171 describe services offered to patients who present with primary physical illnesses, diagnoses, or symptoms and may benefit from assessments and interventions that focus on the psychological and/or psychosocial factors related to the patient's health status. These services do not represent preventive medicine counseling and risk factor reduction interventions.

For patients that require psychiatric services (90785-90899), adaptive behavior services (97151, 97152, 97153, 97154, 97155, 97156, 97157, 97158, 0362T, 0373T) as well as health behavior assessment and intervention (96156, 96158, 96159, 96164,

96165, 96167, 96168, 96170, 96171), report the predominant service performed. Do not report 96156, 96158, 96159, 96164, 96165, 96167, 96168, 96170, 96171 in conjunction with 90785-90899 on the same date.

Evaluation and management services codes (including counseling risk factor reduction and behavior change intervention [99401-99412]) should not be reported on the same day as health behavior assessment and intervention codes 96156, 96158, 96159, 96164, 96165, 96167, 96168, 96170, 96171 by the same provider.

Health behavior assessment and intervention services (96156, 96158, 96159, 96164, 96165, 96167, 96168, 96170, 96171) can occur and be reported on the same date of service as evaluation and management services (including counseling risk factor reduction and behavior change intervention [99401, 99402, 99403, 99404, 99406, 99407, 99408, 99409, 99411, 99412]), as long as the health behavior assessment and intervention service is reported by a physician or other qualified health care professional and the evaluation and management service is performed by a physician or other qualified health care professional who may report evaluation and management services.

Do not report 96158, 96164, 96167, 96170 for less than 16 minutes of service.

> (For health behavior assessment and intervention services [96156, 96158, 96159, 96164, 96165, 96167, 96168, 96170, 96171] performed by a physician or other qualified health care professional who may report evaluation and management services, see Evaluation and Management or Preventive Medicine Services codes)

> (Do not report 96156, 96158, 96159, 96164, 96165, 96167, 96168, 96170, 96171 in conjunction with 97151, 97152, 97153, 97154, 97155, 97156, 97157, 97158, 0362T, 0373T)

(**96150**   deleted 2019 [2020 Edition]. To report, see 96156, 96158, 96159)

(**96151**   deleted 2019 [2020 Edition]. To report, see 96156, 96158, 96159)

(**96152**   deleted 2019 [2020 Edition]. To report, see 96156, 96158, 96159)

(**96153**   deleted 2019 [2020 Edition]. To report, see 96164, 96165)

(**96154**   deleted 2019 [2020 Edition]. To report, see 96167, 96168)

(**96155**   deleted 2019 [2020 Edition]. To report, see 96170, 96171)

96156   Health behavior assessment, or re-assessment (ie, health-focused clinical interview, behavioral observations, clinical decision making)

96158   Health behavior intervention, individual, face-to-face; initial 30 minutes

+ **96159**   each additional 15 minutes (List separately in addition to code for primary service)

> (Use 96159 in conjunction with 96158)

96164   Health behavior intervention, group (2 or more patients), face-to-face; initial 30 minutes

+ **96165**   each additional 15 minutes (List separately in addition to code for primary service)

> (Use 96165 in conjunction with 96164)

96167   Health behavior intervention, family (with the patient present), face-to-face; initial 30 minutes

+ **96168**   each additional 15 minutes (List separately in addition to code for primary service)

> (Use 96168 in conjunction with 96167)

96170   Health behavior intervention, family (without the patient present), face-to-face; initial 30 minutes

+ **96171**   each additional 15 minutes (List separately in addition to code for primary service)

> (Use 96171 in conjunction with 96170)

96160 Administration of patient-focused health risk assessment instrument (eg, health hazard appraisal) with scoring and documentation, per standardized instrument

96161 Administration of caregiver-focused health risk assessment instrument (eg, depression inventory) for the benefit of the patient, with scoring and documentation, per standardized instrument

96164 This code is out of order. See page 964

96165 This code is out of order. See page 964

96167 This code is out of order. See page 964

96168 This code is out of order. See page 964

96170 This code is out of order. See page 964

96171 This code is out of order. See page 964

HYDRATION, THERAPEUTIC, PROPHYLACTIC, DIAGNOSTIC INJECTIONS AND INFUSIONS, AND CHEMOTHERAPY AND OTHER HIGHLY COMPLEX DRUG OR HIGHLY COMPLEX BIOLOGIC ADMINISTRATION

Coding Rules

1. *If a significant E/M service is performed, report the E/M service code with modifier -25 in addition to the infusion/injection codes.*

2. *Local anesthesia, IV start, access to indwelling IV, subcutaneous catheter or port, fFlush at the conclusion of infusion and standard tubing, syringes and supplies are included and not reported separately if performed to facilitate the infusion/injection.*

3. *When multiple drugs are administered, the service(s) and specific drugs or materials for each are reported.*

4. *When administering multiple infusions, injections or combinations, report only one "initial" service code unless two IV sites must be used.*

5. *When reported by the physician, report the "initial" code that best describes the primary reason for the encounter regardless of the order in which the infusions or injections are administered.*

6. *When reported by the facility, the "initial" code should reported in the order of chemotherapy services, followed by therapeutic/prophylactic/diagnostic services, followed by hydrationi services, followed by infusions, followed by pushes, and finally injections.*

Physician or other qualified health care professional work related to hydration, injection, and infusion services predominantly involves affirmation of treatment plan and direct supervision of staff.

Codes 96360-96379, 96401, 96402, 96409-96425, 96521-96523 are not intended to be reported by the physician in the facility setting. If a significant, separately identifiable office or other outpatient evaluation and management (E/M) service is performed, the appropriate E/M service (99202-99215, 99241-99245, 99354-99355) should be reported using modifier 25 in addition to 96360-96549. For same day E/M service, a different diagnosis is not required.

If performed to facilitate the infusion or injection, the following services are included and are not reported separately:

a. Use of local anesthesia

b. IV start

c. Access to indwelling IV, subcutaneous catheter or port

d. Flush at conclusion of infusion

| Separate Procedure | Unlisted Procedure | CCI Comp. Code | Non-specific Procedure | **965** |

e. Standard tubing, syringes, and supplies

> (For declotting a catheter or port, use 36593)

When multiple drugs are administered, report the service(s) and the specific materials or drugs for each.

When administering multiple infusions, injections or combinations, only one "initial" service code should be reported for a given date, unless protocol requires that two separate IV sites must be used. Do not report a second initial service on the same date due to an intravenous line requiring a re-start, an IV rate not being able to be reached without two lines, or for accessing a port of a multi-lumen catheter. If an injection or infusion is of a subsequent or concurrent nature, even if it is the first such service within that group of services, then a subsequent or concurrent code from the appropriate section should be reported (eg., the first IV push given subsequent to an initial one-hour infusion is reported using a subsequent IV push code).

In order to determine which service should be reported as the initial service when there is more than one type of service, hierarchies have been created. These vary by whether they physician or other qualified health care professional or a facility is reporting. The order of selection for reporting is based upon the physician's or other qualified health care professional's knowledge of the clinical condition(s) and treatment(s). The hierarchy that facilities are to use is based upon a structural algorithm. When these codes are reported by the physician or other qualified health care professional, the "initial" code that best describes the key or primary reason for the encounter should always be reported irrespective of the order in which the infusions or injections occur.

When these codes are reported *by the facility,* the following instructions apply: The initial code should be selected using a hierarchy whereby chemotherapy services are primary to therapeutic, prophylactic, and diagnostic services which are primary to hydration services. Infusions are primary to pushes, which are primary to injections. This hierarchy is to be followed by facilities and supersedes parenthetical instructions for add-on codes that suggest an add-on of a higher hierarchical position may be reported in conjunction with a base code of a lower position. (For example, the hierarchy would not permit reporting 96376 with 96360, as 96376 is a higher order code. IV push is primary to hydration.)

When reporting multiple infusions of the same drug/substance on the same date of service, the initial code should be selected. The second and subsequent infusion(s) should be reported based on the individual time(s) of each additional infusion(s) of the same drug/substances using the appropriate add-on code.

When reporting codes for which infusion time is a factor, use the actual time over which the infusion is administered. Intravenous or intra-arterial push is defined as: (a) an injection in which the individual who administers the drug/substance is continuously present to administer the injection and observe the patient; or (b) an infusion of 15 minutes or less. If intravenous hydration (96360, 96361) is given from 11 p.m. to 2 a.m., 96360 would be reported once and 96361 twice. For continuous services that last beyond midnight, use the date in which the service began and report the total units of time provided continuously. However, if instead of a continuous infusion, a medication was given by intravenous push at 10 pm and 2 am, as the service was not continuous, the two administrations would be reported as an initial service (96374) and sequential (96376) as: (1) no other infusion services were performed; and (2) the push of the same drug was performed more than 30 minutes beyond the initial administration. A "keep open" infusion of any type is not separately reported.

HYDRATION

Codes 96360-96361 are intended to report a hydration IV infusion to consist of a pre-packaged fluid and electrolytes (eg., normal saline, D5-1/2 normal saline + 30mEq KCl/liter), but are not used to report infusion of drugs or other substances. Hydration IV infusions typically require direct supervision for purposes of consent, safety oversight, or intraservice supervision of staff. Typically, such infusions require little special handling to prepare or dispose of, and staff that administer these do not typically require advanced practice training. After initial set-up, infusion typically entails little patient risk and thus little monitoring. These codes are not intended to be reported by the physician or other qualified health care profesional in the facility setting.

Some chemotherapeutic agents and other therapeutic agents require pre- and/or post-hydration to be given in order to avoid specific toxicities. A minimum time duration of 31 minutes of hydration infusion is required to report the service. However, the hydration codes 96360 or 96361 are not used when the purpose of the intravenous fluid is to "keep open" and IV line prior or subsequent to a therapeutic infusion, or as a free-flowing IV during chemotherapy or other therapeutic infusion.

96360   Intravenous infusion, hydration; initial, 31 minutes to 1 hour

> (Do not report 96360 if performed as a concurrent infusion service)

> (Do not report intravenous infusion for hydration of 30 minutes or less)

+ 96361   each additional hour (list separately in addition to code for primary procedure)

(Use 96361 in conjunction with 96360)

(Report 96361 for hydration infusion intervals of greater than 30 minutes beyond 1 hour increments)

(Report 96361 to identify hydration if provided as a secondary or subsequent service after a different initial service [96360, 96365, 96374, 96409, 96413] is administered through the same IV access)

THERAPEUTIC, PROPHYLACTIC, AND DIAGNOSTIC INJECTIONS AND INFUSIONS (EXCLUDES CHEMOTHERAPY AND OTHER HIGHLY COMPLEX DRUG OR HIGHLY COMPLEX BIOLOGIC AGENT ADMINISTRATION)

A therapeutic, prophylactic or diagnostic IV infusion or injection (other than hydration) is for the administration of substances/drugs. When fluids are used to administer the drug(s), the administration of the fluid is considered incidental hydration and is not separately reportable. These services typically require direct supervision for any or all purposes of patient assessment, provision of consent, safety oversight, and intra-service supervision of staff. Typically, such infusions require special consideration to prepare, dose or dispose of, require practice training and competency for staff who administer the infusions, and require periodic patient assessment with vital sign monitoring during the infusion. These codes are not intended to be reported by the physician or other qualified health care professional in the facility setting.

See codes 96401-96549 for the administration of chemotherapy or other highly complex drug or highly complex biologic agent services. These highly complex services require advanced practice training and competency for staff who provide these services; special considerations for preparation, dosage or disposal; and commonly, these services entail significant patient risk and frequent monitoring. Examples are frequent changes in the infusion rate, prolonged presence of nurse administering the solution for patient monitoring and infusion adjustments, and frequent conferring with the physician or other qualified health care profesisonal about these issues.

(Do not report 96365-96379 with codes for which IV push or infusion is an inherent part of the procedure [eg, administration of contrast material for a diagnostic imaging study])

96365 Intravenous infusion, for therapy, prophylaxis, or diagnosis (specify substance or drug); initial, up to 1 hour

+ **96366** each additional hour (list separately in addition to code for primary procedure)

(Report 96366 in conjunction with 96365, 96367)

(Report 96366 for additional hour[s] of sequential infusion)

(Report 96366 for infusion intervals of greater than 30 minutes beyond 1 hour increments)

(Report 96366 in conjunction with 96365 to identify each second and subsequent infusions of the same drug/substance)

+ **96367** additional sequential infusion of a new drug/substance, up to 1 hour (list separately in addition to code for primary procedure)

(Report 96367 in conjunction with 96365, 96374, 96409, 96413 to identify the infusion of a new drug/substance provided as a secondary or subsequent service after a different initial service is administered through the same IV access. Report 96367 only once per sequential infusion of same infusate mix)

+ **96368** concurrent infusion (list separately in addition to code for primary procedure)

(Report 96368 only once per date of service)

(Report 96368 in conjunction with 96365, 96366, 96413, 96415, 96416)

96369 Subcutaneous infusion for therapy or prophylaxis (specify substance or drug); initial, up to 1 hour, including pump set-up and establishment of subcutaneous infusion site(s)

(For infusions of 15 minutes or less, use 96372)

+ **96370** each additional hour (list separately in addition to code for primary procedure)

(Use 96370 in conjunction with 96369)

(Use 96370 for infusion intervals of greater than 30 minutes beyond 1 hour increments)

+ 96371 additional pump set-up with establishment of new subcutaneous infusion site(s) (list separately in addition to code for primary procedure)

(Use 96371 in conjunction with 96369)

(Use 96369, 96371 only once per encounter)

96372 Therapeutic, prophylactic, or diagnostic injection (specify substance or drug); subcutaneous or intramuscular

(For administration of vaccines/toxoids, see 90460, 90461, 90471, 90472)

(Report 96372 for non-antineoplastic hormonal therapy injections)

(Report 96401 for antineoplastic nonhormonal injection therapy)

(Report 96402 for antineoplastic hormonal injection therapy)

(Do not report 96372 for injections given without direct physician or other qualified health care professional supervision. To report, use 99211. Hospitals may report 96372 when the physician or other qualified health care professional is not present)

(96372 does not include injections for allergen immunotherapy. For allergen immunotherapy injections, see 95115-95117)

96373 intra-arterial

96374 intravenous push, single or initial substance/drug

+ 96375 each additional sequential intravenous push of a new substance/drug (list separately in addition to code for primary procedure)

(Use 96375 in conjunction with 96365, 96374, 96409, 96413)

(Report 96375 to identify intravenous push of a new substance/drug if provided as a secondary or subsequent service after a different initial sevice is administered through the same IV access)

+ 96376 each additional sequential intravenous push of the same substance/drug provided in a facility (list separately in addition to code for primary procedure)

(Do not report 96376 for a push performed within 30 minutes of a reported push of the same substance or drug)

(96376 may be reported by facilities only)

(Report 96376 in conjunction with 96365, 96374, 96409, 96413)

96377 Application of on-body injector (includes cannula insertion) for timed subcutaneous injection

96379 Unlisted therapeutic, prophylactic, or diagnostic intravenous or intra-arterial injection or infusion

(For allergy immunology, see 95004 et seq)

CHEMOTHERAPY AND OTHER HIGHLY COMPLEX DRUG OR HIGHLY COMPLEX BIOLOGIC AGENT ADMINISTRATION

Chemotherapy administration codes 96401-96549 apply to parenteral administration of non-radionuclide anti-neoplastic drugs; and also to anti-neoplastic agents provided for treatment of noncancer diagnoses (eg, cyclophosphamide for auto-immune conditions) or to substances such as certain monoclonal antibody agents, and other biologic response modifiers. The highly complex infusion of chemotherapy or other drug or biologic agents requires physician or other qualified health care professional work and/or clinical staff monitoring well beyond that of therapeutic drug agents (96360-96379) because the incidence of severe adverse patient reactions are typically greater. These services can be provided by any physician or other qualified health care professional. Chemotherapy services are typically highly complex and require direct supervision for any or all purposes of patient assessment, provision of consent, safety oversight, and intra-service supervision of staff. Typically, such chemotherapy services require advanced practice training and competency for staff who provide these services; special considerations for preparation, dosage, or disposal; and commonly, these services entail significant patient risk and frequent monitoring. Examples are frequent changes in the infusion rate, prolonged presence of the nurse administering the solution for patient monitoring and infusion adjustments, and frequent conferring with the physician or other qualified health care professional about these issues. When performed to facilitate the infusion of injection, preparation of chemotherapy agent(s), highly complex agent(s), or other highly complex drug is included and is not reported separately. To report infusions that do not require this level of complexity, see 96360-96379. Codes 96401-96402, 96409-96425, 96521-96523 are not intended to be reported by the physician or other qualified health care professional in the facility setting.

The term "chemotherapy" in 96401-96549 includes other highly complex drugs or highly complex biologic agents.

Report separate codes for each parenteral method of administration employed when chemotherapy is administered by different techniques. The administration of medications (eg., antibiotics, steroidal agents, antiemetics, narcotics, analgesics) administered independently or sequentially as supportive management of chemotherapy administration, should be separately reported using 96360, 96361, 96365, 96379 as appropriate.

Report both the specific service as well as code(s) for the specific substance(s) or drug(s) provided. The fluid used to administer the drug(s) is considered incidental hydration and is not separately reportable.

Regional (isolation) chemotherapy perfusion should be reported using the codes for arterial infusion (96420-96425). Placement of the intra-arterial catheter should be reported using the appropriate code from the Cardiovascular Surgery section. Placement of arterial and venous cannula(s) for extracorporeal circulation via a membrane oxygenator perfusion pump should be reported using 36823. Code 36823 includes dose calculation and administration of the chemotherapy agent by injection into the perfusate. Do not report 96409-96425 in conjunction with 36823.

(For home infusion services, see 99601-99602)

INJECTION AND INTRAVENOUS INFUSION CHEMOTHERAPY AND OTHER HIGHLY COMPLEX DRUG OR HIGHLY COMPLEX BIOLOGIC AGENT ADMINISTRATION

Intravenous or intra-arterial push is defined as: (a) an injection in which the healthcare professional who administers the substance/drug is continuously present to administer the injection and observe the patient, or (b) an infusion of 15 minutes or less.

96401 Chemotherapy administration, subcutaneous or intramuscular; non-hormonal anti-neoplastic

96402   hormonal anti-neoplastic

96405 Chemotherapy administration; intralesional, up to and including 7 lesions

96406   intralesional, more than 7 lesions

96409   intravenous, push technique, single or initial substance/drug

+ 96411   intravenous, push technique, each additional substance/drug (List separately in addition to code for primary procedure)

(Use 96411 in conjunction with 96409, 96413)

96413 Chemotherapy administration, intravenous infusion technique; up to 1 hour, single or initial substance/drug

(Report 96361 to identify hydration if administered as a secondary or subsequent service in association with 96413 through the same IV access)

(Report 96366, 96367, 96375 to identify therapeutic, prophylactic, or diagnostic drug infusion or injection, if administered as a secondary or subsequent service in association with 96413 through the same IV access)

+ 96415   each additional hour (List separately in addition to code for primary procedure)

(Use 96415 in conjunction with 96413)

(Report 96415 for infusion intervals of greater than 30 minutes beyond 1-hour increments)

96416   initiation of prolonged chemotherapy infusion (more than 8 hours), requiring use of a portable or implantable pump

(For refilling and maintenance of a portable pump or an implantable infusion pump or reservoir for drug delivery, see 96521-96523)

+ 96417   each additional sequential infusion (different substance/drug), up to 1 hour (List separately in addition to code for primary procedure)

(Use 96417 in conjunction with 96413)

(Report only once per sequential infusion. Report 96415 for additional hour(s) of sequential infusion)

INTRA-ARTERIAL CHEMOTHERAPY AND OTHER HIGHLY COMPLEX DRUG OR HIGHLY COMPLEX BIOLOGIC AGENT ADMINISTRATION

96420   Chemotherapy administration, intra-arterial; push technique

96422   infusion technique, up to 1 hour

+ 96423   infusion technique, each additional hour (List separately in addition to code for primary procedure)

(Use 96423 in conjunction with code 96422)

(Report 96423 for infusion intervals of greater than 30 minutes beyond 1-hour increments)

(For regional chemotherapy perfusion via membrane oxygenator perfusion pump to an extremity, use 36823)

96425   infusion technique, initiation of prolonged infusion (more than 8 hours), requiring the use of a portable or implantable pump

(For refilling and maintenance of a portable pump or an implantable infusion pump or reservoir for drug delivery, see 96521-96523)

OTHER INJECTION AND INFUSION SERVICES

Code 96523 does not require direct supervision. Codes 96521-96523 may be reported when these devices are used for therapeutic drugs other than chemotherapy.

(For collection of blood specimen from a completely implantable venous access device, use 36591)

96440   Chemotherapy administration into pleural cavity, requiring and including thoracentesis

96446   Chemotherapy administration into the peritoneal cavity via indwelling port or catheter

96450   Chemotherapy administration, into CNS (eg, intrathecal), requiring and including spinal puncture

(For intravesical (bladder) chemotherapy administration, use 51720)

(For insertion of subarachnoid catheter and reservoir for infusion of drug, see 62350, 62351, 62360, 62361, 62362; for insertion of intraventricular catherter and reservoir, see 61210, 61215)

(If fluoroscopic guidance is performed, use 77003)

96521   Refilling and maintenance of portable pump

96522   Refilling and maintenance of implantable pump or reservoir for drug delivery, systemic (eg, intravenous, intra-arterial)

(For refilling and maintenance of an implantable infusion pump for spinal or brain drug infusion, use 95990-95991)

96523   Irrigation of implanted venous access device for drug delivery systems

---

(Do not report 96523 in conjunction with other services. To report collection of blood specimen, use 36591)

96542 Chemotherapy injection, subarachnoid or intraventricular via subcutaneous reservoir, single or multiple agents

(For radioactive isotope therapy, use 79005)

96549 Unlisted chemotherapy procedure

PHOTODYNAMIC THERAPY

Codes 96573, 96574 should be used to report nonsurgical treatment of cutaneous lesions using photodynamic therapy by external application of light to destroy premalignant lesion(s) of the skin and adjacent mucosa (eg, face, scalp) by activation of photosensitizing drug(s).

A treatment session is defined as an application of photosensitizer to all lesions within an anatomic area (eg, face, scalp), with or without debridement of all premalignant hyperkeratotic lesions in that area, followed by illumination/activation with an appropriate light source to the same area.

Do not report codes for debridement (11000, 11001, 11004, 11005), lesion shaving (11300-11313), biopsy (11102, 11103, 11104, 11105, 11106, 11107), or lesion excision (11400-11471) within the treatment area(s) on the same day as photodynamic therapy (96573, 96574).

(To report ocular photodynamic therapy, use 67221)

96567 Photodynamic therapy by external application of light to destroy premalignant lesions of the skin and adjacent mucosa with application and illumination/activation of photosensitive drug(s), per day

(Use 96567 for reporting photodynamic therapy when physician or other qualified health care professional is not directly involved in the delivery of the photodynamic therapy service)

+ 96570 Photodynamic therapy by endoscopic application of light to ablate abnormal tissue via activation of photosensitive drug(s); first 30 minutes (List separately in addition to code for endoscopy or bronchoscopy procedures of lung and gastrointestinal tract)

(Report 96570 with modifier 52 for service of less than 23 minutes with report)

+ 96571 each additional 15 minutes (List separately in addition to code for endoscopy or bronchoscopy procedures of lung and gastrointestinal tract)

(For 23-27 minutes of service, use 96570. For 38-52 minutes of service, use 96570 in conjunction with 96571)

(96570, 96571 are to be used in addition to bronchoscopy, endoscopy codes)

(Use 96570, 96571 in conjunction with 31641, 43229 as appropriate)

96573 Photodynamic therapy by external application of light to destroy premalignant lesions of the skin and adjacent mucosa with application and illumination/activation of photosensitizing drug(s) provided by a physician or other qualified health care professional, per day

(Do not report 96573 in conjunction with 96567, 96574 for the same anatomic area)

96574 Debridement of premalignant hyperkeratotic lesion(s) (ie, targeted curettage, abrasion) followed with photodynamic therapy by external application of light to destroy premalignant lesions of the skin and adjacent mucosa with application and illumination/activation of photosensitizing drug(s) provided by a physician or other qualified health care professional, per day

(Do not report 96574 in conjunction with 96567, 96573 for the same anatomic area)

SPECIAL DERMATOLOGICAL PROCEDURES

See the **Evaluation and Management coding guidelines** for further instructions on reporting that is appropriate for management of dermatologic illnesses.

(For intralesional injections, see 11900, 11901)

(For Tzanck smear, see 88160-88161)

96900   Actinotherapy (ultraviolet light)

(For rhinophototherapy, intranasal application of ultraviolet and visible light, use 30999)

96902   Microscopic examination of hairs plucked or clipped by the examiner (excluding hair collected by the patient) to determine telogen and anagen counts, or structural hair shaft abnormality

96904   Whole body integumentary photography, for monitoring of high risk patients with dysplastic nevus syndrome or a history of dysplastic nevi, or patients with a personal or familial history of melanoma

96910   Photochemotherapy; tar and ultraviolet B (Goeckerman treatment) or petrolatum and ultraviolet B

96912   psoralens and ultraviolet A (PUVA)

96913   Photochemotherapy (Goeckerman and/or PUVA) for severe photoresponsive dermatoses requiring at least 4 to 8 hours of care under direct supervision of the physician (includes application of medication and dressings)

96920   Laser treatment for inflammatory skin disease (psoriasis); total area less than 250 sq cm

96921   250 sq cm to 500 sq cm

96922   over 500 sq cm

(For laser destruction of premalignant lesions, see 17000-17004)

(For laser destruction of cutaneous vascular proliferative lesions, see 17106-17108)

(For laser destruction of benign lesions, see 17110-17111)

(For laser destruction of malignant lesions, see 17260-17286)

Codes 96931, 96932, 96933, 96934, 96935, 96936 describe the acquisition and/or diagnostic interpretation of the device generated stitched image mosaics related to a single lesion. Do not report 96931, 96932, 96933, 96934, 96935, 96936 for a reflectance confocal microscopy examination that does not produce mosaic images. For services rendered using reflectance confocal microscopy not generating mosaic images, use 96999.

(For optical coherence tomography [OCT] for microstructural and morphological imaging of skin, see 0470T, 0471T)

96931   Reflectance confocal microscopy (RCM) for cellular and sub-cellular imaging of skin; image acquisition and interpretation and report, first lesion

96932   image acquisition only, first lesion

96933   interpretation and report only, first lesion

+ **96934**   image acquisition and interpretation and report, each additional lesion (List separately in addition to code for primary procedure)

(Use 96934 in conjunction with 96931)

+ **96935**   image acquisition only, each additional lesion (List separately in addition to code for primary procedure)

● New Code   ▲ Revised Code   + Add-On Code   ⊘ Modifier -51 Exempt   ★ Telemedicine

(Use 96935 in conjunction with 96932)

+ **96936** interpretation and report only, each additional lesion (List separately in addition to code for primary procedure)

(Use 96936 in conjunction with 96933)

96999 Unlisted special dermatological service or procedure

PHYSICAL MEDICINE AND REHABILITATION

Codes 97010-97763 should be used to report each distinct procedure performed. Do not append modifier 51 to 97010-97763.

The work of the physician or other qualified health care professional consists of face-to-face time with the patient (and caregiver, if applicable) delivering skilled services. For the purpose of determining the total time of a service, incremental intervals of treatment at the same visit may be accumulated.

The meanings of terms in the Physical Medicine and Rehabilitation section are not the same as those in the Evaluation and Management Services section (99202-99350). Do not use the Definitions of Commonly Used Terms in the Evaluation and Management (E/M) Guidelines for physical medicine and rehabilitation services.

(For range of joint motion, see 95851, 95852)

(For biofeedback training by EMG, use 90901)

(For transcutaneous nerve stimulation [TENS], use 97014 for electrical stimulation requiring supervision only, or use 97032 for electrical stimulation requiring constant attendance)

Physical Therapy Evaluations

Physical therapy evaluations include a patient history and an examination with development of a plan of care, conducted by the physician or other qualified health care professional, which is based on the composite of the patient's presentation.

Coordination, consultation, and collaboration of care with physicians, other qualified health care professionals, or agencies is provided consistent with the nature of the problem(s) and the needs of the patient, family, and/or other caregivers.

At a minimum, each of the following components noted in the code descriptors must be documented, in order to report the selected level of physical therapy evaluation. Physical therapy evaluations include the following components:

- History
- Examination
- Clinical decision making
- Development of plan of care

Report 97164 for performance of patient re-evaluation that is based on an established and ongoing plan of care.

Definitions

The level of the physical therapy evaluation performed is dependent on clinical decision making and on the nature of the patient's condition (severity). For the purpose of reporting physical therapy evaluations, the body regions and body systems are defined as follows:

Body regions: head, neck, back, lower extremities, upper extremities, and trunk.

Body systems: musculoskeletal, neuromuscular, cardiovascular pulmonary, and integumentary.

A *review of body systems* include the following:

- For the musculoskeletal system: the assessment of gross symmetry, gross range of motion, gross strength, height, and weight
- For the neuromuscular system: a general assessment of gross coordinated movement (eg, balance, gait, locomotion, transfers, and transitions) and motor function (motor control and motor learning)

- For the cardiovascular pulmonary system: the assessment of heart rate, respiratory rate, blood pressure, and edema

- For the integumentary system: the assessment of pliability (texture), presence of scar formation, skin color, and skin integrity

A review of any of the body systems also includes the assessment of the ability to make needs known, consciousness, orientation (person, place, and time), expected emotional/behavioral responses, and learning preferences (eg, learning barriers, education needs)

Body structures: The structural or anatomical parts of the body, such as organs, limbs, and their components, classified according to body systems.

Personal factors: Factors that include sex, age, coping styles, social background, education, profession, past and current experience, overall behavior pattern, character, and other factors that influence how disability is experienced by the individual. Personal factors that exist but do not impact the physical therapy plan of care are not to be considered, when selecting a level of service.

97161　Physical therapy evaluation: low complexity, requiring these components:

　　—A history with no personal factors and/or comorbidities that impact the plan of care;

　　—An examination of body system(s) using standardized tests and measures addressing 1-2 elements from any of the following: body structures and functions, activity limitations, and/or participation restrictions;

　　—A clinical presentation with stable and/or uncomplicated characteristics; and

　　—Clinical decision making of low complexity using standardized patient assessment instrument and/or measurable assessment of functional outcome. Typically, 20 minutes are spent face-to-face with the patient and/or family.

97162　Physical therapy evaluation: moderate complexity, requiring these components:

　　—A history of present problem with 1-2 personal factors and/or comorbidities that impact the plan of care;

　　—An examination of body systems using standardized tests and measures in addressing a total of 3 or more elements from any of the following: body structures and functions, activity limitations, and/or participation restrictions;

　　—An evolving clinical presentation with changing characteristics; and

　　—Clinical decision making of moderate complexity using standardized patient assessment instrument and/or measurable assessment of functional outcome.

　　Typically, 30 minutes are spent face-to-face with the patient and/or family.

97163　Physical therapy evaluation: high complexity, requiring these components:

　　—A history of present problem with 3 or more personal factors and/or comorbidities that impact the plan of care;

　　—An examination of body systems using standardized tests and measures addressing a total of 4 or more elements from any of the following: body structures and functions, activity limitations, and/or participation restrictions;

　　—A clinical presentation with unstable and unpredictable characteristics; and

　　—Clinical decision making of high complexity using standardized patient assessment instrument and/or measurable assessment of functional outcome.

　　Typically, 45 minutes are spent face-to-face with the patient and/or family.

97164　Re-evaluation of physical therapy established plan of care, requiring these components:

　　—An examination including a review of history and use of standardized tests and measures is required; and

　　—Revised plan of care using a standardized patient assessment instrument and/or measurable assessment of functional outcome

　● New Code　▲ Revised Code　✛ Add-On Code　⊘ Modifier -51 Exempt　★ Telemedicine

Typically, 20 minutes are spent face-to-face with the patient and/or family.

Occupational Therapy Evaluations

Occupational therapy evaluations include an occupational profile, medical and therapy history, relevant assessments, and development of a plan of care, which reflects the therapist's clinical reasoning and interpretation of the data.

Coordination, consultation, and collaboration of care with physicians, other qualified health care professionals, or agencies is provided consistent with the nature of the problem(s) and the needs of the patient, family and/or other caregivers.

At a minimum, each of the following components noted in the code descriptors must be documented, in order to report the selected level of occupational therapy evaluation.

Occupational therapy evaluations include the following components:

- Occupational profile and client history (medical and therapy)
- Assessments of occupational performance
- Clinical decision making
- Development of plan of care

Report 97168 for performance of a re-evaluation that is based on an established and ongoing plan of care.

Definitions

The level of the occupational therapy evaluation performed is determined by patient condition, complexity of clinical decision making, and the scope and nature of the patient's performance deficits relating to physical, cognitive, or psychosocial skills to be assessed. The patient's plan of treatment should reflect assessment of each of the identified performance deficits.

Performance deficits: performance deficits refer to the inability to complete activities due to the lack of skills in one or more of the categories below (ie, relating to physical, cognitive, or psychosocial skills):

Physical skills: Physical skills refer to impairments of body structure or body function (eg, balance, mobility, strength, endurance, fine or gross motor coordination, sensation, dexterity).

Cognitive skills: Cognitive skills refer to the ability to attend, perceive, think, understand, problem solve, mentally sequence, learn, and remember resulting in the ability to organize occupational performance in a timely and safe manner. These skills are observed when: (1) a person attends to and selects, interacts with, and uses task tools and materials; (2) carries out individual actions and steps; and (3) modifies performance when problems are encountered.

Psychosocial skills: Psychosocial skills refer to interpersonal interactions, habits, routines and behaviors, active use of coping strategies, and/or environmental adaptations to develop skills necessary to successfully and appropriately participate in everyday tasks and social situations.b

97165   Occupational therapy evaluation, low complexity, requiring these components:

—An occupational profile and medical and therapy history, which includes a brief history including review of medical and/or therapy records relating to the presenting problem;

—An assessment(s) that identifies 1-3 performance deficits (ie, relating to physical, cognitive, or psychosocial skills) that result in activity limitations and/or participation restrictions; and

—Clinical decision making of low complexity, which includes an analysis of the occupational profile, analysis of data from problem-focused assessment(s), and consideration of a limited number of treatment options. Patient presents with no comorbidities that affect occupational performance. Modification of tasks or assistance (eg, physical or verbal) with assessment(s) is not necessary to enable completion of evaluation component.

Typically, 30 minutes are spent face-to-face with the patient and/or family.

97166   Occupational therapy evaluation, moderate complexity, requiring these components:

—An occupational profile and medical and therapy history, which includes an expanded review of medical and/or therapy records and additional review of physical, cognitive, or psychosocial history related to current functional performance;

—An assessment(s) that identifies 3-5 performance deficits (ie, relating to physical, cognitive, or psychosocial skills) that result in activity limitations and/or participation restrictions; and

—Clinical decision making of moderate analytic complexity, which includes an analysis of the occupational profile, analysis of data from detailed assessment(s), and consideration of several treatment options. Patient may present with comorbidities that affect occupational performance. Minimal to moderate modification of tasks or assistance (eg, physical or verbal) with assessment(s) is necessary to enable patient to complete evaluation component.

Typically, 45 minutes are spent face-to-face with the patient and/or family.

97167   Occupational therapy evaluation, high complexity, requiring these components:

—An occupational profile and medical and therapy history, which includes review of medical and/or therapy records and extensive additional review of physical, cognitive, or psychosocial history related to current functional performance;

—An assessment(s) that identifies 5 or more performance deficits (ie, relating to physical, cognitive, or psychosocial skills) that result in activity limitations and/or participation restrictions; and

—Clinical decision making of high analytic complexity, which includes an analysis of the patient profile, analysis of data from comprehensive assessment(s), and consideration of multiple treatment options. Patient presents with comorbidities that affect occupational performance. Significant modification of tasks or assistance (eg, physical or verbal) with assessment(s) is necessary to enable patient to complete evaluation component.

Typically, 60 minutes are spent face-to-face with the patient and/or family.

97168   Re-evaluation of occupational therapy established plan of care, requiring these components:

—An assessment of changes in patient functional or medical status with revised plan of care;

—An update to the initial occupational profile to reflect changes in condition or environment that affect future interventions and/or goals; and

—A revised plan of care. A formal reevaluation is performed when there is a documented change in functional status or a significant change to the plan of care is required.

Typically, 30 minutes are spent face-to-face with the patient and/or family.

Athletic Training Evaluations

Athletic training evaluations include a patient history and an examination with development of a plan of care, conducted by the physician or other qualified health care professional.

Coordination, consultation, and collaboration of care with physicians, other qualified health care professionals, or agencies is provided consistent with the nature of the problem(s) and the needs of the patient, family, and/or other caregivers.

At a minimum, each of the following components noted in the code descriptors must be documented, in order to report the selected level of athletic training evaluation.

Athletic training evaluations include the following components:

- History and physical activity profile
- Examination
- Clinical decision making
- Development of plan of care

Report 97172 for performance of patient re-evaluation that is based on an established and ongoing plan of care.

Definitions

For the purpose of reporting athletic training evaluations, the body areas and body systems are defined as follows:

Body areas: head, neck, back, lower extremities, upper extremities, and trunk

Body systems: musculoskeletal, neuromuscular, cardiovascular pulmonary, and integumentary.

The body systems review includes the following:

> For the musculoskeletal system: the assessment of gross symmetry, gross range of motion, gross strength, height, and weight

> For the neuromuscular system: a general assessment of gross coordinated movement (eg, balance, gait, locomotion, transfers, and transitions) and motor function (motor control and motor learning)

> For the cardiovascular pulmonary system: the assessment of heart rate, respiratory rate, blood pressure, and edema

> For the integumentary system: the assessment of pliability (texture), presence of scar formation, skin color, and skin integrity

97169 Athletic training evaluation, low complexity, requiring these components:

> —A history and physical activity profile with no comorbidities that affect physical activity;

> —An examination of affected body area and other symptomatic or related systems addressing 1-2 elements from any of the following: body structures, physical activity, and/or participation deficiencies; and

> —Clinical decision making of low complexity using standardized patient assessment instrument and/or measurable assessment of functional outcome.

> Typically, 15 minutes are spent face-to-face with the patient and/or family.

97170 Athletic training evaluation, moderate complexity, requiring these components:

> —A medical history and physical activity profile with 1-2 comorbidities that affect physical activity;

> —An examination of affected body area and other symptomatic or related systems addressing a total of 3 or more elements from any of the following: body structures, physical activity, and/or participation deficiencies; and

> —Clinical decision making of moderate complexity using standardized patient assessment instrument and/or measurable assessment of functional outcome.

> Typically, 30 minutes are spent face-to-face with the patient and/or family.

97171 Athletic training evaluation, high complexity, requiring these components:

> —A medical history and physical activity profile, with 3 or more comorbidities that affect physical activity;

> —A comprehensive examination of body systems using standardized tests and measures addressing a total of 4 or more elements from any of the following: body structures, physical activity, and/or participation deficiencies;

> —Clinical presentation with unstable and unpredictable characteristics; and

> —Clinical decision making of high complexity using standardized patient assessment instrument and/or measurable assessment of functional outcome.

> Typically, 45 minutes are spent face-to-face with the patient and/or family.

97172 Re-evaluation of athletic training established plan of care requiring these components:

> —An assessment of patient's current functional status when there is a documented change; and

---

—A revised plan of care using a standardized patient assessment instrument and/or measurable assessment of functional outcome with an update in management options, goals, and interventions.

Typically, 20 minutes are spent face-to-face with the patient and/or family

MODALITIES

SUPERVISED

The application of a modality that does not require direct (one-on-one) patient contact.

97010   Application of a modality to 1 or more areas; hot or cold packs

97012   traction, mechanical

97014   electrical stimulation (unattended)

            (For acupuncture with electrical stimulation, see 97813, 97814)

97016   vasopneumatic devices

97018   paraffin bath

97022   whirlpool

97024   diathermy (eg, microwave)

97026   infrared

97028   ultraviolet

CONSTANT ATTENDANCE

The application of a modality that requires direct (one-on-one) patient contact.

97032   Application of a modality to 1 or more areas; electrical stimulation (manual), each 15 minutes

            (For transcutaneous electrical modulation pain reprocessing (TEMPR/scrambler therapy], use 0278T)

97033   iontophoresis, each 15 minutes

97034   contrast baths, each 15 minutes

97035   ultrasound, each 15 minutes

97036   Hubbard tank, each 15 minutes

97039   Unlisted modality (specify type and time if constant attendance)

THERAPEUTIC PROCEDURES

A manner of effecting change through the application of clinical skills and/or services that attempt to improve function. Physician or other qualified health care professional (ie, therapist) required to have direct (one-on-one) patient contact.

97110   Therapeutic procedure, 1 or more areas, each 15 minutes; therapeutic exercises to develop strength and endurance, range of motion and flexibility

97112   neuromuscular reeducation of movement, balance, coordination, kinesthetic sense, posture, and/or proprioception for sitting and/or standing activities

97113   aquatic therapy with therapeutic exercises

● New Code   ▲ Revised Code   ✚ Add-On Code   ⊘ Modifier -51 Exempt   ★ Telemedicine

97116   gait training (includes stair climbing)

(Use 96000-96003 to report comprehensive gait and motion analysis procedures)

97124   massage, including effleurage, petrissage and/or tapotement (stroking, compression, percussion)

(For myofascial release, use 97140)

(**97127**   deleted 2019 [2020 Edition]. To report, use 97129)

97129   Therapeutic interventions that focus on cognitive function (eg, attention, memory, reasoning, executive function, problem solving, and/or pragmatic functioning) and compensatory strategies to manage the performance of an activity (eg, managing time or schedules, initiating, organizing, and sequencing tasks), direct (one-on-one) patient contact; initial 15 minutes

(Report 97129 only once per day)

+ **97130**   each additional 15 minutes (List separately in addition to code for primary procedure)

(Use 97130 in conjunction with 97129)

(Do not report 97129, 97130 in conjunction with 97153, 97155)

97139   Unlisted therapeutic procedure (specify)

97140   Manual therapy techniques (eg, mobilization/ manipulation, manual lymphatic drainage, manual traction), 1 or more regions, each 15 minutes

(For needle insertion[s] without injection[s] [eg, dry needling, trigger-point acupuncture], see 20560, 20561)

97150   Therapeutic procedure(s), group (2 or more individuals)

(Report 97150 for each member of group)

(Group therapy procedures involve constant attendance of the physician or other qualified health care professional [ie, therapist], but by definition do not require one-on-one patient contact by the same physician or other qualified health care professional)

(For manipulation under general anesthesia, see appropriate anatomic section in Musculoskeletal System)

(For osteopathic manipulative treatment (OMT), see 98925-98929)

(Do not report 97150 in conjunction with 97154, 97158)

97151   This code is out of order. See page 957

97152   This code is out of order. See page 957

97153   This code is out of order. See page 958

97154   This code is out of order. See page 958

97155   This code is out of order. See page 958

97156   This code is out of order. See page 958

97157   This code is out of order. See page 959

97158   This code is out of order. See page 959

97161   This code is out of order. See page 974

97162   This code is out of order. See page 974

97163	This code is out of order. See page 974
97164	This code is out of order. See page 974
97165	This code is out of order. See page 975
97166	This code is out of order. See page 976
97167	This code is out of order. See page 976
97168	This code is out of order. See page 976
97169	This code is out of order. See page 977
97170	This code is out of order. See page 977
97171	This code is out of order. See page 977
97172	This code is out of order. See page 977

97530 Therapeutic activities, direct (one-on-one) patient contact (use of dynamic activities to improve functional performance), each 15 minutes

(**97532** deleted 2017 [2018 edition]. To report, use 97129)

97533 Sensory integrative techniques to enhance sensory processing and promote adaptive responses to environmental demands, direct (one-on-one) patient contact, each 15 minutes

97535 Self-care/home management training (eg, activities of daily living (ADL) and compensatory training, meal preparation, safety procedures, and instructions in use of assistive technology devices/adaptive equipment) direct one-on-one contact, each 15 minutes

97537 Community/work reintegration training (eg, shopping, transportation, money management, avocational activities and/or work environment/modification analysis, work task analysis, use of assistive technology device/adaptive equipment), direct one-on-one contact, each 15 minutes

(For wheelchair management/propulsion training, use 97542)

97542 Wheelchair management (eg, assessment, fitting, training), each 15 minutes

97545 Work hardening/conditioning; initial 2 hours

+ **97546**   each additional hour (List separately in addition to code for primary procedure)

(Use 97546 in conjunction with code 97545)

ACTIVE WOUND CARE MANAGEMENT

Active wound care procedures are performed to remove devitalized and/or necrotic tissue and promote healing. Chemical cauterization (17250) to achieve wound hemostasis is included in active wound care procedures (97597, 97598, 97602) and should not be separately reported for the same lesion. Services require direct (one-on-one) contact with the patient.

(Do not report 97597-97602 in conjunction with 11042-11047 for the same wound)

(For debridement of burn wounds, see 16020-16030)

97597 Debridement (eg, high pressure waterjet with/without suction, sharp selective debridement with scissors, scalpel and forceps), open wound, (eg, fibrin, devitalized epidermis and/or dermis, exudate, debris, biofilm) including topical application(s), wound assessment, use of a whirlpool, when performed, and instruction(s) for ongoing care, per session, total wound(s) surface area; first 20 square centimeters or less

---

● New Code ▲ Revised Code + Add-On Code ⊘ Modifier -51 Exempt ★ Telemedicine

+ 97598   each additional 20 square centimeters or part thereof (List separately in addition to code for primary procedure)

(Use 97598 in conjunction with 97597)

97602   Removal of devitalized tissue from wound(s), nonselective debridement, without anesthesia (eg, wet-tomoist dressings, enzymatic, abrasion, larval therapy), including topical application(s), wound assessment, and instruction(s) for ongoing care, per session

97605   Negative pressure wound therapy (eg, vacuum assisted drainage collection), utilizing durable medical equipment (DME), including topical application(s), wound assessment, and instruction(s) for ongoing care, per session; total wound(s) surface area less than or equal to 50 square centimeters

97606   total wound(s) surface area greater than 50 square centimeters

97607   Negative pressure wound therapy, (eg, vacuum assisted drainage collection), utilizing disposable, non-durable medical equipment including provision of exudate management collection system, topical application(s), wound assessment, and instructions for ongoing care, per session; total wound(s) surface area less than or equal to 50 square centimeters

97608   total wound(s) surface area less than or equal to 50 square centimeters

(Do not report 97607, 97608 in conjunction with 97605, 97606)

97610   Low frequency, non-contact, non-thermal ultrasound, including topical application(s), when performed, wound assessment, and instruction(s) for ongoing care, per day

TESTS AND MEASUREMENTS

Requires direct one-on-one patient contact.

(For joint range of motion, see 95851, 95852; for electromyography, see 95860-95872, 95885, 95886, 95887; for nerve velocity determination, see 95905, 95907, 95908, 95909, 95910, 95911, 95912, 95913)

97750   Physical performance test or measurement (eg, musculo-skeletal, functional capacity), with written report, each 15 minutes

97755   Assistive technology assessment (eg, to restore, augment or compensate for existing function, optimize functional tasks and/or maximize environmental accessibility), direct one-on-one contact, with written report, each 15 minutes

(To report augmentative and alternative communication devices, use 92605 or 92607)

ORTHOTIC MANAGEMENT AND TRAINING AND PROSTHETIC TRAINING

97760   Orthotic(s) management and training (including assessment and fitting when not otherwise reported), upper extremity(ies), lower extremity(ies) and/or trunk, initial orthotic(s) encounter, each 15 minutes

(Code 97760 should not be reported with 97116 for the same extremity[ies])

97761   Prosthetic(s) training, upper and/or lower extremity(ies), initial prosthetic(s) encounter, each 15 minutes

(97762   deleted 2017 [2018 edition]. To report, use 97763)

97763   Orthotic(s)/prosthetic(s) management and/or training, upper extremity(ies), lower extremity(ies), and/or trunk, subsequent orthotic(s)/prosthetic(s) encounter, each 15 minutes

(Do not report 97763 in conjunction with 97760, 97761)

OTHER PROCEDURES

(For extracorporeal shock wave musculoskeletaltherapy, see 0101T, 0102T)

97799   Unlisted physical medicine/rehabilitation service or procedure

MEDICAL NUTRITION THERAPY

Medical nutrition therapy (MNT) is the assessment of nutritional status followed by nutritional therapy. The nutrition assessment includes review and analysis of 1) medical, nutrition and medication histories, 2) physical examination, 3) anthropometric measurements, and 4) laboratory test values. Nutrition therapy may include 1) diet modification, 2) counseling and education, 3) disease self-management skills training, and 4) administration of specialized therapies such as medical foods, intravenous or tube feedings.

★ 97802   Medical nutrition therapy; initial assessment and intervention, individual, face-to-face with the patient, each 15 minutes

★ 97803   re-assessment and intervention, individual, face-to-face with the patient, each 15 minutes

★ 97804   group (2 or more individual(s)), each 30 minutes

        (Physicians and other qualified health care professional who may report evaluation and management services should use the appropriate E/M codes)

ACUPUNCTURE

Acupuncture refers to the insertion of thin needles through the skin at specific points on the body to control pain and other symptoms. It is a type of complementary and alternative medicine. The acupuncture needle is a stainless steel needle that is slightly thicker than a human hair. The specific spot on the body where a acupuncture needle may be inserted is call an acupuncture point or acupoint.

Acupuncture is reported based on 15-minute increments of personal (face-to-face) contact with the patient, not the duration of acupuncture needle(s) placement.

If no electrical stimulation is used during a 15-minute increment, use 97810, 97811. If electrical stimulation of any needle is used during a 15-minute increment, use 97813, 97814.

Only one code may be reported for each 15-minute increment. Use either 97810 or 97813 for the initial 15-minute increment. Only one initial code is reported per day.

Evaluation and management services may be reported in addition to acupuncture procedures when performed by physicians or other health care professionals, who may report evaluation and management (E/M) services, including new or established patient office or other outpatient services (99202-99215), hospital observation care (99217-99220, 99224-99226), hospital care (99221-99223, 99231-99233), office or other outpatient consultations (99241-99245), inpatient consultations (99251-99255), critical care services (99291, 99292), inpatient neonatal intensive care services and pediatric and neonatal critical care services (99466-99480), emergency department services (99281-99285), nursing facility services (99304-99318), domiciliary, rest home, or custodial care services (99324-99337), and home services (99341-99350) may be reported separately using modifier 25 if the patient's condition requires a significant, separately identifiable E/M service above and beyond the usual preservice and postservice work associated with the acupuncture services. The time of the E/M service is not included in the time of the acupuncture service.

For needle insertion(s) without injection(s) (eg, dry needling, trigger point acupuncture), see 20560, 20561.

97810   Acupuncture, one or more needles; without electrical stimulation, initial 15 minutes of personal one-on-one contact with the patient

        (Do not report 97810 in conjunction with 97813)

+ 97811   without electrical stimulation, each additional 15 minutes of personal one-on-one contact with the patient, with re-insertion of needle(s) (List separately in addition to code for primary procedure)

        (Use 97811 in conjunction with 97810, 97813)

97813   with electrical stimulation, initial 15 minutes of personal one-on-one contact with the patient

        (Do not report 97813 in conjunction with 97810)

● New Code   ▲ Revised Code   + Add-On Code   ⊘ Modifier -51 Exempt   ★ Telemedicine

+ **97814**   with electrical stimulation, each additional 15 minutes of personal one-on-one contact with the patient, with re-insertion of needle(s) (List separately in addition to code for primary procedure)

(Use 97814 in conjunction with 97810, 97813)

(Do not report 97810, 97811, 97813, 97814 in conjunction with 20560, 20561. When both time-based acupuncture services and needle insertion[s] without injection[s] are performed, report only the time-based acupuncture codes)

OSTEOPATHIC MANIPULATIVE TREATMENT

Osteopathic medicine is a system of therapy based on the theory that the body is capable of making its own remedies against disease and other toxic conditions when it is in normal structural relationship and has favorable environmental conditions and adequate nutrition. Osteopathic manipulative treatment (OMT) is a form of manual treatment applied by a physician to eliminate or alleviate somatic dysfunction and related disorders. This treatment may be accomplished by a variety of techniques.

Osteopathic Manipulative Treatment (OMT) is subject to Global Surgery Rules. Per Medicare Anesthesia Rules a provider performing OMT cannot separately report anesthesia services such as nerve blocks or epidural injections for OMT. In addition, per Medicare Global Surgery Rules, postoperative pain management after OMT (e.g., nerve block, epidural injection) is not separately reportable. Epidural or nerve block injections performed on the same date of service as OMT and unrelated to the MT may be reported with OMT using modifier -59.

Coding Rules

1. *Evaluation and management services may be reported separately, if, and only if the patient's condition requires a significant separately identifiable evaluation and management service, above and beyond the usual pre-service and post service work associated with the osteopathic manipulation.*

2. *CPT codes in this section are used to report OMT services provided in any location.*

Evaluation and management (E/M) services including new or established patient office or other outpatient services (99202-99215), hospital observation care (99217-99220, 99224-99226), hospital care (99221-99223, 99231-99233), critical care services (99291, 99292), observation or inpatient care services (99234-99236), office or other outpatient consultations (99241-99245), emergency department services (99281-99285), nursing facility services (99304-99318), domiciliary, rest home, or custodial care services (99324-99337), and home services (99341-99350) may be reported separately using modifier 25 if the patient's condition requires a significant, separately identifiable E/M service above and beyond the usual preservice and postservice work associated with the procedure. The E/M service may be caused or prompted by the same symptoms or condition for which the OMT service was provided. As such, different diagnoses are not required for the reporting of the OMT and E/M service on the same date.

98925   Osteopathic manipulative treatment (OMT); 1-2 body regions involved

98926   3-4 body regions involved

98927   5-6 body regions involved

98928   7-8 body regions involved

98929   9-10 body regions involved

CHIROPRACTIC MANIPULATIVE TREATMENT

Chiropractic medicine is a system of diagnosis and treatment based on the theory that irritation of the nervous system by mechanical, chemical or psychic factors is the cause of disease. Chiropractic services may include office visits, diagnostic tests, physical therapy, and/or chiropractic manipulation. Chiropractic manipulation treatment (CMT) is a form of manual treatment applied by a chiropractic physician to eliminate or alleviate somatic dysfunction and related disorders.

Coding Rules

1. *Chiropractic manipulation treatment includes a pre-manipulation patient assessment.*

Separate Procedure   Unlisted Procedure   CCI Comp. Code   Non-specific Procedure   **983**

2. Evaluation and management services provided in conjunction with CMT may be reported separately with the addition of CPT modifier -25, along with any diagnostic tests or other therapy provided.

REPORTING CHIROPRACTIC MANIPULATION TO MEDICARE

Medicare restricts the number of times the CMT code may be reported, provides a maximum reimbursement amount per year, and requires extensive supporting documentation as described below:

Documentation of Treatment Phase

Proper documentation of the treatment phase is extremely important when submitting claims for chiropractic services to Medicare. The treatment phase consists of the date the course of treatment was initiated and the number of treatments rendered to date. Proper documentation enables Medicare to process your claims quickly and accurately. For payment of chiropractic claims, the following information must be on the CMS1500 claim form:

1. The service must be manual manipulation of the spine. This service is reported by CPT codes 98940-98943.

2. The primary diagnosis must be subluxation of the spine, either so stated or identified by a term descriptive of the subluxation. The following diagnoses are acceptable because they would always involve a subluxation:

Intervertebral disc disorders	722.0-722.9
Curvatures of the spine	737.0-737.9
Spondylolisthesis	738.4, 756.12
Nonallopathic lesions	739.1-739.4
Spondylolysis	756.11

3. The level of subluxation must be stated.

4. The symptoms related to the level of subluxation must be given.

5. The date of the confirming x-ray must be on the claim. Note that the x-ray must have been taken within 12 months prior to or 3 months after the course of treatment was initiated.

6. The date this course of treatment was initiated and the number of treatments rendered since the start of this course must be on the claim.

Special Situations

If a patient returns with a new condition or injury, this represents a new treatment phase. The treatment phase information should reflect when you first saw the patient for this condition. Do not use the date you first saw the patient for an earlier course of treatment. Note on your CMS1500 claim form that this is a new condition. Remember that a new documenting x-ray may be required.

In the case of chronic conditions, an x-ray older than 12 months may be acceptable. For coverage of chronic conditions such as scoliosis, spondylolysis, and spondylolisthesis, there must be a reasonable expectation that there is a restorative potential. Remember that maintenance care is not covered by Medicare.

Chiropractic Manipulative Treatment Medicare covers chiropractic manipulative treatment (CMT) of five spinal regions. Physical therapy services described by CPT codes 97112, 97124 and 97140 are not separately reportable when performed in a spinal region undergoing CMT. If these physical therapy services are performed in a different region than CMT and the provider is eligible to report physical therapy codes under the Medicare program, the provider may report CMT and the above physical therapy codes using modifier -59.

The chiropractic manipulative treatment codes include a pre-manipulation patient assessment. Additional evaluation and management (E/M) services including office or other outpatient services (99202-99215), subsequent observation care (99224-99226), subsequent hospital care (99231-99233), office or other outpatient consultations (99241-99245), subsequent nursing facility services (99307-99310), domiciliary, rest home, or custodial care services (99324-99337), and home services (99341-99350) may be reported separately using modifier 25 if the patient's condition requires a significant, separately identifiable E/M service above and beyond the usual preservice and postservice work associated with the procedure. The E/M service may be caused or prompted by the same symptoms or condition for which the CMT service was provided. As such, different diagnoses are not required for the reporting of the CMT and E/M service on the same date.

For purposes of CMT, the five spinal regions referred to are: cervical region (includes atlanto-occipital joint); thoracic region (includes costovertebral and costotransverse joints); lumbar region; sacral region; and pelvic (sacro-iliac joint) region. The five

● New Code ▲ Revised Code + Add-On Code ⊘ Modifier -51 Exempt ★ Telemedicine

extraspinal regions referred to are: head (including temporomandibular joint, excluding atlanto-occipital) region; lower extremities; upper extremities; rib cage (excluding costotransverse and costovertebral joints) and abdomen.

98940 Chiropractic manipulative treatment (CMT); spinal, 1-2 regions

98941 spinal, 3-4 regions

98942 spinal, 5 regions

98943 extraspinal, 1 or more regions

EDUCATION AND TRAINING FOR PATIENT SELF-MANAGEMENT

The following codes are used to report educational and training services prescribed by a physician or other qualified health care professional and provided by a qualified, nonphysician health care professional using a standardized curriculum to an individual or group of patients for the treatment of established illness/disease(s) or to delay comorbidity(s). Education and training for patient self-management may be reported with these codes only when using a standardized curriculum as described below. This curriculum may be modified as necessary for the clinical needs, cultural norms and health literacy of the patient(s).

(For counseling and education provided by a physician to an individual, see the appropriate evaluation and management codes including office or other outpatient services [99202-99215], hospital observation care [99217-99220, 99224-99226], hospital care [99221-99223, 99231-99233], new or established patient office or other outpatient consultations [99241-99245], inpatient consultations [99251-99255], emergency department services [99281-99285], nursing facility services [99304-99318], domiciliary, rest home, or custodial care services [99324-99337], home services [99341-99350], and counseling risk factor reduction and behavior change intervention [99401-99429]. See also Instructions for Use of the CPT Codebook for definition of reporting qualifications)

(For counseling and education provided by a physician to a group, use 99078)

(For counseling and/or risk factor reduction intervention provided by a physician to patient(s) without symptoms or established disease, see 99401-99412)

(For medical nutrition therapy, see 97802-97804)

(For health behavior assessment and intervention that is not part of a standardized curriculum, see 96156, 96158, 96159, 96164, 96165, 96167, 96168, 96170, 96171)

(For education provided as genetic counseling services, use 96040. For education to a group regarding genetic risks, see 98961, 98962)

★ **98960** Education and training for patient self-management by a qualified, nonphysician health care professional using a standardized curriculum, face-to-face with the patient (could include caregiver/family) each 30 minutes; individual patient

★ **98961** 2-4 patients

★ **98962** 5-8 patients

NON-FACE-TO-FACE NONPHYSICIAN SERVICES

TELEPHONE SERVICES

Telephone services are non-face-to-face assessment and management services provided by a qualified health care professional to a patient via telephone. If the telephone call results in a decision to see the patient within 24 hours, the telephone call is not reported.

Telephone services are non-face-to-face assessment and management services provided by a qualified health care professional to a patient using the telephone. These codes are used to report episodes of care by the qualified health care professional initiated by an established patient or guardian of an established patient. If the telephone service ends with a decision to see the patient within 24 hours or the next available urgent visit appointment, the code is not reported; rather the encounter is considered part of the preservice work of the subsequent assessment and management service, procedure, and visit. Likewise, if the telephone call refers to a service performed and reported by the qualified health care professional within the previous seven days (either qualified health care professional requested or unsolicited patient follow-up) or within the postoperative period of the previously completed procedure, then the service(s) are considered part of that previous service or procedure. (Do not report 98966-98968 if reporting 98966-98968 performed in the previous seven days.)

(For telephone services provided by a physician, see 99441-99443)

98966 Telephone assessment and management service provided by a qualified nonphysician health care professional to an established patient, parent, or guardian not originating from a related assessment and management service provided within the previous 7 days nor leading to an assessment and management service or procedure within the next 24 hours or soonest available appointment; 5-10 minutes of medical discussion

98967 11-20 minutes of medical discussion

98968 21-30 minutes of medical discussion

(Do not report 98966-98968 during the same month with 99439, 99487, 99489, 99490, 99491)

(Do not report 98966, 98967, 98968 in conjunction with 93792, 93793)

QUALIFIED NONPHYSICIAN HEALTH CARE PROFESSIONAL ONLINE DIGITAL EVALUATION AND MANAGEMENT SERVICE

Qualified nonphysician health care professional online digital evaluation and management (E/M) services are patient-initiated digital services with qualified nonphysician health care professionals that require qualified nonphysician health care professional patient evaluation and decision making to generate an assessment and subsequent management of the patient. These services are not for the nonevaluative electronic communication of test results, scheduling of appointments, or other communication that does not include E/M. While the patient's problem may be new to the qualified nonphysician health care professional, the patient is an established patient. Patients initiate these services through Health Insurance Portability and Accountability Act (HIPAA)-compliant, secure platforms, such as through the electronic health record (EHR) portal, email, or other digital applications, which allow digital communication with the qualified nonphysician health care professional.

Qualified nonphysician health care professional online digital E/M services are reported once for the qualified nonphysician health care professional's cumulative time devoted to the service during a seven-day period. The seven-day period begins with the qualified nonphysician health care professional's initial, personal review of the patient-generated inquiry. Qualified nonphysician health care professional cumulative service time includes review of the initial inquiry, review of patient records or data pertinent to assessment of the patient's problem, personal qualified nonphysician health care professional interaction with clinical staff focused on the patient's problem, development of management plans, including qualified nonphysician health care professional generation of prescriptions or ordering of tests, and subsequent communication with the patient through online, telephone, email, or other digitally supported communication. All qualified nonphysician health care professionals in the same group practice who are involved in the online digital E/M service contribute to the cumulative service time devoted to the patient's online digital E/M service. Qualified nonphysician health care professional online digital E/M services require visit documentation and permanent storage (electronic or hard copy) of the encounter.

If the patient generates the initial online digital inquiry within seven days of a previous treatment or E/M service and both services relate to the same problem, or the online digital inquiry occurs within the postoperative period of a previously completed procedure, then the qualified nonphysician health care professional's online digital E/M service may not be reported separately. If the patient generates an initial online digital inquiry for a new problem within seven days of a previous service that addressed a different problem, then the qualified nonphysician health care professional online digital E/M service is reported separately. If a separately reported evaluation service occurs within seven days of the qualified nonphysician health care professional's initial review of the online digital E/M service, 98970, 98971, 98972 are not reported. If the patient presents a new, unrelated problem during the seven-day period of an online digital E/M service, then the qualified nonphysician health care professional's time spent on the evaluation and management of the additional problem is added to the cumulative service time of the online digital E/M service for that seven-day period.

(For an online digital E/M service provided by a physician or other qualified health care professional, see 99421, 99422, 99423)

(**98969** deleted 2019 [2020 Edition]. To report, see 98970, 98971, 98972)

98970 Qualified nonphysician health care professional online digital evaluation and management service, for an established patient, for up to 7 days, cumulative time during the 7 days; 5-10 minutes

---

● New Code ▲ Revised Code + Add-On Code ⊘ Modifier -51 Exempt ★ Telemedicine

98971   11-20 minutes

98972   21 or more minutes

> (Report 98970, 98971, 98972 once per 7-day period)
>
> (Do not report online digital E/M services for cumulative visit time less than 5 minutes)
>
> (Do not count 98970, 98971, 98972 time otherwise reported with other services)
>
> (Do not report 98970, 98971, 98972 for home and outpatient INR monitoring when reporting 93792, 93793)
>
> (Do not report 98970, 98971, 98972 when using 99091, 99339, 99340, 99374, 99375, 99377, 99378, 99379, 99380, 99439, 99487, 99489, 99490, 99491, for the same communication[s])

SPECIAL SERVICES, PROCEDURES AND REPORTS

The MEDICINE section of CPT includes a subsection Special Services and Reports, with CPT codes 99000-99090 which provides the reporting physician with a means of identifying the completion of special reports and services that are an adjunct to the basic services rendered. The specific special services code reported indicates the special circumstances under which a basic procedure is performed.

The proper use of Special Services CPT codes can result in a significant increase in reimbursement. Most codes in this section are "add on" codes which means that they are used in addition to whatever other CPT codes describe the procedures or services performed.

The procedures with code numbers 99000 through 99082 provide the reporting physician or other qualified health care professional with the means to identify the completion of special reports and services that are an adjunct to the basic services rendered. The specific number assigned indicates the special circumstances under which a basic procedure is performed.

Codes 99050-99060 are reported in addition to an associated basic service. Do not append modifier 51 to 99050-99060. Typically, only a single adjunct code from among 99050-99060 would be reported per patient encounter. However, there may be circumstances in which reporting multiple adjunct codes per patient encounter may be appropriate.

MISCELLANEOUS SERVICES

99000   Handling and/or conveyance of specimen for transfer from the office to a laboratory

99001   Handling and/or conveyance of specimen for transfer from the patient in other than an office to a laboratory (distance may be indicated)

99002   Handling, conveyance, and/or any other service in connection with the implementation of an order involving devices (eg, designing, fitting, packaging, handling, delivery or mailing) when devices such as orthotics, protectives, prosthetics are fabricated by an outside laboratory or shop but which items have been designed, and are to be fitted and adjusted by the attending physician or other qualified health care professional

> (For routine collection of venous blood, use 36415)

99024   Postoperative follow-up visit, normally included in the surgical package, to indicate that an evaluation and management service was performed during a postoperative period for a reason(s) related to the origianl procedure

> (As a component of a surgical "package," see Surgery guidelines)

99026   Hospital mandated on call service; in-hospital, each hour

99027   out-of-hospital, each hour

> (For standby services requiring prolonged attendance, use 99360, as appropriate. Time spent performing separately reportable procedure(s) or service(s) should not be included in the time reported as mandated on call service)

99050 Services provided in the office at times other than regularly scheduled office hours, or days when the office is normally closed (eg, holidays, Saturday or Sunday), in addition to basic service

99051 Service(s) provided in the office during regularly scheduled evening, weekend, or holiday office hours, in addition to basic service

99053 Service(s) provided between 10:00 PM and 8:00 AM at 24-hour facility, in addition to basic service

99056 Service(s) typically provided in the office, provided out of the office at request of patient, in addition to basic service

99058 Service(s) provided on an emergency basis in the office, which disrupts other scheduled office services, in addition to basic service

99060 Service(s) provided on an emergency basis, out of the office, which disrupts other scheduled office services, in addition to basic service

99070 Supplies and materials (except spectacles), provided by the physician or other qualified health care professional over and above those usually included with the office visit or other services rendered (list drugs, trays, supplies, or materials provided)

(For supply of spectacles, use the appropriate supply codes)

99071 Educational supplies, such as books, tapes, and pamphlets, for the patient's education at cost to physician or other qualified health care professional

● **99072** Additional supplies, materials, and clinical staff time over and above those usually included in an office visit or other non-facility service(s), when performed during a Public Health Emergency, as defined by law, due to respiratory-transmitted infectious disease

99075 Medical testimony

99078 Physician or other qualified health care professional qualified by education, training, licensure/regulation (when applicable) educational services rendered to patients in a group setting (eg, prenatal, obesity, or diabetic instructions)

99080 Special reports such as insurance forms, more than the information conveyed in the usual medical communications or standard reporting form

(Do not report 99080 in conjunction with 99455, 99456 for the completion of Workmen's Compensation forms)

99082 Unusual travel (eg, transportation and escort of patient)

(**99090** deleted 2018 [2019 Edition])

99091 This code is out of order. See page 180

QUALIFYING CIRCUMSTANCES FOR ANESTHESIA

(For explanation of these services, see Anesthesia guidelines)

+ **99100** Anesthesia for patient of extreme age, younger than 1 year and older than 70 (List separately in addition to code for primary anesthesia procedure)

(For procedure performed on infants less than 1 year of age at time of surgery, see 00326, 00561, 00834, 00836)

+ **99116** Anesthesia complicated by utilization of total body hypothermia (List separately in addition to code for primary anesthesia procedure)

● New Code   ▲ Revised Code   ✛ Add-On Code   ⊘ Modifier -51 Exempt   ★ Telemedicine

+ 99135 Anesthesia complicated by utilization of controlled hypotension (List separately in addition to code for primary anesthesia procedure)

+ 99140 Anesthesia complicated by emergency conditions (specify) (List separately in addition to code for primary anesthesia procedure)

(An emergency is defined as existing when delay in treatment of the patient would lead to a significant increase in the threat to life or body part)

MODERATE (CONSCIOUS) SEDATION

Moderate (also known as conscious) sedation is a drug induced depression of consciousness during which patients respond purposefully to verbal commands, either alone or accompanied by light tactile stimulation. No interventions are required to maintain cardiovascular function or a patent airway, and spontaneous ventilation is adequate.

Moderate sedation codes 99151, 99152, 99153, 99155, 99156, 99157 are not used to report administration of medications for pain control, minimal sedation (anxiolysis), deep sedation, or monitored anesthesia care (00100-01999).

For purposes of reporting, intraservice time of moderate sedation is used to select the appropriate code(s). The following definitions are used to determine intraservice time (compared to pre- and postservice time). An independent trained observer is an individual who is qualified to monitor the patient during the procedure, who has no other duties (eg, assisting at surgery) during the procedure.

Preservice Work

The preservice activities required for moderate sedation are included in the work described by each of these codes (99151, 99152, 99153, 99155, 99156, 99157) and are not reported separately. The following preservice work components are not included when determining intraservice time for reporting:

- Assessment of the patient's past medical and surgical history with particular emphasis on cardiovascular, pulmonary, airway, or neurological conditions;

- Review of the patient's previous experiences with anesthesia and/or sedation;

- Family history of sedation complications;

- Summary of the patient's present medication list;

- Drug allergy and intolerance history;

- Focused physical examination of the patient with emphasis on:

   —Mouth, jaw, oropharynx, neck and airway for Mallampati score assessment;

   —Chest and lungs;

   —Heart and circulation;

- Vital signs, including heart rate, respiratory rate, blood pressure, and oxygenation with end tidal CO_2 when indicated;

- Review of any pre-sedation diagnostic tests;

- Completion of a pre-sedation assessment form (with an American Society of Anesthesiologists [ASA] Physical Status classification);

- Patient informed consent;

- Immediate pre-sedation assessment prior to first sedating doses; and

- Initiation of IV access and fluids to maintain patency.

Intraservice Work

Intraservice time is used to determine the appropriate CPT code to report moderate sedation services:

- Begins with the administration of the sedating agent(s);

- Ends when the procedure is completed, the patient is stable for recovery status, and the physician or other qualified health care professional providing the sedation ends personal continuous face-to-face time with the patient;

- Includes ordering and/or administering the initial and subsequent doses of sedating agents;

- Requires continuous face-to-face attendance of the physician or other qualified health care professional;

- Requires monitoring patient response to the sedating agents, including:

   —Periodic assessment of the patient;

   —Further administration of agent(s) as needed to maintain sedation; and

   —Monitoring of oxygen saturation, heart rate, and blood pressure.

If the physician or other qualified health care professional who provides the sedation services also performs the procedure supported by sedation (99151, 99152, 99153), the physician or other qualified health care professional will supervise and direct an independent trained observer who will assist in monitoring the patient's level of consciousness and physiological status throughout the procedure.

Postservice Work

The postservice activities required for moderate sedation are included in the work described by each of these codes (99151, 99152, 99153, 99155, 99156, 99157) and are not reported separately. Once continuous face-to-face time with the patient has ended, additional face-to-face time with the patient is not added to the intraservice time, however, it is considered as part of the postservice work. The following postservice work components are not included, when determining intraservice time for reporting:

- Assessment of the patient's vital signs, level of consciousness, neurological, cardiovascular, and pulmonary stability in the post-sedation recovery period;

- Assessment of the patient's readiness for discharge following the procedure;

- Preparation of documentation regarding sedation service; and

- Communication with family/caregiver regarding sedation service.

Postservice work/times are not used to select the appropriate code.

Do not report 99151, 99152, 99153, 99155, 99156, 99157 in conjunction with 94760, 94761, 94762.

Codes 99151, 99152, 99155, 99156 are reported for the first 15 minutes of intraservice time providing moderate sedation. Codes 99153, 99157 are reported for each additional 15 minutes, in addition to the code for the primary service.

		Moderate sedation (MS) provided by physician or other qualified health care professional (same physician or qualified health care professional also performing the procedure MS is supporting)	MS provided by different physician or other qualified health care professional (not the physician or qualified health care professional who is performing the procedure MS is supporting)
Total Intraservice Time for MS	**Patient Age**	**Code(s)**	**Code(s)**
Less than 10 minutes	Any age	Not reported separately	Not reported separately
10-22 minutes	< 5 years	99151	99155
10-22 minutes	5 years or older	99152	99156
23-37 minutes	< 5 years	99151 + 99153 x 1	99155 + 99157 x 1
23-37 minutes	5 years or older	99152 + 99153 x 1	99156 + 99157 x 1
38-52 minutes	< 5 years	99151 + 99153 x 2	99155 + 99157 x 2
38-52 minutes	5 years or older	99152 + 99153 x 2	99156 + 99157 x 2
53-67 minutes (53 min. to 1 hr. 7 min.)	< 5 years	99151 + 99153 x 3	99155 + 99157 x 3
53-67 minutes (53 min. to 1 hr. 7 min.)	5 years or older	99152 + 99153 x 3	99156 + 99157 x 3
68-82 minutes (1 hr. 8 min. to 1 hr. 22 min.)	< 5 years	99151 + 99153 x 4	99155 + 99157 x 4

68-82 minutes (1 hr. 8 min. to 1 hr. 22 min.)	5 years or older	99152 + 99153 x 4	99156 + 99157 x 4
83 minutes or longer	< 5 years	99153	Add 99157
83 minutes or longer	5 years or older	Add 99153	Add 99157

(99143, 99144, 99145 have been deleted. To report moderate sedation services provided by the same physician or other qualified health care professional performing the diagnostic or therapeutic service that the sedation supports, see 99151, 99152, 99153)

(99148, 99149, 99150 have been deleted. To report moderate sedation services provided by a physician or other qualified health care professional other than the physician or other qualified health care professional performing the diagnostic or therapeutic service that the sedation supports, see 99155, 99156, 99157)

⊘ **99151** Moderate sedation services provided by the same physician or other qualified health care professional performing the diagnostic or therapeutic service that the sedation supports, requiring the presence of an independent trained observer to assist in the monitoring of the patient's level of consciousness and physiological status; initial 15 minutes of intraservice time, patient younger than 5 years of age

⊘ **99152** initial 15 minutes of intraservice time, patient age 5 years or older

+ **99153** each additional 15 minutes intraservice time (List separately in addition to code for primary service)

(Use 99153 in conjunction with 99151, 99152)

(Do not report 99153 in conjunction with 99155, 99156)

99155 Moderate sedation services provided by a physician or other qualified health care professional other than the physician or other qualified health care professional performing the diagnostic or therapeutic service that the sedation supports; initial 15 minutes of intraservice time, patient younger than 5 years of age

99156 initial 15 minutes of intraservice time, patient age 5 years or older

+ **99157** each additional 15 minutes intraservice time (List separately in addition to code for primary service)

(Use 99157 in conjunction with 99155, 99156)

(Do not report 99157 in conjunction with 99151, 99152)

OTHER SERVICES AND PROCEDURES

99170 Anogenital examination, magnified, in childhood for suspected trauma, including image recording when performed

(For moderate sedation, see 99151, 99152, 99153, 99155, 99156, 99157

99172 Visual function screening, automated or semi-automated bilateral quantitative determination of visual acuity, ocular alignment, color vision by pseudoisochromatic plates, and field of vision (may include all or some screening of the determination(s) for contrast sensitivity, vision under glare)

(This service must employ graduated visual acuity stimuli that allow a quantitative determination of visual acuity (eg, Snellen chart). This service may not be used in addition to a gernal ophthalmological service or an E/M service)

(Do not report 99172 in conjunction with 99173, 99174, 99177, 0469T)

99173 Screening test of visual acuity, quantitative, bilateral

(The screening test used must employ graduated visual acuity stimuli that allow a quantitative estimate of visual acuity (eg, Snellen chart). Other identifiable services unrelated to this screening test provided at the same time may be reported separately (eg, preventive medicine services). When acuity is measured as part of a general ophthalmological service or of an E/M service of the eye, it is a diagnostic examination and not a screening test.)

(Do not report 99173 in conjunction with code 99172, 99174, 99177)

99174 Instrument-based ocular screening (eg, photoscreening, automated-refraction), bilateral; with remote analysis and report

(Do not report 99174 in conjunction with 92002-92014, 99172, 99173, 99177)

99177 with on-site analysis

(Do not report 99177 in conjunction with 92002-92014, 99172, 99173, 99174)

(For retinal polarization scan, use 0469T)

99175 Ipecac or similar administration for individual emesis and continued observation until stomach adequately emptied of poison

(For diagnostic intubation, see 43754, 43755)

(For gastric lavage for diagnostic purposes, see 43754, 43755)

99177 This code is out of order. See page 992

99183 Physician or other qualified health care professional attendance and supervision of hyperbaric oxygen therapy, per session

(Evaluation and Management services and/or procedures [eg, wound debridement] provided in a hyperbaric oxygen treatment facility in conjunction with a hyperbaric oxygen therapy session should be reported separately)

99184 Initiation of selective head or total body hypothermia in the critically ill neonate, includes appropriate patient selection by review of clinical, imaging and laboratory data, confirmation of esophageal temperature probe location, evaluation of amplitude EEG, supervision of controlled hypothermia, and assessment of patient tolerance of cooling

(Do not report 99184 more than once per hospital stay)

99188 Application of topical fluoride varnish by a physician or other qualified health care professional

99190 Assembly and operation of pump with oxygenator or heat exchanger (with or without ECG and/or pressure monitoring); each hour

99191 45 minutes

99192 30 minutes

99195 Phlebotomy, therapeutic (separate procedure)

99199 Unlisted special service, procedure or report

HOME HEALTH PROCEDURES/SERVICES

Home health procedures/services codes are used by non-physician health care professionals to report services provided in the patient's residence.

Physicians should utilize the home visit codes 99341-99350 and utilize CPT codes other than 99500-99600 for any additional procedure/service provided to a patient living in a residence.

The following codes are used to report services provided in a patient's residence (including assisted living apartments, group homes, nontraditional private homes, custodial care facilities, or schools).

Health care professionals who are authorized to use Evaluation and Management (E/M) Home Visit codes (99341-99350) may report 99500-99600 in addition to 99341-99350 if both services are performed. E/M services may be reported separately, using modifier 25, if the patient's condition requires a significant separately identifiable E/M service, above and beyond the home health service(s)/procedure(s) codes 99500-99600.

99500   Home visit for prenatal monitoring and assessment to include fetal heart rate, non-stress test, uterine monitoring, and gestational diabetes monitoring

99501   Home visit for postnatal assessment and follow-up care

99502   Home visit for newborn care and assessment

99503   Home visit for respiratory therapy care (eg, bronchodilator, oxygen therapy, respiratory assessment, apnea evaluation)

99504   Home visit for mechanical ventilation care

99505   Home visit for stoma care and maintenance including colostomy and cystostomy

99506   Home visit for intramuscular injections

99507   Home visit for care and maintenance of catheter(s) (eg, urinary, drainage, and enteral)

99509   Home visit for assistance with activities of daily living and personal care

     (To report self-care/home management training, see 97535)

     (To report home medical nutrition assessment and intervention services, see 97802-97804)

     (To report home speech therapy services, see 92507-92508)

99510   Home visit for individual, family, or marriage counseling

99511   Home visit for fecal impaction management and enema administration

99512   Home visit for hemodialysis

     (For home infusion of peritoneal dialysis, use 99601, 99602)

99600   Unlisted home visit service or procedure

HOME INFUSION PROCEDURES/SERVICES

Home infusion procedures codes are used to report per diem home visits for the purpose of administering infusions. With the exception of the infusion drug; all materials, equipments and supplies are included in the basic code. Drugs used for the infusion are coded separately.

99601   Home infusion/specialty drug administration, per visit (up to 2 hours)

+ 99602   each additional hour (List separately in addition to code for primary procedure)

     (Use 99602 in conjunction with 99601)

MEDICATION THERAPY MANAGEMENT SERVICES

Medication Therapy Management Services or MTMS describes in-person patient assessment and intervention as appropriate by a pharmacist. The purpose of MTMS is to maximize medication response and/or managed medication interactions or complications. MTMS includes review of history, medication profile, and recommendations regarding outcomes and compliance. MTMS codes are not used to report product information at the point of dispensing or other routine activities related to dispensing.

These codes are not to be used to describe the provision of product-specific information at the point of dispensing or any other routine dispensing-related activities.

99605   Medication therapy management service(s) provided by a pharmacist, individual, face-to-face with patient, with assessment and intervention if provided; initial 15 minutes, new patient

---

99606   initial 15 minutes, established patient

+ 99607 each additional 15 minutes (List separately in addition to code for primary service)

     (Use 99607 in conjunction with 99605, 99606)

CATEGORY II CODES

This section of the CPT coding system is the Category II Performance Measurement section. The primary purpose of this section is to provide classification codes which will allow the collection of data for performance measurement.

The assignment of a Category II code to a given service or procedure does not mean that the particular service or procedure is endorsed, approved, safe or has applicability to clinical practice. The Category II code simply provides a mechanism to identify and review performance measurements.

The most current codes and their implementation dates can be found on the Web at http://www.ama-assn.org/go/cpt.

CPT Category II codes are arranged according to the following categories:

Composite Codes	0001F-0015F
Patient Management	0500F-0584F
Patient History	1000F-1505F
Physical Examination	2000F-2060F
Diagnostic/Screening Processes or Results	3006F-3776F
Therapeutic, Preventive or Other Interventions	4000F-4563F
Follow-up or Other Outcomes	5005F-5250F
Patient Safety	6005F-6150F
Structural Measures	7010F-7025F
Nonmeasure Code Listing	9001F-9007F

MODIFIERS

The following performance measurement modifiers may be used for Category II codes to indicate that a service specified in the associate measure(s) was considered but, due to either medical, patient or system circumstance(s) documented in the medical record, the service was not provided. These modifiers serve as denominator exclusions from the performance measure.

Category II modifiers should only be reported with Category II codes; they should not be reported with Category I or Category III codes. In addition, the modifiers in the Category II section should only be used where specified in the guidelines, reporting instructions, parenthetic notes, or code descriptor language listed in the Cateogry II section.

1P Performance Measure Exclusion Modifier due to Medical Reasons:

Reasons include:
- Not indicated (absence of organ/limb, already received/performed, other)
- Contraindicated (patient allergic history, potential adverse drug interaction, other)
- Other medical reason

2P Performance Measure Exclusion Modifier due to Patient Reason:

Reasons include:
- Patient declined
- Economic, social or religious reasons
- Other patient reasons

3P Performance Measure Exclusion Modifier due to System Reason:

Reasons include:
- Resources to perform the services not available
- Insurance coverage/payor-related limitations
- Other reasons attributable to health care delivery system

Modifier 8P is intended to be used as a "reporting modifier" to allow the reporting of circumstances when an action described in a measure's numerator is not performed and the reason is not otherwise specified.

8P Performance measure reporting modifier—action not performed, reason not otherwise specified

---

COMPOSITE CODES

Composite codes combine several measures grouped within a single code descriptor to facilitate reporting for a clinical condition when all components are met. If only some of the components are met, or if services are provided in addition to those included in the composite code, they may be reported individually using the corresponding CPT Category II codes for those services.

0001F   Heart failure assessed (includes assessment of all the following components) (CAD)[1]:

Blood pressure measured (2000F)[1]
Level of activity assessed (1003F)[1]
Clinical symptoms of volume overload (excess) assessed (1004F)[1]
Weight, recorded (2001F)[1]
Clinical signs of volume overload (excess) assessed (2002F)[1]

(To report blood pressure measured, use 2000F)

0005F   Osteoarthritis assessed (OA)[1]

Includes assessment of all the following components:
Osteoarthritis symptoms and functional status assessed (1006F)[1]
Use of anti-inflammatory or over-the-counter (OTC) analgesic medications assessed (1007F)[1]
Initial examination of the involved joint(s) (includes visual inspection, palpation, range of motion) (2004F)[1]

(To report tobacco use cessation intervention, use 4001F)

0012F   Community-acquired bacterial pneumonia assessment (includes all of the following components) (CAP)[1]:

Co-morbid conditions assessed (1026F)[1]
Vital signs recorded (2010F)[1]
Mental status assessed (2014F)[1]
Hydration status assessed (2018F)[1]

0014F   Comprehensive preoperative assessment performed for cataract surgery with intraocular lens (IOL) placement (includes assessment of all of the following components) (EC)[5]:

Dilated fundus evaluation performed within 12 months prior to cataract surgery (2020F)[5]
Pre-surgical (cataract) axial length, corneal power measurement and method of intraocular lens power calculation documented (must be performed within 12 months prior to surgery) (3073F)[5]
Preoperative assessment of functional or medical indication(s) for surgery prior to the cataract surgery with intraocular lens placement (must be performed within 12 months prior to cataract surgery) (3325F)[5]

0015F   Melanoma follow up completed (includes assessment of all of the following components) (ML)[5]:

History obtained regarding new or changing moles (1050F)[5]
Complete physical skin exam performed (2029F)[5]
Patient counseled to perform a monthly self skin examination (5005F)[5]

PATIENT MANAGEMENT

Patient management codes describe utilization measures or measures of patient care provided for specific clinical purposes (eg, prenatal care, pre- and post-surgical care).

0500F   Initial prenatal care visit (report at first prenatal encounter with health care professional providing obstetrical care. Report also date of visit and, in a separate field, the date of the last menstrual period [LMP]) (Prenatal)[2]

0501F   Prenatal flow sheet documented in medical record by first prenatal visit (documentation includes at minimum blood pressure, weight, urine protein, uterine size, fetal heart tones, and estimated date of delivery). Report also: date of visit and, in a separate field, the date of the last menstrual period [LMP] (Note: if reporting 0501F prenatal flow sheet, it is not necessary to report 0500F initial prenatal care visit) (Prenatal)[1]

0502F   Subsequent prenatal care visit (Prenatal)[2]

[Excludes: patients who are seen for a condition unrelated to pregnancy or prenatal care (eg, an upper respiratory infection; patients seen for consultation only, not for continuing care)]

0503F Postpartum care visit(Prenatal)[2]

0505F Hemodialysis plan of care documented (ESRD, P-ESRD)[1]

0507F Peritoneal dialysis plan of care documented (ESRD)[1]

0509F Urinary incontinence plan of care documented (GER)[5]

0513F Elevated blood pressure plan of care documented (CKD)[1]

0514F Plan of care for elevated hemoglobin level documented for patient receiving Erythropoiesis-Stimulating Agent therapy (ESA) (CKD)[1]

0516F Anemia plan of care documented (ESRD)[1]

0517F Glaucoma plan of care documented (EC)[5]

0518F Falls plan of care documented (GER)[5]

0519F Planned chemotherapy regimen, including at a minimum: drug(s) prescribed, dose, and duration, documented prior to initiation of a new treatment regimen (ONC)[1]

0520F Radiation dose limits to normal tissues established prior to the initiation of a course of 3D conformal radiation for a minimum of 2 tissue/organ (ONC)[1]

0521F Plan of care to address pain documented (COA)[2] (ONC)[1]

0525F Initial visit for episode (BkP)[2]

0526F Subsequent visit for episode (BkP)[2]

0528F Recommended follow up interval for repeat colonoscopy of at least 10 years documented in colonoscopy report (End/Polyp)[5]

0529F Interval of 3 or more years since patient's last colonoscopy, documented (End/Polyp)[5]

0535F Dyspnea management plan of care, documented (Pall Cr)[5]

0540F Glucorticoid Management Plan Documented (RA)[5]

0545F Plan for follow-up care for major depressive disorder, documented (MDD ADOL)[1]

Footnotes

1-Physician Consortium for Performance Improvement (PCPI), www.physicianconsortium.org

2-National Committee on Quality Assurance (NCQA), Health Employer Data Information Set (HEDIS®), www.ncqa.org

3-The Joint Commission (TJC), ORYX Initiative Performance Measures, http://www.jointcommission.org/performancemeasurement.aspx

4-National Diabetes Quality Improvement Alliance (NDQIA), http://www.nationaldiabetesalliance.org

5-Joint measure from The Physician Consortium for Performance Improvement, www.physicianconsortium.org and National Committee on Quality Assurance (NCQA), www.ncqa.org

6-The Society of Thoracic Surgeons, http://www.sts.org, and National Quality Forum, http://www.qualityforum.org

7-Optum, www.optum.com

8-American Academy of Neurology, www.aan.com/go/practice/quality/measurements or quality@aan.com

9-College of American Pathologists (CAP), www.cap.org/apps/docs/advocacy/pathology_performance_measurement.pdf

10-American Gastroenterological Association (AGA), www.gastro.org/quality

11-American Society of Anesthesiologists (ASA), http://www.asahq.org

12-American College of Gastroenterology (ACG), www.gi.org; American Gastroenterology Association (AGA), www.gastro.org; and American Society for Gastrointestinal Endoscopy (ASGE), www. asge.org

| Separate Procedure | Unlisted Procedure | CCI Comp. Code | Non-specific Procedure | **997** |

0550F Cytopathology report on routine nongynecologic specimen finalized within two working days of accession date (PATH)[9]

0551F Cytopathology report on nongynecologic specimen with documentation that the specimen was non-routine (PATH)[9]

0555F Symptom management plan of care documented (HF)[1]

0556F Plan of care to achieve lipid control documented (CAD)[1]

0557F Plan of care to manage anginal symptoms documented (CAD)[1]

0575F HIV RNA control plan of care, documented (HIV)[5]

0580F Multidisciplinary care plan developed or updated (ALS)[8]

0581F Patient transferred directly from anesthetizing location to critical care unit (Peri2)[11]

0582F Patient not transferred directly from anesthetizing location to critical care unit (Peri2)[11]

0583F Transfer of care checklist used (Peri2)[11]

0584F Transfer of care checklist not used (Peri2)[11]

PATIENT HISTORY

Patient history codes describe measures for select aspects of patient history or review of systems.

1000F Tobacco use assessed (CAD, CAP, COPD, PV)[1] (DM)[4]

1002F Anginal symptoms and level of activity, assessed(NMA- No Measure Associated)

1003F Level of activity assessed (NMA-No Measure Associated)

1004F Clinical symptoms of volume overload (excess) assessed (NMA-No Measure Associated)

1005F Asthma symptoms evaluated (includes documentation of numeric frequency of symptoms or patient completion of an asthma assessment tool/survey/questionnaire) (NMA-No Measure Associated)

1006F Osteoarthritis symptoms and functional status assessed (may include the use of a standardized scale or the completion of an assessment questionnaire, such as the SF-36, AAOS Hip & Knee Questionnaire) (OA)[1]

[Instructions: report when osteoarthritis is addressed during the patient encounter]

1007F Use of anti-inflammatory or analgesic over-the-counter (OTC) medications for symptom relief assessed (OA)[1]

1008F Gastrointestinal and renal risk factors assessed for patients on prescribed or OTC non-steroidal anti-inflammatory drug (NSAID) (OA)[1]

1010F Severity of angina assessed by level of activity (CAD)[1]

1011F Angina present (CAD)[1]

1012F Angina absent (CAD)[1]

1015F Chronic obstructive pulmonary disease (COPD) symptoms assessed (Includes assessment of at least one of the following: dyspnea, cough/sputum, wheezing), or respiratory symptom assessment tool completed (COPD)[1]

● New Code ▲ Revised Code + Add-On Code ⊘ Modifier -51 Exempt ★ Telemedicine

1018F Dyspnea assessed, not present (COPD)[1]

1019F Dyspnea assessed, present (COPD)[1]

1022F Pneumococcus immunization status assessed (CAP, COPD)[1]

1026F Co-morbid conditions assessed (eg, includes assessment for presence or absence of: malignancy, liver disease, congestive heart failure, cerebrovascular disease, renal disease, chronic obstructive pulmonary disease, asthma, diabetes, other co-morbid conditions) (CAP)[1]

1030F Influenza immunization status assessed (CAP)[1]

1031F Smoking status and exposure to second hand smoke in the home assessed (Asthma)[1]

1032F Current tobacco smoker OR currently exposed to secondhand smoke (Asthma)[1]

1033F Current tobacco non-smoker AND not currently exposed to secondhand smoke (Asthma)[1]

1034F Current tobacco smoker (CAD, CAP, COPD, PV)[1] (DM)[4]

1035F Current smokeless tobacco user (eg, chew, snuff) (PV)[1]

1036F Current tobacco non-user (CAD, CAP, COPD, PV)[1] (DM)[4] (IBD)[10]

1038F Persistent asthma (mild, moderate or severe) (Asthma)[1]

1039F Intermittent asthma (Asthma)[1]

1040F DSM-5™ criteria for major depressive disorder documented at the initial evaluation (MDD, MDD ADOL)[1]

1050F History obtained regarding new or changing moles (ML)[5]

1052F Type, anatomic location, and activity all assessed (IBD)[10]

1055F Visual functional status assessed (EC)[5]

1060F Documentation of permanent OR persistent OR paroxysmal atrial fibrillation (STR)[5]

1061F Documentation of absence of permanent AND persistent AND paroxysmal atrial fibrillation (STR)[5]

1065F Ischemic stroke symptom onset of less than 3 hours prior to arrival (STR)[5]

1066F Ischemic stroke symptom onset greater than or equal to 3 hours prior to arrival (STR)[5]

1070F Alarm symptoms (involuntary weight loss, dysphagia, or gastrointestinal bleeding) assessed; none present (GERD)[5]

1071F one or more present (GERD)[5]

1090F Presence or absence or urinary incontinence assessed (GER)[5]

1091F Urinary incontinence characterized (eg, frequency, volume, timing, type of symptoms, how bothersome) (GER)[5]

1100F Patient screened for future fall risk; documentation of two or more falls in the past year or any fall with injury in the past year (GER)[5]

1101F documentation of no falls in the past year or only one fall without injury in the past year (GER)[5]

Separate Procedure   Unlisted Procedure   CCI Comp. Code   Non-specific Procedure   **999**

1110F Patient discharged from an inpatient facility (eg hospital, skilled nursing facility, or rehabilitation facility) within the last 60 days (GER)[5]

1111F Discharge medications reconciled with the current medication list in outpatient medical record (COA)[2] (GER)[5]

1116F Auricular or periauricular pain assessed (AOE)[1]

1118F Gerd symptoms assessed after 12 months of therapy (GERD)[5]

1119F Initial evaluation for condition (HEP C)[1] (EPI, DSP)[8]

1121F Subsequent evaluation for condition (HEP C)[1] (EPI)[8]

1123F Advance care planning discussed and documented advance care plan or surrogate decision maker documented in the medical record (DEM)[1] (GER, PallCr)[5]

1124F Advance care planning discussed and documented in the medical record patient did not wish or was not able to name a surrogate decision maker or provide an advance care plan (DEM)[1] (GER, PallCr)[5]

1125F Pain severity quantified; pain present (COA)[2] (ONC)[1]

1126F no pain present (COA)[2] (ONC)[1]

1127F New episode for condition (NMA-No Measure Associated)

1128F Subsequent episode for condition (NMA-No Measure Associated)

1130F Back pain and function assessed, including all of the following: Pain assessment AND functional status AND patient history, including notation of presence or absence of "red flags" (warning signs) AND assessment of prior treatment and response, AND employment status (BkP)[2]

1134F Episode of back pain lasting 6 weeks or less (BkP)[2]

1135F Episode of back pain lasting longer than 6 weeks (BkP)[2]

1136F Episode of back pain lasting 12 weeks or less (BkP)[2]

1137F Episode of back pain lasting longer than 12 weeks (BkP)[2]

1150F Documentation that a patient has a substantial risk of death within 1 year (Pall Cr)[5]

1151F Documentation that a patient does not have a substantial risk of death within one year (Pall Cr)[5]

1152F Documentation of advanced disease diagnosis, goals of care prioritize comfort (Pall Cr)[5]

1153F Documentation of advanced disease diagnosis, goals of care do not prioritize comfort (Pall Cr)[5]

1157F Advance care plan or similar legal document present in the medical record (COA)[2]

1158F Advance care planning discussion documented in the medical record (COA)[2]

1159F Medication list documented in medical record (COA)[2]

1160F Review of all medications by a prescribing practitioner or clinical pharmacist (such as, prescriptions, OTCs, herbal therapies and supplements) documented in the medical record (COA)[2]

1170F Functional status assessed (COA)[2] (RA)[5]

1175F Functional status for dementia assessed and results reviewed (DEM)[1]

● New Code ▲ Revised Code ✛ Add-On Code ⊘ Modifier -51 Exempt ★ Telemedicine

1180F All specified thromboembolic risk factors assessed (AFIB)[1]

1181F Neuropsychiatric symptoms assessed and results reviewed (DEM)[1]

1182F Neuropsychiatric symptoms, one or more present (DEM)[1]

1183F Neuropsychiatric symptoms, absent (DEM)[1]

1200F Seizure type(s) and current seizure frequency(ies) documented (EPI)[8]

1205F Etiology of epilepsy or epilepsy syndrome(s) reviewed and documented (EPI)[8]

1220F Patient screened for depression (SUD)[5]

1400F Parkinson's disease diagnosis reviewed (PRKNS)[8]

1450F Symptoms improved or remained consistent with treatment goals since last assessment (HF)[1]

1451F Symptoms demonstrated clinically important deterioration since last assessment (HF)[1]

1460F Qualifying cardiac event/diagnosis in previous 12 months (CAD)[1]

1461F No qualifying cardiac event/diagnosis in previous 12 months (CAD)[1]

1490F Dementia severity classified, mild (DEM)[1]

1491F Dementia severity classified, moderate (DEM)[1]

1493F Dementia severity classified, severe (DEM)[1]

1494F Cognition assessed and reviewed (DEM)[1]

1500F Symptoms and signs of distal symmetric polyneuropathy reviewed and documented (DSP)[8]

1501F Not initial evaluation for condition (DSP)[8]

1502F Patient queried about pain and pain interference with function using a valid and reliable instrument (DSP)[8]

1503F Patient queried about symptoms of respiratory insufficiency (ALS)[8]

1504F Patient has respiratory insufficiency (ALS)[8]

1505F Patient does not have respiratory insufficiency (ALS)[8]

Footnotes

1-Physician Consortium for Performance Improvement (PCPI), www.physicianconsortium.org

2-National Committee on Quality Assurance (NCQA), Health Employer Data Information Set (HEDIS®), www.ncqa.org

3-The Joint Commission (TJC), ORYX Initiative Performance Measures, http://www.jointcommission.org/performancemeasurement.aspx

4-National Diabetes Quality Improvement Alliance (NDQIA), http://www.nationaldiabetesalliance.org

5-Joint measure from The Physician Consortium for Performance Improvement, www.physicianconsortium.org and National Committee on Quality Assurance (NCQA), www.ncqa.org

6-The Society of Thoracic Surgeons, http://www.sts.org, and National Quality Forum, http://www.qualityforum.org

7-Optum, www.optum.com

8-American Academy of Neurology, www.aan.com/go/practice/quality/measurements or quality@aan.com

9-College of American Pathologists (CAP), www.cap.org/apps/docs/ advocacy/pathology_performance_measurement.pdf

10-American Gastroenterological Association (AGA), www.gastro.org/quality

11-American Society of Anesthesiologists (ASA), http://www.asahq.org

12-American College of Gastroenterology (ACG), www.gi.org; American Gastroenterology Association (AGA), www.gastro.org; and American Society for Gastrointestinal Endoscopy (ASGE), www. asge.org

---

PHYSICAL EXAMINATION

Physical examination codes describe aspects of physical examination or clinical assessment.

2000F Blood pressure measured (CKD)[1] (DM)[2,4]

2001F Weight recorded(PAG)[1]

2002F Clinical signs of volume overload (excess) assessed (NMA-No Measure Associated)

2004F Initial examination of the involved joint(s) (includes visual inspection, palpation, range of motion) (OA)[1]

[Instructions: report only for initial osteoarthritis visit or for visits for new joint involvement]

2010F Vital signs (temperature, pulse, respiratory rate, and blood pressure) documented and reviewed (CAP)[1](EM)[5]

2014F Mental status assessed (CAP)[1](EM)[5]

2015F Asthma impairment assessed (Asthma)[1]

2016F Asthma risk assessed (Asthma)[1]

2018F Hydration status assessed (normal/mildly dehydrated/severely dehydrated) (CAP)[1]

2019F Dilated macular exam performed, including documentation of the presence or absence of macular thickening or hemorrhage AND the level of macular degeneration severity (EC)[5]

2020F Dilated fundus evaluation performed within 12 months prior to cataract surgery (EC)[5]

2021F Dilated macular or fundus exam performed, including documentation of the presence or absence of macular edema AND level of severity of retinopathy (EC)[5]

2022F Dilated retinal eye exam with interpretation by an ophthalmologist or optometrist documented and reviewed; with evidence of retinopathy (DM)[2]

2023F without evidence of retinopathy (DM)[2]

2024F 7 standard field stereoscopic retinal photos with interpretation by an ophthalmologist or optometrist documented and reviewed; with evidence of retinopathy (DM)[2]

2025F without evidence of retinopathy (DM)[2]

2026F Eye imaging validated to match diagnosis from 7 standard field stereoscopic retinal photos results documented and reviewed; with evidence of retinopathy (DM)[2]

2033F without evidence of retinopathy (DM)[2]

2027F Optic nerve head evaluation performed (EC)[5]

2028F Foot examination performed (includes examination through visual inspection, sensory exam with monofilament, and pulse exam — report when any of the 3 components are completed) (DM)[4]

2029F Complete physical skin exam performed (ML)[5]

2030F Hydration status documented, normally hydrated (PAG)[1]

2031F Hydration status documented, dehydrated (PAG)[1]

2033F This code is out of order. See page

2035F Tympanic membrane mobility assessed with pneumatic otoscoopy or tympanometry (OME)[1]

2040F Physical examination on the date of the initial visit for low back pain performed, in accordance with specifications (BkP)[2]

2044F Documentation of mental health assessment prior to intervention (back surgery or epidural steroid injection) or for back pain episode lasting longer than 6 weeks (BkP)[2]

2050F Wound characteristics including size AND nature of wound base tissue AND amount of drainage prior to debridement documented (CWC)[5]

2060F Patient interviewed directly on or before date of diagnosis of major depressive disorder (MDD ADOL)[1]

DIAGNOSTIC/SCREENING PROCESSES OR RESULTS

Diagnostic/screening processes or results codes describe results of tests ordered (clinical laboratory tests, radiological or other procedural examinations and conclusions of medical decision-making).

(To report blood pressure, use the corresponding systolic codes [3074F, 3075F, 3077F] and diastolic codes [3078F, 3079F, 3080F])

3006F Chest X-ray results documented and reviewed (CAP)[1]

3008F Body mass index (BMI), documented (PV)[1]

3011F Lipid panel results documented and reviewed (must include total cholesterol, HDL-C, triglycerides and calculated LDL-C) (CAD)[1]

3014F Screening mammography results documented and reviewed (PV)[1,2]

3015F Cervical cancer screening results documented and reviewed (PV)[1]

3016F Patient screened for unhealthy alcohol use using a systematic screening method (PV)[1](DSP)[8]

3017F Colorectal cancer screening results documented and reviewed (PV) [1,2]

3018F Pre procedure risk assessment AND depth of insertion AND quality of the bowel prep AND complete description of polyp(s) found, including location of each polyp, size, number and gross morphology AND recommendations for follow up in final colonoscopy report documented (End/Polyp)[5]

3019F Left ventricular ejection fracrtion (LVEF) assessment planned post discharge (HF)[1]

3020F Left ventricular function (LVF) assessment (eg, echocardiography, nuclear test, or ventriculography) documented in the medical record (Includes quantitative or qualitative assessment results) (NMA-No Measure Associated)

3021F Left ventricular ejection fraction (LVEF) 40% or documentation of moderately or severely depressed left ventricular systolic function (CAD, HF)[1]

3022F Left ventricular ejection fraction (LVEF) 40% or documentation as normal or mildly depressed left ventricular systolic function (CAD, HF)[1]

3023F Spirometry results documented and reviewed (COPD)[1]

3025F Spirometry test results demonstrate FEV1/FVC70% with COPD symptoms (eg, dyspnea, cough/sputum, wheezing) (CAP, COPD)[1]

3027F Spirometry test results demonstrate FEV1/FVC greater than or equal to 70% or patient does not have COPD symptoms (COPD)[1]

3028F Oxygen saturation results documented and reviewed (Includes assessment through pulse oximetry or arterial blood gas measurement) (CAP, COPD)[1] (EM)[5]

3035F Oxygen saturation less than or equal to 88 % or a PaO_2 less than or equal to 55 mm Hg (COPD)[1]

3037F Oxygen saturation greater than 88% or PaO_2 greater than 55 mmHg (COPD)[1]

3038F Pulmonary function test performed within 12 months prior to surgery (Lung/Esop Cx)[6]

3040F Functional expiratory volume (FEV_1) < 40% of predicted value (COPD)[1]

3042F Functional expiratory volume (FEV_1) greater than or equal to 40% of predicted value (COPD)[1]

3044F Most recent hemoglobin A1c (HbA1c) level < 7.0% (DM)[2,4]

(**3045F** deleted 2019 [2020 Edition]. To report, control of HbA1c, see 3051F, 3052F)

3051F Most recent hemoglobin A1c (HbA1c) level greater than or equal to 7.0% and less than 8.0% (DM)[2]

3052F Most recent hemoglobin A1c (HbA1c) level greater than or equal to 8.0% and less than or equal to 9.0% (DM)2 3046F Most recent hemoglobin A1c level greater than 9.0% (DM)[4]

3046F Most recent hemoglobin A1c level greater than 9.0% (DM)[4]

(To report most recent hemoglobin A1c level less than or equal to 9.0%, see 3044F, 3051F, 3052F)

3048F Most recent LDL-C < 100 mg/dL (CAD)[1] (DM)[4]

3049F Most recent LDL-C 100-129 mg/dL (CAD)[1] (DM)[4]

3050F Most recent LDL-C≥ 130 mg/dL (CAD)[1] (DM)[4]

3051F Code is out order. See page 1004

3052F Code is out order. See page 1004

3055F Left ventricular ejection fraction (LVEF) less than or equal to 35% (HF)[1]

3056F Left ventricular ejection fraction (LVEF) greater than 35% or no LVEF result available (HF)[1]

3060F Positive microalbuminuria test result documented and reviewed (DM)[2,4]

3061F Negative microalbuminuria test result documented and reviewed (DM)[2,4]

3062F Positive macroalbuminuria test result documented and reviewed (DM)[2,4]

3066F Documentation of treatment for nephropathy (eg, patient receiving dialysis, patient being treated for ESRD, CRF, ARF, or renal insufficiency, any visit to a nephrologist) (DM)[2,4]

3072F Low risk for retinopathy (no evidence of retinopathy in the prior year) (DM)[2,4]

3073F Pre-surgical (cataract) axial length, corneal power measurement and method of intraocular lens power calculation documented within 12 months prior to surgery (EC)[5]

3074F Most recent systolic blood pressure less than 130mm Hg (DM)[2,4](HTN,CKD, CAD)[1]

3075F Most recent systolic blood pressure 130-139 mm Hg (DM)[2,4](HTN,CKD, CAD)[1]

(To report most recent systolic blood pressure less than 140 mm Hg, see codes 3047F-3075F)

3077F Most recent systolic blood pressure greater than or equal to 140 mmHg (HTN,CKD, CAD)[1] (DM)[2,4]

3078F Most recent diastolic blood pressure less than 80 mm Hg (HTN,CKD, CAD)[1] (DM)[2,4]

3079F Most recent diastolic blood pressure 80-89 mm Hg (HTN,CKD, CAD)[1] (DM)[2,4]

3080F Most recent diastolic blood pressuregreater than or equal to 90 mmHg (HTN,CKD, CAD)[1] (DM)[2,4]

3082F Kt/V less than 1.2 (Clearance of urea [Kt]/volume [V]) (ESRD, P-ESRD)[1]

3083F Kt/V equal to or greater than 1.2 and less than 1.7 (Clearance of urea [Kt]/volume [V]) (ESRD, P-ESRD)[1]

3084F Kt/V greater than or equal to 1.7 (Clearance of urea [Kt]/volume [V]) (ESRD, P-ESRD)[1]

3085F Suicide risk assessed (MDD, MDD ADOL)[1]

3088F Major depressive disorder, mild (MDD)[1]

3089F Major depressive disorder, moderate (MDD)[1]

3090F Major depressive disorder, severe without psychotic features (MDD)[1]

3091F Major depressive disorder, severe with psychotic features (MDD)[1]

3092F Major depressive disorder, in remission (MDD)[1]

3093F Documentation of new diagnosis of initial or recurrent episode of major depressive disorder (MDD)[1]

3095F Dual-energy X-ray Absorptiometry (DXA) results documented (OP)[5](IBD)[10]

3096F Central dual-energy X-ray Absorptiometry (DXA) ordered (OP)[5](IBD)[10]

3100F Carotid imaging study report (includes direct or indirect reference to measurements of distal internal carotid diameter as the denominator for stenosis measurement) (STR, RAD)[5]

3110F Documentation in final CT or MRI report of presence or absence of hemorrhage and mass lesion and acute infarction (STR)[5]

3111F CT or MRI of the brain performed in the hospital within 24 hours of arrival OR performed in an outpatient imaging center, to confirm initial diagnosis of stroke, TIA, or intracranial hemorrhage (STR)[5]

3112F CT or MRI of the brain performed greater than 24 hours after arrival to the hospital OR performed in an outpatient imaging center for purpose other than confirmation of initial diagnosis of stroke, TIA, or intracranial hemorrhage (STR)[5]

Footnotes

1-Physician Consortium for Performance Improvement (PCPI), www.physicianconsortium.org

2-National Committee on Quality Assurance (NCQA), Health Employer Data Information Set (HEDIS®), www.ncqa.org

3-The Joint Commission (TJC), ORYX Initiative Performance Measures, http://www.jointcommission.org/performancemeasurement.aspx

4-National Diabetes Quality Improvement Alliance (NDQIA), http://www.nationaldiabetesalliance.org

5-Joint measure from The Physician Consortium for Performance Improvement, www.physicianconsortium.org and National Committee on Quality Assurance (NCQA), www.ncqa.org

6-The Society of Thoracic Surgeons, http://www.sts.org, and National Quality Forum, http://www.qualityforum.org

7-Optum, www.optum.com

8-American Academy of Neurology, www.aan.com/go/practice/quality/measurements or quality@aan.com

9-College of American Pathologists (CAP), www.cap.org/apps/docs/ advocacy/pathology_performance_measurement.pdf

10-American Gastroenterological Association (AGA), www.gastro.org/quality

11-American Society of Anesthesiologists (ASA), http://www.asahq.org

12-American College of Gastroenterology (ACG), www.gi.org; American Gastroenterology Association (AGA), www.gastro.org; and American Society for Gastrointestinal Endoscopy (ASGE), www. asge.org

---

Separate Procedure　　　Unlisted Procedure　　　CCI Comp. Code　　　Non-specific Procedure　　**1005**

3115F Quantitative results of an evaluation of current level of activity and clinical symptoms (HF)[1]

3117F Heart Failure disease specific structured assessment tool completed (HF)[1]

3118F New York Heart Association (NYHA) Class documented (HF)[1]

3119F No Evaluation of level of activity or clinical symptoms (HF)[1]

3120F 12-Lead ECG Performed (EM)[5]

3126F Esophageal bipsy report with a statement about dysplasia (present, absent, or indefinite, and if present, contains appropriate grading) (PATH)[9]

3130F Upper gastrointestinal endoscopy performed (GERD)[5]

3132F Documentation of referral for upper gastrointestinal endoscopy (GERD)[5]

3140F Upper gastrointestinal endoscopy report indicates suspicion of Barrett's esophagus (GERD)[5]

3141F Upper gastrointestinal endoscopy report indicates no suspicion of Barrett's esophagus (GERD)[5]

3142F Barium swallow test ordered (GERD)[1]

(To report documentation of barium swallow study, use code 3142F)

3150F Forceps esophageal biopsy performed (GERD)[5]

3155F Cytogenetic testing performed on bone marrow at time of diagnosis or prior to initiating treatment (HEM)[1]

3160F Documentation of iron stores prior to initiating erythropoietin therapy (HEM)[1]

▲ **3170F** Baseline flow cytometry studies performed at time of diagnosis or prior to initiating treatment (HEM)[1]

3200F Barium swallow test not ordered (GERD)[5]

3210F Group A Strep Test Performed (PHAR)[2]

3215F Patient has documented immunity to Hepatitis A (HEP-C)[1]

3216F Patient has documented immunity to Hepatitis B (HEP-C)[1] (IBD)[10]

3218F RNA testing for Hepatitis C documented as performed within 6 months prior to initiation of antiviral treatment for Hepatitis C (HEP-C)[1]

3220F Hepatitis C quantitative RNA testing documented as performed at 12 weeks from initiation of antiviral treatment (HEP-C)[1]

3230F Documentation that hearing test was performed within 6 months prior to tympanostomy tube insertion (OME)[1]

3250F Specimen site other than anatomic location of primary tumor (PATH)[1]

3260F pT category (primary tumor), pN category (regional lymph nodes), and histologic grade documented in pathology report (PATH)[1]

3265F Ribonucleic acid (RNA) testing for Hepatitis C viremia ordered or results documented (HEP C)[1]

3266F Hepatitis C genotype testing documented as performed prior to initiation of antiviral treatment for Hepatitis C (HEP C)[1]

● New Code   ▲ Revised Code   ✛ Add-On Code   ⊘ Modifier -51 Exempt   ★ Telemedicine

3267F   Pathology report includes pT category, pN category, Gleason score, and statement about margin status (PATH)[9]

3268F   Prostate-specific antigen (PSA), AND primary tumor (T) stage, AND Gleason score documented prior to initiation of treatment (PRCA)[1]

3269F   Bone scan performed prior to initiation of treatment or at any time since diagnosis of prostate cancer (PRCA)[1]

3270F   Bone scan not performed prior to initiation of treatment nor at any time since diagnosis of prostate cancer (PRCA)[1]

3271F   Low risk of recurrence, prostate cancer (PRCA)[1]

3272F   Intermediate risk of recurrence, prostate cancer (PRCA)[1]

3273F   High risk of recurrence, prostate cancer (PRCA)[1]

3274F   Prostate cancer risk of recurrence not determined or neither low, intermediate nor high (PRCA)[1]

3278F   Serum levels of calcium, phosphorus, intact parathyroid hormone (PTH) and lipid profile ordered (CKD)[1]

3279F   Hemoglobin level greater than or equal to 13 g/dl (CKD, ESRD)[1]

3280F   Hemoglobin level 11 g/dl to 12.9 g/dl (CKD, ESRD)[1]

3281F   Hemoglobin level less than 11 g/dl (CKD, ESRD)[1]

3284F   Intraocular pressure (IOP) reduced by a value of greater than or equal to 15% from the pre-intervention level (EC)[5]

3285F   Intraocular pressure (IOP) reduced by a value less than 15% from the pre-intervention level (EC)[5]

3288F   Falls risk assessment documented (GER)[5]

3290F   Patient is D (Rh) negative and unsensitized (Pre-Cr)[1]

3291F   Patient is D (Rh) positive or sensitized (Pre-Cr)[1]

3292F   HIV testing ordered or documented and reviewed during the first or second prenatal visit (Pre-Cr)[1]

3293F   ABO and Rh blood typing documented as performed (Pre-Cr)[7]

3294F   Group B streptococcus (GBS) screening documented as performed during week 35-37 gestation (Pre-Cr)[7]

3300F   American Joint Committee on Cancer (AJCC) stage documented and reviewed (ONC)[1]

3301F   Cancer stage documented in medical record as metastatic and reviewed (ONC)[1]

(To report measures for cancer staging, see 3321F-3390F)

3315F   Estrogen receptor (ER) or progesterone receptor (PR) positive breast cancer (ONC)[1]

3316F   Estrogen receptor (ER) and progesterone receptor (PR) negative breast cancer (ONC)[1]

3317F   Pathology report confirming malignancy documented in the medical record and reviewed prior to the initiation of chemotherapy (ONC)[1]

3318F   Pathology report confirming malignancy documented in the medical record and reviewed prior to the initiation of radiation therapy (ONC)[1]

Separate Procedure   Unlisted Procedure   CCI Comp. Code   Non-specific Procedure   **1007**

3319F 1 of the following diagnostic imaging studies ordered: chest X-ray, CT, ultrasound, MRI, PET, or nuclear medicine scans (ML)[5]

3320F None of the following diagnostic imaging studies ordered: chest X-ray, CT, ultrasound, MRI, PET, or nuclear medicine scans (ML)[5]

3321F AJCC Cancer Stage 0 or IA Melanoma, documented (ML)[5]

3322F Melanoma greater than AJCC Stage 0 or IA (ML)[5]

3323F Clinical tumor, node and metastases (TNM) staging documented and reviewed prior to surgery (Lung/Esop Cx)[6]

3324F MRI or CT scan ordered, reviewed or requested (EPI)[8]

3325F Preoperative assessment of functional or medical indication(s) for surgery prior to the cataract surgery with intraocular lens placement (must be performed within twelve months prior to cataract surgery) (EC)[5]

3328F Performance status documented and reviewed within 2 weeks prior to surgery (Lung/Esop Cx)[6]

3330F Imaging study ordered (BkP)[2]

3331F Imaging study not ordered (BkP)[2]

3340F Mammogram assessment category of "incomplete: need additional imaging evaluation", documented (RAD)[5]

3341F Mammogram assessment category of "negative", documented (RAD)[5]

3342F Mammogram assessment category of "benign", documented (RAD)[5]

3343F Mammogram assessment category of "probably benign", documented (RAD)[5]

3344F Mammogram assessment category of "suspicious", documented (RAD)[5]

3345F Mammogram assessment category of "highly suggestive of malignancy", documented (RAD)[5]

3350F Mammogram assessment category of "known biopsy proven malignancy", documented (RAD)[5]

3351F Negative screen for depressive symptoms as categorized by using a standardized depression screening/assessment tool (MDD)[2]

3352F No significant depressive symptoms as categorized by using a standardized depression assessment tool (MDD)[2]

3353F Mild to moderate depressive symptoms as categorized by using a standardized depression screening/assessment tool (MDD)[2]

3354F Clinically significant depressive symptoms as categorized by using a standardized depression screening/assessment tool (MDD)[2]

3370F AJCC Breast Cancer Stage 0 documented (ONC)[1]

3372F AJCC Breast Cancer Stage I: T1mic, T1a or T1b (tumor size <= 1 cm) documented (ONC)[1]

3374F AJCC Breast Cancer Stage I: T1c (tumor size > 1 cm to 2 cm) documented (ONC)[1]

3376F AJCC Breast Cancer Stage II documented (ONC)[1]

3378F AJCC Breast Cancer Stage III documented (ONC)[1]

3380F AJCC Breast Cancer Stage IV documented (ONC)[1]

3382F AJCC colon cancer, Stage 0 documented (ONC)[1]

3384F AJCC colon cancer, Stage I documented (ONC)[1]

3386F AJCC colon cancer, Stage II documented (ONC)[1]

3388F AJCC colon cancer, Stage III documented (ONC)[1]

3390F AJCC colon cancer, Stage IV documented (ONC)[1]

3394F Quantitative HER2 immunohistochemistry (IHC) evaluation of breast cancer consistent with the scoring system defined in the ASCO/CAP guidelines (PATH)[9]

3395F Quantitative non-HER2 immunohistochemistry (IHC) evaluation of breast cancer (eg, testing for estrogen or progesterone receptors [ER/PR]) performed (PATH)[9]

3450F Dyspnea screened, no dyspnea or mild dyspnea (Pall Cr)[5]

3451F Dyspnea screened, moderate or severe dyspnea (Pall Cr)[5]

3452F Dyspnea not screened (Pall Cr)[5]

3455F TB screening performed and results interpreted within six months prior to initiation of first time biologic disease modifying anti rheumatic drug therapy for RA (RA)[5]

3470F Rheumatoid arthritis (RA) disease activity, low (RA)[5]

3471F Rheumatoid arthritis (RA) disease activity, moderate (RA)[5]

3472F Rheumatoid arthritis (RA) disease activity, high (RA)[5]

3475F Disease prognosis for rheumatoid arthritis assessed, poor prognosis documented (RA)[5]

3476F Disease prognosis for rheumatoid arthritis assessed, good prognosis documented (RA)[5]

3490F History of AIDS defining condition (HIV)[5]

3491F HIV indeterminate (infants of undetermined HIV status born of HIV infected mothers) (HIV)[5]

3492F History of nadir CD4+ cell count <350 cells/mm (HIV)[5]

3493F No history of nadir CD4+ cell count <350 cells/mm AND no history of AIDS defining condition (HIV)[5]

Footnotes

1-Physician Consortium for Performance Improvement (PCPI), www.physicianconsortium.org

2-National Committee on Quality Assurance (NCQA), Health Employer Data Information Set (HEDIS®), www.ncqa.org

3-The Joint Commission (TJC), ORYX Initiative Performance Measures, http://www.jointcommission.org/performancemeasurement.aspx

4-National Diabetes Quality Improvement Alliance (NDQIA), http://www.nationaldiabetesalliance.org

5-Joint measure from The Physician Consortium for Performance Improvement, www.physicianconsortium.org and National Committee on Quality Assurance (NCQA), www.ncqa.org

6-The Society of Thoracic Surgeons, http://www.sts.org, and National Quality Forum, http://www.qualityforum.org

7-Optum, www.optum.com

8-American Academy of Neurology, www.aan.com/go/practice/quality/measurements or quality@aan.com

9-College of American Pathologists (CAP), www.cap.org/apps/docs/ advocacy/pathology_performance_measurement.pdf

10-American Gastroenterological Association (AGA), www.gastro.org/quality

11-American Society of Anesthesiologists (ASA), http://www.asahq.org

12-American College of Gastroenterology (ACG), www.gi.org; American Gastroenterology Association (AGA), www.gastro.org; and American Society for Gastrointestinal Endoscopy (ASGE), www. asge.org

3494F CD4+ cell count <200 cells/mm (HIV)[5]

3495F CD4+ cell count 200 - 499 cells/mm (HIV)[5]

3496F CD4+ cell count >=500 cells/mm (HIV)[5]

3497F CD4+ cell percentage <15% (HIV)[5]

3498F CD4+ cell percentage >=15% (HIV)[5]

3500F CD4+ cell count or CD4+ cell percentage documented as performed (HIV)[5]

3502F HIV RNA viral load below limits of quantification (HIV)[5]

3503F HIV RNA viral load not below limits of quantification (HIV)[5]

3510F Documentation that tuberculosis (TB) screening test performed and results interpreted (HIV)[5] (IBD)[10]

3511F Chlamydia and gonorrhea screenings documented as performed (HIV)[5]

3512F Syphilis screening documented as performed (HIV)[5]

3513F Hepatitis B screening documented as performed (HIV)[5]

3514F Hepatitis C screening documented as performed (HIV)[5]

3515F Patient has documented immunity to Hepatitis C (HIV)[5]

3517F Hepatitis B Virus (HBV) status assessed and results interpreted within one year prior to receiving a first course of anti-TNF (tumor necrosis factor) therapy (IBD)[10]

3520F Clostridium difficile testing performed (IBD)[10]

3550F Low risk for thromboembolism (AFIB)[1]

3551F Intermediate risk for thromboembolism (AFIB)[1]

3552F High risk for thromboembolism (AFIB)[1]

3555F Patient had International Normalized Ratio (INR) measurement performed (AFIB)[1]

3570F Final report for bone scintigraphy study includes correlation with existing relevant imaging studies (eg, x ray, MRI, CT) corresponding to the same anatomical region in question (NUC_MED)[1]

3572F Patient considered to be potentially at risk for fracture in a weight bearing site (NUC_MED)[1]

3573F Patient not considered to be potentially at risk for fracture in a weight bearing site (NUC_MED)[1]

3650F Electroencephalogram (EEG) ordered, reviewed or requested (EPI)[8]

3700F Psychiatric disorders or disturbances assessed (Prkns)[8]

3702F Cognitive impairment or dysfunction assessed (Prkns)[8]

3725F Screening for depression performed (DEM)[1]

3750F Patient not receiving dose of corticosteroids greater than or equal to 10 mg/day for 60 or greater consecutive days (IBD)[10]

● New Code   ▲ Revised Code   + Add-On Code   ⊘ Modifier -51 Exempt   ★ Telemedicine

3751F Electrodiagnostic studies for distal symmetric polyneuropathy conducted (or requested), documented, and reviewed within 6 months of initial evaluation for condition (DSP)[8]

3752F Electrodiagnostic studies for distal symmetric polyneuropathy **not** conducted (or requested), documented, or reviewed within 6 months of initial evaluation for condition (DSP)[8]

3753F Patient has clear clinical symptoms and signs that are highly suggestive of neuropathy AND cannot be attributed to another condition, AND has an obvious cause for the neuropathy (DSP)[8]

3754F Screening tests for diabetes mellitus reviewed, requested, or ordered (DSP)[8]

3755F Cognitive and behavioral impairment screening performed (ALS)[8]

3756F Patient has pseudobulbar affect, sialorrhea, or ALS-related symptoms (ALS)[8]

3757F Patient does not have pseudobulbar affect, sialorrhea, or ALS-related symptoms (ALS)[8]

3758F Patient referred for pulmonary function testing or peak cough expiratory flow (ALS)[8]

3759F Patient screened for dysphagia, weight loss, and impaired nutrition, and results documented (ALS)[8]

3760F Patient exhibits dysphagia, weight loss, or impaired nutrition (ALS)[8]

3761F Patient does not exhibit dysphagia, weight loss, or impaired nutrition (ALS)[8]

3762F Patient is dysarthric (ALS)[8]

3763F Patient is not dysarthric (ALS)[8]

3775F Adenoma(s) or other neoplasm detected during screening colonoscopy (SCADR)[12]

3776F Adenoma(s) or other neoplasm not detected during screening colonoscopy (SCADR)[12]

THERAPEUTIC, PREVENTIVE OR OTHER INTERVENTIONS

Therapeutic, preventive or other interventions codes describe pharmacologic, procedural, or behavioral therapies, including preventive services such as patient education and counseling.

4000F Tobacco use cessation intervention, counseling (COPD, CAP, CAD, Asthma)[1](DM)[4](PV)[2]

4001F Tobacco use cessation intervention, pharmacologic therapy (COPD, CAD, CAP, PV, Asthma)[1] (DM)[4] (PV)[2]

4003F Patient education, written/oral, appropriate for patients with heart failure performed (NMA-No Measure Associated)

4004F Patient screened for tobacco use AND received tobacco cessation intervention (counseling, pharmacotherapy, or both), if identified as a tobacco user (PV, CAD)[1]

4005F Pharmacologic therapy (other than minerals/vitamins) for osteoporosis prescribed (OP)[5] (IBD)[10]

4008F Beta-blocker therapy prescribed or currently being taken (CAD,HF)[1]

4010F Angiotensin converting enzyme (ACE) inhibitor or angiotensin receptor blocker (ARB) therapy prescribed or currently being taken (CAD, CKD, HF)[1] (DM)[2]

4011F Oral antiplatelet therapy prescribed (CAD)[1]

4012F Warfarin therapy prescribed (NMA-No Measure Associated)

4013F Statin therapy prescrived or currently being taken (CAD)[1]

4014F Written discharge instructions provided to heart failure patients discharged home. (Instructions include all of the following components: activity level, diet, discharge medications, follow-up appointment, weight monitoring, what to do if symptoms worsen) (NMA-No Measure Associated)

4015F Persistent asthma, preferred long term control medication or an acceptable alternative treatment, prescribed (NMA-No Meausre Associated)

(Note: There are no medical exclusion criteria)

(Do not report modifier 1P with 4015F)

(To report patient reasons for not prescribing, use modifier 2P)

4016F Anti-inflammatory/analgesic agent prescribed (OA)[1]

(Use for prescribed or continued medication(s), including over-the-counter medication[s])

4017F Gastrointestinal prophylaxis for NSAID use prescribed (OA)[1]

4018F Therapeutic exercise for the involved joint(s) instructed or physical or occupational therapy prescribed (OA)[1]

4019F Documentation of receipt of counseling on exercise AND either both calcium and vitamin D use or counseling regarding both calcium and vitamin D use (OP)[5]

4025F Inhaled bronchodilator prescribed (COPD)[1]

4030F Long term oxygen therapy prescribed (more than fifteen hours per day) (COPD)[1]

4033F Pulmonary rehabilitation exercise training recommended (COPD)[1]

(Report 4033F with 1019F)

4035F Influenza immunization recommended (COPD)[1](IBD)[10]

4037F Influenza immunization ordered or administered (COPD, PV, CKD, ESRD)[1](IBD)[10]

4040F Pneumococcal vaccine administered or previously received (COPD)[1] (IBD)[10](PV)[1,2]

4041F Documentation of order for cefazolin OR cefurozime for antimicrobial prophylaxis (PERI 2)[5]

4042F Documentation that prophylactic antibiotics were neither given within 4 hours prior to surgical incision nor given intraoperatively (PERI 2)[5]

4043F Documentation that an order was given to discontinue prophylactic antibiotics within 48 hours of surgical end time, cardiac procedures (PERI 2)[5]

4044F Documentation that an order was given for venous thromboembolism (VTE) prophylaxis to be given within 24 hours prior to incision time or 24 hours after surgery end time (PERI 2)[5]

4045F Appropriate empiric antibiotic prescribed (CAP)[1] (EM)[5]

4046F Documentation that prophylactic antibiotics were given within 4 hours prior to surgical incision or given intraoperatively (PERI 2)[5]

4047F Documentation of order for prophylactic parenteral antibiotics to be given within 1 hour (if fluoroquinolone or vancomycin, 2 hours) prior to surgical incision (or start of procedure when no incision is required) (PERI 2)[5]

● New Code   ▲ Revised Code   ＋ Add-On Code   ⊘ Modifier -51 Exempt   ★ Telemedicine

4048F Documentation that administration of prophylactic parenteral antibiotic was initiated within 1 hour (if fluoroquinolone or vancomycin, 2 hours) prior to surgical incision (or start of procedure when no incision is required), as ordered (PERI 2)[5]

4049F Documentation that order was given to discontinue prophylactic antibiotics within 24 hours of surgical end time, non-cardiac procedure (PERI 2)[5]

4050F Hypertension plan of care documented as appropriate (NMA-No Measure Associated)

4051F Referred for an arterio-venous (AV) fistula (ESRD, CKD)[1]

4052F Hemodialysis via functioning arteriovenous (AV) fistula (ESRD)[1]

4053F Hemodialysis via functioning arteriovenous (AV) graft (ESRD)[1]

4054F Hemodialysis via catheter (ESRD)[1]

4055F Patient receiving peritoneal dialysis (ESRD)[1]

4056F Appropriate oral rehydration solution recommended (PAG)[1]

4058F Pediatric gastroenteritis education provided to caregiver (PAG)[1]

4060F Psychotherapy services provided (MDD, MDD ADOL)[1]

4062F Patient referral for psychotherapy documented (MDD, MDD ADOL)[1]

4063F Antidepressant pharmacotherapy considered and not prescribed (MDD ADOL)[1]

4064F Antidepressant pharmacotherapy prescribed (MDD, MDD ADOL)[1]

4065F Antipsychotic pharmacotherapy prescribed (MDD)[1]

4066F Electroconvulsive therapy (ECT) provided (MDD)[1]

4067F Patient referral for electroconvulsive therapy (ECT) documented (MDD)[1]

4069F Venous thromboembolism (VTE) prophylaxis received (IBD)[10]

4070F Deep vein thrombosis (DVT) prophylaxis received by end of hospital day 2 (STR)[5]

4073F Oral antiplatelet therapy prescribed at discharge (STR)[5]

4075F Anticoagulant therapy prescribed at discharge (STR)[5]

Footnotes

1-Physician Consortium for Performance Improvement (PCPI), www.physicianconsortium.org

2-National Committee on Quality Assurance (NCQA), Health Employer Data Information Set (HEDIS®), www.ncqa.org

3-The Joint Commission (TJC), ORYX Initiative Performance Measures, http://www.jointcommission.org/performancemeasurement.aspx

4-National Diabetes Quality Improvement Alliance (NDQIA), http://www.nationaldiabetesalliance.org

5-Joint measure from The Physician Consortium for Performance Improvement, www.physicianconsortium.org and National Committee on Quality Assurance (NCQA), www.ncqa.org

6-The Society of Thoracic Surgeons, http://www.sts.org, and National Quality Forum, http://www.qualityforum.org

7-Optum, www.optum.com

8-American Academy of Neurology, www.aan.com/go/practice/quality/measurements or quality@aan.com

9-College of American Pathologists (CAP), www.cap.org/apps/docs/ advocacy/pathology_performance_measurement.pdf

10-American Gastroenterological Association (AGA), www.gastro.org/quality

11-American Society of Anesthesiologists (ASA), http://www.asahq.org

12-American College of Gastroenterology (ACG), www.gi.org; American Gastroenterology Association (AGA), www.gastro.org; and American Society for Gastrointestinal Endoscopy (ASGE), www. asge.org

4077F Documentation that tissue plasminogen activator (t-PA) administration was considered (STR)[5]

4079F Documentation that rehabilitation services were considered (STR)[5]

4084F Aspirin received within 24 hours before emergency department arrival or during emergency department stay (EM)[5]

4086F Aspirin or clopidogrel prescribed or currently being taken (CAD)[1]

4090F Patient receiving erythropoietin therapy (HEM)[1]

4095F Patient not receiving erythropoietin therapy (HEM)[1]

4100F Bisphosphonate therapy, intravenous, ordered or received (HEM)[1]

4110F Internal mammary artery graft performed for primary, isolated coronary artery bypass graft procedure (CABG)[6]

4115F Beta blocker administered within 24 hours prior to surgical incision (CABG)[6]

4120F Antibiotic prescribed or dispensed (URI, PHAR)[2] , (A-BRONCH)[2]

4124F Antibiotic neither prescribed nor dispensed (URI, PHAR)[2] , (A-BRONCH)[2]

4130F Topical preparations (including OTC) prescribed for acute otitis externa (AOE)[1]

4131F Systemic antimicrobial therapy prescribed (AOE)[1]

4132F Systemic antimicrobial therapy not prescribed (AOE)[1]

4133F Antihistamines or decongestants prescribed or recommended (OME)[1]

4134F Antihistamines or decongestants neither prescribed nor recommended (OME)[1]

4135F Systemic corticosteroids prescribed (OME)[1]

4136F Sysemic corticosteroids not prescribed (OME)[1]

4140F Inhalded corticosteroids prescribed (Asthma)[1]

4142F Corticosteroid sparing therapy prescribed (IBD)[10]

4144F Alternative long-term control medication prescribed (Asthma)[1]

4145F Two or more anti-hypertensive agents prescribed or currently being taken (CAD, HTN)[1]

4148F Hepatitis A vaccine injection administered or previously received (Hep-C)[1]

4149F Hepatitis B vaccine injection administered or previously received (Hep-C, HIV)[1] (IBD)[10]

4150F Patient receiving antiviral treatment for Hepatitis C (Hep-C)[1]

4151F Patient did not start or is not receiving antiviral treatment for Hepatitis C during the measurement period (Hep-C)[1]

4153F Combination peginterferon and ribavirin therapy prescribed (HEP-C)[1]

4155F Hepatitis A vaccine series previously received (Hep-C)[1]

● New Code ▲ Revised Code + Add-On Code ⊘ Modifier -51 Exempt ★ Telemedicine

4157F   Hepatitis B vaccine series previously received (Hep-C)[1]

4158F   Patient counseled about risk of alcohol use (Hep-C)[1]

4159F   Counseling regarding contraception received prior to initiation of antiviral treatment (Hep-C)[1]

4163F   Patient counseling at a minimum on all of the following treatment options for clinically localized prostate cancer: active surveillance, AND interstitial prostate brachytherapy, AND external beam radiotherapy, AND radical prostatectomy, provided prior to initiation of treatment (PRCA)[1]

4164F   Adjuvant (ie, in combination with external beam radiotherapy to the prostate for prostate cancer) hormonal therapy (gonadotropin-releasing hormone [GNRH] agonist or antagonist) prescribed/administered (PRCA)[1]

4165F   Three-dimensional conformal radiotherapy (3D-CRT) or intensity modulated radiation therapy (IMRT) received (PRCA)[1]

4167F   Head of bed elevation (30-45 degrees) on first ventilator day ordered (CRIT)[1]

4168F   Patient receiving care in the intensive care unit (ICU) and receiving mechanical ventilation, 24 hours or less (CRIT)[1]

4169F   Patient either not receiving care in the intensive care unit (ICU) OR not receiving mechanical ventilation OR receiving mechanical ventilation greater than 24 hours (CRIT)[1]

4171F   patient receiving erythropoiesis-stimulating agents (ESA) therapy (CKD)[1]

4172F   Patient not receiving erythropoiesis-stimulating agents (ESA) therapy (CKD)[1]

4174F   Counseling about the potential impact of glaucoma on visual functioning and quality of life, and importance of treatment adherence provided to patient and/or caregiver(s) (EC)[5]

4175F   Best-corrected visual acuity of 20/40 or better (distance or near) achieved within the 90 days following cataract surgery (EC)[5]

4176F   Counseling about value of protection from UV light and lack of proven efficacy of nutritional supplements in prevention or progression of cataract development provided to patient and/or caregiver(s) (NMA-No Measure Associated)

4177F   Counseling about the benefits and/or risks of the age-related eye disease study (AREDS) formulation for preventing progression of age-related macular degeneration (AMD) provided to patient and/or caregiver(s) (EC)[5]

4178F   Anti-D immune globulin received between 26 and 30 weeks gestation (Pre-Cr)[1]

4179F   Tamoxifen or aromatase inhibitor (AI) prescribed (ONC)[1]

4180F   Adjuvant chemotherapy referred, prescribed or previously received for Stage III colon cancer (ONC)[1]

4181F   Conformal radiation therapy received (NMA-No Measure Assoc.)

4182F   Conformal radiation therapy not received (NMA-No Measure Assoc.)

4185F   Continuous (12-months) therapy with proton pump inhibitor (PPI) or histamine H2 receptor antagonist (H2RA) received (GERD)[5]

4186F   no continuous (12-months) therapy with either proton pump inhibitor (PPI) or histamine H2 receptor antagonist (H2RA) received (GERD)[5]

4187F   Disease modifying anti-rheumatic drug therapy prescribed or dispensed (RA)[2]

4188F Appropriate angiotensin converting enzyme (ACE)/angiotensin receptor blockers (ARB) therapeutic monitoring test ordered or performed (AM)[2]

4189F Appropriate digoxin therapeutic monitoring test ordered or performed (AM)[2]

4190F Appropriate diuretic therapeutic monitoring test ordered or performed (AM)[2]

4191F Appropriate anticonvulsant therapeutic monitoring test ordered or performed (AM)[2]

4192F Patient not receiving glucocorticoid therapy (RA)[5]

4193F Patient receiving <10 mg daily prednisone (or equivalent), or RA activity is worsening, or glucocorticoid use is for less than 6 months (RA)[5]

4194F Patient receiving >=10 mg daily prednisone (or equivalent) for longer than 6 months, and improvement or no change in disease activity (RA)[5]

4195F Patient receiving first time biologic disease modifying anti rheumatic drug therapy for rheumatoid arthritis (RA)[5]

4196F Patient not receiving first time biologic disease modifying anti rheumatic drug therapy for rheumatoid arthritis (RA)[5]

4200F External beam radiotherapy as primary therapy to prostate with or without nodal irradiation (PRCA)[1]

4201F External beam radiotherapy with or without nodal irradiation as adjuvant or salvage therapy for prostate cancer patient (PRCA)[1]

4210F Angiotensin converting enzyme (ACE) or angiotensin receptor blockers (ARB) medication therapy for 6 months or more (MM)[2]

4220F Digoxin medication therapy for 6 months or more (MM)[2]

4221F Diuretic medication therapy for 6 months or more (MM)[2]

4230F Anticonvulsant medication therapy for 6 months or more (MM)[2]

4240F Instruction in therapeutic exercise with follow-up provided to patients during episode of back pain lasting longer than 12 weeks (BkP)[2]

4242F Counseling for supervised exercise program provided to patients during episode of back pain lasting longer than 12 weeks (BkP)[2]

4245F Patient counseled during the initial visit to maintain or resume normal activities (BkP)[2]

4248F Patient counseled during the initial visit for an episode of back pain against bed rest lasting 4 days or longer (BkP)[2]

4250F Active warming used intraoperatively for the purpose of maintaining normothermia, OR at least one body temperature equal to or greater than 36 degrees Centigrade (or 96.8 degrees Fahrenheit) recorded within the 30 minutes immediately before or the 15 minutes immediately after anesthesia end time (CRIT)[1]

4255F Duration of general or neuraxial anesthesia 60 minutes or longer, as documented in the anesthesia record (CRIT)[5] (Peri2)[11]

4256F Duration of general or neuraxial anesthesia less than 60 minutes, as documented in the anesthesia record (CRIT)[5] (Peri2)[11]

4260F Wound surface culture technique used (CWC)[5]

● New Code ▲ Revised Code + Add-On Code ⊘ Modifier -51 Exempt ★ Telemedicine

4261F Technique other than surface culture of the wound exudate used (eg, Levine/deep swab technique, semi quantitative or quantitative swab technique) OR wound surface culture technique not used (CWC)[5]

4265F Use of wet to dry dressings prescribed or recommended (CWC)[5]

4266F Use of wet to dry dressings neither prescribed nor recommended (CWC)[5]

4267F Compression therapy prescribed (CWC)[5]

4268F Patient education regarding the need for long term compression therapy including interval replacement of compression stockings received (CWC)[5]

4269F Appropriate method of offloading (pressure relief) prescribed (CWC)[5]

4270F Patient receiving potent antiretroviral therapy for 6 months or longer (HIV)[5]

4271F Patient receiving potent antiretroviral therapy for less than 6 months or not receiving potent antiretroviral therapy (HIV)[5]

4274F Influenza immunization administered or previously received (HIV)[5] (P ESRD)[1]

4276F Potent antiretroviral therapy prescribed (HIV)[5]

4279F Pneumocystis jiroveci pneumonia prophylaxis prescribed (HIV)[5]

4280F Pneumocystis jiroveci pneumonia prophylaxis prescribed within 3 months of low CD4+ cell count or percentage (HIV)[5]

4290F Patient screened for injection drug use (HIV)[5]

4293F Patient screened for high risk sexual behavior (HIV)[5]

4300F Patient receiving warfarin therapy for nonvalvular atrial fibrillation or atrial flutter (AFIB)[1]

4301F Patient not receiving warfarin therapy for nonvalvular atrial fibrillation or atrial flutter (AFIB)[1]

4305F Patient education regarding appropriate foot care AND daily inspection of the feet received (CWC)[5]

4306F Patient counseled regarding psychosocial AND pharmacologic treatment options for opioid addiction (SUD)[1]

4320F Patient counseled regarding psychosocial AND pharmacologic treatment options for alcohol dependence (SUD)[5]

Footnotes

1-Physician Consortium for Performance Improvement (PCPI), www.physicianconsortium.org

2-National Committee on Quality Assurance (NCQA), Health Employer Data Information Set (HEDIS®), www.ncqa.org

3-The Joint Commission (TJC), ORYX Initiative Performance Measures, http://www.jointcommission.org/performancemeasurement.aspx

4-National Diabetes Quality Improvement Alliance (NDQIA), http://www.nationaldiabetesalliance.org

5-Joint measure from The Physician Consortium for Performance Improvement, www.physicianconsortium.org and National Committee on Quality Assurance (NCQA), www.ncqa.org

6-The Society of Thoracic Surgeons, http://www.sts.org, and National Quality Forum, http://www.qualityforum.org

7-Optum, www.optum.com

8-American Academy of Neurology, www.aan.com/go/practice/quality/measurements or quality@aan.com

9-College of American Pathologists (CAP), www.cap.org/apps/docs/ advocacy/pathology_performance_measurement.pdf

10-American Gastroenterological Association (AGA), www.gastro.org/quality

11-American Society of Anesthesiologists (ASA), http://www.asahq.org

12-American College of Gastroenterology (ACG), www.gi.org; American Gastroenterology Association (AGA), www.gastro.org; and American Society for Gastrointestinal Endoscopy (ASGE), www. asge.org

---

Separate Procedure   Unlisted Procedure   CCI Comp. Code   Non-specific Procedure   **1017**

4322F Caregiver provided with education and referred to additional resources for support (DEM)[1]

4324F Patient (or caregiver) queried about parkinson's disease medication related motor complications (Prkns)[8]

4325F Medical and surgical treatment options reviewed with patient (or caregiver) (Prkns)[8]

4326F Patient (or caregiver) queried about symptoms of autonomic dysfunction (Prkns)[8]

4328F Patient (or caregiver) queried about sleep disturbances (Prkns)[8]

4330F Counseling about epilepsy specific safety issues provided to patient (or caregiver(s)) (EPI)[8]

4340F Counseling for women of childbearing potential with epilepsy (EPI)[8]

4350F Counseling provided on symptom management, end of life decisions, and palliation (DEM)[1]

4400F Rehabilitative therapy options discussed with patient (or caregiver) (Prkns)[8]

4450F Self-care education provided to patient (HF)[1]

4470F Implantable cardioverter-defibrillator (ICD) counseling provided (HF)[1]

4480F Patient receiving ACE inhibitor/ARB therapy and beta-blocker therapy for 3 months or longer (HF)[1]

4481F Patient receiving ACE inhibitor/ARB therapy and beta-blocker therapy for less than 3 months or patient not receiving ACE inhibitor/ARB therapy and beta blocker therapy (HF)[1]

4500F Referred to an outpatient cardiac rehabilitation program (CAD)[1]

4510F Previous cardiac rehabilitation for qualifying cardiac event completed (CAD)[1]

4525F Neuropsychiatric intervention ordered (DEM)[1]

4526F Neuropsychiatric intervention received (DEM)[1]

4540F Disease modifying pharmacotherapy discussed (ALS)[8]

4541F Patient offered treatment for pseudobulbar affect, sialorrhea, or ALS-related symptoms (ALS)[8]

4550F Options for noninvasive respiratory support discussed with patient (ALS)[8]

4551F Nutritional support offered (ALS)[8]

4552F Patient offered referral to a speech language pathologist (ALS)[8]

4553F Patient offered assistance in planning for end of life issues (ALS)[8]

4554F Patient received inhalational anesthetic agent (Peri2)[11]

4555F Patient did not receive inhalational anesthetic agent (Peri2)[11]

4556F Patient exhibits 3 or more risk factors for post-operative nausea and vomiting (Peri2)[11]

4557F Patient does not exhibit 3 or more risk factors for post-operative nausea and vomiting (Peri2)[11]

4558F Patient received at least 2 prophylactic pharmacologic anti-emetic agents of different classes preoperatively and intraoperatively (Peri2)[11]

4559F At least 1 body temperature measurement equal to or greater than 35.5 degrees Celsius (or 95.9 degrees Fahrenheit) recorded within the 30 minutes immediately before or the 15 minutes immediately after anesthesia end time (Peri2)[11]

4560F Anesthesia technique did not involve general or neuraxial anesthesia (Peri2)[11]

4561F Patient has a coronary artery stent (Peri2)[11]

4562F Patient does not have a coronary artery stent (Peri2)[11]

4563F Patient received aspirin within 24 hours prior to anesthesia start time (Peri2)[11]

FOLLOW-UP OR OTHER OUTCOMES

Follow-up or other outcomes codes describe review and communication of test results to patients, patient satisfaction or experience with care, patient functional status, and patient morbidity and mortality.

5005F Patient counseled on self-examination for new or changing moles (ML)[5]

5010F Findings of dilated macular or fundus exam communicated to the physician or other qualified health care professional managing the diabetes care (EC)[5]

5015F Documentation of communication that a fracture occurred and that the patient was or should be tested or treated for osteoporosis (OP)[5]

5020F Treatment summary report communicated to physician(s) or other qualified health care professional(s) managing continuing care and to the patient within 1 month of completing treatment (ONC)[1]

5050F Treatment plan communicated to provider(s) managing continuing care within 1 month of diagnosis (ML)[5]

5060F Findings from diagnostic mammogram communicated to practice managing patient's ongoing care within 3 business daysof exam interpretation(RAD)[5]

5062F Findings from diagnostic mammogram communicated to practic managingthe patient's on-going care within 5 business days of exam interpretation (RAD)[5]

5100F Potential risk for fracture communicated to the referring physician or other qualified health care professional within 24 hours of completion of the imaging study (NUC_MED)[1]

5200F Consideration of referral for a neurological evaluation of appropriateness for surgical therapy for intractable epilepsy within the past 3 years (EPI)[8]

5250F Asthma discharge plan provided to patient (Asthma)[1]

PATIENT SAFETY

Patient safety codes that describe patient safety practices.

6005F Rationale (eg, severity of illness and safety) for level of care (eg, home, hospital) documented (CAP)[1]

6010F Dysphagia screening conducted prior to order for or receipt of any foods, fluids or medication by mouth (STR)[5]

6015F Patient receiving or eligible to receive foods, fluids or medication by mouth (STR)[5]

6020F NPO (nothing by mouth) ordered (STR)[5]

| | Separate Procedure | | Unlisted Procedure | | CCI Comp. Code | | Non-specific Procedure | **1019** |

6030F All elements of maximal sterile barrier technique followed including: cap AND mask AND sterile gown AND sterile gloves AND a large sterile sheet AND hand hygiene AND 2% chlorhexidine for cutaneous antisepsis (or acceptable alternative antiseptics, per current guideline) (CRIT)[1]

6040F Use of appropriate radiation dose reduction devices or manual techniques for appropriate moderation of exposure, documented (RAD)[5]

6045F Radiation exposure or exposure time in final report for procedure using fluoroscopy, documented (RAD)[5]

6070F Patient queried and counseled about anti-epileptic drug (AED) side effects (EPI)[8]

6080F Patient (or caregiver) queried about falls (Prkns, DSP)[8]

6090F Patient (or caregiver) counseled about safety issues appropriate to patient's stage of disease (Prkns)[8]

6100F Timeout to verify correct patient, correct site, and correct procedure, documented (PATH)[9]

6101F Safety counseling for dementia provided (DEM)[1]

6102F Safety counseling for dementia ordered (DEM)[1]

6110F Counseling provided regarding risks of driving and the alternatives to driving (DEM)[1]

6150F Patient not receiving a first course of anti-TNF (tumor necrosis factor) therapy (IBD)[10]

STRUCTURAL MEASURES

Structural measures codes are used to identify measures that address the setting or system of the delivered care. These codes also address aspects of the capabilities of the organization or health care professional providing the care.

7010F Patient information entered into a recall system that includes: target date for the next exam specified AND a process to follow up with patients regarding missed or unscheduled appointments (ML)[5]

7020F Mammogram assessment category [eg, Mammography Quality Standards Act (MQSA), Breast Imaging Reporting and Data System (BI-RADS®), or FDA approved equivalent categories] entered into an internal database to allow for analysis of abnormal interpretation (recall) rate (RAD)5

7025F Patient information entered into a reminder system with a target due date for the next mammogram (RAD)[5]

NONMEASURE CODE LISTING

The following codes are included for reporting of certain aspects of care. These factors are not represented by measures developed by existing measures organizations or recognized measures-development processes at the time they are placed in the CPT code set, but may ultimately be associated with measures approved by an appropriate quality improvement organization.

9001F Aortic aneurysm less than 5.0 cm maximum diameter on centerline formatted CT or minor diameter on axial formatted CT (NMA-No Measure Associated)

9002F Aortic aneurysm 5.0-5.4 cm maximum diameter on centerline formatted CT or minor diameter on axial formatted CT (NMA-No Measure Associated)

9003F Aortic aneurysm 5.5-5.9 cm maximum diameter on centerline formatted CT or minor diameter on axial formatted CT (NMA-No Measure Associated)

9004F Aortic aneurysm 6.0 cm or greater maximum diameter on centerline formatted CT or minor diameter on axial formatted CT (NMA-No Measure Associated)

9005F Asymptomatic carotid stenosis: No history of any transient ischemic attack or stroke in any carotid or vertebrobasilar territory (NMA-No Measure Associated)

● New Code ▲ Revised Code + Add-On Code ⦸ Modifier -51 Exempt ★ Telemedicine

9006F Symptomatic carotid stenosis: Ipsilateral carotid territory TIA or stroke less than 120 days prior to procedure (NMA-No Measure Associated)

9007F Other carotid stenosis: Ipsilateral TIA or stroke 120 days or greater prior to procedure or any prior contralateral carotid territory or vertebrobasilar TIA or stroke (NMA-No Measure Associated)

This page intentionally left blank.

● New Code   ▲ Revised Code   ✛ Add-On Code   ⊘ Modifier -51 Exempt   ★ Telemedicine

CATEGORY III CODES

CATEGORY III SECTION OVERVIEW

The following section contains a set of temporary codes for emerging technology, services, procedures, and service paradigms. Category III codes allow data collection for these services/procedures. Use of unlisted codes does not offer the opportunity for the collection of specific data. If a Category III code is available, this code must be reported instead of a Category I unlisted code. This is an activity that is critically important in the evaluation of health care delivery and the formation of public and private policy. The use of the codes in this section allows physicians and other qualified health care professionals, insurers, health services researchers, and health policy experts to identify emerging technology, services, procedures, and service paradigms for clinical efficacy, utilization and outcomes.

The inclusion of a service or procedure in this section does not constitute a finding of support, or lack thereof, with regard to clinical efficacy, safety, applicability to clinical practice, or payer coverage. The codes in this section may not conform to the usual requirements for CPT Category I codes established by the Editorial Panel. For Category I codes, the Panel requires that the service/procedure be performed by many health care professionals in clinical practice in multiple locations and that FDA approval, as appropriate, has already been received. The nature of emerging technology, services, procedures, and service paradigms is such that these requirements may not be met. For these reasons, temporary codes for emerging technology, services, procedures, and service paradigms have been placed in a separate section of the CPT code set and the codes are differentiated from Category I CPT codes by the use of alphanumeric characters.

Services and procedures described in this section make use of alphanumeric characters. These codes have an alpha character as the 5th character in the string (ie, four digits followed by the letter T). The digits are not intended to reflect the placement of the code in the Category I section of CPT nomenclature. Codes in this section may or may not eventually receive a Category I CPT code. In either case, in general, a given Category III code will be archived five years from the date of initial publication or extension unless a modification of the archival date is specifically noted at the time of a revision or change to a code (eg, addition of parenthetical instructions, reinstatement). Services and procedures described by Category III codes which have been archived after five years, without conversion, must be reported using the Category I unlisted code unless another specific cross-reference is established at the time of archiving. New codes or revised codes in this section are released semi-annually via the AMA CPT website to expedite dissemination for reporting. Codes approved for deletion are published annually with the full set of temporary codes for emerging technology, services, procedures, and service paradigms in the CPT code set. See the Introduction section of the CPT code set for a complete list of the dates of release and implementation.

CATEGORY III CODES

(For destruction of localized lesion of choroid by transpupillary thermotherapy, use 67299)

(For destruction of macular drusen, photocoagulation, use 67299)

(For extracorporeal shock wave involving musculoskeletal system, not otherwise specified, low energy, use 20999)

(For application of high energy extracorporeal shock wave involving musculoskeletal system not otherwise specified, use 0101T)

(For application of high energy extracorporeal shock wave involving lateral humeral epicondyle, use 0102T)

(For non-surgical reduction therapy, use 93799)

(For lipoprotein, direct measurement, intermediate density lipoproteins [IDL] [remnant lipoprotein], use 84999)

(For endoscopic lysis of epidural adhesions with direct visualization using mechanical means or solution injection [eg, normal saline], use 64999)

(For dual x-ray absorptiometry [DEXA] body composition study, use 76499)

(For pulsed magnetic neuromodulation incontinence treatment, use 53899)

(To report antiprothrombin [phospholipid cofactor] antibody, use 86849)

(0031T, 0032T have been deleted)

(For speculoscopy, including sampling, use 58999)

(For urinalysis infectious agent detection, semi-quantitative analysis of volatile compounds, use 81099)

0042T Cerebral perfusion analysis using computed tomography with contrast administration, including post-processing of parametric maps with determination of cerebral blood flow, cerebral blood volume, and mean transit time (Sunset January 2024)

(For carbon monoxide, expired gas analysis [eg, ETC0/hemolysis greath test], use 84999)

(0046T, 0047T have been deleted)

(For mammary duct[s] catheter lavage, use 19499)

(**0051T** deleted 2017 [2018 edition]. To report, see 33927, 33928, 33929)

(**0052T** deleted 2017 [2018 edition]. To report, see 33927, 33928, 33929)

(**0053T** deleted 2017 [2018 edition]. To report, see 33927, 33928, 33929)

+ **0054T** Computer-assisted musculoskeletal surgical navigational orthopedic procedure, with image-guidance based on fluoroscopic images (list separately in addition to code for primary procedure) (Sunset January 2024)

+ **0055T** Computer-assisted musculoskeletal surgical navigational orthopedic procedure, with image-guidance based on ct/mri images (list separately in addition to code for primary procedure) (Sunset January 2024)

(When CT and MRI are both performed, report 0055T only once)

(**0058T** deleted 2020 [2021 Edition])

(For cryopreservation, reproductive tissue, ovarian, use 89398)

(For cryopreservation of mature oocytes, use 89337)

(**0357T** deleted 2019 [2020 Edition])

(For cryopreservation of immature oocyte(s), use 89398)

(For cryopreservation of embryos, sperm and testicular reproductive tissue, see 89258, 89259, 89335)

(For electrical impedance breast scan, use 76499)

(For destruction/reduction of malignant breast tumor, microwave phased array thermotherapy, use 19499)

(0062T, 0063T have been deleted)

(For percutaneous intradiscal annuloplasty, any method other than electrothermal, use 22899)

(For intradiscal electrothermal annuloplasty, see 22526-22527)

(To report CT colon, screening, use 74263)

(To report CT colon, diagnostic, use 74261-74262)

(0068T-0070T have been deleted)

(For acoustic heart sound recording and computer analysis, use 93799)

0071T Focused ultrasound ablation of uterine leiomyomata, including MR guidance; total leiomyomata volume less than 200 cc of tissue (Sunset January 2020)

0072T total leiomyomata volume greater or equal to 200 cc of tissue (Sunset January 2020)

(Do not report 0071T, 0072T in conjunction with 51702 or 77022)

0075T   Transcatheter placement of extracranial vertebral arteru stemt(s). including radiologic supervision and interpretation, open or percutaneous; initial vessel (Sunset January 2020)

+ 0076T   each additional vessel (List separately in addition to code for primary procedure) (Sunset January 2020)

(Use 0076T in conjunction with 0075T)

(When the ipsilateral extracranial vertebral arteriogram (including imaging and selective catheterization) confirms the need for stenting, then 0075T and 0076T include all ipsilateral extracranial vertebral catheterization, all diagnostic imaging for ipsilateral extracranial vertebral artery stenting, and all related radiologic supervision and interpretation. If stenting is not indicated, then the appropriate codes for selective catheterization and imaging should be reported in lieu of code 0075T or 0076T.)

(0085T   deleted 2020 [2021 Edition])

(For breath test for heart transplant rejection, use 84999)

(To report total disc lumbar arthroplasty, use 22857)

+ 0095T   Removal of total disc arthroplasty (artificial disc), anterior approach, each additional interspace, cervical (List separately in addition to code for primary procedure) (Sunset January 2024)

(Use 0095T in conjunction with 22864)

(To report revision of total disc lumbar arthroplasty, use 22862)

+ 0098T   Revision including replacement of total disc arhtroplasty (artificial disc), anterior approach, each additional interspace, cervical (List separately in addition to code for primary procedure) (Sunset January 2024)

(Use 0098T in conjunction with 22861)

(Do not report 0098T in conjunction with 0095T)

(Do not report 0098T in conjunction with 22853, 22854, 22859 when performed at the same level)

(For decompression, see 63001-63048)

0100T   Placement of a subconjunctival retinal prosthesis receiver and pulse generator, and implantation of intra-ocular retinal electrode array, with vitrectomy (Sunset January 2021)

(For initial programming of implantable intraocular retinal electrode array device, use 0472T)

0101T   Extracorporeal shock wave involving musculoskeletal system, not otherwise specified, high energy (Sunset January 2021)

(For extracorporeal shock wave therapy involving integumentary system not otherwise specified, see 0512T, 0513T)

(Do not report 0101T in conjunction 0512T, 0513T, when treating same area)

0102T   Extracorporeal shock wave, high energy, performed by a physician, requiring anesthesia other than local, involving lateral humeral epicondyle (Sunset January 2021)

0512T   Extracorporeal shock wave for integumentary wound healing, high energy, including topical application and dressing care; initial wound (Sunset January 2024)

+ 0513T   each additional wound (List separately in addition to code for primary procedure) (Sunset January 2024)

(Use 0513T in conjunction with 0512T)

(For holotranscobalamin, quantitative, use 84999)

(For inert gas rebreathing for cardiac output measurement during rest, use 93799)

(For intert gas rebreathing for cardiac output measurement during exercise, use 93799)

| | Separate Procedure | | Unlisted Procedure | | CCI Comp. Code | | Non-specific Procedure | **1025** |

0106T Quantitative sensory testing (QST), testing and interpretation per extremity; using touch pressure stimuli to assess large diameter sensation (Sunset January 2021)

0107T using vibration stimuli to assess large diameter fiber sensation (Sunset January 2021)

0108T using cooling stimuli to assess small nerve fiber sensation and hyperalgesia (Sunset January 2021)

0109T using heat-pain stimuli to assess small nerve fiber sensation and hyperalgesia (Sunset January 2021)

0110T using other stimuli to assess sensation (Sunset January 2021)

(0111T deleted 2020 [2021 Edition])

(For very long chain fatty acids, use 82726)

(For long-chain [C20-22] omega-3 fatty acids in red blood cell [RBC] membranes, use 84999)

(For fistulization of sclera for glaucoma, through ciliary body, use 66999)

(For conjunctival incision with posterior extrascleral placement of pharmacological agent, use 68399)

(0126T deleted 2020 [2021 Edition])

(For common carotid intima-media thickness [IMT] study for evaluation of atherosclerotic burden or coronary heart disease risk factor assessment, use 93998)

(For bilateral quantitative carotid intima media thickness and carotid atheroma evaluation that includes all required elements, use 93895)

(For validated, statistically reliable, randomized, controlled, single-patient clinical investigation of FDA approved chronic care drugs, provided by a pharmacist, interpretation and report to the prescribing health care professional, use 99199)

(0144T Deleted 2009 [2010 edition]. To report, see 75571-75574.)

(0145T Deleted 2009 [2010 edition]. To report, see 75571-75574.)

(0146T Deleted 2009 [2010 edition]. To report, see 75571-75574.)

(0147T Deleted 2009 [2010 edition]. To report, see 75571-75574.)

(0148T Deleted 2009 [2010 edition]. To report, see 75571-75574.)

(0149T Deleted 2009 [2010 edition]. To report, see 75571-75574.)

(0150T Deleted 2009 [2010 edition]. To report, see 75571-75574.)

(0151T Deleted 2009 [2010 edition]. To report, see 75571-75574.)

(For laparoscopic implantation, replacement, revision or removal of gastric stimulation electrodes, lesser curvature, use 43659)

(For open implantation, replacement, revision, or removal of gastric stimulation electrodes, lesser curvature, use 43999)

(0159T deleted 2018 [2019 Edition]. To report, see 77048, 77049)

+ 0163T Total disc arthroplasty (artificial disc), anterior approach, including discectomy to prepare interspace (other than for decompression), each additional interspace, lumbar (List separately in addition to code for primary procedure) (Sunset January 2024)

(Use 0163T in conjunction with 22857)

● New Code ▲ Revised Code + Add-On Code ⊘ Modifier -51 Exempt ★ Telemedicine

+ 0164T Removal of total disc arthroplasty, (artificial disc), anterior approach, each additional interspace, lumbar (List separately in addition to code for primary procedure) (Sunset January 2024)

(Use 0164T in conjunction with 22865)

+ 0165T Revision including replacement of total disc arthroplasty, (artificial disc), anterior approach, each additional interspace, lumbar (List separately in addition to code for primary procedure) (Sunset January 2024)

(Use 0165T in conjunction with 22862)

(Do not report 0163T, 0164T, 0165T in conjunction with 22853, 22854, 22859, 49010, when performed at the same level)

(For decompression, see 63001-63048)

(For transmyocardial transcatheter closure of ventricular septal defect, with implant, including cadiopulmonary bypass if performed, use 33999)

(For rhinophototherapy, intranasal application of ultraviolet and visible light, use 30999)

(For stereotactic placement of infusion catheter[s] in the brain for delivery of therapeutic agent[s], use 64999)

(To report insertion of interlaminar/interspinous process stabilization/distraction device, without fusion, including image guidance when performed, with openm decompression, lumbar, single level, use 22867. To report insertion of interlaminar/interspinous process stabilization/distraction device, without open decompression or fusion, including image guidance when performed, lumbar, single level, use 22869)

(To report insertion of interlaminar/interspinous process stabilization/distraction device, without fusion, including image guidance when performed, with open decompression, lumbar, second level, use 22868. To report insertion of interlaminar/interspinous process stabilization/distraction device, without open decompression or fusion, including image guidance when performed, lumbar, second level use, 22870)

+ 0174T Computer-aided detection (CAD) (computer algorithm analysis of digital image data for lesion detection) with further physician review for interpretation and report, with or without digitization of film radiographic images, chest radiograph(s), performed concurrent with primary interpretation (List separately in addition to code for primary procedure) (Sunset January 2022)

(Use 0174T in conjunction with 71045, 71046, 71047, 71048)

0175T Computer-aided detection (CAD) (computer algorithm analysis of digital image data for lesion detection) with further physician review for interpretation and report, with or without digitization of film radiographic images, chest radiograph(s), performed remote from primary interpretation (Sunset January 2022)

(Do not report 0175T in conjunction with 71045, 71046, 71047, 71048)

(0178T deleted 2017 [2018 edition])

(0179T deleted 2017 [2018 edition])

(0180T deleted 2017 [2018 edition])

(For electrocardiogram, 64 leads or greater, with graphic presentation and analysis, use 93799)

(For electrocardiogram, routine, with at least 12 leads separately performed, see 93000-93010)

(0182T deleted 2015 [2016 edition]. To report, see 0394T, 0395T)

0184T Excision of rectal tumor, transanal endoscopic microsurgical approach (ie, TEMS), including muscularis propria (ie, full thickness) (Sunset January 2024)

(For non-endoscopic excision of rectal tumor, see 45160, 45171, 45172)

(Do not report 0184T in conjunction with 45300, 45308, 45309, 45315, 45317, 45320, 69990)

(For multivariate analysis of patient-specific findings with quantifiable computer probability assessment, including report, use 99199)

(For suprachoroidal delivery of pharmacologic agent, use 67299)

(**0188T** deleted 2018 [2019 Edition])

(**0189T** deleted 2018 [2019 Edition])

(For remote real-time interactive video-conferenced critical care, evaluation and management of the critically ill or critically injured patient, use 99499)

(**0190T** deleted 2018 [2019 Edition])

(For placement of intraocular radiation source applicator, use 67299)

(For application of the source by radiation oncologist, see Clinical Brachytherapy section)

0191T Insertion of anterior segment aqueous drainage device, without extraocular resevoir; internal approach, into the trabecular meshwork; initial insertion (Sunset January 2024)

+ **0376T** each additional device insertion {List separately in addition to code for primary procedure) (Sunset January 2024)

(Use 0376T in conjunction with 0191T)

0253T Insertion of anterior segment aqueous drainage device, without extraocular resevoir; internal approach, into the suprachoroidal space (Sunset January 2024)

(To report insertion of drainage device by external approach, use 66183)

(**0195T** deleted 2018 [2019 Edition])

(**0196T** deleted 2018 [2019 Edition])

(For arthrodesis, pre-sacral interbody technique, disc space preparation, discectomy, without instrumentation, with image guidance, includes bone graft when performed, L4-L5 interspace, L5-S1 interspace, use 22899)

0198T Measurement of ocular blood flow by repetitive intraocular pressure sampling, with interpretation and report (Sunset January 2020)

(For tremor measurement with accelerometer(s) and/or gyroscope(s), use 95999)

0200T Percutaneous sacral augmentation (sacroplasty), unilateral injection(s), including the use of a balloon or mechanical device, when used, 1 or more needles, includes imaging guidance and bone biopsy, when performed (Sunset January 2020)

0201T Percutaneous sacral augmentation (sacroplasty), bilateral injections, including the use of a balloon or mechanical device, when used, 2 or more needles includes imaging guidance and bone biopsy, when performed (Sunset January 2020)

(Do not report 0200T, 0201T in conjunction with 20225 when performed at the same level)

0202T Posterior vertebral joint(s) arthroplasty (eg, facet joint[s] replacement), including facetectomy, laminectomy, foraminotomy, and vertebral column fixation, injection of bone cement, when performed, including fluoroscopy, single level, lumbar spine (Sunset January 2020)

(Do not report 0202T in conjunction with 22511, 22514, 22840, 22853, 22854, 22857, 22859, 63005, 63012, 63017, 63030, 63042, 63047, 63056 at the same level)

(**0205T** deleted 2019 [2020 Edition])

(For intravascular catheter-based coronary vessel or graft spectroscopy [eg, infrared] during diagnostic evaluation and/or therapeutic intervention including imaging supervision, interpretation, and report, each vessel, use 93799)

(**0206T** deleted 2019 [2020 Edition])

● New Code   ▲ Revised Code   **+** Add-On Code   ⊘ Modifier -51 Exempt   ★ Telemedicine

(For computerized database analysis of multiple cycles of digitized cardiac electrical data from 2 or more ECG leads, including transmission to a remote center, application of multiple nonlinear mathematical transformations, with coronary artery obstruction severity assessment, use 93799)

0207T Evacuation of meibomian glands, automated, using heat and intermittent pressure, unilateral (Sunset January 2020)

(For evacuation of meibomian glands using heat delivered through wearable, open-eye eyelid treatment devices and manual gland expression, use 0563T. For evacuation of meibomian gland using manual gland expression only, use the appropriate evaluation and management code)

0563T Evacuation of meibomian glands, using heat delivered through wearable, open-eye eyelid treatment devices and manual gland expression, bilateral (Sunset January 2025)

(For evacuation of meibomian gland using manual gland expression only, use the appropriate evaluation and management code)

0208T Pure tone audiometry (threshold), automated; air only (Sunset January 2021)

0209T   air and bone (Sunset January 2021)

0210T Speech audiometry threshold, automated; (Sunset January 2021)

0211T   with speech recognition (Sunset January 2021)

0212T Comprehensive audiometry threshold evaluation and speech recognition (0209T, 0211T combined), automated (Sunset January 2021)

(For audiometric testing using audiometers performed manually by a qualified health care professional, see 92551-92557)

0213T Injection(s), diagnostic or therapeutic agent, paravertebral facet (zygapophyseal) joint (or nerves innervating that joint) with ultrasound guidance, cervical or thoracic; single level (Sunset January 2021)

(To report bilateral procedure, use 0213T with modifier 50)

+ 0214T   second level (list separately in addition to code for primary procedure) (Sunset January 2021)

(Use 0214T in conjunction with 0213T)

(For bilateral procedure, report 0214T twice. Do not report modifier 50 in conjunction with 0214T)

+ 0215T   third and any additional level(s) (list separately in addition to code for primary procedure) (Sunset January 2021)

(Do not report 0215T more than once per day)

(Use 0215T in conjunction with 0214T)

(For bilateral procedure, report 0215T twice. Do not report modifier 50 in conjunction with 0215T)

0216T Injection(s), diagnostic or therapeutic agent, paravertebral facet (zygapophyseal) joint (or nerves innervating that joint) with ultrasound guidance, lumbar or sacral; single level (Sunset January 2021)

(To report bilateral procedure, use 0216T with modifier 50)

+ 0217T   second level (list separately in addition to code for primary procedure) (Sunset January 2021)

(Use 0217T in conjunction with 0216T)

(For bilateral procedure, report 0217T twice. Do not report modifier 50 in conjunction with 0217T)

+ 0218T   third and any additional level(s) (list separately in addition to code for primary procedure) (Sunset January 2021)

(Do not report 0218T more than once per day)

(Use 0218T in conjunction with 0216T, 0217T)

(If injection(s) are performed using fluoroscopy or CT, see 64490-64495)

(For bilateral procedure, report 0218T twice. Do not report modifier 50 in conjunction with 0218T)

0219T Placement of a posterior intrafacet implant(s), unilateral or bilateral, including imaging and placement of bone graft(s) or synthetic device(s), single level; cervical (Sunset January 2021)

0220T thoracic (Sunset January 2021)

0221T lumbar (Sunset January 2021)

(Do not report 0219T-0221T in conjunction with any radiological service)

(Do not report 0219T, 0220T, 0221T in conjunction with 20930, 20931, 22600-22614, 22840, 22853, 22854, 22859 at the same level)

+ 0222T each additional vertebral segment (list separately in addition to code for primary procedure) (Sunset January 2021)

(Use 0222T in conjunction with 0219T-0221T)

(For posterior or posterolateral arthrodesis technique, see 22600-22614)

(0228T deleted 2020 [2021 Edition])

(0229T deleted 2020 [2021 Edition])

(0230T deleted 2020 [2021 Edition])

(0231T deleted 2020 [2021 Edition])

(For injection[s], anesthetic agent and/or steroid, transforaminal epidural, with ultrasound guidance, cervical or thoracic, single level, use 64999)

(For transforaminal epidural injections performed under fluoroscopy or CT, see 64479-64484)

0232T Injection(s), platelet rich plasma, any site, including image guidance, harvesting and preparation when performed (Sunset January 2022)

(Do not report 0232T in conjunction with 15769, 15771, 15772, 15773, 15774, 20550, 20551, 20600, 20604, 20605, 20606, 20610, 20611, 36415, 36592, 76942, 77002, 77012, 77021, 86965, 0481T)

(Do not report 38220-38230 for bone marrow aspiration for platelet rich stem cell injection. For bone marrow aspiration for platelet rich stem cell injection, use 0232T)

Atherectomy (Open or Percutaneous) for Supra-Inguinal Arteries

Codes 0234T-0238T describe atherectomy performed by any method (eg, directional, rotational, laser) in arteries above the inguinal ligaments. These codes are structured differently than the codes describing atherectomy performed below the inguinal legaments (37225, 37227, 37229, 37231, 37233, 37235).

These supra-inguinal atherectomy codes all include the surgical work of performing the atherectomy plus the radiological supervision and interpretation of the atherectomy. Unlike the atherectomy codes for infra-inguinal arteries, this set of Category III codes does not include accessing and selectively catheterizing the vessel, traversing the lesion, embolic protection if used, other intervention used to treat the same or other vessels, or closure of the arteriotomy by any method. These codes describe endovascular procedures performed percutaneously and/or through an open surgical exposure.

0234T Transluminal peripheral atherectomy, open or percutaneous, including radiological supervision and interpretation; renal artery (Sunset January 2021)

0235T visceral artery (except renal), each vessel (Sunset January 2021)

● New Code ▲ Revised Code + Add-On Code ⊘ Modifier -51 Exempt ★ Telemedicine

0236T abdominal aorta (Sunset January 2021)

0237T brachiocephalic trunk and branches, each vessel (Sunset January 2021)

0238T iliac artery, each vessel (Sunset January 2021)

(To report esophageal motility studies without high-resolution esophageal pressure topography, use 91010 and with stimulant or perfusion, use 91013)

(**0249T** deleted 2019 [2020 Edition]. To report, use 46948)

0253T This code is out of order. See page 1028

(**0254T** deleted 2019 [2020 Edition]. To report, see 34717, 34718)

(**0255T** deleted 2017 [2018 edition]. To report, use 34717, 34718)

0263T Intramuscular autologous bone marrow cell therapy, with preparation of harvested cells, multiple injections, one leg, including ultrasound guidance, if performed; complete procedure including unilateral or bilateral bone marrow harvest (Sunset January 2022)

(Do not report 0263T in conjunction with 38204-38242, 76942, 93925, 93926)

0264T complete procedure excluding bone marrow harvest (Sunset January 2022)

(Do not report 0264T in conjunction with 38204-38242, 76942, 93925, 93926, 0265T)

0265T unilateral or bilateral bone marrow harvest only for intramuscular autologous bone marrow cell therapy (Sunset January 2022)

(Do not report 0265T in conjunction with 38204-38242, 0264T. For complete procedure, use 0263T)

0266T Implantation or replacement of carotid sinus baroreflex activation device; total system (includes generator placement, unilateral or bilateral lead placement, intra-operative interrogation, programming, and repositioning, when performed) (Sunset January 2022)

0267T lead only, unilateral (includes intra-operative interrogation, programming, and repositioning, when performed) (Sunset January 2022)

(For bilateral lead implantation or replacement, use 0267T with modifier 50)

0268T pulse generator only (includes intra-operative interrogation, programming, and repositioning, when performed) (Sunset January 2022)

(Do not report 0267T, 0268T in conjunction with 0266T, 0269T-0273T)

0269T Revision or removal of carotid sinus baroreflex activation device; total system (includes generator placement, unilateral or bilateral lead placement, intra-operative interrogation, programming, and repositioning, when performed) (Sunset January 2022)

(Do not report 0269T in conjunction with 0266T-0268T, 0270T-0273T)

0270T lead only, unilateral (includes intra-operative interrogation, programming, and repositioning, when performed) (Sunset January 2022)

(Do not report 0270T in conjunction with 0266T-0269T, 0271T-0273T)

(For bilateral lead removal, use 0270T with modifier 50)

(For removal of total carotic sinus baroreflex activation device, use 0269T)

0271T pulse generator only (includes intra-operative interrogation, programming, and repositioning, when performed) (Sunset January 2022)

(Do not report 0271T in conjunction with 0266T-0270T, 0272T, 0273T)

Separate Procedure   Unlisted Procedure   CCI Comp. Code   Non-specific Procedure   **1031**

(For removal and replacement, see 0266T, 0267T, 0268T)

0272T Interrogation device evaluation (in person), carotid sinus baroreflex activation system, including telemetric ineractive communication with the implantable device to monitor device diagnostics and programmed therapy values, with interpretation and report (eg, battery status, lead impedance, pulse amplitude, pulse width, therapy frequency, pathway mode, burst mode, therapy start/stop times each day); (Sunset January 2022)

(Do not report 0272T in conjunction with 0266T-0271T, 0273T)

0273T with programming (Sunset January 2022)

(Do not report 0273T in conjunction with 0266T-0272T)

0274T Percutaneous laminotomy/laminectomy (interlaminar approach) for decompression of neural elements, (with or without ligamentous resection, discectomy, facetectomy and/or foraminotomy), any method, under indirect image guidance (eg, fluoroscopic, CT), single or multiple levels, unilateral or bilateral; cervical or thoracic (Sunset January 2022)

0275T lumbar (Sunset January 2022)

(For percutaneous decompression of the nucleus pulposus of intervertebral disc utilizing needle based technique, use 62287)

0278T Transcutaneous electrical modulation pain reprocessing (eg, scrambler therapy), each treatment session (includes placement of electrodes) (Sunset January 2022)

(For implantation of trial or permanent electrode arrays or pulse generators for peripheral subcutaneous field stimulation, use 64999)

(For delivery of thermal energy to the muscle of the anal canal, use 46999)

+ 0290T Corneal incisions in the recipient cornea created using a laser, in preparation for penetrating or lamellar keratoplasty (List separately in addition to code for primary procedure) (Sunset January 2022)

(Use 0290T in conjunction with 65710, 65730, 65750, 65755)

(**0295T** deleted 2020 [2021 Edition])

(**0296T** deleted 2020 [2021 Edition])

(**0297T** deleted 2020 [2021 Edition])

(**0298T** deleted 2020 [2021 Edition])

(For extracorporeal shock wave for integumentary wound healing, high energy, use 28899)

(For greater than 48 hours of monitoring of external electrocardiographic recording, see 93241, 93242, 93243, 93244, 93245, 93246, 93247, 93248)

(**0301T** deleted 2017 [2018 edition])

(For focused microwave thermotherapy of the breast, use 19499)

(**0302T** deleted 2017 [2018 edition])

(**0303T** deleted 2017 [2018 edition])

(**0304T** deleted 2017 [2018 edition])

(**0305T** deleted 2017 [2018 edition])

(**0306T** deleted 2017 [2018 edition])

● New Code   ▲ Revised Code   + Add-On Code   ⊘ Modifier -51 Exempt   ★ Telemedicine

(**0307T** deleted 2017 [2018 edition])

0308T Insertion of ocular telescope prosthesis including removal of crystalline lens or intraocular lens prosthesis (Sunset January 2021)

(Do not report 0308T in conjunction with 65800-65815, 66020, 66030, 66600-66635, 66761, 66825, 66982-66986, 69990)

(For arthrodesis, pre-sacral interbody technique, including disc space preparation, discectomy, with posterior instrumentation, with image guidance, including bone graft, when performed, lumbar, L4-L5 interspace, use 22899)

(**0310T** deleted 2017 [2018 edition])

(For motor function mapping using non-invasive navigated transcranial magnetic stimulation [nTMS] for therapeutic treatment planning, upper and lower extremity, use 64999)

0312T Vagus nerve blocking therapy (morbid obesity); laparoscopic implantation of neurostimulator electrode array, anterior and posterior vagal trunks adjacent to esophagogastric junction (EGJ), with implantation of pulse generator, includes programming (Sunset January 2023)

0313T laparoscopic revision or replacement of vagal trunk neurostimulator electrode array, including connection to existing pulse generator (Sunset January 2023)

0314T laparascopic removal of vagal trunk neurostimulator (Sunset January 2023)

0315T removal of pulse generator (Sunset January 2023)

0316T replacement of pulse generator (Sunset January 2023)

(Do not report 0315T in conjunction with 0316T)

0317T neurostimulator pulse generator electronic analysis, includes reprogramming when performed (Sunset January 2023)

(For implantation, revision, replacement, and/or removal of vagus [cranial] nerve neurostimulator electrode array and/or pulse generator for vagus nerve stimulation performed other than at the ECJ [eg, epilepsy], see 64568-64570)

(For electronic analysis with programming, when performed, of vagal nerve neurostimulators, see 95970, 95976, 95977. Test stimulation to confirm correct target site placement of the electrode array[s] and/or to confirm the functional status of the system is inherent to placement, and is not separately reported as electronic analysis or programming of the neurostimulator system. Electronic analysis [95970] at the time of implantation is not separately reported.)

0329T Monitoring of intraocular pressure 24 hours or longer, unilateral or bilateral, with interpretation and report (Sunset January 2024)

0330T Tear film imaging, unilateral or bilateral, with interpretation adn report (Sunset January 2024)

0331T Myocardial sympathetic innervation imaging, planar qualitative and quantitative assessment; (Sunset January 2024)

0332T with tomographic SPECT (Sunset January 2024)

(For myocardial infarct avid imaging, see 78466, 78468, 78469)

0333T Visual evoked potential, screening of visual acuity, automated, with report (Sunset January 2024)

(For visual evoked potential testing for glaucoma, use 0464T)

0464T Visual evoked potential, testing for glaucoma, with interpretation and report (Sunset January 2023)

(To report percutaneous/minimally invasive [indirect visualization] arthrodesis of the sacroiliac joint with image guidance, use 27279)

(For visual evoked potential screening of visual acuity, use 0333T)

0335T Insertion of sinus tarsi implant (Sunset January 2024)

(Do not report 0335T in conjunction with 28585, 28725, 29907)

0510T Removal of sinus tarsi implant (Sunset January 2024)

0511T Removal and reinsertion of sinus tarsi implant (Sunset January 2024)

(**0337T** deleted 2018 [2019 Edition])

(For unilateral or bilateral endothelial function assessments, using peripheral vascular response to reactive hyperemia, noninvasive [eg, brachial artery ultrasound, peripheral artery tonometry], use 93998)

0338T Transcatheter renal sympathetic denervation, percutaneous approach including arterial puncture, selective catheter placement(s) renal artery(ies), fluoroscopy, contrast injection(s), intraprocedural roadmapping and radiological supervision and interpretation, including pressure gradient measurements, flush aortogram and diagnostic renal angiography when performed; unilateral (Sunset January 2024)

0339T   bilateral (Sunset January 2024)

(Do not report 0338T, 0339T in conjunction with 36251, 36252, 36253, 36254)

(**0340T** deleted 2017 [2018 edition]. To report, use 32994)

(**0341T** deleted 2019 [2020 edition])

(For quantitative pupillometry with interpretation and report, unilateral or bilateral, us 92499)

0342T Therapeutic apheresis with selective HDL delipidation and plasma reinfusion (Sunset January 2024)

Fluoroscopy (76000) and radiologic supervision and interpretation are inherent to the transcatheter mitral valve repair (TMVR) procedure and are not separately reportable. Diagnostic cardiac catheterization (93451, 93452, 93453, 93454, 93455, 93456, 93457, 93458, 93459, 93460, 93461, 93530, 93531, 93532, 93533) should not be reported with transcatheter mitral valve repair (0345T) for:

- Contrast injections, angiography, roadmapping, and/or fluoroscopic guidance for the transcatheter mitral valve repair (TMVR),
- Left ventricular angiography to assess mitral regurgitation, for guidance of TMVR, or
- Right and left heart catheterization for hemodynamic measurements before, during, and after TMVR for guidance of TMVR.

Diagnostic right and left heart catheterization, (93451, 93452, 93453, 93456, 93457, 93458, 93459, 93460, 93461, 93530, 93531, 93532, 93533) and diagnostic coronary angiography (93454, 93455, 93456, 93457, 93458, 93459, 93460, 93461, 93563, 93564) not inherent to the TMVR, may be reported with 0345T, appended with modifier 59 if:

1. No prior study is available and a full diagnostic study is performed, or

2. A prior study is available, but as documented in the medical record:

  a. There is inadequate visualization of the anatomy and/or pathology, or

  b. The patient's condition with respect to the clinical indication has changed since the prior study, or

  c. There is a clinical change during the procedure that requires new evaluation.

Percutaneous coronary interventional procedures may be reported separately, when performed.

Other cardiac catheterization services may be reported separately, when performed for diagnostic purposes not intrinsic to the TMVR.

● New Code   ▲ Revised Code   ✛ Add-On Code   ⊘ Modifier -51 Exempt   ★ Telemedicine

When transcatheter ventricular support is required, the appropriate code may be reported with the appropriate ventricular assist device (VAD) procedure (33990, 33991, 33992, 33993, 33995, 33997) or balloon pump insertion (33967, 33970, 33973).

0345T   Transcatheter mitral valve repair percutaneous approach via the coronary sinus (Sunset January 2020)

(For transcatheter mitral valve repair percutaneous approach including transseptal puncture when performed, see 33418, 33419)

(Do not report 0345T in conjunction with 93451, 93452, 93453, 93456, 93457, 93458, 93459, 93460, 93461 for diagnostic left and right heart catheterization procedures intrinsic to the valve repair procedure)

(Do not report 0345T in conjunction with 93453, 93454, 93563, 93564 for coronary angiography intrinsic to the valve repair procedure)

(For transcatheter mitral valve implantation/ replacement [TMVI], see 0483T, 0484T)

(For transcatheter mitral valve annulus reconstruction, use 0544T)

(0346T   deleted 2018 [2019 Edition]. To report, see 76981, 76982, 76983)

0347T   Placement of interstitial device(s) in bone for radiostereometric analysis (RSA) (Sunset January 2020)

0348T   Radiologic examination, radiostereometric analysis (RSA); spine, (includes cervical, thoracic and lumbosacral, when performed) (Sunset January 2020)

0349T   upper extremity(ies), (includes shoulder, elbow, and wrist, when performed) (Sunset January 2020)

0350T   lower extremity(ies), (includes hip, proximal femur, knee, and ankle, when performed) (Sunset January 2020)

0351T   Optical coherence tomography of breast or axillary lymph node, excised tissue, each specimen; real-time intraoperative (Sunset January 2020)

0352T   interpretation and report, real-time or referred (Sunset January 2020)

(Do not report 0352T in conjunction with 0351T, when performed by the same physician)

0353T   Optical coherence tomography of breast, surgical cavity; real-time intraoperative (Sunset January 2020)

(Report 0353T once per session)

0354T   interpretation and report, real-time or referred (Sunset January 2020)

(Do not report 0354T in conjunction with 0353T, when performed by the same physician)

0355T   Gastrointestinal tract imaging, intraluminal (e.g. capsule endoscopy), colon, with interpretation and report (Sunset January 2020)

(Use 0355T for imaging of distal ileum, when performed)

(Do not report 0355T in conjunction with 91110, 91111)

0356T   Insertion of drug-eluting implant (including punctal dilation and implant removal when performed) into lacrimal canaliculus, each (Sunset January 2020)

(For placement of drug-eluting insert under the eyelid[s], see 0444T, 0445T)

0358T   Bioelectrical impedance analysis whole body composition assessment, with interpretation and report (Sunset January 2020)

(For bioimpedance-derived physiological cardiovascular analysis, use 93701)

(For bioimpedance spectroscopy use 93702)

ADAPTIVE BEHAVIOR ASSESSMENT AND TREATMENT

Behavior identification supporting assessment (0362T) and adaptive behavior treatment with protocol modification (0373T) include the following required components:

- administration by the physician or other qualified health care professional who is on-site but not necessarily face-to-face with the patient;

- with the assistance of two or more technicians;

- for a patient with destructive behavior that requires the presence of a team;

- completion in an environment that is customized to the patient's behavior.

"On-site" is defined as immediately available and interruptible to provide assistance and direction throughout the performance of the procedure, however, the physician or other qualified health care professional does not need to be present in the room when the procedure is performed.

Typical patients for 0362T and 0373T present with one or more specific destructive behavior(s) (ie, maladaptive behaviors associated with high risk of medical consequences or property damage [eg, elopement, pica, or self-injury requiring medical attention, aggression with injury to other{s}, or breaking furniture, walls, or windows]). Code 0362T may include functional behavior assessment, functional analysis, other structured observations, and standardized and/or nonstandardized instruments and procedures to determine levels of adaptive and maladaptive behavior as well as other impairments in functioning.

Only count the time of one technician when two or more are present. For assistance with code selection of 97152, 0362T, see the Guide to Selection of Codes 97152 and 0362T on page 711. For assistance with code selection of 97153, 97155, 0373T, see Guide to Selection of Codes 97153, 97155, 0373T on page 712.

(**0359T**   deleted 2018 [2019 Edition]. To report, see 97151, 97152)

(**0360T**   deleted 2018 [2019 Edition]. To report, see 97151, 97152)

(**0361T**   deleted 2018 [2019 Edition]. To report, see 97151, 97152)

0362T   Behavior identification supporting assessment, each 15 minutes of technicians' time face-to-face with a patient, requiring the following components:

■ administration by the physician or other qualified health care professional who is on site;
■ with the assistance of two or more technicians;
■ for a patient who exhibits destructive behavior;
■ completion in an environment that is customized to the patient's behavior.
(Sunset January 2024)

(0362T is reported based on a single technician's face-to-face time with the patient and not the combined time of multiple technicians [eg, one hour with three technicians equals one hour of service])

(0362T may be repeated on different days until the behavior identification assessment [97151] and, if necessary, supporting assessment[s] [97152, 0362T], is complete)

(For psychiatric diagnostic evaluation, see 90791, 90792)

(For speech evaluations, see 92521, 92522, 92523, 92524)

(For occupational therapy evaluation, see 97165, 97166, 97167, 97168)

(For medical team conference, see 99366, 99367, 99368)

(For health behavior assessment and intervention, see 96156, 96158, 96159, 96164, 96165, 96167, 96168, 96170, 96171)

(For neurobehavioral status examination, see 96116, 96121)

(For neuropsychological testing, see 96132, 96133, 96136, 96137, 96138, 96139, 96146)

(0363T, 0364T, 0365T, 0366T, 0367T, 0368T, 0369T, 0370T, 0371T, 0372T have been deleted. To report, see 97153, 97154, 97155, 97156, 97157, 97158, 0373T)

(**0363T**   deleted 2018 [2019 Edition]. To report, see 97153, 97154, 97155, 97156, 97157, 97158, 0373T)

● New Code   ▲ Revised Code   + Add-On Code   ⊘ Modifier -51 Exempt   ★ Telemedicine

(0364T   deleted 2018 [2019 Edition]. To report, see 97153, 97154, 97155, 97156, 97157, 97158, 0373T)

(0365T   deleted 2018 [2019 Edition]. To report, see 97153, 97154, 97155, 97156, 97157, 97158, 0373T)

(0366T   deleted 2018 [2019 Edition]. To report, see 97153, 97154, 97155, 97156, 97157, 97158, 0373T)

(0367T   deleted 2018 [2019 Edition]. To report, see 97153, 97154, 97155, 97156, 97157, 97158, 0373T)

(0368T   deleted 2018 [2019 Edition]. To report, see 97153, 97154, 97155, 97156, 97157, 97158, 0373T)

(0369T   deleted 2018 [2019 Edition]. To report, see 97153, 97154, 97155, 97156, 97157, 97158, 0373T)

(0370T   deleted 2018 [2019 Edition]. To report, see 97153, 97154, 97155, 97156, 97157, 97158, 0373T)

(0371T   deleted 2018 [2019 Edition]. To report, see 97153, 97154, 97155, 97156, 97157, 97158, 0373T)

(0372T   deleted 2018 [2019 Edition]. To report, see 97153, 97154, 97155, 97156, 97157, 97158, 0373T)

0373T   Adaptive behavior treatment with protocol modification, each 15 minutes of technicians' time face-to-face with a patient, requiring the following components:

■ administration by the physician or other qualified health care professional who is on site;
■ with the assistance of two or more technicians;
■ for a patient who exhibits destructive behavior;
■ completion in an environment that is customized to the patient's behavior.
(Sunset January 2024)

(0373T is reported based on a single technician's face-to-face time with the patient and not the combined time of multiple technicians)

(Do not report 0373T in conjunction with 90785-90899, 96105, 96110, 96116, 96121, 96156, 96158, 96159, 96164, 96165, 96167, 96168, 96170, 96171)

(0374T   deleted 2018 [2019 Edition]. To report, use 0373T)

(0375T   deleted 2019 [2020 Edition])

(For total disc arthroplasty [artificial disc], anterior approach, including discectomy with end-plate preparation [includes osteophytectomy for nerve root or spinal cord decompression and microdissection], cervical, 3 or more levels, use 22899)

0376T   This code is out of order. See page 1028

(0377T   deleted 2019 [2020 Edition])

(For anoscopy with directed submucosal injection of bulking agent for fecal incontinence, use 46999)

0378T   Visual field assessment, with concurrent real time data analysis and accessible data storage with patient initiated data transmitted to a remote surveillance center for up to 30 days; review and interpretation with report by a physician or other qualified health care professional (Sunset January 2020)

0379T   technical support and patient instructions, surveillance, analysis, and transmission of daily and emergent data reports as prescribed by a physician or other qualified health care professional (Sunset January 2020)

(0380T   deleted 2019 [2020 Edition])

(For computer-aided animation and analysis of time series retinal images for the monitoring of disease progression, unilateral or bilateral, with interpretation and report, use 92499)

(0381T   deleted 2020 [2021 Edition])

(0382T   deleted 2020 [2021 Edition])

Separate Procedure   Unlisted Procedure   CCI Comp. Code   Non-specific Procedure   **1037**

(**0383T** deleted 2020 [2021 Edition])

(**0384T** deleted 2020 [2021 Edition])

(**0385T** deleted 2020 [2021 Edition])

(**0386T** deleted 2020 [2021 Edition])

(For external heart rate and 3-axis accelerometer data recording up to 14 days to assess changes in heart rate and to monitor motion analysis for the purposes of diagnosing nocturnal epilepsy seizure events, including report, scanning analysis with report, review and interpretation by a physician or other qualified health care professional, use 95999)

PACEMAKER—LEADLESS AND POCKETLESS SYSTEM

(**0387T** deleted 2018 [2019 Edition]. To report, see 33274, 33275)

(**0388T** deleted 2018 [2019 Edition]. To report, see 33274, 33275)

(**0389T** deleted 2018 [2019 Edition]. To report, see 33274, 33275, 93279, 93286, 93288, 93294, 93296)

(**0390T** deleted 2018 [2019 Edition]. To report, see 33274, 33275, 93279, 93286, 93288, 93294, 93296)

(**0391T** deleted 2018 [2019 Edition]. To report, see 33274, 33275, 93279, 93286, 93288, 93294, 93296)

(Electronic brachytherapy is a form of radiation therapy in which an electrically generated X-ray source of ionizing radiation is placed inside or in close proximity to the tumor or target tissue to deliver therapeutic radiation dosage)

0394T High dose rate electronic brachytherapy, skin surface application, per fraction, includes basic dosimetry, when performed (Sunset January 2021)

(Do not report 0394T in conjunction with 77261, 77262, 77263, 77300, 77306, 77307, 77316, 77317, 77318, 77332, 77333, 77334, 77336, 77427, 77431, 77432, 77435, 77469, 77470, 77499, 77761, 77762, 77763, 77767, 77768, 77770, 77771, 77772, 77778, 77789)

(For high dose rate radionuclide surface brachytherapy, see 77767, 77768)

(For non-brachytherapy superficial [eg, =200 kV] radiation treatment delivery, use 77401)

0395T High dose rate electronic brachytherapy, interstitial or intracavitary treatment, per fraction, includes basic dosimetry, when performed (Sunset January 2021)

(Do not report 0395T in conjunction with 77261, 77262, 77263, 77300, 77306, 77307, 77316, 77317, 77318, 77332, 77333, 77334, 77336, 77427, 77431, 77432, 77435, 77469, 77470, 77499, 77761, 77762, 77763, 77767, 77768, 77770, 77771, 77772, 77778, 77789)

(For skin surface application of high dose rate electronic brachytherapy, use 0394T)

(**0396T** deleted 2020 [2021 Edition])

(For intraoperative use of kinetic balance sensor for implant stability during knee replacement arthroplasty, use 27599)

+ **0397T** Endoscopic retrograde cholangiopancreatography (ERCP), with optical endomicroscopy (List separately in addition to code for primary procedure) (Sunset January 2021)

(Use 0397T in conjunction with 43260, 43261, 43262, 43263, 43264, 43265, 43274, 43275, 43276, 43277, 43278)

(Do not report 0397T in conjunction with 88375)

(Do not report optical endomicroscopy more than once per session)

● New Code   ▲ Revised Code   ✛ Add-On Code   ⃠ Modifier -51 Exempt   ★ Telemedicine

0398T Magnetic resonance image guided high intensity focused ultrasound (MRgFUS), stereotactic ablation lesion, intracranial for movement disorder including stereotactic navigation and frame placement when performed (Sunset January 2021)

(Do not report 0398T in conjunction with 61781, 61800)

(**0399T** deleted 2019 [2020 Edition]. To report, use 93356)

(**0400T** deleted 2020 [2021 Edition])

(**0401T** deleted 2020 [2021 Edition])

(For multispectral digital skin lesion analysis of clinically atypical cutaneous pigmented lesions for detection of melanomas and high risk melanocytic atypia, use 96999)

0402T Collagen cross-linking of cornea, including removal of the corneal epithelium and intraoperative pachymetry, when performed (Report medication separately) (Sunset January 2025)

(Do not report 0402T in conjunction with 65435, 69990, 76514)

A diabetes prevention program consists of intensive behavioral counseling that is provided in person, online, or via electronic technology, or a combination of both modalities.

Intensive behavioral counseling consists of care management, lifestyle coaching, facilitation of a peersupport group, and provision of clinically validated educational lessons based on a standardized curriculum that is focused on nutrition, exercise, stress, and weight management. Lifestyle coaches must complete a nationally recognized training program. The lifestyle coach is available to interact with the participants.

Codes 0403T and 0488T describe diabetes prevention programs that use a standardized diabetes prevention curriculum. For educational services that use a standardized curriculum provided to patients with an established illness/disease, see 98960, 98961, 98962. Use 0403T for diabetes prevention programs that are provided only in person. Use 0488T for programs that are provided online or via electronic technology. Code 0488T includes in-person components, if provided.

0403T Preventive behavior change, intensive program of prevention of diabetes using a standardized diabetes prevention program curriculum, provided to individuals in a group setting, minimum 60 minutes, per day (Sunset January 2021)

(Do not report 0403T in conjunction with 98960, 98961, 98962, 0488T)

0488T Preventive behavior change, online/electronic structured intensive program for prevention of diabetes using a standardized diabetes prevention program curriculum, provided to an individual, per 30 days (Sunset January 2023)

(Do not report 0488T in conjunction with 98960, 98961, 98962, 0403T)

0404T Transcervical uterine fibroid(s) ablation with ultrasound guidance, radiofrequency (Sunset January 2021)

(**0405T** deleted 2020 [2021 Edition])

(For oversight of the care of an extracorporeal liver-assist system patient requiring review of status, review of laboratory and other studies, and revision of orders and liver-assist care plan [as appropriate], within a calendar month, 30 minutes or more of non-face-to-face time, use 99499)

(**0406T** deleted 2018 [2019 Edition].)

(**0407T** deleted 2018 [2019 Edition].)

(To report endoscopic placement of a drug-eluting implant in the ethmoid sinus without any other nasal/sinus endoscopic surgical service, use 31299. To report endoscopic placement of a drug-eluting implant in the ethmoid sinus in conjunction with biopsy, polypectomy, or debridement, use 31237)

Codes 0408T-0418T describe procedures related to cardiac contractility modulation systems (CCM). These systems consist of a pulse generator plus one atrial and two ventricular pacemaker electrodes (leads). In contrast to a pacemaker or a defibrillator,

---

| | Separate Procedure | | Unlisted Procedure | | CCI Comp. Code | | Non-specific Procedure | **1039** |

which modulate the heart's rhythm, the CCM systems' impulses are designed to modulate the strength of contraction of the heart muscle. Unlike pacemakers, these systems stimulate for specific time intervals in order to improve myocardial function.

All catheterization and imaging guidance required to complete a CCM procedure are included in the work of each code. Left heart catheterization with a high fidelity transducer is intrinsic to the CCM procedure. Left heart catheterization codes (93452, 93453, 93458, 93459, 93460, 93461) at the time of CCM placement, replacement, or revision may not be reported separately. Removal of only the CCM pulse generator is reported with 0412T. If only the pulse generator is removed and replaced at the same session without any right atrial and/or right ventricular lead(s) inserted or replaced, report 0414T. For removal and replacement of the pulse generator and leads, individual codes for removal of the generator (0412T) and removal of the leads (0413T for each lead removed) are used in conjunction with the insertion/replacement system code (0408T). When individual transvenous electrodes are inserted or replaced, report using 0410T and 0411T, as appropriate. When the entire system is inserted or replaced, report with 0408T. (For oversight of the care of an extracorporeal liver-assist system patient requiring review of status, review of laboratory and other studies, and revision of orders and liver-assist care plan [as appropriate], within a calendar month, 30 minutes or more of non-face-to-face time, use 99499)Revision of the CCM generator skin pocket is included in 0408T, 0412T, 0414T. Relocation of a skin pocket for a CCM may be necessary for various clinical situations such as infection or erosion. Relocation is reported with 0416T, and follows conventions for pacemaker skin pocket relocation.

Repositioning of a CCM electrode is reported using 0415T.

CCM device evaluation codes 0417T, 0418T may not be reported in conjunction with pulse generator and lead insertion or revision codes.

0408T Insertion or replacement of permanent cardiac contractility modulation system, including contractility evaluation when performed, and programming of sensing and therapeutic parameters; pulse generator with transvenous electrodes (Sunset January 2022)

0409T pulse generator only (Sunset January 2022)

0410T atrial electrode only (Sunset January 2022)

0411T ventricular electrode only (Sunset January 2022)

(Report 0410T, 0411T once for each transvenous electrode inserted or replaced)

(If the entire system is inserted or replaced, report 0408T)

0412T Removal of permanent cardiac contractility modulation system; pulse generator only (Sunset January 2022)

0413T transvenous electrode (atrial or ventricular) (Sunset January 2022)

(Report 0413T once for each transvenous electrode removed)

(For removal of the pulse generator and all 3 leads, use 0412T plus 0413T once for each electrode removed)

(If transvenous electrodes are removed and replaced, report 0413T once for each electrode removed in conjunction with 0410T, 0411T, as appropriate)

0414T Removal and replacement of permanent cardiac contractility modulation system pulse generator only (Sunset January 2022)

(For removal and replacement of the pulse generator plus all three electrodes, report 0408T in conjunction with 0412T, 0413T once for each transvenous electrode removed)

0415T Repositioning of previously implanted cardiac contractility modulation transvenous electrode (atrial or ventricular lead) (Sunset January 2022)

(Do not report 0408T, 0409T, 0410T, 0411T, 0414T, 0415T in conjunction with 93286, 93287, 93452, 93453, 93458, 93459, 93460, 93461)

(Do not report 0415T in conjunction with 0408T, 0410T, 0411T)

0416T Relocation of skin pocket for implanted cardiac contractility modulation pulse generator (Sunset January 2022)

0417T Programming device evaluation (in person) with iterative adjustment of the implantable device to test the function of the device and select optimal permanent programmed values with analysis, including review and report, implantable cardiac contractility modulation system (Sunset January 2022)

(Do not report 0417T in conjunction with 0408T, 0409T, 0410T, 0411T, 0412T, 0413T, 0414T, 0415T, 0418T)

0418T Interrogation device evaluation (in person) with analysis, review and report, includes connection, recording and disconnection per patient encounter, implantable cardiac contractility modulation system (Sunset January 2022)

(Do not report 0418T in conjunction with 0408T, 0409T, 0410T, 0411T, 0412T, 0413T, 0414T, 0415T, 0417T)

0419T Destruction of neurofibroma, extensive (cutaneous, dermal extending into subcutaneous); face, head and neck, greater than 50 neurofibromas (Sunset January 2022)

(For excision of neurofibroma, use 64792)

(Report 0419T once per session regardless of the number of lesions treated)

0420T trunk and extremities, extensive, greater than 100 neurofibromas (Sunset January 2022)

(For excision of neurofibroma, use 64792)

(Report 0420T once per session regardless of the number of lesions treated)

0421T Transurethral waterjet ablation of prostate, including control of post-operative bleeding, including ultrasound guidance, complete (vasectomy, meatotomy, cystourethroscopy, urethral calibration and/or dilation, and internal urethrotomy are included when performed) (Sunset January 2022)

(Do not report 0421T in conjunction with 52500, 52630, 76872)

0422T Tactile breast imaging by computer-aided tactile sensors, unilateral or bilateral (Sunset January 2022)

0423T Secretory type II phospholipase A2 (sPLA2-IIA) (Sunset January 2022)

(For lipoprotein-associated phospholipase A2 [Lp-PLA2], use 83698)

Phrenic Nerve Stimulation System

A phrenic nerve stimulation system includes a pulse generator (containing electronics and a battery), one stimulation lead (electrode), and one sensing lead (electrode). Pulse generators are placed in a submuscular or subcutaneous "pocket" in the pectoral region. The stimulation lead is placed transvenously into the right brachiocephalic vein or left pericardiophrenic vein. The sensing lead is placed transvenously into the azygos vein.

If replacing less than a complete system, report 0425T, 0426T, and/or 0427T (for sensing lead, stimulation lead or pulse generator respectively). If all three components are replaced, report only 0424T in conjunction with codes for removal of each of the components (0428T, 0429T, 0430T).

Codes 0424T-0433T include vessel catheterization, all image guidance required for the procedure, and interrogation and programming, when performed. Interrogation device evaluation and programming device evaluation include parameters of rate, pulse amplitude, pulse duration, configuration of waveform, battery status, electrode selectability, output modulation, cycling, impedance, and patient compliance measurements. For patients that require programming during an overnight sleep study, report 0436T once, regardless of how many programming changes are made during the sleep study.

0424T Insertion or replacement of neurostimulator system for treatment of central sleep apnea; complete system (transvenous placement of right or left stimulation lead, sensing lead, implantable pulse generator) (Sunset January 2022)

0425T sensing lead only (Sunset January 2022)

0426T stimulation lead only (Sunset January 2022)

0427T   pulse generator only (Sunset January 2022)

(Do not report 0425T, 0426T, 0427T in conjunction with 0424T)

0428T Removal of neurostimulator system for treatment of central sleep apnea; pulse generator only (Sunset January 2022)

0429T   sensing lead only (Sunset January 2022)

0430T   stimulation lead only (Sunset January 2022)

(Report 0429T, 0430T once for each transvenous sensing or stimulation lead removed)

(For removal of the entire system, report 0428T for pulse generator removal plus 0429T or 0430T for each transvenous lead removal)

0431T Removal and replacement of neurostimulator system for treatment of central sleep apnea, pulse generator only (Sunset January 2022)

(For removal and replacement of the pulse generator plus all three leads, report 0424T in conjunction with 0428T, 0429T, 0430T)

0432T Repositioning of neurostimulator system for treatment of central sleep apnea; stimulation lead only (Sunset January 2022)

0433T   sensing lead only (Sunset January 2022)

(Do not report 0432T, 0433T in conjunction with 0424T, 0425T, 0426T, 0427T)

0434T Interrogation device evaluation implanted neurostimulator pulse generator system for central sleep apnea (Sunset January 2022)

0435T Programming device evaluation of implanted neurostimulator pulse generator system for central sleep apnea; single session (Sunset January 2022)

0436T   during sleep study (Sunset January 2022)

(Do not report 0434T, 0435T, 0436T in conjunction with 0424T, 0425T, 0426T, 0427T, 0428T, 0429T, 0430T, 0431T, 0432T, 0433T)

(Do not report 0436T in conjunction with 0435T)

(Report 0436T once per sleep study)

+ 0437T Implantation of non-biologic or synthetic implant (eg, polypropylene) for fascial reinforcement of the abdominal wall (List separately in addition to code for primary procedure) (Sunset January 2022)

(For implantation of mesh or other prosthesis for open incisional or ventral hernia repair, use 49568 in conjunction with 49560, 49561, 49565, 49566)

(For insertion of mesh or other prosthesis for closure of a necrotizing soft tissue infection wound, use 49568 in conjunction with 11004, 11005, 11006)

(**0438T** deleted 2017 [2018 edition]. To report, use 55874)

+ 0439T Myocardial contrast perfusion echocardiography, at rest or with stress, for assessment of myocardial ischemia or viability (List separately in addition to code for primary procedure) (Sunset January 2022)

(Use 0439T in conjunction with 93306, 93307, 93308, 93350, 93351)

0440T Ablation, percutaneous, cryoablation, includes imaging guidance; upper extremity distal/peripheral nerve (Sunset January 2022)

0441T   lower extremity distal/peripheral nerve (Sunset January 2022)

● New Code   ▲ Revised Code   + Add-On Code   ⊘ Modifier -51 Exempt   ★ Telemedicine

0442T   nerve plexus or other truncal nerve (eg, brachial plexus, pudendal nerve) (Sunset January 2022)

+ 0443T   Real-time spectral analysis of prostate tissue by fluorescence spectroscopy, including imaging guidance (List separately in addition to code for primary procedure) (Sunset January 2022)

           (Use 0443T in conjunction with 55700)

           (Report 0443T only once per session)

0444T   Initial placement of a drug-eluting ocular insert under one or more eyelids, including fitting, training, and insertion, unilateral or bilateral (Sunset January 2022)

0445T   Subsequent placement of a drug-eluting ocular insert under one or more eyelids, including re-training, and removal of existing insert, unilateral or bilateral (Sunset January 2022)

           (For insertion and removal of drug-eluting implant into lacrimal canaliculus, use 0356T)

0446T   Creation of subcutaneous pocket with insertion of implantable interstitial glucose sensor, including system activation and patient training (Sunset January 2022)

           (Do not report 0446T in conjunction with 95251, 0447T, 0448T)

0447T   Removal of implantable interstitial glucose sensor from subcutaneous pocket via incision (Sunset January 2022)

0448T   Removal of implantable interstitial glucose sensor with creation of subcutaneous pocket at different anatomic site and insertion of new implantable sensor, including system activation (Sunset January 2022)

           (Do not report 0448T in conjunction with 0446T, 0447T)

           (For placement of non-implantable interstitial glucose sensor without pocket, use 95250)

0449T   Insertion of aqueous drainage device, without extraocular reservoir, internal approach, into the subconjunctival space; initial device (Sunset January 2022)

+ 0450T   each additional device (List separately in addition to code for primary procedure) (Sunset January 2022)

           (Use 0450T in conjunction with 0449T)

           (For removal of aqueous drainage device without extraocular reservoir, placed into the subconjunctival space via internal approach, use 92499)

Codes 0451T-0463T describe a family of services related to the placement and maintenance of permanent aortic counterpulsation ventricular assistance devices. These devices are used to treat congestive heart failure, and they employ a counterpulsation device that is implanted in the aorta, which inflates during diastole to reduce end diastolic ventricular pressure on a long-term basis without rerouting blood flow. The counterpulsation assistance device implantation is achieved by surgically placing a subclavian arterial graft and creating of a subcutaneous pocket to implant a mechano-electrical interface, without requiring access to the heart. The counterpulsation device's mechano-electrical skin interface receives ECG signals from the subcutaneous electrodes and digitizes and transmits a signal through an external driveline to an external "driver," which is carried by the patient. The "driver" receives the ECG signal and determines the location of the dichrotic notch. The "driver" then activates a bellows, which sends compressed air through the external driveline to the mechanoelectrical skin interface in which the compressed air enters the internal driveline and inflates the balloon. After diastole, the bellows creates suction that deflates the balloon through the same pathway.

These services differ from those performed for the implantation, revision, and removal of existing aortic balloon pumps in several ways in that they: (1) use a permanently implanted balloon that is intended for longterm use; (2) require surgical placement of a vascular graft; (3) use a vascular hemostatic seal; (4) implant a mechano-electrical skin interface that contains a programmable processor; and (5) implant subcutaneous electrodes. In addition, they also differ from procedures to insert, revise, and remove extracorporeal and intracorporeal ventricular assist devices because these procedures require access to the heart and include inflow or outflow grafts into the heart, which divert blood flow from either the left and/or right cardiac chambers into a pump that then pumps blood directly into the corresponding artery (either aorta and/or pulmonary artery).

Codes 0451T-0463T are inclusive of all vessel catheterization, diagnostic angiography, radiological supervision and interpretation, and imaging guidance. Removal of a counterpulsation assistance device at the same session as insertion is not separately reportable.

0451T Insertion or replacement of a permanently implantable aortic counterpulsation ventricular assist system, endovascular approach, and programming of sensing and therapeutic parameters; complete system (counterpulsation device, vascular graft, implantable vascular hemostatic seal, mechano-electrical skin interface and subcutaneous electrodes) (Sunset January 2022)

(Do not report 0451T in conjunction with 33973, 33979, 33990, 33991, 33995, 33997, 0452T, 0453T, 0454T, 0455T, 0456T, 0457T, 0458T)

(For insertion of intra-aortic balloon assist device, see 33967, 33970, 33973)

(For insertion or replacement of extracorporeal ventricular assist device, see 33975, 33976, 33981)

(For insertion or replacement of intracorporeal ventricular assist device, see 33979, 33982, 33983)

(For percutaneous insertion of ventricular assist device, see 33990, 33991, 33995)

0452T aortic counterpulsation device and vascular hemostatic seal (Sunset January 2022)

(Do not report 0452T in conjunction with 33973, 33979, 33990, 33991, 33995, 33997, 0451T, 0455T, 0456T)

(For insertion or replacement of intracorporeal ventricular assist device, see 33979, 33982, 33983)

0453T mechano-electrical skin interface (Sunset January 2022)

(Do not report 0453T in conjunction with 33973, 33979, 33990, 33991, 33995, 33997, 0451T, 0455T, 0457T)

(For insertion or replacement of intracorporeal ventricular assist device, see 33979, 33982, 33983)

0454T subcutaneous electrode (Sunset January 2022)

(Report 0454T once for each subcutaneous electrode inserted or replaced)

(If the entire system is inserted or replaced, use 0451T)

(Do not report 0454T in conjunction with 33973, 33979 33990, 33991, 33995, 33997, 0451T, 0455T, 0458T)

(For insertion or replacement of intracorporeal ventricular assist device, see 33979, 33982, 33983)

0455T Removal of permanently implantable aortic counterpulsation ventricular assist system; complete system (aortic counterpulsation device, vascular hemostatic seal, mechano-electrical skin interface and electrodes) (Sunset January 2022)

(Do not report 0455T in conjunction with 33974, 33980, 33992, 0451T, 0452T, 0453T, 0454T, 0456T, 0457T, 0458T)

(For removal of intra-aortic balloon assist device, see 33968, 33971, 33974)

(For removal of extracorporeal ventricular assist device, see 33977, 33978)

(For removal of intracorporeal ventricular assist device, use 33980)

(For removal of percutaneous ventricular assist device, use 33992)

0456T aortic counterpulsation device and vascular hemostatic seal (Sunset January 2022)

(Do not report 0456T in conjunction with 33974, 33980, 33992, 0451T, 0452T, 0455T)

0457T mechano-electrical skin interface (Sunset January 2022)

(Do not report 0457T in conjunction with 33974, 33980, 33992, 0451T, 0453T, 0455T)

0458T   subcutaneous electrode (Sunset January 2022)

(Report 0458T once for each subcutaneous electrode removed)

(Do not report 0458T in conjunction with 33974, 33980, 33992, 0451T, 0454T, 0455T)

0459T Relocation of skin pocket with replacement of implanted aortic counterpulsation ventricular assist device, mechano-electrical skin interface and electrodes (Sunset January 2022)

(Do not report 0459T in conjunction with 33993)

(For repositioning of percutaneous ventricular assist device, use 33993)

0460T Repositioning of previously implanted aortic counterpulsation ventricular assist device; subcutaneous electrode (Sunset January 2022)

(Report 0460T once for each subcutaneous electrode repositioned)

(Do not report 0460T in conjunction with 33993, 0451T, 0454T)

(For repositioning of percutaneous ventricular assist device, use 33993)

0461T   aortic counterpulsation device (Sunset January 2022)

(Do not report 0461T in conjunction with 33993)

(For repositioning of percutaneous ventricular assist device, use 33993)

0462T Programming device evaluation (in person) with iterative adjustment of the implantable mechano-electrical skin interface and/or external driver to test the function of the device and select optimal permanent programmed values with analysis, including review and report, implantable aortic counterpulsation ventricular assist system, per day (Sunset January 2022)

(Do not report 0462T in conjunction with 0451T-0461T, 0463T)

0463T Interrogation device evaluation (in person) with analysis, review and report, includes connection, recording and disconnection per patient encounter, implantable aortic counterpulsation ventricular assist system, per day (Sunset January 2022)

(Do not report 0463T in conjunction with 0451T-0462T)

(Do not report 0451T-0463T in conjunction with 36000, 36002, 36005, 36010, 36200-36228, 75600-75774, 76000, 76936, 76937, 77001, 77002, 77011, 77012, 77021, 93451-93533, 93561-93572)

0464T This code is out of order. See page 1033

0465T Suprachoroidal injection of a pharmacologic agent (does not include supply of medication) (Sunset January 2023)

(To report intravitreal injection/implantation, see 67025, 67027, 67028)

+ 0466T Insertion of chest wall respiratory sensor electrode or electrode array, including connection to pulse generator (List separately in addition to code for primary procedure) (Sunset January 2023)

(Use 0466T in conjunction with 64568)

0467T Revision or replacement of chest wall respiratory sensor electrode or electrode array, including connection to existing pulse generator (Sunset January 2023)

(Do not report 0467T in conjunction with 0466T, 0468T)

(For revision or replacement of cranial nerve [eg, vagus nerve] neurostimulator electrode array, including connection to existing pulse generator, use 64569)

0468T Removal of chest wall respiratory sensor electrode or electrode array (Sunset January 2023)

(Do not report 0468T in conjunction with 0466T, 0467T)

(For removal of cranial nerve [eg, vagus nerve] neurostimulator electrode array and pulse generator, use 64570)

0469T Retinal polarization scan, ocular screening with on-site automated results, bilateral (Sunset January 2023)

(Do not report 0469T in conjunction with 92002, 92004, 92012, 92014)

(For ocular photoscreening, see 99174, 99177)

0470T Optical coherence tomography (OCT) for microstructural and morphological imaging of skin, image acquisition, interpretation, and report; first lesion (Sunset January 2023)

+ 0471T each additional lesion (List separately in addition to code for primary procedure) (Sunset January 2023)

(Use 0471T in conjunction with 0470T)

(For optical coherence tomography for coronary vessel or graft, see 92978, 92979)

(For reflectance confocal microscopy [RCM] of the skin, see 96931, 96932, 96933, 96934, 96935, 96936)

0472T Device evaluation, interrogation, and initial programming of intraocular retinal electrode array (eg, retinal prosthesis), in person, with iterative adjustment of the implantable device to test functionality, select optimal permanent programmed values with analysis, including visual training, with review and report by a qualified health care professional (Sunset January 2023)

0473T Device evaluation and interrogation of intraocular retinal electrode array (eg, retinal prosthesis), in person, including reprogramming and visual training, when performed, with review and report by a qualified health care professional (Sunset January 2023)

(For implantation of intraocular electrode array, use 0100T)

(For reprogramming of implantable intraocular retinal electrode array device, use 0473T)

0474T Insertion of anterior segment aqueous drainage device, with creation of intraocular reservoir, internal approach, into the supraciliary space (Sunset January 2023)

0475T Recording of fetal magnetic cardiac signal using at least 3 channels; patient recording and storage, data scanning with signal extraction, technical analysis and result, as well as supervision, review, and interpretation of report by a physician or other qualified health care professional (Sunset January 2023)

0476T patient recording, data scanning, with raw electronic signal transfer of data and storage (Sunset January 2023)

0477T signal extraction, technical analysis, and result (Sunset January 2023)

0478T review, interpretation, report by physician or other qualified health care professional (Sunset January 2023)

0479T Fractional ablative laser fenestration of burn and traumatic scars for functional improvement; first 100 cm2 or part thereof, or 1% of body surface area of infants and children (Sunset January 2023)

+ 0480T each additional 100 cm2, or each additional 1% of body surface area of infants and children, or part thereof (List separately in addition to code for primary procedure) (Sunset January 2023)

(Use 0480T in conjunction with 0479T)

(Report 0479T, 0480T only once per day)

(Do not report 0479T, 0480T in conjunction with 0492T)

(For excision of cicatricial lesion[s] [eg, full thickness excision, through the dermis], see 11400-11446)

0481T Injection(s), autologous white blood cell concentrate (autologous protein solution), any site, including image guidance, harvesting and preparation when performed (Sunset January 2023)

● New Code ▲ Revised Code + Add-On Code ⊘ Modifier -51 Exempt ★ Telemedicine

(Do not report 0481T in conjunction with 15769, 15771, 15772, 15773, 15774, 20550, 20551, 20600, 20604, 20605, 20606, 20610, 20611, 36415, 36592, 76942, 77002, 77012, 77021, 86965, 0232T)

(Do not report 38220, 38221, 38222, 38230 for bone marrow aspiration for autologous white blood cell concentrate [autologous protein solution] injection. For bone marrow aspiration for autologous white blood cell concentrate [autologous protein solution] injection, use 0481T)

(0482T   deleted 2019 [2020 Edition])

(For absolute quantitation of myocardial blood flow [AQMBF] for cardiac PET, use 78434)

Codes 0483T, 0484T include vascular access, catheterization, balloon valvuloplasty, deploying the valve, repositioning the valve as needed, temporary pacemaker insertion for rapid pacing, and access site closure, when performed.

Angiography, radiological supervision and interpretation, intraprocedural roadmapping (eg, contrast injections, fluoroscopy) to guide the TMVI, left ventriculography (eg, to assess mitral regurgitation for guidance of TMVI), and completion angiography are included in codes 0483T, 0484T.

Diagnostic right and left heart catheterization codes (93451, 93452, 93453, 93456, 93457, 93458, 93459, 93460, 93461, 93530, 93531, 93532, 93533) should not be used with 0483T, 0484T to report:

1. contrast injections, angiography, road-mapping, and/or fluoroscopic guidance for the transcatheter mitral valve implantation (TMVI),

2. left ventricular angiography to assess or confirm valve positioning and function,

3. right and left heart catheterization for hemodynamic measurements before, during, and after TMVI for guidance of TMVI.

Diagnostic right and left heart catheterization codes (93451, 93452, 93453, 93456, 93457, 93458, 93459, 93460, 93461, 93530, 93531, 93532, 93533) and diagnostic coronary angiography codes (93454, 93455, 93456, 93457, 93458, 93459, 93460, 93461, 93563, 93564) performed at the time of TMVI may be separately reportable, if:

1. no prior study is available and a full diagnostic study is performed, or

2. a prior study is available, but as documented in the medical record:

   a. there is inadequate visualization of the anatomy and/or pathology, or

   b. the patient's condition with respect to the clinical indication has changed since the prior study, or

   c. there is a clinical change during the procedure that requires new evaluation.

For same session/same day diagnostic cardiac catheterization services, report the appropriate diagnostic cardiac catheterization code(s) appended with modifier 59, indicating separate and distinct procedural service from TMVI.

When cardiopulmonary bypass is performed in conjunction with TMVI, 0483T, 0484T may be reported with the appropriate add-on code for percutaneous peripheral bypass (33367), open peripheral bypass (33368), or central bypass (33369).

For percutaneous transcatheter tricuspid valve annulus reconstruction, with implantation of adjustable annulus reconstruction device, use 0545T.

0483T   Transcatheter mitral valve implantation/replacement (TMVI) with prosthetic valve; percutaneous approach, including transseptal puncture, when performed (Sunset January 2023)

(For transcatheter mitral valve annulus reconstruction, use 0544T)

(For transcatheter mitral valve repair percutaneous approach including transseptal puncture when performed, see 33418, 33419)

(For transcatheter mitral valve repair percutaneous approach via the coronary sinus, use 0345T)

0484T   transthoracic exposure (eg, thoracotomy, transapical) (Sunset January 2023)

0485T   Optical coherence tomography (OCT) of middle ear, with interpretation and report; unilateral (Sunset January 2023)

0486T   bilateral (Sunset January 2023)

0487T   Biomechanical mapping, transvaginal, with report (Sunset January 2023)

0488T   This code is out of order. See page 1039

0489T   Autologous adipose-derived regenerative cell therapy for scleroderma in the hands; adipose tissue harvesting, isolation and preparation of harvested cells including incubation with cell dissociation enzymes, removal of non-viable cells and debris, determination of concentration and dilution of regenerative cells (Sunset January 2023)

(Do not report 0489T in conjunction with 15769, 15771, 15772, 15773, 15774, 15876, 15877, 15878, 15879, 20600, 20604)

0490T   multiple injections in one or both hands (Sunset January 2023)

(Do not report 0490T in conjunction with 15769, 15771, 15772, 15773, 15774, 15876, 15877, 15878, 15879, 20600, 20604)

(Do not report 0490T for a single injection)

(For complete procedure, use 0490T in conjunction with 0489T)

0491T   Ablative laser treatment, non-contact, full field and fractional ablation, open wound, per day, total treatment surface area; first 20 sq cm or less (Sunset January 2023)

+ 0492T   each additional 20 sq cm, or part thereof (List separately in addition to code for primary procedure) (Sunset January 2023)

(Use 0492T in conjunction with 0491T)

(Do not report 0492T in conjunction with 0479T, 0480T)

0493T   Near-infrared spectroscopy studies of lower extremity wounds (eg, for oxyhemoglobin measurement) (Sunset January 2023)

0494T   Surgical preparation and cannulation of marginal (extended) cadaver donor lung(s) to ex vivo organ perfusion system, including decannulation, separation from the perfusion system, and cold preservation of the allograft prior to implantation, when performed (Sunset January 2023)

0495T   Initiation and monitoring marginal (extended) cadaver donor lung(s) organ perfusion system by physician or qualified health care professional, including physiological and laboratory assessment (eg, pulmonary artery flow, pulmonary artery pressure, left atrial pressure, pulmonary vascular resistance, mean/peak and plateau airway pressure, dynamic compliance and perfusate gas analysis), including bronchoscopy and X ray when performed; first two hours in sterile field (Sunset January 2023)

+ 0496T   each additional hour (List separately in addition to code for primary procedure) (Sunset January 2023)

(Report 0496T in conjunction with 0495T

0497T   External patient-activated, physician- or other qualified health care professional-prescribed, electrocardiographic rhythm derived event recorder without 24 hour attended monitoring; in-office connection (Sunset January 2023)

0498T   review and interpretation by a physician or other qualified health care professional per 30 days with at least one patient-generated triggered event (Sunset January 2023)

(Do not report 0497T, 0498T in conjunction with 93040, 93041, 93042, 93228, 93229, 93268, 93271, 93272)

0499T   Cystourethroscopy, with mechanical dilation and urethral therapeutic drug delivery for urethral stricture or stenosis, including fluoroscopy, when performed (Sunset January 2023)

(Do not report 0499T in conjunction with 52281, 52283)

0500T Infectious agent detection by nucleic acid (DNA or RNA), human papillomavirus (HPV) for five or more separately reported high-risk HPV types (eg, 16, 18, 31, 33, 35, 39, 45, 51, 52, 56, 58, 59, 68) (ie, genotyping) (Sunset January 2023)

(For reporting four or fewer separately reported highrisk HPV types, see 87624, 87625)

(For reporting of separately reported high-risk HPV types 16, 18 and 45, if performed, use 87625)

(Do not report 0500T in conjunction with 87624 or 87625 for the same procedure)

0501T Noninvasive estimated coronary fractional flow reserve (FFR) derived from coronary computed tomography angiography data using computation fluid dynamics physiologic simulation software analysis of functional data to assess the severity of coronary artery disease; data preparation and transmission, analysis of fluid dynamics and simulated maximal coronary hyperemia, generation of estimated FFR model, with anatomical data review in comparison with estimated FFR model to reconcile discordant data, interpretation and report (Sunset January 2023)

0502T   data preparation and transmission (Sunset January 2023)

0503T   analysis of fluid dynamics and simulated maximal coronary hyperemia, and generation of estimated FFR model (Sunset January 2023)

0504T   anatomical data review in comparison with estimated FFR model to reconcile discordant data, interpretation and report (Sunset January 2023)

(Report 0501T, 0502T, 0503T, 0504T one time per coronary CT angiogram)

(Do not report 0501T in conjunction with 0502T, 0503T, 0504T, 0523T)

(For automated quantification and characterization of coronary plaque using coronary computed tomographic angiography data, see 0623T, 0624T, 0625T, 0626T)

● **0623T** Automated quantification and characterization of coronary atherosclerotic plaque to assess severity of coronary disease, using data from coronary computed tomographic angiography; data preparation and transmission, computerized analysis of data, with review of computerized analysis output to reconcile discordant data, interpretation and report

● **0624T**   data preparation and transmission

● **0625T**   computerized analysis of data from coronary computed tomographic angiography

● **0626T** Review of computerized analysis output to reconcile discordant data, interpretation and report

(Use 0623T, 0624T, 0625T, 0626T one time per coronary computed tomographic angiogram)

(Do not report 0623T in conjunction with 0624T, 0625T, 0626T)

(Do not report 0623T, 0624T, 0625T, 0626T in conjunction with 76376, 76377)

(For noninvasive estimated coronary fractional flow reserve [FFR] derived from coronary computed tomography angiography data, see 0501T, 0502T, 0503T, 0504T)

+ **0523T** Intraprocedural coronary fractional flow reserve (FFR) with 3D functional mapping of color-coded FFR values for the coronary tree, derived from coronary angiogram data, for real-time review and interpretation of possible atherosclerotic stenosis(es) intervention (List separately in addition to code for primary procedure) (Sunset January 2024)

(Use 0523T in conjunction with 93454, 93455, 93456, 93457, 93458, 93459, 93460, 93461)

(Do not report 0523T more than once per session)

(Do not report 0523T in conjunction with 76376, 76377, 93571, 93572, 0501T, 0502T, 0503T, 0504T)

0505T Endovenous femoral-popliteal arterial revascularization, with transcatheter placement of intravascular stent graft(s) and closure by any method, including percutaneous or open vascular access, ultrasound guidance for vascular access when performed, all catheterization(s) and intraprocedural roadmapping and imaging guidance necessary to complete the intervention, all associated radiological supervision and interpretation, when performed, with crossing of the occlusive lesion in an extraluminal fashion (Sunset January 2024)

(0505T includes all ipsilateral selective arterial and venous catheterization, all diagnostic imaging for ipsilateral, lower extremity arteriography, and all related radiological supervision and interpretation)

(Do not report 0505T in conjunction with 37224, 37225, 37226, 37227, 37238, 37239, 37248, 37249, within the femoral-popliteal segment)

(Do not report 0505T in conjunction with 76937, for ultrasound guidance for vascular access)

● **0620T** Endovascular venous arterialization, tibial or peroneal vein, with transcatheter placement of intravascular stent graft(s) and closure by any method, including percutaneous or open vascular access, ultrasound guidance for vascular access when performed, all catheterization(s) and intraprocedural roadmapping and imaging guidance necessary to complete the intervention, all associated radiological supervision and interpretation, when performed

(0620T includes all ipsilateral selective arterial and venous catheterization, all diagnostic imaging for ipsilateral, lower extremity arteriography, and all related radiological supervision and interpretation)

(Do not report 0620T in conjunction with 37228, 37229, 37230, 37231, 37238, 37239, 37248, 37249 within the tibial-peroneal segment)

0506T Macular pigment optical density measurement by heterochromatic flicker photometry, unilateral or bilateral, with interpretation and report (Sunset January 2024)

0507T Near infrared dual imaging (ie, simultaneous reflective and transilluminated light) of meibomian glands, unilateral or bilateral, with interpretation and report (Sunset January 2024)

(For external ocular photography, use 92285)

(For tear film imaging, use 0330T)

0508T Pulse-echo ultrasound bone density measurement resulting in indicator of axial bone mineral density, tibia

Electroretinography (ERG) is used to evaluate function of the retina and optic nerve of the eye, including photoreceptors and ganglion cells. A number of techniques that target different areas of the eye, including full field (flash and flicker) (92273) for a global response of photoreceptors of the retina, multifocal (92274) for photoreceptors in multiple separate locations in the retina, including the macula, and pattern (0509T) for retinal ganglion cells are used. Multiple additional terms and techniques are used to describe various types of ERG. If the technique used is not specifically named in the code descriptors for 92273, 92274, 0509T, use the unlisted procedure code 92499.

0509T Electroretinography (ERG) with interpretation and report, pattern (PERG) (Sunset January 2024)

(For full-field ERG, use 92273)

(For multifocal ERG, use 92274)

0510T This code is out of order. See page 1034

0511T This code is out of order. See page 1034

0512T This code is out of order. See page 1025

0513T This code is out of order. See page 1025

+ **0514T** Intraoperative visual axis identification using patient fixation (List separately in addition to code for primary procedure) (Sunset January 2024)

(Use 0514T in conjunction with 66982, 66984)

WIRELESS CARDIAC STIMULATION SYSTEM FOR LEFT VENTRICULAR PACING

A wireless cardiac stimulator system provides biventricular pacing by sensing right ventricular pacing output from a previously implanted conventional device (pacemaker or defibrillator, with univentricular or biventricular leads), and then transmitting an ultrasound pulse to a wireless electrode implanted on the endocardium of the left ventricle, which then emits a left ventricular pacing pulse.

The complete system consists of two components: a wireless endocardial left ventricle electrode and a pulse generator. The pulse generator has two components: a transmitter and a battery. The electrode is implanted transarterially into the left ventricular wall and powered wirelessly using ultrasound delivered by a subcutaneously implanted transmitter. Two subcutaneous pockets are created on the chest wall, one for the battery and one for the transmitter, and these two components are connected by a subcutaneously tunneled cable.

Patients with a wireless cardiac stimulator require programming/interrogation of their existing conventional device, as well as the wireless device. The wireless cardiac stimulator is programmed and interrogated with its own separate programmer and settings.

Code 0515T describes insertion of a complete wireless cardiac stimulator system (electrode and pulse generator, which includes transmitter and battery), including interrogation, programming, pocket creation, revision and repositioning, and all echocardiography and other imaging to guide the procedure, when performed. Use 0516T only when insertion of the electrode is a standalone procedure. For insertion of only a new generator or generator component (battery and/or transmitter), use 0517T.

For removal of only the generator or a generator component (battery and/or transmitter) without replacement, use 0518T. For removal and replacement of a generator or a generator component (battery and/or transmitter), use 0519T. For battery and/or generator removal and reinsertion performed together with a new electrode insertion, use 0520T.

All catheterization and imaging guidance (including transthoracic or transesophageal echocardiography) required to complete a wireless cardiac stimulator procedure is included in 0515T, 0516T, 0517T, 0518T, 0519T, 0520T. Do not report 76000, 76998, 93303-93355 in conjunction with 0515T, 0516T, 0517T, 0518T, 0519T, 0520T.

Do not report left heart catheterization codes (93452, 93453, 93458, 93459, 93460, 93461, 93531, 93532, 93533) for delivery of a wireless cardiac stimulator electrode into the left ventricle.

0515T Insertion of wireless cardiac stimulator for left ventricular pacing, including device interrogation and programming, and imaging supervision and interpretation, when performed; complete system (includes electrode and generator [transmitter and battery]) (Sunset January 2024)

0516T electrode only (Sunset January 2024)

0517T pulse generator component(s) (battery and/or transmitter) only (Sunset January 2024)

(Do not report 0515T, 0516T, 0517T in conjunction with 0518T, 0519T, 0520T, 0521T, 0522T)

0518T Removal of only pulse generator component(s) (battery and/or transmitter) of wireless cardiac stimulator for left ventricular pacing (Sunset January 2024)

(Do not report 0518T in conjunction with 0515T, 0516T, 0517T, 0519T, 0520T, 0521T, 0522T)

0519T Removal and replacement of wireless cardiac stimulator for left ventricular pacing; pulse generator component(s) (battery and/or transmitter) (Sunset January 2024)

0520T pulse generator component(s) (battery and/or transmitter), including placement of a new electrode (Sunset January 2024)

(Do not report 0519T, 0520T in conjunction with 0515T, 0516T, 0517T, 0518T, 0521T, 0522T)

0521T Interrogation device evaluation (in person) with analysis, review and report, includes connection, recording, and disconnection per patient encounter, wireless cardiac stimulator for left ventricular pacing (Sunset January 2024)

(Do not report 0521T in conjunction with 0515T, 0516T, 0517T, 0518T, 0519T, 0520T, 0522T)

0522T Programming device evaluation (in person) with iterative adjustment of the implantable device to test the function of the device and select optimal permanent programmed values with analysis, including review and report, wireless cardiac stimulator for left ventricular pacing (Sunset January 2024)

(Do not report 0522T in conjunction with 0515T, 0516T, 0517T, 0518T, 0519T, 0520T, 0521T)

0523T This code is out of order. See page 1049

0524T   Endovenous catheter directed chemical ablation with balloon isolation of incompetent extremity vein, open or percutaneous, including all vascular access, catheter manipulation, diagnostic imaging, imaging guidance and monitoring (Sunset January 2024)

0525T   Insertion or replacement of intracardiac ischemia monitoring system, including testing of the lead and monitor, initial system programming, and imaging supervision and interpretation; complete system (electrode and implantable monitor) (Sunset January 2024)

0526T   electrode only (Sunset January 2024)

0527T   implantable monitor only (Sunset January 2024)

(Do not report 0525T, 0526T, 0527T in conjunction with 93000, 93005, 93010, 0528T, 0529T)

(For removal and replacement of intracardiac ischemia monitoring system or its components, see 0525T, 0526T, 0527T in conjunction with 0530T, 0531T, 0532T, as appropriate)

0528T   Programming device evaluation (in person) of intracardiac ischemia monitoring system with iterative adjustment of programmed values, with analysis, review, and report (Sunset January 2024)

(Do not report 0528T in conjunction with 93000, 93005, 93010, 0525T, 0526T, 0527T, 0529T, 0530T, 0531T, 0532T)

0529T   Interrogation device evaluation (in person) of intracardiac ischemia monitoring system with analysis, review, and report (Sunset January 2024)

(Do not report 0529T in conjunction with 93000, 93005, 93010, 0525T, 0526T, 0527T, 0528T, 0530T, 0531T, 0532T)

0530T   Removal of intracardiac ischemia monitoring system, including all imaging supervision and interpretation; complete system (electrode and implantable monitor) (Sunset January 2024)

0531T   electrode only (Sunset January 2024)

0532T   implantable monitor only (Sunset January 2024)

(Do not report 0530T, 0531T, 0532T in conjunction with 0528T, 0529T)

0533T   Continuous recording of movement disorder symptoms, including bradykinesia, dyskinesia, and tremor for 6 days up to 10 days; includes set-up, patient training, configuration of monitor, data upload, analysis and initial report configuration, download review, interpretation and report (Sunset January 2024)

0534T   set-up, patient training, configuration of monitor (Sunset January 2024)

0535T   data upload, analysis and initial report configuration (Sunset January 2024)

0536T   download review, interpretation and report (Sunset January 2024)

CELLULAR AND GENE THERAPY

Cellular and gene therapies involve the collection, processing and handling of cells or other tissues, genetic modification of those cells or tissues, and administration of the genetically modified cells or tissues with the intent to treat, modify, reverse or cure a serious or lifethreatening disease or condition.

Codes 0537T, 0538T, 0539T, 0540T describe the various steps required to collect, prepare, transport, receive, and administer genetically modified T cells. The collection and handling code (0537T) may be reported only once per day, regardless of the number of collections or quantity of cells collected. Similarly, the administration code (0540T) may only be reported once per day, regardless of the number of units administered. The development of genetically modified cells is not reported with this family of codes.

   ● New Code   ▲ Revised Code   + Add-On Code   ⊘ Modifier -51 Exempt   ★ Telemedicine

Chimeric antigen receptor therapy (CAR-T) with genetically modified T cells begins with the collection of cells from the patient by peripheral blood leukocyte cell harvesting. The cells are then cryopreserved and/or otherwise prepared for processing or shipping to a manufacturing or cell processing facility, if applicable, where gene modification and expansion of the cells is performed. When gene modification and expansion of the cells by the manufacturer is complete, the genetically modified cells are returned to the physician or other qualified health care professional in which additional preparation occurs, including thawing of the cryopreserved CAR-T cells, if necessary, before the cells are administered to the patient.

The procedure to administer CAR-T cells includes physician monitoring of multiple physiologic parameters, physician verification of cell processing, evaluation of the patient during, as well as immediately before and after the administration of the CAR-T cells, physician presence during the administration and direct supervision of clinical staff, and management of any adverse events during the administration. Care on the same date of service that is not directly related to the service of administration of the CAR-T cells (eg, care provided after the administration is complete, care for the patient's underlying condition or for other medical problems) may be separately reported using the appropriate evaluation and management code with modifier 25. Management of uncomplicated adverse events (eg, nausea, urticaria) during the infusion is not reported separately.

The fluid used to administer the cells and other infusions for incidental hydration (eg, 96360, 96361) are not reported separately. Similarly, infusion(s) of any supportive medication(s) (eg, steroids) concurrently with the CAR-T cell administration are not reported separately. However, hydration or administration of medications (eg, antibiotics, opioids) unrelated to the CAR-T administration may be reported separately with modifier 59.

0537T Chimeric antigen receptor T-cell (CAR-T) therapy; harvesting of blood-derived T lymphocytes for development of genetically modified autologous CAR-T cells, per day (Sunset January 2024)

0538T preparation of blood-derived T lymphocytes for transportation (eg, cryopreservation, storage) (Sunset January 2024)

0539T receipt and preparation of CAR-T cells for administration (Sunset January 2024)

0540T CAR-T cell administration, autologous (Sunset January 2024)

0541T Myocardial imaging by magnetocardiography (MCG) for detection of cardiac ischemia, by signal acquisition using minimum 36 channel grid, generation of magnetic-field time-series images, quantitative analysis of magnetic dipoles, machine learning-derived clinical scoring, and automated report generation, single study; (Sunset January 2024)

0542T interpretation and report (Sunset January 2024)

(For transesophageal echocardiography image guidance, use 93355)

Codes 0544T and 0545T include vascular access, catheterization, deploying and adjusting the reconstruction device(s), temporary pacemaker insertion for rapid pacing if required, and access site closure, when performed.

Angiography, radiological supervision and interpretation, intraprocedural roadmapping (eg, contrast injections, fluoroscopy) to guide the device implantation, ventriculography (eg, to assess target valve regurgitation for guidance of device implantation and adjustment), and completion angiography are included in 0544T and 0545T.

Diagnostic right and left heart catheterization codes (93451, 93452, 93453, 93454, 93455, 93456, 93457, 93458, 93459, 93460, 93461, 93530, 93531, 93532, 93533, 93565, 93566) may not be used in conjunction with 0544T, 0545T to report:

1. contrast injections, angiography, road-mapping, and/or fluoroscopic guidance for the implantation and adjustment of the transcatheter mitral or tricuspid valve annulus reconstruction device, or

2. right or left ventricular angiography to assess or confirm transcatheter mitral or tricuspid valve annulus reconstruction device positioning and function, or

3. right and left heart catheterization for hemodynamic measurements before, during, and after transcatheter mitral or tricuspid valve annulus reconstruction for guidance.

Diagnostic right and left heart catheterization codes (93451, 93452, 93453, 93456, 93457, 93458, 93459, 93460, 93461, 93530, 93531, 93532, 93533) and diagnostic coronary angiography codes (93454, 93455, 93456, 93457, 93458, 93459, 93460, 93461, 93563, 93564) performed at the time of transcatheter mitral or tricuspid valve annulus reconstruction may be separately reportable if:

---

1. no prior study is available and a full diagnostic study is performed, or

2. a prior study is available, but as documented in the medical record:

    a. there is inadequate visualization of the anatomy and/or pathology, or

    b. the patient's condition with respect to the clinical indication has changed since the prior study, or

    c. there is a clinical change during the procedure that requires new evaluation.

Other cardiac catheterization services may be reported separately, when performed for diagnostic purposes not intrinsic to the transcatheter mitral valve annulus reconstruction.

For same session/same day diagnostic cardiac catheterization services, report the appropriate diagnostic cardiac catheterization code(s) appended with modifier 59 indicating separate and distinct procedural service from transcatheter mitral or tricuspid valve annulus reconstruction.

Percutaneous coronary interventional procedures may be reported separately, when performed.

When cardiopulmonary bypass is performed in conjunction with transcatheter mitral valve or tricuspid valve annulus reconstruction, 0544T, 0545T should be reported with the appropriate add-on code for percutaneous peripheral bypass (33367), open peripheral bypass (33368), or central bypass (33369).

When transcatheter ventricular support is required, the appropriate code may be reported with the appropriate ventricular assist device (VAD) procedure (33990, 33991, 33992, 33993) or balloon pump insertion (33967, 33970, 33973).

For percutaneous transcatheter mitral valve repair, use 0345T. For percutaneous transcatheter mitral valve implantation/replacement (TMVI) with prosthetic valve, use 0483T.

0544T   Transcatheter mitral valve annulus reconstruction, with implantation of adjustable annulus reconstruction device, percutaneous approach including transseptal puncture (Sunset January 2025)

    (For transcatheter mitral valve repair percutaneous approach including transseptal puncture when performed, see 33418, 33419)

    (For transcatheter mitral valve repair percutaneous approach via the coronary sinus, use 0345T)

    (For transcatheter mitral valve implantation/ replacement [TMVI] with prosthetic valve percutaneous approach, use 0483T)

0545T   Transcatheter tricuspid valve annulus reconstruction with implantation of adjustable annulus reconstruction device, percutaneous approach (Sunset January 2025)

    (Do not report 0544T, 0545T in conjunction with 76000)

    (Do not report 0544T, 0545T in conjunction with 93451, 93452, 93453, 93456, 93457, 93458, 93459, 93460, 93461, 93530, 93531, 93532, 93533, 93565, 93566 for diagnostic left and right heart catheterization procedures intrinsic to the annular repair procedure)

    (Do not report 0544T, 0545T in conjunction with 93454, 93455, 93456, 93457, 93458, 93459, 93460, 93461, 93563, 93564 for coronary angiography procedures intrinsic to the annular repair procedure)

0546T   Radiofrequency spectroscopy, real time, intraoperative margin assessment, at the time of partial mastectomy, with report (Sunset January 2025)

    (Use 0546T only once for each partial mastectomy site)

    (Do not report 0546T for re-excision)

0547T   Bone material quality testing by microindentation(s) of the tibia(s), with results reported as a score (Sunset January 2025)

0548T   Transperineal periurethral balloon continence device; bilateral placement, including cystoscopy and fluoroscopy (Sunset January 2025)

0549T   unilateral placement, including cystoscopy and fluoroscopy (Sunset January 2025)

   ● New Code   ▲ Revised Code   ＋ Add-On Code   ⊘ Modifier -51 Exempt   ★ Telemedicine

0550T   removal, each balloon (Sunset January 2025)

0551T   adjustment of balloon(s) fluid volume (Sunset January 2025)

     (Do not report 0551T in conjunction with 0548T, 0549T, 0550T)

0552T   Low-level laser therapy, dynamic photonic and dynamic thermokinetic energies, provided by a physician or other qualified health care professional (Sunset January 2025)

0553T   Percutaneous transcatheter placement of iliac arteriovenous anastomosis implant, inclusive of all radiological supervision and interpretation, intraprocedural roadmapping, and imaging guidance necessary to complete the intervention (Sunset January 2025)

     (Do not report 0553T in conjunction with 36005, 36011, 36012, 36140, 36245, 36246, 37220, 37221, 37224, 37226, 37238, 37248, 75710, 75820)

0554T   Bone strength and fracture risk using finite element analysis of functional data and bone-mineral density utilizing data from a computed tomography scan; retrieval and transmission of the scan data, assessment of bone strength and fracture risk and bone-mineral density, interpretation and report (Sunset January 2025)

     (Do not report 0554T in conjunction with 0555T, 0556T, 0557T)

0555T   retrieval and transmission of the scan data (Sunset January 2025)

0556T   assessment of bone strength and fracture risk and bone-mineral density (Sunset January 2025)

0557T   interpretation and report (Sunset January 2025)

0558T   Computed tomography scan taken for the purpose of biomechanical computed tomography analysis (Sunset January 2025)

     (Do not report 0558T in conjunction with 71250, 71260, 71270, 71275, 72125, 72126, 72127, 72128, 72129, 72130, 72131, 72132, 72133, 72191, 72192, 72193, 72194, 74150, 74160, 74170, 74174, 74175, 74176, 74177, 74178, 74261, 74262, 74263, 75571, 75572, 75573, 75574, 75635, 78816)

Codes 0559T, 0560T represent production of 3D-printed models of individually prepared and processed components of structures of anatomy. These individual components of structures of anatomy include, but are not limited to, bones, arteries, veins, nerves, ureters, muscles, tendons and ligaments, joints, visceral organs, and brain. Each 3D-printed anatomic model of a structure can be made up of one or more separate components. The 3D anatomic printings can be 3D printed in unique colors and/or materials.

Codes 0561T, 0562T represent the production of 3D-printed cutting or drilling guides using individualized imaging data. 3D-printed guides are cutting or drilling tools used during surgery and are 3D printed so that they precisely fit an individual patient's anatomy to guide the surgery. A cutting guide does not have multiple parts, but instead is a unique single tool. It may be necessary to make a 3D-printed model and a 3D-printed cutting or drilling guide on the same patient to assist with surgery.

0559T   Anatomic model 3D-printed from image data set(s); first individually prepared and processed component of an anatomic structure (Sunset January 2025)

+ 0560T   each additional individually prepared and processed component of an anatomic structure (List separately in addition to code for primary procedure) (Sunset January 2025)

     (Use 0560T in conjunction with 0559T)

     (Do not report 0559T, 0560T in conjunction with 76376, 76377)

0561T   Anatomic guide 3D-printed and designed from image data set(s); first anatomic guide (Sunset January 2025)

+ 0562T   each additional anatomic guide (List separately in addition to code for primary procedure) (Sunset January 2025)

     (Use 0562T in conjunction with 0561T)

     (Do not report 0561T, 0562T in conjunction with 76376, 76377)

    Separate Procedure   Unlisted Procedure   CCI Comp. Code   Non-specific Procedure   **1055**

0563T This code is out of order. See page 1029

0564T Oncology, chemotherapeutic drug cytotoxicity assay of cancer stem cells (CSCs), from cultured CSCs and primary tumor cells, categorical drug response reported based on percent of cytotoxicity observed, a minimum of 14 drugs or drug combinations (Sunset January 2025)

0565T Autologous cellular implant derived from adipose tissue for the treatment of osteoarthritis of the knees; tissue harvesting and cellular implant creation (Sunset January 2025)

(Do not report 0565T in conjunction with 15769, 15771, 15772, 15773, 15774)

0566T injection of cellular implant into knee joint including ultrasound guidance, unilateral (Sunset January 2025)

(Do not report 0566T in conjunction with 20610, 20611, 76942, 77002)

(For bilateral procedure, report 0566T with modifier 50)

0567T Permanent fallopian tube occlusion with degradable biopolymer implant, transcervical approach, including transvaginal ultrasound (Sunset January 2025)

(Do not report 0567T in conjunction with 58340, 58565, 74740, 74742, 76830, 76856, 76857)

0568T Introduction of mixture of saline and air for sonosalpingography to confirm occlusion of fallopian tubes, transcervical approach, including transvaginal ultrasound and pelvic ultrasound (Sunset January 2025)

(Do not report 0568T in conjunction with 58340, 74740, 74742, 76830, 76831, 76856, 76857)

TRICUSPID VALVE REPAIR

Codes 0569T, 0570T include the work of percutaneous vascular access, placing the access sheath, cardiac catheterization, advancing the repair device system into position, repositioning the prosthesis as needed, deploying the prosthesis, and vascular closure. Code 0569T may only be reported once per session. Add-on code 0570T is reported in conjunction with 0569T for each additional prosthesis placed.

For open tricuspid valve procedures, see 33460, 33463, 33464, 33465, 33468.

Angiography, radiological supervision and interpretation performed to guide transcatheter tricuspid valve repair (TTVr) (eg, guiding device placement and documenting completion of the intervention) are included in these codes.

Intracardiac echocardiography (93662), when performed, is included in 0569T, 0570T. Transesophageal echocardiography (93355) performed by a separate operator for guidance of the procedure may be separately reported.

Fluoroscopy (76000) and diagnostic right and left heart catheterization codes (93451, 93452, 93453, 93456, 93457, 93458, 93459, 93460, 93461, 93530, 93531, 93532, 93533, 93566) may not be used with 0569T, 0570T to report the following techniques for guidance of TTVr:

1. Contrast injections, angiography, roadmapping, and/or fluoroscopic guidance for the TTVr,

2. Right ventricular angiography to assess tricuspid regurgitation for guidance of TTVr, or

3. Right and left heart catheterization for hemodynamic measurements before, during, and after TTVr for guidance of TTVr.

Diagnostic right and left heart catheterization codes (93451, 93452, 93453, 93456, 93457, 93458, 93459, 93460, 93461, 93530, 93531, 93532, 93533, 93566) and diagnostic coronary angiography codes (93454, 93455, 93456, 93457, 93458, 93459, 93460, 93461, 93563, 93564) may be reported with 0569T, 0570T, representing separate and distinct services from TTVr, if:

1. No prior study is available, and a full diagnostic study is performed, or

2. A prior study is available, but as documented in the medical record:

a. There is inadequate evaluation of the anatomy and/or pathology, or

b. The patient's condition with respect to the clinical indication has changed since the prior study, or

c. There is a clinical change during the procedure that requires new diagnostic evaluation.

● New Code ▲ Revised Code **+** Add-On Code ⊘ Modifier -51 Exempt ★ Telemedicine

Other cardiac catheterization services may be reported separately when performed for diagnostic purposes not intrinsic to TTVr.

For same session/same day diagnostic cardiac catheterization services, report the appropriate diagnostic cardiac catheterization code(s) with modifier 59 indicating separate and distinct procedural service from TTVr.

Diagnostic coronary angiography performed at a separate session from an interventional procedure may be separately reportable.

Percutaneous coronary interventional procedures may be reported separately, when performed.

When transcatheter ventricular support is required in conjunction with TTVr, the procedure may be reported with the appropriate ventricular assist device (VAD) procedure code (33990, 33991, 33992, 33993) or balloon pump insertion code (33967, 33970, 33973).

When cardiopulmonary bypass is performed in conjunction with TTVr, 0569T, 0570T may be reported with the appropriate add-on code for percutaneous peripheral bypass (33367), open peripheral bypass (33368), or central bypass (33369).

0569T   Transcatheter tricuspid valve repair, percutaneous approach; initial prosthesis (Sunset January 2025)

+ 0570T   each additional prosthesis during same session (List separately in addition to code for primary procedure) (Sunset January 2025)

(Use 0570T in conjunction with 0569T)

(Do not report 0569T, 0570T in conjunction with 93451, 93452, 93453, 93456, 93457, 93458, 93459, 93460, 93461, 93566 for diagnostic left and right heart catheterization procedures intrinsic to the valve repair procedure)

(Do not report 0569T, 0570T in conjunction with 93454, 93563, 93564 for coronary angiography intrinsic to the valve repair procedure)

IMPLANTABLE CARDIOVERTER-DEFIBRILLATOR WITH SUBSTERNAL ELECTRODE

An implantable cardioverter-defibrillator system with substernal electrode (substernal implantable cardioverter-defibrillator) consists of a pulse generator and at least one substernal electrode. The generator is placed in a subcutaneous pocket over the lateral rib cage. The electrode is tunneled subcutaneously and placed into the substernal anterior mediastinum, without entering the pericardial cavity. The electrode performs defibrillation and antitachycardia pacing, but not chronic pacing. The system requires programming and interrogation of the device.

All imaging guidance (eg, fluoroscopy) required to complete the substernal implantable defibrillator procedure is included in 0571T, 0572T, 0573T, 0574T. The work of implantation, removal, repositioning, interrogation, or programming of substernal implantable cardioverter-defibrillator systems, generators, or leads may not be reported using 33202-33275, 93260-93298, 93640, 93641, 93642, 93644.

0571T   Insertion or replacement of implantable cardioverterdefibrillator system with substernal electrode(s), including all imaging guidance and electrophysiological evaluation (includes defibrillation threshold evaluation, induction of arrhythmia, evaluation of sensing for arrhythmia termination, and programming or reprogramming of sensing or therapeutic parameters), when performed (Sunset January 2025)

(Use 0571T in conjunction with 0573T, 0580T for removal and replacement of an implantable defibrillator pulse generator and substernal electrode)

(Do not report 0571T in conjunction with 93260, 93261, 93644, 0572T, 0575T, 0576T, 0577T)

(For insertion or replacement of permanent subcutaneous implantable defibrillator system with subcutaneous electrode, use 33270)

0572T   Insertion of substernal implantable defibrillator electrode (Sunset January 2025)

(Do not report 0572T in conjunction with 93260, 93261, 93644, 0571T, 0575T, 0576T, 0577T, 0580T)

(For insertion of subcutaneous implantable defibrillator electrode, use 33271)

0573T   Removal of substernal implantable defibrillator electrode (Sunset January 2025)

(Use 0573T in conjunction with 0580T for removal of substernal electrode in conjunction with removal of implantable defibrillator pulse generator without replacement)

(Do not report 0573T in conjunction with 93260, 93261, 93644, 0575T, 0576T, 0577T)

(For removal of subcutaneous implantable defibrillator electrode, use 33272)

0574T Repositioning of previously implanted substernal implantable defibrillator-pacing electrode (Sunset January 2025)

(Do not report 0574T in conjunction with 93260, 93261, 93644, 0572T, 0575T, 0576T, 0577T)

(For repositioning of previously implanted subcutaneous implantable defibrillator electrode, use 33273)

0575T Programming device evaluation (in person) of implantable cardioverter-defibrillator system with substernal electrode, with iterative adjustment of the implantable device to test the function of the device and select optimal permanent programmed values with analysis, review and report by a physician or other qualified health care professional (Sunset January 2025)

(Do not report 0575T in conjunction with pulse generator or lead insertion, removal or repositioning codes 0571T, 0572T, 0573T, 0574T, 0580T, 0614T)

(Do not report 0575T in conjunction with 93260, 93282, 93287, 0576T)

0576T Interrogation device evaluation (in person) of implantable cardioverter-defibrillator system with substernal electrode, with analysis, review and report by a physician or other qualified health care professional, includes connection, recording and disconnection per patient encounter (Sunset January 2025)

(Do not report 0576T in conjunction with pulse generator or lead insertion, removal or repositioning codes 0571T, 0572T, 0573T, 0574T, 0580T, 0614T)

(Do not report 0576T in conjunction with 93261, 93289, 0575T)

▲ **0577T** Electrophysiologic evaluation of implantable cardioverter- defibrillator system with substernal electrode (includes defibrillation threshold evaluation, induction of arrhythmia, evaluation of sensing for arrhythmia termination, and programming or reprogramming of sensing or therapeutic parameters)

(Do not report 0577T in conjunction with 93640, 93641, 93642, 93644, 0571T at the time of insertion or replacement of implantable defibrillator system with substernal lead)

(Do not report 0577T in conjunction with 0580T, 0614T)

(For electrophysiologic evaluation of subcutaneous implantable defibrillator system with subcutaneous electrode, use 93644)

0578T Interrogation device evaluation(s) (remote), up to 90 days, substernal lead implantable cardioverter-defibrillator system with interim analysis, review(s) and report(s) by a physician or other qualified health care professional (Sunset January 2025)

(Do not report 0578T in conjunction with 93294, 93295, 93297, 93298, 0576T)

(Report 0578T only once per 90 days)

0579T Interrogation device evaluation(s) (remote), up to 90 days, substernal lead implantable cardioverter-defibrillator system, remote data acquisition(s), receipt of transmissions and technician review, technical support and distribution of results (Sunset January 2025)

(Do not report 0579T in conjunction with 93296, 0576T)

(Report 0579T only once per 90 days)

0580T Removal of substernal implantable defibrillator pulse generator only (Sunset January 2025)

(Use 0580T in conjunction with 0573T for removal of substernal electrode in conjunction with removal of implantable defibrillator pulse generator without replacement)

(Use 0580T in conjunction with 0571T, 0573T for removal and replacement of an implantable cardioverterdefibrillator and substernal electrode[s])

● New Code ▲ Revised Code ✛ Add-On Code ⊘ Modifier -51 Exempt ★ Telemedicine

(Do not report 0580T in conjunction with 0575T, 0576T, 0577T, 0614T)

● **0614T** Removal and replacement of substernal implantable defibrillator pulse generator

(Do not report 0614T in conjunction with 33262, 0571T, 0572T, 0575T, 0576T, 0577T, 0580T)

0581T Ablation, malignant breast tumor(s), percutaneous, cryotherapy, including imaging guidance when performed, unilateral (Sunset January 2025)

(Report 0581T only once per breast treated)

(Do not report 0581T in conjunction with 76641, 76642, 76940, 76942)

(For cryoablation of breast fibroadenoma[s], use 19105)

0582T Transurethral ablation of malignant prostate tissue by high-energy water vapor thermotherapy, including intraoperative imaging and needle guidance (Sunset January 2025)

(Do not report 0582T in conjunction with 52000, 72195, 72196, 72197, 76376, 76377, 76872, 76940, 76942, 77021, 77022)

(For transurethral destruction of prostate tissue by radiofrequency-generated water vapor thermotherapy for benign prostatic hypertrophy [BPH], use 53854)

0583T Tympanostomy (requiring insertion of ventilating tube), using an automated tube delivery system, iontophoresis local anesthesia (Sunset January 2025)

(Do not report 0583T in conjunction with 69209, 69210, 69420, 69421, 69433, 69436, 69990, 92504, 97033)

(For bilateral procedure, report 0583T with modifier 50)

0584T Islet cell transplant, includes portal vein catheterization and infusion, including all imaging, including guidance, and radiological supervision and interpretation, when performed; percutaneous (Sunset January 2025)

0585T laparoscopic (Sunset January 2025)

0586T open (Sunset January 2025)

0587T Percutaneous implantation or replacement of integrated single device neurostimulation system including electrode array and receiver or pulse generator, including analysis, programming, and imaging guidance when performed, posterior tibial nerve (Sunset January 2025)

(Do not report 0587T in conjunction with 64555, 64566, 64575, 64590, 95970, 95971, 95972, 0588T, 0589T, 0590T)

0588T Revision or removal of integrated single device neurostimulation system including electrode array and receiver or pulse generator, including analysis, programming, and imaging guidance when performed, posterior tibial nerve (Sunset January 2025)

(Do not report 0588T in conjunction with 64555, 64566, 64575, 64590, 95970, 95971, 95972, 0587T, 0589T, 0590T)

0589T Electronic analysis with simple programming of implanted integrated neurostimulation system (eg, electrode array and receiver), including contact group(s), amplitude, pulse width, frequency (Hz), on/off cycling, burst, dose lockout, patient-selectable parameters, responsive neurostimulation, detection algorithms, closed-loop parameters, and passive parameters, when performed by physician or other qualified health care professional, posterior tibial nerve, 1-3 parameters (Sunset January 2025)

(Do not report 0589T in conjunction with 43647, 43648, 43881, 43882, 61850-61888, 63650, 63655, 63661, 63662, 63663, 63664, 63685, 63688, 64553-64595, 95970, 95971, 95972, 95976, 95977, 95983, 95984, 0587T, 0588T, 0590T)

0590T Electronic analysis with complex programming of implanted integrated neurostimulation system (eg, electrode array and receiver), including contact group(s), amplitude, pulse width, frequency (Hz), on/off cycling, burst, dose lockout, patient-selectable parameters, responsive neurostimulation, detection algorithms, closed-loop parameters, and passive parameters, when performed by physician or other qualified health care professional, posterior tibial nerve, 4 or more parameters (Sunset January 2025)

(Do not report 0590T in conjunction with 43647, 43648, 43881, 43882, 61850-61888, 63650, 63655, 63661, 63662, 63663, 63664, 63685, 63688, 64553-64595, 95970, 95971, 95972, 95976, 95977, 95983, 95984, 0587T, 0588T, 0589T)

HEALTH AND WELL-BEING COACHING

Health and well-being coaching is a patient-centered approach wherein patients determine their goals, use selfdiscovery or active learning processes together with content education to work toward their goals, and selfmonitor behaviors to increase accountability, all within the context of an interpersonal relationship with a coach.

The coach is a nonphysician health care professional certified by the National Board for Health and Wellness Coaching or National Commission for Health Education Credentialing, Inc. Coaches' training includes behavioral change theory, motivational strategies, communication techniques, health education and promotion theories, which are used to assist patients to develop intrinsic motivation and obtain skills to create sustainable change for improved health and well-being.

0591T Health and well-being coaching face-to-face; individual, initial assessment (Sunset January 2025)

0592T individual, follow-up session, at least 30 minutes (Sunset January 2025)

(Do not report 0592T in conjunction with 96156, 96158, 96159, 98960, 0488T, 0591T)

(For medical nutrition therapy, see 97802, 97803, 97804)

0593T group (2 or more individuals), at least 30 minutes (Sunset January 2025)

(Do not report 0593T in conjunction with 96164, 96165, 97150, 98961, 98962, 0403T)

● **0594T** Osteotomy, humerus, with insertion of an externally controlled intramedullary lengthening device, including intraoperative imaging, initial and subsequent alignment assessments, computations of adjustment schedules, and management of the intramedullary lengthening device

(Do not report 0594T in conjunction with 20696, 24400, 24410, 24420, 24516)

(For revision of externally controlled intramedullary lengthening device, use 24999)

(0595T has been deleted)

● **0596T** Temporary female intraurethral valve-pump (ie, voiding prosthesis); initial insertion, including urethral measurement

● **0597T** replacement

(Do not report 0596T, 0597T in conjunction with 51610, 51700, 51701, 51702, 51703, 51705)

● **0598T** Noncontact real-time fluorescence wound imaging, for bacterial presence, location, and load, per session; first anatomic site (eg, lower extremity)

●+**0599T** each additional anatomic site (eg, upper extremity) (List separately in addition to code for primary procedure)

(Use 0599T in conjunction with 0598T)

● **0600T** Ablation, irreversible electroporation; 1 or more tumors per organ, including imaging guidance, when performed, percutaneous

(Do not report 0600T in conjunction with 76940, 77002, 77013, 77022)

● **0601T** 1 or more tumors per organ, including fluoroscopic and ultrasound guidance, when performed, open

(Do not report 0601T in conjunction with 76940, 77002)

● **0602T** Glomerular filtration rate (GFR) measurement(s), transdermal, including sensor placement and administration of a single dose of fluorescent pyrazine agent

---

● New Code ▲ Revised Code + Add-On Code ⊘ Modifier -51 Exempt ★ Telemedicine

● **0603T** Glomerular filtration rate (GFR) monitoring, transdermal, including sensor placement and administration of more than one dose of fluorescent pyrazine agent, each 24 hours

(Do not report 0603T in conjunction with 0602T)

● **0604T** Optical coherence tomography (OCT) of retina, remote, patient-initiated image capture and transmission to a remote surveillance center, unilateral or bilateral; initial device provision, set-up and patient education on use of equipment

● **0605T**   remote surveillance center technical support, data analyses and reports, with a minimum of 8 daily recordings, each 30 days

● **0606T**   review, interpretation and report by the prescribing physician or other qualified health care professional of remote surveillance center data analyses, each 30 days

(Do not report 0604T, 0605T, 0606T in conjunction with 99457, 99458)

● **0607T** Remote monitoring of an external continuous pulmonary fluid monitoring system, including measurement of radiofrequency-derived pulmonary fluid levels, heart rate, respiration rate, activity, posture, and cardiovascular rhythm (eg, ECG data), transmitted to a remote 24-hour attended surveillance center; set-up and patient education on use of equipment

(Do not report 0607T in conjunction with 93224, 93225, 93226, 93227, 93228, 93229, 93264, 93268, 93270, 93271, 93272, 93297, 99453, for same monitoring period)

● **0608T**   analysis of data received and transmission of reports to the physician or other qualified health care professional

(Report 0608T only once per 30 days)

(Do not report 0608T in conjunction with 93224, 93225, 93226, 93227, 93228, 93229, 93264, 93268, 93270, 93271, 93272, 93297, 99454, for same monitoring period)

● **0609T** Magnetic resonance spectroscopy, determination and localization of discogenic pain (cervical, thoracic, or lumbar); acquisition of single voxel data, per disc, on biomarkers (ie, lactic acid, carbohydrate, alanine, laal, propionic acid, proteoglycan, and collagen) in at least 3 discs

● **0610T**   transmission of biomarker data for software analysis

● **0611T**   postprocessing for algorithmic analysis of biomarker data for determination of relative chemical differences between discs

● **0612T**   interpretation and report

(Do not report 0609T, 0610T, 0611T, 0612T in conjunction with 72141, 72142, 72146, 72147, 72148, 72149, 72156, 72157, 72158, 72159, 76390)

● **06113T** Percutaneous transcatheter implantation of interatrial septal shunt device, including right and left heart catheterization, intracardiac echocardiography, and imaging guidance by the proceduralist, when performed

(Do not report 0613T in conjunction with 76937, 93313, 93314, 93318, 93355, 93451, 93452, 93453, 93456, 93457, 93458, 93459, 93460, 93461, 93462, 93530, 93531, 93532, 93533, 93662)

(For transcatheter atrial septostomy for congenital cardiac abnormality, use 33741)

(For transcatheter intracardiac shunt creation by stent placement for congenital cardiac abnormality, see 33745, 33746)

(For transvenous atrial balloon septectomy or septostomy, see 33741, 33745, 33746)

0614T Code is out of order. See page 1059

● **0615T** Eye-movement analysis without spatial calibration, with interpretation and report

(Do not report 0615T in conjunction with 92540, 92541, 92542, 92544, 92545, 92546, 92547)

● **0616T** Insertion of iris prosthesis, including suture fixation and repair or removal of iris, when performed; without removal of crystalline lens or intraocular lens, without insertion of intraocular lens

---

● **0617T**   with removal of crystalline lens and insertion of intraocular lens

(Do not report 0617T in conjunction with 66982, 66983, 66984)

● **0618T**   with secondary intraocular lens placement or intraocular lens exchange

(Do not report 0618T in conjunction with 66985, 66986)

(Do not report 0616T, 0617T, 0618T in conjunction with 66600, 66680, 66682)

● **0619T**   Cystourethroscopy with transurethral anterior prostate commissurotomy and drug delivery, including transrectal ultrasound and fluoroscopy, when performed

(Do not report 0619T in conjunction with 52000, 52441, 52442, 52450, 52500, 52601, 52630, 52640, 52647, 52648, 52649, 53850, 53852, 53854, 76872, 0499T)

0620T   This code is out of order. See page 1050

● **0621T**   Trabeculostomy ab interno by laser;

● **0622T**   with use of ophthalmic endoscope

(Do not report 0621T, 0622T in conjunction with 92020)

0623T   This code is out of order. See page 1049

0624T   This code is out of order. See page 1049

0625T   This code is out of order. See page 1049

0626T   This code is out of order. See page 1049

● **0627T**   Percutaneous injection of allogeneic cellular and/or tissue-based product, intervertebral disc, unilateral or bilateral injection, with fluoroscopic guidance, lumbar; first level

●+**0628T**   each additional level (List separately in addition to code for primary procedure)

(Use 0628T in conjunction with 0627T)

(Do not report 0627T, 0628T in conjunction with 77003)

● **0629T**   Percutaneous injection of allogeneic cellular and/or tissue-based product, intervertebral disc, unilateral or bilateral injection, with CT guidance, lumbar; first level

●+**0630T**   each additional level (List separately in addition to code for primary procedure)

(Use 0630T in conjunction with 0629T)

(Do not report 0629T, 0630T in conjunction with 77012)

● **0631T**   Transcutaneous visible light hyperspectral imaging measurement of oxyhemoglobin, deoxyhemoglobin, and tissue oxygenation, with interpretation and report, per extremity

(Do not report 0631T in conjunction with 94760, 94761, 94762, 0061U)

● **0632T**   Percutaneous transcatheter ultrasound ablation of nerves innervating the pulmonary arteries, including right heart catheterization, pulmonary artery angiography, and all imaging guidance

(Do not report 0632T in conjunction with 36013, 36014, 36015, 75741, 75743, 75746, 93451, 93453, 93456, 93460, 93503, 93505, 93568)

● **0633T**   Computed tomography, breast, including 3D rendering, when performed, unilateral; without contrast material

● **0634T**   with contrast material(s)

● **0635T**   without contrast, followed by contrast material(s)

(Do not report 0633T, 0634T, 0635T in conjunction with 76376, 76377, 76380, 76497)

● **0636T** Computed tomography, breast, including 3D rendering, when performed, bilateral; without contrast material(s)

● **0637T** with contrast material(s)

● **0638T** without contrast, followed by contrast material(s)

(Do not report 0636T, 0637T, 0638T in conjunction with 76376, 76377, 76380, 76497)

● **0639T** Wireless skin sensor thermal anisotropy measurement(s) and assessment of flow in cerebrospinal fluid shunt, including ultrasound guidance, when performed

(Do not report 0639T in conjunction with 76998, 76999)

This page intentionally left blank.

● New Code   ▲ Revised Code   ✚ Add-On Code   ⊘ Modifier -51 Exempt   ★ Telemedicine

ALPHABETICAL INDEX

The alphabetical index includes listings by procedure, CPT® headings and sub-headings and anatomic site. Procedures and services commonly known by their acronyms, eponyms, homonyms or other designations are also included. The alphabetical index of CPT® PLUS is unique in that both indexes to specific page numbers and indexes to CPT code numbers are included.

HOW TO USE THE ALPHABETICAL INDEX

When using the alphabetical index to locate CPT codes, use the following search sequence:

- *Look for the CPT HEADING for the general category of surgical procedure(s) or medical service(s) or TOPIC for instructional and/or explanatory information.*

- *Look for the CPT Sub-heading for the organ system(s) involved or service(s) performed or the TOPIC sub-heading for the instructional or explanatory issue. Scan the index listings to determine if the specific procedure or service or topic is listed.*

- *For CPT codes, use the thumb-tab indexes to locate the appropriate CPT code section. If the specific procedure or service was listed in the index, locate the procedure or service in the CPT code section and verify the full description of the CPT code before using. If the specific procedure or service was not listed in the index, first locate the organ system and/or medical service sub-heading and then review the CPT code section until you locate the specific procedure and/or service.*

- *For instructional and/or explanatory topics, turn to the page number specified in the alphabetical index.*

- *Alternately, look for SYNONYMS, HOMONYMS, EPONYMS or ACRONYMS.*

The alphabetic index is NOT a substitute for the main text of CPT. Even if codes are found in the index, the user must refer to the main text to ensure that the code selection is accurate.

This page intentionally left blank.

A

Abbe-Estlander procedure ~ 40527, 40761
Abdomen
  abdominal aorta, angiography ~ 75635
  abdominal wall
    debridement, infected~ 11005, 11006
    fascial reinforcement with implant ~ 0437T
    implantation, non-biologic or synthetic implant ~ 0437T
    removal, mesh/prosthesis ~ 11008
    repair hernia ~ 49491-49496, 49501, 49507, 49521, 49590
    tumor, excision ~ 22900-22905
      radical resection ~ 22904, 22905
    unlisted services and procedures ~ 22999
  abscess
    incision and drainage ~ 49020, 49040
  angiography ~ 74174, 74175, 75635
  artery ligation ~ 37617
  biopsy ~ 49000
  bypass graft ~ 35907
  catheter removal ~ 49422
  celiotomy, exploratory ~ 49000
  CT scan ~ 74150-74178, 75635
  cyst destruction/excision ~ 49203-49205
  drainage fluid ~ 49082-49083
  ectopic pregnancy ~ 59130
  endometrioma destruction/excision ~ 49203-49205
  exploration ~ 49000-49002
    blood vessel ~ 35840
    staging ~ 58960
  incision ~ 49000-49084
    staging ~ 58960
  incision and drainage pancreatitis ~ 48000
  infraumbilical panniculectomy ~ 15830
  injection
    air ~ 49400
    contrast material ~ 49400
  insertion
    catheter ~ 49324, 49418-49419, 49421
    venous shunt ~ 49425
  intraperitoneal
    catheter exit site ~ 49436
    catheter insertion ~ 49418-49421, 49435
    catheter removal ~ 49422
    catheter revision ~ 49325
    shunt
      insertion ~ 49425
      ligation ~ 49428
      removal ~ 49429
      revision ~ 49426
  laparoscopy ~ 49320-49327, 49329
  laparotomy
    reopening ~ 49002
    staging ~ 58960
  magnetic resonance imaging (MRI) ~ 74181-74183
  needle biopsy, mass ~ 49180
  paracentesis ~ 49082-49083
  peritoneal lavage ~ 49084
  radical resection ~ 51597
  radiation therapy, guidance ~ 49411-49412
  repair
    blood vessel ~ 35221
      with other graft ~ 35281
      with vein graft ~ 35251
    hernia ~ 49491-49525, 49560-49587
    suture ~ 49900
  revision venous shunt ~ 49426
  suture ~ 49900
  tumor destruction/excision ~ 49203-49205
  ultrasound ~ 76700-76705
  unlisted services and procedures ~ 49999
  wound exploration penetrating ~ 20102
  X-ray ~ 74018, 74019, 74021, 74022
Abdominal aorta ~ *see* aorta, abdominal
Abdominal deliveries ~ *see* cesarean delivery
Abdominal hysterectomy ~ *see* hysterectomy, abdominal

Abdominal lymphangiogram ~ 75805, 75807
Abdominal paracentesis ~ *see* abdomen, drainage
Abdominal wall
  debridement, infected ~ 11005-11006
  reconstruction ~ 49905
  removal
    mesh ~ 11008
    prosthesis ~ 11008
  surgery ~ 22999
  tumor excision ~ 22900-22905
Abdominopelvic amputation ~ 27290
Abdominoplasty
  excision ~ 15847
Ablation
  anal polyp or tumor ~ 46615
  bone tumor ~ 20982, 20983
  breast, malignant tumor ~ 0581T
  colon tumor ~ 44401, 45346, 45388
  cryosurgical
    breast tumor ~ 0581T
    fibroadenoma ~ 19105
    liver tumor ~ 47381
    renal mass ~ 50250
    renal tumor, percutaneous ~ 50593
  CT scan guidance ~ 77013
  electroporation ~ 0600T-0601T
  endometrial ~ 58353, 58356, 58563
    with ultrasound guidance ~ 58356
  heart
    arrhythmogenic focus ~ 33250-33251, 33261, 93653, 93654, 93655
    atrioventricular ~ 93650, 93653, 93654
  high intensity focused ultrasound (HIFU) ~ 55880
  larynx, lesion ~ 31572
  laser, wound ~ 0491T, 0492T
  liver tumor
    cryosurgical ~ 47381, 47383
    laparoscopic ~ 47370, 47371
    radiofrequency ~ 47380-47382
  lung tumor
    radiofrequency ~ 32998
  nerve
    percutaneous ~ 0440T-0442T
    radiofrequency ~ 64625
    ultrasound ~ 0632T
  parenchymal tissue
    CT scan guidance ~ 77013
    magnetic resonance guidance ~ 77022
    ultrasound guidance ~ 76940
  prostate
    cryosurgical ~ 55873
    high intensity focused ultrasound (HIFU) ~ 55880
    transurethral water vapor thermotherapy ~ 0582T
    watrejet ~ 0421T
  pulmonry tumor ~ 32994, 32998
  radiofrequency
    liver tumor ~ 47382
    lung tumor ~ 32998
    renal tumor ~ 50592
    tongue base ~ 41530
    uterine fibroid ~ 0404T
  rectum, polyp or tumor ~ 45346
  renal
    cyst ~ 50541
    mass ~ 50542
    tumor, percutaneous cryotherapy ~ 50593
  stereotactic, intracranial lesion, MRI-guided intensity focused ultrasound ~ 0398T
  tongue base, radiofrequency ~ 41530
  transurethral water vapor thermotherapy ~ 0582T
  turbinate mucosa ~ 30801-30802
  uterine fibroids
    laparoscpic ~ 58674
    radiofrequency ~ 0404T
  uterine tumor, ultrasound, focused ~ 0071T-0072T
  vein, endovenous
    chemical adhesive ~ 36482, 36483
    laser ~ 36478, 36479
    mechanochemical ~ 36473, 36474
    radiofrequency ~ 36475, 36476

Abortion

incomplete ~ 59812
induced by
  dilation and curettage ~ 59840
  dilation and evacuation ~ 59841
  saline ~ 59850-59851
  vaginal suppositories ~ 59855-59856
missed
  first trimester ~ 59820
  second trimester ~ 59821
septic ~ 59830
spontaneous ~ 59812
therapeutic, by saline ~ 59850
  with dilation and curettage ~ 59851
  with hysterectomy ~ 59852
with hysterectomy ~ 59100, 59852, 59857

Abrasion (skin)

chemical peel ~ 15788-15793
dermabrasion ~ 15780-15783
lesion ~ 15786-15787
salabrasion ~ 15810-15811

Abscess

abdomen ~ 49040
  incision and drainage ~ 49040
anal, incision and drainage ~ 46045-46050
ankle ~ 27603, 27607
appendix, incision and drainage ~ 44900
  open ~ 44900
arm, lower ~ 25028
  excision ~ 25145
  incision and drainage ~ 25035
arm, upper, incision and drainage ~ 23930-23935
auditory canal, external ~ 69020
Bartholin's gland, incision and drainage ~ 56420
bladder, incision and drainage ~ 51080
brain
  drainage ~ 61150-61151
  excision ~ 61514, 61522
  incision and drainage ~ 61320-61321
breast, incision and drainage ~ 19020
carpals, incision, deep ~ 25035
clavicle sequestrectomy ~ 23170
drainage, with X-ray ~ 75989
ear, external
  complicated ~ 69005
  simple ~ 69000
elbow, incision and drainage ~ 23930-23935
epididymis, incision and drainage ~ 54700
excision
  olecranon process ~ 24138
  radius ~ 24136
  ulna ~ 24138
eyelid, incision and drainage ~ 67700
facial bones, excision ~ 21026
femur ~ 27303
finger ~ 26010-26011
  incision and drainage ~ 26034
foot, incision ~ 28005
gums, incision and drainage ~ 41800
hand, incision and drainage ~ 26034
hematoma, incision and drainage ~ 27603
hip, incision and drainage ~ 26990-26992
humeral head ~ 23174
humerus
  excision ~ 24134
  incision and drainage ~ 23935
kidney incision and drainage ~ 50020
leg, lower,incision and drainage ~ 27603
liver ~ 47010
  drainage, open ~ 47010
  injection ~ 47015
  repair ~ 47300
localization, nuclear medicine ~ 78800-78804, 78830-78832
lung, percutaneous drainage ~ 32200
lymph node, incision and drainage ~ 38300-38305
lymphocele drainage ~ 49062
mandible, excision ~ 21025
mouth, incision and drainage ~ 40800-40801, 41005-41009, 41015-41018
nasal septum, incision and drainage ~ 30020
neck, incision and drainage ~ 21501-21502

Abscess ~ *continued*

ovarian incision and drainage ~ 58820-58822
  abdominal approach ~ 58822
  vaginal approach ~ 58820
palate, incision and drainage ~ 42000
paraurethral gland, incision and drainage ~ 53060
parotid gland drainage ~ 42300-42305
pelvis, incision and drainage ~ 26990-26992, 45000
perineum, incision and drainage ~ 56405
perirenal or renal
  drainage ~ 50020
peritoneum
  incision and drainage ~ 49020
prostate
  incision and drainage ~ 55720-55725
  transurethral drainage ~ 52700
radius, incision, deep ~ 25035
rectum, incision and drainage ~ 45005-45020, 46040, 46060
retroperitoneal ~ 49060
  drainage ~ 49060
salivary gland, drainage ~ 42300-42320
scapula, sequestrectomy ~ 23172
scrotum, incision & drainage ~ 54700, 55100
shoulder, drainage ~ 23030
Skene's gland, incision and drainage ~ 53060
skin
  incision and drainage ~ 10060-10061
  puncture aspiration ~ 10160
subdiaphragmatic ~ 49040
sublingual gland, drainage ~ 42310-42320
submaxillary gland, drainage ~ 42310-42320
subphrenic ~ 49040
testis, incision and drainage ~ 54700
thoracostomy ~ 32551
thorax, incision and drainage ~ 21501-21502
throat, incision and drainage ~ 42700-42725
tongue, incision and drainage ~ 41000-41006
tonsil, incision and drainage ~ 42700
ulna, incision, deep ~ 25035
urethra, incision and drainage ~ 53040
uvula, incision and drainage ~ 42000
vagina, incision and drainage ~ 57010
vulva, incision and drainage ~ 56405
wrist
  excision ~ 25145
  incision and drainage ~ 25028, 25035
X-ray ~ 76080

Absorptiometry

dual energy ~ 3095F-3096F
bone
  appendicular ~ 77081
  axial skeleton ~ 77080
  vertebral ~ 77086
dual photon, bone ~ 78351
single photon, bone ~ 78350

Absorption spectrophotometry, atomic ~ 82190
Accessory nerve, spinal ~ 63191
Accessory, toes ~ 28344
ACE (angiotensin converting enzyme) ~ 82164
Acetabuloplasty ~ 27120-27122

Acetabulum

fracture
  closed treatment ~ 27220-27222
  open treatment ~ 27226-27228
  with manipulation ~ 27222
  without manipulation ~ 27220
reconstruction ~ 27120
  with resection, femoral head ~ 27122
tumor, excision ~ 27076

Acetaminophen, urine ~ 80329-80331
Acetic anhydrides ~ 84600
Acetone, blood or urine ~ 82009-82010
Acetone body ~ 82009-82010
Acetylcholinesterase, blood or urine ~ 82013
AcG ~ 85220

Achilles tendon

incision ~ 27605-27606
lengthening ~ 27612
repair ~ 27650-27654
Achillotomy ~ 27605-27606

Acid(s)
  adenylic ~ 82030
  amino ~ 82127-82139
  aminolevulinic ~ see aminolevulinic acid (ALA)
  ascorbic ~ 82180
  bile ~ 82239
  deoxyribonucleic ~ 86225-86226
  fatty ~ see fatty acid
  folic ~ 82747
  glycocholic ~ 82240
  lactic ~ 83605
  n-acetylneuraminic ~ 84275
  n-acetylneuraminic ~ 84275
  phenylethylbarbituric ~ 80345
  uric ~ see uric acid
Acidity/alkalinity ~ *see* pH
Acid fast bacilli (AFB), culture ~ 87116
Acid fast stain ~ 88312
Acid perfusion test, esophagus ~ 91030
Acid phosphatase ~ 84060-84066
Acid probes, nucleic ~ *see* nucleic acid probes
Acid reflux test, esophagus ~ 91034-91038
Acne surgery
  incision and drainage
    abscess ~ 10060-10061
    comedones ~ 10040
    cyst ~ 10040
    milia, multiple ~ 10040
    pustules ~ 10040
Acne treatment
  abrasion ~ 15786-15787
  chemical peel ~ 15788-15793
  cryotherapy ~ 17340
  dermabrasion ~ 15780-15783
  exfoliation, chemical ~ 17360
  salabrasion ~ 15810-15811
Acoustic neuroma (*see also* **brainstem, skull base surgery) ~** 61510,
    61518, 61520-61521, 61526-61530, 61545, 62164
Acoustic recording, heart sounds, with computer analysis ~ 93799
Acromioclavicular joint, arthrocentesis ~ 20605
  arthrotomy ~ 23044
    with biopsy ~ 23101
  dislocation ~ 23540-23552
  open treatment ~ 23550-23552
  X-ray ~ 73050
Acromion,excision, shoulder ~ 23130
Acromionectomy, partial ~ 23130
Acromioplasty ~ 23415-23420
  partial ~ 23130
ACTH releasing factor ~ 80412
Actigraphy, sleep study ~ 95803
Actinomyces, antibody ~ 86602
Actinomycosis ~ 86000
Actinomycotic infection ~ 86000
Actinotherapy ~ see dermatology ~ 96900
Activated factor X ~ 85260
Activated partial thromboplastin time ~ 85730-85732
Activation, lymphocyte ~ 86353
Activities of daily living ~ *see* physical medicine/therapy/occupational
    therapy
Activity, glomerular procoagulant ~ *see* thromboplastin
Acupuncture
  with electrical stimulation ~ 97813-97814
  without electrical stimulation ~ 97810-97811
Acute poliomyelitis ~ *see* polio
Acylcarnitines ~ 82016-82017
Adamantinoma, pituitary ~ *see* craniopharyngioma
Adaptive Behavior Services
  Assessment
    Administered by Physician/QHP ~ 0362T, 97151
    Supporting, Administered by Technician ~ 0362T, 97152
  Treatment
    Group ~ 97154, 97158
    Individual ~ 0373T, 97153, 97155
    Treatment Guidance ~ 97156, 97157
Addam operation ~ 26040-26045
Adductor tenotomy of hip ~ 27000-27003
Adenoidectomy ~ 42820-42821, 42830-42836

Adenoids
  excision ~ 42830-42836
    with tonsils ~ 42820-42821
  unlisted services and procedures ~ 42999
Adenoma
  pancreas, excision ~ 48120
  thyroid gland excision ~ 60200
Adenosine 3'5' monophosphate ~ 82030
Adenosine diphosphate, blood ~ 82030
Adenosine monophosphate (AMP), blood ~ 82030
Adenovirus
  antibody ~ 86603
  antigen detection
    enzyme immunoassay ~ 87301
    immunofluorescense ~ 87260
Adenovirus vaccine ~ *see* vaccines
Adenylic acid ~ *see* adenosine monophosphate (AMP)
ADH (antidiuretic hormone) ~ 84588
Adhesions
  epidural ~ , 62263-62264
  eye
    corneovitreal ~ 65880
    incision
      anterior segment ~ 65860-65870
      posterior segment ~ 65875
    intermarginal, construction ~ 67880
      transposition of tarsal plate ~ 67882
  intestinal, enterolysis ~ 44005
    laparoscopic ~ 44180
  intracranial, dissection ~ 62161
  intrauterine, lysis ~ 58559
  labial, lysis ~ 56441
  liver, lysis ~ 58660
  lungs, pneumolysis ~ 32124, 32940
  nose, lysis ~ 30560
  pelvic, lysis ~ 58660, 58740
  penile, lysis, post-circumcision ~ 54162
  preputial, lysis ~ 54450
  urethral, lysis ~ 53500
Adipectomy ~ *see* lipectomy
ADL ~ *see* activities of daily living
Administration
  immunization
    each additional vaccine/toxoid ~ 90472, 90474
      with counseling ~ 90461
    one vaccine/toxoid ~ 90471, 90473
      with counseling ~ 90460
  occlusive substance ~ 31634
  pharmacologic agent ~ 93463
ADP ~ *see* adenosine diphosphate
ADP phosphocreatine phosphotransferase ~ *see* CPK
Adrenal cortex hormone ~ *see* corticosteroids
Adrenal gland
  biopsy ~ 60540-60545
  excision ~ 60540
    laparoscopy ~ 60650
    retroperitoneal tumor ~ 60545
  exploration ~ 60540-60545
  nuclear medicine, imaging ~ 78075
Adrenal medulla ~ *see* medulla
Adrenalectomy ~ 60540
  anesthesia ~ 00866
  laparoscopic ~ 50545
Adrenalin ~ 80424, 82382-82384
  blood ~ 82383
  urine ~ 82382, 82384
Adrenaline-noradrenaline
  testing ~ 82382-82384
Adrenocorticotropic hormone (ACTH) ~ 80400-80406, 80412, 80418,
    82024
  blood or urine ~ 82024
  stimulation panel ~ 80400-80406
Adrenogenital syndrome ~ 56805, 57335
Adult T cell leukemia lymphoma virus I ~ *see* HTLV I
Advanced life support ~ 99281-99288
  physician direction ~ 99288
Advancement
  genioglossus ~ 21199
  tendon foot ~ 28238
Advancement flap ~ 14000-14350

Aerosol inhalation ~ *see* pulmonology, therapeutic
  pentamidine ~ 94642
AFB ~ *see* acid fast bacilli
Afferent nerve ~ *see* sensory nerve
AFP ~ *see* alpha-fetoprotein
After hours medical services ~ 99050
Agents, anticoagulant ~ 85300-85305, 85307
Agglutinin
  cold ~ 86156-86157
  febrile ~ 86000
Aggregation, platelet ~ 85576
AHG ~ 85210-85293
AICD (pacing cardioverter-defibrillator) ~ *see* defibrillator, heart;
  pacemaker, heart
Aid, hearing ~ *see* hearing aid
AIDS antibodies ~ 86689, 86701-86703
AIDS virus ~ *see* HIV-1
Akin operation ~ 28296-28299
ALA ~ *see* aminolevulinic acid
Alanine 2 oxoglutarate aminotransferase ~ 84460
Alanine amino (ALT) ~ 84460
Alanine transaminase ~ 84460
Albumin
  ischemia modified ~ 82045
  serum ~ 82040
  urine ~ 82042-82044
Alcohol
  breath ~ 82075
    ethylene glycol ~ 82693
  ethanol
    any specimen except breath, urine ~ 82077
    breath ~ 82075
  dehydrogenase
    gene analysis ~ 81205, 81400, 81401
  methyl
    definitive drug identification ~ 80320
Aldolase, blood ~ 82085
Aldosterone
  blood ~ 82088
  suppression evaluation ~ 80408
  urine ~ 82088
Alimentary canal ~ *see* gastrointestinal tract
Alkaline phosphatase ~ 84075-84080
  leukocyte ~ 85540
  WBC ~ 85540
Alkaloids ~ *see* specific drug
  urine ~ 80323
Allergen bronchial provocation tests ~ 95070
Allergen challenge, endobronchial ~ 95070
Allergen immunotherapy
  allergen
    IgE ~ 86003, 86005, 86008
    IgG ~ 86001
    multiallergen screen ~ 86005
  allergenic extracts
    injection ~ 95115, 95117
    injection and provision ~ 95120-95134
    insect venom ~ 95130-95134
  antigens ~ 95144-95165
    insect venom ~ 95145-95149
  insect, whole body extract ~ 95170
  rapid desensitization ~ 95180
Allergy services/procedures ~ 95004-95199
  unlisted services and procedures ~ 95199
Allergy tests
  challenge test
    bronchial ~ 95070
    ingestion ~ 95076, 95079
  eye allergy ~ 95060
  food allergy ~ 95076, 95079
  intradermal
    allergen extract ~ 95024-95028
    biologicals ~ 95018
    drugs ~ 95018
    incremental ~ 95027
    venoms ~ 95017
  nasal mucous membrane test ~ 95065
  nose allergy ~ 95065

Allergy tests ~ *continued*
  patch
    application tests ~ 95044
    photo patch ~ 95052
  photosensitivity ~ 95056
  skin tests
    allergen extract ~ 95004, 95024, 95027
    biologicals ~ 95018
    drugs ~ 95018
    venoms ~ 95017
Allogeneic donor, lymphocyte infusion ~ 38242
Allogeneic transplantation ~ *see* homograft
Allograft
  aortic valve ~ 33406, 33413
  bone
    elbow joint ~ 24370, 24371
    shoulder joint ~ 23473-23474
    spine surgery
      morselized ~ 20930
      structural ~ 20931
  cartilage, knee ~ 27415
  cornea
    amniotic membrane ~65780
    endothelial ~ 65756
    lamellar ~ 65710
    penetrating ~ 65730, 65750, 65755
    for Aphakia ~ 65750
  lung transplant ~ 32850
  nerve ~ 64910, 64912, 64913
  skin ~ 15350-15351
  skin substitute graft ~ 15271-15278
  spine surgery
    morselized ~ 20930
    structural ~ 20931
Allograft preparation
  cornea ~ 65757
  heart ~ 33933, 33944
  intestines ~ 44715-44721
  kidney ~ 50323-50329
  liver ~ 47143-47147
  lung ~ 32855-32856, 33933
  pancrease ~ 48551-48552
  renal ~ 50323-50329
Allotransplantation
  intestines ~ 44135-44137
  renal ~ 50360-50365
    removal ~ 50370
Almen test ~ 82270
Alpha-1 antitrypsin ~ 82103-82104
Alpha-2 antiplasmin ~ 85410
Alpha-fetoprotein
  amniotic fluid ~ 82106
  serum ~ 82105, 82107
Alphatocopherol ~ 84446
ALT ~ 84460
Altemeier procedure ~ (*see* anus) 45130-45135
Aluminum, blood ~ 82108
Alveolafracture
  closed treatment ~ 21421
  open treatment ~ 21422-21423
Alveolar cleft
  ungrafted bilateral ~ 21147
  ungrafted unilateral ~ 21146
Alveolar nerve
  avulsion ~ 64738
  incision ~ 64738
  transection ~ 64738
Alveolar ridge fracture
  closed treatment ~ 21440
  open treatment ~ 21445
Alveolectomy ~ 41830
Alveoloplasty ~ 41874
Alveolus, excision ~ 41830
Amide, procaine ~ *see* procainamide
Amikacin, assay ~ 80150
Amine, vaginal fluid ~ 82120
Amino acids ~ 82127-82139
Aminolevulinic acid (ALA), blood or urine ~ 82135
Aminotransferase ~ *see* transaminase
Aminotransferase, alanine ~ 84460
Aminotransferase, aspartate ~ 84450

Amitriptyline, assay ~ 80335, 80336, 80337
Ammonia
  blood ~ 82140
  urine ~ 82140
Amniocenteses ~ 59000
  with amniotic fluid reduction ~ 59001
  induced abortion ~ 59850
    with dilation and curettage ~ 59851
    with dilation and evacuation ~ 59851
    with hysterectomy ~ 59852
Amnioinfusion, transabdominal ~ 59070
Amnion ~ 59001
  amniocentesis ~ 59000
    with amniotic fluid reduction ~ 59001
  amnioinfusion, transabdominal ~ 59070
Amniotic fluid
  alpha-fetoprotein ~ 82106
  scan ~ 82143
  testing ~ 83661, 83663-83664
Amniotic membrane ~ 59001
  ocular wound healing ~ 65778-65779
Amobarbital ~ 80345
AMP ~ 82030
AMP, cyclic ~ 82030
Amphetamine, blood or urine ~ 80324-80326
Amputation ~ *see* radical resection; replantation
  ankle ~ 27888
  arm, lower ~ 25900-25905, 25915
    revision ~ 25907-25909
  arm, upper ~ 24900-24920
    and shoulder ~ 23900-23921
    revision ~ 24925-24930
      with implant ~ 24931-24935
  cervix, total ~ 57530
  ear
    partial ~ 69110
    total ~ 69120
  finger ~ 26910-26952
  foot ~ 28800-28805
  hand at metacarpal ~ 25927
    at wrist ~ 25920
      revision ~ 25922
    revision ~ 25924, 25929-25931
  interpelviabdominal ~ 27290
  interthoracoscapular ~ 23900
  leg, lower ~ 27598, 27880-27882
    revision ~ 27884-27886
  leg, upper ~ 27590-27592
    at hip ~ 27290-27295
    revision ~ 27594-27596
  metacarpal ~ 26910
  metatarsal ~ 28810
  nose ~ *see* resection, nose
  penis
    partial ~ 54120
    radical ~ 54130-54135
    total ~ 54125
  thumb ~ 26910-26952
  toe ~ 28810-28825
  upper extremity ~ 24900-24940
    cineplasty ~ 24940
    revision ~ 24925, 24930, 24935
    with implant ~ 24931-24935
Amylase
  blood ~ 82150
  urine ~ 82150
ANA ~ 86038-86039
Anabolic steroid ~ *see* androstenedione
Anal abscess ~ *see* abscess, anal
Anal bleeding ~ *see* anus, hemorrhage
Anal fistula ~ *see* fistula, anal
Anal fistulectomy ~ 46288, 46706
Anal fistulotomy ~ 46270, 46280
Anal sphincter
  dilation ~ 45905
  incision ~ 46080
Anal ulceration ~ *see* anus, fissure
Analgesia ~ *see* anesthesia; sedation 99141-99142

Analysis
  computer data ~ 99090
    cardiovascular monitoring ~ 93290, 93297
    implantable defibrillator ~ 93260, 93261, 93282-93284, 93287,
      93295, 93296, 93640, 93641
    leadless pacemaker system ~ 0388T-0391T
    loop recorder ~ 93285, 93291, 93298
    pacemaker ~ 93279-93281, 93288, 93293-93294
  electroencephalogram, digital ~ 95957
  electronic
    drug infusion pump ~ 62367-62370
    neurostimulator pulse generator system
      brain ~ 95970, 95983, 95984
      cranial nerve ~ 95970, 95976, 95977
      gastric ~ 95980-95982
      peripheral nerve ~ 95970-95972
      spinal cord ~ 95970-95972
      with programming ~ 95971, 95972, 95976, 95977, 95980,
        95982-95984
      without reprogramming ~ 95970, 95981
      with vagus nerve blocking therapy ~ 0317T
  multianalyte assays with algorithmic analysis (MAAA)
    endocrinology analytes ~ 81506
    fetal aneuploidy DNA sequence ~ 81507
    fetal congenital abnormal ~ 81508-81512
    gene expression for oncology ~ 81504
    ovarian oncology proteins ~ 81500, 81503
    unlisted assay ~ 81599
  physiologic data, remote ~ 99091
    proprietary laboratory ~ 0001U-003U, 0005U-0014U, 0016U-0061U
  protein, tissue western blot ~ 88372
  semen ~ 89320-89322
    sperm isolation ~ 89260-89261
  spectrum ~ *see* spectrophotometry
  waveform, central arterial pressure ~ 93050
Anaspadias ~ *see* epispadias
Anastomosis
  aorta-pulmonary artery ~ 33606
  arteriovenous fistula
    direct ~ 36821
    with bypass graft ~ 35686
    with graft ~ 36825-36830, 36832
  artery
    extracranial-intracranial ~ 61711
    iliac arteriovenous implant placement ~ 0553T
    pulmonary artery to aorta ~ 33606
  atria to pulmonary arter ~ 33615
  bile duct
    to bile duct ~ 47800
    to intestines ~ 47760, 47780
  bile duct to gastrointestinal ~ 47785
  bladder, to intestine ~ 51960
  broncho-bronchial ~ 32486
  caval to mesenteric ~ 37160
  colorectal ~ 44620
  epididymis
    to vas deferens
      bilateral ~ 54901
      unilateral ~ 54900
  excision trachea ~ 31780-31781
  fallopian tube ~ 58750
  gallbladder to intestines ~ 47720-47740
  hepatic duct ~ *see* hepatic duct, anastomosis
  Anastomosis ~ *continued*
  hepatic duct to intestines ~ 47765, 47802
  ileo-anal ~ 45113
  intestines
    colo-anal ~ 45119
    cystectomy ~ 51590
    enterocystoplasty ~ 51960
    resection, laparoscopic ~ 44202-44205
  intestine to intestine ~ 44130
  intrahepatic portosystemic ~ 37182-37183
  jejunum ~ 43825
  lacrimal sac to conjunctival sac ~ *see* conjunctivorhinostomy
  microvascular, free transfer, jejunum ~ 43496
  nerve
    facial to hypoglossal ~ 64868

Anastomosis ~ *continued*
- oviduct ~ 58750
- pancreas ~ see pancreas, anastomosis
- pancreas to intestines ~ 48520-48540, 48548
- portocaval ~ 37140
- pulmonary ~ 33606
- renoportal ~ 37145
- splenorenal ~ 37180-37181
- stomach ~ 43825
  - to duodenum ~ 43810, 43855
    - revision ~ 43850
  - to jejunum ~ 43820, 43860-43865
- tubotubal ~ 58750
- ureter
  - to bladder ~ 50780-50785
  - to colon ~ 50810-50815
    - removal ~ 50830
  - to intestine ~ 50800, 50820-50825
    - removal ~ 50830
  - to kidney ~ 50727-50750
  - to ureter ~ 50727, 50760-50770
- vein, saphenopopliteal ~ 34530
- vein to vein ~ 37140-37160, 37182-37183

Anatomic pathology services ~ 88000-88099
Anderson tibial lengthening ~ *see* ankle 27715
Androstanediol glucuronide ~ 82154
Androstanolone ~ 80327, 80328
Androstenedione, blood or urine ~ 82157
Androstenolone ~ 82626
Androsterone, blood or urine ~ 82160
Anesthesia ~ 00100-01999
- Abbe-Estlander procedure ~ 00102
- abdomen
  - abdominal wall ~ 00700, 00730, 00800-00802, 00820, 00836
    - Halsted repair ~ 00750-00756
  - blood vessels ~ 00770, 00880-00882
  - endoscopy ~ 00731, 00732, 00811-00813
  - extraperitoneal ~ 00860-00870
  - hernia repair ~ 00830-00836
    - Halsted repair ~ 00750-00756
  - intraperitoneal ~ 00790-00797, 00840-00851
- abdominoperineal resection ~ 00844
- abortion, induced ~ 01964
- Achilles tendon repair ~ 01472
- acromioclavicular joint ~ 01620
- adrenalectomy ~ 00866
- amniocentesis ~ 00842
- aneurysm
  - axillary-brachial ~ 01652
  - knee ~ 01444
  - popliteal artery ~ 01444
- angiography ~ 01920
- ankle ~ 00400, 01462-01522
- anorectal procedure ~ 00902
- anus ~ 00902
- arm
  - lower ~ 00400, 01810-01820, 01830-01860
  - upper ~ 00400, 01710-01782
- arrhythmias ~ 00410
- arteriography ~ 01916
- arteriovenous fistula ~ 01432, 01784
- arthroplasty
  - hip ~ 01214-01215
  - knee ~ 01402
- arthroscopic procedures
  - ankle ~ 01464
  - elbow ~ 01732-01740
  - foot ~ 01464
  - hip ~ 01202
  - knee ~ 01382, 01400
  - shoulder ~ 01622-01630
  - wrist ~ 01829-01830
- auditory canal, external, removal foreign body ~ 69205
- axilla ~ 00400, 01610, 01650, 01652, 01654, 01656, 01670
- back skin ~ 00300
- Batch-Spittler-McFaddin operation ~ 01404
- biopsy ~ 00100
  - liver ~ 00702
- bladder ~ 00870, 00912
- brain ~ 00210-00218, 00220-00222

Anesthesia ~ *continued*
- breast ~ 00402-00406
- bronchi ~ 00542
  - intrathoracic repair of trauma ~ 00548
  - reconstruction ~ 00539
- bronchoscopy ~ 00520
- burns
  - debridement and/or excision ~ 01951-01953
  - dressings and/or debridement ~ 16010-16015
- burr hole ~ 00214
- bypass graft
  - leg, lower ~ 01500
  - leg, upper ~ 01270
  - shoulder, axillary ~ 01654-01656
- cardiac catheterization ~ 01920
- cast, knee ~ 01420
- cast application
  - forearm, wrist and hand ~ 01860
  - leg ~ 01490
  - pelvis ~ 01130
  - shoulder ~ 01680
- central venous circulation ~ 00532
- cervical cerclage ~ 00948
- cervix ~ 00948
- cesarean delivery ~ 01961, 01963
- chest ~ 00400-00406, 00410, 00470-00474, 00522, 00530-00539, 00542, 00546-00550
- chest skin ~ 00400
- childbirth
  - cesarean delivery ~ 01961, 01963, 01968-01969
  - external cephalic version ~ 01958
  - vaginal delivery ~ 01960, 01967
- clavicle ~ 00450-00454
- cleft lip repair ~ 00102
- cleft palate repair ~ 00172
- colonoscopy, screening ~ 00812
- colpectomy ~ 00942
- colporrhaphy ~ 00942
- colpotomy ~ 00942
- corneal transplant ~ 00144
- cranioplasty ~ 00215
- culdoscopy ~ 00950
- cystectomy ~ 00864
- cystolithotomy ~ 00870
- cystourethroscopy
  - local ~ 52265
  - spinal ~ 52260
- decortication ~ 00542
- defibrillator ~ 00534, 00560
- diaphragm ~ 00540-00541
- disarticulation
  - hip ~ 01212
  - knee ~ 01404
  - shoulder ~ 01634
- diskography ~ 01935, 01936
- dressing change ~ 15852
- drug administration, epidural or subarachnoid ~ 01996
- ear ~ 00120-00126
- elbow ~ 00400, 01710-01782
- electrocoagulation, intracranial nerve ~ 00222
- electroconvulsive therapy ~ 00104
- embolectomy
  - arm, upper ~ 01772
  - femoral ~ 01274
  - femoral artery ~ 01274
  - forearm, wrist and hand ~ 01842
  - leg, lower ~ 01502
- endoscopy
  - arm, lower ~ 01830
  - gastrointestinal ~ 00731, 00732, 00813
  - intestines ~ 00811-00812
  - uterus ~ 00952
  - vagina ~ 00950
- esophagus ~ 00320, 00500
- external cephalic version ~ 01958
- external fixation system
  - adjustment/revision ~ 20693
  - removal ~ 20694

Anesthesia ~ *continued*

eye ~ 00140-00148
   cornea ~ 00144
   iridectomy ~ 00147
   iris ~ 00147
eyelid ~ 00103
facial bones ~ 00190-00192
fallopian tube, ligation ~ 00851
femoral artery, ligation ~ 01272
femur ~ 01220-01234, 01340-01360
fibula ~ 01390-01392
foot ~ 00400, 01462-01522
forearm ~ 00400, 01810-01820, 01830-01860
Fowler-Stephens orchiopexy ~ 00930
gastrocnemius recession ~ 01474
gastrointestinal endoscopy ~ 00731, 00732, 00813
genitalia
   female ~ 00940-00952, 01958-01969
   male ~ 00920-00938
great vessels of chest ~ 00560-00563
hand ~ 00400, 01810-01820, 01830-01860
Harrington rod technique ~ 00670
head ~ 00222, 00300
   muscles ~ 00300
   nerves ~ 00300
heart ~ 00560-00567, 00580
   coronary artery bypass grafting ~ 00566-00567
   electrophysiology/ablation ~ 00537
   transplant ~ 00580
hepatectomy, partial ~ 00792
hernia repair, abdomen
   lower ~ 00830-00836
   upper ~ 00750-00752, 00756
hip ~ 01200-01215
humerus ~ 01620, 01730, 01742-01744, 01758
hysterectomy ~ 01962
   cesarean ~ 01963, 01969
   radical ~ 00846
   vaginal ~ 00944
hysterosalpingography ~ 00952
hysteroscopy ~ 00952
induced abortion ~ 01964
inferior vena cava ligation ~ 00882
injections, nerve ~ 01991-01992
integumentary system
   anterior trunk ~ 00400
   arm, upper ~ 00400
   axilla ~ 00400
   elbow ~ 00400
   extremity ~ 00400
   forearm ~ 00400
   hand ~ 00400
   head ~ 00300
   knee ~ 00400
   leg, lower ~ 00400
   leg, upper ~ 00400
   neck ~ 00300
   perineum ~ 00400
   popliteal area ~ 00400
   posterior pelvis ~ 00300
   posterior trunk ~ 00300
   shoulder ~ 00400
   wrist ~ 00400
intestines, endoscopy ~ 00811-00813
intracranial procedures ~ 00210-00218, 00220-00222
intraoral procedures ~ 00170-00176
intrathoracic procedures
   bronchi ~ 00539, 00548
   trachea ~ 00539, 00548
intrathoracic system ~ 00500, 00520-00529, 00530-00539, 00540-00548, 00550, 00560-00567, 00580
iridectomy ~ 00147
Keen operation ~ 00604
kidney ~ 00862, 00868, 00872-00873
knee ~ 00400, 01320-01444
knee skin ~ 00400
laminectomy ~ 00604
laparoscopy ~ 00790-00792, 00840
larynx ~ 00320, 00326

Anesthesia ~ *continued*

leg
   lower ~ 00400, 01462-01522
   upper ~ 01200-01274
lens ~ 00142
life support for organ donor ~ 01990
ligation, fallopian tube ~ 00851
lithotripsy ~ 00872-00873
liver ~ 00702, 00796
   transplant ~ 00796
liver hemorrhage ~ 00792
lumbar puncture ~ 00635
lungs ~ 00522, 00539, 00540-00548
   transplant ~ 00580
lymphadenectomy ~ 00934-00936
lymphatic system ~ 00320
mammoplasty ~ 00402
marcellation operation ~ 00944
mediastinoscopy ~ 00528-00529
mediastinum ~ 00528-00529, 00540-00541
mouth ~ 00170-00172
myelography ~ 01935, 01936
myringotomy ~ 69421
neck ~ 00300, 00320-00322, 00350-00352
nephrectomy ~ 00862
neuraxial
   cesarean delivery ~ 01968-01969
   labor ~ 01967-01969
   vaginal delivery ~ 01967
nose ~ 00160-00164
   removal, foreign body ~ 30310
omphalocele ~ 00754
ophthalmoscopy ~ 00148
orchiectomy ~ 00926-00928
orchiopexy ~ 00930
   Torek procedure ~ 00930
organ harvesting, brain dead patient ~ 01990
osteoplasty, tibia/fibula ~ 01484
osteotomy
   humerus ~ 01742
   tibia/fibula ~ 01484
other procedures ~ 01990, 01996-01999
otoscopy ~ 00124
pacemaker insertion ~ 00530
pacing cardioverter/defibrillator ~ 00534
pancreas ~ 00794
pancreatectomy ~ 00794
panniculectomy ~ 00802
patella ~ 01390-01392
pectus excavatum ~ 00474
pelvic exenteration ~ 00848
pelvis ~ 00400, 00865, 01112
   amputation ~ 01140
   bone ~ 01120
   bone marrow ~ 01112
   examination ~ 57400
   extraperitoneal ~ 00864
   intraperitoneal ~ 00844-00848
   repair ~ 01173
   skin ~ 00300, 00400
penis ~ 00932-00938
pericardial sac ~ 00560-00563
perineum ~ 00904-00908
pharynx ~ 00174-00176
phleborrhaphy
   arm, upper ~ 01782
   forearm, wrist, and hand ~ 01852
pleura ~ 00540-00541
   needle biopsy ~ 00522
pneumocentesis ~ 00524
popliteal area ~ 00400, 01320, 01430-01444
prognathism ~ 00192
prostate ~ 00865, 00908, 00914
prostatectomy
   perineal ~ 00908
   radical ~ 00865
   Walsh modified radical ~ 00865
radiologic procedures ~ 01916-01936
   arterial, therapeutic ~ 01924-01926
   venous/lymphatic, therapeutic ~ 01930-01933

Anesthesia ~ continued
renal procedures ~ 00862
repair of skull ~ 00215
replacement
   ankle ~ 01486
   elbow ~ 01760
   hip ~ 01212-01215
   knee ~ 01402
   shoulder ~ 01638
   wrist ~ 01832
restriction, gastric
   for obesity ~ 00797
retropharyngeal tumor excision ~ 00174
rib resection ~ 00470-00474
sacroiliac joint ~ 01160-01170, 27096
salivary glands ~ 00100
Scheie procedure ~ 00147
sedation, moderate ~ 99151-99153, 99155-99157
   with independent observation ~ 99151-99153
seminal vesicles ~ 00922
shoulder ~ 00400, 00450-00454, 01610, 01620, 01622, 01630, 01634,
   01636, 01638
   dislocation, closed treatment ~ 23655
shunt, spinal fluid ~ 00220
sinuses, accessory ~ 00160-00164
skull ~ 00190
skull fracture, elevation ~ 00215
special circumstances
   emergency ~ 99140
   extreme age ~ 99100
   hypotension ~ 99135
   hypothermia ~ 99116
spinal instrumentation ~ 00670
spinal manipulation ~ 00640
spine and spinal cord ~ 00600-00604, 00620, 00670
   cervical ~ 00600-00604, 00640, 00670
   injection ~ 62320-62327
   lumbar ~ 00630-00635, 00640, 00670
   percutaneous image guided ~ 01935, 01936
   thoracic ~ 00620-00626, 00640, 00670
   vascular ~ 00670
sternoclavicular joint ~ 01620
sternum ~ 00550
stomach, restriction, for obesity ~ 00797
Strayer procedure ~ 01474
subdural taps ~ 00212
suture removal ~ 15850-15851
sympathectomy
   lumbar ~ 00632
symphysis pubis ~ 01160-01170
tenodesis ~ 01716
tenoplasty ~ 01714
tenotomy ~ 01712
testis ~ 00924-00930
thoracoplasty ~ 00472
thoracoscopy ~ 00528-00529, 00540-00541
thoracotomy ~ 00540-00541
thorax ~ 00400-00406, 00410, 00450-00454, 00470-00474
thromboendarterectomy ~ 01442
thyroid ~ 00320-00322
tibia ~ 01390-01392, 01484
trachea ~ 00320, 00326, 00542
   reconstruction ~ 00539
transplantation
   cornea ~ 00144
   heart ~ 00580
   kidney ~ 00868
   liver ~ 00796, 01990
   lungs ~ 00580
   organ harvesting ~ 01990
transurethral procedures ~ 00910-00918
tubal ligation ~ 00851
tuffier vaginal hysterectomy ~ 00944
TURP ~ 00914
tympanostomy ~ 00120
tympanotomy ~ 00126
unlisted services and procedures ~ 01999
urethra ~ 00910, 00918-00920, 00942
urethrocystoscopy ~ 00910
urinary bladder ~ 00864, 00870, 00912

Anesthesia ~ continued
urinary tract ~ 00860
uterus ~ 00952
vagina ~ 00940-00942, 00950
   dilation ~ 57400
   removal, foreign body ~ 57415
vaginal delivery ~ 01960
vas deferens, excision ~ 00921
vascular access ~ 00532
vascular shunt ~ 01844
vascular surgery
   abdomen, lower ~ 00880-00882
   abdomen, upper ~ 00770
   arm, lower ~ 01840-01852
   arm, upper ~ 01770-01782
   brain ~ 00216
   elbow ~ 01770-01782
   hand ~ 01840-01852
   knee ~ 01430-01444
   leg, lower ~ 01500-01522
   leg, upper ~ 01260-01274
   neck ~ 00350-00352
   shoulder ~ 01650-01670
   wrist ~ 01840-01852
vasectomy ~ 00921
venography ~ 01916
ventriculography ~ 00214, 01920
vertebral process, fracture/dislocation, closed treatment ~ 22315
vertebroplasty ~ 01935, 01936
vitrectomy ~ 00145
vitreoretinal surgery ~ 00145
vitreous body ~ 00145
vulva ~ 00906
vulvectomy ~ 00906
Wertheim operation ~ 00846
wrist ~ 00400, 01810-01860
Aneurysm repair
abdominal aorta ~ 34830-34832, 34845-34848, 35081-35103
axillary artery ~ 35011-35013
basilar artery ~ 61698, 61702
brachial artery ~ 35011-35013
carotid artery ~ 35001-35002, 61613, 61697, 61700, 61703
celiac artery ~ 35121-35122
femoral artery ~ 35141-35142
hepatic artery ~ 35121-35122
iliac artery ~ 34703-34708, 34717, 34718, 35131, 35132
infrarenal artery ~ 34701-34706, 34709-34711
innominate artery ~ 35021, 35022
intracranial artery ~ 61705-61708
mesenteric artery ~ 35121-35122
popliteal artery ~ 35151-35152
radial artery ~ 35045
renal artery ~ 35121-35122
splenic artery ~ 35111-35112
subclavian artery ~ 35001-35002, 35021-35022
thoracoabdominal aorta ~ 33877
ulnar artery ~ 35045
vascular malformation or carotid-cavernous fistula ~ 61710
vertebral artery ~ 61698, 61702
Angel dust ~ 83992
Angina assessment ~ *see* performance measure
Angiocardiographies ~ *see* heart, angiography
Angiography
abdomen ~ 74174-74175, 74185, 75635, 75726
adrenal ~ 75731-75733
arm artery ~ 73206, 75710, 75716
brain ~ 70496
bypass graft ~ 93455, 93457, 93459-93461
carotid artery ~ 36221-36228
cervicocerebral arch ~ 36221-36226
chest ~ 71275, 71555
congenital heart ~ 93563-93564
common carotid, selective catheterization ~ 36222, 36223
endovascular repair ~ 75956, 75957
extracranial carotid
   non-selective ~ 36221
   selective ~ 36222-36224
extremity, lower ~ 73725
extremity, upper ~ 73225
fluorescein ~ 92235, 92242

Angiography~*continued*
head ~ 70496, 70544-70546
heart
    abdominal aorta ~ 75635
    aorta, injection ~ 93567
    atrial ~ 93565, 93566
    congenital heart ~ 93563, 93564
    coronary artery ~ 93454-93461, 93563
      flow velocity measurement ~ 93571, 93572
    left heart injection ~ 93565
    right heart injection ~ 93566
injection ~ 93454-93461, 93563, 93565, 93566
indocyanine-green ~ 92240, 92242
innominate artery ~ 36222, 36223, 36225
intracranial ~ 36221, 36223, 36224
    with endovascular infusion ~ 61640, 61650, 61651
    with thrombectomy ~ 61645
left heart, injection ~ 93565
leg artery ~ 73706, 75635, 75710-75716
lung, injection ~ 93568
mammary artery ~ 75756
neck ~ 70498, 70547-70549
    artery ~ 36221-36226
nuclear medicine ~ 78445
other artery ~ 75774
pelvic artery ~ 72198, 75736
pelvis ~ 72191, 74174
pulmonary ~ 75741-75746, 93568
renal artery ~ 36251-36254
right heart, injection ~ 93566
spinal artery ~ 75705
spinal canal ~ 72159
thorax ~ 71275
transcatheter therapy
    embolization ~ 75894, 75898
    infusion ~ 75894, 75898
ventricular ~ 93565-93566
vertebral ~ 36211, 36225-36226, 36228
Angioma ~ see lesion, skin
Angioplasties, coronary balloon ~ see percutaneous transluminal
    angioplasty
Angioplasty
aorta
    intraoperative ~ 37246, 37247
    percutaneous ~ 37246, 37247
axillary artery, intraoperative ~ 37246, 37247
brachiocephalic artery
    intraoperative ~ 37246, 37247
    percutaneous ~ 37246, 37247
coronary artery
    percutaneous transluminal ~ 92920, 92921
    with atherectomy ~ 92937, 92938, 92941, 92943, 92944
    with stent placement ~ 92928, 92929, 92937, 92938, 92941, 92943, 92944
femoral artery, intraoperative ~ 37224
iliac artery, intraoperative ~ 37220, 37222
intracranial, percutaneous ~ 61630
patch
    blood vessel ~ 35201-35286
    vein ~ 35879
percutaneous transluminal angioplasty ~ see percutaneous transluminal
    angioplasty
perineal artery ~ 37228
popliteal artery, intraoperative ~ 37224
pulmonary artery, percutaneous transluminal ~ 92997, 92998
renal artery
    open ~ 37246-37249
    percutaneous ~ 37246-37249
subclavian artery, intraoperative ~ 37246, 37247
tibioperoneal artery, intraoperative ~ 37228
    balloon ~ 37246-37249
    dialysis circuit ~ 36902, 36907
    venous ~ 37248, 37249
venous
    open ~ 37248, 37249
    percutaneous ~ 37248, 37249
visceral artery
    open ~ 37246, 37247
    percutaneous ~ 37246, 37247
with endovascular repair ~ 34841-34848
with intravascular stent placement ~ 37215-37218, 37236-37239

Angioscopy, non-coronary vessels ~ 35400
Angiotensin converting enzyme (ACE) ~ 82164
Angiotensin forming enzyme ~ 80408, 80416, 84244
Angiotensin I ~ 84244
    riboflavin ~ 84252
Angiotensin II, blood or urine ~ 82163
Angle deformity, reconstruction toe ~ 28313
Anhydride, carbonic ~ 82374
Anhydrides, acetic ~ 84600
Animal inoculation ~ 87003, 87250
Ankle
(see also fibula; leg, lower; tibia; tibiofibular joint)
abscess, incision and drainage ~ 27603
amputation ~ 27888
arthrocentesis ~ 20605
arthrodesis ~ 27870
arthrography ~ 73615
arthroplasty ~ 27700-27703
arthroscopy, surgical ~ 29891-29899
arthrotomy ~ 27610-27612, 27620-27626
biopsy ~ 27613-27614, 27620
bursa, incision and drainage ~ 27604
disarticulation ~ 27889
dislocation
    closed treatment ~ 27840-27842
    open treatment ~ 27846-27848
exploration ~ 27610, 27620
fracture
    bimalleolar ~ 27808-27814
    lateral ~ 27786-27814, 27792
    medial ~ 27760-27766, 27808-27814
    posterior ~ 27767-27769, 27808-27814
    trimalleolar ~ 27816-27823
fusion ~ 27870
hematoma, incision and drainage ~ 27603
incision ~ 27607
injection, radiologic ~ 27648
lesion excision ~ 27630
magnetic resonance imaging (MRI) ~ 73721-73723
manipulation ~ 27860
removal
    foreign body ~ 27610, 27620
    implant ~ 27704
    loose body ~ 27620
repair
    Achilles tendon ~ 27650-27654
    ligament ~ 27695-27698
    tendon ~ 27612, 27680-27687
strapping ~ 29540
synovium, excision ~ 27625-27626
tenotomy ~ 27605-27606
tumor, excision ~ 27615-27619, 27632, 27634
unlisted services and procedures ~ 27899
X-ray ~ 73600-73610
    with contrast ~ 73615
Ankylosis (surgical) ~ see arthrodesis
Annuloplasty
percutaneous, intradiscal ~ 22526-22527
Anogenital region ~ see perineum
Anoplasty, stricture ~ 46700-46705
Anorectal biofeedback ~ 90912, 90913
Anorectal exam (surgical) ~ 45990
Anorectal fistula, repair ~ 46706, 76707
Anorectal myectomy ~ 45108
Anorectovaginoplasty ~ 46744-46746
Anoscopy
ablation, polyp/tumor ~ 46615
biopsy ~ 46606
collection of specimen ~ 46600, 46601
dilation ~ 46604
exploration ~ 46600
hemorrhage ~ 46614
high resolution anoscopy (HRA)
    diagnostic ~ 46601
    with biopsies ~ 46607
removal
    foreign body ~ 46608
    polyp/tumor ~ 46610-46612
Antebrachium ~ 20805
Antecedent, plasma thromboplastin ~ 85270

Antepartum care
  vaginal delivery ~ 59400, 59425-59426
  with cesarean delivery ~ 59510
    previous ~ 59610, 59618
Anterior ramus of thoracic nerve ~ see intercostal nerve
Anthrax vaccine ~ 90476-90749
Anthrogon ~ 80418, 80426, 83001
Anti Australia antigens ~ see antibody, hepatitis B
Anti D immunoglobulin ~ 90384-90386
Anti-human globulin consumption test ~ 86880
Anti-phospholipid antibody ~ 86147
Antiactivator, plasmin ~ 85410
Antibiotic administration
  injection ~ 96372
  prescribed or dispensed ~ 4120F-4124F
Antibiotic sensitivity ~ 87181-87184, 87188
  enzyme detection ~ 87185
  minimum bactericidal concentration ~ 87187
  minimum inhibitory concentration ~ 87186
Antibody detection
  actinomyces ~ 86602
  adenovirus ~ 86603
  antinuclear ~ 86038-86039
  antiphosphatidylserine (phospholipid) ~ 86148
  antistreptolysin O ~ 86060-86063
  aspergillus ~ 86606
  bacterium ~ 86609
  bartonella ~ 86611
  beta 2 glycoprotein 1 ~ 86146
  blastomyces ~ 86612
  blood crossmatch ~ 86920-86923
  bordetella ~ 86615
  borrelia ~ 86618-86619
  brucella ~ 86622
  campylobacter ~ 86625
  candida ~ 86628
  cardiolipin ~ 86147
  chlamydia ~ 86631-86632
  coccidioides ~ 86635
  coxiella burnetii ~ 86638
  c-reactive protein (CRP) ~ 86140-86141
  cryptococcus ~ 86641
  cyclic citrullinated peptide (CCP)~ 86200
  cytomegalovirus ~ 86644-86645
  cytotoxic screen ~ 86807-86808
  deoxyribonuclease ~ 86215
  deoxyribonucleic acid (DNA) ~ 86225-86226
  diphtheria ~ 86648
  ehrlichia ~ 86666
  encephalitis ~ 86651-86654
  enterovirus ~ 86658
  Epstein-Barr virus ~ 86663-86665
  fluorescent ~ 86255-86256
  francisella tularensis ~ 86668
  fungus ~ 86671
  giardia lamblia ~ 86674
  growth hormone ~ 86277
  helicobacter pylori ~ 86677
  helminth ~ 86682
  hemophilus influenza ~ 86684
  hepatitis, delta agent ~ 86692
  hepatitis A ~ 86708-86709
  hepatitis B
    core ~ 86704
    IgM ~ 86705
    surface ~ 86706
  hepatitis Be ~ 86707
  hepatitis C ~ 86803-86804
  herpes simplex ~ 86694-86696
  heterophile ~ 86308-86310
  histoplasma ~ 86698
  HIV ~ 86689, 86701-86703
  HIV 1 ~ 86701, 86703
  HIV 2 ~ 86702-86703
  HTLV I ~ 86687, 86689
  HTLV II ~ 86688
  human leukocyte antigens (HLA) ~ 86828-86835
  infectious agent, other ~ 86317
  influenza virus ~ 86710
  insulin ~ 86337

Antibody detection ~ *continued*
  intrinsic factor ~ 86340
  islet cell ~ 86341
  JC (John Cunningham) virus ~ 86711
  legionella ~ 86713
  leishmania ~ 86717
  leptospira ~ 86720
  listeria monocytogenes ~ 86723
  Lyme disease ~ 86617
  lymphocytic choriomeningitis ~ 86727
  malaria ~ 86750
  microsomal ~ 86376
  mucormycosis ~ 86732
  mumps ~ 86735
  mycoplasma ~ 86738
  neisseria meningitidis ~ 86741
  nocardia ~ 86744
  nuclear antigen ~ 86235
  parvovirus ~ 86747
  phospholipid ~ 85597, 85598, 86147
  plasmodium ~ 86750
  platelet ~ 85597-85598, 86022-86023
  protozoa ~ 86753
  red blood cell ~ 86850, 86860, 86870
  respiratory syncytial virus (RSV) ~ 86756
  rickettsia ~ 86757
  rotavirus ~ 86759
  rubella ~ 86762
  rubeola ~ 86765
  salmonella ~ 86768
  shigella ~ 86771
  sperm ~ 89325
  streptokinase ~ 86590
  tetanus ~ 86774
  thyroglobulin ~ 86800
  toxoplasma ~ 86777-86778
  treponema pallidum ~ 86780
  trichinella ~ 86784
  varicella-zoster ~ 86787
  virus, other ~ 86790
  West Nile virus ~ 86788-86789
  white blood cell ~ 86021
  yersinia ~ 86793
  Zika virus, IgM ~ 86794
Antibody identification
  fluorescent ~ 86255-86256
  immunoassay ~ 83516, 83518-83520
  immunocytochemistry ~ 88342, 88344
  immunoelectrophoresis ~ 86320, 86325, 86327, 86334-86335
  leukocyte antibodies ~ 86021, 86828-86835
  platelet ~ 86022-86023
  red blood cell ~ 86850, 86860, 86870
    pretreatment ~ 86970-86972, 86975-86978
  solid phase assay ~ 86828-86835
Antibody neutralization test ~ 86382
Antibody screening
  fluorescent noninfectious ~ 86255
  cytotoxic percent reactive antibody (PRA) ~ 86807-86808
Anticoagulant ~ 85300-85305, 85307
Antidiabetic hormone ~ 82943
Antidiuretic hormone measurement~ 84588
AntiDNA autoantibody ~ 86038-86039
Antigen(s)
  allergen immunotherapy ~ 95144-95149, 95165, 95170
  carcinoembryonic ~ 82378
  prostate specific ~ 84152-84153
Antigen detection
  direct fluorescence
    cytomegalovirus ~ 87271
    enterovirus ~ 87267
  immunoassay
    adenovirus ~ 87301
    aspergillus ~ 87305
    chlamydia trachomatis ~ 87320
    clostridium difficile ~ 87324
    cryptococcus neoformans ~ 87327
    cryptosporidium ~ 87328
    cytomegalovirus ~ 87332
    entomoeba histolytica dispar group ~ 87336
    entomoeba histolytica group ~ 87337

Antigen detection ~ *continued*
  escherichia coli 0157 ~ 87335
  giardia ~ 87329
  helicobacter pylori ~ 87338, 87339
  hepatitis Be antigen (HBeAg) ~ 87350
  hepatitis B surface antigen (HBsAg) ~ 87340
  hepatitis B surface antigen (HBsAg) neutralization ~ 87341
  hepatitis delta agent ~ 87380
  histoplasma capsulatum ~ 87385
  HIV 1 ~ 87389-87390
  HIV 2 ~ 87391
  infectious agent, otherwise ~ 87449, 87451
  influenza A ~ 87400
  influenza B ~ 87400
  polyvalent ~ 87451
  not otherwise specified ~ 87449, 87451
  respiratory syncytial virus ~ 87420
  rotavirus ~ 87425
  shigella-like toxin ~ 87427
  streptococcus, group A ~ 87430
  immunoassay, direct optical
    clostridium difficile toxin A ~ 87803
    influenza ~ 87804
    respiratory syncytial virus ~ 87807
    streptococcus, group B ~ 87802
    trichomonas vaginalis ~ 87808
  immunofluorescence
    adenovirus ~ 87260
    bordetella pertussis ~ 87265
    chlamydia trachomatis ~ 87270
    cryptosporidium ~ 87272
    giardia ~ 87269
    herpes simplex ~ 87273, 87274
    influenza A ~ 87276
    influenza B ~ 87275
    legionella pneumophila ~ 87278
    not otherwise specified ~ 87299
    parainfluenza virus ~ 87279
    pneumocystis carinii ~ 87281
    polyvalent ~ 87300
    respiratory syncytial virus ~ 87280
    rubeola ~ 87283
    treponema pallidum ~ 87285
    varicella-zoster ~ 87290
Antihemophilic factor B ~ 85250
Antihemophilic factor C ~ 85250
Antihemophilic globulin (AHG) ~ 85240
Antihuman globulin ~ 86880-86886
Antimony ~ 83015
Antinuclear antibodies (ANA) ~ 86038-86039
Antiplasmin, alpha 2 ~ Antigen detection
Antiplatelet therapy ~ see performance measures
Antiprotease, alpha 1 ~ 82103-82104, 99565
Antistreptococcal antibody ~ 86215
Antistreptokinase titer ~ 86590
Antistreptolysin O ~ 86060-86063
Antithrombin III ~ 85300-85301
Antithrombin VI (six) ~ 85362-85380
Antitoxin assay ~ 87230
Antiviral antibody ~ 86280
Antrostomy, sinus, maxillary ~ 31256-31267
Antrotomy, sinus
  maxillary ~ 31020-31032
  transmastoid ~ 69501
Antrum puncture, sinus
  maxillary ~ 31000
  sphenoid ~ 31002
Anus ~ see also hemorrhoids; rectum
  ablation ~ 46615
  abscess, incision and drainage ~ 46045-46050
  biofeedback ~ 90912, 90913
  biopsy, endoscopy ~ 46606
  crypt, excision ~ 46999
  dilation, endoscopy ~ 46604
  endoscopy
    biopsy ~ 46606
    dilation ~ 46604
    exploration ~ 46600
    hemorrhage ~ 46614

Anus ~ *continued*
  removal
    foreign body ~ 46608
    polyp ~ 46610, 46612
    tumor ~ 46610, 46612
  excision, tag ~ 46220, 46230
  exploration, endoscopy ~ 46600
  fissure
    destruction ~ 46940-46942
    excision ~ 46200
  fistula
    excision ~ 46270-46285
    repair ~ 46706
  hemorrhage, endoscopic control ~ 46614
  hemorrhoids
    clot excision ~ 46320
    destruction ~ 46930
    excision ~ 46250-46262
    injection ~ 46500
    ligation ~ 46221, 46945, 46946, 46948
    stapling ~ 46947
    suture ~ 46945, 46946, 46948
    transanal hemorrhoidal dearterialization (THD) ~ 46948
  imperforated, repair ~ 46715-46742
  incision, septum ~ 46070
  lesion
    destruction ~ 46900-46917, 46924
    excision ~ 45108, 46922
  manometry ~ 91122
  placement, seton ~ 46020
  reconstruction ~ 46742
    congenital absence ~ 46730-46740
    sphincter ~ 46750-46751, 46760
    with graft ~ 46753
  removal
    foreign body ~ 46608
    seton ~ 46030
    suture ~ 46754
    wire ~ 46754
  repair
    anovaginal fistula ~ 46715-46716
    cloacal anomaly ~ 46748
    fistula ~ 46706
    stricture ~ 46700-46705
  sphincter
    electromyography ~ 51784-51785
    needle ~ 51785
  unlisted services and procedures ~ 46999
Aorta
  abdominal
    aneurysm
      endovascular repair ~ 34845-34848
      screening ~ 76706
    angiography ~ 75635
    thromboendarterectomy ~ 35331
  anastomosis, to pulmonary artery ~ 33606
  angiogram, radiologic injection ~ 93567
  angioplasty ~ 37246, 37247
  aortography ~ 75600-75630
  ascending, graft ~ 33858, 33859, 33864
  balloon ~ 33967, 33970
  catheterization
    catheter ~ 36200
    intracatheter/needle ~ 36160
  circulation assist
    insertion ~ 33967, 33970, 33973
    removal ~ 33968, 33971, 33974
  conduit to heart ~ 33404
  endograft, fenestrated ~ 34839, 34841-34848
  excision, coarctation ~ 33840-33851
  graft
    descending thoracic ~ 33875
    hemiarch ~ 33866
    transverse arch ~ 33871
  implantable counterpulsation ventricular assist system
    insertion ~ 0451T-0454T
    interrogation device evaluation ~ 0463T
    programming device evaluation ~ 0462T
    relocation ~ 0459T
    removal ~ 0455T-0458T

Aorta~*continued*
   replacement ~ 0451T-0454T
   repositioning ~ 0460T, 0461T
  infrarenal abdominal repair
    endovascular ~ 34701-34706, 34709-34711, 34845-34848
  insertion
    balloon device ~ 33967, 33970, 33973
    catheter ~ 36200
    graft ~ 33330-33335, 33864
    intracatheter/needle ~ 36160
  removal, balloon assist device ~ 33968, 33971, 33974
  repair ~ 33320-33322, 33802, 33803
    aneurysm
      ascending ~ 33859, 33863, 33864
      sinus of valsalva ~ 33720
      thoracic ~ 33875, 33877
      transverse arch ~ 33871
    coarctation ~ 33840-33851
    hypoplastic or interrupted aortic arch
      with cardiopulmonary bypass ~ 33853
      without cardiopulmonary bypass ~ 33852
    sinus of Valsalva ~ 33702-33720
  suspension ~ 33800
  suture ~ 33320-33322
  thoracic repair ~ 75956-75959
    endovascular ~ 33880-33891
  translocation, aortic root ~ 33782-33783
  valve
    implantation ~ 33361-33369
    incision ~ 33415
    repair ~ 33390, 33391
      left ventricle ~ 33414
      supravalvular stenosis ~ 33417
  X-ray with contrast ~ 75600-75630
Aortic sinus ~ 33702-33720
Aortic stenosis
  repair ~ 33415
  supravalvular ~ 33417
Aortic valve
  closure, paravalvular leak ~ 93591, 93592
  construction, apical-aortic conduit ~ 33404
  implantation, transcatheter ~ 33361-33369
  occlusion, paravalvular leak ~ 93591, 93592
  repair
    Gusset aortoplasty ~ 33417
    outflow tract obstruction, left ventricle ~ 33414
    stenosis
      idiopathic hypertrophic ~ 33416
      subvalvular ~ 33415
      supravalvular ~ 33417
    valvuloplasty
      open with cardiopulmonary bypass ~ 33390, 33391
Aortic valve replacement
  open
    with allograft valve ~ 33406
    with cardiopulmonary bypass ~ 33405, 33406, 33410
    with prosthesis ~ 33405
    with stentless tissue valve ~ 33410
  Ross procedure ~ 33413
  transcatheter ~ see transcatheter aortic valve replacement
  with allograft valve ~ 33406
  with aortic annulus enlargement ~ 33411, 33412
  with cardiopulmonary bypass ~ 33367-33369, 33405, 33406, 33410
  with prosthesis ~ 33405, 33361-33369
  with stentless tissue valve ~ 33410
  with translocation, pulmonary valve ~ 33413
Aortocoronary bypass ~ 33503-33505, 33510-33516
Aortography ~ (see angiography) 75600-75605, 75630, 93567
  serial ~ 75625
  with iliofemoral artery ~ 75630
Aortoiliac
  embolectomy ~ 34151-34201
  thrombectomy ~ 34151-34201
Aortopexy ~ 33800
Aortoplasty, supravalvular stenosis ~ 33417
AP ~ see voiding pressure studies
Apert-Gallais syndrome ~ see adrenogenital syndrome
Aphasia testing ~ (see neurology, diagnostic) 96105
Apheresis, therapeutic ~ 36511-36516
Apical-aortic conduit ~ 33404
Apoaminotransferase, aspartate ~ see transaminase, glutamic oxaloacetic

Apolipoprotein, blood or urine ~ 82172
Appendectomy ~ 44950-44960
  laparoscopic ~ 44970
Appendiceal abscess ~ see abscess, appendix
Appendico-vesicostomy, cutaneous ~ 50845
Appendix
  abscess
    incision and drainage
      open ~ 44900
  excision ~ 44950, 44955, 44960, 44970
Application
  allergy tests ~ 95044
  bone fixation device
    multiplane ~ 20692
      stereotactic computer assisted ~ 20696-20697
    uniplane ~ 20690
  caliper ~ 20660
  cranial tongs ~ 20660
  fixation device, shoulder ~ 23700
  halo
    cranial ~ 20661
      thin skull osteology ~ 20664
    femoral ~ 20663
    maxillofacial fixation ~ 21100
    pelvic ~ 20662
  injector device for timed subcutaneous injection ~ 96377
  interdental fixation device ~ 21110
  neurostimulation ~ 64566
  radioelement
    infusion or instillation ~ 77750
    interstitial ~ 77770-77772, 77778
    intracavitary ~ 77761-77763, 77770-77772, 77790, 77799
    surface ~ 77767, 7776877789
    with ultrasound ~ 76965
  stereotactic frame ~ 20660
    headframe ~ 61800
  strapping, multi-layer compession system
    arm ~ 29584
    leg ~ 29581
Application of external fixation device ~ see fixation device, application, external
APPT ~ see thromboplastin, partial, time
Aquatic therapy ~ 97113
Aqueous shunt
  to extraocular reservoir ~ 66180
  revision ~ 66185
Arch, zygomatic ~ see zygomatic arch
Arm
  see also radius; ulna; wrist
  lower
    abscess ~ 25028
      excision ~ 25145
      incision and drainage, bone ~ 25035
    amputation ~ 24900-24920, 25900-25905, 25915
      cineplasty ~ 24940
      revision ~ 25907-25909
    angiography ~ 73206
    artery ligation ~ 37618
    biopsy ~ 25065-25066
    bursa, incision and drainage ~ 25031
    bypass graft ~ 35903
    cast ~ 29075
    CT scan ~ 73200-73206
    decompression ~ 25020-25025
    exploration, blood vessel ~ 35860
    fasciotomy ~ 24495, 25020-25025
    hematoma ~ 25028
    lesion, tendon sheath, excision ~ 25110
    magnetic resonance imaging (MRI) ~ 73218-73220, 73223
    reconstruction, ulna ~ 25337
    removal, foreign body ~ 25248
    repair
      blood vessel with other graft ~ 35266
      blood vessel with vein graft ~ 35236
      decompression ~ 24495
      muscle ~ 25260-25263, 25270
      secondary muscle or tendon ~ 25272-25274
      tendon ~ 25260-25263, 25270, 25280-25295, 25310-25316
        secondary ~ 25265
      tendon sheath ~ 25275

Arm ~ *continued*
    replantation ~ 20805
    splint ~ 29125-29126
    tenotomy ~ 25290
    tumor, excision ~ 25071-25078
    unlisted services and procedures ~ 25999
    X-ray ~ 73090
        with upper arm ~ 73092
    removal, foreign body, forearm or wrist ~ 25248
    repair
        muscle ~ 24341
        tendon ~ 24341
    upper
        abscess, incision and drainage ~ see elbow; humerus ~ 23930
        amputation ~ 23900-23921, 24900-24920
            cineplasty ~ 24940
            revision ~ 24925-24930
            with implant ~ 24931-24935
        anesthesia ~ 00400, 01710-01782
        angiography ~ 73206
        artery, ligation ~ 37618
        biopsy ~ 24065-24066
        bypass graft ~ 35903
        cast ~ 29065
        CT scan ~ 73200-73206
        exploration, blood vessel ~ 35860
        hematoma, incision and drainage ~ 23930
        magnetic resonance imaging (MRI) ~ 73218-73220, 73223
        muscle revision ~ 24330-24331
        removal
            cast ~ 29705
            foreign body ~ 24200-24201
        repair
            blood vessel with other graft ~ 35266
            blood vessel with vein graft ~ 35236
            muscle transfer ~ 24301, 24320
            tendon ~ 24332
            tendon lengthening ~ 24305
            tendon revision ~ 24320
            tendon transfer ~ 24301
            tenotomy ~ 24310
        replantation ~ 20802
        splint ~ 29105
        tumor, excision ~ 24071-24079
        unlisted services and procedures ~ 24999
        wound exploration, penetrating ~ 20103
        X-ray, with lower arm, infant ~ 73092
Arnold-Chiari malformation repair ~ 61343
Arrest, epiphyseal ~ see epiphyseal arrest
Arrhythmogenic focus, heart
    ablation ~ 33250-33251, 33261, 93653-93654, 93656
        catheter ~ 93655
Arsenic
    blood or urine ~ 82175
    detection ~ 83015
    measurement ~ 82175, 83018
ART (syphilis test) ~ 86592, 86593
Arterial
    catheterization ~ see cannulation, arterial
    dilation, transluminal ~ see angioplasty, transluminal
    grafting for coronary artery bypass ~ see bypass graft, coronary artery, arterial
    pressure ~ see also blood pressure
        noninvasive waveform analysis ~ 93050
    puncture ~ 36600
Arterialization, venous
    transcatheter stent placement
        peroneal vein ~ 0620T
        tibial vein ~ 0620T
Arteriography, aorta ~ see aortography
Arteriosus, ductus ~ see ductus arteriosus
Arteriosus, truncus ~ see truncus arteriosus
Arteriotomy ~ see incision, artery; transection, artery
Arteriovenous anastomosis ~ 36818-36820
Arteriovenous fistula
    cannulization vein ~ 36815
    creation ~ 36825-36830
    hemodialysis via fistula ~ 4052F
    referral ~ 4051F

Arteriovenous fistula ~ *continued*
    repair
        abdomen ~ 35182
            acquired or traumatic ~ 35189
        head ~ 35180
            acquired or traumatic ~ 35188
        lower extremity ~ 35184
            acquired or traumatic ~ 35190
        neck ~ 35180
            acquired or traumatic ~ 35188
        thorax ~ 35182
            acquired or traumatic ~ 35189
        upper extremity ~ 35184
            acquired or traumatic ~ 35190
    revision
        with thrombectomy ~ 36833
        without thrombectomy ~ 36832
    thrombectomy
        dialysis graft, without revision ~ 36831
        graft ~ 36830-36833
Arteriovenous malformation
    carotid
        obliteration ~ 61613
        occlusion ~ 61705
    cranial, repair
        carotid artery occlusion ~ 61705
        dural ~ 61690, 61692
        electrothrombosis ~ 61708
        infratentorial ~ 61684, 61686
        supratentorial ~ 61680, 61682
    iliac artery repair ~ 34707, 34708, 34717, 34718
    spinal
        excision ~ 63250-63252
        injection ~ 62294
        repair ~ 63250-63252
Arteriovenous shunt
    aorta to pulmonary artery ~ 33755, 33762
    Blalock-Taussig shunt ~ 33750
    intrahepatic portosystemic ~ 37182, 37183
    patency ~ 78291
    peritoneal venous
        evaluation ~ 49427
        insertion ~ 49425
        ligation ~ 49428
        removal ~ 49429
        revision ~ 49426
    Potts-Smith shunt ~ 33762
    subclavian to pulmonary artery ~ 33750
    Thomas shunt ~ 36835
    Waterston shunt ~ 33755
Artery
    abdomen
        angiography ~ 75726
        catheterization ~ 36245-36248
        ligation ~ 37617
    adrenal, angiography ~ 75731-75733
    anastomosis, cranial ~ 61711
    angioplasty ~ see angioplasty
    aorta
        angioplasty ~ 37246, 37247
        aortobi-iliac bypass graft ~ 35538, 35638
        aortobifemoral bypass graft ~ 35540
        aortocarotid bypass graft ~ 35526, 35626
        aortofemoral bypass graft ~ 35539
        aortoiliac
            bypass graft ~ 35537, 35637
            embolectomy/thrombectomy ~ 34151-34201
        aortoiliofemoral ~ 35363
        aortoinnominate bypass graft ~ 35526, 35626
        aortosubclavian bypass graft ~ 35526, 35626
    arm
        angiography ~ 75710-75716
        harvest of artery for coronary artery bypass graft ~ 35600
    atherectomy
        brachiocephalic ~ 0237T
        coronary ~ 92924-92925, 92933-92934, 92937-92938, 92941, 92943-92944
        femoral ~ 37225, 37227

Artery ~ *continued*
  iliac ~ 0238T
  peroneal ~ 37229, 37231, 37333, 37335
  popliteal ~ 37225, 37227
  renal ~ 0234T
  tibial ~ 37229, 37231, 37333, 37335
  visceral ~ 0235T
  transluminal ~ 0234T-0238T, 92924-92925, 92933-92934, 92937-92938, 92941, 92943-92944
  axillary
    aneurysm ~ 35011-35013
    angioplasty ~ 37246, 37247
    bypass graft ~ 35616, 35621, 35623, 35650, 35654
    embolectomy ~ 34101
    exploration ~ 35702
    thrombectomy ~ 34101
    thromboendarterectomy ~ 35321
  basilar, aneurysm ~ 61698, 61702
  biopsy, transcatheter ~ 75970
  brachial
    aneurysm ~ 35011-35013
    bypass graft ~ 35510, 35512, 35522-35525
    embolectomy ~ 34101
    exploration ~ 24495, 35702
    exposure ~ 34834
    thrombectomy ~ 34101
    thromboendarterectomy ~ 35321
  brachiocephalic
    angioplasty ~ 37246, 37247
    catheterization ~ 36215-36218
  bypass graft, with composite graft ~ 35681-35683
  cannulization
    for extra corporeal circulation ~ 36823
    to vein ~ 36810-36815
  carotid
    aneurysm ~ 35001-35002, 61697, 61700, 61703, 61705, 61708, 61710
    bypass graft ~ 33891, 35501-35510, 35601-35606, 35642
    carotid-cavernous fistula ~ 61705, 61708, 61710
    catheterization ~ 36100, 36221-36224, 36227-36228
    decompression ~ 61590-61591, 61596
    embolectomy ~ 34001
    exploration ~ 35701
    ligation ~ 37600-37606, 61611
    reimplantation ~ 35691, 35694-35695
    stenosis, imaging study measurement ~ 3100F
    stent placement, transcatheter ~ 37217
    thrombectomy ~ 34001
    thromboendarterectomy ~ 35301, 35390
    transection ~ 61611
    transposition ~ 33889, 35691, 35694-35695
    vascular malformation ~ 61705, 61708, 61710
  celiac
    aneurysm ~ 35121-35122
    bypass graft ~ 35531, 35631
    embolectomy ~ 34151
    endoprosthesis ~ 34841-34848
    thrombectomy ~ 34151
    thromboendarterectomy ~ 35341
  chest, ligation ~ 37616
  coronary
    angiography ~ 93454-93461, 9292492925, 92933-92934
    atherectomy ~ 92924-92925, 92933-92934
    bypass ~ 33510-33536
      internal mammary artery graft ~ 4110F
    fractional flow reserve ~ 0501T-0504T
    graft ~ 33503-33504
    ligation ~ 33502
    repair ~ 33500-33507
    thrombectomy, percutaneous ~ 92973
    thrombolysis ~ 92975, 92977
    translocation ~ 33506-33507
    unroofing ~ 33507
  digital, sympathectomy ~ 64820
  ethmoidal, ligation ~ 30915
  extracorporeal circulation, for regional chemotherapy of extremity ~ 36823
  extracranial anastomosis ~ 61711

Artery ~ *continued*
  extremities
    vascular studies ~ 93922-93931
      bypass grafts ~ 93925-93931
    bypass graft revision ~ 35879-35884
    catheterization ~ 36140, 36245-36248
    ligation ~ 37618
  femoral
    aneurysm ~ 35141-35142
    angiography ~ 73706
    angioplasty ~ 37224
    approach
      transcatheter aortic valve replacement ~ 33361-33366
    bypass graft ~ 35521, 35533, 35556-35558, 35566, 35621, 35646-35647, 35654-35661, 35666, 35700
    bypass graft revision ~ 35883-35884
    bypass in-situ ~ 35583-35585
    embolectomy ~ 34201
    exploration ~ 35703
    exposure ~ 34812
    thrombectomy ~ 34201
    thromboendarterectomy ~ 35371-35372
  great vessel, repair ~ 33770-33781
  hepatic
    aneurysm ~ 35121-35122
    bypass graft ~ 35535
  iliac
    anastomosis implant placement ~ 0553T
    aneurysm
      direct repair ~ 35001, 35131, 35132
      endovascular repair ~ 34703-34711, 34717, 34718
    angioplasty ~ 37220, 37222
    atherectomy ~ 0238T
    bypass graft ~ 35563, 35632-35634, 35637, 35663
    embolectomy ~ 34151-34201
    endograft ~ 34717, 34718
    exposure ~ 34820, 34833
    occlusion device ~ 34808
    revascularization ~ 37220-37222
    thrombectomy ~ 34151-34201
    thromboendarterectomy ~ 35351, 35361-35363
  ilio-celiac bypass graft ~ 35632
  iliofemoral
    bypass graft ~ 35565
    thromboendarterectomy ~ 35355, 35363
    X-ray with contrast ~ 75630
  ilio-mesenteric bypass graft ~ 35633
  iliorenal bypass graft ~ 35634
  innominate
    aneurysm ~ 35021-35022
    catheterization ~ 36222-36223, 36225
    embolectomy ~ 34001-34101
    stent placement, trasncatheter ~ 37217
    thrombectomy ~ 34001-34101
    thromboendarterectomy ~ 35311
  intracranial
    anastomosis ~ 33606
    aneurysm ~ 61705, 61708
    angiography, with thrombectomy ~ 61645
    angioplasty ~ 61630
    infusion
      for other than thrombolysis ~ 61650, 61651
      for thrombolysis ~ 61645
    thrombectomy ~ 61645
  leg
    angiography ~ 73706, 75710-75716
    catheterization ~ 36245-36248
  mammary, angiography ~ 75756
  maxillary, ligation ~ 30920
  mesenteric
    aneurysm ~ 35121-35122
    bypass graft ~ 35531, 35631
    embolectomy ~ 34151
    thrombectomy ~ 34151
    thromboendarterectomy ~ 35341
  middle cerebral artery
    fetal, vascular studies ~ 76821
    ligation ~ 37615

Artery ~ *continued*
  neck
    angiography ~ 36221-36226
    ligation ~ 37615
  nose, incision ~ 30915-30920
  other angiography ~ 75774
  other artery
    angiography ~ 75774
  pelvic
    angiography ~ 72198, 75736
    catheterization ~ 36245-36248
  peripheral arterial rehabilitation ~ 93668
  peroneal
    angioplasty ~ 37228-37235
    atherectomy ~ 37229, 37231, 37333, 37335
    bypass graft ~ 35566-35571, 35666-35671
    bypass in-situ ~ 35585-35587
    embolectomy ~ 34203
    thrombectomy ~ 34203
    thromboendarterectomy ~ 35305-35306
  popliteal
    aneurysm ~ 35151-35152
    angioplasty ~ 37224
    atherectomy ~ 37225, 37227
    bypass graft ~ 35556, 35571, 35623, 35656, 35671, 35700
    bypass in-situ ~ 35583, 35587
    embolectomy ~ 34201-34203
    exploration ~ 35703
    thrombectomy ~ 34201-34203
    thromboendarterectomy ~ 35303
  pressure
    waveform analysis ~ 93050
  pulmonary
    anastomosis ~ 33606
    angiography ~ 75741-75746
    angioplasty ~ 92997-92998
    banding ~ 33620, 33622, 33690
    embolectomy ~ 33910, 33915-33916
    endarterectomy ~ 33916
    ligation ~ 33924
    repair ~ 33917, 33920, 33925-33926
  radial
    aneurysm ~ 35045
    bypass graft ~ 35523
    embolectomy ~ 34111
    exploration ~ 35702
    sympathectomy ~ 64821
    thrombectomy ~ 34111
  rehabilitation ~ 93668
  reimplantation
    carotid ~ 35691, 35694-35695
    subclavian ~ 35693-35695
    vertebral ~ 35691-35693
    visceral ~ 35697
  renal
    aneurysm ~ 35121-35122
    angiography ~ 36251-36254
    angioplasty ~ 37246, 37247
    atherectomy ~ 0234T
    bypass graft ~ 35631, 35634, 35636
    catheterization ~ 36251-36254
    embolectomy ~ 34151
    endoprosthesis ~ 34841-34848
    fluoroscopy ~ 36251-36254
    thrombectomy ~ 34151
    thromboendarterectomy ~ 35341
  repair
    aneurysm ~ 61697-61708
    angioplasty
      radiological supervision ~ 37246, 37247
  revision
    hemodialysis graft or fistula~ 36831-36833
  spine, angiography ~ 75705
  splenic
    aneurysm ~ 35111-35112
    bypass graft ~ 35536, 35636

Artery ~ *continued*
  subclavian
    aneurysm ~ 35001-35002, 35021-35022
    angioplasty ~ 37246, 37247
    bypass graft ~ 35506, 35511-35516, 35606-35616, 35626, 35645
    catheterization ~ 36225
    embolectomy ~ 34001-34101
    reimplantation ~ 35693-35695
    thrombectomy ~ 34001-34101
    thromboendarterectomy ~ 35301, 35311
    transposition ~ 33889, 35693-35695
    unlisted services and procedures ~ 37799
  superficial palmar arch, sympathectomy ~ 64823
  temporal biopsy/ligation ~ 37609
  thoracic, catheterization ~ 33621, 36215-36218
  thrombectomy
    coronary ~ 92973
    dialysis circuit ~ 36904-36906
    intracranial ~ 61645
    noncoronary ~ 37184-37186
    hemodialysis graft or fistula ~ 36831
    other than hemodialysis graft or fistula ~ 35875, 36830-36833
  thrombolysis
    intracranial ~ 61645
    non-coronary ~ 37211, 37213, 37214
  tibial
    angiography ~ 73706
    angioplasty ~ 37228
    atherectomy ~ 37229, 37231
    bypass graft ~ 35566-35571, 35623, 35666-35671
    bypass in-situ ~ 35585-35587
    embolectomy ~ 34203
    exploration ~ 35703
    thrombectomy ~ 34203
    thromboendarterectomy ~ 35305-35306
    tibial/peroneal trunk-tibial bypass graft ~ 35570
  tibioperoneal
    angioplasty ~ 37228-37235
    atherectomy ~ 37233-37235
  transcatheter therapy, with angiography ~ 75894-75898
  transposition
    carotid ~ 33889, 35691, 35694-35695
    subclavian ~ 33889, 35693-35695
    vertebral ~ 35691-35693
  ulnar
    aneurysm ~ 35045
    bypass graft ~ 35523
    embolectomy ~ 34111
    exploration ~ 35702
    sympathectomy ~ 64822
    thrombectomy ~ 34111
  umbilical vascular study ~ 76820
  unlisted services and procedures ~ 37799
  upper extremity exploration ~ 35702
  vertebral
    aneurysm ~ 35005, 61698, 61702
    bypass graft ~ 35508, 35515, 35642-35645
    catheterization ~ 36100, 36221, 36225-36226, 36228
    decompression ~ 61597
    reimplantation ~ 35691-35693
    thromboendarterectomy ~ 35301
    transposition ~ 35691-35693
  visceral
    angioplasty ~ 37246, 37247
    atherectomy ~ 0235T
    reimplantation ~ 35697
Artery catheterization, pulmonary ~ see catheterization, pulmonary artery
Arthrectomy, elbow ~ 24155
Arthrocentesis
  intermediate joint ~ 20605
  large joint ~ 20610
  small joint ~ 20600
Arthrodesis
  ankle ~ 27870
    tibiotalar and fibulotalar joints ~ 29899
  anterior interbody ~ 22551-22552
  carpometacarpal joint
    hand ~ 26843-26844
    thumb ~ 26841-26842

Arthrodesis ~ *continued*
cervical anterior, with discectomy ~ 22554
elbow ~ 24800-24802
finger joint ~ 26852
  interphalangeal ~ 26860-26863
  metacarpophalangeal ~ 26850
foot joint ~ 28730-28735, 28740
  pantalar ~ 28705
  subtalar ~ 28725
  triple ~ 28715
  with advancement ~ 28737
  with lengthening ~ 28737
hand joint ~ 26843-26844
hip joint ~ 27284-27286
intercarpal joint ~ 25820
  with autograft ~ 25825
interphalangeal joint ~ 26860-26863
  great toe ~ 28755
    with tendon transfer ~ 28760
knee ~ 27580
metacarpophalangeal joint ~ 26850-26852
metatarsophalangeal joint, great toe ~ 28750
pubic symphysis ~ 27282
radioulnar joint, with resection of ulna ~ 25830
sacroiliac joint ~ 27280
shoulder joint ~ 23800-23802
talus
  pantalar ~ 28705
  subtalar ~ 28725
  triple ~ 28715
tarsal joint ~ 28730-28735, 28740
  with advancement ~ 28737
  with lengthening ~ 28737
tarsometatarsal joint ~ 28730-28735, 28740
thumb joint ~ 26841-26842
tibiofibular joint ~ 27871
vertebra
  additional interspace
    anterior/anterolateral approach ~ 22585
    lateral extracavitary ~ 22534
    posterior ~ 22614, 22634
  cervical
    anterior/anterolateral approach ~ 22548
    posterior/posterolateral and/or lateral traverse process ~ 22590-22600
  lumbar
    anterior/anterolateral approach ~ 22558
    lateral extracavitary ~ 22533, 22534
    pre-sacral interbody ~ 0195T, 0196T, 22586
    posterior/interbody ~ 22630
    posterior/posterolateral and/or lateral transverse process ~ 22612, 22633, 22634
  sacroiliac, presacral interbody ~ 0195T
  spinal deformity
    anterior approach ~ 22808-22812
    posterior approach ~ 22800-22804
  spinal fusion, exploration ~ 22830
  thoracic
    anterior/anterolateral approach ~ 22556
    lateral extracavitary ~ 22532, 22534
    posterior/posterolateral and/or lateral traverse process ~ 22610
  with insertion of biomechanical device ~ 22853, 22854
with bunionectomy ~ 28295, 28296, 28298, 28299
wrist ~ 25800
  with graft ~ 25810
  with sliding graft ~ 25805
Arthrography
ankle ~ 73615
  injection ~ 27648
elbow ~ 73085
  injection ~ 24220
hip ~ 73525
  injection ~ 27093-27095
knee ~ 73580
  injection ~ 27369
sacroiliac joint
  injection ~ 27096
shoulder ~ 73040
  injection ~ 23350

Arthrography ~ *continued*
temporomandibular joint (TMJ) ~ 70328-70332
  injection ~ 21116
wrist ~ 73115
  injection ~ 25426
Arthroplasties, knee replacement ~ 27438, 27445
Arthroplasty
ankle ~ 27700-27703
elbow ~ 24360
  total replacement ~ 24363
  with implant ~ 24361-24362
hip ~ 27132
  partial replacement ~ 27125
  revision ~ 27134-27138
  total replacement ~ 27130
interphalangeal joint ~ 26535-26536
intervertebral disc
  removal ~ 0164T, 22864-22865
  revision ~ 0165T, 22861-22862
  total replacement ~ 0163T, 22856-22857
    with osteophytectomy ~ 22856
knee ~ 27437-27443, 27446-27447
  revision ~ 27486-27487
  with prosthesis ~ 27438, 27445
metacarpophalangeal joint ~ 26530-26531
radius ~ 24365
  with implant ~ 24366
reconstruction, prosthesis, hip ~ 27125
shoulder joint ~ 23470, 23472-23474
temporomandibular joint ~ 21240-21243
vertebral joint, lumbar spine ~ 0202T
wrist ~ 25447
  carpal ~ 25443
  lunate ~ 25444
  navicular ~ 25443
  radius ~ 25441
  revision ~ 25449
  total replacement ~ 25446
  trapezium ~ 25445
  ulna ~ 25442
  with implant ~ 25441-25445
  wrist (pseudarthrosis type) ~ 25332
Arthropods, examination ~ 87168
Arthroscopy
diagnostic
  elbow ~ 29830
  hip ~ 29860
  knee ~ 29870
  metacarpophalangeal joint ~ 29900
  shoulder ~ 29805
  temporomandibular joint ~ 29800
  wrist ~ 29840
surgical
  ankle ~ 29891-29899
  elbow ~ 29834-29838
  hip ~ 29861-29863, 29914
  knee ~ 29871-29889
    cartilage allograft ~ 29867
    cartilage autograft ~ 29866
    meniscal transplantation ~ 29868
    metacarpophalangeal joint ~ 29901-29902
    shoulder ~ 29806-29828
      biceps tenodesis ~ 29828
    subtalar joint ~ 29904-29907, 29915-29916
      arthrodesis ~ 29907
      debridement ~ 29906
      with labral repair ~ 29916
      removal of loose or foreign body ~ 29904
      synovectomy ~ 29905
    temporomandibular joint ~ 29804
    wrist ~ 29843-29848
unlisted services and procedures ~ 29999
Arthrotomy
acromioclavicular joint ~ 23044
ankle ~ 27610-27612, 27620
ankle joint ~ 27625-27626
carpometacarpal joint ~ 26070
  with biopsy, synovium
    with synovial biopsy ~ 26100

Arthrotomy~_continued_
- elbow ~ 24000
  - capsular release ~ 24006
  - with joint exploration ~ 24101
  - with synovectomy ~ 24102
  - with synovial biopsy ~ 24100
- finger joint ~ 26075
  - interphalangeal
    - with synovial biopsy ~ 26110
  - metacarpophalangeal
    - with biopsy, synovium ~ 26105
- glenohumeral joint ~ 23040
- hip ~ 27033
  - for infection
    - with drainage ~ 27030
  - with synovectomy ~ 27054
- interphalangeal joint ~ 26080, 26110
  - toe ~ 28024, 28054
- intertarsal joint ~ 28020, 28050
- knee ~ 27310, 27330-27335, 27403, 29868
- metacarpophalangeal joint ~ 26075, 26105
- metatarsophalangeal joint ~ 28022, 28052
- shoulder ~ 23044, 23105-23107
- shoulder joint ~ 23100-23101
  - exploration and/or removal of loose or foreign body ~ 23107
- sternoclavicular joint ~ 23044
- tarsometatarsal joint ~ 28020, 28050
- temporomandibular joint ~ 21010
- with biopsy
  - acromioclavicular joint ~ 23101
  - glenohumeral joint ~ 23100
  - hip joint ~ 27052
  - knee joint ~ 27330
  - sacroiliac joint
    - hip joint ~ 27050
  - sternoclavicular joint ~ 23101
- with synovectomy
  - glenohumeral joint ~ 23105
  - sternoclavicular joint ~ 23106
- wrist ~ 25040, 25100-25107

Articular ligament ~ see ligament
Artificial abortion ~ see abortion
Artificial cardiac pacemaker ~ see heart, pacemaker
Artificial eye ~ see prosthesis
Artificial genitourinary sphincter ~ see prosthesis, urethral sphincter
Artificial insemination ~ 58976
- intra-cervical ~ 58321
- intra-uterine ~ 58322
- sperm washing ~ 58323

Artificial knee joints ~ 27438, 27445
Artificial penis ~ see penile prosthesis
Artificial pneumothorax ~ 32960
Arytenoid, excision, endoscopic ~ 31560-31561
Arytenoid cartilage
- excision ~ 31400
- repair ~ 31400

Arytenoidectomy ~ 31400
- endoscopic ~ 31560

Arytenoidopexy ~ 31400
Ascorbic acid, blood ~ 82180
Aspartate aminotransferase ~ 84450
Aspergillus
- antibody ~ 86606
- antigen detection
  - enzyme immunoassay ~ 87305

Aspiration ~ see puncture aspiration
- abdomen ~ 49322
- amniotic fluid
  - diagnostic ~ 59000
  - therapeutic ~ 59001
- bladder ~ 51100-51102
- bone marrow ~ 38220, 38222
  - spine surgery ~ 20939
- brain lesion ~ 61750-61751
- bronchi ~ 31629, 31633, 31645, 31646, 31725
- bursa ~ 20600-20611
- catheter
  - nasotracheal ~ 31720
  - tracheobronchial ~ 31725
- chest ~ 32554-32555

Aspiration ~ _continued_
- lcyst
  - bone ~ 20615
  - ganglion ~ 20612
  - kidney ~ 50390
  - pelvis ~ 50390
  - spinal cord ~ 62268
  - thyroid.~ 60300
- disc ~ 62267
- duodenal ~ 43756-43757
- evaluation ~ 88172, 88173, 88177
- fetal fluid ~ 59074
- ganglion cyst ~ 20612
- gastric ~ 43753-43755
- hydrocele, tunica vaginalis ~ 55000
- joint ~ 20600-20610
- aryngoscopy
  - direct ~ 31515
- lens material ~ 66840
- liver ~ 47015
- nail ~ 11740
- nucleus of disk, lumbar ~ 62287
- orbital contents ~ 67415
- pelvis, endoscopy ~ 49322
- pericardium ~ 33016
- pleural cavity ~ 32554-32555
- puncture, cyst, breast ~ 19000-19001
- spinal puncture ~ see spinal tap
- syrinx, spinal cord ~ 62268
- thyroid ~ 60300
- trachea
  - nasotracheal ~ 31720
  - puncture ~ 31612
- tunica vaginalis, hydrocele ~ 55000
- vitreous ~ 67015

Aspiration lipectomies ~ 15876-15879
Aspiration of bone marrow from donor for transplant ~ 38230
Assay, very long chain fatty acids ~ 82726
Assay tobramycin ~ 80200
Assisted circulation ~ see circulation assist
AST ~ 84450
Astragalectomy ~ 28130
Astragalus ~ see talus
Asymmetry, face ~ 21247
Ataxia telangiectasia, chromosome analysis ~ 88248
Ataxy, telangiectasia ~ 88248
Atherectomy
- abdominal aorta ~ 0236T
- brachiocephalic ~ 0237T
- coronary ~ 92924-92925, 92937-92938, 92941, 92943-92944
- femoral ~ 37225, 37227
- iliac ~ 0238T
- peroneal ~ 37229, 37231, 37333, 37335
- popliteal ~ 37225, 37227
- renal ~ 0234T
- tibial ~ 37229, 37231, 37333, 37335
- visceral ~ 0235T

Athletic training
- evaluation ~ 97169-97171
- re-evaluation ~ 97172

ATLV ~ see HTLV I
ATLV antibodies ~ 86688
Atomic absorption spectroscopy ~ 82190
ATP creatine phosphotranferase ~ 82550-82552
Atresia
- choanal ~ 30540-30545
- congenital
  - auditory canal, external ~ 69320
  - bile duct ~ 47700
  - small intestine ~ 44126-44127
- pulmonary artery ~ 33920
- tetralogy of fallot ~ 33697
- tricuspid ~ 33615

Atria
- ablation ~ 33254-33256, 33265-33266
- Baffle procedure ~ 33774
- Blalock-Hanlon operation ~ 33735
- cor triatriatum repair ~ 33732
- cuff preparation ~ 32855-32856
- electrogram ~ 93615-93616

Atria ~ *continued*
  endoscopy, surgical ~ 33265-33266
  left atrial appendage closure ~ 33340
  membrane resection ~ 33732
  pacemaker
    electrode removal ~ 33229, 33236
    electrode repositioning ~ 33215
    insertion ~33206, 33208
  Rashkind procedure ~ 33741
  reconstruction ~ 33254-33256, 33265-33266
  septum
    interatrial septal shunt device implantation ~ 0613T
    septectomy ~ 33735-33737
    septostomy ~ 33735-33737
      transcatheter, for congenital anomaly ~ 33741
  shunt ~ 62190, 62220
  thrombus ~ 33310
Atrial electrogram ~ see cardiology, diagnostic
  esophageal recording ~ 93615-93616
Atrial fibrillation ~ see fibrillation, atrial
Atrioseptopexy ~ see heart, repair, atrial septum
Atrioseptoplasty ~ see heart, repair, atrial septum
Attachment ~ see fixation
Atticotomy ~ 69631, 69635
Audiologic function tests ~ 92590-92595
  acoustic reflex ~ 92568
  acoustic reflex decay ~ 92570
  audiometry
    Bekesy ~ 92560-92561
    comprehensive ~ 0212T, 92557
    conditioning play ~ 92582
    groups ~ 92559
    pure tone ~ 0208T-0209T, 92552-92553
    select picture ~ 92583
    speech ~ 0210T-0211T, 92555-92556
    visual reinforcement ~ 92579
  auditory brainstem implant ~ 92640
  auditory processing treatment ~ 92507-92508
  central auditory function ~ 92620-92621
  ear protector attenuation ~ 92596
  electrocochleography ~ 92584
  evoked otoacoustic emission ~ 92558, 92587-92588
  filtered speech ~ 92571
  hearing aid evaluation ~ 92590-92595
  loudness balance ~ 92562
  screening ~ 92551
  sensorineural acuity ~ 92575
  short increment sensitivity index ~ 92564
  staggered spondaic word test ~ 92572
  Stenger test ~ 92565, 92577
  synthetic sentence test ~ 92576
  tinnitus assessment ~ 92625
  tone decay ~ 92563
  tympanometry ~ 92550, 92567, 92570
Audiometry
  Bekesy ~ 92560-92561
  comprehensive ~ 0212T, 92557
  conditioning play ~ 92582
  groups ~ 92559
  pure tone ~ 92552-92553
    automated 0208T-0209T
  select picture ~ 92583
  speech ~ 0210T-0211T, 92555-92556
  tympanometry ~ 92550, 92567, 92570
Auditory canal
  decompression ~ 61591
  external
    abscess, incision and drainage ~ 69020
    biopsy ~ 69105
    lesion, excision ~ 69140-69155
    reconstruction
      for congenital atresia ~ 69320
      for stenosis ~ 69310
    removal
      cerumen ~ 69209, 69210
      ear wax ~ 69209, 69210
      foreign body ~ 69200-69205
  internal, decompression ~ 69960
Auditory atresia, external ~ 69320
Auditory evoked otoacoustic emission ~ 92587-92588
Auditory evoked potentials ~ 92590-92595

Auditory labyrinth ~ see ear, inner
Auditory meatus, X-ray ~ 70134
Auditory system surgical procedures ~ 69000-69990
Auditory tube ~ see eustachian tube
Augmentation
  chin ~ 21120, 21123
  cruciate ligament ~ 29888, 29889
  facial bones ~ 21208
  knee ligament ~ 27427, 27556-27558
  larynx ~ 31574
  malar ~ 21210, 21270
  mandibular body
    with bone graft ~ 21127
    with prosthesis ~ 21125
  palate ~ 21082
  pulmonary valve outflow ~ 33478
  spine
    lumbar ~ 22514, 22515
    thoracic ~ 22513, 22515
Aural rehabilitation ~ 92510
Auricle (heart) ~ see atria
Auricular fibrillation ~ fibrillation, atria
Auricular prosthesis ~ 21086
Australia antigen ~ 87340-87341
Autograft
  adipose cellular implant for knee osteoarthritis ~ 0565T, 0566T
  bone ~ 20936-20938
  bone marrow ~ 20939
  chondrocytes, knee ~ 27412
  fat ~ 15771-15774
  osteochondral
    knee ~ 27416
    talus ~ 28446
  skin
    dermal ~ 15130-15136
    epidermal ~ 15110-15116
    soft tissue ~ 15769
    tissue culture ~ 15150-15157
      harvesting ~ 15040
  spine ~ 20936-20939
Autologous blood transfusion ~ 86890-86891
Autologous transplantation ~ see autograft
Autonomic nervous system function ~ see neurology, diagnostic;
  neurophysiologic testing
Autoprothrombin
  C ~ 85260
  I ~ 85230
  II ~ 85250
  III ~ 85260
Autopsy
  coroner's exam ~ 88045
  forensic exam ~ 88040
  gross and micro exam ~ 88020-88029
  gross exam ~ 88000-88016
  organ ~ 88037
  regional ~ 88036
  unlisted services and procedures ~ 88099
Autotransfusion, blood ~ 86890-86891
Autotransplant ~ see autograft
Autotransplantation, renal ~ 50380
Avulsion
  nails ~ 11730-11732
  nerve ~ 64732-64772
AV fistula ~ see arteriovenous fistula
AV shunt ~ see arteriovenous shunt
Axillary arteries ~ see artery, axillary
Axillary nerve, injection, anesthetic ~ 64417
Axis, dens ~ 22548

B

B antibodies, hepatitis ~ see antibody, hepatitis B
B antigens, hepatitis ~ 87516, 87517
B-DNA ~ 86225-86226
B-hexosaminidase ~ 83080
B1 vitamin ~ see 84425
B6 vitamin ~ 84207

B12 vitamin ~ 82607-82608
Babcock operation ~ 37700-37735, 37780
Bacillus Calmette Guerin vaccine ~ see BCG vaccine
Back/ flank
  biopsy ~ 21920-21925
  repair, hernia ~ 49540
  strapping ~ 29799
  tumor
    excision ~ 21930-21936
    radical resection ~ 21935, 21936
  wound exploration
    penetrating ~ 20102
Backbone ~ see spine
Bacteria culture
  additional methods ~ 87077
  aerobic ~ 87040-87071
  anaerobic ~ 87073-87076
  blood ~ 87040
  other source ~ 87070-87075
  screening ~ 87081
  stool ~ 87045-87046
  typing ~ 87140, 87143, 87147, 87149-87150, 87152-87153, 87158
  urine ~ 87086-87088
Bacterial endotoxins ~ 87176, 87205
Bacterial overgrowth breath test ~ 91065
Bactericidal titer, serum ~ 87197
Bacterium, antibody ~ 86609
Baker's cyst ~ 27345
Baker tube, intestine decompression ~ 44021
Balanoplasty ~ see penis, repair
Baldy-Webster operation ~ 58400
Balkan grippe ~ 86000, 86638
Balloon
  angioplasty ~ *see* angioplasty
  assisted device
    aorta ~ 33967-33974
    bronchoscopy ~ 31647-31649, 31651
Band, pulmonary artery ~ 33690
Banding, artery
  fistula ~ 37607
  pulmonary ~ 33610, 33620, 33690
Bank, blood ~ see blood banking
Bankart procedure ~ 23450-23462
Barany caloric test ~ 92533
Barbiturates, blood or urine ~ 80345
Bardenheurer operation ~ 37616
Bariatric surgery
  gastric bypass ~ 43644-43645, 43846-43847
  gastric restriction ~ 43644-43645, 43842-43843, 43845-43846,
    43847-43848
    device placement ~ 43770
    device removal ~ 43772-43774
    device replacement ~ 43773
    device revision ~ 43771
    port component ~ 43886-43888
  sleeve gastrectomy ~ 43775
  surgically altered stomach ultrasound examination ~ 43242
Barium ~ 83015
Barium enema ~ 74270-74280
Barker operation ~ 28120, 28130
Barr bodies ~ 88130
Barr procedure ~ 27690-27692
Bartholin's gland
  abscess, incision and drainage ~ 56420
  cyst, repair ~ 56440
  excision ~ 56740
  marsupialization ~ 56440
Bartonella
  antibody ~ 86611
  detection ~ 87472
Basic life services ~ 99450
Basic proteins, myelin ~ 83873
Basilar arteries ~ 61698, 61702
Batch-Spittler-McFaddin operation ~ 27598
BCG vaccine ~ 90585, 90586
Be antigens, hepatitis ~ 87350
Bed sores ~ see debridement; skin graft and flap; 15920-15999
Bed testing ~ 94780, 94781
Bekesy audiometry ~ 92560-92561
Belsey IV procedure ~ see fundoplasty
Bender-Gestalt test ~ 96100

Benedict test for urea ~ 81005
Benign cystic mucinous tumour ~ see ganglion
Benign neoplasm of cranial nerves ~ see cranial nerve
Bennett fracture ~ see phalanx, finger; 26720-26727
Bennett procedure ~ see revision; 27385-27386, 27400, 27430
Benzidine test ~ 82270, 82272
Benzodiazepine, assay ~ 80346, 80347
Benzoyl cholinesterase ~ 82480-82482
Bernstein test ~ 91030
Beryllium ~ 83015
Beta-2 -microglobulin
  blood ~ 82232
  urine ~ 82232
Beta-hydroxydehydrogenase ~ 80406
Beta 2 glycoprotein 1 antibody ~ 86146
Beta blocker therapy ~ see performance measures
Beta glucosidase ~ 82963
Beta hypophamine ~ 84588
Beta lipoproteins ~ 83700-83704, 83721
Beta test ~ see psychiatric diagnosis ~ 96100
Bethesda system ~ 88164-88167
Bicarbonate ~ 82374
Biceps tendon, insertion ~ 24342
Bichloride, methylene ~ 84600
Bicuspid valve ~ see mitral valve
Bifrontal craniotomy ~ 61557
Bilaminate skin substitute/ neodermis ~ see tissue
  repair ~ see tissue, culture; 15100-15101, 15120-15121
Bile acids ~ 82239
  blood ~ 82240
Bile duct ~ see gallbladder
  anastomosis
    with intestines ~ 47760, 47780-47785
  biopsy
    endoluminal ~ 47543
    endoscopy ~ 47553
  cholangiography
    injection ~ 47531, 47532
    with catheterization ~ 47533-47537
    with placement of access to small bowel ~ 47541
    with stent placement ~ 47538-47540
  cyst, excision ~ 47715
  destruction
    calculi (stone) ~ 43265, 47544
  dilation
    endoscopy ~ 43277, 47555, 47556
    percutaneous ~ 47542
    X-ray ~ 74360
  drainage
    catheter
      change ~ 75984
      conversion of external to internal-external ~ 47535
      exchange ~ 47536
      placement ~ 47533, 47534
      removal ~ 47537
  endoscopic retrograde cholangiopancreatography (ERCP) with optical
    endomicroscopy ~ 0397T
  endoscopy
    biopsy ~ 47553
    cannulation ~ 43273
    destruction, calculi (stone) ~ 43265
    dilation ~ 43277, 47555-47556
    exploration ~ 47552
    intraoperative ~ 47550
    placement, stent ~ 43274
    removal
      calculi (stone) ~ 43264, 47554
      foreign body ~ 43275
    specimen collection ~ 43260
    sphincterotomy ~ 43262, 43274
    sphincter pressure ~ 43263
  exploration
    atresia ~ 47700
    endoscopy ~ 47552
  incision, sphincter ~ 43262, 47460
  incision and drainage ~ 47420-47425
  insertion
    stent ~ 47801
  nuclear medicine, imaging ~ 78226-78227
  pharmacologic intervention ~ 78227

Bile duct ~ *continued*
  placement
    access to small bowel ~ 47541
    catheter, drainage ~ 47533, 47534
    stent ~ 43274, 47801
  reconstruction, anastomosis ~ 47800
  removal
    calculi (stone) ~ 43264, 47420, 47425, 47544
    foreign body ~ 43275
    stent ~ 43275
  repair ~ 47701
    gastrointestinal tract ~ 47785
    with intestines ~ 47760, 47780
  stent placement ~ 47538-47540, 47801
  tumor
    ablation ~ 43278
    excision ~ 47711-47712
  unlisted services and procedures ~ 47999
  X-ray
    guide dilation ~ 74360
    with contrast ~ 47532, 74300, 74301
      calculus removal ~ 47544
    guide catheter ~ 74328, 74330
Bilirubin
  blood ~ 82247-82248
  feces ~ 82252
  total
    direct ~ 82247-82248
    transcutaneous ~ 88720
Billroth I or II ~ 43631-43635, 43845
Bilobectomy ~ 32482
Bimone ~ 84402
Binding globulin, testosterone-estradiol ~ 84270
Binet-Simon test ~ 96100
Binet test ~ 96100
Binet-Simon test, binocular microscopy ~ 92504
Biofeedback training
  anorectal ~ 90912, 90913
  psychiatric treatment ~ 90875, 90876
Bioimpedance
  thorax ~ 93701
Biometry, eye ~ 76516-76519, 92136
Biomechanical mapping
  transvaginal ~ 0487T
Biopsies, needle ~ see needle biopsy
Biopsy ~ see brush biopsy; needle biopsy
  abdomen ~ 49000
  adrenal gland ~ 60540-60545
  anal, endoscopy ~ 46606
  ankle ~ 27613-27614, 27620
  arm, lower ~ 25065-25066
  arm, upper ~ 24065-24066
  artery, temporal ~ 37609
  auditory canal, external ~ 69105
  back/flank ~ 21920-21925
  bile duct
    endoluminal ~ 47543
    endoscopy ~ 47553
    with transhepatic guided cholangiography, laparoscopic ~ 47579
  bladder ~ 52354
    cystourethroscope ~ 52204
    cystourethroscopy ~ 52224, 52250
  blood vessel, transcatheter ~ 75970
  bone ~ 0200T, 0201T, 20220-20245, 22510-22512
  bone marrow ~ 38221, 38222, 88305
  brain ~ 61140
    stereotactic ~ 61750-61751
  brainstem ~ 61575-61576
  breast ~ 19100-19101
    with localization device placement ~ 19081-19086
      with magetic resonance guidance ~ 19085-19086
      with stereotactic guidance ~ 19081-19082
      with ultrasound guidance ~ 19083-19084
    with imaging of specimen ~ 19081-19086
  bronchi
    catheterization ~ 31717
    endoscopic ~ 31625-31629, 31632-31633

Biopsy ~ *continued*
  brush
    bronchi ~ 31717
    renal pelvis ~ 52007
    ureter ~ 52007
    with cystourethroscopy ~ 52204
  carpometacarpal joint, synovium ~ 26100
  cervix ~ 57454-57455, 57460, 57500, 57520
  chorionic villus ~ 59015
  colon ~ 44025, 44100
    endoscopy ~ 44389, 45380, 45391, 45392
    multiple, with colostomy, cecostomy ~ 44322
  colon-sigmoid, endoscopy ~ 45305, 45331
  conjunctiva ~ 68100
  core needle
    lung ~ 32408
    mediastinum ~ 32408
    thyroid ~ 60100
  cornea ~ 65410
  duodenum ~ 44010
  ear, external ~ 69100
  elbow ~ 24065-24066, 24101
    synovium ~ 24100
  embryo blastomere ~ 89290-89291
  endometrium ~ 58100, 58558
  epididymis ~ 54800-54865
  esophagus, endoscopy ~ 43202
    forceps ~ 3150F
  eye muscle ~ 67346
  eyelid ~ 67810
  forearm, soft tissue ~ 25065-25066
  gallbladder, endoscopy ~ 43261
  gastrointestinal, upper, endoscopy ~ 43239
  hand joint, synovium ~ 26100
  heart ~ 93505
  hip ~ 27040-27041
    joint ~ 27052
  hypopharynx ~ 31510, 31535, 31536, 31576
  ileum, endoscopy ~ 44382
  interphalangeal joint
    finger ~ 26110
    toe ~ 28054
  intertarsal joint, toe ~ 28050
  intestines, small ~ 44020, 44100
    endoscopy ~ 44361, 44377
  kidney ~ 50200-50205
    endoscopic ~ 50555-50557, 50574-50576, 52354
  knee ~ 27323-27324
    synovium ~ 27330
  knee joint, synovium ~ 27330
  lacrimal gland ~ 68510
  lacrimal sac ~ 68525
  larynx, endoscopy ~ 31510, 31576
  leg
    lower ~ 27613-27614
    upper ~ 27323-27324
  lip ~ 40490
  liver ~ 47000-47001, 47100
  lung
    thoracoscopy ~ 32607-32608
    thoracotomy ~ 32096-32097
  lymph nodes ~ 38500-38530
    endobronchial ultrasound (EBUS) guided ~ 31652, 31653
    injection procedure, radioactive tracer ~ 38792
    laparoscopic ~ 38570-38573
    needle ~ 38505
    open ~ 38500, 38510, 38520, 38525, 38530
      superficial ~ 38500
    para-aortic ~ 57109, 57531, 58210, 58548
    prostate ~ 55812, 55842, 55862
    transbronchial ~ 31652, 31653
    transtracheal ~ 31652, 31653
  mediastinum
    mediastinoscopy ~ 39401, 39402
    mediastinotomy ~ 39000, 39010
  metacarpophalangeal joint ~ 26105
  metatarsophalangeal joint ~ 28052
  mouth ~ 40808, 41108
  muscle ~ 20200-20206

Biopsy ~ *continued*
nail ~ 11755
nasopharynx ~ 42804-42806
neck ~ 21550
nerve ~ 64795
nose
  endoscopic ~ 31237
  intranasal ~ 30100
oocyte polar body ~ 89290-89291
orbit
  exploration ~ 67400, 67450
oropharynx ~ 42800
ovary ~ 58900
palate ~ 42100
pancreas ~ 48100
pelvis ~ 27040-27041
penis ~ 54100
  deep structures ~ 54105
percutaneous needle, spinal cord ~ 62269
perineum ~ 56605-56606
pharynx ~ 42800-42806
pleura
  needle ~ 32400
  thoracoscopy ~ 32609
  thoracotomy ~ 32098, 32400
prostate
  incisional ~ 55705
  needle or punch ~ 55700, 55706
  stereotactic ~ 55706
  lymph nodes ~ 55812, 55842, 55862
rectum ~ 45100, 45305, 45331
renal pelvis ~ 50606
retroperitoneal area ~ 49010
sacroiliac joint ~ 27050
salivary gland ~ 42405
shoulder
  deep ~ 23066
  soft tissue ~ 23065
shoulder joint ~ 23100-23101
sinus, sphenoid ~ 31050-31051
skin ~ see skin, biopsy
skin lesion
  fine needle aspiration (FNA) ~ 10004-10012, 10021
  incisional ~ 11106, 11107
  punch ~ 11104, 11105
  tangential ~ 11102, 11103
spinal cord ~ 63275-63290
  percutaneous ~ 62269
stomach ~ 43605
tarsometatarsal joint, synovial ~ 28050
testis ~ 54500-54505
thorax ~ 21550
throat ~ 42800-42806
tongue ~ 41100-41105
transcatheter ~ 37200
ureter ~ 52354
  endoluminal, non-endoscopic ~ 50606
  endoscopic ~ 50955-50957, 50974-50976
urethra ~ 52204, 52354, 53200
uterus
  endometrial ~ 58100
  endoscopic ~ 58558
uvula ~ 42100
vagina ~ 57100-57105, 57421
vein ~ 75970
vertebral body ~ 20250-20251
vulva ~ 56605-56606, 56821
with arthrotomy
  acromioclavicular joint ~ 23101
  glenohumeral joint ~ 23100
  sternoclavicular joint ~ 23101
with cystourethroscopy ~ 52354
wrist ~ 25065-25066, 25100-25101
Biostatistics ~ 76516-76519, 92136
Biosterol ~ 84590
Biotinidase ~ 82261
Birthing room, newborn care ~ 99465
Bischof procedure ~ 63170-63172
Bismuth ~ 83015
Bizzozero's corpuscle/cell ~ see blood, platelet

Bladder
abscess, incision and drainage ~ 51080
anastomosis ~ 51960
aspiration ~ 51100-51102
biopsy ~ 52204
catheterization ~ 51045, 51701-51703
change tube ~ 51705-51710
creation, stoma ~ 51980
cyst, urachal, excision ~ 51500
destruction, endoscopic ~ 52214-52224, 52354
dilation, ureter ~ 52260-52265, 52341-52342, 52344-52345
diverticulum
  excision ~ 51525
  incision ~ 52305
  resection ~ 52305
endoscopy ~ 52000
  biopsy ~ 52204, 52354
  catheterization ~ 52005, 52010
  destruction ~ 52214-52224, 52400
  dilation ~ 52260-52265
  diverticulum ~ 52305
  evacuation, clot ~ 52001
  excision, tumor ~ 52234-52240, 52355
  exploration ~ 52351
  injection ~ 52283
  lithotripsy ~ 52353
  radiotracer ~ 52250
  removal
    calculus ~ 52310-52315, 52352
    foreign body ~ 52310-52315
  sphincter surgery ~ 52277
  tumor, excision ~ 52355
  ureter surgery ~ 52290-52300
  urethral syndrome ~ 52285
  with urethrotomy ~ 52270-52276
excision
  partial ~ 51550-51565
  total ~ 51570, 51580, 51590-51597
    with nodes ~ 51575, 51585, 51595
  transurethral ~ 52640
  tumor ~ 52234-52240
incision
  catheter ~ 51045
  with destruction ~ 51020-51030
  with radiotracer ~ 51020
incision and drainage ~ 51040
injection, radiologic ~ 51600-51610
insertion, stent ~ 51045, 52334
instillation, drugs ~ 51720
irrigation ~ 51700
lesion, destruction ~ 51030
neck, endoscopy, injection of implant material ~ 51715
  excision ~ 51520
  micro-remodeling ~ 53860
nuclear medicine, residual study ~ 78730
radiotracer ~ 52250
reconstruction, and urethra ~ 51800-51820
  with intestines ~ 51960
removal
  calculus ~ 51050, 52310-52315
  foreign body ~ 52310-52315
  urethral stent ~ 52310-52315
repair
  diverticulum ~ 52305
  exstrophy ~ 51940
  fistula ~ 44660-44661, 45800-45805, 51880-51925
  neck ~ 51845
  wound ~ 51860-51865
  resection ~ 52500
  sphincter surgery ~ 52277
  suspension ~ 51990
suture
  fistula ~ 44660-44661, 45800-45805, 51880-51925
  wound ~ 51860-51865
tumor, excision ~ 51530
iunlisted services and procedures ~ 53899
urethrocystography ~ 74450-74455
urethrotomy ~ 52270-52276

Bladder ~ *continued*
  urinary incontinence procedures
    laparoscopy ~ 51990-51992
    plan of care documented ~ 0509F
  X-ray ~ 74430
    with contrast ~ 74450-74455
Bladder voiding pressure studies ~ 51728-51729
Blalock-Hanlon procedure ~ 33735-33737
Blalock-Taussig procedure ~ see shunt, great vessel
Blastocyst implantation ~ see implantation
Blastocyst transfer ~ see embryo transfer
Blastogenesis ~ 86353
Blastomyces, antibody ~ 86612
Blastomycosis, european ~ see cryptococcus
Blast cells ~ see stem cell
Blast transformation ~ 86353
Bleeding ~ see also hemorrhage
  anal ~ 46614
  disorder ~ 85390
  time ~ 85002
  tube, passage and placement ~ 43460
  uterine ~ 59160
  vaginal ~ 57180
Blepharoplasty ~ 15820-15823, 67950
  anesthesia ~ 00103
Blepharoptosis
  repair ~ 67901-67909
    frontalis muscle technique ~ 67901
      with fascial sling ~ 67902
    superior rectus technique with fascial sling ~ 67906
    tarso levator resection/advancement
      external approach ~ 67904
      internal approach ~ 67903
Blepharorrhaphy ~ 67875
Blepharospasm, chemodenervation ~ 64612
Blepharotomy ~ 67700
Blister ~ see bulla
Blom-Singer prosthesis ~ 31611
Blood ~ 85025-85027
  bleeding time ~ 85002
  collection, for autotransfusion
    intraoperative ~ 86891
    preoperative ~ 86890
  feces ~ 82270
    by hemoglobin immunoassay ~ 82274
  hemoglobin A1c (HbA1c) level ~ 3044F
  hemoglobin concentration ~ 85046
  nuclear medicine
    flow imaging ~ 78445
    plasma iron ~ 78160
    red cell ~ 78140
    red cell survival ~ 78130
  osmolality ~ 83930
  plasma, exchange ~ 36514-36516
  platelet
    aggregation ~ 85576
    automated count ~ 85049
    count ~ 85008
    manual count ~ 85032
  stem cell
    count ~ 86587
    donor search ~ 38204
    erythropoietin therapy ~ 3160F, 4090F-4095F
    harvesting ~ 38205-38206
    transplantation ~ 38240-38242
      cell concentration ~ 38215
      cryopreservation ~ 38207, 88240
      plasma depletion ~ 38214
      platelet depletion ~ 38213
      red blood cell depletion ~ 38212
      T-cell depletion ~ 38210
      thawing ~ 38208-38209, 88241
      tumor cell depletion ~ 38211
      washing ~ 38209
  transfusion ~ 36430
    exchange ~ 36455
      newborn ~ 36450, 36456
    fetal ~ 36460
    push, infant ~ 36440

Blood ~ *continued*
  unlisted services and procedures ~ 85999
  urine ~ 83491
  viscosity ~ 85810
Blood, occult ~ 82270-82272
Blood banking
  frozen blood preparation ~ 86930-86932
  frozen plasma preparation ~ 86927
  physician services ~ 86077-86079
Blood cell
  CD4 and CD8, including ratio ~ 86360
  enzyme activity ~ 82657
  exchange ~ 36511-36513
  red ~ see red blood cell (RBC)
  sedimentation rate
    automated ~ 85652
    manual ~ 85651
  white ~ see leukocyte
Blood cell count
  automated ~ 85049
  B-cells ~ 86064
  blood smear ~ 85007-85008
  differential WBC count ~ 85004-85007, 85009
  hematocrit ~ 85014
  hemoglobin ~ 85018
  hemogram
    added indices ~ 85025-85027
    automated ~ 85025-85027
    manual ~ 85032
  microhematocrit ~ 85013
  natural killer (NK) cells ~ 86379
  red ~ 85032-85041
  red blood cells ~ 85032-85041
  reticulocyte ~ 85044-85046
  stem cells ~ 86587
  T-cells ~ 86359-86361
  white ~ 85032, 85048, 89055
  white blood cells ~ 85032, 85048, 89055
Blood clot
  assay ~ 85396
  clotting factor ~ 85250-85293
  clotting factor test ~ 85210-85244
  clotting inhibitors ~ 85300-85302, 85305, 85307
  clot lysis time ~ 85175
  clot retraction ~ 85170
  coagulation time ~ 85345-85348
  thrombolytic agent(s), tissue plasminogen activator (tPA) ~ 4077F
Blood coagulation
  defect ~ 85390
  disorders ~ 34401-34490, 35875-35876, 50230
  factor ~ 85210-85293
  factor I ~ 85384-85385
  factor II ~ 85210
  factor III ~ see thromboplastin
  factor IV ~ see calcium
  factor VII ~ 85230
  factor VIII ~ 85210-85293
  factor IX ~ 85250
  factor X ~ 85260
  factor X, activated ~ 85260
  factor XI ~ 85270
  factor XIII ~ 85290-85291
  test ~ 85999
Blood component removal ~ 36511-36516
Blood count, complete ~ 85025-85027
Blood flow
  graft check ~ 15860, 90940
  myocardial absolute quantitation ~ 78343
Blood gases
  CO2 ~ 82803
  HCO3 ~ 82803
  O2 saturation ~ 82805-82810
  pCO2 ~ 82803
  pH ~ 82800-82803
  pO2 ~ 82803
Blood letting ~ 99195
Blood lipoprotein ~ see lipoprotein
Blood pool imaging ~ 78472-78473, 78481-78483, 78494-78496

Blood pressure
  baroreflex activation device ~ 0266T-0273T
  determination
    central arterial noninvasive waveform analysis ~ 93050
    patient self-measurement ~ 99473, 99474
  monitoring, 24 hour ~ 93784, 93786, 93788, 93790
  ocular
    measurement ~ 0198T
    monitoring ~ 0329T
  performance measures
    chronic kidney disease ~ 0513F, 2000F, 3074F, 3075F, 3077F-3080F
    coronary artery disease ~ 0001F, 3074F
    hypertension ~ 3074F, 3075F, 3077F-3080F
  venous ~ 93770
Blood products
  irradiation ~ 86945
  pooling ~ 86965
  splitting ~ 86985
Blood sample, fetal ~ 59030
Blood serum ~ see serum
Blood smear ~ 85060
Blood syndrome, chromosome analysis ~ 88245-88248
Blood tests
  iron stores ~ 3160F
  Kt/V ~ 3082F-3084F
  nuclear medicine
    iron, chelatable ~ 78172
    iron absorption ~ 78162
    iron utilization ~ 78170
    plasma volume ~ 78110-78111
    platelet survival ~ 78191
    red cell volume ~ 78120-78121
    whole blood volume ~ 78122
  panels
    acute hepatitis ~ 80074
    electrolyte ~ 80051
    general health panel ~ 80050
    hepatic function ~ 80076
    hepatitis, acute ~ 80074
    lipid panel ~ 80061
    metabolic
      basic, total calcium ~ 80048
      basic, ionized calcium ~ 80047
      comprehensive ~ 80053
    obstetric panel ~ 80055, 80081
    renal function ~ 80069
  volume determination ~ 78122
Blood transfusion, autologous ~ 86890-86891
Blood typing, serologic
  ABO only ~ 86900
  antigen screen ~ 86904
  antigen testing, donor blood ~ 86902
  compatibility ~ 86920-86923
  crossmatch ~ 86920-86923
  other RBC antigens ~ 86905
  paternity testing ~ 86910-86911
  Rh (D) ~ 86901
  Rh phenotype ~ 86906
Blood urea nitrogen ~ 84520-84525
Blood vessels ~ see also artery; vein
  angioscopy, non-coronary ~ 35400
  endoscopy, surgical ~ 37500, 37501
  endothelial function assessment, noninvasive ~ 93998
  excision, arteriovenous malformation ~ 63250-63252
  exploration
    abdomen ~ 35840
    carotid artery ~ 35701
    chest ~ 35820
    extremity ~ 35860, 35702, 35703
    femoral artery ~ 35703
    neck ~ 35800
    popliteal artery ~ 35703
  great vessel, suture ~ 33320-33322
  harvest
    endoscopic ~ 33508
    lower extremity vein ~ 35572
    upper extremity artery ~ 35600
    upper extremity vein ~ 35500

Blood vessels ~ *continued*
  repair
    aorta ~ 33320-33322
    direct ~ 35201-35226
    finger ~ 35207
    hand ~ 35207
    intra-abdominal ~ 35221, 35281
    intra-thoracic ~ 35211, 35216, 35271, 35276
    kidney ~ 50100
    lower extremity ~ 35226, 35288
    neck ~ 35201, 35231, 35261
    upper extremity ~ 35236, 35266
  shunt creation, direct ~ 36818, 36821
    thomas shunt ~ 36835
    with bypass graft ~ 35686
    with graft ~ 36825-36830
    with transposition ~ 36818-36820
  shunt revision, with graft ~ 36832
Blood, occult ~ see occult blood
Bloom syndrome, chromosome analysis ~ 88245
Blotting, western ~ see western blot
Blot test, ink ~ 96100
Blow-out fracture, orbital floor ~ 21385-21395
Blue, dome cyst ~ 19000-19001
BMT ~ 38240-38242
Boarding home care
  established patient ~ 99334-99337
  new patient ~ 99324-99328
Bodies
  acetone ~ 82009-82010
  Barr ~ 88130
  carotid ~ see carotid body
  ciliary ~ see ciliary body
  Heinz ~ 85441-85445
  inclusion ~ see inclusion bodies
  ketone ~ 82009-82010
Body cast
  halo ~ 29000
  removal ~ 29700, 29710
  repair ~ 29720
  Risser jacket ~ 29010-29015
  upper body and head ~ 29040
  upper body and legs ~ 29046
  upper body and one leg ~ 29044
  upper body only ~ 29035
Body fluid, crystal identification ~ 89060
Body of vertebra ~ see vertebral, body
Body section
  X-ray ~ 76100
  motion ~ 76101-76102
Body system, neurologic ~ *78699*
Boil ~ 10060-10061
Boil, vulva ~ 56405
Bone ~ see also specific bone***
  ablation, tumor ~ 20982
  biopsy ~ 20220-20245
  carpal ~ see carpal bone
  cheek ~ see cheekbone
  CT scan, density study ~ 77078
  cyst
    drainage ~ 20615
    injection ~ 20615
  dual energy X-ray absorptiometry ~ 77080-77081
  excision
    epiphyseal bar ~ 20150
    facial bones ~ 21026
    mandible ~ 21025
  facial ~ see facial bone
  fixation
    caliper ~ 20660
    cranial tong ~ 20660
    halo ~ 20661-20663, 21100
    interdental ~ 21110
    multiplane ~ 20692
      stereotactic computer assisted ~ 20696-20697
    pin/wire ~ 20650
    skeletal, humeral epicondyle, percutaneous ~ 24566
    stereotactic frame ~ 20660
    uniplane ~ 20690

Bone ~ continued
   fracture, osteoporosis screening ~ 5015F
   insertion
      needle ~ 36680
      osseointegrated implant, for external speech processor/cochlear
         stimulator ~ 69714-69718
   marrow, cytogenic testing ~ 3155F
   metatarsal ~ see metatarsal
   nasal ~ see nasal bone
   navicular ~ see navicular
   nuclear medicine
      density study ~ 78350, 78351
      imaging ~ 78300, 78305, 78306, 78315
      SPECT ~ 78803
      unlisted services and procedures ~ 78399
   osetoporosis, pharmacologic therapy ~ 4005F
   protein ~ 83937
   quality testing, microindentation ~ 0547T
   removal, fixation device ~ 20670-20680
   replacement, osseointegrated implant, for external speech
      processor/cochlear stimulator ~ 69717-69718
   scan ~ see bone, nuclear medicine; nuclear medicine
   semilunar ~ see lunate
   sesamoid ~ see sesamoid bone
   tarsal ~ see ankle
   temporal ~ see temporal bone
   X-ray
      age study ~ 77072
      dual energy absorptiometry ~ 77080-77081
      length study ~ 77073
      osseous survey ~ 77074-77077
Bone analysis
   CT scan for fracture risk/strength assessment ~ 0554T-0557T
   microindentation for quality testing ~ 0547T
Bone 4-carboxyglutamic protein ~ 83937
Bone conduction hearing device, electromagnetic
   implantation/replacement ~ 69710
   removal/repair ~ 69711
Bone density study
   appendicular skeleton ~ 77081
   axial skeleton ~ 77078, 77080
   CT scan ~ 0554T-0557T
   dual energy X-ray absorptiometry (DXA) ~ 77080, 77081, 77085
   ultrasound ~ 76977, 0508T
   vertebral fracture assessment ~ 77085, 77086
Bone graft
   any donor area ~ 20900, 20902
   clavicle ~ 23485
   craniofacial separation ~ 21436
   cranium ~ 61316, 61559, 62146-62148
   femur ~ 27170, 27177, 27470
   harvesting ~ 20900-20902
   knee drilling ~ 29885
   malar area ~ 21210, 21366
   mandible ~ 21127, 21194, 21215
   mandibular ramus ~ 21194
   maxilla ~ 21210
   metacarpal nonunion ~ 26546
   metatarsal nonunion ~ 28322
   microvascular anastomosis
      fibula ~ 20955
      iliac crest ~ 20956
      metatarsal ~ 20957
      other ~ 20962
   nasal area ~ 21210
   nasomaxillary complex fracture ~ 21348
   osteocutaneous flap ~ 20969-20973
   palate, cleft ~ 42210
   spine surgery ~ 0195T, 0196T, 20930, 20931, 22586, 22899
      bone marrow aspiration ~ 20939
   toe transfer ~ 26551
   ulna ~ 25830
   vertebra ~ 0222T
      cervical ~ 0219T, 63051
      lumbar ~ 0221T
      thoracic ~ 0220T
   wrist ~ 25810, 25825

Bone healing
   electrical stimulation
      invasive ~ 20975
      noninvasive ~ 20974
   ultrasound stimulation ~ 20979
Bone marrow
   aspiration ~ 38220, 38222
   biopsy ~ 38221, 38222, 88305
   cell therapy ~ 0263T-0265T
   harvesting
      allogenic ~ 38230
      autologous ~ 38232
   magnetic resonance imaging (MRI) ~ 77084
   needle biopsy ~ 38221
   nuclear medicine, imaging ~ 78102-78104
   smear ~ 85097
   T-cell transplantation ~ 38240-38242
   trocar biopsy ~ 38221
Bone plate, mandible ~ 21244
Bone scan ~ see bone, nuclear medicine; nuclear medicine
Bone spur ~ 69140
Bone wedge reversal, osteotomy ~ 21122
Bordetella
   antibody ~ 86615
   antigen detection, direct fluorescence ~ 87265
Borrelia, antibody ~ 86618-86619
Borrelia burgdorferi ab ~ 86617
Borreliosis, Lyme ~ 86617-86618
Bost fusion ~ 25800
Bosworth operation ~ see arthrodesis, vertebrae; fasciotomy; 23540-23552
Bottle type procedure ~ 55060
Botulinum toxin ~ see chemodenervation
Boutonniere deformity ~ 26426-26428
Bowel ~ see intestine
Bowleg repair ~ 27455-27457
Boyce operation ~ 50040-50045
Boyd hip disarticulation ~ see radical resection; replantation; 27590-27592
Brace ~ see cast for leg cast ~ 29358
Brachial arteries ~ see artery, brachial
Brachial plexus
   decompression ~ 64713
   injection anesthetic ~ 64415-64416
   neuroplasty ~ 64713
   release ~ 64713
   repair/suture ~ 64861
Brachiocephalic artery ~ see artery, brachiocephalic
Brachycephaly ~ 21175
Brachytherapy
   device placement
      breast ~ 19296-19298
      genitalia ~ 55920
      head~ 41019
      intraocular ~ 0190T
      neck ~ 41019
      pelvis ~ 55920
      uterus ~ 57155
      vagina ~ 57155, 57156
   dose plan ~ 77316-77318
   high dose electronic ~ 0394T, 0395T
   interstitial application ~ 0395T, 77778
   planning
      isodose plan ~ 77316-77318
      prostate volume study ~ 76873
   radioelement solution ~ 77750
   remote afterloading
      interstitial ~ 77770-77772
      intracavitary ~ 77770-77772
      surface ~ 77767, 77768
   surface application ~ 0394T, 77789
      remote afterloading ~ 77767, 77768
   unlisted clinical procedures ~ 77799
Bradykinin, blood or urine ~ 82286
Brain ~ see also brainstem; skull base surgery;
   abscess
      drainage ~ 61150-61151
      excision ~ 61514, 61522
      incision and drainage ~ 61320-61321
   adhesions, lysis ~ 62161
   anesthesia ~ 00210-00218, 00220-00222
   angiography ~ 70496

Brain ~ continued
biopsy ~ 61140
  stereotactic ~ 61750-61751
catheter
  irrigation ~ 62194, 62225
  replacement ~ 62160, 62194, 62225
cisternography ~ 70015
cortex, magnetic stimulation ~ 90867-90868
craniopharyngioma, excision ~ 61545
CT scan ~ 0042T, 70450-70470, 70496
cyst
  drainage ~ 61150-61151, 62161-62162
  excision ~ 61516, 61524, 62162
Doppler, transcranial ~ 93886-93893
epileptogenic focus, excision ~ 61534, 61536
excision
  amygdala ~ 61566
  choroid plexus ~ 61544
  hemisphere ~ 61543
  hippocampus ~ 61566
  other lobe ~ 61323, 61539-61540
  temporal lobe ~ 61537-61538
exploration
  infratentorial ~ 61305
  supratentorial ~ 61304
hematoma
  drainage ~ 61154
  incision and drainage ~ 61312-61315
implantation
  chemotherapy agent ~ 61517
  electrode ~ 61210, 61533, 61850, 61860, 61863-61864, 61867, 61868
  pulse generator ~ 61885-61886
  reservoir ~ 61210, 61215
incision
  corpus callosum ~ 61541
  subpial ~ 61567
insertion, catheter ~ 61210
  electrode ~ 61531-61533, 61850
  pulse generator ~ 61885-61886
  receiver ~ 61885-61886
  reservoir ~ 61210-61215
lesion
  aspiration stereotactic ~ 61750-61751
  excision ~ 61600, 61601, 61605-61608, 61615, 61616
meningioma, excision ~ 61512, 61519
myelography ~ 70010
positron emission tomography ~ 78608-78609
removal
  electrode ~ 61535, 61880
  foreign body ~ 61570
  pulse generator ~ 61888
  receiver ~ 61888
  shunt ~ 62256-62258
repair
  dura ~ 61618
  wound ~ 61571
shunt
  creation ~ 62180-62192, 62200-62223
  removal ~ 62256-62258
  replacement ~ 62160, 62194, 62225-62230, 62256-62258
  reprogramming ~ 62252
skull
  transcochlear approach ~ 61596
  transcondylar approach ~ 61597
  transpetrosal approach ~ 61598
  transtemporal approach ~ 61595
skull base
  craniofacial approach ~ 61580-61585
  infratemporal approach ~ 61590-61591
  orbitocranial-zygomatic approach ~ 61592
stereotaxis-aided procedures
  aspiration ~ 61750-61751
  biopsy ~ 61750-61751
  catheter placement ~ 61770
  create lesion ~ 61720-61735, 61790-61791
  localization for placement of therapy fields ~ 61770
  navigation ~ 61781, 61782
  procedure ~ 61781, 61782
  radiation treatment ~ 77432
  radiosurgery ~ 61796-61800, 77371-77373
  trigeminal tract ~ 61791

Brain ~ continued
transection, subpial ~ 61567
tumor, excision ~ 61510, 61518, 61520-61521, 61526-61530, 61545, 62164
X-ray, with contrast ~ 70010-70015
Brainstem ~ see also brain
biopsy ~ 61575-61576
decompression ~ 61575-61576
lesion, excision ~ 61575-61576
Brain coverings ~ 61512, 61519
Brain death, determination ~ 95824
Brain surface electrode, stimulation ~ 95961-95962
Brain tumor
acoustic neuroma ~ 61510, 61518, 61520-61521, 61526-61530, 61545, 62164
craniopharyngioma ~ 61545
meningioma ~ 61512, 61519
Brain ventriculography ~ see ventriculography
Branchial cleft cyst excision ~ 42810-42815
Branchioma ~ 42810-42815
Breast
ablation
  fibroadenoma ~ 19105
  malignant tumor ~ 0581T
abscess
  incision and drainage ~ 19020
augmentation with implant ~ 19325
biopsy ~ 19100-19101
  with imaging of specimen ~ 19081-19086
  with localization device palcement
    magnetic resonance guided ~ 19085-19086
    stereotactic guidance ~ 19081-19082
    ultrasound guided ~ 19083-19084
cancer gene analysis
  BRCA1 variants ~ 81212
    duplication/deletion ~ 81162, 81164
    full sequence ~ 81162, 81165
    known familial variant ~ 81215
  BRCA2 variants ~ 81212
    duplication/deletion ~ 81162, 81167
    full sequence ~ 81162, 81216
    known familial variant ~ 81217
  ERBB2 (HER2) ~ 0009U
cyst
  excision ~ 19120
  puncture aspiration ~ 19000-19001
diagnostic imaging
  axillary lymph node ~ 0351T, 0352T
  CT scan ~ 0633T-0638T
  ductogram ~ 19030, 77053, 77054
  galactobram ~ 77053, 77054
  injection ~ 19030
  MRI
    with computer-aided detection ~ 77048, 77049
    without contrast ~ 77046, 77047
  mammography, diagnostic ~ 77065, 77066
  mammogram, screening ~ 3014F, 77067
  ultrasound ~ 76641, 76642
excision
  biopsy ~ 19100-19101
  capsules ~ 19371
  chest wall tumor ~ 21601-21603
  cyst ~ 19120
  lactiferous duct ~ 19110
    fistula ~ 19112
  lesion ~ 19120, 19125-19126, 19301
    by needle localization ~ 19125-19126
  mastectomy ~ 19300-19307
  tissue ~ 19120
  tumor ~ 19120, 21601-61203
exploration
  abscess ~ 19020
  nipple ~ 19110
implants
  insertion ~ 19325, 19340, 19342
  preparation of moulage ~ 19396
  removal ~ 19328, 19330
  supply ~ 19396

1091

Breast ~ *continued*

lesion, localizatiion device placement
    with magetnic resonance guidance ~ 19287-19288
    with mammographic guidance ~ 19281-19282
    with stereotactic guidance ~ 19283-19284
    with ultrasound guidance ~ 19285-19286
mammogram screening ~ 3014F, 77067
mammoplasty
    augmentation with implant ~ 19325
    reduction ~ 19318
mastectomy
    complete ~ 19303
    gynecomastia ~ 19300
    modified radical ~ 19307
    partial ` 19301-19302
    radical ~ 19303-19306
    with axillary lymphadenectomy ~ 19302
mastopexy ~ 19316
periprosthetic capsulectomy ~ 19371
periprosthetic capsulotomy ~ 19370
radiation therapy
    catheter placement, for interstitial radioelement application ~
      19296-19298
    preparation of tumor cavity ~ 19294
reduction ~ 19318
reconstruction
    augmentation ~ 19325
    mammoplasty ~ 19318-19325
    nipple ~ 19350, 19355
      areola ~ 19350
    revision ~ 19380
    with free flap ~ 19364
    with latissimus dorsi flap ~ 19361
    with tissue expander ~ 19357
    with transverse rectus abdominis myocutaneous flap ~ 19367-19369
reduction ~ 19318
removal
    capsules ~ 19371
    modified radical ~ 19307
    partial ~ 19300-19302
    radical ~ 19305-19306
    simple, complete ~ 19303
suspension ~ 19316
tissue expander
    removal w/o implant insertion ~ 11971
    replacement with implant ~ 11970
tumor
    ablation ~ 0581T
    destruction/reduction microwave thermotherapy ~ 19499
    excision
      benign ~ 19120
      chest wall ~ 21601-21603
      involving ribs ~ 21601-21603
      malignant ~ 19120
unlisted services and procedures ~ 19499

Breath odor alcohol ~ 82075

Breath test

alcohol, ethyl ~ 82075
helicobacter pylori ~ 78267-78268, 83013-83014
hydrogen ~ 91065

Bricker procedure, intestines anastomosis ~ 50820

Bristow procedure ~ 23450-23462

Brock operation ~ 33470-33474

Broken, nose ~ see fracture, nasal bone

Bronchi

allograft preparation ~ 32855, 32856
aspiration
    catheter ~ 31720, 31725
    endoscopic ~ 31629, 31633, 31645, 31646
biopsy ~ 31625-31629, 31632, 31633
bronchial valve
    insertion ~ 31647, 31651
    removal ~ 31648, 31649
bronchodilator
    home care ~ 99503
    spirometry ~ 94012, 94060
bronchoscopy
    alveolar lavage ~ 31624
    aspiration ~ 31629, 31633, 31645, 31646
    biopsy ~ 31625-31629, 31632, 31633

Bronchi ~ *continued*

catheter placement for radiotherapy ~ 31643
cell brushing ~ 31623
cell washing ~ 31622
computer assisted/image guided navigation ~ 31627
dilation ~ 31630, 31631, 31636, 31638
endobronchial ultrasound (EBUS) ~ 31652-31654
exploration ~ 31622
    with balloon occlusion ~ 31634, 31647, 31651
foreign body removal ~ 31635
stenosis relief ~ 31641
stent placement ~ 31631, 31636-31638
thermoplasty ~ 31660, 31661
tumor destruction ~ 31641
tumor excision ~ 31640
catheterization
    aspiration ~ 31725
    bronchial brush biopsy ~ 31717
endoscopy
    ablation, photodynamic therapy ~ 96570, 96571
exploration ~ 31622, 31634, 31647, 31651
fracture reduction ~ 31630
insertion, bronchial valve ~ 31647, 31651
needle biopsy ~ 31629, 31633
reconstruction
    anastomosis ~ 31775, 32486
    graft repair ~ 31770
    stenosis ~ 31775
removal, foreign body ~ 31635
repair ~ 32501
    fistula ~ 32815, 32906
stenosis ~ 31641, 96570, 96571
stent
    placement ~ 31636, 31637
    revision ~ 31638
tests
    air leak assessment ~ 31647, 31651
    bronchospasm evaluation ~ 94070, 94617, 94619
    wheeze rate ~ 94799
thermoplasty ~ 31660, 31661
tumor
    destruction ~ 31641
    excision ~ 31640
unlisted services and procedures ~ 31899

Bronchial

alveolar lavage ~ 31624
brushings/protected brushing ~ 31623
brush biopsy, with catheterization ~ 31717
challenge test
    bronchospasm evaluation ~ 94070, 94617, 94619
    for wheeze rate ~ 94799
    with chemicals ~ 95070
    with histamine ~ 95070
    with methacholine ~ 95070
lavage ~ 31624

Broncho-bronchial anastomosis ~ 32486

Bronchoalveolar lavage ~ 31624

Bronchography ~ 76499

injection, transtracheal ~ 31899
segmental, injection ~ 31899

Bronchoplasty ~ 32501

excision stenosis and anastomosis ~ 31775
graft repair ~ 31770

Bronchopneumonia, hiberno-vernal ~ 86000, 86638

Bronchopulmonary lavage ~ 31624

Bronchoscopy

ablation ~ 96570, 96571
alveolar lavage ~ 31624
aspiration ~ 31629, 31633, 31645, 31646
balloon occlusion ~ 31634, 31647, 31651
biopsy ~ 31625-31629, 31632, 31633
brushing/protected brushing ~ 31623
catheter placement
    aspiration ~ 31725
    intracavitary radioelement ~ 31643
computer assisted navigation ~ 31627
dilation ~ 31630-31631, 31636-31638
exploration ~ 31622, 31634, 31647, 31651
fiducial marker placement ~ 31626
fracture ~ 31630

Bypass graft ~ *continued*
    common carotid-ipsilateral internal carotid ~ 35501, 35601
    coronary ~ 33510-33514, 33516
    femoral-popliteal ~ 35556, 35572, 35656
    femoral-femoral ~ 35558, 35661
    femoral-tibial ~ 35566, 35666
    femoral-peroneal ~ 35566
    hepatorenal ~ 35535
    ilioceliac ~ 35632
    iliofemoral ~ 35565, 35665
    ilioiliac ~ 35563, 35663
    ilimesenteric ~ 35633
    iliorenal ~ 35634
    mesenteric ~ 35531, 35631
    peroneal ~ 35556-35571, 35666-35671
    peroneal-tibial ~ 35570
    popliteal-peroneal ~ 35571, 35671
    popliteal-tibial ~ 35571, 35671
    splenorenal ~ 35536, 35636
    subclavian-axillary ~ 35516, 35616
    subclavian-brachial ~ 35512
    subclavian-carotid ~ 35506
    subclavian-subclavian ~ 35511, 35612
    subclavian-vertebral ~ 35515, 35645
    tibial/peroneal trunk-tibial ~ 35570
    tibial-tibial ~ 35570
   with composite graft ~ 35681
Bypass in-situ
    femoral artery ~ 35583-35585
    peroneal artery ~ 35585-35587
    popliteal artery ~ 35583, 35587
    tibial artery ~ 35585-35587
   ventricular restoration ~ 33548

C

C vitamin ~ 82180
C-13
    urea breath test ~ 83013-83014
    urease activity ~ 83013-83014
C-14
    urea breath test ~ 78267-78268
    urease activity ~ 83013-83014
C-peptide ~ 80432, 84681
C-reactive protein ~ 86140-86141
C-section ~ see cesarean delivery
CABG ~ see coronary artery bypass graft (CABG) ~ 33503-33505, 33510-33516
Cadmium, urine ~ 82300
Calcaneal spur ~ 28119
Calcaneus
    craterization ~ 28120
    cyst, excision ~ 28100-28103
    diaphysectomy ~ 28120
    excision ~ 28118-28120
    fracture
        open treatment ~ 28415-28420
        percutaneous fixation ~ 28406
        without manipulation ~ 28400
        with manipulation ~ 28405-28406
    repair, osteotomy ~ 28300
    saucerization ~ 28120
    tumor, excision ~ 27647, 28100-28103
    X-ray ~ 73650
Calcareous deposits, subdeltoid, removal ~ 23000
Calcifediol, blood or urine ~ 82306
Calciferol, blood or urine ~ 82306
Calcification ~ see calcium, deposits
Calciol ~ 82306
Calcitonin
    blood or urine ~ 82308
    stimulation panel ~ 80410
Calcium, blood, infusion test ~ 82331
    deposits ~ see removal, calculi (stone) ~ 65205-65265
    ionized ~ 82330
    total ~ 82310
    urine ~ 82340

Calcium-binding protein, vitamin K-dependent ~ 83937
Calcium-pentagastrin stimulation ~ 80410
Calculus
    analysis ~ 82355-82370
    destruction
        bile duct ~ 43265, 47544
        extracorporeal shock wave lithotripsy ~ 50590
        gallbladder ~ 47544
        pancreatic duct ~ 43265
    removal
        bile duct ~ 43264, 47544, 47554
        biliary tract ~ 47400, 47420, 47425, 47480
        bladder ~ 51050, 52310, 52315, 52352
        gallbladder ~ 74544
        kidney ~ 50060-50081, 50130, 50561, 50580, 52352
        liver ~ 47400
        pancreatic duct ~ 43264, 48020
        renal pelvis ~ 50075, 50080, 50081, 50130
        ureter ~ 50610-50630, 50945, 50961, 50980, 52310, 52315, 52320, 52352
Calculus of kidney ~ 50060-50081, 50130, 50561, 50580, 52352
Caldwell-Luc procedure ~ 21385
    sinusotomy ~ 31030-31032
Caliper, application/removal ~ 20660
Callander knee disarticulation ~ 27598
Callosum, corpus ~ 61541
Calmette Guerin Bacillus vaccine ~ see BCG vaccine
Caloric vestibular test ~ 92533
Calprotectin, fecal ~ 83993
Calycoplasty ~ 50405
Camey enterocystoplasty ~ 50825
Campbell procedure ~ 27422
Campylobacter, antibody ~ 86625
Campylobacter pylori ~ see helicobacter pylori
Canal, ear ~ see auditory canal
Canalith repositioning ~ 95992
Canaloplasty ~ 69631, 69635
Candida
    antibody ~ 86628
    skin test ~ 86485
Cannulation ~ 36821
    arterial ~ 36620-36625
    sinus
        maxillary ~ 31000
        sphenoid ~ 31002
    thoracic duct ~ 38794
Cannulation, renoportal ~ 37145
Cannulization ~ see catheterization
    arteriovenous ~ 36810-36815
    declotting ~ 36593, 36860-36861
    diaysis circuit ~ 36901-36903
    external, declotting ~ 36860, 36861
    vas deferens ~ 55200
    vein to vein ~ 36800
Canthocystostomy ~ 68745, 68750
Canthopexy
    lateral ~ 21282
    medial ~ 21280
Canthoplasty ~ 67950
Canthorrhaphy ~ 67880-67882
Canthotomy ~ 67715
Canthus, reconstruction ~ 67950
Cap, cervical ~ 57170
Capsule ~ 26516-26518
    ankle ~ 27612, 27630
    elbow ~ 24006, 24149
    eye ~ 66830
    finger ~ 26160, 26520
    foot ~ 28090, 28264, 28289, 28291
    hand ~ 26160, 26520
    heyman ~ 58346
    hip ~ 27036
    interphalangeal joint ~ 26525, 28272
    knee ~ 27347, 27405, 27435
    leg ~ 27630
    shoulder ~ 23020
    Tenon's ~ 67515
    toe ~ 28270, 28272
    wrist, excision ~ 25320
Capsulectomy, breast, periprosthetic ~ 19371

Capsulodesis
metacarpophalangeal joint ~ 26516-26518
wrist ~ 25320
Capsulorrhaphy
anterior ~ 23450-23462
glenohumeral joint ~ 23465-23466
multi-directional instability ~ 23466
posterior ~ 23465
shoulder ~ 29806
wrist ~ 25320
Capsulotomy
breast, periprosthetic ~ 19370
eye ~ 66830
foot ~ 28260-28262, 28264
hip, with release, flexor muscles ~ 27036
interphalangeal joint ~ 28272
knee ~ 27435
leg ~ 27630
metacarpophalangeal joint ~ 26520
metatarsophalangeal joint ~ 28270
shoulde ~ 23020
toe ~ 28270-28272
wrist ~ 25085, 25320
Captopril ~ 80416-80417
Car seat testing ~ 94780, 94781
Carbamazepine, assay ~ 80156-80157
Carbazepin ~ 80156-80157
Carbinol ~ 84600
Carbohydrate deficient transferrin ~ 82373
Carbon dioxide, blood or urine ~ 82374
Carbon monoxide, blood ~ 82375-82376
Carbon tetrachloride ~ 84600
Carboxycathepsin ~ 82164
Carboxyhemoglobin ~ 82375-82376, 88740
Carbuncle, incision and drainage ~ 10060-10061
Carcinoembryonal antigen ~ 82378
Carcinoembryonic antigen ~ 82378
Cardiac ~ *see* coronary
Cardiac anomoly, reconstruction ~ 33622
Cardiac arrhythmia, tachycardia ~ 93609
Cardiac Assist Devices
cardiac contractility modulation system
device evaluation ~ 0417T, 0418T
insertion.~ 0408T-0411T
relocation of skin pocket ~ 0416T
removal ~ 0412T, 0413T
replacement ~ 0414T
repositioning. ~ 0415T
cardiovascular physiologic monitor system device evaluation ~ 93290, 93297
implantable defibrillators
subcutaneous implantable defibrillator (SICD)
device evaluation.~ 93260, 93261, 93287,93295, 93296, 93644
insertion
electrode ~ 33202, 33203, 33271
pulse generator ~ 33230, 33231, 33240
system ~ 33270
relocation of skin pocket.~ 33223
removal ~ 33241, 33262, 33272
repair, electrode ~ 33218, 33220
replacement, pulse generator.~ 33262
repositioning, electrode ~ 33215, 33273
transvenous implantable pacing defibrillator (ICD)
device evaluation ~ 93282-93284, 93287, 93289, 93295, 93296
insertion
electrode ~ 33202, 33203, 33216, 33217, 33224, 33225
pulse generator ~ 33230, 33231, 33249
system ~ 33249
relocation of skin pocket ~ 33223
removal
electrodes ~ 33244
pulse generator ~ 33241, 33262-33264
replacement, pulse generator ~ 33262-33264
repositioning, electrode ~ 33215, 33273
ischemia monitoring system
device evaluation ~ 0528T, 0529T
insertion or replacement ~ 0525T-0527T
removal ~ 0530T-0532T

Cardiac Assist Devices ~ *continued*
pacemaker system
device evaluation ~ 93279-93281, 93286, 93288, 93293, 93294, 93296, 93724
insertion
electrode/lead ~ 33202, 33203, 33210, 33211, 33216, 33217, 33224, 33225, 33230, 33231, 33243, 33244, 33249, 93583
pulse generator ~ 33212, 33213, 33221
system ~ 33206-33208
relocation of skin pocket ~ 33222
removal ~ 33233-33237
repair, electrode ~ 33218-33220
replacement
catheter/electrode ~ 33210, 33211
pulse generator ~ 33227-33229
repositioning, electrode ~ 33215, 33226
single-to-dual chamber system upgrade ~ 33214
pacemaker system, leadless
device evaluation ~ 93279, 93286, 93288, 93294, 93296
transcatheter insertion ~ 33274
transcatheter removal ~ 33275
transcatheter replacement ~ 33274
subcutaneous cardiac rhythm monitor system
device evaluation ~ 93285, 93291, 93298
insertion ~ 33285
removal ~ 33286
substernal implantable cardioverter-defibrillator
electrophysiological evaluation ~ 0577T
insertion ~ 0571T, 0572T
interrogation device evaluation ~ 0576T, 0578T, 0579T
programming device evaluation ~ 0575T
removal and replacement of pulse generator ~ 0614T
removal of electrode ~ 0573T
removal of pulse generator ~ 0580T
replacement ~ 0571T
repositioning of electrode ~ 0574T
wireless cardiac stimulation system
device evaluation ~ 0521T, 0522T
insertion ~ 0515T-0517T
removal ~ 0518T
replacement ~ 0519T, 0520T
Cardiac catheterization
combined left and right heart ~ 93460, 93461
with left ventriculography ~ 93453, 93460, 93461
combined right and retrograde left congenital cardiac anomalies ~ 93531
combined right and transseptal left congenital cardiac anomalies ~ 93532, 93533
congenital cardiac anomalies ~ 93530-93533
for angiography
bypass graft(s) ~ 93455, 93457, 93459, 93461
congenital heart ~ 93563, 93564
coronary ~ 93454-93461, 93563, 93571
left atrial ~ 93565
left ventricular ~ 93565
pulmonary ~ 93568
right atrial ~ 93566
right ventricular ~ 93566
for biopsy ~ 93505
for congenital prosthetic valve implantation ~ 33477
for dilution studies ~ 93561, 93562
for flow measurement ~ 93571, 93572
for measurement of O2, cardiac output ~ 93451

Cardiac catheterization ~ *continued*
for supravalvular aortography ~ 93567
imaging ~ 93452-93461, 93563-93568
injection ~ 93454-93461, 93563-93568
left heart
by transapical puncture ~ 93462
with ventriculography ~ 93452, 93458, 93459, 93565
pacemaker ~ 33210
right heart ~ 93451, 93456, 93503
congenital cardiac anomalies ~ 93530
Cardiac electroversion ~ 92960-92961
Cardiac magnetic resonance imaging (CMRI) ~ 75557-75563, 75565
Cardiac massage, thoracotomy ~ 32160
Cardiac muscle ~ see myocardium
Cardiac neoplasm ~ 33120-33130
Cardiac output, indicator dilution ~ 93561-93562
Cardiac pacemaker ~ see heart, pacemaker
Cardiac rehabilitation ~ 93797-93798

1095

Cardiac septal defect ~ 33813-33814
Cardiac transplantation ~ 33935, 33945
Cardiectomy, donor ~ 33930, 33940
Cardioassist ~ 92970-92971
Cariography
  acoustic ~ 93799
  arterial pressure waveform analysis ~ 93050
Cardiolipin antibody ~ 86147
Cardiology
  diagnostic
    acoustic cardiography ~ 93799
    arrhythmia induction ~ 93618-93624, 93640, 93641, 93653-93656
    arterial pressure waveform analysis ~ 93050
    atrial electrogram ~ 93615, 93616
      esophageal recording ~ 93615, 93616
    bioimpedence derived analysis ~ 93701
    echocardiography
      Doppler ~ 76827-76828, 93306-93308, 93320-93350
        intracardiac ~ 93662
        transesophageal ~ 93318
        transthoracic ~ 93303-93317
      congenital cardiac anomoly
        fetal ~ 76825, 76826
        doppler, fetal ~ 76827, 76828
        transesophageal ~ 93315-93317
        transthoracic ~ 93303, 93304
    ergonovine provocation test ~ 93024
    intracardiac pacing and mapping
      3-D mapping ~ 93613, 93654
      follow-up study ~ 93624
      localization ~ 93631
      stimulation and pacing ~ 93623
    intracardiac pacing and recording
      arrhythmia induction ~ 93618-93624, 93653-93654, 93656
      bundle of His ~ 93600, 93619-93620, 93653-93654, 93656
      comprehensive ~ 93619-93622
      intra-atrial ~ 93602, 93610, 93616, 93656
      left ventricular ~ 93654
      right ventricle ~ 93603, 93653, 93656
      tachycardia sites ~ 93609
      ventricular ~ 93612
    intravascular ultrasound ~ 92978-92979
    perfusion imaging ~ 78451-78454, 78430-78433
    stress tests
      cardiovascular ~ 93015-93018
      drug induced ~ 93024
      multiple gated acquisition (MUGA) ~ 78473
    temperature gradient studies ~ 93740
    tilt table evaluation ~ 93660
    venous pressure determination ~ 93784, 93786, 93788, 93790
  therapeutic
    ablation ~ 93650, 93653-93656
    cardioassist ~ 92970-92971
    cardioversion ~ 92960-92961
    intravascular ultrasound ~ 92978-92979
    pacing, transcutaneous, temporary ~ 92953
    rehabilitation ~ 93668, 93797-93798
    thrombolysis ~ 92975-92977
    thrombolysis, coronary ~ 92977
    valvuloplasty, percutaneous ~ 92986-92990
Cardiomyotomy ~ 32665, 43330-43331
Cardioplasty ~ 43320
Cardiopulmonary bypass
  establishment ~ 34714, 34716, 34833
  with transcatheter aortic valve replacement ~ 33367-33369
Cardiopulmonary resuscitation ~ 92950
Cardiotomy ~ 33310-33315
Cardiovascular stress test ~ 93015-93018
Cardiovascular system
  medical services ~ 92950-93799
  surgical procedures ~ 33000-39599
Cardioversion ~ 92960-92961
Care, custodial ~ see nursing facility services
Care, neonatal intensive ~ see intensive care, neonatal
Care, self ~ see self care
Care plan oversight services ~ 99339-99340, 99374-99380
Carneous mole ~ see abortion
Carnitine ~ 82379
Carotene ~ 82380
Caroticum, glomus ~ 60605, 60600

Carotid artery
  aneurysm repair
    vascular malformation or carotid-cavernous fistula ~ 61710
  bypass graft ~ 33891, 35501-35510, 35601-35606, 35642
  catheterization ~ 36100, 36221-36224, 36227-36228
  decompression ~ 61590-61591, 61596
  embolectomy ~ 34001
  evauation ~ 93895
  excision ~ 60605
  ligation ~ 37600-37606, 61611
  stenosis imaging ~ 3100F
  stent placement ~ 37217, 37218
  thrombectomy ~ 34001
  thromboendarterectomy ~ 35301, 35390
  transection ~ 61611
  transposition ~ 33889, 35691, 35694-35695
Carotid body
  lesion
    carotid artery ~ 60605
    excision ~ 60600
Carpals, incision and drainage ~ 25035
Carpal bone ~ see wrist
  arthroplasty, with implant ~ 25443
  cyst, excision ~ 25130-25136
  dislocation
    closed treatment ~ 25690
    open treatment ~ 25695
  excision ~ 25210-25215
    partial ~ 25145
  fracture
    closed treatment ~ 25622, 25630
    open treatment ~ 25628, 25645
    without manipulation ~ 25630
    with manipulation ~ 25624, 25635
  incision and drainage ~ 26034
  insertion, vascular pedicle ~ 25430
  osteoplasty ~ 25394
  repair ~ 25431-25440
  sequestrectomy ~ 25145
  tumor, excision ~ 25130-25136
Carpal tunnel, injection, therapeutic ~ 20526
Carpal tunnel syndrome, decompression ~ 64721
Carpectomy ~ 25210-25215
Carpometacarpal joint
  arthrodesis
    hand ~ 26843-26844
    thumb ~ 26841-26842
  arthrotomy ~ 26070
  biopsy, synovium ~ 26100
  dislocation
    closed treatment ~ 26670
      with manipulation ~ 26675-26676
    open treatment ~ 26685-26686
  exploration ~ 26070
  fusion
    hand ~ 26843-26844
    thumb ~ 26841-26842
  removal, foreign body ~ 26070
  repair ~ 25447
  synovectomy ~ 26130
Cartilage, arytenoid ~ 31560-31561
Cartilage, ear ~ 21235
Cartilage graft
  ear to face ~ 21235
  harvesting ~ 20910-20912
  rib to face ~ 21230
Cartilaginous exostoses ~ 69140
Case management services
  online ~ 98970-98972, 99421-99423
  team conferences ~ 99366-99368
  telephone calls ~ 98966-98968, 99441-99443
Cast ~ see also splint ~ 29358
  body, Risser jacket ~ 29010-29015
  body cast
    halo ~ 29000
    upper body and head ~ 29040
    upper body and legs ~ 29046
    upper body and one leg ~ 29044
    upper body only ~ 29035
  clubfoot ~ 29450

Cast ~ continued
cylinder ~ 29365
finger ~ 29086
hand ~ 29085
hip ~ 29305-29325
leg, rigid total contact ~ 29445
long arm ~ 29065
long leg ~ 29345-29355, 29365, 29450
long leg brace ~ 29358
patellar tendon bearing (PTB) ~ 29435
removal ~ 29700
repair ~ 29720
short arm ~ 29075
short leg ~ 29405-29435, 29450
shoulder ~ 29049-29058
walking ~ 29355, 29425
   revision ~ 29440
wedging ~ 29740-29750
windowing ~ 29730
wrist ~ 29085
Casting, unlisted services and procedures ~ 29799
Castration ~ see orchiectomy
Castration, female ~ 58262-58263, 58291-58292, 58552, 58554, 58661, 58940-58943
Cat scan ~ see CT scan
Cataract
discission ~ 66820, 66821
excision ~ 66830
   dilated fundus evaluation ~ 2021F
incision ~ 66820-66821
   laser ~ 66821
   stab incision ~ 66820
removal/extraction
   extracapsular ~ 66982, 66984
      with endoscopic cyclophotocoagulation ~ 66987, 66988
   intracapsular ~ 66983
   presurgical measurement/calculation ~ 3073F
Catecholamines ~ 80424, 82382-82384
blood ~ 82383
urine ~ 82382
Cathepsin-D ~ 82387
Catheter ~ see also cannulization; venipuncture
aspiration
   nasotracheal ~ 31720
   tracheobronchial ~ 31725
bladder ~ 51701-51703
   irrigation ~ 51700
blood specimen collection ~ 36592, 37799
conversion
   biliary drainage, external to internal- external~ 47535
   nephrostomy to nephroureteral ~ 50434
declotting ~ 36593, 36861
drainage
   biliary
      conversion ~ 47535
      exchange ~ 47536
      placement ~ 47533, 47534
      removal ~ 47537
   pericardial ~ 33017-33019
   peritoneal ~ 49406, 49407
   pleural ~ 32556, 32557
   retroperitoneal ~ 49406, 49407
   spinal ~ 62272
   ureteral ~ 50693
   ventricular ~ 62162, 62164
   visceral ~ 49405
electrode array ~ 63650
embolization ~ 61624, 61626
   peritoneal ~ 49423
exchange
   nephrostomy ~ 50435
   with biliary stent placement ~ 47538-47540
flow directed ~ 93503
for cystourethroscopy ~ 52320-52356
for embolectomy ~ 34001, 34051, 34101-34111, 34151, 34201, 34203
intraperitoneal, tunneled
   insertion
      laparoscopic ~ 49324
      open ~ 49421
      percutaneous ~ 49418-49419

Catheter ~ continued
obstruction clearance ~ 36595-36596
occlusion ~ 61624, 61626
removal
   central venous ~ 36589
   foreign body ~ 37197
   peritoneal ~ 49422
   spinal cord ~ 62355
   with biliary stent placement ~ 47538-47540
repair
   central venous ~ 36575
   intraperitoneal ~ 49325
replacement
   central venous ~ 36580-36581, 36584
   shunt system ~ 62230
   subarachnoid ~ 62194
   subdural ~ 62194
   ventricular ~ 62225
repositioning ~ 36597
transcatheter therapy
   arterial for chemotherapy ~ 36640
   arterial, intracranial ~ 61650, 61651
   epidural or subarachnoid ~ 62320-62327
   newborn ~ 36660
   thrombolysis ~ 37211-37214
ureteral
   manometric studies ~ 50396, 50686
   ureterography ~ 50684
Catheterization ~ see also catheter
abdomen ~ 49421
abdominal artery ~ 36245-36248
aorta ~ 36160, 36200
arterial system ~ 36215, 36245-36248
   cutdown ~ 36625
   intracatheter/needle ~ 36100-36140
   percutaneous ~ 36620
bile duct, percutaneous
   conversion ~ 47535
   exchange ~ 47536
   placement ~ 47533, 47534
   removal ~ 47537
bladder ~ 51045, 51102, 51702-51703
brachiocephalic artery ~ 36215-36218
brain ~ 61210
   replacement ~ 62160, 62194, 62225
breast ~ 19296-19298, 20555, 41019
bronchus ~ 31643, 31710
cardiac ~ see cardiac catheteriztaion
carotid artery ~ 36100, 36221-36224, 36227-36228
cerebral artery ~ 36215
cholecystostomy ~ 47490
coronary artery ~ 93455
cystourethroscopy, ejaculatory duct ~ 52010
   ureteral ~ 52005
dialysis ~ 36901-36903, 49418, 49419, 49421
ear, middle ~ 69799
electrode array ~ 63650
eustachian tube ~ 69799
extremity, artery ~ 36140
fallopian tube ~ 58345, 74742
gastrointestinal ~ 43241
hepatic vein ~ 37182-37183
innominate artery ~ 36222-36223, 36225
intracardiac, ablation ~ 93650, 93653-93657
intraperitoneal, tunneled ~ 49324, 49421
jejunum, for enteral ~ 44015
kidney, percutaneous
   for nephrostomy ~ 50432
   nephroureteral ~ 50433
legs ~ 36245-36248
nasotracheal ~ 31720
newborn, umbilical vein ~ 36510
pelvic artery ~ 36245-36248
pericardium ~ 33017-33019
peripheral ~ 36568-36571
pleural cavity ~ 32550-32552
portal vein ~ 36481, 37182-37183
pulmonary artery ~ 36013-36015
radioelement application ~ 519296-19297, 20555, 31643, 41019, 55875, 55920

1097

Catheterization ~ *continued*
  removal
    fractured catheter ~ 37197
    obstructive material
      intracatheter ~ 36596
      pericatheter ~ 36595
  renal artery ~ 36251-36254
  salivary duct ~ 42660
  skull ~ 61107
  spinal cord ~ 62350-62351
  subclavian artery ~ 36225
  thoracic artery ~ 36215-36218
  tracheobronchi ~ 31725
  umbilical artery ~ 36660
  umbilical vein ~ 36510
  ureter
    endoscopic ~ 50553, 50572, 50953, 50972, 52005
    injection ~ 50684
    manometric studies ~ 50396, 50686
    via kidney ~ 50693
  uterus, radiology ~ 58340
  vena cava ~ 36010
  venous
    central line ~ see Central venous catheter
    first order ~ 36011
    intracatheter/needle ~ 36000
    organ blood ~ 36500
    second order ~ 36012
    umbilical vein ~ 36510
  vertebral artery ~ 36100, 36221, 36225-36226, 36228
  ventricular ~ 61020-61026, 61210-61215, 62160-62162, 62164, 62225
Cauda equina ~ see spinal cord
  decompression ~ 63005-63011, 63017, 63047-63048, 63055-63057, 63087-63091
  exploration ~ 63005-63011, 63017
Cauterization
  anal fissure ~ 46940-46942
  cervix ~ 57522
    cryocautery ~ 57511
    electro or thermal ~ 57510
    laser ablation ~ 57513
  chemical, granulation tissue ~ 17250
  everted punctum ~ 68705
  lower esophageal sphincter, thermal, via endoscopy ~ 0057T
  nasopharyngeal hemorrhage ~ 42970
  nose, hemorrhage ~ 30901-30906
  skin lesion ~ 11055-11057, 17000-17004
  skin tags ~ 11200-11201
  turbinate mucosa ~ 30801-30802
Cavernitides, fibrous ~ see Peyronie disease
Cavernosography, corpora ~ 54230
Cavernosometry ~ 54231
Cavities, pleural ~ see pleural cavity
Cavus foot correction ~ 28309
CBC ~ see blood cell count ~ 85025-85027
CCL4 ~ 84600
CCU visit ~ see Critical Care Services
CD142 antigens ~ see thromboplastin
CD143 antigens ~ 82164
CD4 ~ 86360
CD8 ~ 86360
CEA ~ 82378
Cecil repair ~ 46744-46746
Cecostomy ~ 44300
  contrast ~ 49465
  insertion of tube ~ 49442
  laparoscopic ~ 44188
  obstructive material removal ~ 49460
  radiological evaluation of tube ~ 49465
  tube replacement ~ 49450
Celiac plexus
  destruction ~ 64680
  injection
    anesthetic ~ 64530
    neurolytic ~ 64680
Celiac trunk artery ~ see artery, celiac
Celioscopy ~ see endoscopy, peritoneum
Celiotomy ~ 49000
Cell count, body fluid ~ 89050-89051

Cell, blood ~ see blood cell
Cell, islet ~ 86341
Cell, mother ~ see stem cell
Cell-stimulating hormone, interstitial ~ 80418, 80426, 83002
Cellobiase ~ 82963
Cellular function assay ~ 86352
Cellular inclusion ~ see inclusion bodies
Central shunt ~ 33764
Central nervous system assessments or tests ~ 96101-96120
Central venous catheter placement
  insertion
    central ~ 36555-36558
    peripheral ~ 36568-36569
  repair ~ 36575
  replacement ~ 36580-36585
  repositioning ~ 36597
Central venous catheter removal ~ 36589
Cephalic version, of fetus, external ~ 59412
Cephalocele ~ 62120-62121
Cephalogram, orthodontic ~ 70350
Cerclage, cervix ~ 57700
  abdominal ~ 59325
  removal under anesthesia ~ 59871
  vaginal ~ 59320
Cerebellopontine angle tumor ~ see brainstem; skull base surgery ~ , 61510, 61518, 61520-61521, 61526-61530, 61545, 62164
Cerebral cortex decortication ~ see decortication
Cerebral death ~ 95824
Cerebral hernia ~ 62120-62121
Cerebral perfusion analysis ~ 0042T
Cerebral ventriculographies ~ see ventriculography
Cerebral vessels, occlusion ~ 61623
Cerebrose ~ 82760
Cerebrospinal fluid ~ 86325
  nuclear imaging ~ 78630-78650
Cerebrospinal fluid leak ~ 63744
  brain, repair ~ 61618-61619, 62100
  nasal/sinus endoscopy, repair ~ 31290-31291
  spinal cord, repair ~ 63707-63709
Cerebrospinal fluid shunt ~ 63740, 63746
  creation ~ 62190, 62192, 62220, 62223
  lumbar ~ 63740, 63741
  flow monitoring skin sensor ~ 0639T
  irrigation ~ 62194, 62225
  removal ~ 62256, 62258, 63746
  replacement ~ 62160, 62258, 63744
    catheter ~ 62194, 62225, 62230
    valve ~ 62230
  reprogramming ~ 62252
  torkidsen operation ~ 62180
  ventriculocisternostomy ~ 62180, 62200, 62201
Ceruloplasmin ~ 82390
Cerumen
  removal
    with instrumentation ~ 69210
    with irrigation/lavage ~ 69209
Cervical cap ~ 57170
Cervical lymphadenectomy ~ 38720-38724
Cervical mucus penetration test ~ 89330

Cervical plexus
  nerve conduction studies~ 64999
Cervical pregnancy ~ 59140
Cervical puncture ~ 61050-61055
Cervical smears ~ 88141, 88155, 88164-88167, 88174-88175
Cervical spine ~ see vertebra, cervical
Cervical sympathectomy ~ 64802
Cervicectomy ~ 57530
Cervicography ~ 0003T
Cervicoplasty ~ 15819
Cervicothoracic ganglia ~ 64510
Cervix ~ see cytopathology
  acetwhitening effect imaging/quantification ~ 57465
  amputation, total ~ 57530
  biopsy ~ 57500, 57520
    colposcopy ~ 57454-57455, 57460
  cauterization ~ 57522
    cryocautery ~ 57511
    electro or thermal ~ 57510
    laser ablation ~ 57513

Cervix ~ *continued*
cerclage ~ 57700
  abdominal ~ 59325
  removal under anesthesia ~ 59871
  vaginal ~ 59320
cervicography ~ 0003T
colposcopy ~ 57452, 57454-57456, 57460, 57461
  with computer-aided mapping ~ 57465
conization ~ 57461, 57520-57522
curettage, endocervical ~ 57454, 57456, 57505
dilation
  canal ~ 57800
  stump ~ 57558
dilation and curettage ~ 57558
ectopic pregnancy ~ 59140
excision
  radical ~ 57531
  stump
    abdominal approach ~ 57540-57545
    vaginal approach ~ 57550-57556
  total ~ 57530
exploration, endoscopy ~ 57452
insertion
  dilation ~ 59200
  laminaria ~ 59200
  prostaglandin ~ 59200
  sensor, fetal oximetry ~ 0021T
repair, cerclage ~ 57700
  abdominal ~ 59325
  suture ~ 57720
  vaginal ~ 59320
unlisted services and procedures ~ 58999
Cesarean delivery
antepartum care ~ 59610, 59618
delivery
  after attempted vaginal delivery ~ 59618
    delivery only ~ 59620
    postpartum care ~ 59622
    routine care ~ 59610, 59618
delivery only ~ 59514
postpartum care ~ 59515
routine care ~ 59510
tubal ligation at time of ~ 58611
with hysterectomy ~ 59525
Chalazion, excision ~ 67805
  multiple
    different lids ~ 67805
    same lid ~ 67801
  single ~ 67800
  under anesthesia ~ 67808
Challenge tests, bronchial/ingestion ~ 95070, 95076-95079
Chambers procedure ~ 28300
Change
catheter
  bile duct ~ 75984
fetal position
  by manipulation ~ 59412
tube or stent
  endoscopic
    bile or pancreatic duct ~ 43275-43276
Change of, dressing ~ 15852
Cheek
bone
  excision ~ 21030, 21034
  fracture
    closed treatment with manipulation ~ 21355
    open treatment ~ 21360-21366
  reconstruction ~ 21270
fascia graft ~ 15840
muscle graft ~ 15841-15845
muscle transfer ~ 15845
Cheilectomy, metatarsophalangeal joint release ~ 28289, 28291
Cheiloplasty ~ 40650-40654
Cheiloschisis ~ 30460-30462, 40700-40761
Cheilotomy ~ 40806
Chemical cauterization, granulation tissue ~ 17250
Chemical exfoliation ~ 17360
Chemical peel ~ 15788-15793
Chemiluminescent assay ~ 82397
Chemistry tests ~ 84999

Chemocauterization
corneal epithelium ~ 65435
  with chelating agent ~ 65436
Chemodenervation
anal sphincter ~ 46505
bladder ~ 52287
eccrine glands
  axillae ~ 64650
  other area ~ 64653
extraocular muscle ~ 67345
extremity muscle ~ 64642-64645
facial muscle ~ 64612, 64615
guidance
  electrical stimulation ~ 95873
  needle electromyography ~ 64617, 95874
neck muscle ~ 64615, 64616
salivary gland ~ 64611
trunk muscle ~ 64646-64647
Chemonucleolysis ~ 62292
Chemosurgery
destruction of benign lesion ~ 17110-17111
skin lesion ~ 17000-17004, 17110-17111, 17270, 17280
Chemotaxis assay ~ 86155
Chemotherapy
administration ~ 96401-96549
arterial catheterization ~ 36640
bladder instillation ~ 51720
brain ~ 61517
CNS ~ 61517, 96450
extracorporeal circulation, extremity ~ 36823
home infusion procedures ~ 99601-99602
intra-arterial ~ 96420-96425
intralesional ~ 96405-96406
intramuscular ~ 96401-96402
intravenous ~ 96409-96417
kidney instillation ~ 50391
peritoneal cavity ~ 96446
  catheterization ~ 49418
pleural cavity ~ 96440
pump services
  implantable ~ 96530
  maintenance ~ 95990-95991
  portable ~ 96520
reservoir filling ~ 96542
response assessment
  cytotoxicity assay of cancer stem cells (CSCs) ~ 0564T
subcutaneous ~ 96400
supply of agent ~ 96545
unlisted services and procedures ~ 96549
ureteral instillation ~ 50391
venous cannulation ~ 36823
Chest ~ see mediastinum; thorax
angiography ~ 71275
artery, ligation ~ 37616
CT scan ~ 71250-71275
exploration, blood vessel ~ 35820
magnetic resonance imaging (MRI) ~ 71550-71552
repair, blood vessel ~ 35211-35216
  with other graft ~ 35271-35276
  with vein graft ~ 35241-35246
ultrasound ~ 76604
wound exploration, penetrating ~ 20101
X-ray ~ 71045-71048
  with computer-aided detection ~ 0174T, 0175T
Chest, funnel ~ 21740, 21742-21743
Chest cavity, bypass graft ~ 35905
endoscopy
  exploration ~ 32601-32606
  surgical ~ 32650-32665
Chest wall
debridement ~ 11044, 11047
manipulation ~ 94667, 94668
mechanical oscillation ~ 94669
reconstruction ~ 49904
  with lung tumor resection ~ 32504
  trauma ~ 32820
repair ~ 32905
  closure ~ 32810
  fistula ~ 32906
  lung hernia ~ 32800

Chest wall ~ *continued*
resection ~ 32503
tumor
cryoablation ~ 32994
excision ~ 21601-21603
unlisted services and procedures ~ 32999
Chest wall fistula ~ 32906
Chevron procedure ~ 28296
Chiari osteotomy of the pelvis ~ 27158
Chicken pox vaccine ~ 90716
Child procedure ~ 48140-48146, 48150, 48153-48154, 48160
Chin
repair
augmentation ~ 21120
osteotomy ~ 21121-21123
Chinidin ~ 80194
Chiropractic manipulation (CMT) ~ 98940-98943
Chiropractic treatment
spinal
extraspinal ~ 98940-98943
Chlamydia
antibody ~ 86631-86632
antigen detection
amplified nucleic acid probe ~ 87486, 87491
direct nucleic acid probe ~ 87485, 87490
direct optical ~ 87810
enzyme immunoassay ~ 87320
immunofluorescence ~ 87270
nucleic acid quantification ~ 87487, 87492
culture ~ 87110
Chloramphenicol ~ 82415
Chloride
blood ~ 82435
other source ~ 82438
spinal fluid ~ 82438
urine ~ 82436
Chloride, methylene ~ 84600
Chlorinated hydrocarbons ~ 82441
Chlorohydrocarbon ~ 82441
Chlorpromazine ~ 80342-80344
Choanal atresia, repair ~ 30540-30545
Cholangiography
injection ~ 47531, 47532
intraoperative ~ 74300-74301
postoperative ~ 47531
repair
with bile duct exploration ~ 47700
with cholecystectomy ~ 47563, 47605, 47620
transhepatic, laparoscopically guided ~ 47579
with
conversion of drainage catheter ~ 47535
exchange of drainage catheter ~ 47536
placement
of access to small bowel ~ 47541
of drainage catheter ~ 47533, 47534
of stent ~ 47538-47540
removal of drainage catheter ~ 47537
Cholangiopancreatography ~ see bile duct; pancreatic duct
endoscopic retrograde (ERCP)
with ablation
lesion/polyp/tumor ~ 43278
with biopsy ~ 43261
with collection of specimen(s) ~ 43260
with exchange stent ~ 43276
with optical endomciroscopy ~ 0397T
with papillotomy ~ 43262
with placement stent ~ 43274
with pressure measurement, sphincter of Oddi ~ 43263
with removal, foreign body ~ 43275
with removal, stent ~ 43275, 43276
with removal/destruction of calculus ~ 43264-43265
with sphincterotomy ~ 43262, 43274, 43276, 43277
with transendoscopic balloon dilation ~ 43277
intraoperative ~ 74300, 74301
postoperative ~ 47531
Cholangiostomy ~ 47400
Cholangiotomy ~ 47400
Cholecalciferol ~ 82306

Cholecystectomy
any method
with cholangiography ~ 47563, 47605, 47620
with choledochoenterostomy ~ 47612
with exploration common duct ~ 47564, 47610
donor liver ~ 47143
excision ~ 47600-47620
laparoscopic ~ 47562-47564
Cholecystenterostomy
direct ~ 47720
with gastroenterostomy ~ 47721, 47741
laparoscopic ~ 47570
Roux-en-Y ~ 47740-47741
Cholecystography ~ 47490, 74290-74291
Cholecystostomy
open ~ 47480
percutaneous ~ 47490
with peripancreatic drain placement ~ 48000
Choledochoplasty ~ 47701
Choledochoscopy ~ 47550
Choledochostomy ~ 47420-47425
Choledochotomy ~ 47420-47425
Choledochus, cyst ~ see cyst, choledochal
Cholera vaccine
live, for oral use ~ 90625
Cholesterol
measurement ~ 83721
serum ~ 82465
testing ~ 83718-83719
Cholinesterase, blood ~ 82480-82482
Choline esterase I ~ 82013
Choline esterase II ~ 82480-82482
Cholylglycine, blood ~ 82240
Chondroitin sulfate ~ 82485
Chondromalacia patella, repair ~ 27418
Chondropathia patellae ~ 27418
Chondrosteoma ~ 69140
Chopart procedure ~ see radical resection; replantation ~ 28800-28805
Chordotomies ~ 63194-63199
Chorioangioma ~ see lesion, skin
Choriogonadotropin ~ 80414-80415, 84702-84703
Choriomeningitides, lymphocytic ~ 86727
Chorionic gonadotropin ~ 80414, 84702-84704
stimulation ~ 80414-80415
Chorionic growth hormone ~ 83632
Chorionic tumor ~ 59100, 59870
Chorionic villi ~ 59015
Chorionic villus, biopsy ~ 59015
Choroid, destruction, lesion ~ 67220-67225
Choroid plexus, excision ~ 61544
Christmas factor ~ 85250
Chromaffinoma, medullary ~ 80424
Chromatin, sex ~ 88130
Chromatography
column ~ see specific analyte in Drug Assay, Pathology and Laboratory
unspecified non-drug analyte(s) ~ 82542
column/mass spectrometry ~ see specific analyte in Drug Assay, Pathology and Laborary
unspecified non-drug analyte(s) ~ 82542
drug screen ~ 80305-80307, 80320-80377
gas liquid or HPLC
typing ~ 87143
unspecified non-drug analyte(s) ~ 82542
hemoglobin ~ 83021, 83036
paper
sugars ~ 84375
unlisted chemistruy procedure ~ 84999
thin layer
unlisted chemistry procedure ~ 84999
Chromium ~ 82495
Chromogenic substrate assay ~ 85130
Chromosome analysis
added study ~ 88280-88289
amniotic fluid ~ 88267, 88269
culture ~ 88235
biopsy culture, tissue ~ 88233
bone marrow culture ~ 88237
breakage syndromes ~ 88245, 88248, 88249

Chromosome analysis ~ *continued*
  chorionic villus ~ 88267
    5 cells ~ 88261
    15-20 cells ~ 88262
    20-25 cells ~ 88264
    45 cells ~ 88263
    culture ~ 88235
  cytogenomic constitutional microarray ~ 81228, 81229
  cytogenomic neoplasia microarray ~ 81277
  fragile-X ~ 88248
  in-situ hybridization ~ 88272, 88273
  lymphocyte culture ~ 88230
  molecular pathology, level 5 ~ 81404
  pregnancy associated plasma protein-A ~ 84163
  skin culture, tissue ~ 88233
  tissue culture
    amniotic fluid cells ~ 88325
    blood cells ~ 88237
    bone marrow cells ~ 88237
    chorionic villus cells ~ 88235
    skin ~ 88233
    tumor ~ 88239
  unlisted cytogenic study ~ 88299
Chromotubation ~ 58350
  oviduct ~ 58350
Chronic erection ~ see priapism
Chronic interstitial cystitides ~ 52260-52265
Ciliary body
  cyst
    destruction
      cryotherapy ~ 66720
      cyclodialysis ~ 66740
      cyclophotocoagulation ~ 66710, 66711
      diathermy ~ 66700
      nonexcisional ~ 66770
    destruction ~ 66770
      cyclophotocoagulation ~ 66710, 66711
      endoscopic ~ 66711
  lesion, destruction ~ 66770
  repair ~ 66680
Cimino type procedure ~ 36821
Cinefluorographies ~ see cineradiography
Cineplasty, arm, lower or upper ~ 24940
Cineradiography
  esophagus ~ 74230
  pharynx ~ 70371, 74230
  speech evaluation ~ 70371
  swallowing evaluation ~ 74230
  unlisted services and procedures ~ 76120-76125
Circulation, extracorporeal ~ 33946-33949
Circulation assist
  aortic ~ 33967, 33970
  balloon ~ 33967, 33970
  external ~ 33946-33949
Circulatory assist ~ see circulation assist
Circumcision
  repair ~ 54163
  surgical excision ~ 54161
    newborn ~ 54160
  with clamp or other device ~ 54150
    newborn ~ 54150
Cisternal puncture ~ 61050-61055
Cisternography ~ 70015
  nuclear ~ 78630
Citrate, blood or urine ~ 82507
Clagett procedure ~ 32810
Clavicle
  craterization ~ 23180
  cyst
    excision ~ 23140
      with allograft ~ 23146
      with autograft ~ 23145
  diaphysectomy ~ 23180
  dislocation
    acromioclavicular joint
      closed treatment ~ 23540-23545
      open treatment ~ 23550-23552
    sternoclavicular joint
      closed treatment ~ 23520-23525
      open treatment ~ 23530-23532
    without manipulation ~ 23540

Clavicle ~ *continued*
  excision ~ 23170
    partial ~ 23120, 23180
    total ~ 23125
  fracture
    closed treatment
      without manipulation ~ 23500
      with manipulation ~ 23505
    open treatment ~ 23515
  pinning, wiring ~ 23490
  prophylactic treatment ~ 23490
  repair osteotomy ~ 23480-23485
  saucerization ~ 23180
  sequestrectomy ~ 23170
  tumor, excision ~ 23140, 23146, 23200
    with autograft ~ 23145
    radical resection ~ 23200
  X-ray ~ 73000
Clavicula ~ see clavicle
Claviculectomy
  partial ~ 23120
  total ~ 23125
Claw finger repair ~ 26499
Cleft, branchial ~ see branchial cleft
Cleft cyst, branchial ~ 42810-42815
Cleft foot, reconstruction ~ 28360
Cleft hand, repair ~ 26580
Cleft lip
  repair ~ 40700-40761
  rhinoplasty ~ 30460-30462
Cleft palate
  repair ~ 42200-42225
  rhinoplasty ~ 30460-30462
Clinical act of insertion ~ see insertion
Clinical chemistry test ~ 84999
Clinical pathology ~ 80500-80502
Clitoroplasty, intersex state ~ 56805
Closed [transurethral] biopsy of bladder ~ 52224, 52250
Clostridial tetanus ~ 86280
Clostridium botulinum toxin ~ see chemodenervation
Clostridium difficile
  antigen detection
    enzyme immunoassay ~ 87324
  by immunoassay
    with direct optical observation ~ 87803
Clostridium tetani AB ~ 86774
Closure
  anal fistula ~ 46288
  atrioventricular valve ~ 33600
  cystostomy ~ 51880
  enterostomy ~ 44227, 44620, 44625, 44626
    laparoscopic ~ 44227
  lacrimal fistula ~ 68770
  lacrimal punctum
    plug ~ 68761
    thermocauterization, ligation or laser surgery ~ 68760
  left atrial appendage, with implant ~ 33340
  paravalvular leak, percutaneous transcatheter
    aortic valve ~ 93591, 93592
    mitral valve ~ 93590, 93592
  rectovaginal fistula ~ 57300-57308
  semilunar valve ~ 33602
  septal defect
    ventricular ~ 33776, 33780, 93581
    ventricular tunnel ~ 33722
Clot ~ 34401-34490, 35875, 35876, 50230
Clotting disorder ~ 85390
Clotting factor
  factor I (fibrinogen) ~ 85384, 85385
  factor II (prothrombin) ~ 85210
  factor III (thromboplastin) ~ 85730, 85732
  factor IV (calcium) ~ 82310
  factor VII (proconvertin) ~ 85230
  factor VIII (AHG) ~ 85240-85247
    AHG ~ 85240
    related antigen ~ 85244
    von Willebrand factor ~ 85247
    VW factor ~ 85245, 85246
  factor IX (Christmas factor) ~ 85250
  factor X (thrombokinase) (Stuart-Prower factor) ~ 85260

Clotting factor ~ *continued*
factor XI (plasma thromboplastin, antecedent [PTA]) ~ 85270
factor XII (Hageman factor) ~ 85280
factor XIII (fibrin stabilizing) ~ 85290, 85291
inhibition ~ 85705
inhibition test ~ 85347
partial time ~ 85730-85732
Clotting operation ~ 11765
Clotting test
protein C ~ 85303, 85307
protein S ~ 85306
Clotting time ~ 85345-85348
Clot lysis time ~ 85175
Clot retraction ~ 85170
Clubfoot cast ~ 29450
wedging ~ 29750
CMG ~ 51725-51726
CMRI ~ see cardiac magnetic resonance imaging
CMV ~ see cytomegalovirus
CNPB (continuous negative pressure breathing) ~ 94662
Co-factor I , heparin ~ 85300-85301
CO2 ~ 82374
Coagulation
blood ~ see blood clot
defect ~ 85390
light ~ see photocoagulation
time ~ 85345-85348
unlisted services and procedures ~ 85999
Coagulin ~ see thromboplastin
Coagulopathy ~ 85390
assay ~ 85130
Cocaine
blood or urine ~ 80353
Coccidioides, antibody ~ 86635
Coccidioidin test ~ 86590
Coccidioidomycosis, skin test ~ 86490
Coccygeal spine fracture ~ 27200, 27202
Coccygectomy ~ 15920-15922, 27080
Coccyx
excision ~ 27080
fracture
closed treatment ~ 27200
open treatment ~ 27202
tumor, excision ~ 49215
X-ray ~ 72220
Cochlear device
insertion ~ 69930
programming ~ 92601-92604
Codeine, alkaloid screening ~ 80323
Cofactor protein S ~ 85305, 85306
Coffey operation ~ 58400
Cognitive function tests ~ 96101-96125 (see also neurology, diagnostic)
Cognitive skills development
one-on-one patient contact ~ 97129, 97130
Cold agglutinin ~ 86156-86157
Cold pack treatment ~ 97010
Cold preservation ~ see cryopreservation
Colectomy
partial ~ 44140
laparoscopic ~ 44213
with anastomosis ~ 44140
laparoscopic ~ 44204, 44207-44208
with coloproctostomy ~ 44145-44146
with colostomy ~ 44141-44144
laparoscopic ~ 44206, 44208
with ileocolostomy, laparoscopic ~ 44205
with ileostomy ~ 44144
with ileum removal ~ 44160
with splenic flexure mobilization ~ 44139
laparoscopic ~ 44213
with transcanal approach ~ 44147
total
laparoscopic ~ 44210-44212
with creation of ileal reservoir ~ 44211
with ileoanal anastomosis ~ 44211
with ileoproctostomy ~ 44210
with ileostomy ~ 44210-44212
with protectomy ~ 44211--44212
with rectal mucosectomy ~ 44211
without protectomy ~ 44210

Colectomy ~ *continued*
open
with complete proctectomy ~ 45121
with ileoproctostomy ~ 44150
with ileostomy ~ 44150-44151
with protectomy ~ 44155-44158
Collagen cross links
any method ~ 82523
cornea ~ 0402T
Collagen injection ~ 11950-11954
Collar bone ~ see clavicle
Collateral ligament
ankle repair ~ 27695-27698
interphalangeal joint ~ 26545
knee
joint repair ~ 27409
repair ~ 27405
metacarpophalangeal joint ~ 26540-26542
Collection and processing
allogeneic blood harvesting of stem cells ~ 38205
autologous blood
harvesting of stem cells ~ 38206
intraoperative ~ 86891
preoperative ~ 86890
brushings and washings
abdomen ~ 49320
anus ~ 46600, 46601
biliary tract ~ 47552
colon ~ 44388, 45300, 45330, 45378
duodenum ~ 43235, 44360, 44376
esophagus ~ 43197, 43200, 43235
hepatobiliary system ~ 43260
ileum ~ 44376, 44380
jejunum ~ 43235
omentum ~ 49320
peritoneum ~ 49320
rectum ~ 45300, 45330
small intestine ~ 44385
stomach ~ 43235
radiologic guidance ~ 75989
specimen
capillary blood ~ 36416
duodenum ~ 43756-43757
for dark field examination ~ 87164
ear ~ 36416
hematoma ~ 10140
sputum ~ 89220
stomach ~ 43754
sweat ~ 89230
tears ~ 83861
venous blood ~ 36415, 36591-36592
venous catheter ~ 36592
stem cells
harvesting
allogenic blood ~ 38205
autologous blood ~ 38206, 86890-86891
processing ~ 38210-38215
Colles fracture ~ 25600-25605
Colles fracture reversed ~ see Smith fracture
Collins syndrome, Treacher ~ 21150-21151
Collis procedure ~ 43283, 43842-43843
Colon ~ see also colon-sigmoid
biopsy ~ 44025, 44100, 44322
endoscopic ~ 44389, 45380, 45391, 45392
colostomy, revision ~ 44340-44346
colotomy ~ 44322
colostomy ~ 44320
CT scan
colonography ~ 74261-74263
destruction
lesion ~ 44401, 45383
tumor ~ 44401, 45383
endoscopy
biopsy ~ 44389, 45380, 45391, 45392
destruction
lesion ~ 44401
tumor ~ 44401, 45383
dilation ~ 45386
exploration ~ 44388, 45378, 45381, 45386
hemorrhage ~ 44391, 45382

Colposcopy ~ continued
  perineum ~ 99170
  vagina ~ 57420-57421
  vulva ~ 56820
    biopsy ~ 56821
Colpotomy
  drainage, abscess ~ 57010
  exploration ~ 57000
Colprosterone ~ 84144
Columna vertebralis ~ see spine
Combined heart-lung transplantation ~ 33935
Combined right and left heart cardiac catheterization ~ 93453
Comedones, removal ~ 10040
Commissurotomy, right ventricle ~ 33476-33478
Common sensory nerve, repair/suture ~ 64834
Common truncus ~ 33786
Communication device
  non-speech-generating ~ 92605-92606
  speech-generating ~ 92606-92609
Community/work reintegration training ~ 97537
Compatibility test, blood ~ 86920
Complement
  antigen ~ 86160
  fixation test ~ 86171
  functional activity ~ 86161
  hemolytic, total ~ 86162
  total ~ 86162
Complete blood count (CBC) ~ see also blood cell count ~ 85025-85027
Complete colectomy ~ see colectomy, total
Complete pneumonectomy ~ 32488
Complete transposition of great vessels ~ 33770-33781
Complex, factor IX ~ 85250
Component removal, blood ~ 36511-36516
Composite graft ~ 15760-15770, 35681-35683
Compound B ~ 82528
Compound F ~ 80400-80406, 80418-80420, 80436, 82530
Compression, nerve, median ~ 64721
Computed tomographic angiography (CTA)
  abdomen ~ 74174, 74175
  abdominal aorta ~ 75635
  arm ~ 73206
  chest ~ 71275
  coronary artery ~ 75574
    automated data analysis for atherosclerotic plaque ~ 0623T-0626T
    software analysis for fractional flow reserve (FFR) ~ 0501T-0504T
  head ~ 70496
  heart ~ 75571-75574
  leg ~ 73076
  neck ~ 70498
  pelvis ~ 72191, 74174
Computed tomography (CT) ~ see CT scan; specific anatomic site
Computer assisted navigation, orthopedic surgery ~ 0054T-0055T, 20985
Computer analysis
  acoustic recording, heart sounds ~ 93799
  digital image data, mammography ~ 77065-77067
  electrocardiographic data ~ 93228
  motion analysis ~ 96000-96004
  pediatric home apnea monitor ~ 94776
Computer-aided detection
  lesion, chest radiograph ~ 0174T, 0175T
  mammography ~ 77065-77067
    MRI ~ 0159T
Concentration, hydrogen ion ~ see pH
Concentration, minimum inhibitory ~ 87186
Concentration of specimen ~ 87015
Concentric procedure ~ 28296
Conchae nasale ~ 30930
Concha Bullosa resection
  with nasal/sinus endoscopy ~ 31240
Conduction, nerve ~ see nerve conduction
Conduit, ileal ~ 50690
Condyle
  humerus, fracture
    closed treatment ~ 24576-24577
    open treatment ~ 24579
    percutaneous ~ 24582
  mandibular ~ 21247, 21465
  metatarsal, excision ~ 28288
  phalanges, toe, excision ~ 28126

Condylectomy
  temporomandibular joint ~ 21050
  with skull base surgery ~ 61596-61597
Condyloma, destruction ~ 54050-54065
Conference, medical, with interdisciplinary team ~ 99366-99368
Congenital arteriovenous malformation ~ see arteriovenous malformation
Congenital cardiac anomaly
  atrial septostomy ~ 33741
  catheterization ~ 93530-93533
    injection ~ 93563, 93564
  closure ~ 93580, 93581
  echocardiography
    for congenital anomalies ~ 93303, 93304, 93315-93317
    Doppler, fetal ~ 76827, 76828
    fetal ~ 76825, 76826
  ectopy, ventricular treatment ~ 93654
  transcatheter intracardiac shunt (TIS) ~ 33745, 33746
Congenital elevation of scapula ~ 23400
Congenital heart septum defect ~ 33813-33814
Congenital kidney abnormality
  nephrolithotomy ~ 50070
  pyeloplasty ~ 50405
  pyelotomy ~ 50135
Congenital laryngocele ~ 31300
Congenital vascular anomaly ~ see vascular malformation
Conisation ~ 57461, 57520-57522
Conization, cervix ~ 57461, 57520-57522
Conjoint psychotherapy ~ 90846-90849, 99510
Conjunctiva
  biopsy ~ 68100
  cyst, incision and drainage ~ 68020
  fistulize for drainage, with tube ~ 68750
    without tube ~ 68745
  follicle expression ~ 68040
  graft ~ 65150, 65782
    harvesting ~ 68371
  injection ~ 68200
  insertion
    aqueous drainage device ~ 0449T, 0450T, 0474T
    stent ~ 68750
  lesion
    destruction ~ 68135
    excision ~ 68110, 68115
      with adjacent sclera ~ 68130
  reconstruction ~ 68320, 68325, 68326, 68328
    with flap ~ 67971, 68360, 68362
  removal, foreign body ~ 65205, 65210
  repair
    eyelid wound ~ 67961, 67966
      direct closure ~ 65270, 67930, 67935
      mobilization and rearrangement ~ 65272, 65273
    symblepharon
      division ~ 68340
      with graft ~ 68335
      without graft ~ 68330
  unlisted services and procedures ~ 68399
Conjunctivo-tarso-Muller resection ~ 67908
Conjunctivocystorhinostomy ~ 68745-68750
Conjunctivodacryocystostomy ~ 68745-68750
Conjunctivoplasty ~ 68320-68330
  reconstruction cul de sac, with extensive rearrangement ~ 68326
    with graft ~ 68326
      buccal mucous membrane ~ 68328
  with extensive rearrangement ~ 68320
  with graft ~ 68320
    buccal mucous membrane ~ 68325
Conjunctivorhinostomy
  with tube ~ 68750
  without tube ~ 68745
Conscious sedation ~ see sedation
Construction
  finger, toe to hand transfer ~ 26551-26556
  neobladder ~ 51596
  vagina
    with graft ~ 57292
    without graft ~ 57291
Consultation(s) ~ 99241-99255
  clinical pathology ~ 80500-80502
  initial inpatient ~ 99251-99255
    new or established patient ~ 99251-99255

Consultation(s) ~ *continued*
  office and/or other outpatient ~ 99241-99245
    new or established patient ~ 99241-99245
  psychiatric, with family ~ 90887
  radiation therapy, radiation physics ~ 77336-77370
  surgical pathology ~ 88321-88325
    intraoperation ~ 88329-88332
  X-ray ~ 76140
Consumption test, antiglobulin ~ 86880
Contact lens services
  fittings and prescription ~ 92071-92072, 92310-92313
  modification ~ 92325
  prescription ~ 92314-92317
  replacement ~ 92326
Continuous negative pressure breathing (CNPD) ~ 94662
Continuous positive airway pressure (CPAP) ~ 94660
Contouring
  silicone injections ~ 11950-11954
  tumor, facial bone ~ 21029
Contraception
  cervical cap
    fitting ~ 57170
  diaphragm
    fitting ~ 57170
  intrauterine device (IUD)
    insertion ~ 58300
    removal ~ 58301
Contraceptive capsules, implantable
  removal ~ 11976
Contraceptive device, intrauterine ~ 58300-58301
Contracture
  elbow, release
    with radical resection of capsule ~ 24149
  palm, release ~ 26121-26125
  thumb, release ~ 26508
Contracture of palmar fascia ~ 26040-26045
Contralateral ligament repair, knee ~ 27405
Contrast aortogram ~ 75600-75605, 75630, 93567
Contrast bath therapy ~ see also physical medicine/therapy/occupational
  therapy ~ 97034
Contrast material
  injection via peritoneal catheter ~ 49424
Contrast phlebogram ~ see venography
Contusion ~ see hematoma
Converting enzyme, angiotensin ~ 82164
Coombs test ~ 86880
Copper ~ 82525
Coprobilinogen, feces ~ 84577
Coproporphyrin ~ 84120
Coracoacromial ligament release ~ 23415
Coracoid process transfer ~ 23462
Cord
  spermatic ~ see spermatic cord
  spinal ~ see spinal cord
  vocal ~ see vocal cords
Cordectomy ~ 31300
Cordocentesis ~ 59012
Cordotomy ~ 63194-63199
Corectomy ~ see excision, iris
Coreoplasty ~ 66762
Cornea
  astigmatism
    relaxing incision ~ 65772
    wedge resection ~ 65775
  biopsy ~ 65410
  collagen cross links ~ 0402T
  curettage ~ 65435-65436
    with chelating agent ~ 65436
  epithelium, excision ~ 65435-65436
    with chelating agent ~ 65436
  hysteresis determination ~ 92145
  implantation, corneal ring segments ~ 65785
  incision
    for astigmatism correction ~ 65772
  lesion
    destruction ~ 65450
    excision ~ 65400
      with graft ~ 65426
      without graft ~ 65420
  pachymetry ~ 76514

Cornea ~ *continued*
  prosthesis ~ 65770
  pterygium, excision ~ 65420
  puncture ~ 65600
  relaxing incisions ~ 65772-65775
  repair
    astigmatism ~ 65772-65775
    wedge resection ~ 65775
    with glue ~ 65286
    wound
      nonperforating ~ 65275
      perforating ~ 65280-65285
      tissue glue ~ 65286
  reshape
    epikeratoplasty ~ 65765
    keratomileusis ~ 65760
    keratoprosthesis ~ 65767
  scraping, smear ~ 65430
  tattoo ~ 65600
  thickness measurement ~ 76514
  transplantation
    amniotic membrane ~ 65780
    autograft or homograft
      allograft preparation ~ 0290T, 65757
      endothelial ~ 65756
      lamellar ~ 65710
      penetrating ~ 65730-65755
    for aphakia ~ 65750
  unlisted procedure ~ 66999
Coronary
  atherectomy, percutaneous ~ 92995-92996
  thrombectomy, percutaneous ~ 92973
Coronary angioplasty, transluminal balloon ~ see percutaneous
  transluminal angioplasty
Coronary artery
  angiography ~ 93454-93461
  angioplasty ~ 92920, 92921
    with atherectomy ~ 92933, 92934, 92937, 92938, 92941, 92943, 92944
    with stent placement ~ 92928, 92929, 92933, 92934, 92937, 92938, 92941, 92943, 92944
  atherectomy ~ 92924-92295
    with angioplasty ~ 92933, 92934, 92937, 92938, 92941, 92943, 92944
    with stent ~ 92933, 92934, 92937, 92938, 92941, 92943, 92944
  computed tomographic angiography (CTA)
    automated data analysis for atherosclerotic plaque ~ 0623T-0626T
  endarterectomy ~ 33572
  fractional flow reserve ~ 0501T-0504T
  graft
    anomaly ~ 33503, 33504
    arterial bypass ~ 33533-33536
      harvest ~ 35600
    arterial-venous bypass ~ 33517-33519, 33521-33523
    internal mammary artery graft ~ 4110F
    venous bypass ~ 33510-33516
      harvest ~ 35500
  insertion, stent ~ 92928, 92929
  ligation ~ 33502
  placement, radiation delivery device ~ 92974
  reconstruction ~ 33863, 33864
  repair, anomaly ~ 33500-33507
  revascularization ~ 92937, 92938, 92941, 92943, 92944
  thrombectomy ~ 92973
  thrombolysis ~ 92975, 92977
  translocation ~ 33506, 33507
  ventricular restoration ~ 33548
Coronary artery bypass graft (CABG) ~ 33503-33505, 33510-33516
  arterial ~ 33533-33536
  arterial-venous ~ 33517-33523
  beta-blocker administration ~ 4115F
  harvest, upper extremity artery ~ 35600
  internal mammary artery graft ~ 4110F
  reoperation ~ 33530
  venous ~ 33510-33516
Coronary endarterectomy ~ 33572
Coronavirus Disease (COVID 19)
  antibody detection
    immunoassay, multiple-step ~ 86769
    immunoassay, single-step ~ 86328
  infectious agent detection, nucleic acid probe ~ 87635
  pathogen detection, pathogen-specific nucleic acid ~ 0202U

Coroner's exam ~ 88045
Coronoidectomy, temporomandibular joint ~ 21070
Corpectomy ~ 63101-63103
Corpora cavernosa
  corpus spongiosum shunt ~ 54430
  glans penis fistulization ~ 54435
  injection ~ 54235
  irrigation, priapism ~ 54220
  saphenous vein shunt ~ 54420
  X-ray with contrast ~ 74445
Corpora cavernosography ~ 74445
Corpus callosum, transection ~ 61541
Corpus vertebrae (vertebrae) ~ see vertebral body
Correction (of)
  cleft palate ~ 42200-42225
  lid retraction ~ 67911
  malrotation of duodenum ~ 44055
  syndactyly ~ 26560-26562
  ureteropelvic junction ~ 50400-50405, 50544
Cortex decortication, cerebral ~ see decortication
Cortical mapping
  transection, by electric stimulation ~ 95961-95962
Corticoids ~ 83491
Corticoliberin ~ 80412
Corticosteroids
  blood ~ 83491
  urine ~ 83491
Corticosteroid-binding globulin ~ 84449
Corticosteroid-binding protein ~ 84449
Corticosterone, blood or urine ~ 82528
Corticotropic releasing hormone (CRH) ~ 80412
Cortisol ~ 80400-80406, 80418-80420, 80436, 82530
  stimulation ~ 80412
  total ~ 82533
Cortisol binding globulin ~ 84449
Costectomy ~ see rib, excision
Costen syndrome ~ see temporomandibular joint (TMJ)
Costotransversectomy ~ 21610
Cothromboplastin ~ 85230
Cotte operation ~ see revision ~ 58400-58410
Cotton procedure, Bohler procedure ~ 28405
Counseling and/or risk factor reduction intervention ~ 99401-99429
  alcohol and/or substance abuse ~ 99408-99409
  behavior change ~ 99406-99409
  smoking and tobacco use ~ 99406-99407
Count
  blood cell ~ see blood cell count
  blood platelet ~ 85008
  cell ~ 89050-89051
  complete blood ~ 85025-85027
  erythrocyte ~ 85032-85041
  leukocyte ~ 85032, 85048, 89055
  reticulocyte ~ 85044-85045
Counters, cell ~ 89050-89051
Countershock, electric ~ 92960-92961
Coventry tibial wedge osteotomy ~ 27455-27457, 27705, 27709-27712
COVID-19 (Coronavirus Disease)
  antibody detection
    immunoassay, multiple-step ~ 86769
    immunoassay, single-step ~ 86328
  infectious agent detection, nucleic acid probe ~ 87635
  pathogen detection, pathogen-specific nucleic acid ~ 0202U
Cowper's gland, excision ~ 53250
Coxiella burnetii, antibody ~ 86638
Coxsackie, antibody ~ 86658
CPAP ~ 94660
CPK, blood ~ 82550-82552
CPR (cardiopulmonary resuscitation) ~ 92950
Cranial bone
  halo, thin skull osteology ~ 20664
  reconstruction, extracranial ~ 21181-21184
  tumor, excision ~ 61563-61564
Cranial halo ~ 20661
Cranial nerve ~ see specific nerve
  avulsion ~ 64732-64760, 64771
  decompression ~ 61458, 61460, 64716
  implantation ~ 64568-64569
    electrode ~ 64553

Cranial nerve ~ *continued*
  injection
    anesthetic ~ 64400, 64408
    neurolytic ~ 64600, 64605, 64610
  insertion, electrode ~ 64553
  neuroplasty ~ 64716
  release ~ 64716
  removal, neurostimulator ~ 64570
  repair, suture, with or without graft ~ 64864-64865
  section ~ 61460
  transection ~ 64732-64760, 64771
  transposition ~ 64716
Cranial nerve II ~ see optic nerve
Cranial nerve V (five) ~ see trigeminal nerve
Cranial nerve VII (seven) ~ see facial nerve
Cranial nerve X (ten) ~ see vagus nerve
Cranial nerve XI ~ see accessory nerve
Cranial nerve XII (twelve) ~ 64868
Cranial tongs
  application/removal ~ 20660
  removal ~ 20665
Craniectomy ~ see also craniotomy ~ 61501
  abscess drainage ~ 61320-61321
  anesthesia ~ 00211
  decompression ~ 61322-61323, 61340, 61343
  drainage ~ 61320-61321
  evacuation of hematoma ~ 61312-61315
  excision
    abscess ~ 61514, 61522
    bone lesion ~ 61500
    fenestration of cyst ~ 61516, 61524
    meningioma ~ 60512, 61519
    tumor ~ 61500, 61518, 61520, 61521
  exploratory ~ 61304-61305, 61458
  extensive, for multiple suture craniosynostosis ~ 61558, 61559
  for electrode ~ 61860-61868
  release stenosis ~ 61550-61552
  section ~ 61450, 61460
  with craniotomy ~ 61316, 61530
  wound treatment ~ 61571
Craniofacial, unlisted procedures ~ 21299
Craniofacial separation
  closed treatment ~ 21431
  open treatment ~ 21432-21436
  wire fixation ~ 21431
Craniomegalic skull, reduction ~ 62115-62117
Craniopharyngioma, excision ~ 61545
Cranioplasty ~ 62120
  autograft ~ 62146-62147
  bone graft ~ 61316, 62146-62147
  bone graft retrieval ~ 62148
  encephalocele repair ~ 62120
  skull defect ~ 62140-62141, 62145
Craniostenosis ~ see craniosynostosis
Craniosynostosis
  bifrontal craniotomy ~ 61557
  extensive craniectomy ~ 61558-61559
Craniotomy ~ see burr hole; drill hole; puncture ~ 61501
  bifrontal ~ 61557
  decompression ~ 61322-61323
  exploratory ~ 61304-61305
  for craniosynostosis ~ 61556-61557
  for encephalocele ~ 62121
  for implant of neurostimulators ~ 61850
  frontal ~ 61556
  parietal ~ 61556
  surgery ~ 61312-61315, 61320-61323, 61546, 61570-61571, 61582-61583, 61590, 61592, 61760, 62120
  with bone flap ~ 61510-61516, 61526-61530, 61533-61545, 61566-61567
Cranium ~ see skull
Craterization
  calcaneus ~ 28120
  clavicle ~ 23180
  femur ~ 27070-27071, 27360
  fibula ~ 27360, 27641
  hip ~ 27070
  humerus ~ 23184, 24140
  ileum ~ 27070
  metacarpal ~ 26230
  metatarsal ~ 28122

Craterization ~ *continued*
 olecranon process ~ 24147
 phalanges
  finger ~ 26235-26236
  toe ~ 28124
 pubis ~ 27070
 radius ~ 24145, 25151
 scapula ~ 23182
 talus ~ 28120
 tarsal ~ 28122
 tibia ~ 27360, 27640
 ulna ~ 24147, 25150
Creatine ~ 82553-82554
 blood or urine ~ 82540
Creatine kinase, total ~ 82550
Creatine phosphokinase
 blood ~ 82552
 total ~ 82550
Creatinine
 blood ~ 82565
 clearance ~ 82575
 other source ~ 82570
 urine ~ 82570-82575
Creation
 arteriovenous fistula ~ 35686, 36825, 36830
 catheter exit site ~ 49436
 cavopulmonary anastomosis ~ 33622
 colonic reservoir ~ 45119, 45397
 complete heart block ~ 93650
 defect ~ 40720
 ileal reservoir ~ 44158, 44211, 45113
 iliac artery conduit ~ 34833
 lesion ~ 61720, 61735, 61790, 63600
 mucofistula ~ 44144
 pericardial window ~ 32659, 33025
 recipient site ~ 15002-15005
 shunt
  cerebrospinal fluid ~ 62200
  subarachnoid, lumbar-peritoneal ~ 63740
  subarachnoid-subdural ~ 62190
  ventriculo ~ 62200
 sigmoid bladder ~ 50810
 speech prosthesis ~ 31611
 stoma
  bladder ~ 51980
  tympanic membrane ~ 69433, 69436, 0583T
  ureter ~ 50860
 subcutaneous pocket with glucose sensor insertion ~ 0446T, 0448T
 ventral hernia ~ 39503
 vertebral cavity ~ 22513-22515
CRH ~ see corticotropic releasing hormone (CRH)
Cricoid cartilage split, larynx ~ 31587
Cricothyroid membrane, incision ~ 31605
Cristobalite ~ 84285
Critical care services
 cardiopulmonary resuscitation ~ 92950
 evaluation and management ~ 99291-99292
 interfacility transport ~ 99466-99467
 ipecac administration for poison ~ 99175
 neonatal
  initial ~ 99468
  intensive ~ 99477
  low birth weight infant ~ 99478-99479
  subsequent ~ 99469
 pediatric
  initial ~ 99471, 99475
  interfacility transport ~ 99466-99467
   supervision ~ 99485-99486
  subsequent ~ 99472, 99476
 remote ~ 0188T-0189T
Cross finger flap ~ 15574
Crossmatch ~ 86920-86922
Crossmatching, tissue ~ 86812-86817, 86821
Cruciate ligament
 arthroscopic repair ~ 29888-29889
 repair ~ 27407-27409
  knee, with collateral ligament ~ 27409
Cryoablation
 nerve, percutaneous ~ 0440T-0442T
Cryofibrinogen ~ 82585
Cryofixation ~ see cryopreservation

Cryoglobulin ~ 82595
Cryopreservation
 cells ~ 38207-38209, 88240-88241
 embryo ~ 89258
 for transplantation ~ 32850, 33930, 33940, 44132, 47133, 47140, 48550, 50300-50320, 50547
 freezing and storage ~ 38207, 88240
 sperm ~ 89259
 testes ~ 89335
 thawing
  embryo ~ 89352
  oocytes ~ 89353
  reproductive tissue ~ 89354
  sperm ~ 89356
Cryosurgery ~ 17000-17286, 47371, 47381
 ablation
  fibroadenoma, breast ~ 19105
  lesion/tumor
   chest wall ~ 32994
   liver ~ 47371, 47381, 47383, 50250
   pleura ~ 32994
 bladder ~ 52214
  tumor ~ 52234, 52235, 52240
 hemorrhoids ~ 46999
 lesion
  anus ~ 46916, 46924
  bladder ~ 51030, 52224
  ear ~ 17280-17284, 17286
  eyelid ~ 17280-17284, 17286
  face ~ 17280-17284, 17286
  lips ~ 17280-17284, 17286
  kidney ~ 50250
  mouth ~ 17280-17284, 17286, 40820
  nose ~ 17280-17284, 17286
  penis ~ 54056, 54065
  skin ~ 17000, 17003, 17004, 17106-17108, 17110, 17111
  urethra ~ 52224
  vagina ~ 57061, 57065
  vulva ~ 56501, 56515
 prostate ~ 52214, 55873
 trichiasis ~ 67825
 urethra ~ 52214
Cryotherapy
 ablation, renal tumor ~ 50593
 acne ~ 17340
 bronchial stenosis ~ 31641
 destruction
  bronchial tumor ~ 31641
  ciliary body ~ 66720
  retinopathy ~ 67227
 lesion
  cornea ~ 65450
  retina ~ 67208
 retinal detachment
  prophylaxis ~ 67141
  repair ~ 67101, 67107, 67108, 67113
 trichiasis, correction ~ 67825
Cryptectomy ~ 46999
Cryptococcus
 antibody ~ 86641
 antigen detection, enzyme immunoassay ~ 87327
Cryptococcus neoformans, antigen detection, enzyme immunoassay ~ 87327
Cryptorchism ~ 54550-54560
Cryptosporidium
 antigen detection
  direct fluorescence ~ 87272
  enzyme immunoassay ~ 87328
Crystal identification, any body fluid ~ 89060
CSF ~ see cerebrospinal fluid leak
CT angiography ~ 75574
CT scan
 3-D rendering ~ 76376, 76377
 abdomen ~ 74150-74178, 75635
 arm ~ 73200-73206
 biomedical CT analysis ~ 0558T
 bone
  density study ~ 77078, 0554T-0557T
  fracture risk assessment ~ 0554T-0557T
  strength assessment ~ 0554T-0557T

CT scan ~ *continued*

brain ~ 70450-70470
  stroke diagnosis ~ 3110F-3112F
breast ~ 0633T-0638T
drainage ~ 75989
follow-up study ~ 76380
guidance
  localization ~ 77011
  needle placement ~ 77012
  parenchymal tissue ablation ~ 77013
  radiation therapy ~ 77014
  vertebroplasty ~ 72292
  visceral tissue ablation ~ 77013
heart ~ 75571-75574
optical coherence tomography (OCT)
  axillary lymph node ~ 0351T, 0352T
  breast ~ 0351T-0354T
  intravascular ~ 92978, 92979
parathyroid gland ~ 78072
radiopharmaceutical localization
  of inflammation ~ 78830, 78832
  of tumor ~ 78830, 78832
unlisted services and procedures ~ 76497
with contrast ~ 70460
  abdomen ~ 74160, 74177
  arm ~ 73201
  brain ~ 0042T, 70460
  cerebral blood flow/volume ~ 0042T
  ear ~ 70481
  face ~ 70487
  head ~ 70460
  leg ~ 73701
  maxilla ~ 70487
  neck ~ 70491
  orbit ~ 70481
  pelvis ~ 72193, 74177
  sella tucica ~ 70481
  spine
    cervical ~ 72126
    lumbar ~ 72132
    thoracic ~ 72129
  thorax ~ 71260
without and with contrast
  abdomen ~ 74170, 74174-74175, 74178, 75635
  arm ~ 73202
  brain ~ 70470, 70496
  chest ~ 71275
  ear ~ 70482
  face ~ 70488
  head ~ 70470, 70496
  leg ~ 73702-73706, 75635
  maxilla ~ 70488
  neck ~ 70492, 70498
  orbit ~ 70482
  pelvis ~ 72194, 74174, 74178
  sella turcica ~ 70482
  spine, cervical ~ 72127
    lumbar ~ 72133
    thoracic ~ 72130
  thorax ~ 71270
without contrast ~ 70450
  abdomen ~ 74150, 74176, 74178
  arm ~ 73200
  brain ~ 70450
  colonography ~ 74261-74263
  ear ~ 70480
  face ~ 70486
  head ~ 70450
  leg ~ 73700
  maxilla ~ 70486
  neck ~ 70490
  orbit ~ 70480
  pelvis ~ 72192, 74176, 74178
  sella turcica ~ 70480
  spine
    cervical ~ 72125
    lumbar ~ 72131
    thoracic ~ 72128
  thorax ~ 71250, 71271
Cuff, rotator ~ 23410-23420
Culdocentesis ~ 57020

Culture

acid fast bacilli ~ 87116
amniotic fluid, chromosome analysis ~ 88235
bacteria
  aerobic ~ 87040-87071, 87077
  anaerobic ~ 87073-87076
  blood ~ 87040
  other ~ 87070-87075
  screening ~ 87081
  stool ~ 87045-87046
  urine ~ 87086-87088
bone marrow, chromosome analysis ~ 88237
cancer stem cells (CSCs) cytotoxicity assay ~ 0564T
chlamydia ~ 87110
chorionic villus, chromosome analysis ~ 88235
fertilized oocyte for in vitro fertilization ~ 89250
  co-culture of embryo ~ 89251
fungus
  blood ~ 87103
  hair ~ 87101
  identification ~ 87106
  nail ~ 87101
  other ~ 87102
  skin ~ 87101
lymphocyte
  chromosome analysis ~ 88230
  HLA typing ~ 86821
mold ~ 87107
mycobacteria ~ 87118
mycoplasma ~ 87109
oocyte/embryo ~ 89250
  co-culture of oocyte/embryo ~ 89251
  extended culture ~ 89272
pathogen ~ 87081-87084
skin, chromosome analysis ~ 88233
tissue
  homogenization ~ 87176
  infectious agent drug resistance ~ 87903-87904
  toxin/antitoxin ~ 87230
  virus ~ 87252-87253
tubercle bacilli ~ 87116
typing ~ 87140-87158
unlisted services and procedures ~ 87999
yeast ~ 87106
Curettage ~ 59840
cervix, endocervical ~ 57454, 57456, 57505
cornea ~ 65435-65436
  chelating agent ~ 65436
hydatidiform mole ~ 59870
postpartum ~ 59160
uterus ~ 58356
Curettage and dilatation ~ 59840
Curettement, skin lesion ~ 11055-11057, 17004, 17110, 17270, 17280
Curietherapy ~ 77761-77778, 77789
Custodial care ~ see domiciliary services; nursing facility services
Cutaneolipectomy ~ *see* lipectomy
Cutaneous-vesicostomy ~ 51980
Cutaneous tag ~ 11200-11201
Cutaneous tissue ~ see integumentary system
CVS ~ 59015
Cyanacobalamin ~ 82607-82608
Cyanide
blood ~ 82600
tissue ~ 82600
Cyanocobalamin ~ 82607-82608
Cyclic AMP ~ 82030
Cyclic somatostatin ~ 84307
Cyclocryotherapy ~ 66720
Cyclodialysis, destruction ciliary body ~ 66740
Cyclophotocoagulation, destruction ciliary body ~ 66710
Cyclosporine, assay ~ 80158
Cyst
abdomen, destruction/excision ~ 49203-49205
ankle
  capsule ~ 27630
  tendon sheath ~ 27630
Bartholin's gland excision ~ 56740
  repair ~ 56440
bile duct ~ 47715
bladder, excision ~ 51500

Cyst ~ *continued*

bone
  drainage ~ 20615
  injection ~ 20615
brain
  drainage ~ 61150-61151, 61156, 62161-62162
  excision ~ 61516, 61524, 62162
branchial cleft, excision ~ 42810-42815
breast
  incision and drainage ~ 19020
  puncture aspiration ~ 19000-19001
calcaneus ~ 28100-28103
carpal ~ 25130-25136
choledochal ~ 47715
ciliary body, destruction ~ 66770
clavicle, excision ~ 23140-23146
conjunctiva ~ 68020
dermoid, nose, excision ~ 30124-30125
drainage
  contrast injection ~ 49424
    with X-ray ~ 76080
excision
  cheekbone ~ 21030
  clavicle ~ 23140
    with allograft ~ 23146
    with autograft ~ 23145
  femur ~ 27355-27358
  ganglion ~ see ganglion
  humerus
    with allograft ~ 23156
    with autograft ~ 23155
  hydatid ~ 86171, 86280
  lymphatic ~ 49062, 49323
  maxilla ~ 21030
  mediastinum ~ 32662
  olecranon process
    with allograft ~ 24126
    with autograft ~ 24125
  pericardial ~ 32661
  pilonidal ~ 11770-11772
  radius
    with allograft ~ 24126
    with autograft ~ 24125
  scapula ~ 23140
    with allograft ~ 23146
    with autograft ~ 23145
  ulna
    with allograft ~ 24126
    with autograft ~ 24125
  zygoma ~ 21030
facial bones
  excision ~ 21030
femur ~ 27065-27067
fibula ~ 27635-27638
ganglion, aspiration/injection ~ 20612
gums, incision and drainage ~ 41800
hip ~ 27065-27067
humerus
  excision ~ 23150-23156, 24110
    with allograft ~ 24116
    with autograft ~ 24115
ileum ~ 27065-27067
incision and drainage ~ 10060-10061
  pilonidal ~ 10080-10081
iris, destruction ~ 66770
kidney
  ablation ~ 50541
  aspiration ~ 50390
  excision ~ 50280-50290
  injection ~ 50390
  X-ray ~ 74470
knee
  Baker's ~ 27345
  excision ~ 27347
leg, lower
  capsule ~ 27630
  tendon sheath ~ 27630
liver ~ 47010
  drainage ~ 47010
    open ~ 47010
  repair ~ 47300

Cyst ~ *continued*

lung
  incision and drainage ~ 32200
  removal ~ 32140
lymph node
  axillary/cervical
    excision ~ 38550-38555
mandible, excision ~ 21040, 21046-21047
maxilla, excision ~ 21030, 21048-21049
mediastinal, excision ~ 39200
metacarpal ~ 26200-26205
metatarsal ~ 28104-28107
mouth ~ 41005-41009, 41015-41018
  incision and drainage ~ 40800-40801
mullerian duct, excision ~ 55680
nose, excision ~ 30124-30125
olecranon ~ 24120
ovarian
  excision ~ 58925
  incision and drainage ~ 58800-58805
pancreas ~ 48500
  anastomosis ~ 48520-48540
  excision ~ 48120
pelvis
  aspiration ~ 50390
  injection ~ 50390
pericardial, excision ~ 33050
phalanges
  finger ~ 26210-26215
  toe ~ 28108
pilonidal
  excision ~ 11770-11772
  incision and drainage ~ 10080-10081
pubis ~ 27065-27067
radius ~ 24120, 25120-25126
Rathke's pouch ~ 61545
removal, skin ~ 10040
retroperitoneal, destruction/excision ~ 49203-49205, 58957, 58958
salivary gland creation
  destruction/excision, fistula ~ 42325-42326
  drainage ~ 42409
  excision ~ 42408
scapula, excision ~ 23140-23146
seminal vesicle, excision ~ 55680
skin, puncture aspiration ~ 10160
spinal cord
  aspiration ~ 62268
  incision and drainage ~ 63172-63173
sublingual gland drainage ~ 42409
  excision ~ 42408
talus ~ 28100-28103
tarsal ~ 28104-28107
thyroglossal duct
  excision ~ 60280-60281
  incision and drainage ~ 60000
thyroid gland aspiration ~ 60300
  excision ~ 60200
  injection ~ 60300
tibia ~ 27635-27638
tongue ~ 41000-41006, 41015
ulna ~ 24120, 25120-25126
urachal, bladder, excision ~ 51500
vaginal, excision ~ 57135
wrist ~ 25130-25136
  excision ~ 25111-25112
zygoma
  excision ~ 21030
Cyst ovary ~ see ovary, cyst
Cystatin C ~ 82610
Cystatins, kininogen ~ 85293
Cystectomy
complete ~ 51570
  with bilateral pelvic lymphadenectomy ~ 51575, 51585, 51595
  with continent diversion ~ 51596
  with ureteroileal conduit ~ 51590
  with ureterosigmoidostomy ~ 51580
ovarian ~ 58925
  laparoscopic ~ 58661

Cystectomy ~ *continued*
  partial
    complicated ~ 51555
    reimplantation of ureters ~ 51565
    simple ~ 51550
Cystic hygroma ~ 38550-38555
Cystine, urine ~ 82615
Cystitis, interstitial ~ 52260-52265
Cystography ~ 74430
  injection ~ 52281
  radiologic ~ 51600
Cystolithotomy ~ 51050
Cystometrogram ~ 51725-51726
Cystoplasty ~ 51800
Cystorrhaphy ~ 51860-51865
Cystoscopy ~ 52000
Cystoscopy, with biopsy ~ 52224, 52250
Cystostomy
  change tube ~ 51705-51710
  closure ~ 51880
  home visit ~ 99505
  with fulguration ~ 51020
  with insertion radioactive material ~ 51020
  with urethrectomy
    female ~ 53210
    male ~ 53215
Cystotomy
  excision
    bladder diverticulum ~ 51525
    bladder tumor ~ 51530
    repair of ureterocele ~ 51535
    vesical neck ~ 51520
  repair of ureterocele ~ 51535
  with calculus basket extraction ~ 51065
  with destruction intravesical lesion ~ 51030
  with drainage ~ 51040
  with fulguration ~ 51020
  with insertion
    radioactive material ~ 51020
    ureteral catheter ~ 51045
  with removal calculus ~ 51050, 51065
Cystourethrogram, retrograde ~ 51610
Cystourethropexy ~ 51840-51841
Cystourethroplasty ~ 51800-51820
Cystourethroscopy
  biopsy ~ 52204, 52224, 52250, 52354
  brush ~ 52007
  calibration and/or dilation
    urethral stricture or stenosis ~ 52281, 52630, 52647-52649
  catheterization
    ejaculatory duct ~ 52010
    ureteral ~ 52005, 52320
  chemodenervation, bladder ~ 52287
  dilation
    bladder ~ 52260, 52265
    intra-renal stricture ~ 52343, 52346
    ureter ~ 52341-52342, 52344-52345
    urethra ~ 52281, 52285, 0499T
  drug delivery, urethra ~ 0499T
  evacuation, clot ~ 52001
  examination ~ 52000
  female urethral syndrome ~ 52285
  incision, ejaculatory duct ~ 52402
  injection of implant material ~ 52327
  insertion
    indwelling ureteral stent ~ 50947, 52332
    radioactive substance ~ 52250
    transprostatic implant ~ 52441, 52442
    ureteral guide wire ~ 52334
    urethral stent ~ 52282
  lithotripsy ~ 52353
  lysis
    urethra ~ 53500
    urethrovaginal septal fibrosis ~ 52285
  manipulation of ureteral calculus ~ 52330
  meatotomy, ureteral ~ 52290-52305

Cystourethroscopy ~ *continued*
  prostate
    laser coagulation ~ 52647
    laser enucleation ~ 52649
    laser vaporization ~ 52648
    transurethral commissurotomy ~ 0619T
  removal
    calculus ~ 52310-52315, 52320-52325, 52352
    foreign body ~ 52310-52315
    urethral stent ~ 52310-52315
  resection
    ejaculatory duct ~ 52402
    external sphincter ~ 52277
    tumor ~ 52355
  urethral syndrome ~ 52285
  vasectomy, transurethral ~ 52402
  vasotomy
    transurethral ~ 52402
  with direct vision internal urethromtomy ~ 52276
  with ejaculatory duct catheterization ~ 52010
  with fulguration ~ 52214, 52354
    lesion ~ 52224
    tumor ~ 52234-52240
  with internal urethrotomy
    female ~ 52270
    male ~ 52275
  with steroid injection ~ 52283
  with ureteral catheterization ~ 52005
  with ureteral meatotomy ~ 52290-52305
Cytochrome reductase, lactic ~ 83615-83625
Cytogenetic studies
  bone marrow
    diagnostic ~ 3155F
    neoplastic disorder ~ 88237
  interpretation and report ~ 88291
  molecular, DNA probe ~ 88271-88275, 88364-88366
  neoplastic disorders
    bone marrow ~ 88237
    tumor ~ 88239
  non-neoplastic disorders
    amniotic fluid ~ 88235
    chorionic villus cells ~ 88235
    lymphocyte ~ 88230
    skin or tissue biopsuy ~ 88233
  unlisted services and procedures ~ 88299
Cytogenomic neoplasia (genome-wide) microarray analysis
  interrogation of genomic regions ~ 81277
Cytomegalovirus
  antibody ~ 86644-86645
  antigen detection
    direct fluorescence ~ 87271
    enzyme immunoassay ~ 87332
    nucleic acid ~ 87495-87497
Cytometries, flow ~ 88184-88189
Cytopathology
  cervical or vaginal
    definitive hormone evaluationi ~ 88155
    Pap ~ 88164-88167
    requiring interpretation by physician ~ 88141
    thin layer prep ~ 88142-88143, 88174-88175
  evaluation ~ 88172, 88177
  fluids, washings, brushings ~ 88104, 88106
  forensic ~ 88125
  other source ~ 88160-88162
  sex chromatin identification ~ 88130, 88140
  selective cellular enhancement technique ~ 88112
  smears
    any other source ~ 88160-88162
    brushings ~ 88104
    cervical or vaginal
      automated screen ~ 88174
      hormone evaluation ~ 88155
      manual screen ~ 88150, 88153, 88164-88165
    washings ~ 88104
  unlisted services and procedures ~ 88199
  urinary tract specimen ~ 88120-88121
Cytoscopy ~ 52000
Cytosol aminopeptidase ~ 83670

Cytotoxic screen
  lymphocyte ~ 86805-86806
  percent reactive antibody (PRA) ~ 86807-86808
  serum antibodies ~ 86807-86808

D

D and C ~ 59840
D and E ~ 59841
D-xylose absorption test ~ 84620
Dacryoadenectomy
  partial ~ 68505
  total ~ 68500
Dacryocystectomy ~ 68520
Dacryocystogram ~ 68850, 70170
Dacryocystography ~ 68850, 70170
  nuclear imaging ~ 78660
Dacryocystorhinostomy ~ 68720
  total, with nasal/sinus endoscopy ~ 31239
Dacryocystostomies ~ 68420
Dacryocystotomy ~ 68420
Daily living activities ~ 97535, 99509
Damus-Kaye-Stansel procedure ~ 33606
Dana operation ~ 63185-63190
Dandy operation ~ 62180, 62200-62201
Dark adaptation examination ~ 92284
Dark field examination ~ 87164-87166
Darrach procedure ~ 25150-25151, 25240
Day test ~ 82270, 82272
De Quervain's disease treatment ~ 25000
Death, brain ~ 95824
Debridement
  ankle ~ 29897, 29898
  bone ~ 11044, 11047
    with open fracture or dislocation ~ 11012
  brain ~ 62010
  burns ~ 01951-01953, 16010-16030
  cartilage ~ 29862, 29877, 29880, 29881, 29885
  elbow ~ 29837, 29838
    with prosthesis removal ~ 24160, 24164
  forearm ~ 25023, 25025
  knee ~ 27441, 27443, 27497, 27499
  leg ~ 27892, 27894
  lesion, premalignant ~ 96574
  liver ~ 47361
  mastoid cavity
    complex ~ 69222
    simple ~ 69220
  metatarsophalangeal joint ~ 28289, 28291, 29901, 29902
  muscle ~ 11043, 11044, 11046, 11047
    infected ~ 11004-11006, 11008
  nails ~ 11720, 11721
  nonviable tissue ~ 25023, 25025, 27497, 27892-27894
  nose
    endoscopic ~ 31237
  pancreatic tissue ~ 48105
  shoulder ~ 29822, 29823
    with prosthesis removal ~ 23334, 23335
  skin
    eczematous ~ 11000, 11001
    excision ~ 15920-15999
    infected ~ 11000-11006
    with open fracture and/or dislocation ~ 11010-11012
    subcutaneous tissue ~ 11042-11047
      infected ~ 11004-11006
  sternum ~ 21627, 21750
  wound
    non-selective ~ 97602
    selective ~ 97597, 97598
  wrist joint ~ 29846
    nonviable tissue ~ 25023, 25025
Debulking procedure
  ovary/pelvis ~ 58952-58954

Decompression ~ see section
  arm, lower ~ 24495, 25020-25025
  auditory canal, internal ~ 69960
  brainstem ~ 61575-61576
  cauda equina ~ 63011, 63017, 63047-63048, 63056-63057, 63087-63091
  cranial nerve ~ 61458
  esophagogastric varices ~ 37181
  facial nerve ~ 61590
    intratemporal
      lateral to geniculate ganglion ~ 69720, 69740
      medial to geniculate ganglion ~ 69725, 69745
    total ~ 69955
  finger ~ 26035
  gasserian ganglion
    sensory root ~ 61450
  hand ~ 26035-26037
  intestines
    small ~ 44021
  jejunostomy
    laparoscopic ~ 44201
  leg, fasciotomy ~ 27600-27602
  nerve ~ 64702-64727
    root ~ 63020-63048, 63055-63103
  nucleus of disk
    lumbar ~ 62287
  optic nerve ~ 67570
  orbit ~ 61330
    removal of bone ~ 67414, 67445
  skull ~ 61322-61323, 61340-61345
  spinal cord ~ 22856, 22858, 62287, 62380, 63001-63017, 63045-63103
    cauda equina ~ 63005
  tarsal tunnel release ~ 28035
  volvulus ~ 45321, 45337
  with nasal/sinus endoscopy
    optic nerve ~ 31294
    orbit wall ~ 31292-31293
  wrist ~ 25020-25025
Decortication
  lung
    endoscopic ~ 32651-32652
    with parietal pleurectomy ~ 32320
    partial ~ 32225
    total ~ 32220
Decubiti ~ see pressure ulcer (decubitus)
Decubitus ulcers ~ see debridement; pressure ulcer (decubitus); skin graft and flap
Deetjeen's body ~ see blood, platelet
Defect, coagulation ~ 85390
Defect, heart septal ~ 33813-33814
Defect, septal closure, atrial ~ see heart, repair, atrial septum
Deferens, ductus ~ see vas deferens
Defibrillation ~ 92960-92961
Defibrillator, implantable
  device evaluation
    electrophysiologic ~ 93644
    interrogation
      in-person
        subcutaneous ~ 93261
        transvenous ~ 93289
      remote ~ 93295, 93296
    peri-procedural ~ 93287
    programming device evaluation
      subcutaneous ~ 93260
      transvenous ~ 93282-93284
  insertion
    electrodes ~ 33202, 33203, 33216, 33217, 33224, 33225, 33271
    pulse generator ~ 33230, 33231, 33240
    system ~ 33249, 33270
  removal
    electrodes ~ 33238, 33243, 33244, 33272
    pulse generator ~ 33241, 33262-33264
  repair, electrodes ~ 33218, 33220
  replacement
    pulse generator ~ 33224, 33262-33264
    system ~ 33249, 33270
  repositioning, electrode ~ 33215, 33273
  wearable device ~ 93745
    data analysis ~ 93292
Deformity, boutonniere ~ 26426-26428
Deformity, Sprengel's ~ 23400
Degenerative, articular cartilage, patella ~ 27418

Degradation products, fibrin ~ 85362-85380
Dehydroepiandrosterone ~ 82626
Dehydroepiandrosterone sulfate ~ 82627
Dehydrogenase, 6-phosphogluconate ~ 84085
Dehydrogenase, alcohol ~ 84588
Dehydrogenase, glucose-6-phosphate ~ 82955-82960
Dehydrogenase, glutamate ~ 82965
Dehydrogenase, isocitrate ~ 83570
Dehydrogenase, lactate ~ 83615-83625
Dehydrogenase, malate ~ 83775
Dehydroisoandrosterone sulfate ~ 82626
Delay of flap, skin graft ~ 15600-15630
Deligation, ureter ~ 50940
Deliveries, abdominal ~ see cesarean delivery
Delivery ~ see cesarean delivery; vaginal delivery
Delorme operation ~ see pericardiectomy
Denervation
  hip
    femoral ~ 27035
    obturator ~ 27035
    sciatic ~ 27035
Denervation, sympathetic ~ 64802-64818
Dens axis ~ 22548
Denver developmental screening test ~ 96100
  Denver shuntpatency test ~ 78291
Denver Krupic procedure ~ 66180
Denver-Krupin procedure ~ 66180
Deoxycorticosterone ~ 82633
Deoxycortisol ~ 80436, 82634
Deoxyephedrine ~ 80324-80326
Deoxyribonuclease antibody ~ 86215
Deoxyribonuclease I ~ 86215
Deoxyribonucleic acid antibody ~ 86225-86226
Depilation ~ see removal, hair
Depletion
  plasma ~ 38214
  platelet ~ 38213
  T-cell ~ 38210
  tumor cell ~ 38211
Deposit calcium ~ 82310, 82330, 82340
Depth electrode
  insertion ~ 61760
Derma-fat-fascia graft ~ 15770
Dermabrasion ~ 15780-15783
Dermatology
  actinotherapy ~ 96900
  microscopic examination of hair ~ 96902
  photochemotherapy
    ultraviolet A treatment ~ 96912, 96913
    ultraviolet B treatment ~ 96910, 96913
  psoriasis laser treatment ~ 96920-96922
  reflectance confocal microscopy (RCM) skin imaging ~ 96931-96936
  unlisted services and procedures ~ 96999
  whole body photography ~ 96904
Dermatoplasty, septal ~ 30620
Dermoid ~ 30124-30125
Derrick-Burnet disease ~ 86000, 86638
Descending abdominal aorta ~ see aorta, abdominal
Desipramine, assay ~ 80335-80337
Desmotomy ~ 23415, 29848
Desoxycorticosterone ~ 82633
Desoxycortone ~ 82633
Desoxyephedrine ~ 80324-80326
Desoxynorephedrin ~ 80324-80326
Desoxyphenobarbital ~ 80188
Desquamation ~ 17360
Destruction
  acne ~ 17340-17360
    cryotherapy ~ 17340
  arrhythmogenic focus, heart ~ 33250-33251, 33261
  bladder ~ 51020, 52214-52224, 52354
  calculus
    bile duct ~ 43265
    kidney ~ 50590
    pancreatic duct ~ 43265
  chemical cauterization, granulation tissue ~ 17250
  chemosurgery ~ 17110-17111

Destruction ~ *continued*
  ciliary body
    cryotherapy ~ 66720
    cyclodialysis ~ 66740
    cyclophotocoagulation ~ 66710-66711
    diathermy ~ 66700
    endoscopic ~ 66711
  cryosurgery ~ 17110-17111
  cyst
    abdomen ~ 49203-49205
    ciliary body ~ 66770
    iris ~ 66770
  endometrial ablation ~ 58356
  endometriomas
    abdomen ~ 49203-49205
  fissure, anal ~ 46940-46942
  hemorrhoids, thermal ~ 46930
  kidney ~ 52354
    endoscopic ~ 50557, 50576
  laser surgery ~ 17110-17111
  lesion
    anal ~ 46900-46917, 46924
    bladder ~ 51030
    choroid ~ 67220-67225
    ciliary body ~ 66770
    conjunctiva ~ 68135
    cornea ~ 65450
    eyelid ~ 67850
    facial ~ 17000-17004, 17280-17286
    gums ~ 41850
    iris ~ 66770
    larynx ~ 31572
    mouth ~ 40820
    nerve plantar ~ 64632
    nose, intranasal ~ 30117-30118
    palate ~ 42160
    penis
      cryosurgery ~ 54056
      electrodesiccation ~ 54055
      extensive ~ 54065
      laser surgery ~ 54057
      simple ~ 54050-54060
      surgical excision ~ 54060
    pharynx ~ 42808
    prostrate ~ 45320
      thermotherapy ~ 53850-53852
        microwave ~ 53850
        radio frequency ~ 53852
    retina
      cryotherapy, diathermy ~ 67208-67218, 67227
      photocoagulation ~ 67210, 67228-67229
      radiation by implantation of source ~ 67218
    skin
      benign ~ 17110-17111
      malignant ~ 17260-17286, 96567
      premalignant ~ 17000-17004, 96567
    spinal cord ~ 62280-62282
    ureter ~ 52341-52342, 52344-52345
    urethra ~ 52400, 53265
    uvula ~ 42160
    vagina
      extensive ~ 57065
      simple ~ 57061
    vascular, cutaneous ~ 17106-17108
    vulva
      extensive ~ 56515
      simple ~ 56501
  nerve ~ 64600-64610, 64620-64640, 64680-64681
  neurofibroma, extensive ~ 0419T, 0420T
  polyp
    aural ~ 69540
    nose ~ 30110-30115
    urethra ~ 53260
  prostate ~ 55873
  prostate tissue, transurethral thermotherapy ~ 53850-53852
  sinus, frontal ~ 31080-31085
  Skene's gland ~ 53270

Destruction ~ *continued*
  skin lesion
    benign ~ 17110, 17111
    malignant ~ 17260-17286
      by photodynamic therapy ~ 96567
    premalignant ~ 17000-17004, 96567, 96573, 96574
  tonsil, lingual ~ 42870
  tumor
    abdomen ~ 49203-49205
    breast, microwave thermotherapy ~ 19499
    colon ~ 45383
    intestines
      large ~ 44401
      small ~ 44369
    mesentery ~ 49203-49205
    pancreatic duct ~ 43272
    rectum ~ 45190, 46937-46938
    retroperitoneal ~ 49203-49205
    urethra ~ 53220
  tumor or polyp, rectum ~ 45320
  turbinate mucosa ~ 30801-30802
  ureter ~ 52354
    endoscopic ~ 50957, 50976
  urethra ~ 52214-52224, 52354
    prolapse ~ 53275
  warts, flat ~ 17110-17111
  with cystourethroscopy ~ 52354
Determination, blood pressure ~ see blood pressure
Developmental testing ~ 96110-96111
Device
  adjustable gastric band ~ 43770-43774
  annulus reconstruction device ~ 0544T, 0545T
  balloon continence device
    placement ~ 0548T, 0549T
    removal ~ 0550T
    volume adjustment ~ 0551T
  iliac artery occlusion device insertion ~ 34808
  subcutaneous port for gastric restrictive procedure ~ 43770, 43774, 43886-43888
  venous access
    collection of blood specimen ~ 36591, 36592
    fluoroscopic guidance ~ 36598, 77001
    insertion
      central ~ 36560-36566
      peripheral ~ 36570-36571
    irrigation ~ 96523
    obstruction clearance ~ 36595-36596
      imaging ~ 75901-75902
    removal ~ 36590
    repair ~ 36576
    replacement ~ 36582-36583, 36585
      catheter ~ 36578
  ventricular assist
    extracorporeal
      removal ~ 33990-33993
      replacement ~ 33981
    implantable
      removal ~ 33980
      replacement ~ 33982-33983
Device, intrauterine ~ 58300-58301
Device, orthotic ~ 97760
Device handling ~ 99002
Dexamethasone suppression test ~ 80420
DHA sulfate ~ 82627
Dhea ~ 82626
Dhea sulfate ~ 82627
Diagnosis, psychiatric ~ see psychiatric diagnosis
Diagnostic amniocentesis ~ 59000
Diagnostic aspiration of anterior chamber of eye ~ 65800
Diagnostic radiology ~ 70010-76499
Diagnostic skin and sensitization tests ~ see allergy tests
Diagnostic ultrasound ~ 76506-76999
Diagnostic ultrasound of heart ~ see echocardiography
Dialysis
  anesthesia ~ 01844
  arteriovenous fistula ~ 36831-36833
  end stage renal disease ~ 90951-90970
  hemodialysis ~ 90935-90937, 4051F-4054F
    blood flow study ~ 90940
    plan of care documented ~ 0505F

Dialysis ~ *continued*
  hemoperfusion ~ 90997
  hepatitis B vaccine (HepB) ~ 90740, 90747
  introduction
    dialysis circuit ~ 36901-36903
      with transcatheter placement of stent ~ 36906
  Kt/V level ~ 3082F-3084F
  patient training
    completed course ~ 90989
    per session ~ 90993
  peritoneal ~ 90945, 90947, 4055F
    catheter insertion ~ 49418, 49419, 49421
    catheter removal ~ 49422
    home infusion ~ 99601, 99602
    plan of care documented ~ 0507F
  thrombectomy
    dialysis circuit ~ 36904-36906
  with transcatheter stent placemehnt via dialysis circuit ~ 36908
  with transluminal balloon angioplasty via dialysis circuit ~ 36907
  with vascular embolization/occlusion ~ 36909
  unlisted services and procedures ~ 90999
Dialysis, extracorporeal ~ 90935-90937
Diaphragm
  repair
    for eventration ~ 39545
    hernia ~ 39503-39541
    laceration ~ 39501
  resection ~ 39560-39561
  unlisted procedures ~ 39599
  vagina
    fitting ~ 57170
Diaphragm contraception ~ 57170
Diaphysectomy
  calcaneus ~ 28120
  clavicle ~ 23180
  femur ~ 27360
  fibula ~ 27360, 27641
  humerus ~ 23184, 24140
  metacarpal ~ 26230
  metatarsal ~ 28122
  olecranon process ~ 24147
  phalanges
    finger ~ 26235-26236
    toe ~ 28124
  radius ~ 24145, 25151
  scapula ~ 23182
  talus ~ 28120
  tarsal ~ 28122
  tibia ~ 27360, 27640
  ulna ~ 24147, 25150
Diastase ~ 82150
Diastasis ~ see separation
  pelvic ring, closed treatment ~ 27197, 27198
Diathermy ~ 97024
  destruction ciliary body ~ 66700
  lesion retina ~ 67208, 67227
  retinal detachment
    prophylaxis ~ 67141
    repair ~ 67101
  surgical ~ 17000-17286
Dibucaine number ~ 82638
Dichloride, methylene ~ 84600
Dichlorides, ethylene ~ 84600
Dichloroethane ~ 84600
Dichloromethane ~ 84600
Diethylether ~ 84600
Differential count ~ 85032, 85048, 89055
Differentiation reversal factor ~ 85210
Diffusion test, gel ~ 86329-86331
Digestive system, surgical procedures ~ 40490-49999
Digestive tract ~ see gastrointestinal tract
Digit replantation ~ 20816-20822
Digital artery sympathectomy ~ 64820
Digital slit-beam radiograph ~ see scanogram
Digits pinch graft ~ 15050
Digoxin assay ~ 80162
Dihydrocodeinone ~ 80361
Dihydroepitestosterone ~ 80327, 80328
Dihydromorphinone ~ 80361
Dihydrotestosterone ~ 80327, 80328
Dihydroxyethanes ~ 82693

Dihydroxyvitamin D ~ 82652
Dilation ~ 59840
  anal
    endoscopy ~ 46604
    sphincter ~ 45905, 46940
  aortic valve ~ 33930, 33931
  bile duct
    balloon ~ 47542
    endoscopy ~ 43277, 47555, 47556
    stricture ~ 74363
    with stent placement ~ 47538-47540
  biliary ampulla, balloon ~ 47542
  bladder, cystourethroscopy ~ 52260, 52265
  bronchi, endoscopy ~ 31630, 31636
  cerebral vessels ~ 61640-61642
  cervix
    canal ~ 57800
    stump ~ 57558
  colon endoscopy ~ 45386
  colon-sigmoid endoscopy ~ 45340
  esophagus ~ 43450, 43453
    balloon ~ 43195, 43213-43214, 43220, 43233, 43249
    endoscopy ~ 43195-43196, 43212-43213, 43220, 43226, 43229, 43233, 43453
  eustachian tube ~ 69705, 69706
  gastric/duodenol stricture ~ 43245
    surgical ~ 43510
  intestines~ 44615
    endoscopy ~ 44370
    stent placement ~ 44379, 44384, 44402
  kidney ~ 50080-50081
    intra-renal stricture ~ 52343, 52346
  lacrimal punctum ~ 68801
  larynx
    endoscopy ~ 31528-31529
  nasal/sinus endoscopy ~ 31295-31297
  nasolacrimal duct ~ 68816
  pancreatic duct
    endoscopy ~ 43277
  rectum
    endoscopy ~ 45303, 45327, 45340, 45347, 45386-45389
    sphincter ~ 45910
  salivary duct ~ 42650, 42660
  sclera, aqueous outflow canal ~ 66174-66175
  sinus ostium ~ 31295-31297
  sphincter of Oddi, balloon ~ 47542
  trachea
    endoscopy ~ 31630, 31631, 31636, 31638
  ureter
    balloon ~ 50706
    endoscopy ~ 50553, 50572, 50575, 50953, 50972
    with cystourethroscopy ~ 52341-52343
      with ureteroscopy ~ 52344-52346
  urethra ~ 52285, 52601, 52630, 52647-52649, 53660, 53661, 53665, 55801, 55821
    stenosis ~ 52281
    stricture ~ 52281, 53600-53601, 53605, 53620-53621, 53655
  vagina ~ 57400
Dilation and curettage ~ 59840
  cervix ~ 57558, 57800
  corpus uteri ~ 58120
  hysteroscopy ~ 58558
  postpartum ~ 59160
  with amniotic injections ~ 59851
  with vaginal suppositories ~ 59856
Dilation and evacuation ~ 59841
  with amniotic injections ~ 59851
Dimethadione ~ 80339-80341
Dioxide, carbon ~ 82374
Dioxide, silicon ~ 84285
Dipeptidyl peptidase A ~ 82164
Diphenylhydantoin ~ 80185-80186
Diphosphate, adenosine ~ 82030
Diphtheria ~ 86648
Dipropylacetic acid assay ~ 80164
Direct pedicle flap formation ~ 15570-15576
Disability evaluation services
  basic life and/or disability evaluation ~ 99450
  work-related or medical disability evaluation ~ 99455-99456

Disarticulation
  ankle ~ 27889
  hip ~ 27295
  knee ~ 27598
  shoulder ~ 23920-23921
  wrist ~ 25920, 25924
    revision ~ 25922
Disc, intervertebral ~ see intervertebral disk
Discectomies ~ 63075-63078
  percutaneous ~ 62287
Discectomy
  additional segment ~ 22226
  arthrodesis
    additional interspace ~ 22534, 22585, 22634
    cervical ~ 22551, 22552, 22554, 22585
    lumbar ~ 0195T, 0196T, 22533, 22534, 22558, 22585, 22630, 62380
    sacral ~ 0195T, 22586
    thoracic ~ 22532, 22534, 22556, 22585, 63077, 63078
  cervical ~ 22220, 22551, 22552, 22554, 22856-22858, 63075, 63076
  lumbar ~ 0163T, 0164T, 0195T, 0196T, 22224, 22630, 22633, 22634, 22857
  percutaneous ~ 0274T, 0275T
  sacral ~ 0195T, 22586
  thoracic ~ 22222
  with end plate preparation ~ 22856, 22858
Discharge services
  hospital ~ 99238, 99239
  newborn ~ 99463
  nursing facility ~ 99315, 99316
  observation care ~ 99217, 99234, 99236
Discission
  cataract
    laser surgery ~ 66821
    stab incision ~ 66820
  vitreous strands ~ 67030
Discography
  cervical disk ~ 72285
  injection ~ 62290-62291
  lumbar disk ~ 62287, 72295
  thoracic ~ 72285
Discolysis ~ 62292
Disease
  Erb-Goldflam ~ 95857
  Heine-Medin ~ see polio
  hydatid ~ see echinococcosis
  Lyme ~ see Lyme disease
  Ormond ~ see retroperitoneal fibrosis
  Peyronie ~ see Peyronie disease
  Posada-Wernicke ~ 86490
Disease/organ panel ~ see organ or disease oriented panel
Disk chemolyses, intervertebral ~ 62292
Dislocated joint ~ see dislocation
Dislocation
  acromioclavicular joint, open treatment ~ 23550-23552
  ankle
    closed treatment ~ 27840-27842
    open treatment ~ 27846-27848
  carpal
    closed treatment ~ 25690
    open treatment ~ 25695
  carpometacarpal joint ~ 26670
    closed treatment
      with manipulation ~ 26675-26676
    open treatment ~ 26685-26686
    percutaneous fixation ~ 26676
  clavicle
    closed treatment ~ 23540-23545
    open treatment ~ 23550-23552
    without manipulation ~ 23540
    with manipulation ~ 23545
  closed treatment
    carpometacarpal joint ~ 26670-26675
    metacarpophalangeal ~ 26700-26706
    thumb ~ 26641
  elbow
    closed treatment ~ 24600-24605, 24640
    open treatment ~ 24615

Domiciliary services ~ 99324-99340
  discharge services ~ 99315-99316
  established patient ~ 99331-99333
  new patient ~ 99321-99323
Donor procedures
  conjunctival graft ~ 68371
  heart/lung excision ~ 33930
  heart excision ~ 33940
  liver segment ~ 47140-47142
  stem cells
    donor search ~ 38204
Dopamine ~ 80424, 82382-82384
  blood ~ 82383-82384
  urine ~ 82382, 82384
Doppler echocardiography ~ 76827-76828, 93306-93308, 93320-93350
  intracardiac ~ 93662
  transesophageal ~ 93318
  transthoracic ~ 93303-93317
Doppler scan
  arterial studies
    coronary flow reserve ~ 93571, 93572
    extremities ~ 93922-93924
    fetal
      middle cerebral artery ~ 76821
      umbilical artery ~ 76820
  duplex, transplanted kidney ~ 76776
  intracranial arteries
    complete study ~ 93886
    emboli detection ~ 93892, 93893
    limited study ~ 93888
    vasoreactivity study ~ 93890
  saline infusion sonohysterography (SIS) ~ 76831
  transplanted kidney ~ 76776
Dorsal vertebra ~ 22101, 22112
Dosimetry
  radiation therapy ~ 77300, 77331
    brachytherapy ~ 77316-77318
    intensity modulation IMRT ~ 77301, 77338, 77385, 77386
    special ~ 77331
    teletherapy ~ 77306, 77307, 77321
  Unlisted procedure ~ 77399
Double-stranded DNA ~ 86225-86226
Doxepin
  assay ~ 80335-80337
DPH ~ 80185-80186
Drainage ~ see also excision; incision; incision and drainage
  abdomen
    abdomen fluid ~ 49082-49083
  abscess
    appendix ~ 44900
    brain ~ 61150, 61151, 61320, 61321
    breast ~ 19020
    elbow ~ 23930
    eyelid ~ 67700
    knee ~ 27301
    lef ~ 27603
    liver ~ 47010
    lung ~ 31645, 31646, 32200
    lymph node ~ 38300, 38305
    mouth
      lingual ~ 41000
      masticator space ~ 41009, 41018
      sublingual ~ 41005, 41006, 41015, 42310
      submandibular space ~ 41008, 41017
      submaxillary ~ 42310, 42320
      submental space ~ 41007, 41016
    neck ~ 21501, 21502
    nasal ~ 30000
    nasal septum ~ 30020
    ovary ~ 58820, 58822
    palate ~ 42000
    parotid ~ 42300, 42305
    pelvic ~ 45000, 45020
    perineal ~ 56405
    peri-renal or renal ~ 50020
    peritoneal ~ 49020
    peritonsillar ~ 42700
    pharyngeal ~ 42720, 42725
    prostate ~ 52700, 55720, 55725
    rectum ~ 45005, 45020, 46040

Drainage ~ *continued*
  retroperitoneal ~ 49060, 49323
  shoulder ~ 23030
  skene's gland ~ 53060
  soft tissue
    percutaneous ~ 10030
    subfascial ~ 22010, 22015
  subdiaphragmatic or subphrenic ~ 49040
  urethra ~ 53040
  uvula ~ 42000
  vestible of mouth ~ 40800, 40801
  with X-ray ~ 75989
  wrist ~ 25028
  amniotic fluid
    diagnostic aspiration ~ 59000
    therapeutic aspiration ~ 59001
  bile duct ~ 47533-47540
  biliary tract ~ 47400, 47420, 47425, 47480
    catheterization ~ 47533, 47534
  bladder ~ 51040, 51080
  brain ~ 62160, 62162, 62164
  bursa
    arm, upper ~ 23930
    foot ~ 28001-28003
    forearm ~ 25028
    hip ~ 26990
    knee ~ 27301
    leg ~ 27604
    palm ~ 26025, 26030
    pelvis ~ 26990
    shoulder ~ 23031
    thigh ~ 27301
    wrist ~ 25028
  cerebrospinal fluid ~ 62272
  cyst
    brain ~ 61150, 61151, 62162
    breast ~ 19000, 19001
    conjunctiva ~ 68020
    dentoalveolar structures ~ 41800
    intramedullary ~ 63172
    liver ~ 47010
    lung ~ 32200
    ovary ~ 58800, 58805
    pilondial ~ 10080, 10081
    skene's gland ~ 53060
    vestible of mouth ~ 40800, 40801
  empyema, chest ~ 32036, 32810
  elbow ~ 23930
  eye ~ 0191T, 0253T, 0376T, 66183
    lacrimal gland ~ 68400
    lacrimal sac ~ 68420
  fetal fluid ~ 59074
  ganglion cyst ~ 20612
  hematoma
    brain ~ 61108, 61154, 61156
    subungual ~ 11740
    superficial ~ 10140
    vagina ~ 57022, 57023
  joint
    ankle ~ 27610
    carpometacarpal ~ 26070
    hip ~ 26990, 27030
    interphalangeal ~ 26080, 28024
    intertarsal ~ 28022
    knee ~ 29871
    metacarpophalangeal ~ 26075
    metatarsophalangeal ~ 28022
    midcarpal ~ 25040
    pelvis ~ 26990
    radiocarpal ~ 25040
    sternoclavicular ~ 23044
    thigh ~ 27301
    wrist ~ 29843
  liver
    abscess or cyst ~ 47010
  lymphocele, endoscopic ~ 49323
  onychia ~ 10060-10061
  orbit ~ 67405, 67440
  pancreas
    pseudocyst ~ 48510

Drainage ~ continued
  paronychia ~ 10060-10061
  pericardial sac ~ 32659
  pericardium ~ 33017-33019, 33025
  pseudocyst
    gastrointestinal, upper
      transmural endoscopic ~ 43240
    pancreas ~ 48510
  puncture
    chest ~ 32554-32555
    skin ~ 10040-10180
  spinal cord
    cerebrospinal fluid ~ 62272
    subdural fluid ~ 61000-61001
  urethra
    extravasation ~ 53080-53085
  ventricular fluid ~ 61020
Drainage implant, glaucoma ~ 66180, 66185
Dressings
  burns ~ 16010-16030
  change
    anesthesia ~ 15852
Drez procedure ~ see incision, spinal cord ~ 63200
Dril ~ 36838
Drill hole, skull
  catheter ~ 61107
  drain hematoma ~ 61108
  exploration ~ 61105
  implant electrode ~ 61850, 61863-61868
Drug ~ see drug assay; specific drug
  aspirin ~ 4084F
  infusion ~ 62360-62362
Drugs, anticoagulant ~ 85300-85305, 85307
Drug assay (testing)
  Presumptive Drug Class ~ 80305-80307
  Definitive Drug Class
    alcohols ~ 80320
    alcohol biomarkers ~ 80321, 80322
    alkaloids, NOS ~ 80323
    amphetamines ~ 80324-80326
    anabolic steroids ~ 80327, 80328
    analgesics, non-opioid ~ 80329-80331
    antidepressants
      not otherwise specified ~ 80338
      serotonergic class ~ 80332-80334
      tricyclic and other cyclicals ~ 80335-80337
    antiepileptics ~ 80339-80341
    antipsychotics, NOS ` 80342-80344
    barbiturates ~ 80345
    benzodiazepines ~ 80346, 80347
    buprenorphine ~ 80348
    cannabinoids ~ 80349, 80350-80352
    cocaine ~ 80353
    codeine ~ 80361
    fentanyl ~ 80354
    gabapentin, non-blood ~ 80355
    heroin metabolite ~ 80356
    ketamine and norketamine ~ 80357
    methadone ~ 80358
    methylenedioxyamphetamines (MDMA) ~ 80359
    methylphenidate ~ 80360
    opiates ~ 80361
    opioids and other analogs ~ 80362-80364
    oxycodone ~ 80365
    pregabalin ~ 80366
    propoxyphene ~ 80367
    sedative hypnotics ~ 80368
    skeletal muscle relaxants ~ 80369, 80370
    stimulants ~ 80371
    tapentadol ~ 80372
    tramadol ~ 80373
  Therapeutic Drug Assay
    amikacin ~ 80150
    amitriptyline ~ 80335-80337
    benzodiazepine ~ 80346, 80347
    caffeine ~ 80155
    carbamazepine ~ 80156-80157
    clozapine ~ 80159
    cyclosporine ~ 80158
    desipramine ~ 80335-80337

Drug Assay ~ continued
  digoxin ~ 80162, 80163
  dipropylacetic acid ~ 80164, 80165
  doxepin ~ 80335-80337
  ethosuximide ~ 80168
  everolimus ~ 80169
  gabapentin ~ 80171
  gentamicin ~ 80170
  gold ~ 80375
  haloperidol ~ 80173
  imipramine ~ 80335-80337
  lamotrigine ~ 80175
  levetiracetam ~ 80177
  lidocaine ~ 80176
  lithium ~ 80178
  nortriptyline ~ 80335-80337
  oxcarbazepine ~ 80183
  phenobarbital ~ 80184
  phenytoin ~ 80185-80186
  primidone ~ 80188
  procainamide ~ 80190-80192
  quantitative, other ~ 80299
  quinidine ~ 80194
  salicylate ~ 80329-80331
  sirolimus ~ 80195
  tacrolimus ~ 80197
  theophylline ~ 80198
  tiagabine ~ 80199
  tobramycin ~ 80200
  topiramate ~ 80201
  vancomycin ~ 80202
  zonisamide ~ 80203
Drug delivery system
  drug delivery device, muscular
    insertion ~ 20700, 20702, 20704
    removal ~ 20701, 20703, 20705
  implantation
    contraceptive ~ 11976
    intravitreal ~ 67027
  insertion ~ 11981
    for clinical brachytherapy ~ 58346
  irrigation ~ 96523
  maintenance and refill
    brain ~ 95990-95991
    epidural ~ 95990-95991
    intra-arterial ~ 96522
    intrathecal ~ 95990-95991
    intravenous ~ 96522
    intraventricular ~ 95990-95991
    spinal ~ 95990, 95991
  removal
    device ~ 20701, 20703, 20705
    implant ~ 11982, 11983
    with reinsertion ~ 11983
Drug instillation ~ see instillation, drugs
Drug management
  by pharmacist ~ 99605-99607
  psychiatric ~ 90863
Drug screen ~ see Drug assay
Drug testing ~ see Drug assay
DST ~ 80420
DT shots
  diphtheria and tetanus toxoids (DT) ~ 90702
  diphtheria and tetanus toxoids, acellular pertussis, haemophilus influenza type b, and inactivated poliovirus (DTaP-IPV/Hib) ~ 90698
  diphtheria and tetanus toxoids, acellular pertussis, inactivated poliovirus, haemophilus influenzae type b PRP-OMP conjugate, an Hepatitis B (DTaP-IPV-Hib- HepB) ~ 60697
DTaP-HepB-IPV immunization ~ 90723
DTaP immunization ~ 90700
Dual X-ray absorptiometry (DXA) ~ 3095F-3096F
  appendicular ~ 77081
  axial skeleton ~ 77080
  vertebral fracture ~ 77086
Dual photon absorptiometry ~ 78351
Duct
  bile ~ see bile duct
  hepatic ~ see hepatic duct
  nasolacrimal ~ see nasolacrimal duct
  omphalomesenteric ~ 44800

Duct ~ *continued*
pancreatic ~ see pancreatic duct
salivary ~ see salivary duct
Stensen's ~ see parotid duct
thoracic ~ see thoracic duct
Ductogram, mammary ~ galactogram
Ductus arteriosus repair ~ 33820-33824
Ductus deferens ~ see vas deferens
Duhamel procedure ~ 45110, 45112, 45119-45120
Dunn operation ~ 28730-28735, 28740
Duodenostomy
contrast ~ 49465
insertion ~ 49441
obstructive material removal ~ 49460
radiological evaluation ~ 49465
replacement ~ 49451
Duodenotomy ~ 44010
Duodenum
biopsy ~ 44010
exclusion ~ 48547
exploration ~ 44010
incision ~ 44010
intubation and aspiration ~ 43756-43757
removal, foreign body ~ 44010
Duplex scan ~ see vascular studies
arterial studies
aorta ~ 93978-93979
extracranial ~ 93880-93882
lower extremity ~ 93925-93926
penile ~ 93980-93981
upper extremity ~ 93930-93931
visceral ~ 93975-93979
hemodialysis
access ~ 93990
preoperative assessment ~ 93985, 93986
venous studies
extremity ~ 93970-93971
penile ~ 93980-93981
Dupuy-Dutemp operation ~ see reconstruction, eyelid; revision
Dupuytren's contracture
fasciotomy ~ 26040-26045
injection, enzyme ~ 20527
manipulation ~ 26341
Dust, Angel ~ 83992
Duvries operation ~ 01714
Dwyer procedure ~ 28300
DXA ~ see dual X-ray absorptiometry (DXA)
Dynamometry ~ 28300
venous studies ~ 28300
with ophthalmoscopy ~ 92260
D & C yellow no. 7 (seven) ~ see fluorescein
D 2, vitamin ~ 82306
D galactose ~ 82760
D glucose ~ 80422-80424, 80430-80435, 95250-95251
D vitamin ~ 82306, 82652

E

E1 ~ 82679
E2 ~ 82670
E3 ~ 82677
Ear
collection of blood ~ 36415-36416
drum ~ 69420-69421, 69433-69436, 69450, 69610-69620
external
abscess incision and drainage
complicated ~ 69005
simple ~ 69000
biopsy ~ 69100
excision
partial ~ 69110
total ~ 69120
hematoma, incision and drainage ~ 69000-69005
reconstruction ~ 69300

Ear ~ *continued*
removal
foreign body ~ 69200, 69205
impacted cerumen ~ 69209, 69210
unlisted services and procedures ~ 69399
inner
CT scan ~ 70480-70482
endolymphatic sac ~ 69805-69806
insertion cochlear device ~ 69930
labyrinth
excision ~ 69905, 69910
incision for perfusion ~ 69801
unlisted services and procedures ~ 69949
meatoplasty ~ 69310
for congenital atresia ~ 69320
middle
CT scan ~ 70480-70482
eustachian tube dilation ~ 69705, 69706
exploration ~ 69440
excision
polyp ~ 69540
glomus tumor ~ 69550, 69552, 69554
facial nerve decompression ~69720, 69725
facial nerve suture ~ 69740, 69745
nasopharyngoscopy, surgical ~ 69705, 69706
optical coherence tomography ~ 0485T, 0486T
repair, fistula ~ 69666, 69667
stapedectomy ~ 69660-69662
tumor excision ~ 69550, 69552, 69554
tympanostomy ~ 69433, 69436, 0583T
temporal bone
bone conduction hearing device ~ 69710, 69711
osseointegrated implant ~ 69714, 69715, 69717
resection ~ 69535
unlisted services and procedures ~ 69799
Ear canal ~ see auditory canal
Ear cartilage graft to face ~ 21235
Ear lobes, pierce ~ 69090
Ear, nose, and throat ~ see also hearing aid services ~ 92700
audiologic function tests
acoustic reflex ~ 92568
acoustic reflex decay ~ 92570
audiometry
Bekesy ~ 92560-92561
comprehensive ~ 92557
conditioning play ~ 92582
groups ~ 92559
pure tone ~ 92552-92553
select picture ~ 92583
speech ~ 92555-92556
central auditory function ~ 92620-92621
ear protector evaluation ~ 92596
electrocochleography ~ 92584
filtered speech ~ 92571
hearing aid evaluation ~ 92590-92595
Lombard test ~ 92700
loudness balance ~ 92562
screening test ~ 92551
sensorineural acuity ~ 92575
short increment sensitivity index (SISI) ~ 92564
staggered spondaic word test ~ 92572
Stenger test ~ 92565, 92577
synthetic sentence test ~ 92576
tone decay ~ 92563
tympanometry ~ 92567
audiometry
evoked otoacoustic emissions ~ 92587-92588
visual reinforcement ~ 92579
binocular microscopy ~ 92504
diagnostic analysis
auditory brainstem implant ~ 92640
cochlear implant ~ 92601-92604
evaluation
auditory rehabilitation status ~ 92626-92627, 92630, 92633
language comprehension/expression ~ 92523
laryngeal sensory testing ~ 92614-92617
prescription of communication device
non-speech generating ~ 92605, 92618
speech generating ~ 92607-92608

Ear, nose, and throat ~ *continued*
    speech fluency ~ 92521
    speech sound production ~ 92522
    swallowing ~ 92610-92613, 92616
    voice resonance analysis ~ 92524
  examination under anesthesia ~ 92502
  facial nerve function study ~ 92516
  laryngeal function study ~ 92520
  nasal function study ~ 92512
  nasopharyngoscopy ~ 92511
  treatment
    hearing, language and speech disorder ~ 92507-92508
    oral function for feeding ~ 92526
    swallowing dysfunction ~ 92526
  vestibular function tests
    additional electrodes ~ 92547
    basic ~ 92540
    caloric tests ~ 92533
    nystagmus
      optokinetic ~ 92534, 92544
      positional ~ 92532, 92542
      spontaneous ~ 92531, 92541
    posturography ~ 92548
    torsion swing test ~ 92546
    tracking tests ~ 92545
Ear protector attenuation ~ see also hearing aid services ~ 92596
Ear wax ~ 69210
Ebstein anomaly repair ~ 33468
ECG ~ see electrocardiography
Echinococcosis ~ 86171, 86280
Echocardiography
  cardiac ~ 93320-93350
    intracardiac ~ 93662
    transesophageal ~ 93318
    transthoracic ~ 93303-93317
      with stress test ~ 93350-93352
  Doppler ~ 93303-93317, 93320-93321, 93662
  fetal heart ~ 76825-76826
    Doppler
      complete ~ 76827
      follow-up or repeat study ~ 76828
  for congenital anomalies
    transesophageal ~ 93315-93317
    transthoracic ~ 93303-93304
  intracardiac ~ 93662
  myocardial
    contrast perfusion ~ 0439T
    strain imaging ~ 93356
  speckle tracking assessment ~ 93356
  transesophageal ~ 93312-93318, 93355
  transthoracic ~ 93306-93308, 93350-93352
    for congenital anomalies ~ 93303, 93304
    with stress test ~ 93350-93352
Echoencephalography ~ 76506
Echography
  abdomen ~ 76700-76705
  arm ~ 76881, 76882
  breast ~ 76641, 76642
  cardiac ~ 93303-93317, 93320-93321, 93350-93352, 93662
    guidance ~ 76932
  chest ~ 76604
  extracranial arteries ~ 93880-93882
  eyes ~ 76510-76529
  head ~ 76536
  heart imaging guidance ~ 76932
  hip infant ~ 76885-76886
  intracranial arteries ~ 93886-93893
  intraoperative ~ 76998
  kidney transplant ~ 76776
  leg ~ 76881, 76882
  neck ~ 76536
  pelvis ~ 76856-76857
  placement therapy fields ~ 77387
  pregnant uterus ~ 76801-76828
  prostate ~ 76872-76873
  retroperitoneal ~ 76770-76775
  scrotum ~ 76870
  spine ~ 76800
  transvaginal ~ 76817, 76830
  unlisted services and procedures ~ 76999
  vagina ~ 76817, 76830

Echotomography ~ see echography
ECMO ~ see extracorporeal membrane oxygenation
ECS ~ see emission computerized tomography
ECSF (erythrocyte colony stimulating factor) ~ 82668
ECT ~ see emission computerized tomography
Ectasia ~ see dilation
Ectopic pregnancy ~ see obstetrical care
  abdominal ~ 59130
  cervix ~ 59140
  interstitial
    partial resection uterus ~ 59136
    total hysterectomy ~ 59135
  laparoscopy ~ 59150
    with salpingectomy and/or oophorectomy ~ 59151
  tubal ~ 59121
    with salpingectomy and/or oophorectomy ~ 59120
Ectropion, repair
  excision tarsal wedge ~ 67916
  extensive ~ 67917
  suture ~ 67914
  thermocauterization ~ 67915
Education services
  group ~ 98961-98962, 99078
  individual, pediatric gastroenteritis ~ 4058F
Education supplies ~ 99071
EEG ~ see electroencephalography (EEG)
Egg (ova) ~ 87177
Ehrlichia antibody ~ 86666
EKG ~ see electrocardiogram
Elastase ~ 82656
Elbow ~ see also humerus; radius; ulna
  abscess, incision and drainage ~ 23930, 23935
  anesthesia ~ 00400, 01710-01782
  arthrectomy ~ 24155
  arthrocentesis ~ 20605
  arthrodesis ~ 24800-24802
  arthroplasty ~ 24360
    with implant ~ 24361-24362
    prosthesis removal ~ 24160, 24164
    revision ~ 24370-24371
    total replacement ~ 24361-24363, 24365-24366
  arthroscopy
    diagnostic ~ 29830
    surgical ~ 29834-29838
  arthrotomy ~ 24000
    capsular release ~ 24006
    removal of foreign body ~ 24000
    with joint exploration ~ 24000, 24101
    with synovectomy ~ 24102
  biopsy ~ 24065-24066, 24101
  bursa, incision and drainage ~ 23931
  dislocation
    closed treatment ~ 24600-24605, 24640
    open treatment ~ 24615
    subluxate ~ 24640
  excision ~ 24155
    bursa ~ 24105
    synovium ~ 24102, 29835-29836
  exploration ~ 24000, 24101
  fracture
    Monteggia ~ 24620-24635
      open treatment ~ 24586-24587
  hematoma, incision and drainage ~ 23930
  implant, removal ~ 24164
  incision and drainage ~ 24000
  injection, arthrography, radiologic ~ 24220
  magnetic resonance imaging (MRI) ~ 73221
  manipulation ~ 24300
  radical resection, capsule, soft tissue and bone with contracture release ~ 24149
  removal
    foreign body ~ 24000, 24101, 24200-24201, 29834
    implant ~ 24160
    loose body ~ 24101, 29834
  repair
    epicondylitis ~ 24357-24359
    flexorplasty ~ 24330
    graft ~ 24320
    hemiepiphyseal arrest ~ 24470
    ligament ~ 24343-24346

Elbow ~ *continued*
  muscle ~ 24341
  muscle transfer ~ 24301
  tendon ~ 24340-24342, 24357-24359
    lengthening ~ 24305
    transfer ~ 24301
  tennis elbow ~ 24357-24359
  Steindler advancement ~ 24330
  strapping ~ 29260
  tumor excision ~ 24071-24079
  unlisted services and procedures ~ 24999
  X-ray ~ 73070-73080
    with contrast ~ 73085
Elbow, golfer ~ 24357-24359
Elbows, tennis ~ 24357-24359
Electrical stimulation
  bone healing
    invasive ~ 20975
    noninvasive ~ 20974
  brain surface ~ 95961-95962
  physical therapy
    attended, manual ~ 97032
    unattended ~ 97014
Electric countershock ~ 92960-92961
Electro-hydraulic procedure ~ 52325
Electro-oculography ~ 92270
Electrocardiography
  12-lead ~ 3120F, 93000
  evaluation ~ 93000, 93010, 93660
  external recording
    auto-activated ~ 93268, 93270-93272
    duration
      more than 48 hours up to 7 days ~ 93241, 93244
      more than 7 days up to 15 days ~ 93245-93248
      up to 30 days ~ 93268, 93270-93272
      up to 48 hours ~ 93224-93227
    mobile
      more than 24 hours ~ 93228, 93229
    patient-activated ~ 0497T, 0498T, 93268, 93270-93272
    transmission and evaluation ~ 93268, 93270-93272
  interpretation
    auto activated ~ 93268, 93272
    external recording
      more than 7 days up to 15 days ~ 93245, 93248
      more than 48 hours up to 7 days ~ 93241, 93244
      up to 48 hours ~ 93224, 93227
  rhythm
    evaluation ~ 93042
    microvolt T-wave alternans ~ 93025
    tracing ~ 93041
    tracing and evaluation ~ 93040
  signal averaged ~ 93278
  symptom-activated memory loop ~ 93268, 93270-93272
Electrocautery ~ see also destruction ~ 17000-17285
  inferior turbinates soft tissue ~ 30801-30802
  prostate resection ~ 52601
  ureteral stricture ~ 52341-52346
Electrochemistry ~ 17380
Electroconvulsive therapy ~ 90870-90871
Electrocortiogram, intraoperative ~ 95829
Electrode, depth ~ 61760
Electrodesiccation ~ 17000-17286
  lesion, penis ~ 54055
Electroejaculation ~ 55870
Electroencephalography (EEG)
  activation scenarios
    with data review ~ 95705-95716
    digital analysis for epileptic spike ~ 95957
    by health professional ~ 95954
    wada ~ 95958
  electrode placement ~ 95830
  monitoring
    continuous ~ 95707, 95710, 95713
    extended ~ 95812, 95813
    in-person administration by technologist ~ 95700
    intermittent ~ 95706, 95709
    unmonitored ~ 95705, 95708
    with wada activation ~ 95958

Electroencephalography (EEG) ~ *continued*
  recording
    awake and asleep ~ 95819
    awake and drowsy ~ 95816
    for brain death evaluation ~ 95824
    coma only ~ 95822
    complete study ~ 95721-95726
    continuous for seizure detection ~ 95717-95726
  sleep only ~ 95822
Electroencephalography with Video (VEEG)
  data review ~ 95711-95715
    with in-person administration by technologist ~ 95700
  monitoring
    continuous ~ 95713, 95716
    intermittent ~ 95712, 95715
    unmonitored ~ 95711, 95714
  recording
    complete study ~ 95722, 95724, 95726
    continuous for seizure detection ~ 95718, 95720, 95722, 95724, 95726
Electrogastrography ~ 91132-91133
Electrogram, atrial esophageal recording ~ 93615-93616
Electrolysis ~ 17380
Electromyography
  anorectal with biofeedback ~ 90912, 90913
  fine wire dynamic ~ 96004
  needle
    extremities ~ 95860-95864
    extremity ~ 95860, 95885-95886
    face and neck muscles ~ 95867-95868
    ocular ~ 92265
    other than thoracic paraspinal ~ 95870
    single fiber electrode ~ 95872
    thoracic paraspinal muscles ~ 95869
  sphincter muscles
    anus ~ 51784-51785
      needle ~ 51785
    urethra ~ 51784-51785
      needle ~ 51785
  surface dynamic ~ 96002-96004
Electron microscopy ~ 88348
Electronic analysis
  cardioverter-defibrillator, implantable
    data analysis ~ 93289, 93295-93296
    evaluation of programming ~ 93282-94284, 93287, 93640, 93642
  drug infusion pump ~ 62367-62368
  loop recorder, implantable
    data analysis ~ 93291, 93298
    evaluation of programming ~ 93285
  neurostimulator pulse generator ~ 95970-95982
Electrophoresis
  hemoglobin ~ 83020
  hight resolution ~ 83701
  immuno- ~ 86320, 86325, 86327
  immunofixation ~ 86334-86335
  protein ~ 84165-84166
  unlisted services and procedures ~ 82664
Electrophysiology procedure ~ 93600-93660
Electroretinogram ~ 92275
Electroretinography ~ 92275
Electrosurgery, trichiasis correction ~ 67825
Electroversion, cardiac ~ 92960-92961
Elevation, scapula, congenital ~ 23400
Elliot operation ~ 66130
Eloesser procedure ~ 32035-32036
Eloesser thoracoplasty ~ 32905
Embolectomy
  aortoiliac artery ~ 34151, 34201
  axillary artery ~ 34101
  brachial artery ~ 34101
  carotid artery ~ 34001
  celiac artery ~ 34151
  femoral ~ 34201
  iliac ~ 34151, 34201
  innominate artery ~ 34001-34101
  mesentery artery ~ 34151
  peroneal artery ~ 34203
  popliteal artery ~ 34201, 34203
  pulmonary artery ~ 33910, 33915-33916
  radial artery ~ 34111

Embolectomy ~ continued
renal artery ~ 34151
subclavian artery ~ 34001, 34101
tibial artery ~ 34203
ulnar artery ~ 34111
Embolization
central nervous system ~ 61624
non-central nervous system, head or neck ~ 61626
intra-arterial
for aneurysm ~ 61710
for carotid-cavernous fistula ~ 61710
for vascular malformation ~ 61710
ureteral ~ 50705
vascular
arterial ~ 37242
dialysis circuit ~ 36909
for hemorrhage ~ 37244
for infarction ~ 37243
for lymphatic extravasation ~ 37244
for organ ischemia ~ 37243
for tumors ~ 37243
venous ~ 37241
Embryo
biopsy ~ 89290-89291
cryopreservation ~ 89258
cryopreserved preparation thawing ~ 89352
culture ~ 89250
with co-culture oocyte ~ 89251
hatching assisted microtechnique ~ 89253
preparation for transfer ~ 89255
storage ~ 89342
Embryonated eggs inoculation ~ 87250
Embryo/fetus monitoring ~ 59050-59051, 99500
Embryo transfer
in vitro fertilization ~ 58974-58976
intrafallopian transfer ~ 58976
intrauterine transfer ~ 58974
Emergency department services ~ 99281-99288
anesthesia ~ 99140
physician direction of advanced life support ~ 99288
Emesis induction ~ 99175
EMG ~ see electromyography, needle
EMI scan ~ see CAT scan
Emmet operation ~ 59300
Empyema
closure, chest wall ~ 32810
lung ~ 21501-21502
thoracostomy ~ 32035-32036, 32551
Empyemectomy ~ 32540
Encephalitis
antibody ~ 86651-86654
Encephalocele
repair ~ 62120
craniotomy ~ 62121
Encephalon ~ see brain
End stage renal disease services ~ 90951-90970
End-expiratory pressure, positive ~ 94660
Endarterectomy
coronary artery ~ 33572
pulmonary ~ 33916
Endemic flea-borne typhus ~ 86000
Endobronchial challenge tests ~ 95070
Endobronchial Ultrasound (EBUS)
with bronchoscopy ~ 31652-31654
Endocavitary fulguration ~ 17000-17286
Endocrine, pancreas ~ 86341
Endocrine system surgical procedures 60000-60699
Endolymphatic sac
exploration
with shunt ~ 69806
without shunt ~ 69805
Endometrial ablation ~ 0009T, 58353
exploration via hysteroscopy ~ 58563
Endometrioma
abdomen
destruction/excision ~ 49203-49205, 58957, 58958
retroperitoneal
destruction/excision ~ 49203-49205, 58957, 58958
Endometriosis, adhesive ~ 58559

Endometrium
ablation ~ 58356
biopsy ~ 58100, 58558
Endonuclease, DNA ~ 86215
Endoscopic retrograde cannulation of pancreatic duct (ERCP) ~ 43260
Endoscopies, pleural ~ see thoracoscopy
Endoscopy ~ see arthroscopy; thoracoscopy
adrenal gland
biopsy ~ 60650
excision ~ 60650
anus
biopsy ~ 46606
dilation ~ 46604
exploration ~ 46600
hemorrhage ~ 46614
removal
foreign body ~ 46608
polyp ~ 46610, 46612
tumor ~ 46610, 46612
atria ~ 33265-33266
bile duct ~ 43273
biopsy ~ 47553
cannulation ~ 43273
catheterization ~ 47533-47537, 74328, 74330
destruction, calculi (stone) ~ 43265
dilation ~ 43277, 47555-47556
exploration ~ 47552
intraoperative ~ 47550
percutaneous ~ 47552-47556
placement, stent ~ 43274
removal
calculi (stone) ~ 43264, 47554
foreign body ~ 43275
stent ~ 43275
specimen collection ~ 43260
sphincter pressure ~ 43263
sphincterotomy ~ 43262
tube placement ~ 43274
bladder ~ 52000
biopsy ~ 52204, 52354
catheterization ~ 52005, 52010
destruction ~ 52354
lesion ~ 52400
evacuation clot ~ 52001
excision tumor ~ 52355
exploration ~ 52351
lithotripsy ~ 52353
removal calculus ~ 52352
urethral stent ~ 52282
bladder neck
injection of implant material ~ 51715
brain shunt creation ~ 62201
bronchi
aspiration ~ 31645-31646
biopsy ~ 31625-31629, 31632-31633
destruction
lesion ~ 31641
tumor ~ 31641
dilation ~ 31630-31631, 31636-31638
exploration ~ 31622
injection ~ 31899
lesion destruction ~ 31641
needle biopsy ~ 31629, 31633
placement stent ~ 31631, 31636-31637
revision stent ~ 31638
specimen collection ~ 31623-61324
stenosis ~ 31641
tumor destruction ~ 31641
with endobronchial ultrasound (EBUS) ~ 31652, 31653
cervix
biopsy ~ 57454-57455, 57460
curettage ~ 57454, 57456
exploration ~ 57452
loop electrode biopsy ~ 57460
loop electrode conization ~ 57461
chest cavity
exploration ~ 32601-32606
surgical ~ 32650-32665

Endoscopy ~ *continued*
colon
  biopsy ~ 44389, 45380, 45392
  destruction
    lesion ~ 44401, 45383
    tumor ~ 44401, 45383
  exploration ~ 45378
  hemorrhage ~ 44391, 45382
  injection ~ 45381
  placement stent ~ 45389
  removal
    foreign body ~ 44390, 45379
    polyp ~ 44392, 45384-45385
    tumor ~ 44392, 45384-45385
  specimen collection ~ 45380
  ultrasound ~ 45391-45392
  via colotomy ~ 45399
  via stoma ~ 44401, 44402
colon-sigmoid
  ablation
    polyp ~ 45346
    tumor ~ 45346
  biopsy ~ 45331
  dilation ~ 45340
  exploration ~ 45330, 45335
  hemorrhage ~ 45334
  needle biopsy ~ 45342
  placement stent ~ 45327, 45347
  removal
    foreign body ~ 45332
    polyp ~ 45333, 45338
    tumor ~ 45333, 45338
  specimen collection ~ 45331
  ultrasound ~ 45341-45342
  volvulus ~ 45337
cyclophotocoagulation ~ 66987, 66988
esophagus
  biopsy ~ 43202
  dilation ~ 43220-43226
  exploration ~ 43200
  hemorrhage ~ 43227
  injection ~ 43201, 43204
  insertion stent ~ 43212
  needle biopsy ~ 43232
  removal
    foreign body ~ 43215
    polyp ~ 43216-43217, 43229
    tumor ~ 43216, 43229
  ultrasound ~ 43231-43232
  vein ligation ~ 43205
eye ~ 66990
foot, plantar fasciotomy ~ 29893
gastrointestinal, upper ~ 3130F-3132F, 3140F-3141F
  biopsy ~ 43239
  catheterization ~ 43241
  destruction of lesion ~ 43270
  dilation ~ 43245, 43248-43249
  drainage of pseudocyst ~ 43240
  exploration ~ -43235
  foreign body ~ 43247
  gastric bypass ~ 43644-43645
  gastroenterostomy ~ 43644-43645
  hemorrhage ~ 43255
  inject varices ~ 43243
  injection ~ 43236
  needle biopsy ~ 43238, 43242
  referral ~ 3132F
  removal ~ 43247, 43250-43251
  roux-en-y ~ 43644
  stent placement ~ 43266
  thermal radiation ~ 43257
  tube placement ~ 43246
  ultrasound ~ 43237-43242, 43259, 76975
  vein ligation ~ 43244
ileum via stoma ~ 44384

Endoscopy ~ *continued*
intestines, small
  biopsy ~ 44361, 44377
  destruction
    lesion ~ 44369
    tumor ~ 44369
  diagnostic ~ 44376
  exploration ~ 44360
  hemorrhage ~ 44366, 44378
  insertion
    stent ~ 44370, 44379
    tube ~ 44379
  pelvic pouch ~ 44385-44386
  removal
    foreign body ~ 44363
    lesion ~ 44365
    polyp ~ 44364-44365
  tube placement ~ 44372
  tube revision ~ 44373
  via stoma ~ 44380-44384
    tumor ~ 44364-44365
intracranial ~ 62160-62165
kidney
  biopsy ~ 50555, 50574-50576, 52354
  catheterization ~ 50553, 50572
  destruction ~ 50557, 50576, 52354
  dilation of ureter ~ 50553
  excision tumor ~ 52355
  exploration ~ 52351
  lithotripsy ~ 52353
  removal
    calculus ~ 50561, 50580, 52352
    foreign body ~ 50561, 50580
  via incision ~ 50562-50580
  via stoma ~ 50551-50561
larynx
  ablation, lesion ~ 31572
  aspiration ~ 31515
  biopsy ~ 31510, 31535-31536
  dilation ~ 31528, 31529
  direct ~ 31515, 31520, 31525-31529
    diagnostic ~ 31520, 31525, 31526
    operative ~ 31530, 31531, 31535, 31536, 31540, 31541, 31545, 31546, 31560, 31561
  epiglottis stripping ~ 31540, 31541
  excision, tumor ~ 31540
  flexible ~ 31575-31579
  indirect ~ 31505-31513
  laser destruction, lesion ~ 31572
  operative ~ 31530-31561
  reconstruction ~ 31545, 31546
  removal
    foreign body ~ 31511, 31530-31531
    lesion ~ see endoscopic ~ 31512, 31545-31546
mediastinoscopy
  biopsy ~ 39401, 39402
nose
  diagnostic ~ 31231-31235
  surgical ~ 31237-31241, 31253-31257, 31259, 31267, 31276, 31287, 31288, 31290-31298
  unlisted services and procedures ~ 31299
pancreatic duct
  cannulation ~ 43273
  destruction
    calculi (stone) ~ 43265
    tumor ~ 43272
  dilation ~ 43277
  removal
    calculi (stone) ~ 43264
    foreign body ~ 43275-43276
    stent ~ 43275-43276
  specimen collection ~ 43260
  sphincter pressure ~ 43263
  sphincterotomy ~ 43262
  tube placement ~ 43274

Endoscopy ~ *continued*
pelvis
  aspiration ~ 49322
  destruction of lesion ~ 58662
  lysis of adhesions ~ 58660
  oviduct surgery ~ 58670-58671
  removal of adnexal structures ~ 58661
peritoneum
  drainage lymphocele ~ 49323, 54690
rectum
  biopsy ~ 45305
  destruction tumor ~ 45320
  dilation ~ 45303
  exploration ~ 45300
  hemorrhage ~ 45317
  removal
    foreign body ~ 45307
    polyp ~ 45308-45315
    tumor ~ 45308-45315
  volvulus ~ 45321
spinal cord, nerve root decompression ~ 62380
spleen, removal ~ 38120
testis, removal ~ 54690
trachea
  dilation ~ 31630-31631, 31636-31638
  via tracheostomy ~ 31615
ureter
  biopsy ~ 50955-50957, 50974-50976, 52354
  catheterize ~ 50953, 50972
  destruction ~ 50957, 50976, 52354
  excision tumor ~ 52355
  exploration ~ 52351
  injection of implant material ~ 52327
  lithotripsy ~ 52353
  manipulation of ureteral calculus ~ 52330
  placement stent ~ 50947
  removal
    calculus ~ 50961, 50980, 52352
    foreign body ~ 50961, 50980
  resection ~ 52355
  via incision ~ 50970-50980
  via stoma ~ 50951-50961
ureteral
  biopsy ~ 52007
  catheterization ~ 52005
urethra ~ 52000
  biopsy ~ 52204, 52354
  catheterization ~ 52010
  destruction ~ 52354
    lesion ~ 52400
  evacuation clot ~ 52001
  excision tumor ~ 52355
  exploration ~ 52351
  incision ejaculatory duct ~ 52402
  injection of implant material ~ 51715
  lithotripsy ~ 52353
  removal calculus ~ 52352
  resection ejaculatory duct ~ 52402
  vasectomy ~ 52402
  vasotomy ~ 52402
uterus
  anesthesia ~ 00952
  hysteroscopy
    diagnostic ~ 58555
    with division/resection intrauterine septum ~ 58560
    with lysis of intrauterine adhesions ~ 58559
  placement fallopian tube ~ 58565
  removal
    endometrial ~ 58563
    impacted foreign body ~ 58562
    leiomyomata ~ 58561
  surgical with biopsy ~ 58558
vagina ~ 57420
  anesthesia ~ 00950
  biopsy ~ 57421, 57454
  exploration ~ 57452
vascular, surgical ~ 33508, 37500-37501
vulva ~ 56820
  biopsy ~ 56821

Endosteal implant
reconstruction
  mandible ~ 21248-21249
  maxilla ~ 21248-21249
Endothelioma, dural ~ 61512, 61519
Endotracheal intubation ~ 31500
Endotracheal tube
intubation ~ 31500
Endovascular repair
angiography ~ 75956-75959
delivery of endograft ~ 34712, 34713
delivery of endovascular prosthesis ~ 34714-34716
iliac artery
  with endograft ~ 34703-34708, 34717, 34718
  with prosthesis ~ 34709-34711
infrarenal abdominal aorta
  with endograft ~ 34701-34706, 34845-34848
vena cava ~ 37191-37193
visceral aorta, with fenestrated endograft ~ 34839, 34841-34848
Endovascular revascularization ~ 37220-37235
Endovascular therapy
ablation, vein ~ 36473-36479, 36482, 36483
balloon angioplasty ~ 61630
intracranial
  dilatation ~ 61640-61642
  infusion
    for other than thrombolysis ~ 61650, 61651
    for thrombolysis ~ 61645
  injection ~ 61645
  thrombectomy ~ 61645
occlusion
  arterial balloon ~ 61623
  transcatheter ~ 61624, 61626
vascular catheterization ~ 61630, 61635
Enema
home visit for fecal impaction ~ 99511
intussusception ~ 74283
therapeutic, for intussusception ~ 74283
Energies, electromagnetic ~ 86945
ENT ~ see ear nose and throat ~ 92700
Entamoeba histolytica
antigen detection
  enzyme immunoassay ~ 87336-87337
Enterectomy ~ 44120-44121, 44126-44128, 44137, 44202
donor ~ 44132-44133
with enterostomy ~ 44125
Enterocele
repair ~ 57556
  hysterectomy
    with colpectomy ~ 58280
Enterocystoplasty ~ 51960
Camey ~ 50825
Enteroenterostomy ~ see anastomosis, intestines
Enterolysis ~ 44005
laparoscopic ~ 44200
Enteropancreatostomy ~ see anastomosis, pancreas to intestines
Enterorrhaphy ~ 44602-44603, 44615
Enterostomy ~ 44300
closure ~ 44625-44626
with enterectomy
  intestine, small ~ 44125
Enterotomy ~ 44615
Enterovirus
antibody ~ 86658
Entropion
repair ~ 67921-67924
  excision tarsal wedge ~ 67923
  suture ~ 67921
  thermocauterization ~ 67922
Enucleation
eye
  with implant ~ 65103
    muscles attached ~ 65105
  without implant ~ 65101
pleural ~ 32540
Enucleation, cyst, ovarian ~ 58925
Environmental intervention
for psychiatric patients ~ 90882
Enzyme
angiotensin converting ~ 82164
angiotensin-forming ~ 80408, 80416, 84244

1123

Enzyme activity ~ 82657
  radioactive substrate ~ 82658
EOG ~ 92270
Eosinocyte ~ 89190
Eosinophils
  nasal smear ~ 89190
Epiandrosterone ~ 80327, 80328
Epicondylitides, lateral humeral ~ 24357-24359
Epicondylitis, radiohumeral ~ 24357-24359
Epidemic parotitis ~ see mumps
Epididymectomy
  bilateral ~ 54861
  unilateral ~ 54860
Epididymis
  abscess, incision and drainage ~ 54700
  anastomosis
    to vas deferens
      bilateral ~ 54901
      unilateral ~ 54900
  biopsy ~ 54800, 54865
  epididymography ~ 74440
  excision
    bilateral ~ 54861
    unilateral ~ 54860
  exploration biopsy ~ 54865
  hematoma, incision and drainage ~ 54700
  lesion
    excision
      local ~ 54830
      spermatocele ~ 54840
  needle biopsy ~ 54800
  spermatocele excision ~ 54840
  unlisted services and procedures ~ 55899
  X-ray with contrast ~ 74440
Epididymograms ~ 55300
Epididymography ~ 74440
Epididymoplasty ~ 54900-54901
Epididymovasostomy
  bilateral ~ 54901
  unilateral ~ 54900
Epidural
  administration
    device ~ 62360-62362, 62365
      analysis ~ 62367
    drug ~ 62320-62327
      hospital management ~ 01996
  catheterization ~ 62350, 62351
    removal ~ 62355
  electrode
    insertion ~ 61531, 63650, 63655
    removal ~ 61535
  injection ~ 62281, 62282, 62320-62327
    blood or clot patch ~ 62273
    neurolytic substance ~ 62281, 62282
    transforaminal ~ 64479, 64480, 64483, 64484
    with disc decompression ~ 62287
  lysis ~ 62263-62264
Epidural anesthesia
  Infusion
    with imaging guidance ~ 62325, 62327
    without imaging guidance ~ 62324, 62326
  Injection
    with imaging guidance ~ 62321, 62323
    without imaging guidance ~ 62320, 62322
Epidurography ~ 72275
Epigastric hernia repair ~ 49572
Epiglottidectomy ~ 31420
Epiglottis excision ~ 31420
Epikeratoplasty ~ 65767
Epilation ~ 17380
Epinephrine ~ 80424, 82382-82384
  blood ~ 82383-82384
  urine ~ 82384
Epiphysis ~ see bone; specific bone
Epiphyseal arrest
  femur ~ 20150, 27185, 27475, 27479-27485, 27742
  fibula ~ 20150, 27477-27485, 27730-27742
  radius ~ 20150, 25450-25455
  tibia ~ 20150, 27477-27485, 27730, 27734-27742
  ulna ~ 20150, 25450-25455

Epiphyseal separation
  radius
    closed treatment ~ 25600
    open treatment ~ 25607-25609
Epiphysiodesis ~ see epiphyseal arrest
Epiploectomy ~ 49255
Episiotomy ~ 59300
Epispadias
  penis reconstruction ~ 54385
  repair ~ 54380-54390
    with extrophy of bladder ~ 54390
    with incontinence ~ 54380-54390
Epistaxis ~ 30901-30906
  with nasal/sinus endoscopy ~ 31238
EPO ~ see erythropoietin
Epstein-Barr virus
  antibody ~ 86663-86665
Equina, cauda ~ see cauda equina
ERCP ~ see bile duct; pancreatic duct ~ 43260
ERG ~ 92275
Ergocalciferol ~ 82306
Ergocalciferols ~ 82306
Ergonovine provocation test ~ 93024
Erythrocyte ~ see red blood cell (RBC)
Erythrocyte AB ~ see antibody, red blood cell
Erythrocyte count ~ 85032-85041
Erythropoietin ~ 82668
Escharotomy, burns ~ 16035-16036
Escherichia coli 0157
  antigen detection, enzyme immunoassay ~ 87335
ESD ~ see endoscopy, gastrointestinal, upper
Esophageal
  acid infusion test ~ 91030
  lengthening ~ 43283, 43338
  polyp ~ 43229
  tumor ~ 43229
  varices
    decompression ~ 37181
    ligation ~ 43205, 43244, 43400
    sclerosis injection ~ 43204, 43243
Esophagectomy
  Ivor Lewis ~ 43287
  laparoscopic thoracoscopic ~ 43287
  McKeown ~ 43112, 43288
  partial ~ 43116-43118, 43121-43124, 43287
  total ~ 43107, 43108, 43112, 43113, 43124, 43286, 43288
  tri-incisional ~ 43112, 43288
Esophagoenterostomy with total gastrectomy ~ 43620
Esophagogastroduodenoscopy
  flexible transoral
    ablation ~ 43270
    band ligation ~ 43244
    biopsy ~ 43239
    collection of specimen ~ 43235
    control of bleeding ~ 43255
    delivery of thermal energy ~ 43257
    dilation of esophagus ~ 43233, 43249
    dilation of gastric/duodenal stricture ~ 43245
    drainage of pseudocyst ~ 43240
    esophagogastric fundoplasty ~ 43210
    examination, ultrasound guided ~ 43237, 43238, 43253, 43259
    injection ~ 43236, 43243, 43253
    insertion
      catheter or tube ~ 43241
      guide wire ~ 43248
    needle aspiration/biopsy ~ 43238, 43242
    placement
      gastrostomy tube ~ 43246
      stent ~ 43266
    removal
      foreign body ~ 43247
      lesion/polyp/tumor ~ 43250, 43251
    resection, mucosal ~ 43254
    with optical endomicroscopy ~ 43252
Esophagogastromyotomy ~ 32665, 43330-43331
Esophagogastrostomy ~ 43320
Esophagojejunostomy ~ 43340-43341
Esophagomyotomy ~ 32665, 43330-43331
  with fundoplasty ~ 43279

Esophagorrhaphy ~ 43405
Esophagoscopies ~ see endoscopy, esophagus
Esophagostomy ~ 43352
  closure ~ 43420-43425
Esophagotomy ~ 43020, 43045
Esophagotracheal fistula ~ see fistula, tracheoesophageal
Esophagus
  ablation ~ 43229
  acid perfusion test ~ 91030
  acid reflux tests ~ 91034-91035, 91037-91038
  balloon distention provocation study ~ 91040
  biopsy
    endoscopy ~ 43198, 43202
    forceps ~ 3150F
  cricopharyngeal myotomy ~ 43030
  dilation ~ 43450, 43453
    endoscopic ~ 43195-43196, 43212-43214, 43220, 43226, 43229, 43233, 43248-43249
    surgical ~ 43510
  excision
    diverticula ~ 43130, 43135
    Ivor Lewis ~ 43287
    laparascopic Thoracoscopic ~ 43287
    laparascopic Transhiatal ~ 43286
    McKeown ~ 43112, 43288
    partial ~ 43116-43118, 43121-43124, 432
    total ~ 43107, 43108, 43112, 43113, 43124, 43286, 43288
    tri-incisional ~ 43112, 43288
  exploration endoscopy ~ 43200
  hemorrhage ~ 43227
  incision ~ 43020, 43045
    muscle ~ 43030
  imaging studies ~ 91110-91111
    motility ~ 78258
    obstructions ~ 74360
    reflux ~ 78262
    removal of foreign body ~ 74235
    strictures ~ 74360
    swallowing cineradiography ~ 74230
    X-ray ~ 74210, 74220, 74221
  injection
    sclerosing agent ~ 43204
    submucosal ~ 43192, 43201
  insertion
    stent ~ 43212
    tamponade ~ 43460
    tube ~ 43510
  lengthening ~ 43283, 43338
  lesion excision ~ 43100-43101
  ligation ~ 43405
  motility study ~ 78258, 91010, 91013
  mucosal resection ~ 43211
  needle biopsy endoscopy ~ 43232
  nuclear medicine
    imaging (motility) ~ 78258
    reflux study ~ 78262
  reconstruction ~ 43300, 43310, 43313
    creation stoma ~ 43352
    esophagostomy ~ 43352
    fistula ~ 43305, 43312, 43314
    gastrointestinal ~ 43360-43361
  removal
    foreign bodies ~ 43020, 43045, 43194, 43215, 74235
    lesion ~ 43216
    polyp ~ 43216-43217
  repair ~ 43300, 43310, 43313
    esophagogastroduodenoscopy ~ 43235-43239
    esophagogastric fundoplasty ~ 43325, 43327-43328
      esophagogastroduodenoscopic ~ 43210
      laparoscopic ~ 43280
    esophagogastrostomy ~ 43320
    esophagojejunostomy ~ 43340, 43341
    esophagomyotomy ~ 43279
    esophagoplasty ~ 43300, 43305, 43310, 43312
    fistula ~ 43305, 43312, 43314, 43420-43425
    Heller esophagomyotomy ~ 32665
    muscle ~ 43330-43331
    Nissen procedure ~ 43280

Esophagus ~ *continued*
  paraesophageal hernia
    laparoscopic ~ 43281-43282
    via laparotomy ~ 43332-43333
    via thoracoabdominal incision ~ 43336-43337
    via thoracotomy ~ 43334-43335
    pre-existing perforation ~ 43405
    Thal-Nissen procedure ~ 43325
    Toupet procedure ~ 43280
    wound ~ 43410, 43415
  sphincter augmentation
    device placement ~ 43284
    device removal ~ 43285
  suture ~ 43405
    wound ~ 43410, 43415
  ultrasound endoscopy ~ 43231-43232
  unlisted services and procedures ~ 43289, 43499
  vein ligation ~ 43205, 43400
Esophagus, varix ~ 43205, 43400
Esophagus neoplasm ~ 43229
Established patient
  critical care ~ 99291, 99292
  domiciliary or rest home visit ~ 99334-99337, 99339, 99340
  emergency department services ~ 99281-99285
  evaluation services
    basic life and/or disability ~ 99450
    work-related or medical disability ~ 99455
  home services ~ 99347-99350, 99606
  hospital inpatient services ~ 99221-99239
  hospital observation services ~ 99217-99220, 99224-99226, 99235, 99236
  initial inpatient consultations ~ 99251-99255
  nursing facility ~ 99304-99310, 99315, 99316, 99318
  office and/or other outpatient consultations ~ 99241-99245
  office visit ~ 99211-99215
  online medical evaluation ~ 98970-98972, 99421-99423
  ophthalmological services ~ 92012, 92014
  outpatient visit ~ 99211-99215
  preventive medicine ~ 99391-99397
  prolonged services
    with patient contact ~ 99354-99357
      with physician supervision ~ 99415, 99416
    without patient contact ~ 99358, 99359
  telephone services ~ 98966-98968, 99441-99443
Establishment
  colostomy
    abdominal ~ 50810
    perineal ~ 50810
Estes operation ~ 58825
Estlander procedure ~ 40525
Estradiol ~ 82670
  free ~ 82681
  response, total ~ 80415
  total ~ 82670
Estriol
  blood or urine ~ 82677
Estrogen
  blood or urine ~ 82671-82672
  receptor ~ 84233
Estrone blood or urine ~ 82679
Ethanediols ~ 82693
Ethanol
  any specimen, except breath, urine ~ 82077
  breath ~ 82075
Ethchlorovynol ~ 80320
Ethchlorvinol ~ 80320
Ethchlorvynol
  blood ~ 80320
  urine ~ 80320
Ethmoid fracture with fixation ~ 21340
Ethmoid, sinus ~ see sinus, ethmoid
Ethmoidectomy ~ 31200-31205
  endoscopic ~ 31254-31255
  skull base surgery ~ 61580-61581
  with nasal/sinus endoscopy ~ 31254-31255
Ethosuccimid ~ 80168
Ethosuximide ~ 80168
  assay ~ 80168
Ethylene dichlorides ~ 84600
Ethyl alcohol ~ 80321-80322, 82075
Ethylene glycol ~ 82693
Ethylmethylsuccimide ~ 80168

1125

Etiocholanolone ~ 82696
Etiocholanolone measurement ~ 82696
ETOH ~ 80321-80322
Euglobulin lysis ~ 85360
Eustachian tube
  catheterization ~ 69799
  inflation
    myringotomy ~ 69420
      anesthesia ~ 69421
  insertion, catheter ~ 69799
Eutelegenesis ~ 58976
Evacuation
  cervical pregnancy ~ 59140
  clots, endoscopic ~ 52001
  hematoma
    brain ~ 61108, 61154, 61312-61315
      anesthesia ~ 00211
    subungual ~ 11740
  hydatidiform mole ~ 59870
  intraspinal lesion ~ 63265
  meibomian glands ~ 0207T, 0563T
  stomach ~ 43753
Evaluation
  athletic training ~ 97169-97172
    evaluation ~ 97169-97171
    re-evaluation ~ 97172
  carotid artery
    atheroma ~ 93895
    intima media thickness ~ 93895
  cine ~ 74230
  electrophysiologic ~ 93653, 93654, 93656
  implantable defibrillator device ~ 93287, 93289, 93295, 93296
  physical therapy ~ 97161-97164
  treatment ~ 92526
  video ~ 74230
Evaluation and management services
  advance care planning ~ 99497, 99498
  assistive technology, assessment ~ 97755
  basic life and/or disability evaluation services ~ 99450
  care management
    behavioral health conditions ~ 99484
    psychiatric collaborative care ~ 99492-99494
  care plan oversight services ~ 99339, 99340, 99374-99380
    home health agency care ~ 99374-99375
    home or rest home ~ 99339-99340
    hospice ~ 99377-99378
    nursing facility ~ 99379-99380
  care planning, cognitive impairment ~ 99483
  case management services ~ 99366-99368
  chronic care ~ 99439, 99490, 99491
  consultation ~ 99241-99255
    interprofessional ~ 99446-99449
  critical care ~ 99291-99292
    interfacility pediatric transport ~ 99466-99467, 99485-99486
  domiciliary or rest home
    established patient ~ 99334-99337
    new patient ~ 99324-99328
  emergency department ~ 99281-99288
  health behavior
    assessment ~ 96156
    family intervention ~ 96167, 96168, 96170, 96171
    group intervention ~ 96164, 96165
    individual intervention ~ 96158, 96159
  home services ~ 99341-99350
  hospital ~ 99221-99233
    discharge ~ 99238-99239
    observation care ~ 99217-99220, 99224-99226, 99234-99236
  hyperbaric oxygen treatment facility ~ 99183
  insurance exam ~ 99455-99456
  internet communication ~ 98970-98972, 99421-99423
  low birthweight infant ~ 99478-99479
  medical team conferences ~ 99366-99368
  neonatal critical care ~ 99468-99469
  newborn care ~ 99460-99465
  nursing facility ~ see nursing facility services ~ 99304-99318
  occupation therapy evaluation ~ 97166, 97167
    re-evaluation ~ 97168
  office and other outpatient ~ 99202-99215
    prolonged services ~ 99417
  online services ~ 98970-98972, 99421-99423

Evaluation and management services ~ *continued*
  pediatric critical care ~ 99471, 99472
  pediatric interfacility transport ~ 99466-99467, 99485, 99486
  post-discharge transitional care ~ 99495, 99496
  preventive services ~ 99381-99429
  prolonged services ~ 99415, 99416, 99417
  remote
    physiologic monitoring of physiologic paramters ~ 99453, 99454
    physiologic monitoring treatment services ~ 99457, 99458
  standby services ~ 99360
  team conferences ~ 99366-99368
  telephone services ~ 98966-98968, 99441-99443
  unlisted services and procedures ~ 99499
  with psychotherapy ~ 90833, 90836, 90838
  work-related and/or medical disability evaluation ~ 99455
Evisceration
  ocular contents
    with implant ~ 65093
    without implant ~ 65091
  pelvic ~ 45126, 58240
Evocative/suppression testing ~ 80400-80439, 84146
  stimulation panel ~ 80410
Evoked potentials
  auditory ~ *see* Evoked potentials, auditory
  central nervous system
    somatosensory testing ~ 95925-95927, 95938
    transcranial motor stimulation ~ 95928, 95929, 95939
    visual ~ 95930
  visual
    acuity ~ 0333T
    central nervous system ~ 95930
    glaucoma test ~ 0464T
Evoked potentials, auditory
  evoked otoacoustic emissions
    evaluation ~ 92587, 92588
    screening ~ 92558
  frequency threshold estimations ~ 92652
  hearing status determination ~ 92651
  neurodiagnostic testing ~ 92653
  screening of auditory potential ~ 92650
  vestibular evoked myogenic potential (VEMP) testing ~ 92517-92519
Ewart procedure ~ 42226-42227
Excavatum, pectus ~ 21740-21743
Exchange
  arterial catheter ~ 37211-37214
  drainage catheter
    under radiologic guidance ~ 49423
  intraocular lens ~ 66986
  transfusion ~ 36455
Excision ~ see debridement; destruction
  abscess
    brain ~ 61514, 61522
    olecranon process ~ 24138
    radius ~ 24136
    ulna ~ 24138
  acromion
    shoulder ~ 23130
  adenoids ~ 42830-42836
  adenoma thyroid gland ~ 60200
  adrenal gland ~ 60540
    with excision retroperitoneal tumor ~ 60545
    laparoscopic ~ 60650
  alveolus ~ 41830
  anal crypt ~ 46999
  anal fissure ~ 46200
  anal tag ~ 46220, 46230
  aorta coarctation ~ 33840-33851
  appendix ~ 44950-44960
  arteriovenous malformation
    spinal ~ 63250-63252
  arytenoid cartilage ~ 31400
    endoscopic ~ 31560-31561
  atrial septum ~ 33735-33737
  Bartholin's gland ~ 56740
  bladder
    diverticulum ~ 51525
    neck ~ 51520
    partial ~ 51550-51565
    total ~ 51570, 51580, 51590-51597
      with nodes ~ 51575, 51585, 51595

Excision ~ *continued*

bladder
  transurethral ~ 52640
  tumor ~ 51530
bladder neck contracture, postoperative ~ 52640
bone
  facial ~ 21026
  mandible ~ 21025
  postoperative
    femur ~ 20150
    fibula ~ 20150
    radius ~ 20150
    tibia ~ 20150
    ulna ~ 20150
bone abscess
  facial ~ 21026
  mandible ~ 21025
brain
  amygdala ~ 61566
  epileptogenic focus ~ 61536
  hemisphere ~ 61543
  hippocampus ~ 61566
  other lobe ~ 61323, 61539-61540
  temporal lobe ~ 61537-61538
brain lobe ~ 61323, 61537-61540
breast
  biopsy ~ 19100-19101
  chest wall tumor ~ 21601-21603
  cyst ~ 19120-19126
  lactiferous duct fistula ~ 19112
  lesion ~ 19120-19126
    by needle localization ~ 19125-19126
  mastectomy ~ 19300-19307
  nipple exploration ~ 19110
bulbourethral gland ~ 53250
bullae
  lung ~ 32141
    endoscopic ~ 32655
burns ~ 01951-01953, 15002-15005
bursa
  elbow ~ 24105
  femur ~ 27062
  ischial ~ 27060
  knee ~ 27340
  wrist ~ 25115-25116
bypass graft ~ 35901-35907
calcaneus ~ 28118-28120
calculi (stone)
  parotid gland ~ 42330, 42340
  salivary gland ~ 42330-42340
  sublingual gland ~ 42330
  submandibular gland ~ 42330-42335
carotid artery ~ 60605
carpal ~ 25145, 25210-25215
cartilage
  knee joint ~ 27332-27333
  shoulder joint ~ 23101
  temporomandibular joint ~ 21060
  wrist ~ 25107
caruncle
  urethra ~ 53265
cataract
  secondary ~ 66830
cervix
  radical ~ 57531
  stump
    abdominal approach ~ 57540-57545
    vaginal approach ~ 57550-57556
  total ~ 57530
chalazion
  multiple
    different lids ~ 67805
    same lid ~ 67801
  single ~ 67800
  with anesthesia ~ 67808
chest wall tumor ~ 21601-21603
choroid plexus ~ 61544
clavicle
  partial ~ 23120, 23180
  sequestrectomy ~ 23170
  total ~ 23125

Excision ~ *continued*

tumor
  radical resection ~ 23200
coccyx ~ 27080
colon
  excision
    partial ~ 44140-44147, 44160
      with anastomosis ~ 44140
    total ~ 44150-44158
  laparoscopic
    with anastomosis ~ 44204, 44207-44208
    with colostomy ~ 44206, 44208
      with ileocolostomy ~ 44205
condyle, temporomandibular joint ~ 21050
constricting ring
  finger ~ 26596
cornea
  epithelium ~ 65435
    with chelating agent ~ 65436
  scraping ~ 65430
coronoidectomy ~ 21070
Cowper's gland ~ 53250
cranial bone tumor ~ 61563-61564
cyst ~ see also ganglion cyst
  bile duct ~ 47715
  bladder ~ 51500
  brain ~ 61516, 61524, 62162
  branchial ~ 42810-42815
  calcaneus ~ 28100-28103
  carpal ~ 25130-25136
  cheekbone ~ 21030
  clavicle ~ 23140
    with allograft ~ 23146
    with autograft ~ 23145
  facial bone ~ 21030
  femur ~ 27065-27067, 27355-27358
  fibula ~ 27635-27638
  finger ~ 26160
  foot ~ 28090
  hand ~ 26160
  hip ~ 27065-27067
  humerus ~ 23150, 24110
    with allograft ~ 23156, 24116
    with autograft ~ 23155, 24115
  ileum ~ 27065-27067
  kidney ~ 50280-50290
  knee ~ 27345-27347
  lung ~ 32140
  mandible ~ 21040, 21046-21047
  maxilla ~ 21030, 21048-21049
  mediastinal ~ 39200
  mediastinum ~ 32662
  metacarpal ~ 26200-26205
  metatarsal ~ 28104-28107
  mullerian duct ~ 55680
  nose ~ 30124-30125
  olecranon ~ 24120
  olecranon process
    with allograft ~ 24126
    with autograft ~ 24125
  ovarian ~ 58925
  pericardial ~ 33050
    endoscopic ~ 32661
  phalanges ~ 26210-26215
    toe ~ 28108
  pilonidal ~ 11770-11772
  pubis ~ 27066-27067
  radius ~ 24120, 25120-25126
    with allograft ~ 24126
    with autograft ~ 24125
  salivary gland ~ 42408
  scapula ~ 23140
    with allograft ~ 23146
    with autograft ~ 23145
  seminal vesicle ~ 55680
  sublingual gland ~ 42408
  talus ~ 28100-28103
  tarsal ~ 28104-28107
  thyroglossal duct ~ 60280-60281
  thyroid gland ~ 60200

Excision ~ continued

- tibia ~ 27635-27638
- toe ~ 28092
- ulna ~ 24120, 25120-25126
  - with allograft ~ 24126
  - with autograft ~ 24125
- urachalbladder ~ 51500
- vaginal ~ 57135
- destruction of the vestibule of the mouth ~ 40808-40820
- diverticulum, Meckel's ~ 44800
- ear, external
  - partial ~ 69110
  - total ~ 69120
- elbow joint ~ 24155
- electrode ~ 57522
- embolectomy/thrombectomy
  - aortoiliac artery ~ 34151-34201
  - axillary artery ~ 34101
  - brachial artery ~ 34101
  - carotid artery ~ 34001
  - celiac artery ~ 34151
  - femoral artery ~ 34201
  - heart ~ 33310-33315
  - iliac artery ~ 34151-34201
  - innominate artery ~ 34001-34101
  - mesentery artery ~ 34151
  - peroneal artery ~ 34203
  - popliteal artery ~ 34203
  - radial artery ~ 34111
  - renal artery ~ 34151
  - subclavian artery ~ 34001-34101
  - tibial artery ~ 34203
  - ulnar artery ~ 34111
- embolism, pulmonary artery ~ 33910-33916
- empyema
  - lung ~ 32540
  - pleural ~ 32540
- epididymis
  - bilateral ~ 54861
  - unilateral ~ 54860
- epiglottis ~ 31420
- esophagus
  - diverticula ~ 43130-43135
  - partial ~ 43116-43124
  - total ~ 43107-43113, 43124
- eye ~ 65101, 65103, 65109
- fallopian tube
  - salpingectomy ~ 58700
  - salpingo-oophorectomy ~ 58720
- fascia ~ see fasciectomy
- femur ~ 27360
  - partial ~ 27070-27071
- fibula ~ 27360, 27455-27457, 27641
- fistula
  - anal ~ 46270-46285
- foot
  - fasciectomy ~ 28060
    - radical ~ 28060-28062
- gallbladder ~ 47600-47620
  - cholecystectomy ~ 47562-47564
    - with cholangiography ~ 47563
    - with exploration common duct ~ 47564
- ganglion cyst
  - knee ~ 27347
  - wrist ~ 25111-25112
- gingiva ~ 41820
- gums ~ 41820
  - alveolus ~ 41830
  - operculum ~ 41821
- heart
  - donor ~ 33940
- heart/lung
  - donor ~ 33930
- hemangioma ~ 11400-11446
- hemorrhoids ~ 46221, 46250
  - clot ~ 46320
  - complex ~ 46260-46262
  - with fissurectomy ~ 46257-46258
  - simple ~ 46255
- hip, partial ~ 27070-27071

Excision ~ continued

- hippocampus ~ 61566
- humeral head
  - resection ~ 23195
  - sequestrectomy ~ 23174
- humerus ~ 23184, 23220, 24134, 24140, 24150
- hydrocele
  - spermatic cord ~ 55500
  - tunica vaginalis ~ 55040-55041
    - bilateral ~ 55041
    - unilateral ~ 55040
- hygroma, cystic, axillary/cervical ~ 38550-38555
- hymenotomy ~ 56700
- ileum
  - ileoanal reservoir ~ 45136
  - partial ~ 27070-27071
- inner ear ~ 69905-69910
- interphalangeal joint
  - toe ~ 28160
- intervertebral disk
  - decompression ~ 63075-63078
  - hemilaminectomy ~ 63040, 63043-63044
  - herniated ~ 63020-63044, 63055-63066
- intestine
  - laparoscopic
    - with anastomosis ~ 44202-44203
  - donor ~ 44132-44133
- intestines, small ~ 44120-44128
  - transplantation ~ 44137
- iris
  - iridectomy
    - with corneoscleral or corneal section ~ 66600
    - with cyclectomy ~ 66605
    - optical ~ 66635
    - peripheral ~ 66625
    - sector ~ 66630
- kidney
  - donor ~ 50300-50320, 50547
  - partial ~ 50240
  - recipient ~ 50340
  - transplantation ~ 50370
  - with ureters ~ 50220-50236
- kneecap ~ 27350
- labyrinth
  - with mastoidectomy ~ 69910
  - transcanal ~ 69905
- lacrimal gland
  - partial ~ 68505
  - total ~ 68500
- lacrimal sac ~ 68520
- larynx
  - partial ~ 31367-31382
  - with pharynx ~ 31390-31395
  - total ~ 31360-31365
- lesion
  - anal ~ 45108, 46922
  - ankle ~ 27630
    - arthroscopic ~ 29891
  - auditory canal, external
    - exostosis ~ 69140
    - radical with neck dissection ~ 69155
    - radical without neck dissection ~ 69150
    - soft tissue ~ 69145
  - bladder ~ 52224
  - brain ~ 61534, 61536-61540
  - brainstem ~ 61575-61576
  - carotid body ~ 60600-60605
  - colon ~ 44110-44111
  - conjunctiva ~ 68110-68130
    - over 1cm ~ 68115
    - with adjacent sclera ~ 68130
  - cornea ~ 65400
    - without graft ~ 65420
  - ear, middle ~ 69540
  - epididymis
    - local ~ 54830
    - spermatocele ~ 54840
  - esophagus ~ 43100-43101
  - eye ~ 65900

Excision ~ *continued*

eyelid
    multiple, different lids ~ 67805
    multiple, same lid ~ 67801
    single ~ 67800
    under anesthesia ~ 67808
    without closure ~ 67840
femur ~ 27062
finger ~ 26160
foot ~ 28080, 28090
gums ~ 41822-41828
hand ~ 26160
intestines ~ 44110
    small ~ 43250, 44111
intraspinal ~ 63265-63273
knee ~ 27347
larynx, endoscopic ~ 31545-31546
leg, lower ~ 27630
meniscus ~ 27347
mesentery ~ 44820
mouth ~ 40810-40816, 41116
nerve ~ 64774-64792
neuroma ~ 64778
nose, intranasal ~ 30117-30118
orbit ~ 61333
    lateral approach ~ 67420
palate ~ 42104-42120
pancreas ~ 48120
penis ~ 54060
    surgical excision penile plaque ~ 54110-54112
pharynx ~ 42808
rectum ~ 45108
sclera ~ 66130
skin
    benign ~ 11400-11471
    malignant ~ 11600-11646
skull ~ 61500, 61615-61616
spermatic cord ~ 55520
spinal cord ~ 63300-63308
stomach ~ 43611
talus, arthroscopic ~ 29891
testis ~ 54512
tibia, arthroscopic ~ 29891
toe ~ 28092
tongue ~ 41110-41114
urethra ~ 52224, 53265
uterus ~ 59100
    leiomyomata ~ 58140, 58545-58546, 58561
uvula ~ 42104-42107
wrist tendon ~ 25110
lesion, arthroscopic
    ankle ~ 29891
    talus ~ 29891
    tibia ~ 29891
lesion, tendon sheath
    arm, lower ~ 25110
lip ~ 40500-40530
    frenum ~ 40819
liver
    extensive ~ 47122
    lobectomy ~ 47125-47130
    partial ~ 47120, 47125-47130, 47140-47142
    total ~ 47133
lung
    bronchus resection ~ 32486
    bullae, completion ~ 32488
    lobe ~ 32480-32482
    pleurectomy ~ 32310, 32320
    pneumonectomy 32440-32445
    segment ~ 32484
    tumor, apical ~ 32503-32504
lung/heart donor ~ 33930
lymph nodes ~ 38500, 38510-38530
    abdominal ~ 38747
    inguinofemoral ~ 38760-38765
    limited, for staging
        para-aortic ~ 38562
        pelvic ~ 38562
        retroperitoneal ~ 38564
    pelvic ~ 38770

Excision ~ *continued*

radical
    axillary ~ 38740-38745
    cervical ~ 38720-38724
    suprahyoid ~ 38700
retroperitoneal transabdominal ~ 38780
thoracic ~ 38746
mandibular exostosis ~ 21031
mastoid
    complete ~ 69502
    radical ~ 69511
        modified ~ 69505
        petrous apicectomy ~ 69530
    simple ~ 69501
maxilla exostosis ~ 21032
maxillary torus palatinus ~ 21032
meningioma, brain ~ 61512, 61519
meniscectomy, temporomandibular joint ~ 21060
metacarpal ~ 26230
metatarsal ~ 28110-28114, 28122, 28140
    condyle ~ 28288
mouth, frenum ~ 40819
mucosa
    gums ~ 41828
    mouth ~ 40818
nail fold ~ 11765
nails ~ 11750
nerve
    foot ~ 28055
    leg, upper ~ 27325
    sympathetic ~ 64802-64818
neurofibroma ~ 64788-64790
neurolemmoma ~ 64788-64792
neuroma ~ 64774-64786
nose
    cyst ~ 30124-30125
    lesion ~ 30117-30118
    polyp ~ 30110-30115
    rhinectomy ~ 30150, 30160
    skin ~ 30120
    turbinate ~ 30130, 30140
odontoid process ~ 22548
olecranon process ~ 24147
omentum ~ 49255
ovary ~ 58720
    cystectomy ~ 58925
    oophorectomy ~ 58940, 58943
    salpingo-oophorectomy ~ 58720
    wedge resection/bisection ~ 58920
oviduct ~ 58700, 58720
palate ~ 42120, 42145
    lesion ~ 42104, 42106-42107
pancreas
    ampulla of Vater ~ 48148
    duct ~ 48148
    partial ~ 48140-48146, 48150, 48153-48154, 48160
    peripancreatic tissue ~ 48105
    total ~ 48155-48160
parathyroid gland ~ 60500-60502
parotid gland ~ 42340
    partial ~ 42410-42415
    total ~ 42420-42426
patella ~ 27350, 27424
penile adhesions, post-circumcision ~ 54162
penis
    amputation ~ 54120, 54125, 54130, 54135
    circumcision ~ 54150, 54160-54161, 54163
    frenulum ~ 54164
    partial ~ 54120
    post circumcision adhesion ~ 54162
    prepuce ~ 54150-54161, 54163
    radical ~ 54130-54135
    total ~ 54125
pericardium ~ 33030-33031
    endoscopic ~ 32659
petrous temporal
    apex ~ 69530
phalanges
    fingers ~ 26235-26236
    toe ~ 28124-28126, 28150-28160

Excision ~ *continued*

pharynx ~ 42145
  with larynx ~ 31390-31395
  partial ~ 42890
  resection ~ 42892-42894
pituitary gland ~ 61546-61548
pleura ~ 32310-32320
  endoscopic ~ 32656
polyp
  nose
    endoscopic ~ 31237
    extensive ~ 30115
    simple ~ 30110
  urethra ~ 53260, 53265
pressure ulcers ~ see also skin graft and flap ~ 15920-15999
prostate
  abdominoperineal ~ 45119
  partial ~ 55801, 55821-55831
  perineal ~ 55801-55815
  radical ~ 55810-55815, 55840-55845
  regrowth ~ 52630
  residual obstructive tissue ~ 52630
  retropubic ~ 55831-55845
  suprapubic ~ 55821
  transurethral ~ 52601, 52630
pterygium, with graft ~ 65426
pubis, partial ~ 27070-27071
radical synovium wrist ~ 25115-25116
radius ~ 24130, 24136, 24145, 24152, 25145
  styloid process ~ 25230
rectum
  with colon ~ 45121
  partial ~ 45111, 45113-45116, 45123
  prolapse ~ 45130-45135
  stricture ~ 45150
  total ~ 45119-45120
redundant skin of eyelid ~ 15820-15823
ribs ~ 21600-21616, 32900
scapula
  ostectomy ~ 23190
  partial ~ 23182
  sequestrectomy ~ 23172
  tumor/cyst ~ 23140, 23145, 23146
sclera ~ 66150, 66155, 66160, 66170
scrotum ~ 55150
semilunar cartilage of knee ~ 27332-27333
seminal vesicle ~ 55650
sesamoid bone
  foot ~ 28315
sinus
  ethmoid ~ 31200-31205
  maxillary ~ 31225-31230
Skene's gland ~ 53270
skin
  excess ~ 15830-15839, 15847
  lesion
    benign ~ 11400-11471
    malignant ~ 11600-11646
  nose ~ 30120
skin graft, preparation of site ~ 15000
skull ~ 61501
spermatic veins ~ 55530-55540
  abdominal approach ~ 55535
  hernia repair ~ 55540
spleen ~ 38100-38102
  laparoscopic ~ 38120
stapes
  with footplate drill out ~ 69661
  without foreign material ~ 69660
sternum ~ 21620, 21630-21632
stomach
  partial ~ 43631-43639, 43845
  total ~ 43620-43622
sublingual gland ~ 42450
submandibular gland ~ 42440

Excision ~ *continued*

sweat glands
  axillary ~ 11450-11451
  inguinal ~ 11462-11463
  perianal ~ 11470-11471
  perineal ~ 11470-11471
  umbilical ~ 11470-11471
synovium
  ankle ~ 27625-27626
  carpometacarpal joint ~ 26130
  elbow ~ 24102
  hip joint ~ 27054
  interphalangeal joint ~ 26140
  intertarsal joint ~ 28070
  knee joint ~ 27334-27335
  metacarpophalangeal joint ~ 26135
  metatarsophalangeal joint ~ 28072
  shoulder ~ 23105-23106
  tarsometatarsal joint ~ 28070
  wrist ~ 25105, 25118-25119
talus ~ 28120, 28130
tarsal ~ 28116, 28122
temporal bone ~ 69535
temporal, petrous apex ~ 69530
tendon
  arm
    lower ~ 25109
  finger ~ 26180, 26390, 26415
  hand ~ 26390, 26415
  palm ~ 26170
tendon sheath
  finger ~ 26145
  foot ~ 28086-28088
  palm ~ 26145
  wrist ~ 25115-25116
testis
  laparoscopic ~ 54690
  partial ~ 54522
  radical ~ 54530-54535
  simple ~ 54520
  tumor ~ 54530-54535
thrombectomy
  axillary vein ~ 34490
  bypass graft ~ 35875-35876
  femoropopliteal vein ~ 34401-34451
  iliac vein ~ 34401-34451
  subclavian vein ~ 34471-34490
  vena cava ~ 34401-34451
thromboendarterectomy
  aorta, abdominal ~ 35331
  aortoiliofemoral ~ 35363
  axillary artery ~ 35321
  brachial artery ~ 35321
  carotid artery ~ 35301, 35390
  celiac artery ~ 35341
  femoral artery ~ 35371-35372
  iliac ~ 35361-35363
  iliac artery ~ 35351
  iliofemoral artery ~ 35355, 35363
  innominate artery ~ 35311
  mesenteric artery ~ 35341
  peroneal artery ~ 35305-35306
  popliteal artery ~ 35303
  renal artery ~ 35341
  subclavian artery ~ 35301-35311
  tibial artery ~ 35305-35306
  vertebral artery ~ 35301
thymus gland ~ 60521
thyroid gland for malignancy
  partial ~ 60210-60225
  removal all thyroid tissue ~ 60260
  secondary ~ 60260
  total ~ 60240
    cervical approach ~ 60271
    sternal split/transthoracic approach ~ 60270
      limited neck dissection ~ 60252
      radical neck dissection ~ 60254
tibia ~ 27360, 27640

Excision ~ *continued*
 tongue
  complete ~ 41140-41155
  frenum ~ 41115
   with mouth resection ~ 41150-41153
  partial ~ 41120-41135
  with radical neck ~ 41135, 41145-41155
 tonsils ~ 42825-42826
  lingual ~ 42870
  radical ~ 42842-42845
  tag ~ 42860
  with adenoids ~ 42820-42821
 torus mandibularis ~ 21031
 trachea stenosis ~ 31780-31781
 transcervical approach ~ 60520
 tricuspid valve ~ 33460
 tumor
  abdominal wall ~ 22900-22905
  acetabulum ~ 27076
  ankle ~ 27615-27619, 27632, 27634
  arm, lower ~ 25071-25078
  arm, upper ~ 24071-24079
  back/flank ~ 21930
  bile duct ~ 47711-47712
  bladder ~ 51530, 52234-52240, 52355
  brain ~ 61510, 61518, 61520-61521, 61526-61530, 61545, 62164
  breast ~ 19120, 19125, 19126
   chest wall ~ 21601-21603
  bronchi ~ 31640
  calcaneus ~ 27647, 28100-28103
  carpal ~ 25130-25136
  cheekbone ~ 21030, 21034, 21048-21049
  clavicle ~ 23140
   with allograft ~ 23146
   with autograft ~ 23145
  ear, middle
   extended ~ 69554
   transcanal ~ 69550
   transmastoid ~ 69552
  elbow ~ 24071-24079
  esophagus endoscopic ablation ~ 43229
  facial bones ~ 21029-21030, 21034-21040, 21046-21049
  facial tissue ~ 21011-21016
  femur ~ 27065-27067, 27355-27358, 27365
  fibula ~ 27635-27638, 27646
  finger ~ 26111-26118
  foot ~ 28039-28047
  gums ~ 41825-41827
  hand ~ 26111-26118
  heart ~ 33120-33130
  hip ~ 27043-27045, 27049, 27059, 27065-27067
   radical ~ 27075-27076
  humerus ~ 23150, 23220, 24110-24115
   with allograft ~ 23156, 24116
   with autograft ~ 23155, 24116
   radial head or neck ~ 24152
  ileum ~ 27065-27067
  innominate ~ 27077
  intestines, small ~ 43250
  ischial ~ 27078
  kidney ~ 52355
  knee ~ 27327-27328, 27337-27339, 27365
  lacrimal gland
   frontal approach ~ 68540
   involving osteotomy ~ 68550
  larynx ~ 31300
   endoscopic ~ 31540-31541, 31578
  leg, lower ~ 27615-27619, 27632, 27634
  leg, upper ~ 27327-27329, 27337-27339, 27365
  mandible ~ 21040-21047
  maxilla ~ 21030, 21034, 21048-21049
  mediastinal ~ 39220
  mediastinum ~ 32662
  metacarpal ~ 26200-26205, 26250
  metatarsal ~ 28104-28107, 28173
  neck ~ 21552-21558
  olecranon process ~ 24120
   with allograft ~ 24126
   with autograft ~ 24125
  parotid gland ~ 42410-42426

Excision ~ *continued*
 pelvis ~ 27043-27045, 27049, 27059
 pericardial ~ 33050
 pericardium ~ 32661
 phalanges ~ 26210-26215, 26260-26262
  toe ~ 26215, 28108, 28175
 pituitary gland ~ 61546-61548, 62165
 presacral ~ 49215
 pubis ~ 27065-27067
 radius ~ 24120-24125, 25120-25126, 25170
 rectum ~ 45160-45172
 sacrococcygeal ~ 49215
 scapula ~ 23140
  with allograft ~ 23146
  with autograft ~ 23145
 shoulder ~ 23071-23078
 skull ~ 61500
 spermatocele ~ 54840
 spinal cord ~ 63275-63290
 spleen, total ~ 38100
 sternum ~ 21630
 stomach ~ 43610
 talus ~ 27647, 28100-28103
 tarsal ~ 28104-28107, 28171
 thorax ~ 21552-21558
 thyroid ~ 60200
 tibia ~ 27635-27638, 27645-27646
 trachea
  cervical ~ 31785
  thoracic ~ 31786
 ulna ~ 24120-24125, 25120-25126, 25170
 ureter ~ 52355
 urethra ~ 52234-52240, 52355, 53220
 uterus
  abdominal approach ~ 58140, 58146
   vaginal approach ~ 58145
 vagina ~ 57135
 vertebra, lumbar ~ 22102
 vertebra, thoracic ~ 22101
 wrist ~ 25071-25078
 zygoma ~ 21030, 21034
 turbinate ~ 30130-30140
 tympanic nerve ~ 69676
 ulcer
  stomach ~ 43610
 ulna ~ 24147, 25145
  complete ~ 25240
  partial ~ 25150-25151, 25240
 umbilicus ~ 49250
 ureter ~ 50650-50660
 ureterocele ~ 51535
 urethra
  diverticulum ~ 53230-53235
  prolapse ~ 53275
  total
   female ~ 53210
   male ~ 53215
 uterus
  laparoscopic ~ 58550
  leiomyomata ~ 58546
  partial ~ 58180
  radical ~ 58210, 58285
  removal tubes and/ or ovaries ~ 58262-58263, 58291, 58552, 58554
  total ~ 58150-58152, 58200
  vaginal ~ 58260, 58290-58294, 58550, 58553
   with colpectomy ~ 58275-58280
   with colpo-urethrocystopexy ~ 58267
   with repair of enterocele ~ 58270, 58292, 58294
 uvula ~ 42140-42145
 vagina
  cyst ~ 57135
  lumen ~ 57120
  repair of enterocele ~ 58280
  septum ~ 57130
  total ~ 57110
   with hysterectomy ~ 58275-58280
 varicocele
  spermatic cord ~ 55530-55540
   abdominal approach ~ 55535
   hernia repair ~ 55540

Excision ~ *continued*
  vas deferens ~ 55250
  vascular malformation
    finger ~ 26115
    hand ~ 26115
  vein, varicose ~ 37765-37766
  vertebra
    additional segment ~ 22103, 22116
    cervical ~ 22110
    for tumor ~ 22100, 22110
    lumbar ~ 22102
      for tumor ~ 22114
    thoracic ~ 22112
      for tumor ~ 22101
  vertebral body
    decompression ~ 63081-63103
    lesion ~ 63300-63308
  vitreous ~ 67039
    with retinal surgery ~ 67041-67043
    total
      pars plana approach ~ 67036
      with epiretinal membrane stripping ~ 67041-67043
  vulva
    radical
      complete ~ 56633-56640
      partial ~ 56630-56632
    simple
      complete ~ 56625
      partial ~ 56620
Exclusion
  duodenum ~ 48547
  small intestine ~ 44700
Exenteration
  eye
    removal orbital contents ~ 65110
    therapeutic removal of bone ~ 65112
    with muscle or myocutaneous flap ~ 65114
  pelvis ~ 45126, 58240
Exercise stress tests
  cardiovascular ~ 93015-93018, 93464
  pulmonary ~ 94617, 94618, 94619
Exercise test ~ see also electromyography, needle
  cardiopulmonary ~ 94621
  ischemic limb ~ 95875
Exercise therapy ~ 97110-97113
Exfoliation, chemical ~ 17360
Exocrine, pancreas ~ see pancreas
Exomphalos ~ 49600-49611
Exostectomy ~ 28288
Exostoses ~ 69140
Exostoses, cartilaginous ~ 69140
Exostosis excision ~ 69140
Expander, skin, inflatable ~ see tissue, expander
Expired gas analysis ~ 94680-94690
  nitric oxide ~ 95012
  spectroscopic ~ 94799
Exploration
  abdomen ~ 49000-49002
    penetrating wound ~ 20102
    staging ~ 58960
  adrenal gland ~ 60540-60545
  anal endoscopy ~ 46600
  ankle ~ 27610, 27620
  arm, lower ~ 25248
  artery
    brachial ~ 24495
    carotid ~ 35701
    femoral ~ 35703
    neck ~ 35701
    popliteal ~ 35703
    upper extremity ~ 35702
  back, penetrating wound ~ 20102
  bile duct
    atresia ~ 47700
    endoscopy ~ 47552-47553
  blood vessel
    abdomen ~ 35840
    chest ~ 35820
    extremity ~ 35860
    neck ~ 35800

Exploration ~ *continued*
  brain
    via burr hole
      infratentorial ~ 61253
      supratentorial ~ 61250
    infratentorial ~ 61305
    supratentorial ~ 61304
  breast ~ 19020
  bronchi endoscopy ~ 31622
  bronchoscopy ~ 31622
  cauda equina ~ 63005-63011, 63017
  chest penetrating wound ~ 20101
  colon endoscopic ~ 44388, 45378
  colon-sigmoid endoscopic ~ 45330, 45335
  common bile duct with cholecystectomy ~ 47610
  duodenum ~ 44010
  ear, inner
    endolymphatic sac
      with shunt ~ 69806
      without shunt ~ 69805
  ear, middle ~ 69440
  elbow ~ 24000, 24101
  epididymis ~ 54865
  esophagus endoscopy ~ 43200
  extremity penetrating wound ~ 20103
  finger joint ~ 26075-26080
  flank penetrating wound ~ 20102
  gallbladder ~ 47480
  gastrointestinal tract, upper endoscopy ~ 43235-43236
  hand joint ~ 26070
  heart ~ 33310-33315
  hepatic duct ~ 47400
  hip ~ 27033
  interphalangeal joint toe ~ 28024
  intertarsal joint ~ 28020
  intestines, small
  endoscopy ~ 44360
  enterotomy ~ 44020
  kidney ~ 50010, 50045, 50120
  knee ~ 27310, 27331
  lacrimal duct ~ 68810
    canaliculi ~ 68840
    with anesthesia ~ 68811
    with insertion tube or stent ~ 68815
  liver wound ~ 47361-47362
  mediastinum ~ 39000-39010
  metatarsophalangeal joint ~ 28022
  nasolacrimal duct ~ 68810
    with anesthesia ~ 68811
    with insertion tube or stent ~ 68815
  neck
    lymph nodes ~ 38542
    penetrating wound ~ 20100
  nipple ~ 19110
  nose endoscopy ~ 31231-31235
  orbit ~ 61333
    with/without biopsy ~ 67450
    without bone flap ~ 67400
  parathyroid gland ~ 60500-60505
  pelvis ~ 49320
    wound ~ 49014
  preperitoneal area ~ 49014
  prostate ~ 55860
    with nodes ~ 55862-55865
  rectum
    endoscopic ~ 45300
    injury ~ 45562-45563
  retroperitoneal area ~ 49010
  scrotum ~ 55110
  shoulder joint ~ 23040-23044, 23107
  sinus
    frontal ~ 31070-31075
    maxillary ~ 31020-31030
  skull ~ 61105
  spinal cord ~ 63001-63011, 63015-63017, 63040-63044
  spine fusion ~ 22830
  stomach ~ 43500
  tarsometatarsal joint ~ 28020
  testis, undescended ~ 54550-54560
  toe joint ~ 28024

Exploration ~ *continued*
ureter ~ 50600
vagina ~ 57000
   endocervical ~ 57452
wrist ~ 25101, 25248
   joint ~ 25040
Exploratory laparotomy ~ 49000-49002
Expression lesion, conjunctiva ~ 68040
Exteriorization, small intestine ~ 44300
External cephalic version ~ 59412
External ear ~ see ear, external
External extoses ~ 69140
External fixation
adjustment/revision ~ 20693
application ~ 20690-20692
   stereotactic computer assisted ~ 20696-20697
mandibular fracture
open treatment ~ 21454
percutaneous treatment ~ 21452
removal ~ 20694
Extirpation, lacrimal sac ~ 68520
Extracorporeal circulation
cannulation
   chemotherapy perfusion ~ 36823
Extracorporeal dialyses ~ 90935-90937
Extracorporeal membrane oxygenation cannulization (ECMO)
arterial exposure with graft creation ~ 33987
insertion of cannula(e)
   open ~ 33953, 33954
   percutaneous ~ 33951, 33952
   sternotomy/thoracotomy ~ 33955, 33956
daily management
   veno-arterial ~ 33947
   veno-venous ~ 33946
left heart valve
   insertion ~ 33988
   removal ~ 33989
removal of cannula(e)
   open ~ 33969, 33984
   percutaneous ~ 33965, 33966
   sternotomy/thoracotomy ~ 33985, 33986
repositioning of cannula(e)
   open ~ 33959, 33962
   percutaneous ~ 33957, 33958
   sternotomy/thoracotomy ~ 33963, 33964
Extracorporeal photochemotherapies ~ 36522
Extracorporeal shock wave therapy ~ see lithotripsy
plantar fascia ~ 0020T
Extracranial intracranial ~ 61623
Extraction lens
extracapsular ~ 66940
intracapsular ~ 66920
   for dislocated lens ~ 66930
Extraction, cataract ~ 66830
Extradural injection
Infusion
   with imaging guidance ~ 62325, 62327
   without imaging guidance ~ 62324, 62326
Injection
   with imaging guidance ~ 62321, 62323
   without imaging guidance ~ 62320, 62322
Extraocular muscle ~ 67340
Extrauterine pregnancy ~ see ectopic pregnancy
Extravasation blood ~ see hemorrhage
Extremity
lower
   harvest of vein for bypass graft ~ 35500
   harvest of vein for vascular reconstruction ~ 35572
   revision ~ 35879-35881
   ultrasound ~ 76881-76882
upper
   harvest of artery for coronary artery bypass graft ~ 35600
   harvest of vein for bypass graft ~ 35500
   repair blood vessel ~ 35206
wound exploration penetrating wound ~ 20103
Eye
age-related eye disease study (AREDS) ~ 4177F
aspiration, orbital contents ~ 67415

Eye ~ *continued*
biopsy
   cornea ~ 65410, 65430
   extraocular muscle ~ 67346
   orbit ~ 67400
chemodenervation, extraocular muscle ~ 67345
computerized corneal topography ~ 92025
diagnostic and monitoring studies
   biometry ~ 76516, 76519, 92136
   blood flow measurement ~ 0198T
   computerized corneal topography ~ 92025
   corneal hysteresis determination ~ 92145
   corneal pachymetry ~ 76514
   dilated fundus evaluation ~ 2020F, 2021F
   dilated macular exam ~ 2019F, 2021F
   dilated retinal exam ~ 2022F
   field stereoscopic photos ~ 2024F
      eye imaging validation ~ 2026F
   foreign body localization ~ 76529
   heterochromatic flicker photometry ~ 0506T
   interferometry biometry ~ 92136
   intraocular pressure
      measurement ~ 0198T, 92100
      monitoring ~ 0329T
   movement analysis ~ 0615T
   optic nerve head evaluation ~ 2027F
   tear film imaging ~ 0330T
   tear osmolarity ~ 83861
   ultrasound ~ 76510-76514
      biometry ~ 76516-76519
      foreign body ~ 76529
   visual field
      assessment ~ 0378T, 0379T
      exam ~ 92081-92083
   x-ray ~ 70030
dilation outflow canal ~ 66174-66175
discission of anterior hyaloid membrane ~ 65810
drainage, anterior chamber
   with diagnostic aqueous aspiration ~ 65800
   with removal of blood ~ 65815
   with removal of vitreous ~ 65810
   with therapeutic aqueous release ~ 65800
endoscopy ~ 66990
evacuation, meibomian glands ~ 0207T, 0563T
evaluation
   dilated fundus ~ 2020F-2021F
   dilated macular ~ 2019F
goniotomy ~ 65820
incision
   adhesions
      anterior synechiae ~ 65860, 65870
      corneovitreal adhesions ~ 65880
      goniosynechiae ~ 65865
      posterior synechiae ~ 65875
   anterior chamber ~ 65820
   trabeculae ~ 65850
injection
   air ~ 66020
   medication ~ 66030, 67500
   pharmacologic agent ~ 0465T, 67028
insertion
   aqueous drainage device ~ 66179, 66180
   drug eluting ocular inseert, eyelid ~ 0444T, 0445T
implantation
   corneal ring segments ~ 65785
   drainage device ~ 0191T, 0253T
   drug delivery system ~ 67027
   electrode array ~ 0100T
   foreign material for reinforcement ~ 65155
   muscles attached ~ 65140
   muscles, not attached ~ 65135
   reinsertion ~ 65150
   scleral shell ~ 65130
interferometry biometry ~ 92136
lesion excision ~ 65900
meibomian glands
   evacuation ~ 0207T, 0563T
   near infrared dual imaging ~ 0507T

Eye ~ continued

nerve
  destruction ~ 67345
  optic, head evaluation ~ 2027F
paracentesis anterior chamber
  with diagnostic aspiration of aqueous ~ 65800
  removal of blood ~ 65815
  removal of vitreous and/or discission anterior hyaloid membrane ~
    65810
  with therapeutic release of aqueous ~ 65800
prosthesis
  custom preparation ~ 21077
  intraocular lens
    exchange ~ 66986
    insertion ~ 66985
    removal ~ 0308T
    repositioning ~ 66825
  iris ~ 0616T-0618T
  ocular telescope ~ 0308T
  retinal receiver and pulse generator
    implantation electrode array ~ 0100T
    placement ~ 0100T
pterygium
  excision ~ 65420, 65426
  transposition ~ 65420, 65426
puncture, cornea ~ 65600
radial keratotomy ~ 65771
reconstruction
  graft
    conjunctiva ~ 65782
    stem cell ~ 65781
    transplantation
      amniotic membrane ~ 65780
removal
  blood clot ~ 65930
  bone ~ 65112
  foreign body
    conjunctival embedded ~ 65210
    conjunctival superficial ~ 65205
    corneal with slit lamp ~ 65222
    corneal without slit lamp ~ 65220
    intraocular ~ 65235-65265
  implant ~ 65175
    anterior segment ~ 65920
    muscles, not attached ~ 65103
    posterior segment ~ 67120-67121
repair
  amniotic membrane ~ 65778-65779
  conjunctiva
    by mobilization and rearrangement without hospitalization ~ 65272
    by mobilization and rearrangement with hospitalization ~ 65273
    direct closure ~ 65270
  cornea
    nonperforating ~ 65275
    perforating ~ 65280-65285
  muscles ~ 65290
  sclera
    anterior segment ~ 66250
    with graft ~ 66225
    with tissue glue ~ 65286
  trabeculae ~ 65855
  wound
    by mobilization and rearrangement ~ 65272-65273
    direct closure ~ 65270
shunt, aqueous to extraocular reservoir ~ 66180
trabeculostomy ab interno, laser ~ 0621T, 0622T
transluminal dilation, aqueous outflow canal ~ 66174-66175
ultrasound ~ 76510-76514
  biometry ~ 76516-76519
  foreign body ~ 76529
unlisted services and procedures
  anterior segment ~ 66999
  posterior segment ~ 67299
with muscle or myocutaneous flap ~ 65114
  muscles attached ~ 65105
  ocular contents
    without implant ~ 65091
    with implant ~ 65093
    orbital contents ~ 65110
    without implant ~ 65101
X-ray ~ 70030

Eye and ocular adnexa, surgical procedures 65091-68899
Eyebrow repair
  ptosis ~ 67900
Eyeglasses ~ 92340-92342
Eyelashes
  repair trichiasis
    epilation
      by forceps only ~ 67820
      by other than forceps ~ 67825
    incision of lid margin ~ 67830
    with free mucous membrane graft ~ 67835
Eyelid
abscess, incision and drainage ~ 67700
biopsy ~ 67810
blepharoplasty ~ 15820-15823
chalazion
  excision ~ 67805
    with anesthesia ~ 67808
    multiple ~ 67801-67805
    single ~ 67800
closure by suture ~ 67875
evacuation, meibomian glands ~ 0207T, 0563T
incision
  canthus ~ 67715
  sutures ~ 67710
injection, subconjunctival ~ 68200
lesion
  destruction ~ 67850
  excision
    with anesthesia ~ 67808
    without closure ~ 67840
    multiple ~ 67801-67805
    single ~ 67800
meibomian glands
  evacuation ~ 0207T, 0563T
  near infrared dual imaging ~ 0507T
placement, drug-eluting ocular insert ~ 0444T, 0445T
reconstruction
  canthus ~ 67950
  total ~ 67973-67975
  total eyelid
    lower ~ 67973-67975
    second stage ~ 67975
    upper ~ 67974
  transfer of tarsoconjunctival flap from opposing eyelid ~ 67971
removal foreign body ~ 67938
repair ~ 21280-21282
  blepharoptosis
    conjunctivo-tarso-muller's muscle-levator resection ~ 67908
    frontalis muscle technique ~ 67901-67094
    reduction overcorrection of ptosis ~ 67909
    superior rectus technique with fascial sling ~ 67906
  ectropion
    blepharoplasty ~ 67914
    suture ~ 67914
  entropion
    excision tarsal wedge ~ 67923
    extensive ~ 67924
    suture ~ 67921
    thermocauterization ~ 67922
  excisional ~ 67961
    over one-fourth of lid margin ~ 67966
  lagophthalmos ~ 67912
  lashes
    epilation, by forceps only ~ 67820
    epilation, by other than forceps ~ 67825
    lid margin ~ 67830-67835
  wound
    full thickness ~ 67935
    partial thickness ~ 67930
repair with graft retraction ~ 67911
skin graft
  full thickness ~ 67961
  split ~ 67961
suture ~ 67880
  with transposition of tarsal plate ~ 67882
tissue transfer, adjacent ~ 67961
unlisted services and procedures ~ 67999
Eyelid ptoses ~ see blepharoptosis
Eye allergy test ~ 95060
Eye evisceration ~ 65091, 65093

Eye exam
  established patient ~ 92012-92014
  new patient ~ 92002-92004
  with anesthesia ~ 92018-92019
Eye exercises, training ~ 92065
Eye muscles
  biopsy ~ 67346
  repair
    strabismus
      adjustable sutures ~ 67335
      exploration and/or repair detached extraocular muscle ~ 67340
      one vertical muscle ~ 67314
      on patient with previous surgery ~ 67331
      posterior fixation suture ~ 67334
      recession or resection ~ 67311-67312
      release of scar tissue without detaching extraocular muscle ~ 67343
      two or more vertical muscles ~ 67316
      with scarring extraocular muscles ~ 67332
      with superior oblique muscle ~ 67318
    transposition ~ 67320
    unlisted services and procedures ~ 67399
Eye prosthesis ~ see prosthesis
Eye socket ~ see orbit ~ 21385-21395, 21260-21263, 21267-21268, 67415
E antigens ~ 87350
E B virus ~ 86663-86665
E vitamin ~ 84446

F

Face
  CT scan ~ 70486-70488
  lesion
    destruction ~ 17000-17004, 17280-17286
  lift ~ 15824-15828
  magnetic resonance imaging (MRI) ~ 70540-70543
  tumor resection ~ 21015
Facial asymmetries ~ 21247
Facial bones ~ see also mandible; maxilla
  abscess excision ~ 21026
  reconstruction
    secondary ~ 21275
  repair ~ 21208-21209
  tumor
    excision ~ 21029-21034
    resection
      radical ~ 21015
  X-ray ~ 70140-70150
Facial nerve
  anastomosis
    to hypoglossal ~ 64868
    to spinal accessory ~ 64866
  avulsion ~ 64742
  chemodenervation, muscles ~ 64615
  decompression ~ 61590, 61596
    intratemporal
      lateral to geniculate ganglion ~ 69720, 69740
      medial to geniculate ganglion ~ 69725, 69745
    total ~ 69955
  function study ~ 92516
  incision ~ 64742
  injection, anesthetic ~ 64400
  mobilization ~ 61590
  repair
    lateral to geniculate ganglion ~ 69740
    medial to geniculate ganglion ~ 69745
  repair/suture
    with or without graft ~ 64864-64865
  suture
    lateral to geniculate ganglion ~ 69740
    medial to geniculate ganglion ~ 69745
  transection ~ 64742
Facial nerve paralysis
  graft ~ 15840-15845
  repair ~ 15840-15845
Facial prosthesis impression ~ 21088
Facial rhytidectomy ~ 15824-15828

Factor
  ACTH-releasing ~ 80412
  antinuclear ~ 86038-86039
  blood coagulation ~ 85210-85293
  Factor I ~ 85384-85385
  Factor II ~ 85210
  Factor III ~ see thromboplastin
  Factor inhibitor test ~ 85335
  Factor IV ~ see calcium
  Factor IXix ~ 85250
  Factor rheumatoid ~ 86430-86431
  Factor VII ~ 85230
  Factor VIII ~ 85210-85293
  Factor X ~ 85260
  Factor X, activated ~ 85260
  Factor XA inhibitor ~ 85300-85301
  Factor XI ~ 85270
  Factor XII ~ 85280
  Factor XIII ~ 85290-85291
  Fitzgerald ~ 85293
  Fletcher ~ 85293
  hyperglycemic-glycogenolytic ~ 82943
  intrinsic ~ 83528
  sulfation ~ 84305
Fallopian tube
  anastomosis ~ 58750
  biopsy ~ 49321
  cannulation ~ 58565
  catheterization ~ 58345, 74742
  destruction endoscopy ~ 58670
  ectopic pregnancy ~ 59121
    with salpingectomy and/or oophorectomy ~ 59120, 59151
  excision ~ 58661, 58700, 58720, 58943, 58950, 58953, 58956
  imaging
    hysterosalpingography ~ 74740
    sonosalpingography ~ 0568T
  ligation ~ 58600, 58611
  lysis adhesions ~ 58740
  occlusion
    by biopolymer implant ~ 0567T
    by cannulation ~ 58565
    by device ~ 58615, 58671
    endoscopy ~ 58671
    placement, implant for occlusion ~ 58568
    sonosalpingography to confirm ~ 0568T
  pregnancy ~ 59121
  repair ~ 58752
    anastomosis ~ 58750
    create stoma ~ 58770
  tumor resection ~ 58950, 58952-58956
  unlisted services and procedures ~ 58999
  X-ray ~ 74742
Fallot, tetralogy of ~ 33692-33697, 33924
Family psychotherapy ~ 90846-90849, 99510
Fanconi anemia chromosome analysis ~ 88248
Farnsworth-Munsell color test ~ 92283
Farr test ~ 82784-82787
Fasanella-Servat procedure ~ 67908
Fascia graft ~ 15840
Fascia lata graft harvesting ~ 20920-20922
Fascial defect
  leg ~ 27656
  urostomy ~ 50728
Fascial graft
  cheek ~ 15840
  fascia and skin flap ~ 15733, 15734, 15736, 15738
  free microvascular anastomosis ~ 15758
  harvest ~ 20920, 20922
  reconstruction
    collateral ligament ~ 26541
    hamstring muscle ~ 27386
    infrapatellar tendon ~ 27381
    quadriceps muscle ~ 27386
    tendon pulley ~ 26502
  sternoclavicular dislocation ~ 23532
Fasciectomy
  foot ~ 28060
    radical ~ 28060-28062
  palm ~ 26121-26125
Fasciocutaneous flaps ~ 15733-15738

Fasciotomy
  arm, lower ~ 24495, 25020-25025
  buttock, decompression ~ 27027
    with debridement ~ 27057
  foot ~ 28008
  hand decompression ~ 26037
  hip ~ 27025
  knee ~ 27305, 27496-27499
  leg, lower ~ 27600-27602, 27892-27894
  leg, upper ~ 27305, 27496-27499, 27892-27894
  palm ~ 26040-26045
  pelvis, decompression ~ 27027
    with debridement ~ 27057
  plantar endoscopic ~ 29893
  thigh ~ 27025
  toe ~ 28008
  wrist ~ 25020-25023
FAST ~ see allergen immunotherapy
Fat
  feces ~ 82705-82715
  removal, lipectomy ~ 15876-15879
Fatty acid
  blood ~ 82725
  very long chain ~ 82726
Fat stain
  feces ~ 89125
  respiratory secretions ~ 89125
  sputum ~ 89125
  urine ~ 89125
FDP ~ 85362-85380
Fe (iron) ~ 83540
Feedback, psychophysiologic (see biofeedback) ~ 90901-90911
Female castration ~ 58262-58263, 58291-58292, 58552, 58554, 58661, 58940-58943
Female genital system, surgical procedures ~ 56405-58999
Female gonad ~ see ovary
Femoral arteries ~ see artery, femoral
Femoral nerve
  injection, anesthetic ~ 64447-64448
Femoral stem prosthesis ~ 27132
Femoral vein ~ 34501
Femur ~ see hip; knee; leg, upper
  abscess, incision ~ 27303
  bursa, excision ~ 27062
  craterization ~ 27070, 27360
  cyst, excision ~ 27065-27067, 27355-27358
  diaphysectomy ~ 27360
  drainage ~ 27303
  excision ~ 27070, 27360
    epiphyseal bar ~ 20150
  fracture ~ 27244
    closed treatment ~ 27501-27503
    distal ~ 27508, 27510, 27514
    distal, medial or lateral condyle ~ 27509
    epiphysis ~ 27516-27519
    intertrochanteric ~ 27244
    intertrochanteric
      closed treatment ~ 27238
      treatment with implant ~ 27244
      with implant ~ 27245
      with manipulation ~ 27240
    neck
      closed treatment ~ 27230-27232
      open treatment ~ 27236
      percutaneous fixation ~ 27235
    open treatment ~ 27245, 27269, 27506-27507, 27511-27513
    percutaneous fixation ~ 27509
    pertrochanteric ~ 27244
    pertrochanteric
      closed treatment ~ 27238
      treatment with implant ~ 27244
      with implant ~ 27245
      with manipulation ~ 27240
    proximal end, head
      closed treatment ~ 27267-27268
      open treatment ~ 27269
    shaft ~ 27500, 27502, 27506-27507
    subtrochanteric ~ 27244

Femur ~ *continued*
  subtrochanteric
    closed treatment ~ 27238
    treatment with implant ~ 27244
    with implant ~ 27245
    with manipulation ~ 27240
  supracondylar ~ 27501-27503, 27509, 27511-27513
  transcondylar ~ 27501-27503, 27509, 27511-27513
  trochanteric
    closed treatment ~ 27246
    open treatment ~ 27248
  without manipulation ~ 27501
  with manipulation ~ 27503
  halo ~ 20663
  lesion excision ~ 27062
  osteoplasty
    lengthening ~ 27466-27468
    shortening ~ 27465, 27468
  osteotomywithout fixation ~ 27448
  prophylactic treatment ~ 27187, 27495
  realignment ~ 27454
  reconstruction ~ 27468
    at knee ~ 27442-27443, 27446
    lengthening ~ 27466-27468
    shortening ~ 27465, 27468
  repair ~ 27470-27472
    epiphysis ~ 27181, 27475, 27742
      arrest ~ 27185
    muscle transfer ~ 27110
    osteotomy ~ 27140, 27151-27156, 27161-27165, 27450-27454
    with graft ~ 27170
  saucerization ~ 27070, 27360
  tumor excision ~ 27065-27067, 27355-27358, 27365
  X-ray ~ 7355, 73552
Fenestration procedure
  skin, laser ~ 0479T, 0480T
  tracheostomy ~ 31610
Fern test ~ 87210
Ferric chloride, urine ~ 81005
Ferrihemoglobin ~ 83045-83050
Ferritin, blood or urine ~ 82728
Ferroxidase ~ (ceruloplasmin) 82390
Fertility control ~ see contraception
Fertility test
  semen analysis ~ 89300-89321
  sperm analysis
    cervical mucus penetration test ~ 89330
    hamster penetration ~ 89329
Fertilization, assisted
  oocyte ~ 89250, 89251
    microtechnique ~ 89280-89281
    with co-culture ~ 89251
Fertilization in vitro ~ 58321-58322
Fetal biophysical profile ~ 76818-76819
Fetal contraction stress test ~ 59020
Fetal hemoglobin ~ 85461
Fetal lung maturity assessment; lecithin sphingomyelin ratio ~ 83661
Fetal monitoring ~ 59050-59051, 99500
Fetal non-stress test ~ 59025
  ultrasound ~ 76818
Fetal procedure
  amniocentesis ~ 59000
  amnioinfusion ~ 59070
  amniotic fluid reduction ~ 59001
  cord occlusion ~ 59072
  cordocentesis ~ 59012
    ultrasound guidance ~ 76941
  fluid drainage ~ 59074
  intrauterine transfusion ~ 36460
    ultrasound guidance ~ 76941
  magnetic cardiac signal recording ~ 0475T-0478T
  MRI ~ 74712, 74713
  non-stress test ~ 59025
  shunt placement ~ 59076
  stress test ~ 59020
  unlisted fetal invasive procedure ~ 59897
  unlisted laparoscopy procedure ~ 59898
  unlisted procedure, maternity care and delivery ~ 59899

Fetal testing
  amniocentesis ~ 59000
  amniotic fluid lung maturity ~ 83661, 83663-83664
  heart ~ 76825-76826
    Doppler
      complete ~ 76827
      follow-up or repeat study ~ 76828
  hemoglobin ~ 83030-83033, 85460
  MRI ~ 74712, 74713
  non-stess test ~ 59025
    ultrasound ~ 76815-76818
  ultrasound ~ 76801-76828
    biophysical profile ~ 76818, 76819
    fetal ~ 76813-76816
    fetal and maternal ~ 76801, 76802, 76805, 76810-76812, 76817
    heart ~ 76825-76828
    middle cerebral artery ~ 76821
    umbilical artery ~ 76820
Fetuin ~ 82105-82106
Fever, Australian Q ~ 86000, 86638
Fever, Japanese river ~ 86000
Fibrillation, atrial ~ 33254-33256, 33265-33266
  documentation ~ 1060F-1061F
Fibrillation, heart ~ see heart, fibrillation
Fibrin
  degradation products ~ 85362-85380
  deposit removal ~ 32150
  stabilizing factor ~ 85290-85291
Fibrinase ~ 85400
Fibrinogen ~ 85384-85385
Fibrinolysin ~ 85400
Fibrinolysins ~ 85390
Fibrinolysis
  alpha-2 antiplasmin ~ 85410
  assay ~ 85396
    activity ~ 85397
  plasmin ~ 85400
  plasminogen ~ 85420-85421
  plasminogen activator ~ 85415
  pleural cavity, instillation of agent ~ 32561, 32562
Fibroadenoma, excision ~ 19120-19126
  ablation
    cryosurgical ~ 19105
Fibroblastoma, arachnoidal ~ 61512, 61519
Fibrocutaneous tags ~ 11200-11201
Fibromatosis, Dupuytren's ~ 26040-26045
Fibromatosis, penile ~ see Peyronie disease
Fibromyoma ~ 58140, 58545-58546, 58561
Fibronectin, fetal ~ 82731
Fibrosis, penile ~ see Peyronie disease
Fibrosis, retroperitoneal ~ 50715
Fibrous cavernitides ~ see Peyronie disease
Fibrous dysplasia ~ 21029, 21181-21184
Fibula ~ see ankle; knee; tibia
  bone graft with microvascular anastomosis ~ 20955
  craterization ~ 27360, 27641
  cyst excision ~ 27635-27638
  diaphysectomy ~ 27360, 27641
  excision ~ 27360, 27641
    epiphyseal bar ~ 20150
  fracture
    malleolus ~ 27786-27814
    shaft ~ 27780-27784
  incision ~ 27607
  osteoplasty lengthening ~ 27715
  repair
    epiphysis ~ 27477-27485, 27730-27742
    nonunion or malunion ~ 27726
    osteotomy ~ 27707-27712
  saucerization ~ 27360, 27641
  tumor excision ~ 27635-27638, 27646
  X-ray ~ 73590
Figure of eight cast ~ 29049
Filariasis ~ 86280
Filtering operation ~ see incision, sclera, fistulization
Filtration implant, glaucoma ~ 66180, 66185
Fimbrioplasty ~ 58760
  laparoscopic ~ 58672

Fine needle aspiration
  diagnostic ~ 10021
  evaluation ~ 88172, 88173, 88177
  orbital contents ~ 67415
  transendoscopic ~ 43232, 43242
    colon ~ 45392
    esophagus ~ 43238
Fine needle aspiration (FNA) biopsy
  Lesion
    with CT guidance ~ 10009, 10010
    with fluoroscopic guidance ~ 10007, 10008
    with MR guidance ~ 10011, 10012
    with ultrasound guidance ~ 10005, 10006
    without guidance ~ 10004, 10021
Finger ~ see phalanx, finger
  abscess
    bone, incision and drainage ~ 26034
    incision and drainage ~ 26010-26011
  amputation ~ 26951-26952
    with exploration or removal ~ 26910
  arthrocentesis ~ 20600
  arthrodesis
    interphalangeal joint ~ 26860-26863
    metacarpophalangeal joint ~ 26850-26852
  bone, incision and drainage ~ 26034
  cast ~ 29086
  collection of blood ~ 36415-36416
  decompression ~ 26035
  excision
    constricting ring ~ 26596
    tendon ~ 26180, 26390, 26415
  insertion, tendon graft ~ 26392
  magnetic resonance imaging (MRI) ~ 73221
  reconstruction
    extra digit ~ 26587
    toe to hand transfer ~ 26551-26556
  removal
    implantation ~ 26320
    tube ~ 26392, 26416
  repair
    blood vessel ~ 35207
    claw finger ~ 26499
    extra digit ~ 26587
    macrodactylia ~ 26590
    tendon
      extensor ~ 26415-26434, 26445-26449, 26460
      flexor ~ 26356-26358, 26440-26442, 26455
    volar plate ~ 26548
    web finger ~ 26560-26562
  replantation ~ 20816-20822
  reposition ~ 26555
  sesamoidectomy ~ 26185
  splint ~ 29130-29131
  strapping ~ 29280
  tendon sheath
    excision ~ 26145
    incision ~ 26055
    incision and drainage ~ 26020
  tenotomy ~ 26060, 26460
    flexor ~ 26455
  tumor excision ~ 26111-26118

Finger ~ continued
  unlisted services and procedures ~ 26989
  X-ray ~ 73140
Finger flap, tissue transfer ~ 14350
Finger joint ~ see intercarpal joint
Finney operation ~ 43810, 43850-43855
FISH ~ 88365
Fissurectomy, anal ~ 46200
Fissure in ano ~ 46200, 46949-46942
Fistula
  anal, repair ~ 46288, 46706
  autogenous graft ~ 36825
  bronchi, repair ~ 32815
  carotid-cavernous, repair ~ 61710
  chest wall, repair ~ 32906
  conjunctiva
    without tube ~ 68745
    with tube or stent ~ 68750

Fistula ~ *continued*
  enterovesical
    closure ~ 44660-44661
  kidney ~ 50520-50526
  lacrimal gland closure ~ 68770
    dacryocystorhinostomy ~ 68720
  nose repair ~ 30580-30600
  oval window ~ 69666
  postauricular ~ 69700
  rectovaginal
    abdominal approach ~ 57305
    transperineal approach ~ 57308
    with concomitant colostomy ~ 57307
  round window ~ 69667
  sclera
    sclerectomy with punch or scissors with iridectomy ~ 66160
    thermocauterization with iridectomy ~ 66155
    trabeculectomy ab externo in absence previous surgery ~ 66170
    trabeculectomy ab externo with scarring ~ 66172
    trephination with iridectomy ~ 66150
  suture
    kidney ~ 50520-50526
    ureter ~ 50920-50930
    trachea ~ 31755
    tracheoesophageal
      repair ~ 43305, 43312, 43314
      speech prothesis ~ 31611
    ureter ~ 50920-50930
    urethra ~ 53400-53405
    urethrovaginal ~ 57310
      with bulbocavernosus transplant ~ 57311
    vesicouterine closure ~ 51920-51925
    vesicovaginal
      closure ~ 51900
      transvesical and vaginal approach ~ 57330
      vaginal approach ~ 57320
  X-ray ~ 76080
Fistulectomy, anal ~ 46060, 46270-46285
Fistulization
  conjunction to nasal cavity ~ 68745
  esophagus ~ 43352
  intestines ~ 44300-44346
  lacrimal sac to nasal cavity ~ 68720
  penis ~ 54435
  pharynx ~ 42955
  repair salivary cyst, sublingual ~ 42325-42326
  tracheopharyngeal ~ 31755
Fistulization, interatrial ~ 33735-33737
Fistulotomy, anal ~ 46270, 46280
Fitting
  cervical cap ~ 57170
  contact lens ~ 92071-92072, 92310-92313
  diaphragm ~ 57170
  low vision aid ~ 92354-92355
  ocular prosthesis ~ 92330
  spectacles ~ 92340-92342
  spectacle prosthesis ~ 92352-92353
Fitzgerald factor ~ 85293
Fixation, interdental without fracture ~ 21497
Fixation, external ~ see external fixation
Fixation, kidney ~ see nephropexy
Fixation, rectum ~ see proctopexy
Fixation (device) ~ see application; bone, fixation; spinal instrumentation
  application, external ~ 20690-20692, 20696-20697
  pelvic, insertion ~ 22848
  removal
    external ~ 20694
    internal ~ 20670-20680
  sacrospinous ligament, vaginal prolapse ~ 57282
  shoulder ~ 23700
  skeletal, humeral epycondyle, percutaneous ~ 24566
  spinal ~ see spinal instrumentation
Fixation test, complement ~ 86171
Flank ~ see back/flank
Flap ~ see skin graft and flap
  free, breast reconstruction ~ 19364
  grafts ~ 15570-15738, 15842
  latissimus dorsi breast reconstruction ~ 19361
  omentum ~ 49905

Flap ~ *continued*
  omentum, free, with microvascular anastomosis ~ 49906
  transverse rectus abdominis myocutaneous breast reconstruction ~ 19367-19369
Flatfoot correction ~ 28735
Flea typhus ~ 86000
Fletcher factor ~ 85292
Flow cytometry ~ 88182-88189
  diagnostic/pre-treatment ~ 3170F
Flow-volume loop, pulmonary ~ 94375
Fluid
  amniotic ~ see amniotic fluid
  body ~ 89060
  cerebrospinal ~ 86325
  collection, incision and drainage, skin ~ 10140
Fluorescein
  angiography, ocular ~ 92287
  intravenous injection
    vascular flow check, graft ~ 15860
Fluorescein angiography ~ 92235
Fluorescent in situ hybridization ~ 88365
Fluoride
  blood ~ 82735
  urine ~ 82735
Fluoroscopy
  examination
    angiography ~ 36901, 36902, 36903
    central venous access device~ 36598
    GI tract~ 74340
    larynx ~ 70370
    pharynx ~ 70370
  guidance
    abscess drainage~ 75989
    bile duct
      calculus removal~ 47544
      guide catheter~ 74328, 74330
    catheterization
      central venous~ 36597
      dialysis circuit ~ 36901, 36902, 36903
      renal artery~ 36251-36254
      spine/paraspinous~ 77003
    chest
      bronchoscopy~ 31622-31638, 31640, 31641, 31643, 31645, 31646, 31647-31649, 31651, 31660, 31661
    disc decompression~ 62287
    electrothermal annuloplasty~ 22526, 22527
    esophagoscopy~ 43213, 43214
    intubation
      colonic~ 49442, 49450
      duodenostomy~ 49441, 49451
      gastro-jejunostomy~ 49446, 49452
      gastrostomy~ 49440, 49446, 49450
      GI tract~ 74340
      jejunostomy~ 49441, 49446, 49451
      nasogastric~ 43752
      nephrostomy~ 50389
      orogastric~ 43752
    nephroureteral catheter
      replacement~ 50387
    spinal neurostimulator electrode
      removal~ 63661, 63662
      revision/replacement~ 63663, 63664
    stoma
      creation~ 49465
      removal of foreign body~ 49460
    thrombectomy
      arterial
        coronary ~ 92973
        intracranial ~ 61645
        noncoronary ~ 37184-37186
      venous ~ 37187, 37188
    vena cava filter
      insertion ~ 37191
      removal ~ 37193
      repositioning ~ 37192
    venous access device ~ 36598, 77001
  hourly ~ 76000
  needle biopsy ~ 77002
  unlisted services and procedures ~ 76496
Flurazepam, blood or urine ~ 80346, 80347
Flush aortogram ~ 36251-36254

FNA ~ see fine needle aspiration
Foam stability test ~ 83662
Fold, vocal ~ see vocal cords
Foley operation pyeloplasty ~ 50400-50405, 50544
Foley Y-pyeloplasty ~ 50400-50405
Folic acid ~ 82747
   blood ~ 82746
Follicle stimulating hormone (FSH) ~ 80418, 80426, 83001
Folliculin ~ 82679
Follitropin ~ 80418, 80426, 83001
Follow-up inpatient consultations ~ 99251-99255
Follow-up services
   post-op ~ 99024
Fontan procedure ~ 33600-33617
Food allergy test
   allergen-specific IgE ~ 86003, 86005, 86008
   challenge test ~ 95076, 95079
Foot ~ see metatarsal ~ 28456
   amputation ~ 28800-28805
   bursa incision and drainage ~ 28001
   capsulotomy ~ 28260-28264
   cast ~ 29450
   fasciectomy ~ 28060
     radical ~ 28060-28062
   fasciotomy ~ 28008
     endoscopic ~ 29893
   incision ~ 28002-28005
   joint ~ see tarsometatarsal joint ~ 28570-28576, 28585
     magnetic resonance imaging (MRI) ~ 73721-73723
   lesion excision ~ 28080, 28090
   magnetic resonance imaging (MRI) ~ 73718-73720
   nerve
     excision ~ 28055
     incision ~ 28035
   neuroma excision ~ 28080
   reconstruction cleft foot ~ 28360
   removal foreign body ~ 28190-28193
   repair
     muscle ~ 28250
     tendon ~ 28200-28230, 28234-28238
   replantation ~ 20838
   sesamoid excision ~ 28315
   strapping ~ 29540
   suture tendon ~ 28200-28210
   tendon sheath excision ~ 28086-28088
   tenotomy ~ 28230, 28234
   tumor excision ~ 28039-28047
   unlisted services and procedures ~ 28899
   X-ray ~ 73620-73630
Foot abscess ~ 28005
Forearm ~ see arm, lower ~ 20805
Forehead
   flap ~ 15731
   reconstruction ~ 21179, 21180, 21182-21184
     midface ~ 15730, 21159, 21160
   reduction ~ 21137-21139
Forehead and orbital rim
   reconstruction ~ 21172-21180
Foreign body removal
   anal ~ 46608
   arm
     lower ~ 25248
     upper ~ 24200, 24201
   auditory canal, external ~ 69200
     with anesthesia ~ 69205
   bronchi ~ 31635
   colon ~ 44025, 44390, 45332, 45379
   conjunctival, embedded ~ 65210
   cornea ~ 65220, 65222
   duodenum ~ 44010
   external eye ~ 65205
   eyelid ~ 67938
   finger ~ 26075, 26080
   foot ~ 28190, 28193
   gum ~ 41805
   hand ~ 26070
   hip ~ 27033, 27086, 27087
   intraocular ~ 65235
   knee joint ~ 27310, 27331, 27372
   lacrimal duct/gland ~ 68530

Foreign body removal ~ *continued*
   larynx ~ 31511, 31530, 31531, 31577
   leg, upper ~ 27372
   lung ~ 32151
   mandible ~ 41806
   maxillary sinus ~ 31299
   mediastinum ~ 39000, 39010
   mouth ~ 40804, 40805
   nose ~ 30300
     with anesthesia ~ 30310
     lateral rhinotomy ~ 30320
   orbit ~ 67413, 67430
   pancreatic duct ~ 43275-43276
   pelvis ~ 27086, 27087
   penis ~ 54115
   pericardium ~ 33020
     endoscopic ~ 32658
   pharynx ~ 42809
   pleura ~ 32150, 32151
     endoscopic ~ 32653
   rectum ~ 45307, 45915
   scrotum ~ 55120
   shoulder ~ 23040, 23044
     complicated ~ 23335
     deep ~ 23334
   subcutaneous 23330
   skin with debridement ~ 11010-11012
   subcutaneous ~ 10120, 10121
     with debridement ~ 11010-11012
   ureter ~ 50961, 50980
   urethra ~ 52310, 52315
   uterus ~ 58562
   vagina ~ 57415
Forensic exam
   autopsy ~ 88040
   cytopathology ~ 88125
Foreskin of penis ~ 54450
Formycin diphosphate ~ 85362-85380
Fournier's gangrene ~ 11004-11006
Fowler-Stephens orchiopexy ~ 54640, 54650, 54692
Fowler-Stephens procedure ~ 54650
Fox operation ~ 67921-67924
Fraction, factor IX (nine) ~ 85250
Fracture
   acetabulum
     closed treatment ~ 27220-27222
       with manipulation ~ 27222
       without manipulation ~ 27220
     open treatment ~ 27226-27228
   alveola
     closed treatment ~ 21421
     open treatment ~ 21422-21423
   alveolar ridge
     closed treatment ~ 21440
     open treatment ~ 21445
   ankle
     bimalleolar ~ 27808-27814
     closed treatment ~ 27816-27818
     lateral ~ 27786-27814, 27792
     medial ~ 27760-27766, 27808-27814
     posterior ~ 27767-27769, 27808-27814
     trimalleolar ~ 27816-27823
   ankle bone
     medial ~ 27760-27762
   Bennett's thumb fracture
     with dislocation ~ 26645, 26650
     open treatment ~ 26665
   bronchi endoscopy ~ 31630
   calcaneus
     closed treatment ~ 28400-28405
       with manipulation ~ 28405-28406
       without manipulation ~ 28400
     open treatment ~ 28415-28420
     percutaneous fixation ~ 28436
   carpal
     closed treatment
       with manipulation ~ 25624, 25635
       without manipulation ~ 25622, 25630
     open treatment ~ 25628, 25645

Fracture ~ *continued*

carpal scaphoid, closed treatment ~ 25622
cheekbone
  with manipulation ~ 21355
  open treatment ~ 21360-21366
clavicle
  closed treatment
    with manipulation ~ 23505
    without manipulation ~ 23500
  open treatment ~ 23515
  closed treatment ~ 27520
coccyx
  closed treatment ~ 27200
  open treatment ~ 27202
Colles ~ see Colles fracture
Colles-reversed ~ see Smith fracture
elbow
  Monteggia
    closed treatment ~ 24620
    open treatment ~ 24635
  open treatment ~ 24586-24587
femur ~ 27244
  closed treatment ~ 27230, 27238-27240, 27246, 27500-27503, 27508,
    27510, 27516-27517
    with manipulation ~ 27232
  distal ~ 27508, 27510, 27514
  epiphysis ~ 27516-27519
  intertrochanteric ~ 27244
    closed treatment ~ 27238
    intramedullary implant ~ 27245
    open treatment ~ 27244
      with implant ~ 27245
    with manipulation ~ 27240
  neck
    closed treatment ~ 27230
      with manipulation ~ 27232
    open treatment ~ 27236
    percutaneous fixation ~ 27235
  open treatment ~ 27245, 27248, 27506-27507, 27511-27514, 27519
  percutaneous fixation ~ 27235, 27509
  pertrochanteric
    closed treatment ~ 27238
      with manipulation ~ 27240
    intramedullary implant shaft ~ 27245, 27500, 27502, 27506-27507
    open treatment ~ 27245, 27245
  subtrochanteric
    closed treatment ~ 27238
      with manipulation ~ 27240
    intramedullary implant ~ 27245
    open treatment ~ 27245
  supracondylar ~ 27501-27503, 27509, 27511-27513
  transcondylar ~ 27501-27503, 27509, 27511-27513
  trochanteric
    closed treatment ~ 27246
    open treatment ~ 27248
  with manipulation ~ 27232, 27502-27503, 27510
  without manipulation ~ 27230, 27238, 27246, 27500-27501, 27508,
    27516-27517, 27520
fibula
  closed treatment ~ 27780-27781, 27786-27788, 27808-27810
  malleolus ~ 27786-27814
  open treatment ~ 27784, 27792, 27814
  shaft ~ 27780-27786, 27808
  with manipulation ~ 27788, 27810
  without manipulation ~ 27780-27781
frontal sinus, open treatment ~ 21343-21344
great toe
  closed treatment ~ 28490
  without manipulation ~ 28490
heel
  closed treatment
    with manipulation ~ 28405-28406
    without manipulation ~ 28400
  open treatment ~ 28415-28420
humerus
  closed treatment ~ 24500-24505
    with manipulation ~ 23605
    without manipulation ~ 23600

Fracture ~ *continued*

condyle
  closed treatment ~ 24576-24577
  open treatment ~ 24579
  percutaneous ~ 24582
epicondyle
  closed treatment ~ 24560-24565
  open treatment ~ 24575
  skeletal fixation, percutaneous ~ 24566
greater tuberosity fracture
  closed treatment with manipulation ~ 23625
  closed treatment without manipulation ~ 23620
  open treatment ~ 23630
  open treatment ~ 23615-23616
shaft ~ 24500-24505, 24516
  open treatment ~ 24515
supracondylar
  closed treatment ~ 24530-24535
  open treatment ~ 24545-24546
  percutaneous fixation ~ 24538
transcondylar
  closed treatment ~ 24530-24535
  open treatment ~ 24545-24546
  percutaneous fixation ~ 24538
with dislocation
  closed treatment ~ 23665
  open treatment ~ 23670
with shoulder dislocation
  closed treatment ~ 23675
  open treatment ~ 23680
hyoid bone
  closed treatment
    manipulation ~ 21494
    without manipulation ~ 21493
ilium
  open treatment ~ 27215, 27218
  percutaneous fixation ~ 27216
knee ~ 27520
  arthroscopic treatment ~ 29850-29851
  open treatment ~ 27524
larynx
  closed treatment
    with manipulation ~ 31586
    without manipulation ~ 31585
  open treatment ~ 31584
malar area
  open treatment ~ 21360-21366
  with bone graft ~ 21366
  with manipulation ~ 21355
mandible
  closed treatment
    interdental fixation ~ 21453
    with manipulation ~ 21451
    without manipulation ~ 21450
  open treatment ~ 21454-21470
    external fixation ~ 21454
    with interdental fixation ~ 21462
    without interdental fixation ~ 21461
  percutaneous treatment ~ 21452
maxilla
  closed treatment ~ 21421
  open treatment ~ 21422-21423
metacarpal
  closed treatment ~ 26600-26605
    with fixation ~ 26607
    with manipulation ~ 26605-26607
    without manipulation ~ 26600
  open treatment ~ 26615
  percutaneous fixation ~ 26608
metatarsal
  closed treatment ~ 28470-28475
    with manipulation ~ 28475-28476
    without manipulation ~ 28450, 28470
  open treatment ~ 28485
  percutaneous fixation ~ 28476
Monteggia ~ see fracture, ulna ~ 24620-24635
nasal bone
  closed treatment ~ 21310-21320
    with manipulation ~ 21315-21320
    without manipulation ~ 21310
  open treatment ~ 21325-21335

Fracture ~ *continued*
nasal septum
  closed treatment ~ 21337
  open treatment ~ 21336
nasal turbinate therapeutic ~ 30930
nasoethmoid
  open treatment ~ 21338-21339
  percutaneous treatment ~ 21340
  with fixation ~ 21340
nasomaxillary
  closed treatment ~ 21345
  open treatment ~ 21346-21348
  with bone grafting ~ 21348
  with fixation ~ 21345-21347
navicular
  closed treatment ~ 25622
  open treatment ~ 25628
  with manipulation ~ 25624
odontoid
  open treatment
    with graft ~ 22319
    without graft ~ 22318
orbit
  closed treatment
    with manipulation ~ 21401
    without manipulation ~ 21400
  open treatment ~ 21406-21408
    blowout fracture ~ 21385-21395
orbital floor
  blow out ~ 21385-21395
palate
  closed treatment ~ 21421
  open treatment ~ 21422-21423
patella
  closed treatment, without manipulation ~ 27520
  open treatment ~ 27524
pelvic ring
  closed treatment ~ 27197, 27198
  open treatment
    anterior ~ 27217
    posterior ~ 27218
  percutaneous fixation ~ 27216
  with manipulation ~ 27198
  without manipulation ~ 27197
phalanges
  articular
    closed treatment ~ 26740
    open treatment ~ 26746
    with manipulation ~ 26742
  closed treatment ~ 26742, 28510
    articular ~ 26740
    distal ~ 26750
    with manipulation ~ 26755
  distal ~ 26755-26756
    closed treatment ~ 26750
    open treatment ~ 26765
    percutaneous fixation ~ 26756
  finger/thumb
    closed treatment ~ 26720-26725
      with manipulation ~ 26725-26727
    shaft ~ 26720, 26727
  great toe ~ 28490
    closed treatment ~ 28495
      with manipulation ~ 28495-28496
    open treatment ~ 28505
    percutaneous fixation ~ 28496
  open treatment ~ 26735, 26746
    distal ~ 26765
  shaft
    closed treatment ~ 26725
    open treatment ~ 26735
    percutaneous fixation ~ 26727
  toe
    closed treatment ~ 28515
      with manipulation ~ 28515
      without manipulation ~ 28510
    open treatment ~ 28525
  with manipulation ~ 26742, 26755
  without manipulation ~ 26740, 26750

Fracture ~ *continued*
radius
  closed treatment ~ 25560-25565
  Colles ~ 25600-25605
  distal ~ 25600-25606
    open treatment ~ 25607-25609
    Smith ~ 25600-25605
  head/neck
    closed treatment ~ 24650-24655
    open treatment ~ 24665-24666
  open treatment ~ 25515, 25607-25609
  percutaneous fixation ~ 25606
  shaft ~ 25500, 25525-25526
    closed treatment ~ 25500-25505, 25520
    open treatment ~ 25515, 25525-25526, 25574
  with manipulation ~ 25565, 25605
  without manipulation ~ 25560, 25600
  with ulna ~ 25560-25565
    open treatment ~ 25575
rib
  with internal fixation ~ 21811-21813
risk assessment, CT scan ~ 0554T-0557T
scaphoid
  closed treatment ~ 25622
  open treatment ~ 25628
  with dislocation
    closed treatment ~ 25680
    open treatment ~ 25685
  with manipulation ~ 25624
scapula
  closed treatment
    with manipulation ~ 23575
    without manipulation ~ 23570
  open treatment ~ 23585
sesamoid
  closed treatment ~ 28530
  foot ~ 28530-28531
  open treatment ~ 28531
skin debridement ~ 11010-11012
skull ~ 62000-62010
sternum
  closed treatment ~ 21820
  open treatment ~ 21825
talus
  closed treatment ~ 28430-28435
  open treatment ~ 28445
  with manipulation ~ 28435-28436
  without manipulation ~ 28430
tarsal
  open treatment ~ 28465
  percutaneous fixation ~ 28456
  with manipulation ~ 28455-28456
thumb
  open treatment ~ 26665
  with dislocation ~ 26645-26650
tibia ~ 27759
  arthroscopic treatment ~ 29855-29856
  closed treatment ~ 27530-27532, 27538, 27750-27752, 27760-27762, 27808-27810, 27824-27825
  distal ~ 27824-27828
  intercondylar ~ 27538-27540
  malleolus ~ 27760-27766, 27808-27814
  open treatment ~ 27535-27536, 27540, 27758, 27766, 27814, 27826-27828
  percutaneous fixation ~ 27756
  plateau ~ 27530-27536, 29855-29856
  shaft ~ 27750-27759
  with manipulation ~ 27752, 27760-27762, 27810
  without manipulation ~ 27530, 27750, 27760-27762, 27808, 27825
trachea, endoscopy ~ 31630
ulna
  closed treatment ~ 25560-25565
  olecranon
    closed treatment ~ 24670-24675
    open treatment ~ 24685
  open treatment ~ 25574-25575
  shaft
    closed treatment ~ 25530-25535
    open treatment ~ 25545, 25574

Fracture ~ *continued*
   styloid process
     closed treatment ~ 25650
     open treatment ~ 25652
     percutaneous fixation ~ 25651
   with dislocation ~ 24620, 24635
     closed treatment ~ 24620
     Monteggia ~ 24620-24635
     open treatment ~ 24635
   with manipulation ~ 25535, 25565
   with radius ~ 25560-25565
     open treatment ~ 25575
   without manipulation ~ 25530, 25560
   vertebra
     additional segment, open treatment ~ 22328
     cervical, open treatment ~ 22326
     closed treatment
       with manipulation, casting and/or bracing ~ 22315
       without manipulation ~ 22310
     lumbar, open treatment ~ 22325
     posterior, open treatment ~ 22325-22327
     thoracic, open treatment ~ 22327
     with shoulder dislocation
       closed treatment ~ 23675
       open treatment ~ 23680
   wrist, with dislocation
     closed treatment ~ 25680
     open treatment ~ 25685
   zygomatic arch
     open treatment ~ 21356-21366
     with manipulation ~ 21355
Fragile-X chromosome analysis ~ 88248
Fragility
   red blood cell
     mechanical ~ 85547
     osmotic ~ 85555-85557
Frames, stereotactic ~ 20660
Francisella ~ 86000
   antibody ~ 86668
Fredet-Ramstedt procedure ~ 43520
Free E3 ~ 82677
Free skin graft ~ 15050-15157, 15200-15261, 15271-15278, 15757
Free T4 (four) ~ 84439
Frenectomy ~ 40819, 41115
Frenectomy, lingual ~ 41115
Frenotomy ~ 40806, 41010
Frenulectomy ~ 40819
Frenuloplasty ~ 41520
Frenum lip, incision ~ 40806
Frenumectomy ~ 40819
Frickman operation ~ see proctopexy
Frontal craniotomy ~ 61556
Frontal sinus ~ see sinus, frontal
Frontal sinusotomy ~ 31070-31075
Frost suture ~ 67875
Frozen blood preparation ~ 86930-86932
Fructose ~ 84375
   semen ~ 82757
Fructose intolerance breath test ~ 91065
Fruit sugar ~ 84375
FSF ~ 85290-85291
FSH ~ 80418, 80426, 83001
FT-4 ~ 84439
Fulguration ~ see destruction
   bladder ~ 51020
   cystourethroscopy with ~ 52214
     lesion ~ 52224
     tumor ~ 52234-52240
   ureter ~ 50957-50959, 50976-50978
   ureterocele
     ectopic ~ 52301
     orthotopic ~ 52300
Fulguration, endocavitary ~ 17000-17286
Full thickness graft ~ 15200-15261
Function, study, nasal ~ 92512
Function test, lung ~ see pulmonology, diagnostic
Function test, vestibular ~ see vestibular function tests

Fundoplasty
   esophagogastric ~ 43325
   esophagogastroduodenoscopic ~ 43210
     laparoscopic ~ 43279, 43280, 43282
     laparotomy ~ 43327
     via thoracotomy ~ 43328
   esophagomyotomy, laparoscopic ~ 43279
   paraesophageal hiatal hernia repair
     laparoscopic ~ 43281, 43282
     with fundoplication
       laparotomy ~ 43332, 43333
       thoracoabdominal incision ~ 43336, 43337
       thoracotomy ~ 43334, 43335
Fundoplication ~ **43325**
Fungus
   antibody ~ 86671
   culture
     blood ~ 87103
     hair ~ 87101
     identification ~ 87106
     nail ~ 87101
     other ~ 87102
     skin ~ 87101
   tissue exam ~ 87220
Funnel chest ~ 21740-21743
Furuncle
   incision and drainage ~ 10060-10061
   vulva ~ 56405
Fusion ~ see arthrodesis
   pleural cavity ~ 32560
   thumb in opposition ~ 26820
Fusion, epiphyseal-diaphyseal ~ see epiphyseal arrest
Fusion, joint ~ see arthrodesis
Fusion, joint, interphalangeal, finger ~ 26860-26863

G

Gabapentin assay ~ 80171
Gago procedure ~ 33463-33465
Gait training ~ 97116
Galactogram ~ 77053-77054
   injection ~ 19030
Galactokinase, blood ~ 82759
Galactose
   blood ~ 82760
   urine ~ 82760
Galactose-1-phosphate
   uridyl transferase ~ 82775-82776
Gallbladder ~ see also bile duct
   anastomosis with intestines ~ 47720-47741
   biopsy ~ 43261
   diagnostic imaging
     nuclear medicine ~ 78223, 78227
     X-ray with conrast ~ 74290
   destruction, calculi (stone) ~ 47544
   excision ~ 47562-47564, 47600-47620
   exploration ~ 47480
     endoscopic retrograde cholangio- pancreatography (ERCP)~ 43260
   fistulization ~ 47480, 47490
   incision ~ 47490
   incision and drainage ~ 47480
   removal, calculi (stone) ~ 47480, 47544
   repair
     with gastroenterostomy ~ 47741
     with intestines ~ 47720-47740
   unlisted services and procedures ~ 47999
   X-ray with contrast ~ 74290
Galvanocautery ~ 17000-17286
Galvanoionization ~ 97033
Gamete intrafallopian transfer ~ see GIFT
Gamete transfer, in vitro fertilization ~ 58976
Gamma camera imaging ~ see nuclear medicine
Gamma glutamyl transferase ~ 82977
Gamma seminoprotein ~ 84152-84153
Gammacorten ~ 80420
Gammaglobulin, blood ~ 82784-82787
Gamulin Rh ~ 90384-90386

Gastrointestinal, upper ~ continued
  removal
    foreign body ~ 43247
    lesion ~ 43250
    polyp ~ 43250-43251
    tumor ~ 43250
  tube placement, endoscopy ~ 43246
  ultrasound endoscopy ~ 43237-43238, 43242, 43259, 76975
Gastrojejunostomy ~ 43860-43865
  conversion from gastrostomy tube ~ 49446
  contrast injection ~ 49465
  removal of obstructive material ~ 49460
  replacement of tube ~ 49452
  with duodenal exclusion ~ 48547
  with partial gastrectomy ~ 43632
  with vagotomy ~ 43825
  without vagotomy ~ 43820
Gastroplasty
  Collis ~ 43283, 43338
  evision for obesity ~ 43644-43645, 43842-43848
  wedge gastroplasty ~ 43283, 43338
  with esophagogastric fundoplasty ~ 43842-43843
Gastrorrhaphy ~ 43840
Gastroschises ~ 49605
Gastrostomy
  closure ~ 43870
  laparoscopic, temporary ~ 43653
  temporary ~ 43830
    laparoscopic ~ 43653
    neonatal ~ 43831
  with pancreatic drain ~ 48001
  with pyloroplasty ~ 43640
  with vagotomy ~ 43640
Gastrostomy tube
  contrast injection ~ 49465
  conversion to gastro-jejunostomy tube ~ 49446
  directed placement, endoscopic ~ 43246
  insertion ~ 49440
  obstructive material removal ~ 49460
  placement, percutaneous
    endoscopic ~ 43246
    nonendoscopic ~ 49440
  replacement ~ 49450
  repositioning ~ 43761
Gastrotomy ~ 43500-43501, 43510
GDH ~ 82965
Gel diffusion ~ 86331
Gel diffusion test ~ 86329-86331
Gene Analysis
  Analytes
  ABCA4 (ATP-binding cassette, sub-family A [ABC1], member 4) ~ 81408
  ABCC8 (ATP-binding cassette, sub-family C [CFTR/MRP], member 8) ~ 81400, 81401, 81407
  ABCD1 (ATP-binding cassette, sub-family D [ALD], member 1) ~ 81405
  ABL1 (ABL proto-oncogene 1, non-receptor tyrosine kinase) ~ 81170, 81401
  ACADM (acyl-CoA dehydrogenase, C4 to C12 straight chain) ~ 81400, 81401
  ACADS (acyl-CoA dehydrogenase, C2 to C3 short chain) ~ 81404, 81405
  ACADVL (acyl-CoA dehydrogenase, very long chain) ~ 81406
  ACE (angiotensin I converting enzyme [peptidyl-dipeptidase A] 1) ~ 81400
  ACTA2 (actin, alpha 2, smooth muscle, aorta) ~ 81405
  ACTC1 (actin, alpha, cardiac muscle 1) ~ 81405
  ACTN4 (actinin, alpha 4) ~ 81405
  ADRB2 (adrenergic, beta-2-, receptor, surface) ~ 81401
  AFF2 (AF4/FMR2 family, member 2 [FMR2]) ~ 81401, 81404
  AFG3L2 (AFG3 ATPase family gene 3 like 2 [S. cerevisiae]) ~ 81406
  AGL (amylo-alpha-1, 6-glucosidase, 4-alpha-glucanotransferase) ~ 81407
  AHI1 (Abelson helper integration site 1) ~ 81407
  AIRE (autoimmune regulator) ~ 81406
  ALDH7A1 (aldehyde dehydrogenase 7 family, member A1) ~ 81406
  ANG (angiogenin, ribonuclease, RNase A family, 5) ~ 81403
  ANKRD1 (ankyrin repeat domain 1) ~ 81405
  ANO5 (anoctamin 5) ~ 81406
  ANOS1 (anosmin-1) ~ 81406

Gene Analysis ~ *continued*
  APOB (apolipoprotein B) ~ 81401
  APOE (apolipoprotein E) ~ 81401
  APP (amyloid beta [A4] precursor protein) ~ 81406
  AGTR1 (angiotensin II receptor, type 1) ~ 81400
  APC (adenomatous polyposis coli) ~ 81201, 81202
  APTX (aprataxin) ~ 81405
  AQP2 (aquaporin 2 [collecting duct]) ~ 81404
  AR (androgen receptor) ~ 81401, 81405
  ARSA (arylsulfatase A) ~ 81405
  ARX (aristaless related homeobox) ~ 81403, 81404
  ASPA (aspartoacylase) ~ 81200
  ASPM (asp [abnormal spindle] homolog, microcephaly associated [Drosophila]) ~ 81407
  ASS1 (argininosuccinate synthase 1) ~ 81406
  ASXL1 (additional sex combs like 1, transcriptional regulator) ~ 81175, 81176
  ATL1 (atlastin GTPase 1) ~ 81406
  ATM (ataxia telangiectasia mutated) ~ 81408
  ATN1 (atrophin 1) ~ 81401
  ATP1A2 (ATPase, Na+/K+ transporting, alpha 2 polypeptide) ~ 81406
  ATP7B (ATPase, Cu++ transporting, beta polypeptide) ~ 81406
  ATXN1 (ataxin 1) ~ 81401
  ATXN2 (ataxin 2) ~ 81401
  ATXN3 (ataxin 3) ~ 81401
  ATXN7 (ataxin 7) ~ 81401
  ATXN8OS (ATXN8 opposite strand [non-protein coding]) ~ 81401
  ATXN10 (ataxin 10) ~ 81401
  AVPR2 (arginine vasopressin receptor 2) ~ 81404
  BBS1 (Bardet-Biedl syndrome 1) ~ 81406
  BBS2 (Bardet-Biedl syndrome 2) ~ 81406
  BBS10 (Bardet-Biedl syndrome 10) ~ 81404
  BCKDHA (branched chain keto acid dehydrogenase E1, alpha polypeptide) ~ 81400, 81405
  BCKDHB (branched chain keto acid dehydrogenase E1, beta polypeptide) ~ 81205, 81406
  BCL1/IgH, t(11;14) ~ 81401
  BCR/ABL1 (chronic myelogenous leukemia) Translocation ~ 81206-81208
  BCS1L (BCS1-like [S. cerevisiae]) ~ 81405
  BEST1 (bestrophin 1) ~ 81406
  BLM (Bloom syndrome, RecQ helicase-like) ~ 81209
  BMPR2 (bone morphogenetic protein receptor, type II [serine/threonine kinase]) ~ 81405, 81406
  BRAF (B-Raf proto-oncogene , serine/threonine kinase) ~ 81210, 81406
  BRCA1 variants ~ 81212
    duplication/deletion ~ 81162, 81164
    full sequence ~ 81162, 81165
    known familial variant ~ 81215
  BRCA2 variants ~ 81212
    duplication/deletion ~ 81162, 81167
    full sequence ~ 81162, 81216
    known familial variant ~ 81217
  BSCL2 (Berardinelli-Seip congenital lipodystrophy 2 [seipin]) ~ 81406
  BTD (biotinidase) ~ 81404
  BTK (Bruton agammaglobulinemia tyrosine kinase) ~ 81406
  C10orf2 (chromosome 10 open reading frame 2) ~ 81404
  CACNA1A (calcium channel, voltagedependent, P/Q type, alpha 1A subunit) ~ 81401, 81407
  CACNB2 (calcium channel, voltage-dependent, beta 2 subunit) ~ 81406
  CALR (calreticulin) (eg, myeloproliferative disorders) ~ 81219
  CAPN3 (calpain 3) ~ 81406
  CASQ2 (calsequestrin 2 [cardiac muscle]) ~ 81405
  CASR (calcium-sensing receptor) ~ 81405
  CAV3 (caveolin 3) ~ 81404
  CBFB/MYH11 (inv (16)) ~ 81401
  CBS (cystathionine-beta-synthase) ~ 81401, 81406
  CCND1/IGH (t(11;14)) ~ 81168
  CD40LG (CD40 ligand) ~ 81404
  CCND1/IGH (BCL1/IgH, t(11;14)) ~ 81401
  CCR5 (chemokine C-C motif receptor 5) ~ 81400
  CDH1 (cadherin 1, type 1, E-cadherin [epithelial]) ~ 81406
  CDH23 (cadherin-related 23) ~ 81408
  CDKL5 (cyclin-dependent kinase-like 5) ~ 81405, 81406
  CDKN2A (cyclin-dependent kinase inhibitor 2A) ~ 81404
  CEBPA (CCAAT/enhancer binding protein [C/EBP], alpha) ~ 81218
  CEL (carboxyl ester lipase [bile salt stimulated lipase]) ~ 81403
  CEP290 (centrosomal protein 290kDa) ~ 81408

Gene Analysis ~ *continued*

CFH/ARMS2 (complement factor H/age-related maculopathy susceptibility 2) ~ 81401

CFTR (cystic fibrosis transmembrane conductance regulator) ~ 81220-81224

CHD7 (chromodomain helicase DNA binding protein 7) ~ 81407

CHRNA4 (cholinergic receptor, nicotinic, alpha 4) ~ 81405

CHRNB2 (cholinergic receptor, nicotinic, beta 2 [neuronal]) ~ 81405

Chromosome 1p-/19q- ~ 81402

Chromosome 18q- ~ 81402

CLCN1 (chloride channel 1, skeletal muscle) ~ 81406

CLCNKB (chloride channel, voltage-sensitive Kb) ~ 81406

CLRN1 (clarin 1) ~ 81400, 81404

CNBP (CCHC-type zinc finger, nucleic acid binding protein) ~ 81401

CNTNAP2 (contactin associated protein-like 2) ~ 81406

COL1A1 (collagen, type I, alpha 1) ~ 81408

COL1A1/PDGFB (t(17;22)) ~ 81402

COL1A2 (collagen, type I, alpha 2) ~ 81408

COL4A1 (collagen, type IV, alpha 1) ~ 81408

COL4A3 (collagen, type IV, alpha 3 [Goodpasture antigen]) ~ 81408

COL4A4 (collagen, type IV, alpha 4) ~ 81407

COL4A5 (collagen, type IV, alpha 5) ~ 81407, 81408

COL6A1 (collagen, type VI, alpha 1) ~ 81407

COL6A2 (collagen, type VI, alpha 2) ~ 81406, 81407

COL6A3 (collagen, type VI, alpha 3) ~ 81407

COX6B1 (cytochrome c oxidase subunit VIb polypeptide 1) ~ 81404

COX10 (COX10 homolog, cytochrome c oxidase assembly protein) ~ 81405

COX15 (COX15 homolog, cytochrome c oxidase assembly protein) ~ 81405

CPOX (coproporphyrinogen oxidase) ~ 81405

CPT1A (carnitine palmitoyltransferase 1A [liver]) ~81406

CPT2 (carnitine palmitoyltransferase 2) 81404

CRB1 (crumbs homolog 1 [Drosophila]) ~ 81406

CREBBP (CREB binding protein) ~ 81406, 81407

CRX (cone-rod homeobox) ~ 81404

CSTB (cystatin B [stefin B]) ~ 81401, 81404

CTNNB1 (catenin [cadherin-associated protein], beta 1, 88kDa) ~ 81403

CTRC (chymotrypsin C) (eg, hereditary pancreatitis) ~ 81405

CYP1B1 (cytochrome P450, family 1, subfamily B, polypeptide 1) ~ 81404

CYP21A2 (cytochrome P450, family 21, subfamily A, polypeptide 2) ~ 81402, 81405

CYP2C19 (cytochrome P450, family 2, subfamily C, polypeptide 19) ~ 81225

CYP2C9 (cytochrome P450, family 2, subfamily C, polypeptide 9) ~ 81227

CYP2D6 (cytochrome P450, family 2, subfamily D, polypeptide 6) ~ 81226

CYP3A4 (cytochrome P450, family 3, subfamily A member 4) ~ 81230

CYP3A5 (cytochrome P450, family 3, subfamily A member 5) ~ 81231

CYP11B1 (cytochrome P450, family 11, subfamily B, polypeptide 1) ~ 81405

CYP17A1 (cytochrome P450, family 17, subfamily A, polypeptide 1) ~ 81405

CYP21A2 (cytochrome P450, family 21, subfamily A, polypeptide2) ~ 81402, 81405

Constitution ~ 81228, 81229

Neoplasia. ~ 81277, 81406

DAZ/SRY (deleted in azoospermia and sex determining region Y) ~ 81403

DBT (dihydrolipoamide branched chain transacylase E2) ~ 81405, 81406

DCX (doublecortin) ~ 81405

DEK/NUP214 (t(6;9)) ~ 81401

DES (desmin) ~ 81405

DFNB59 (deafness, autosomal recessive 59) ~ 81405

DGUOK (deoxyguanosine kinase) ~ 81405

DHCR7 (7-dehydrocholesterol reductase) ~ 81405

DLAT (dihydrolipoamide S-acetyltransferase) ~ 81406

DLD (dihydrolipoamide dehydrogenase) ~ 81406

DMD (dystrophin) ~ 81161, 81408

DMPK (dystrophia myotonica-protein kinase) ~ 81401, 81404

DNMT3A (DNA [cytosine-5-]-methyltransferase 3 alpha) ~ 81403

DPYD (dihydropyrimidine dehydrogenase) ~ 81232

DSC2 (desmocollin) ~ 81406

DSG2 (desmoglein 2) ~ 81406

DSP (desmoplakin) ~ 81406

Gene Analysis ~ *continued*

DYSF (dysferlin, limb girdle muscular dystrophy 2B [autosomal recessive]) ~ 81408

E2A/PBX1 (t(1;19)) ~ 81401

EFHC1 (EF-hand domain [C terminal] containing 1) ~ 81406

EGFR (epidermal growth factor receptor) 81235

EGR2 (early growth response 2) ~ 81404

EIF2B2 (eukaryotic translation initiation factor 2B, subunit 2 beta, 39kDa) ~ 81405

EIF2B3 (eukaryotic translation initiation factor 2B, subunit 3 gamma, 58kDa) ~ 81406

EIF2B4 (eukaryotic translation initiation factor 2B, subunit 4 delta, 67kDa) ~ 81406

EIF2B5 (eukaryotic translation initiation factor 2B, subunit 5 epsilon, 82kDa) ~ 81406

EMD (emerin) ~ 81404, 81405

EML4/ALK (inv(2)) ~ 81401

ENG (endoglin) ~ 81405, 81406

EPCAM (epithelial cell adhesion molecule) ~ 81403

EPM2A (epilepsy, progressive myoclonus type 2A, Lafora disease [laforin]) ~ 81404

ERBB2 (HER2) ~ 0009U

ESR1/PGR (receptor 1/progesterone receptor) ~ 81402

ETV6/NTRK3 (t(12;15)) ~ 81401

ETV6/RUNX1 (t(12;21)) ~ 81401

EWSR1/ATF1 (t1(2;22)) ~ 81401

EWSR1/ERG (t(21;22)) ~ 81401

EWSR1/FLI1 (t(11;22)) ~ 81401

EWSR1/WT1 (t(11;22)) ~ 81401

EYA1 (eyes absent homolog 1 [Drosophila]) ~ 81405, 81406

F2 (prothrombin, coagulation factor II) ~ 81240, 81400

F5 (coagulation factor V) ~ 81241, 81400

F7 (coagulation factor VII [serum prothrombin conversion accelerator]) ~ 81400

F8 (coagulation factor VIII) ~ 81403, 81406, 81407

F9 (coagulation factor IX) ~ 81238

F11 (coagulation factor XI) ~ 81401

F12 (coagulation factor XII [Hageman factor]) ~ 81403

F13B (coagulation factor XIII, B polypeptide) ~ 81400

FAH (fumarylacetoacetate hydrolase [fumarylacetoacetase]) ~ 81406

FANCC (Fanconi anemia, complementation group C) ~ 81242

FASTKD2 (FAST kinase domains 2) ~ 81406

FBN1 (fibrillin 1) ~ 81408

FGB (fibrinogen beta chain) ~ 81400

FGF23 (fibroblast growth factor 23) ~ 81404

FGFR1 (fibroblast growth factor receptor 1) ~ 81400, 81405

FGFR2 (fibroblast growth factor receptor 2) ~ 81404

FGFR3 (fibroblast growth factor receptor 3) ~ 81400, 81401, 81403, 81404

FH (fumarate hydratase) ~ 81405

FHL1 (four and a half LIM domains 1) ~ 81404

FIG4 (FIG4 homolog, SAC1 lipid phosphatase domain containing [S. cerevisiae]) ~ 81406

FIP1L1/PDGFRA (del(4q12)) ~ 81401

FKRP (fukutin related protein) ~ 81404

FKTN (fukutin) ~ 81400, 81405

FLG (filaggrin) ~ 81401

FLT3 (fms-related tyrosine kinase 3) ~ 81245, 81246

FMR1 (fragile X mental retardation 1) ~ 81243, 81244

FOXG1 (forkhead box G1) ~ 81404

FOXO1/PAX3 (t(2;13)) ~ 81401

FOXO1/PAX7 (t(1;13)) ~ 81401

FSHMD1A (facioscapulohumeral muscular dystrophy 1A) ~ 81404

FTSJ1 (FtsJ RNA methyltransferase homolog 1 [E. coli]) ~ 81405, 81406

FUS (fused in sarcoma) ~ 81406

FUS/DDIT3 (t(12;16)) ~ 81401

FXN (frataxin) ~ 81401, 81404

G6PC (glucose-6-phosphatase, catalytic subunit) ~ 81250

G6PD (glucose-6-phosphate dehydrogenase) ~ 81247-81249

GAA (glucosidase, alpha; acid) ~ 81406

GABRG2 (gamma-aminobutyric acid [GABA] A receptor, gamma 2) ~ 81405

GALC (galactosylceramidase) ~ 81401, 81406

GALT (galactose-1-phosphate uridylyltransferase) ~ 81401, 81406

GARS (glycyl-tRNA synthetase) ~ 81406

GBA (glucosidase, beta, acid) ~ 81251

GCDH (glutaryl-CoA dehydrogenase) ~ 81406

1145

Gene Analysis ~ *continued*

- GCH1 (GTP cyclohydrolase 1) ~ 81405
- GCK (glucokinase [hexokinase 4]) ~ 81406
- GDAP1 (ganglioside-induced differentiationassociated protein 1) ~ 81405
- GFAP (glial fibrillary acidic protein) ~ 81405
- GH1 (growth hormone 1) ~ 81404
- GHR (growth hormone receptor) ~ 81405
- GHRHR (growth hormone releasing hormone receptor) ~ 81405
- GJB1 (gap junction protein, beta 1) ~ 81403
- GJB2 (gap junction protein, beta 2, 26kDa, connexin 26) ~ 81252, 81253
- GJB6 (gap junction protein, beta 6, 30kDa, connexin 30) ~ 81254
- GLA (galactosidase, alpha) ~ 81405
- GLUD1 (glutamate dehydrogenase 1) ~ 81406
- GNAQ (guanine nucleotide-binding protein G[q] subunit alpha) ~ 81403
- GNE (glucosamine [UDP-N-acetyl]-2-epimerase/N-acetylmannosamine kinase) ~ 81400, 81406
- GP1BB (glycoprotein Ib [platelet], beta polypeptide) ~ 81404
- GRN (granulin) ~ 81406
- H19 (imprinted maternally expressed transcript [non-protein coding]) ~ 81401
- HADHA (hydroxyacyl-CoA dehydrogenase/3-ketoacyl-CoA thiolase/enoyl-CoA hydratase [trifunctional protein] alpha subunit) ~ 81406
- HADHB (hydroxyacyl-CoA dehydrogenase/ 3 ketoacyl-CoA thiolase/enoyl-CoA hydratase [trifunctional protein], beta subunit) ~ 81406
- HBA1/HBA2 (alpha globin 1 and alpha globin 2) ~ 81257-81259, 81269
- HBB (hemoglobin, beta, beta-Globin) ~ 81361-81364
- HEXA (hexosaminidase A [alpha polypeptide]) ~ 81255, 81406
- HFE (hemochromatosis) ~ 81256
- HLA Class I and II Typing, Low Resolution ~ 81370, 81371
- HLA Class I Typing, Low Resolution ~ 81372-81374
- HLA Class II Typing, Low Resolution ~ 81375-81377
- HLA Class I and II Typing, High Resolution ~ 81378
- HLA Class I Typing, High Resolution ~ 81379-81381
- HLA Class II Typing,High Resolution ~ 81382, 81383
- HLCS (HLCS holocarboxylase synthetase) ~ 81406
- HMBS (hydroxymethylbilane synthase) ~ 81406
- HNF1A (HNF1 homeobox A) ~ 81405
- HPA (Human Platelet Antigen) ~ 81105-81112
- HNF1B (HNF1 homeobox B) ~ 81404, 81405
- HNF4A (hepatocyte nuclear factor 4, alpha) ~ 81406
- HRAS (v-Ha-ras Harvey rat sarcoma viral oncogene homolog) ~ 81403, 81404
- HSD3B2 (hydroxyl-delta-5-steroid dehydrogenase, 3 beta- and steroid-delta isomerase 2) ~ 81404
- HSD11B2 (hydroxysteroid [11-beta] dehydrogenase 2) ~ 81404
- HSPB1 (heat shock 27kDa protein 1) ~ 81404
- HTRA1 (HtrA serine peptidase 1) ~ 81405
- HTT (huntingtin) ~ 81401
- Human Erythrocyte Antigen. ~ 81403
- Human Platelet Antigen 1 (HPA-1) ~ 81105
- Human Platelet Antigen 2 (HPA-2) ~ 81106
- Human Platelet Antigen 3 (HPA-3) ~ 81107
- Human Platelet Antigen 4 (HPA-4) ~ 81108
- Human Platelet Antigen 5 (HPA-5) ~ 81109
- Human Platelet Antigen 6 (HPA-6w) ~ 81110
- Human Platelet Antigen 9 (HPA-9w) ~ 81111
- Human Platelet Antigen 15 (HPA-15) ~ 81112
- IDH1 (isocitrate dehydrogenase 1 [NADP+], soluble) ~ 81120
- IDH2 (isocitrate dehydrogenase 2 [NADP+], mitochondrial) ~ 81121
- IDS (iduronate 2-sulfatase) ~ 81405
- IDUA (iduronidase, alpha L-) ~ 81406
- IFNL3 (interferon, lambda 3) ~ 81283
- IGH@ (immunoglobulin heavy chain locus) ~ 81261-81263
- IGH@/BCL2 (t(14;18)) ~ 81278, 81401
- IGK@ (immunoglobulin kappa light chain locus) ~ 81264
- IKBKAP (inhibitor of kappa light polypeptide gene enhancer in B-cells, kinase complex-associated protein) ~ 81260
- IL2RG (interleukin 2 receptor, gamma) ~ 81405
- INF2 (inverted formin, FH2 and WH2 domain containing) ~ 81406
- INS (insulin) ~ 81404
- ISPD (isoprenoid synthase domain containing) ~ 81405
- ITPR1 (inositol 1,4,5-trisphosphate receptor, type 1) ~ 81408
- IVD (isovaleryl-CoA dehydrogenase) ~ 81400, 81406
- JAG1 (jagged 1) ~ 81406, 81407
- JAK2 (Janus kinase 2) ~ 81270, 81279

Gene Analysis ~ *continued*

- JUP (junction plakoglobin) ~ 81406
- KCNC3 (potassium voltage-gated channel, Shaw-related subfamily, member 3) ~ 81403
- KCNH2 (potassium voltage-gated channel, subfamily H [eag-related], member 2) ~ 81406
- KCNJ2 (potassium inwardly-rectifying chanel, subfamily J, member 2) ~ 81403
- KCNJ1 (potassium inwardly-rectifying channel, subfamily J, member 1) ~ 81404
- KCNJ10 (potassium inwardly-rectifying channel, subfamily J, member 10) ~ 81404
- KCNJ11 (potassium inwardly-rectifying channel, subfamily J, member 11) ~ 81403
- KCNQ1 (potassium voltage-gated channel, KQT-like subfamily, member 1) ~ 81406
- KCNQ1OT1 (KCNQ1 overlapping transcript 1 [non-protein coding]) ~ 81401
- KCNQ2 (potassium voltage-gated channel, KQT-like subfamily, member 2) ~ 81406
- KDM5C (lysine [K]-specific demethylase 5C) ~ 81407
- KIAA0196 (KIAA0196) ~ 81407
- Killer cell immunoglobulin-like receptor (KIR) gene family ~ 81403
- KIT (v-kit Hardy-Zuckerman 4 feline sarcoma viral oncogene homolog) ~ 81272, 81273
- Known familial variant not otherwise specified. ~ 81403
- KRAS (Kirsten rat sarcoma viral oncogene homolog) ~ 81275, 81276, 81405
- L1CAM (L1 cell adhesion molecule) ~ 81407
- LAMA2 (laminin, alpha 2) ~ 81408
- LAMB2 (laminin, beta 2 [laminin S]) ~ 81407
- LAMP2 (lysosomal-associated membrane protein 2) ~ 81405
- LCT (lactase-phlorizin hydrolase) ~ 81400
- LDB3 (LIM domain binding 3) ~ 81406
- LDLR (low density lipoprotein receptor) ~ 81405, 81406
- LEPR (leptin receptor) ~ 81406
- LHCGR (luteinizing hormone/ choriogonadotropin receptor) ~ 81406
- LINC00518 (long intergenic non-protein coding RNA 518) ~ 81401
- LITAF (lipopolysaccharide-induced TNF factor) ~ 81404
- LMNA (lamin A/C) ~ 81406
- LRP5 (low density lipoprotein receptor-related protein 5) ~ 81406
- LRRK2 (leucine-rich repeat kinase 2) ~ 81401, 81408
- MAP2K1 (mitogen-activated protein kinase 1) ~ 81406
- MAP2K2 (mitogen-activated protein kinase 2) ~ 81406
- MAPT (microtubule-associated protein tau) ~ 81406
- MC4R (melanocortin 4 receptor) ~ 81403
- MCCC1 (methylcrotonoyl-CoA carboxylase 1 [alpha]) ~ 81406
- MCCC2 (methylcrotonoyl-CoA carboxylase 2 [beta]) ~ 81406
- MCOLN1 (mucolipin 1) ~ 81290
- MECP2 (methyl CpG binding protein 2 [Rett syndrome]) ~ 81302-81306
- MED12 (mediator complex subunit 12) ~ 81401
- MEFV (Mediterranean fever) ~ 81402, 81404
- MEG3/DLK1 (maternally expressed 3 [non-protein coding]/delta-like 1 homolog [Drosophila]) ~ 81401
- MEN1 (multiple endocrine neoplasia I) ~ 81404, 81405
- MFN2 (mitofusin 2) ~ 81406
- MGMT (O-6-methylguanine DNA methyltransferase) ~ 81287
- MICA (MHC class I polypeptide-related sequence A) ~ 81403
- MLH1 (mutL homolog 1, colon cancer, nonpolyposis type 2) ~ 81288, 81292-81294
- MLL/AFF1 (t(4;11)) ~ 81401
- MLL/MLLT3 (t(9;11)) ~ 81401
- MMAA (methylmalonic aciduria [cobalamine deficiency] type A) ~ 81405
- MMAB (methylmalonic aciduria [cobalamine deficiency] type B) ~ 81405
- MMACHC (methylmalonic aciduria [cobalamin deficiency] cblC type, with
- homocystinuria) ~ 81404
- MPI (mannose phosphate isomerase) ~ 81405
- MPL (MPL proto-oncogene, thrombopoietin receptor) ~ 81338, 81339
- MPV17 (MpV17 mitochondrial inner membrane protein) ~ 81404, 81405
- MPZ (myelin protein zero) ~ 81405
- MSH2 (mutS homolog 2, colon cancer, nonpolyposis type 1) ~ 81295-81297
- MSH6 (mutS homolog 6 [E. coli]) ~ 81298-81300
- MT-ATP6 (mitochondrially encoded ATP synthase 6) ~ 81401

Gene Analysis ~ *continued*

MT-ND4, MT-ND6 (mitochondrially encoded NADH dehydrogenase 4, mitochondrially encoded NADH dehydrogenase 6) ~ 81401

MT-RNR1 (mitochondrially encoded 12S RNA) ~ 81401, 81403

MT-TK (mitochondrially encoded tRNA lysine) ~ 81401

MT-TL1 (mitochondrially encoded tRNA leucine 1 [UUA/G]) ~ 81401

MT-TL1, MT-ND5 (mitochondrially encoded tRNA leucine 1 [UUA/G], tochondrially encoded NADH dehydrogenase 5) ~ 81401

MT-TS1 (mitochondrially encoded tRNA serine 1) ~ 81403

MT-TS1, MT-RNR1 (mitochondrially encoded tRNA serine 1 [UCN], mitochondrially encoded 12S RNA) ~ 81401

MTM1 (myotubularin 1) ~ 81405, 81406

MTHFR (5, 10-methylenetetrahydrofolate reductase) ~ 81291

MUT (methylmalonyl CoA mutase) ~ 81406

MUTYH (mutY homolog [E. coli]) ~ 81401, 81406

MYBPC3 (myosin binding protein C, cardiac) ~ 81407

MYH6 (myosin, heavy chain 6, cardiac muscle, alpha) ~ 81407

MYH7 (myosin, heavy chain 7, cardiac muscle, beta) ~ ~ 81407

MYH11 (myosin, heavy chain 11, smooth muscle) ~ 81408

MYL2 (myosin, light chain 2, regulatory, cardiac, slow) ~ 81405

MYL3 (myosin, light chain 3, alkali, ventrcular, skeletal, slow) ~ 81405

MYO7A (myosin VIIA) ~ 81407

MYOT (myotilin) ~ 81405

NDP (Norrie disease [pseudoglioma]) ~ 81403, 81404

NDUFA1 (NADH dehydrogenase [ubiquinone] 1 alpha subcomplex, 1, 7.5kDa) ~ 81404

NDUFAF2 (NADH dehydrogenase [ubiquinone] 1 alpha subcomplex, assembly factor 2) ~ 81404

NDUFS1 (NADH dehydrogenase [ubiquinone] Fe-S protein 1, 75kDa [NADH-coenzyme Q reductase]) ~ 81406

NDUFS4 (NADH dehydrogenase [ubiquinone] Fe-S protein 4, 18kDa [NADH-coenzyme Q reductase]) ~ 81404

NDUFS7 (NADH dehydrogenase [ubiquinone] Fe-S protein 7, 20kDa [NADH-coenzyme Q reductase]) ~ 81405

NDUFS8 (NADH dehydrogenase [ubiquinone] Fe-S protein 8, 23kDa [NADH-coenzyme Q reductase]) ~ 81405

NDUFV1 (NADH dehydrogenase [ubiquinone] flavoprotein 1, 51kDa) ~ 81405

NEB (nebulin) ~ 81400, 81408

NEFL (neurofilament, light polypeptide) 81405

NF1 (neurofibromin 1) ~ 81408

NF2 (neurofibromin 2 [merlin]) ~ 81405, 81406

NHLRC1 (NHL repeat containing 1) ~ 81403

NIPA1 (non-imprinted in Prader-Willi/ Angelman syndrome 1) ~ 81404

NLGN3 (neuroligin 3) ~ 81405

NLGN4X (neuroligin 4, X-linked) ~ 81404, 81405

NOD2 (nucleotide-binding oligomerization domain containing 2) ~ 81401

NOTCH1 (notch 1) ~ 81407

NOTCH3 (notch 3) ~ 81406

NPC1 (Niemann-Pick disease, type C1) ~ 81406

NPC2 (Niemann-Pick disease, type C2 [epididymal secretory protein E1]) ~ 81404

NPHP1 (nephronophthisis 1 [juvenile]) ~ 81405, 81406

NPHS1 (nephrosis 1, congenital, Finnish type [nephrin]) ~ 81407

NPHS2 (nephrosis 2, idiopathic, steroid resistant [podocin]) ~ 81405

NPM1 (nucleophosmin [nucleolar phosphoprotein B23, numatrin]) ~ 81310

NPM1/ALK (t(2;5)) ~ 81401

NRAS (neuroblastoma RAS viral [v-ras] oncogene homolog) ~ 81311

NR0B1 (nuclear receptor subfamily 0, group B, member 1) ~ 81404

NSD1 (nuclear receptor binding SET domain protein 1) ~ 81405, 81406

NRTK (neurotrophic-tropomyosin receptor tyrosine kinase 1,2,and3) ~ 81194

NRTK1 (neurotrophic receptor tyrosine kinase 1) ~ 81191

NRTK2 (neurotrophic receptor tyrosine kinase 2) ~ 81192

NRTK3 (neurotrophic receptor tyrosine kinase 3) ~ 81193

NUDT15 (nudix hydrolase 15) ~ 81306

OPA1 (optic atrophy 1) ~ 81406, 81407

OPTN (optineurin) ~ 81406

OTC (ornithine carbamoyltransferase) ~ 81405

PABPN1 (poly[A] binding protein, nuclear 1) ~ 81401

PAFAH1B1 (platelet-activating factor acetylhydrolase 1b, regulatory subunit 1 [45kDa]) ~ 81405, 81406

PAH (phenylalanine hydroxylase) ~ 81406

PALB2 (partner and localizer of BRCA2) 81307, 81308

PARK2 (Parkinson protein 2, E3 ubiquitin protein ligase [parkin]) ~ 81405, 81406

Gene Analysis ~ *continued*

PAX2 (paired box 2) ~ 81406

PAX8/PPARG (t(2;3) (q13;p25)) ~ 81401

PC (pyruvate carboxylase) ~ 81406

PCA3/KLK3 (prostate cancer antigen 3 [non protein coding]/kallikrein related peptidase 3 [prostate specific antigen]) ~ 81313

PCCA (propionyl CoA carboxylase, alpha polypeptide) ~ 81405, 81406

PCCB (propionyl CoA carboxylase, beta polypeptide) ~ 81406

PCDH15 (protocadherin-related 15) ~ 81400, 81406, 81407

PCDH19 (protocadherin 19) ~ 81405

PCSK9 (proprotein convertase subtilisin/kevin type 9) ~ 81406

PDGFRA (platelet-derived growth factor receptor, alpha polypeptide) ~ 81314

PDHA1 (pyruvate dehydrogenase [lipoamide] alpha 1) ~ 81405, 81406

PDHB (pyruvate dehydrogenase [lipoamide] beta) ~ 81405

PDHX (pyruvate dehydrogenase complex, component X) ~ 81406

PDX1 (pancreatic and duodenal homeobox 1) ~ 81404

PHEX (phosphate regulating endopeptidase homolog, X-linked) ~ 81406

PHOX2B (paired-like homeobox 2b) ~ 81403, 81404

PIK3CA (phosphatidylinositol-4,5-bisphosphate 3-kinase, catalytic subunit alpha) ~ 81309

PINK1 (PTEN induced putative kinase 1) ~ 81405

PKD1 (polycystic kidney disease1 [autosomal dominant]) ~ 81407

PKD2 (polycystic kidney disease 2 [autosomal dominant]) ~ 81406

PKHD1 (polycystic kidney and hepatic disease 1) ~ 81408

PKLR (pyruvate kinase, liver and RBC) (eg, pyruvate kinase deficiency) ~ 81405

PKP2 (plakophilin 2) ~ 81406

PLCE1 (phospholipase C, epsilon 1) ~ 81407

PLN (phospholamban) ~ 81403

PLP1 (proteolipid protein 1) ~ 81404, 81405

PML/RARalpha, (t(15;17)) (promyelocytic leukemia/retinoic acid receptor alpha) ~ 81315, 81316

PMP22 (peripheral myelin protein 22) ~ 81324-81326

PMS2 (PMS2 postmeiotic segregation increased 2 [S. cerevisiae]) ~ 81317-81319

PNKD (paroxysmal nonkinesigenic dyskinesia) ~ 81406

POLG (polymerase [DNA directed], gamma) ~ 81406

POMGNT1 (protein O-linked mannose beta1, 2-N-cetylglucosaminyltransferase) ~ 81406

POMT1 (protein-O-mannosyltransferase 1) ~ 81406

POMT2 (protein-O-mannosyltransferase 2) ~ 81406

POU1F1 (POU class 1 homeobox 1) ~ 81405

PPOX (protoporphyrinogen oxidase) ~ 81406

PPP2R2B (protein phosphatase 2, regulatory subunit B, beta) ~ 81401

PQBP1 (polyglutamine binding protein 1) ~ 81404, 81405

PRAME (preferentially expressed antigen in melanoma) ~ 81401

PRKAG2 (protein kinase, AMP-activated, gamma 2 non-catalytic subunit) ~ 81406

PRKCG (protein kinase C, gamma) ~ 81406

PRNP (prion protein) ~ 81404

PROP1 (PROP paired-like homeobox 1) ~ 81404

PRPH2 (peripherin 2 [retinal degeneration slow]) ~ 81404

PRSS1 (protease, serine, 1 [trypsin 1]) ~ 81401, 81404

PRX (periaxin) ~ 81405

PSEN1 (presenilin 1) ~ 81405

PSEN2 (presenilin 2 [Alzheimer disease 4]) ~ 81406

PTEN (phosphatase and tensin homolog) ~ 81321-81323

PTPN11 (protein tyrosine phosphatase, non-receptor type 11) ~ 81406

PYGM (phosphorylase, glycogen, muscle) ~ 81401, 81406

RAB7A (RAB7A, member RAS oncogene family) ~ 81405

RAF1 (v-raf-1 murine leukemia viral oncogene homolog 1) ~ 81404, 81406

RAI1 (retinoic acid induced 1) ~ 81405

REEP1 (receptor accessory protein 1) ~ 81405

RET (ret proto-oncogene) ~ 81404-81406

RHD (Rh blood group, D antigen) ~ 81403

RHO (rhodopsin) ~ 81404

RP1 (retinitis pigmentosa 1) ~ 81404

RPE65 (retinal pigment epithelium specific protein 65kDa) ~ 81406

RPS19 (ribosomal protein S19) ~ 81405

RRM2B (ribonucleotide reductase M2 B [TP53 inducible]) ~ 81405

RUNX1 (runt related transcription factor 1) ~ 81334

RUNX1/RUNX1T1(t(8;21)) ~ 81401

RYR1 (ryanodine receptor 1, skeletal) ~ 81406, 81408

RYR2 (ryanodine receptor 2 [cardiac]) ~ 81408

SCN1A (sodium channel, voltage-gated, type I, alpha subunit) ~ 81407

SCN1B (sodium channel, voltage-gated, type I, beta) ~ ~ 81404

SCN4A (sodium channel, voltage-gated, type IV, alpha subunit) ~ 81406

Gene Analysis ~ *continued*

SCN5A (sodium channel, voltage-gated, type V, alpha subunit) ~ 81407
SCNN1A (sodium channel, nonvoltage-gated 1 alpha) ~ 81406
SCNN1B (sodium channel, nonvoltage-gated 1, beta) ~ ~ 81406
SCNN1G (sodium channel, nonvoltage-gated 1, gamma) ~ 81406
SCO1 (SCO cytochrome oxidase deficient homolog 1) ~ 81405
SCO2 (SCO cytochrome oxidase deficient homolog 2 [SCO1L]) ~ 81404
SDHA (succinate dehydrogenase complex, subunit A, flavoprotein [Fp]) ~ 81406
SDHB (succinate dehydrogenase complex, subunit B, iron sulfur) ~ 81405
SDHC (succinate dehydrogenase complex, subunit C, integral membrane protein, 15kDa) ~ 81404, 81405
SDHD (succinate dehydrogenase complex, subunit D, integral membrane protein) ~ 81404
SEPT9 (septin 9) ~ 81327
SERPINA1 (serpin peptidase inhibitor, clade A [alpha-1 antiproteinase, antitrypsin], member 1) ~ 81332
SERPINE1 (serpine peptidase inhibitor clade E, member 1, plasminogen activator inhibitor 1, PAI 1) ~ 81400
SETX (senataxin) ~ 81406
SF3B1 (splicing factor [3b] subunit B1) ~ 81347
SGCA (sarcoglycan, alpha [50kDa dystrophin-associated glycoprotein]) ~ 81405
SGCB (sarcoglycan, beta [43kDa dystrophinassociated glycoprotein]) ~ 81405
SGCD (sarcoglycan, delta [35kDa dystrophinassociated glycoprotein]) ~ 81405
SGCE (sarcoglycan, epsilon) ~ 81405, 81406
SGCG (sarcoglycan, gamma [35kDa dystrophinassociated glycoprotein]) ~ 81404, 81405
SH2D1A (SH2 domain containing 1A) ~ 81403, 81404
SH3TC2 (SH3 domain and tetratricopeptide repeats 2) ~ 81406
SHOC2 (soc-2 suppressor of clear homolog) ~ 81400, 81405
SHOX (short stature homeobox) ~ 81405
SIL1 (SIL1 homolog, endoplasmic reticulum chaperone [S. cerevisiae]) ~ 81405
SLC9A6 (solute carrier family 9 [sodium/ hydrogen exchanger], member 6) ~ 8406
SLC2A1 (solute carrier family 2 [facilitated glucose transporter], member 1) ~ 81405
SLC12A1 (solute carrier family 12 [sodium/potassium/chloride transporters], member 1) ~ 81407
SLC12A3 (solute carrier family 12 [sodium/ chloride transporters], member 3) ~ 81407
SLC16A2 (solute carrier family 16, member 2 [thyroid hormone transporter]) ~ 81404, 81405
SLC22A5 (solute carrier family 22 organic cation/carnitine transporter], member 5) ~ 81405
SLC25A4 (solute carrier family 25 [mitochondrial carrier; adenine nucleotide translocator], member 4) ~ 81404
SLC25A20 (solute carrier family 25 [carnitine/acylcarnitine translocase], member 20) ~ 81404, 81405
SLC26A4 (solute carrier family 26, member 4) ~ 81404
SLC37A4 (solute carrier family 37 [glucose-6- phosphate transporter], member 4) ~ 81406
SLCO1B1 (solute carrier organic anion transporter family, member 1B1) ~ 81328
SMAD4 (SMAD family member 4) ~ 81405, 81406
SMN1 (survival of motor neuron 1, telomeric) ~ 81400, 81403, 81405
SMN1/SMN2 (survival of motor neuron 1, telomeric/survival of motor neuron 2, centromeric) ~ 81401
SMPD1 (sphingomyelin phosphodiesterase 1, acid lysosomal) ~ 81330
SNRPN/UBE3A (small nuclear ribonucleoprotein polypeptide N/ubiquitin protein ligase E3A) ~ 81331
SOD1 (superoxide dismutase 1, soluble) 81404
SOS1 (son of sevenless homolog 1) ~ 81406
SPAST (spastin) ~ 81405, 81406
SPG7 (spastic paraplegia 7 [pure and complicated autosomal recessive]) ~ 81405, 81406
SPG11 (spastic paraplegia 11 [autosomal recessive]) ~ 81407
SPINK1 (serine peptidase inhibitor, Kazal type 1) ~ 81404
SPRED1 (sprouty-related, EVH1 domain containing 1) ~ 81405
SPTBN2 (spectrin, beta, non-erythrocytic 2) ~ 81407
SRSF2 (serine and arginine-rich splicing factor 2) ~ 81348
SRY (sex determining region Y) ~ 81400
SS18/SSX1 (t(X;18)) ~ 81401
SS18/SSX2 (t(X;18)) ~ 81401

Gene Analysis ~ *continued*

STAT3 (signal transduce and activator of transcription 3 [acute-phase response factor]) ~ 81405
STK11 (serine/threonine kinase 11) ~ 81404, 81405
STXBP1 (syntaxin binding protein 1) ~ 81406
SURF1 (surfeit 1) ~ 81405
TACO1 (translational activator of mitochondrial encoded cytochrome c oxidase ~ 81404
TARDBP (TAR DNA binding protein) ~ 81405
TAZ (tafazzin) ~ 81406
TBP (TATA box binding protein) ~ 81401
TBX5 (T-box 5) ~ 81405
TCF4 (transcription factor 4) ~ 81405, 81406
TGFBR1 (transforming growth factor, beta receptor 1) ~ 81405
TGFBR2 (transforming growth factor, beta receptor 2) ~ 81405
TH (tyrosine hydroxylase) ~ 81406
THAP1 (THAP domain containing, apoptosis associated protein 1) ~ 81404
THRB (thyroid hormone receptor, beta) ~ 81405
TK2 (thymidine kinase 2, mitochondrial) 81405
TMEM43 (transmembrane protein 43) ~ 81406
TMEM67 (transmembrane protein 67) ~ 81407
TNNC1 (troponin C type 1 [slow]) ~ 81405
TNNI3 (troponin I, type 3 [cardiac]) ~ 81405
TNNT2 (troponin T, type 2 [cardiac]) ~ 81406
TOR1A (torsin family 1, member A [torsin A]) ~ 81400, 81404
TP53 (tumor protein 53) ~ 81351-81353
TPM1 (tropomyosin 1 [alpha]) ~ 81405
TPMT (thiopurine S-methyltransferase) 81335
TRB@ (T cell receptor beta locus) 81340, 81341
TRD@ (T cell antigen receptor, delta) Rearrangement ~ 81402
TRG@ (T cell receptor gamma locus) ~ 81342
TRPC6 (transient receptor potential cation channel, subfamily C, member 6) ~ 81406
TSC1 (tuberous sclerosis 1) ~ 81405, 81406
TSC2 (tuberous sclerosis 2) ~ 81406, 81407
TTPA (tocopherol [alpha] transfer protein) ~ 81404
TTR (transthyretin) ~ 81404
TWIST1 (twist homolog 1 [Drosophila]) ~ 81403, 81404
TYMP (thymidine phosphorylase) ~ 81405
TYMS (thymidylate synthetase) ~ 81346
TYR (tyrosinase [oculocutaneous albinism IA]) ~ 81404
U2AF1 (U2 small nuclear RNA auxiliary factor 1) ~ 81357
UBA1 (ubiquitin-like modifier activating enzyme 1) ~ 81403
UBE3A (ubiquitin protein ligase E3A) ~ 81406
UGT1A1 (UDP glucuronosyltransferase 1 family, polypeptide A1) ~ 81350
UMOD (uromodulin) ~ 81406
Uniparental disomy (UPD) ~ 81402
USH1C (Usher syndrome 1C [autosomal recessive, severe]) ~ 81407
USH1G (Usher syndrome 1G [autosomal recessive]) ~ 81404
USH2A (Usher syndrome 2A [autosomal recessive, mild]) ~ 81408
VHL (von Hippel-Lindau tumor suppressor) ~ 81403, 81404
VKORC1 (vitamin K epoxide reductase complex, subunit 1) ~ 81355
VPS13B (vacuolar protein sorting 13 homolog B [yeast]) ~ 81407, 81408
VWF (von Willebrand factor) ~ 81401, 81403-81406, 81408
WAS (Wiskott-Aldrich syndrome [eczemathrombocytopenia]) ~ 81406
WDR62 (WD repeat domain 62) ~ 81407
WT1 (Wilms tumor 1) ~ 81405
ZEB2 (zinc finger E-box binding homeobox 2) ~ 81404, 81405
ZNF41 (zinc finger protein 41) ~ 81404
ZRSR2 (sinc finger CCCH-type, RNA binding motif and serine/arginine-rich 2) ~ 81360
chimerism Analysis ~ 81267, 81268
comparative Analysis Using Short Tandem Repeat (STR) Markers ~ 81265, 81266
cytogenomic Constitutional Targeted Microarray Analysis, Chromosome 22q13 ~ 81425
cytogenomic Microarray Analysis, Neoplasia ~ 81406
HLA Class I and II Typing, Low Resolution. ~ 81370, 81371
HLA Class I Typing, Low Resolution ~ 81372-81374
HLA Class II Typing, Low Resolution ~ 81375-81377
HLA Class I and II Typing, High Resolution ~ 81378
HLA Class I Typing, High Resolution. ~ 81379-81381
HLA Class II Typing, High Resolution. ~ 81382, 81383
human Platelet Antigen Genotyping ~ 81105-81112
microsatellite Instability Analysis ~ 81301
short Tandem Repeat (STR) Analysis. ~ 81265, 81266, 81402

Gene Analysis ~ *continued*
 translocation Analysis
  BCR/ABL1 (t(9;22)) ~ 81206-81208
  CCND1/IGH (t(11;14)) ~ 81168
  COL1A1/PDGFB (t(17;22)) ~ 81402
  E2A/PBX1 (t(1;19)) ~ 81401
  EML4/ALK (inv(2)) ~ 81401
  ETV6/NTRK3 (t(12;15)) ~ 81401
  ETV6/RUNX1 (t(12;21)) ~ 81401
  EWSR1/ATF1 (t(12;22)) ~ 81401
  EWSR1/ERG (t(21;22)) ~ 81401
  EWSR1/FLI1 (t(11;22)) ~ 81401
  EWSR1/WT1 (t(11;22)) ~ 81401
  FOXO1/PAX3 (t(2;13)) ~ 81401
  FOXO1/PAX7 (t(1;13)) ~ 81401
  FUS/DDIT3 (t(12;16)) ~ 81401
  IGH@/BCL2 (t(14;18) ~ 81278
  MLL/AFF1 (t(4;11)) ~ 81401
  MLL/MLLT3 (t(9;11)) ~ 81401
  NPM1/ALK (t(2;5)) ~ 81401
  NTRK ~ 81194
  NTRK1 ~ 81191
  NTRK2 ~ 81192
  NTRK3 ~ 81193
  PAX8/PPARG (t(2;3)) (q13;p25)) ~ 81401
  PML/RARalpha (t(15;17)) ~ 81315, 81316
  RUNX1/RUNX1T1 (t(8;21)) ~ 81401
  SS18/SSX1 (t(X;18)) ~ 81401
  SS18/SSX2 (t(X;18)) ~ 81401
Gene product ~ see protein
Genioplasty ~ 21120-21123
 augmentation ~ 21120, 21123
 osteotomy ~ 21121-21123
Genitourinary sphincter, artificial ~ 53444-53449
Genomic sequencing procedures (GSPs)
 acute myelogenous leukemia ~ 0023U
 aortic dysfunction or dilation ~ 81410, 81411
 Ashkenazi Jewish Associated Disorders ~ 81412
 cardiac ion channelopathies ~ 81413, 81414
 C0MT (catechol-0-methyltransferase) ~ 0032U
 CYP1A2 ~ 0031U
 CYP2D6 ~ 0070U
 drug metabolism ~ 0029U, 0030U
 epilepsy ~ 81419
 exome ~ 0036U, 81415-81417
 fetal chromosomal aneuploidy ~ 81420
 fetal chromosomal microdeletion(s) ~ 81422
 genome ~ 81425-81427
 germline disorders ~ 0012U
 hearing loss ~ 81430, 81431
 helicobacter pylori detection and antibiotic resistance. ~ 0008U
 hematolymphoid neoplasia ~ 0014U, 0016U, 0017U
 hereditary breast cancer-related disorders. ~ 81432, 81433
 hereditary cardiomyopathy ~ 81439
 hereditary colon cancer disorders ~ 81435, 81436
 hereditary neuroendocrine tumor disorders. ~ 81437, 81438
 hereditary peripheral neuropathies. ~ 81448
 hereditary retinal disorders ~ 81434
 HTR2A ~ 0033U
 HTR2C ~ 0033U
 JAK2 ~ 0027U
 non-small cell lung neoplasia ~ 0022U
 NUDT15 ~ 0034U
 Noonan spectrum disorders. ~ 81442
 nuclear encoded mitochondrial genes ~ 81440
 severe inherited conditions ~ 81443
 solid organ neoplasia ~ 0013U, 0037U
 targeted genomic sequence analysis panel ~ 81445, 81450, 81455
 thyroid DNA and RNA ~ 0026U
 TPMT ~ 0034U
 whole mitochondrial genome ~ 81460, 81465
 X-linked intellectual disability (XLID) ~ 81470, 81471
Genotype analysis
 by Nucleic Acid
  hepatitis C Virus ~ 87902
  HIV-1 ~ 87901, 87906
   protease/Reverse Transcriptase Regions. ~ 87901
  vancomycin Resistance ~ 87500
 human Platelet Antigen ~ 81105-81112human platelet antigen ~ 81400
Gentamicin ~ 80170
 assay ~ 80170

Gentamycin level ~ 80170
Gentiobiase ~ 82963
GERD ~ 91034-91038
German measles ~ 86762
Gestational trophoblastic tumor ~ 59100, 59870
GGT ~ 82977
GI tract ~ see gastrointestinal tract
Giardia
 antigen detection
  immunofluorescence ~ 87269
  enzyme immunoassay ~ 87329
Giardia lamblia
 antibody ~ 86674
Gibbons stent ~ 52332
GIF ~ 84307
GIFT (gamete intrafallopian transfer) ~ 58976
Gillies approach
 fracture, zygomatic arch ~ 21356
Gill operation ~ 63012
Gingiva ~ see gums
Gingiva, abscess ~ see abscess
 fracture ~ see 41800 ~ gums
  zygomatic arch ~ 41800
Gingivectomy ~ 41820
Gingivoplasty ~ 41872
Girdlestone laminectomy ~ see laminectomy
Girdlestone procedure ~ 27120
G1A protein (bone) ~ 83937
Gland ~ see specific gland
Glasses ~ see spectacle services
Glaucoma
 counseling ~ 4174F
 cryotherapy ~ 66720
 cyclophotocoagulation ~ 66710, 66711
 diathermy ~ 66700
 fistulization of sclera ~ 66150
  through ciliary body ~ 66999
 iridectomy ~ 66625, 66630
 plan of care ~ 0517F
Glaucoma drainage implant ~ 66180, 66185
Glenn procedure ~ 33766-33767
 bidirectional ~ 33622
Glenohumeral joint
 arthrotomy ~ 23040
  with biopsy ~ 23100
  with synovectomy ~ 23105
 exploration ~ 23107
 removalforeign or loose body ~ 23107
Glenoid Fossa reconstruction ~ 21255
GLN ~ 82127, 82128, 82131
Globulin
 antihuman
  Coombs test, direct ~ 86880, 86885, 86886
  Coombs test, indirect ~ 86850, 86870
  corticosteroid-binding ~ 84449
 immune
  administration ~ 96365-96368
  product
   botulinum antitoxin ~ 90288
   botulism ~ 90288
   cytomegalovirus (CMV-IgIV) ~ 90291
   diphtheria antitoxin ~ 90296
   gammaglobulin ~ 82784-82785
   hepatitis B (HBIg) ~ 90371
   Ig ~ 90281
   IgIV ~ 90281
   rabies (RIg) ~ 90375
   rabies (RIg-HT) ~ 90376
   rabies (RIg-HT S/D) ~ 90377
   respiratory syncytial virus ~ 90378
   Rho(D) (RhIg/RhIgV) ~ 90384-90386
   SCIg ~ 90284
   tetanus (TIg) ~ 90389
   unlisted ~ 90399
   vaccinia ~ 90393
   varicella-zoster ~ 90396
 sex hormone binding ~ 84270
 thyroxine-binding ~ 84442

Glomerular filtration rate (GFR)
  measurement ~ 0602T
  monitoring ~ 0603T
Glomerular procoagulant activity ~ see thromboplastin
Glomus caroticum ~ 60600, 60605
Glossectomies ~ see excision, tongue
Glossorrhaphy ~ see suture, tongue
Glucagon ~ 82943
  tolerance panel ~ 80422-80424
  tolerance test ~ 82946
Glucose
  blood test ~ 82947, 82948, 82950
    home test ~ 82962
  body fluid ~ 82945
  interstitial fluid
    continuous monitoring ~ 95249-95251
    data interpretation ~ 99091
  panel
    basic metabolic ~ 80047, 80048
    comprehensive metabolic ~ 80053
    glucagon tolerance ~ 80422, 80424
    growth hormone suppression ~ 80430
    insulin tolerance ~ 80434, 80435
    insulin-induced C-peptide suppression ~ 80432
    renal function ~ 80069
  sensor
    insertion, subcutaneous pocket ~ 0446T, 0448T
    removal ~ 0447T, 0448T
  tolerance test ~ 82951, 82952
    intravenous push ~ 96374
  urinalysis ~ 81000-81003, 81005
Glucose-6-phosphate dehydrogenase ~ 82955-82960
Glucose phosphate isomerase ~ 84087
Glucosidase ~ 82963
Glucuronide androstanediol ~ 82154
Glue
  cornea wound ~ 65286
  sclera wound ~ 65286
Glukagon ~ see glucagon
Glutamate dehydrogenase, blood ~ 82965
Glutamate pyruvate transaminase ~ 84460
Glutamic
  alanine transaminase ~ 84460
  aspartic transaminase ~ 84450
  dehydrogenase ~ 82965
Glutamine ~ 82127, 82128, 82131
Glutamyltransferase, gamma ~ 82977
Glutathione ~ 82978
Glutathione reductase ~ 82979
Glycanhydrolase, N-acetylmuramide ~ 85549
Glycated hemoglobins ~ 83036
Glycated protein ~ 82985
Glycerol, phosphatidyl ~ 84081
Glycerol, phosphoglycerides ~ 84081
Glycerophosphatase ~ 84075-84080
Glycinate, theophylline sodium ~ 80198
Glycocholic acid ~ 82240
Glycohemoglobin ~ 83036
Glycol, ethylene ~ 82693
Glycosaminoglycan ~ 83864
Goeckerman treatment ~ 96910-96913
Gol-Vernet operation
  pyelotomy, exploration 50120
Gold assay ~ 80375
Goldwaite procedure ~ 27422
Golfer's elbow ~ 24357-24359
Gonadectomy, female ~ 58262-58263, 58291-58292, 58552, 58554, 58661, 58940-58943
Gonadectomy, male ~ 54520, 54522, 54530-54535, 54690
Gonadotropin
  chorionic ~ 84702-84704
  FSH ~ 83001
  ICSH ~ 83002
  LH ~ 83002
  panel ~ 80426
Gonioscopy ~ 92020
Goniotomy ~ 65820
Gonococcus ~ 87590-87592, 87850
Goodenough Harris drawing test ~ 96100
GOTT ~ 84450
GPUT ~ 82775-82776

Graft ~ see bone graft; bypass graft
  anal ~ 46753
  artery
    coronary ~ 33503-33505
  bone ~ 38240-38242
    harvesting ~ 20900-20902
    microvascular anastomosis ~ 20955-20962
    osteocutaneous flap with microvascular anastomosis ~ 20969-20973
    vascular pedicle ~ 25430
  bone marrow, aspiration ~ 20939
  bone and skin ~ 20969-20973
  cartilage
    ear to face ~ 21235
    harvesting ~ 20910-20912
    rib to face ~ 21230
  conjunctiva ~ 65782
    harvesting ~ 68371
  cornea, with lesion excision ~ 65426
  cornea transplant
    allograft preparation ~ 65757
    endothelial ~ 65756
    in aphakia ~ 65750
    lamellar ~ 65710
    penetrating ~ 65730
    in pseudophakia ~ 65755
  dura, spinal cord ~ 63710
  eye
    amniotic membrane ~ 65780
    conjunctiva ~ 65782
    stem cell ~ 65781
  facial nerve paralysis ~ 15840-15845
  fascia, cheek ~ 15840
  fascia lata, harvesting ~ 20920-20922
  fat ~ 15771-15774
  gum mucosa ~ 41870
  heart ~ 33935, 33945
  heart lung ~ 33935
  kidney ~ see kidney, transplantation
  liver ~ 47135
  lung ~ 32851-32854, 33935
  muscle, cheek ~ 15841-15845
  nail bed reconstruction ~ 11762
  nerve ~ 64885-64907
  oral mucosa ~ 40818
  organ ~ see transplantation
  pancreas ~ 48160, 48550, 48554-48556
  skin
    biological—see Allograft, skin substitute
    blood flow check, graft ~ 15860
  tendon
    finger ~ 26392
    hand ~ 26392
    harvesting ~ 20924
  vein cross-over ~ 34520
Grain alcohol ~ see alcohol, ethyl
Granulation tissue cauterization, chemical ~ 17250
Great toe
  flap ~ 20973
  fracture ~ 28490, 28496, 28505
Great vessels
  graft insertion ~ 33330, 33335
  shunt
    aorta to pulmonary artery
      ascending ~ 33755
      descending ~ 33762
    central ~ 33764
    subclavian to pulmonary artery ~ 33750
    vena cava to pulmonary artery ~ 33766-33767
  unlisted services and procedures ~ 33999
Great vessels transposition ~ 33770-33781
Greater tuberosity fracture
  with shoulder dislocation
    closed treatment ~ 23665
    open treatment ~ 23670
Greater vestibular gland ~ see Bartholin's gland
Green operation ~ (scapulopexy) 23400
Gridley stain ~ 88312
Grippe, Balkan ~ 86000, 86638
Gritti operation ~ 27590-27592
Groin repair, hernia ~ 49550-49557

Group health education
  genetic ~ 98961, 98962, 99078
  physical ~ 99078
  preventive medicine ~ 99411
  self-management, condition or treatment ~ 98961, 98962
  well-being coaching ~ 0593T
Grouping, blood ~ see blood typing
Growth factors, insulin-like ~ 84305
Growth hormone ~ 83003
  human ~ 80418, 80428-80430, 86277
Growth hormone release inhibiting factor ~ 84307
GTT (hydatidiform mole) ~ 82951, 82952
Guaiac test, blood in feces ~ 82270
Guard stain ~ 88313
Gullett ~ see esophagus
Gums
  abscess, incision and drainage ~ 41800
  alveolus, excision ~ 41830
  cyst, incision and drainage ~ 41800
  excision
    gingiva ~ 41820
    operculum ~ 41821
  graft, mucosa ~ 41870
  hematoma, incision and drainage ~ 41800
  lesion
    destruction ~ 41850
    excision ~ 41822-41828
  mucosa, excision ~ 41828
  reconstruction
    alveolus ~ 41874
    gingiva ~ 41872
  removal, foreign body ~ 41805
  tumor, excision ~ 41825-41827
  unlisted services and procedures ~ 41899
Gunning-Lieben test ~ 82009-82010
Guthrie test ~ 84030

H

H flu ~ see Hemophilus influenza
HAAb (antibody, hepatitis) ~ 86708, 86709
HAA (hepatitis associated antigen) ~ 87340-87380, 87516-87527
Haemoglobin F ~ see fetal hemoglobin
Haemorrhage ~ see hemorrhage
Haemorrhage rectum ~ see hemorrhage, rectum
Hageman factor ~ 85280
Hair
  electrolysis ~ 17380
  KOH examination ~ 87220
  microscopic evaluation ~ 96902
  removal ~ see removal, hair
  transplant
    punch graft ~ 15775-15776
    strip graft ~ 15220-15221
HAI test ~ see hemagglutination inhibition test
Hallux ~ see great toe
Halo
  body cast ~ 29000
  cranial ~ 20661
    for thin skull osteology ~ 20664
  femur ~ 20663
  maxillofacial ~ 21100
  pelvic ~ 20662
  removal ~ 20665
Haloperidol assay ~ 80173
Halsted mastectomy ~ see mastectomy, radical
Halsted hernia repair ~ 49495
Ham test ~ 85475
Hammertoe repair ~ 28285-28286
Hamster penetration test ~ 89329
Hand ~ see also carpometacarpal joint; intercarpal joint
  amputation
    at metacarpal ~ 25927
    revision ~ 25924, 25929-25931
    at wrist ~ 25920
      revision ~ 25922

Hand ~ *continued*
  arthrodesis
    carpometacarpal joint ~ 26843-26844
    intercarpal joint ~ 25820-25825
  bone, incision and drainage ~ 26034
  cast ~ 29085
  decompression ~ 26035-26037
  fracture metacarpal
    carpometacarpal ~ 26645, 26650
    metacarpal
      closed treatment ~ 26600, 26605, 26607
      open treatment ~ 26615
      skeletal fixation ~ 26608
    metacarpophalangeal ~ 26740-26746
    phalangeal ~ 26720-26735, 26750-26765
  injection, cell therapy for scleroderma ~ 0490T
  insertion tendon graft ~ 26392
  magnetic resonance imaging (MRI) ~ 73218-73223
  reconstruction tendon pulley ~ 26500-26502
  removal
    implantation ~ 26320
      tube/rod ~ 26390-26392, 26416
  repair
    blood vessel ~ 35207
    cleft hand ~ 26580
    muscle ~ 26591-26593
    tendon
      extensor ~ 26410-26416, 26426-26428, 26433-26437
      flexor ~ 26350-26358, 26440
      profundus ~ 26370-26373
  replantation ~ 20808
  strapping ~ 29280
  tendon excision ~ 26390
    extensor ~ 26415
  tenotomy ~ 26450, 26460
  tumor excision ~ 26111-26118
  unlisted services and procedures ~ 26989
  X-ray ~ 73120-73130
Handling
  device ~ 99002
  radioelement ~ 77790
  specimen ~ 99000-99001
Hand abscess ~ see abscess, hand
Hand phalange ~ see finger, bone
Hanganutziu Deicher antibodies ~ see antibody, heterophile
Haptoglobin ~ 83010-83012
Hard palate ~ see palate
Harelip operation ~ see cleft lip, repair
Harii procedure ~ 25430
Harrington rod
  insertion ~ 22840
  removal ~ 22850
Hartmann procedure
  open ~ 44143
  laparoscopic ~ 44206
Harvesting
  adipose tissue cells
    cell therapy for scleroderma ~ 0489T
    for cellular knee implant ~ 0565T
  bone graft ~ 20900-20902
  bone marrow
    allogenic ~ 38230
    autograft ~ 0265T, 20939, 38232
  cartilage graft ~ 20910-20912
  conjunctival graft ~ 68371
  eggs, in vitro fertilization ~ 58970
  endoscopic, vein for bypass graft ~ 33508
  fascia lata graft ~ 20920-20922
  fat, by liposuction ~ 15771-15774, 15876-15879
  intestines ~ 44132-44133
  kidney ~ 50300-50320, 50547
  liver ~ 47133, 47140-47142
  lower extremity vein for vascular reconstruction ~ 35572
  stem cell ~ 38205-38206
  tendon graft ~ 20924
  upper extremity
    artery for coronary artery bypass graft ~ 35600
    vein for bypass graft ~ 35500
Hauser procedure ~ 27420
Haygroves procedure ~ 27120, 27122
HBcAb ~ 86704, 86705

HBeAb ~ 86707
HBeAg ~ 87350
HBsAb ~ 86706
HBsAg (hepatitis B surface antigen) ~ 87340
HCG ~ 84702, 84703
HCO3 ~ see bicarbonate
Hct (hematocrit) ~ 85014
HCV antibodies ~ see antibody, hepatitis C
HDL (high density lipoprotein) ~ 83718
Head
  excision
    bone, facial ~ 21025, 21026
    tumor, soft tissue ~ 21011-21016
  fracture and/or dislocation ~ 21310-21497
  halo appliance ~ 21100
  incision ~ 21010, 61316, 62148
  introduction or removal ~ 21076-21116
  imaging
    angiography ~ 70496, 70544-70546
    CT scan ~ 70450, 70460, 70470, 70496
    magnetic resonance angiography (MRA) ~ 70544-70546
    ultrasound exam ~ 76506, 76536
    X-ray ~ 70350
  lipectomy, suction assisted ~ 15876
  nerve graft ~ 64885-64886
  other procedures ~ 21299, 21499
  positron emission tomography (PET) ~ 78811, 78814
  prosthesis
    cheekbone malar augmentation ~ 21270
    chin ~ 21120
    cornea ~ 65770
    ear ossicle reconstruction ~ 69633, 69637
    facial osteoplasty ~ 21208
    lens ~ 66825, 66982-66985, 66987
    mandible ~ 21125
    ocular ~ 65770, 66982-66985, 66987
      telescope prosthesis ~ 0308T
      temporary ~ 92358
    palate ~ 42280, 42281
    retina ~ 0100T
    speech aid ~ 31611
    temporomandibular joint ~ 21243
  repair/revision and/or reconstruction ~ 21120-21296
  unlisted services and procedures ~ 21499
Head rings, stereotactic ~ see stereotactic frame
Headbrace
  application ~ 21100
  application/removal ~ 20661
Heaf TB test ~ 86580
Health behavior
  assessment ~ 96156
  coaching ~ 0591T-0593T
  intervention
    family ~ 96167, 96168, 96170, 96171
    group ~ 96164, 96165
    individual ~ 96158, 96159
Health risk assessment instrument
  administration
    caregiver-focused ~ 96160
    patient-focused ~ 96161
Hearing aid
  bone conduction
    implantation ~ 69710
    removal ~ 69711
    repair ~ 69711
    replacement ~ 69710
  check ~ 92592-92593
  services
    electroacoustic test ~ 92594-92595
    examination ~ 92590-92591
Hearing evaluation ~ 92510
Hearing tests ~ see audiologic function tests; hearing evaluation
Hearing therapy ~ 92507-92510, 92601-92604
Heart
  ablation
    arrhythmogenic focus ~ 33250-33251, 33261
    atrial tissue ~ 33254-33259
      endoscopic ~ 33265-33266
  anomoly repair ~ 33615, 33617

Heart ~ *continued*
  artificial heart
    implantation ~ 33927
    removal ~ 33929
    replacement ~ 33928
  atria ~ see atria
  balloon device ~ 33973-33974
  biopsy ~ 93505
    ultrasound imaging guidance ~ 76932
  blood vessel repair ~ 33320-33322
  cardiac contractility modulation
    electrode reposition ~ 0415T
  cardiac output measurements ~ 93451, 93561-93562
  cardiac rehabilitation ~ 93797-93798
  cardioassist ~ 92970-92971
  cardiopulmonary bypass
    with aortic aneurysm repair ~ 33877
    with ascending aorta graft ~ 33858, 33859, 33863, 33864
    with atrial septectomy/septostomy ~ 33736
    with chamber fistula repair ~ 33500
    with descending thoracic aorta graft ~ 33875
    with lung transplant ~ 32852, 32854
    with operative ablation ~ 33251, 33256, 33259, 33261
    with pericardiectomy ~ 33031
    with pulmonary artery repair ~ 33910, 33916, 33922, 33926
    with replacement of ventricular assist ~ 33983
    with sinus of valsalva repair ~ 33702, 33720
    with transcatheter aortic valve replacement (TAVR/TAVI) ~ 33367-33369
    with transverse arch graft ~ 33871
    with tumor excision ~ 33120
    with wound repair ~ 33305
  cardioversion ~ 92960-92961
  catheterization ~ see Cardiac catheterization
  chordae tendineae, artificial placement ~ 0543T
  cor triatriatum repair ~ 33732
  CT scan ~ 75571-75573
    angiography ~ 75574
  cyst, pericardial, resection ~ 33050
  diagnostic imaging
    acoustic cardiography ~ 93799
    blood pool ~ 78472-78473, 78481, 78483, 78496
      SPECT ~ 78494
    CT scan ~ 75571-75573
      angiography ~ 75574
    myocardial imaging
      infarct avid ~ 78466, 78468-78469
      magnetocardiography ~ 0541T, 0542T
      perfusion ~ 78451-78454
      perfusion study ~ 78430-78433, 78491-78492
      PET metabolic evaluation ~ 78429, 78432, 78433, 78459
      speckle-tracking assessment of mechanics ~ 93356
      SPECT ~ 0332T, 78451, 78452, 78469
      sympathetic innervation ~ 0331T, 0332T
    shunt detection ~ 78428
    unlisted cardiovascular diagnostic nuclear medicine procedure ~ 78499
  electrophysiologic procedure ~ 93600-93660
  electrode
    insertion ~ 33202-33203, 33210-33211, 33216-33217, 33224-33225
    removal ~ 33238
      single/dual chamber ~ 33243-33244
  exploration ~ 33310-33315
  foreign body removal ~ 33310
  great vessels ~ see great vessels
  heart-lung bypass ~ see cardiopulmonary bypass
  heart-lung transplantation ~ see transplantation, heart-lung
  hemodialysis access ~ 93985, 93986, 93990
  hemodynamic monitoring
    non-invasive ~ 93880, 93882, 93922-93931, 93970-93990, 93998
    with pharmacologic agent ~ 93463
    with physiologic exercise study ~ 93464
  implantation
    artificial heart, intracorporeal ~ 33927
    total replacement heart system, intracorporeal ~ 33928
    ventricular assist device ~ 33975-33976, 33979
  infundibular stenosis ~ 33476-33478
  intraoperative pacing and mapping ~ 93631
  ligation, fistula ~ 37607
  magnetic resonance imaging (MRI) ~ 75557-75565
  mitral valve ~ see mitral valve

Heart ~ continued
  myocardial infarction
    revascularization ~ 92941, 92943-92944
    tissue plasminogen activator (tPA) ~ 4077F
  myocardium
    imaging ~ 78466-78469
    perfusion study ~ 78451-78454
    revascularization ~ 33140-33141
    speckle-tracking assessment of mechanics ~ 93356
  open chest massage ~ 32160
  output ~ see cardiac output
  pacemaker ~ see also Pacemaker, heart
    conversion ~ 33214
    insertion ~ 33206-33208
    pulse generator ~ 33212-33213, 33221
    removal ~ 33233-33237
    replacement
      catheter ~ 33210
      electrode ~ 33210-33211
      insertion ~ 33206-33208
      pulse generator ~ 33227-33229
  pacing
    arrhythmia induction ~ 93618
    atria ~ 93610
    transcutaneous, temporary ~ 92953
    ventricular ~ 33224-33226, 93612
  pacing cardioverter-defibrillator ~ see Cardioverter-defibrillator
  pericardium
    drainage ~ 33017-33019, 33025
    pericardiectomy ~ 33030, 33031
    pericardiocentesis ~ 33016
  reconstruction
    atrial septum ~ 33735-33737
    vena cava ~ 34502
  removal
    balloon device ~ 33974
    electrode ~ 33238
    ventricular assist device ~ 33977-33978
      extracorporeal ~ 33990-33993
      intracorporeal ~ 33980
  removal single/dual chamber
    electrodes ~ 33243-33244
    pulse generator ~ 33241
    repair ~ 33218-33220
  repair
    anomaly ~ 33615-33617
    aortic sinus ~ 33702-33722
    atrial septum ~ 33641, 33647
    atrioventricular canal ~ 33660-33665
      complete ~ 33670
      prosthetic valve ~ 33670
    atrioventricular valve ~ 33660-33665
    cor triatriatum ~ 33732
    electrode ~ 33218
    fenestration ~ 93580
    infundibular ~ 33476-33478
    mitral valve ~ 33420-33430
    myocardium ~ 33542
    outflow tract ~ 33476-33478
    postinfarction ~ 33542-33545
    prosthetic valve dysfunction ~ 33496
    septal defect ~ 33608-33610, 33660, 33813-33814, 93581
    sinus of valsalva ~ 33702-33722
    sinus venosus ~ 33645
    tetralogy of Fallot ~ 33692-33697, 33924
    total replacement heart system
      implantation ~ 33927
      removal ~ 33929
      replacement ~ 33928
    tricuspid valve ~ 33463-33468
    ventricle ~ 33611-33612
      obstruction ~ 33619
    ventricular septum ~ 33545, 33647, 33681-33688, 33692-33697, 93581
    ventricular tunnel ~ 33722
    wound ~ 33300-33305
  replacement
    electrode ~ 33210-33211, 33217
    mitral valve ~ 33430
    total replacement heart system ~ 33928

Heart ~ continued
    tricuspid valve ~ 33465
    ventricular assist device ~ 33981-33983
  repositioning
    electrode ~ 33215, 33217, 33226
    tricuspid valve ~ 33468
  resuscitation ~ 92950
  septal defect ~ see septal defect
  sinus of valsalvus repair ~ 33702-33722
  sinus venosus repair ~ 33645
  tetralogy of fallot repair ~ 33692-33697, 33924
  thrombectomy ~ see thrombectomy
  transplantation ~ 33935, 33945
    allograft preparation ~ 33933, 33944
  tumor excision ~ 33120-33130
  unlisted services and procedures ~ 33999
  valve closure ~ 33600, 33602
  vena cava reconstruction ~ 34502
  ventricle
    commissurotomy, right ventricle ~ 33476-33478
    leadless pacemaker system
      device evaluation, in person
        interrogation ~ 0391T
        peri-procedural ~ 0390T
        programming ~ 0389T
      transcatheter insertion ~ 0387T
      transcatheter removal ~ 0388T
      transcatheter replacement ~ 0387T
    obstruction removal ~ 33619
    pacing ~ 33224-33226, 93612
    repair ~ 33548, 33611-33612
    tunnel repair ~ 33722
    ventriculomyectomy ~ 33416
    wound repair ~ 33300-33305
Heart sounds, acoustic recording, with computer analysis ~ 93799
Heart vessels
  angioplasty, percutaneous ~ 92982-92984
  insertion graft ~ 33330-33335
  thrombolysis ~ 92975-92977
  valvuloplasty, percutaneous ~ 92986-92990
Heat unstable haemoglobin ~ see hemoglobin, thermolabile
Heavy lipoproteins ~ see lipoprotein
Heavy metal ~ 83015-83018
Heel ~ 36415-36416
  X-ray ~ 73650
Heel bone ~ see calcaneus
Heel fracture ~ see calcaneus, fracture
Heel spur excision ~ 28119
Heine-Medin disease ~ see polio
Heine operation ~ see cyclodialysis
Heinz bodies ~ 85441-85445
Helicobacter pylori
  antibody ~ 86677
  antigen detection enzyme immunoassay ~ 87338-87339
  blood test ~ 83009
  breath test ~ 78267-78268, 83013-83014
  stool ~ 87338
  urease activity ~ 83009, 83013-83014
Heller procedure ~ 32665, 43330-43331
Helminth antibody ~ 86682
Hemagglutination inhibition test ~ 86280
Hemangioma ~ 17106-17108
Hemapheresis ~ 36511-36516
Hematochezia ~ 82270, 82274
Hematologic test ~ see blood tests
Hematology and coagulation ~ 85002-85999
Hematoma
  ankle ~ 27603
  arm, lower ~ 25028
  arm, upper, incision and drainage ~ 23930
  brain
    drainage ~ 61154-61156
    evacuation ~ 61312-61315
    incision and drainage ~ 61312-61315
  drain ~ 61108
  ear, external
    complicated ~ 69005
    simple ~ 69000
  elbow, incision and drainage ~ 23930
  epididymis, incision and drainage ~ 54700

Hematoma ~ *continued*
- gums, incision and drainage ~ 41800
- hip ~ 26990
- incision and drainage
  - neck ~ 21501-21502
  - skin ~ 10140
  - thorax ~ 21501-21502
- knee ~ 27301
- leg, lower ~ 27603
- leg, upper ~ 27301
- mouth ~ 41005-41009, 41015-41018
  - incision and drainage ~ 40800-40801
- nasal septum, incision and drainage ~ 30020
- nose, incision and drainage ~ 30000-30020
- pelvis ~ 26990
- scrotum, incision and drainage ~ 54700
- shoulder, drainage ~ 23030
- skin
  - incision and drainage ~ 10140
  - puncture aspiration ~ 10160
- subdural ~ 61108
- subungual, evacuation ~ 11740
- testis, incision and drainage ~ 54700
- tongue ~ 41000-41006, 41015
- vagina, incision and drainage ~ 57022-57023
- wrist ~ 25028

Hematopoietic stem cell transplantation ~ see stem cell, transplantation
Hematopoietin ~ see erythropoietin
Hematuria ~ see blood, urine
Hemic and lymphatic systems, surgical procedures ~ 38100-38999
Hemiepiphyseal arrest, elbow ~ 24470
Hemifacial microsomia, reconstruction, mandibular condyle ~ 21247
Hemilaminectomy ~ 63020-63044
Hemilaryngectomy ~ 31370-31382
Hemipelvectomies ~ see amputation, interpelviabdominal
Hemiphalangectomy, toe ~ 28160
Hemispherectomy
- partial ~ 61543

Hemocytoblast ~ see stem cell
Hemodialysis ~ 90935-90937
- blood flow study ~ 90940
- duplex scan of access ~ 93985, 93986, 93990
- home visit ~ 99512
- Kt/V level ~ 3082F-3084F
- plan of care documented ~ 0505F
- via catheter ~ 4054F
- via functioning arteriovenous
  - fistula 4052F
  - graft 4053F

Hemodynamic monitoring, non-invasive left ventricular ~ 93799
Hemofiltration ~ 90945-90947
Hemoglobin
- A1c (HbA1c) level ~ 3044F, 3051F, 3052F
- analysis, O2 affinity ~ 82820
- carboxyhemoglobin ~ 82375-82376, 88740
- chromatography ~ 83021
- concentration ~ 85046
- electrophoresis ~ 83020
- fetal ~ 83030-83033, 85460-85461
- fractionation and quantitation ~ 83020
- glycosated (A1C) ~ 83036-83037
- methemoglobin ~ 83045-83050
  - transcutaneous ~ 88741
- non-automated ~ 83026
- plasma ~ 83051
- sulfhemoglobin ~ 83060
- thermolabile ~ 83065-83068
- transcutaneous ~ 88738, 88740
- urine ~ 83069

Hemoglobin, glycosylated ~ see glycohemoglobin
Hemoglobin F (fetal)
- chemical ~ 83030
- qualitative ~ 83033

Hemogram
- added indices ~ 85025-85027
- automated ~ 85025-85027
- manual ~ 85014-85018, 85032

Hemolysins ~ 85475
- with agglutinins ~ 86940-86941

Hemolytic complement ~ see complement, hemolytic
Hemolytic complement, total ~ see complement, hemolytic, total

Hemoperfusion ~ 90997
Hemophil ~ see clotting factor
Hemophilus influenza
- antibody ~ 86684
- vaccines ~ 90644-90648, 90748

Hemorrhage
- abdomen ~ 49002
- anal, endoscopic control ~ 46614
- chest cavity, endoscopic control ~ 32654
- colon, endoscopic control ~ 44391, 45382
- colon-sigmoid, endoscopic control ~ 45334
- control
  - gastrointestinal ~ 43753
  - liver ~ 47350
  - lung ~ 32110
  - nasal (epistaxis) ~ 30901, 30903, 30905, 30906
  - nasopharynx ~ 42970-42972
  - neck ~ 35800
  - preperitoneal pelvis ~ 49013, 49014
  - prostate, transurethral fulguration ~ 52214
  - throat ~ 42960-42962
  - uterus, postpartum ~ 59160
  - vagina ~ 57180
- esophagus, endoscopic control ~ 43227
- gastrointestinal, upper, endoscopic control ~ 43255
- intestines, small, endoscopic control ~ 44366, 44378
- liver, control ~ 47350
- lung ~ 32110
- nasal
  - cauterization ~ 30901-30906
  - endoscopic control ~ 31238
- nasopharynx ~ 42970-42972
- oropharynx ~ 42960-42962
- rectum, endoscopic control ~ 45317
- throat ~ 42960-42962
- uterus, postpartum ~ 59160
- vagina ~ 57180

Hemorrhoidectomy
- complex ~ 46260
  - with fissurectomy ~ 46261-46262
- external complete ~ 46250
- ligation ~ 46221, 46945, 46946, 46948
  - with mucopexy ~ 46948
- simple ~ 46255
  - with fissurectomy ~ 46257-46258
- transanal hemorrhoidal dearterialization (THD) ~ 46948

Hemorrhoidopexy ~ 46947
Hemorrhoids
- band ligation
  - with colonoscopy ~ 45398
  - with sigmoidoscopy ~ 45350
- destruction ~ 46930
- excision ~ 46250-46262, 46320
- incision, external ~ 46083
- injection, sclerosing solution ~ 46500
- ligation ~ 46945, 46946, 46948
- stapling ~ 46947
- suture ~ 46945, 46946, 46948
- transanal hemorrhoidal dearterialization (THD) ~ 46948

Hemosiderin ~ 83070
Hemothorax, thoracostomy ~ 32551
Heparin ~ see clotting inhibitors ~ 85520
- neutralization ~ 85525
- protamine tolerance test ~ 85530

Heparin cofactor I ~ see antithrombin III
Hepatectomy
- extensive ~ 47122
- left lobe ~ 47125
- partial
  - donor ~ 47140-47142
  - lobe ~ 47120
- right lobe ~ 47130
- total
  - donor ~ 47133

Hepaticodochotomy ~ see hepaticostomy
Hepaticoenterostomy ~ 47802
Hepaticostomy ~ 47400
Hepaticotomy ~ 47400
Hepatic arteries ~ see artery, hepatic
Hepatic artery aneurysm ~ see artery, hepatic, aneurysm

Hepatic duct
  anastomosis, with intestines ~ 47765, 47802
  exploration ~ 47400
  incision and drainage ~ 47400
  removalcalculi (stone) ~ 47400
  repair, with intestines ~ 47765, 47802
  unlisted services and procedures ~ 47999
Hepatic haemorrhage ~ see hemorrhage, liver
Hepatic portal vein ~ see vein, hepatic portal
Hepatic portoenterostomies ~ see hepaticoenterostomy
Hepatic transplantation ~ see liver, transplantation
Hepatitis A and hepatitis B ~ 90636
Hepatitis antibody
  A ~ 86708-86709
  B core ~ 86704-86705
  B surface ~ 86706
  Be ~ 86707
  C ~ 86803-86804
  delta agent ~ 86692
  IgG ~ 86704, 86708
  IgM ~ 86704, 86705, 86709
  Panel
    acute hepatitis ~ 80074
    obstetric ~ 80055, 80081
Hepatitis antigen
  B ~ 87516, 87517
  B surface ~ 87340-87341
  Be ~ 87350
  C ~ 87520-87522
  delta agent ~ 87380
  G ~ 87525-87527
Hepatitis A vaccine
  adolescent/pediatric
    2 dose schedule ~ 90633
    3 dose schedule ~ 90634
  adult dosage ~ 90632
Hepatitis B and Hib ~ 90748
Hepatitis B vaccine dosage
  adolescent ~ 90743
  adult ~ 90746
  immunosuppressed ~ 90740, 90747
  pediatric/adolescent ~ 90744
Hepatitis B virus e antibody ~ see antibody, hepatitis
Hepatitis B virus surface ab ~ see antibody, hepatitis B, surface
Hepatorrhaphy ~ see liver, repair
Hepatotomy
  abscess ~ 47010
  cyst ~ 47010
Hernia repair
  abdominal ~ 49590
    incisional ~ 49560
    recurrent ~ 49565
  diaphragmatic ~ 39503, 39540--39541
  epigastric ~ 49570
    incarcerated ~ 49572
    laparoscopic ~ 49652-49653
  femoral ~ 49550
    incarcerated ~ 49553
    recurrent ~ 49555
    recurrent incarcerated ~ 49557
  incisional
    incarcerated ~ 49561
    laparoscopic ~ 49654-49657
    thoracoabdominal 43336-43337
  inguinal ~ 49491, 49495-49500, 49505
    incarcerated ~ 49492, 49496, 49501, 49507, 49521
    laparoscopic ~ 49650-49651
    recurrent ~ 49520
    sliding ~ 49525
    strangulated ~ 49492
  lumbar ~ 49540
  lung ~ 32800
  orchiopexy ~ 54640
  paraesophageal hiatal
    via
      laparotomy ~ 43332-43333
      thoracoabdominal incision ~ 43336-43337
      thoractopy ~ 43334-43335

Hernia repair ~ *continued*
  recurrent incisional
    incarcerated ~ 49566
    reducible ~ 49565
  umbilicus
    incarcerated ~ 49582, 49587
    laparoscopic ~ 49652-49653
    reducible ~ 49580, 49585
  with spermatic cord ~ 55540
    spigelian ~ 49590
  ventral, laparoscopic ~ 49652-49653
Hernia, cerebral ~ see encephalocele
Hernia, rectovaginal ~ see rectocele
Hernia, umbilical ~ see omphalocele
Heroin screening ~ see Drug assay
Herpes simplex
  antibody ~ 86696
  antigen detection
    immunofluorescence ~ 87273-87274
    nucleic acid ~ 87528-87530
  identification smear and stain ~ 87207
Herpes smear and stain ~ 87207
Herpes virus-4 (gamma), human ~ see Epstein-Barr virus
Herpes virus-6 (six) detection ~ 87531-87533
Herpetic vesicle destruction ~ 54050-54065
Heteroantibodies ~ see antibody, heterophile
Heterologous transplant ~ see xenograft
Heterologous transplantation ~ see heterograft
Heterophile antibody ~ 86308-86310
Heterotropia ~ see strabismus
Hex b ~ see b-hexosaminidase
Hexadecadrol ~ see dexamethasone
Hexosephosphate isomerase ~ see phosphohexose isomerase
Heyman procedure ~ 27179, 28264
Hgb (hemoglobin) ~ 85018
HGH (human growth hormone) ~ 80418, 80428, 80430, 83003, 86277
Hg factor ~ see glucagon
HHV-4 ~ see Epstein-Barr virus
HIAA (hydroxyindolacetic acid, urine) 83497
Hibb operation ~ 22841
Hib vaccine
  4 dose schedule
    PRP-T ~ 90648
  PRP-OMP
    3 dose schedule ~ 90647
Hickmann catheterization ~ see cannulization; catheterization, venous, central line; venipuncture
Hidradenitis (see also sweat gland)
  excision ~ 11450-11471
  suppurative, incision and drainage ~ 10060-10061
Highly selective vagotomy ~ see vagotomy, highly selective
Highmore antrum ~ see sinuses, maxillary
High altitude simulation test ~ 94452-94453
High density lipoprotein ~ 83718
High intensity focused ultrasound (HIFU)
  ablation, prostate tissue ~ 55880
High molecular weight kininogen ~ 85293
Hill procedure
  laparoscopic ~ 43280
Hinton positive ~ 86592, 86593
Hip joint
  arthroplasty ~ 27132
    revision ~ 27134-27138
  arthrotomy ~ 27052
  biopsy ~ 27052
  capsulotomy, with release, flexor muscles ~ 27036
    dislocation ~ 27250-27252
    congenital ~ 27256-27259
    open treatment ~ 27253-27254
    without trauma ~ 27265-27266
  manipulation ~ 27275
  reconstruction, revision ~ 27134-27138
  synovium
    excision ~ 27054
    arthroscopic ~ 29863
  total replacement ~ 27132

Hip ~ see also femur; pelvis
abscess, incision and drainage ~ 26990
arthrocentesis ~ 20610
arthrodesis ~ 27284-27286
arthrography ~ 73525
arthroplasty ~ 27130-27132
arthroscopy ~ 29860-29863, 29914
arthrotomy ~ 27030-27033
biopsy ~ 27040-27041
bone, drainage ~ 26992
bursa, incision and drainage ~ 26991
capsulectomy with release, flexor muscles ~ 27036
cast ~ 29305-29325
craterization ~ 27070
cyst, excision ~ 27065-27067
denervation ~ 27035
echography, infant ~ 76885-76886
endoprosthesis ~ see prosthesis, hip
excision ~ 27070
exploration ~ 27033
fasciotomy ~ 27025
fusion ~ 27284-27286
hematoma, incision and drainage ~ 26990
injectio, radiologic ~ 27093-27096
reconstruction, total replacement ~ 27130
removal
  cast ~ 29710
  foreign body ~ 27033, 27086-27087
    arthroscopic ~ 29861
  loose body
    arthroscopic ~ 29861
  prosthesis ~ 27090-27091
repair
  muscle transfer ~ 27100-27105, 27111
  osteotomy ~ 27146-27156
  tendon ~ 27097
saucerization ~ 27070
stem prosthesis ~ see arthroplasty, hip
strapping ~ 29520
tenotomy
  abductor tendon ~ 27006
  adductor tendon ~ 27000-27003
  iliopsoas ~ 27005
total replacement ~ 27130-27132
tumor
  excision ~ 27043-27045, 27049, 27059, 27065-27067
    radical ~ 27075-27076
ultrasound, infant ~ 76885-76886
X-ray
  bilateral ~ 73521-73523
  unilateral ~ 73501-73503
  with contrast ~ 73525
Hip stem prostheses ~ see arthroplasty, hip
Hippocampus excision ~ 61566
Histamine ~ 83088
Histamine release test ~ 86343
Histochemistry ~ 88319
Histocompatibility testing ~ see tissue typing
Histoplasma
antibody ~ 86698
antigen ~ 87385
Histoplasma capsulatum, antigen detection, enzyme immunoassay ~ 87385
Histoplasmin test ~ see histoplasmosis, skin test
Histoplasmoses ~ see histoplasmosis
Histoplasmosis skin test ~ 86510
History and physical ~ 57410
HIV
antibody ~ 86701-86703
  confirmation test ~ 86689
HIV-1
antibody detection, enzyme immunoassay ~ 86701, 86703, 87389
antigen detection, enzyme immunoassay ~ 87389-87390
genotype analysis ~ 87901, 87906
infectious agent detection
  amplified probe ~ 87535
  direct probe ~ 87534
  quantification ~ 87536

HIV-2
antibody detection, enzyme immunoassay ~ 86702-86703, 87389
antigen detection
  enzyme immunoassay ~ 87389, 87391
infectious agent detection
  amplified probe ~ 87538
  direct probe ~ 87537
  quantification ~ 87539
HK3 kallikrein ~ see prostate specific antigen
HLA
crossmatch ~ 86825, 86826
molecular pathology ~ 81370-81383
typing ~ 86812-868122
HMRK ~ see Fitzgerald factor
HMW kininogen ~ see Fitzgerald factor
Hoffman apparatus ~ 20690
Hofmeister operation (gastrectomy, total) ~ 43632
Holographic imaging ~ 76375
Holten test ~ 82575
Home health services
activities of daily living ~ 99509
anticoagulant management ~ 93793
apnea monitoring ~ 94774-94777
catheter care ~ 99507
enema administration ~ 99511
established patient ~ 99347-99350
hemodialysis ~ 99512
home infusion procedures ~ 99601, 99602
individual or family counseling ~ 99510
intramuscular injections ~ 99506
mechanical ventilation ~ 99504
newborn care ~ 99502
new patient ~ 99341-99345
postnatal assessment ~ 99501
prenatal monitoring ~ 99500
respiratory therapy ~ 99503
sleep studies ~ 95805-95811
stoma care ~ 99505
unlisted services and procedures ~ 99600
ventilation assist ~ 94005
Home visits ~ 99341-99350
Homocystine ~ 83090
urine ~ 82615
Homogenization, tissue ~ 87176
Homograft, skin ~ 15350
Homologous grafts ~ see graft
Homologous transplantation ~ see homograft
Homovanillic acid, urine ~ 83150
Hormone adrenocorticotrophic (ACTH) ~ 80400-80406, 80412, 80418, 82024
corticotropic-releasing ~ 80412
growth ~ see human growth hormone
human growth ~ 80418, 80428, 80430, 86277, 83003
interstitial cell-stimulating ~ see luteinizing hormone (LH)
luteinizing hormone (LH) ~ 80418, 80426, 83002
parathyroid ~ 83970
pituitary lactogenic (prolactin) ~ 80418, 84146
placental lactogen ~ 83632
somatotropin release-inhibiting (somatostatin) ~ 84307
thyroid-stimulating (TSH) ~ 80418, 80438-80439, 80443, 84146
Hormone-binding globulin, sex ~ see globulin, sex hormone binding
Hormones, adrenal cortex ~ see corticosteroids
Hormones, antidiuretic ~ see antidiuretic hormone
Hormone assay
ACTH ~ 82024
aldosterone, blood or urine ~ 82088
androstenedione, blood or urine ~ 82157
androsterone, blood or urine ~ 82160
angiotensin II ~ 82163
corticosterone ~ 82528
cortisol, total ~ 82533
dehydroepiandrosterone ~ 82626
dihydroelestosterone ~ 80327, 80328
dihydrotestosterone ~ 80327, 80328
epiandrosterone ~ 80327, 80328
estradiol ~ 82670
estriol ~ 82677
estrogen ~ 82671-82672

Hormone assay ~ *continued*
  estrone ~ 82679
  follicle stimulating hormone (FSH) ~ 83001
  growth hormone, human ~ 83003
  hydroxyprogesterone ~ 83498
  luteinizing hormone ~ 83002
  somatotropin ~ 83003
  testosterone
    bioavailable ~ 84410
    free ~ 84402
    total ~ 84403
  vasopressin ~ 84588
Hormone pellet implantation ~ 11980
Hospital discharge services ~ 99238-99239
Hospital services
  inpatient services ~ 99238-99239
    discharge services ~ 99238-99239, 1110F-1111F
    initial care, new or established patient ~ 99221-99223
    initial hospital care ~ 99221-99223
    newborn ~ 99460-99462, 99477
    prolonged services ~ 99356-99357
    subsequent hospital care ~ 99231-99233
  observation
    discharge services ~ 99234-99236
    initial care ~ 99218-99220
      new or established patient ~ 99218-99220
    subsequent ~ 99224-99226
  same day admission, discharges services ~ 99234-99236
  subsequent newborn care ~ 99462
  subsequent observation care ~ 99224-99226
Hot pack treatment ~ 97010
House calls ~ 99341-99350
Howard test ~ 52005
HPL ~ (lactogen, human placental) 83632
HTLV I antibody
  confirmatory test ~ 86689
  detection ~ 86687
HTLV II antibody ~ 86688
HTLV III ~ see HIV
HTLV III antibodies ~ see antibody, HIV
HTLV IV ~ see HIV-2
Hubbard tank therapy ~ 97036
Hue test ~ 92283
Huggin operation ~ 54520
Huhner test ~ 89300, 89320
Human chorionic gonadotropin ~ see chorionic gonadotropin
Human chorionic somatomammotropin ~ see lactogen, human placental
Human epididymus protein ~ 86305
Human growth hormone(HGH) ~ 80418, 80428-80430
Human herpes virus 4 ~ see Epstein-Barr virus
Human immunodeficiency virus ~ see HIV
Human immunodeficiency virus 1 ~ see HIV-1
Human immunodeficiency virus 2 ~ see HIV-2
Human papillomavirus detection
  nucleic acid probe ~ 0500T, 87623-87625
Human placental lactogen ~ 83632
Human T cell leukemia virus I ~ see HTLV I
Human T cell leukemia virus II ~ see HTLV II
Human T cell leukemia virus I antibodies ~ see antibody, HTLV
  I **Human T cell** leukemia virus II antibodies ~ see antibody, HTLV II
Humeral epicondylitides, lateral (tennis elbow) ~ 24357-24359
Humeral fracture ~ see fracture, humerus
Humerus ~ see arm, upper; shoulder
  abscess
    incision and drainage ~ 23935
  craterization ~ 23184, 24140
  cyst
    excision ~ 23150, 24110
      with allograft ~ 23156, 24116
      with autograft ~ 23155, 24115
  diaphysectomy ~ 23184, 24140
  excision ~ 23174, 23184, 23195, 24134, 24140, 24150
  fracture
    closed treatment ~ 24500-24505
      with manipulation ~ 23605
      without manipulation ~ 23600
    condyle
      closed treatment ~ 24576-24577
      open treatment ~ 24579
      percutaneous fixation ~ 24582

Humerus ~ *continued*
  epicondyle
    closed treatment ~ 24560-24565
    open treatment ~ 24575
    skeletal fixation, percutaneous ~ 24566
  greater tuberosity fracture
    closed treatment with manipulation ~ 23625
    closed treatment without manipulation ~ 23620
    open treatment ~ 23630
  open treatment ~ 23615-23616
  shaft ~ 24500-24505, 24516
    open treatment ~ 24515
  supracondylar
    closed treatment ~ 24530-24535
    open treatment ~ 24545-24546
    percutaneous fixation ~ 24538
  transcondylar
    closed treatment ~ 24530-24535
    open treatment ~ 24545-24546
    percutaneous fixation ~ 24538
  with dislocation ~ 23665-23670
  osteomyelitis ~ 24134
  osteotomy
    insertion, intramedullary lengthening device ~ 0594T
    intramedullary rod realignment ~ 24410
    Sofield procedure ~ 24410
  pinning, wiring ~ 23491, 24498
  prophylactic treatment ~ 23491, 24498
  radical resection ~ 23220
  repair ~ 24430
    with graft ~ 24435
    nonunion, malunion ~ 24430-24435
    osteoplasty ~ 24420
    osteotomy ~ 24400-24410
    resection head ~ 23195
  saucerization ~ 23184, 24140
  sequestrectomy ~ 23174, 24134
  tumor
    excision ~ 23150, 23220, 24110
      with allograft ~ 23156, 24116
      with autograft ~ 23155, 24115
      radial head or neck ~ 24152
  X-ray ~ 73060
Hummelshein operation ~ see strabismus, repair
Humor shunt, aqueous ~ 66180, 66185
HVA (homovanillic acid) ~ 83150
Hyaluron binding assay ~ 89398
Hybrid approach
  stage 1 ~ 33620-33621
  stage 2 ~ 33622
Hybridization probes, DNA ~ see nucleic acid probe
Hydatid disease ~ see echinococcosis
Hydatidiform mole
  evacuation and curettage ~ 59870
  excision ~ 59100
Hydration ~ 96360-96361
  rehydration oral solution ~ 4056F
  status ~ 2030F-2031F
Hydrocarbons, chlorinated ~ 82441
Hydrocele
  aspiration ~ 55000
  excision
    bilateral, tunica vaginalis ~ 55041
    unilateral
      spermatic cord ~ 55500
      tunica vaginalis ~ 55040
  repair ~ 55060
Hydrochloric acid, gastric ~ see acid, gastric
Hydrochloride, vancomycin ~ see vancomycin
Hydrocodon ~ see dihydrocodeinone
Hydrogen ion concentration ~ see pH
Hydrolase, acetylcholine ~ see acetylcholinesterase
Hydrolase, triacylglycerol ~ see lipase
Hydrolases, phosphoric monoester ~ see phosphatase
Hydrotherapy (Hubbard tank) ~ 97036, 97113
Hydrotubation ~ 58350
Hydroxyacetanilide ~ see acetaminophen
Hydroxycorticosteroid ~ 83491
Hydroxyindolacetic acid ~ 83497
  urine ~ 83497
Hydroxypregnenolone ~ 80406, 84143

Hydroxyprogesterone ~ 80402-80406, 83498
Hydroxyproline ~ 83500-83505
Hydroxytyramine ~ see dopamine
Hygroma, cystic, axillary/cervical, excision ~ 38550-38555
Hymen
   excision ~ 56700
   incision ~ 56442
Hymenal ring, revision ~ 56700
Hymenectomy ~ 56700
Hymenotomy ~ 56442
Hyoid
   bone, fracture
      closed treatment
         with manipulation ~ 21494
         without manipulation ~ 21493
   muscle, incision and suspension ~ 21685
Hyperbaric oxygen pressurization ~ 99183
Hypercycloidal X-ray ~ 76101-76102
Hyperdactylies ~ see supernumerary digit
Hyperglycemic glycogenolytic factor ~ see glucagon
Hypertelorism of orbit ~ see orbital hypertelorism
Hyperthermia therapy ~ see thermotherapy
Hyperthermia treatment ~ 77600-77620
Hypnotherapy ~ 90880
Hypodermis ~ see subcutaneous tissue
Hypogastric plexus
   destruction ~ 64681
   injection
      anesthetic ~ 64517
      neurolytic ~ 64681
Hypoglossal-facial anastomosis ~ see anastomosis, nerve, facial to
   hypoglossal
Hypoglossal nerve
   anastomosis, to facial nerve ~ 64868
Hypopharynges ~ see hypopharynx
Hypopharynx, biopsy ~ 31510, 31535, 31536, 31576
Hypophysectomy ~ 61546-61548, 62165
Hypophysis ~ see pituitary gland
Hypopyrexia ~ see hypothermia
Hypospadias repair ~ 54300, 54352
   complications ~ 54340-54348
   first stage ~ 54304
      proximal penile or penoscrotal ~ 54332
   one stage
      meatal advancement ~ 54322
      perineal ~ 54336
   urethroplasty
      local skin flaps ~ 54324
      local skin flaps and mobilization of urethra ~ 54326
      local skin flaps, skin graft patch and/or island flap ~ 54328
   urethroplasty for second stage ~ 54308-54316
      free skin graft ~ 54316
   urethroplasty for third stage ~ 54318
Hypoxia
   breathing response ~ 94450
   high altitude simulation test ~ 94452-94453
Hysterectomy
   abdominal
      radical ~ 58210
      resection of ovarian malignancy ~ 58951, 58953-58956
      supracervical ~ 58180
      total ~ 58150, 58200, 58956
         with colpo-urethrocystopexy ~ 58152
         with partial vaginectomy ~ 58200
         with omentectomy ~ 58956
   cesarean
      after cesarean delivery ~ 59525
      with closure of vesicouterine fistula ~ 51925
   laparoscopic ~ 58541-58544
      radical ~ 58548
      total ~ 58570-58573, 58575
   removal lesion ~ 59100
   supracervical
      laparoscopic ~ 58541-58544
   vaginal ~ 58260-58270, 58290-58294, 58550-58554
      with colpectomy ~ 58275-58280
      with colpo-urethrocystopexy ~ 58267
      laparoscopic ~ 58550, 58570-58573, 58575
      radical ~ 58285
      removal tubes/ovaries ~ 58262-58263, 58291-58292, 58552, 58554
      repair of enterocele ~ 58263, 58292, 58294

Hysterolysis ~ 58559
Hysteroplasty ~ 58540
Hysterorrhaphy ~ 58520, 59350
Hysterosalpingography ~ 74740
   catheterization ~ 58345
   injection procedure ~ 58340
Hysterosalpingostomy ~ see implantation, tubouterine
Hysteroscopy
   ablation, endometrial ~ 58563
   diagnostic ~ 58555
   lysis adhesions ~ 58559
   placement fallopian tube implants ~ 58565
   removal
      impacted foreign body ~ 58562
      leiomyomata ~ 58561
   resection of intrauterine septum ~ 58560
   surgical with biopsy ~ 58558
   unlisted services and procedures ~ 58579
Hysterosonography ~ 76831
Hysterotomy ~ 59100
   induced abortion
      with amniotic injections ~ 59852
      with vaginal suppositories ~ 59857
Hysterotrachelectomy ~ 57530

I

I, angiotensin ~ see angiotensin I
1 antibodies, HTLV ~ see antibody, HTLV-1
I, coagulation factor ~ see fibrinogenI, heparin cofactor ~ see antithrombin
IIIICCE ~ see extraction, lens, intracapsular
Ichthyosis, sex linked ~ see syphilis test
ICSH ~ see luteinizing hormone (LH)
Identification
   oocyte, from follicular fluid ~ 89254
   sex chromatin ~ 88130, 88140
   sperm
      from aspiration ~ 89257
      from tissue ~ 89264
      medicolegal ~ 88125
   urate crystal ~ 89060
IDH (isocitric dehydrogenase, blood) ~ 83570
Ig ~ see immune globulins
IgA ~ 82784
IgD ~ 82784
IgE ~ 82785, 86003, 86005, 86008
IgG ~ 82784, 82787, 86001
IgM ~ 82784
II, coagulation factor ~ see prothrombin
II, cranial nerve ~ see optic nerve
Ileal conduit visualization ~ 50690
Ileoscopy via stoma ~ 44384
Ileostomy ~ 44310, 45136
   continent (Kock procedure) ~ 44316
   revision ~ 44312-44314
Iliac arteries ~ see artery, iliac
Iliac crest (free osteocutaneous flap with microvascular anastomosis) ~
   20970
Iliohypogastric nerve, injection anesthetic ~ 64425
Ilioinguinal nerve, injection anesthetic ~ 64425
Ilium
   craterization ~ 27070
   cyst excision ~ 27065-27067
   excision ~ 27070
   fracture, open treatment ~ 27215, 27218
   saucerization ~ 27070
   tumor excision ~ 27065-27067, 27075, 27076
Ilizarov procedure, Monticelli type ~ (see also application, bone fixation
   device) 20692
Imaging
   anatomic model 3D printing ~ 0559T-0562T
Imaging, magnetic resonance ~ see magnetic resonance imaging (MRI)
Imaging, ultrasonic ~ see echography
Imbrication, diaphragm ~ 39545
Imidobenzyle ~ 80335-80337
Imipramine assay ~ 80335-80337
Immune complex assay ~ 86332

Immune globulins
  antitoxin
    botulinum ~ 90287
    diphtheria ~ 90296
  botulism ~ 90288
  cytomegalovirus ~ 90291
  hepatitis B ~ 90371
  human ~ 90281, 90283, 90284
  rabies ~ 90375, 90376, 90377
  respiratory syncytial virus ~ 90378
  Rho (D) ~ 90384-90386
  tetanus ~ 90389
  unlisted immune globulin ~ 90399
  vaccinia ~ 90393
  varicella-zoster ~ 90396
Immune globulin administration ~ 96365-96368, 96372, 96374-96375
Immune globulin E ~ 82785, 86003-86005
Immunization administration
  one vaccine/toxoid ~ 90471, 90473
    with counseling ~ 90460
  each additional vaccine/toxoid ~ 90472, 90474
    with counseling ~ 90461
Immunizations
  active
    acellular pertussis ~ 90700, 90723
    BCG ~ 90585, 90586
    diphtheria ~ 90700-90702, 90723
    diphtheria, tetanus, acellular influenza B and poliovirus inactivated ~ 90698
    hemophilus influenza B ~ 90648, 90748
    hepatitis A ~ 90632-90636
    hepatitis B ~ 90740-90748
    influenza ~ 90655-90660
    influenza B ~ 90647, 90648
    measles, mumps, rubella (MMR) ~ 90707
    measles, mumps, rubella, varicella ~ 90710
    meingococcal ~ 90733, 90734
    pneumococcal ~ 90732
    poliomyelitis ~ 90713
    rabies ~ 90675, 90676
    rotavirus vaccine ~ 90680
    tetanus ~ 90700-90702, 90715, 90723
    typhoid ~ 90690
    varicella (chicken pox) ~ 90716
    yellow fever ~ 90717
  passive
    hyperimmune serum globulin ~ 90287-90399
    immune serum globulin ~ 90281, 90283
  unlisted services and procedures ~ 90749
Immunoassay
  amniotic fluid protein ~ 84112
  analyte ~ 83516, 83518-83520
    calprotectin, fecal ~ 83993
    hemoglobin, fecal ~ 82274
  cellular function, detection of biomarker ~ 86352
  infectious agent ~ 86317-86318, 87449-87451
  nonantibody ~ 83516-83519
  tumor antigen
    human epididymis protein 4 (HE4) ~ 86305
    qualitative/semiqualitative ~ 86294
    quantitative
      CA-125 ~ 86304
      CA 15-3 ~ 86300
      CA 19-9 ~ 86301
      other antigen ~ 86316
Immunoblotting, Western ~ see Western Blot
Immunochemical, lysozyme (muramidase) ~ see lysozyme
Immunocytochemistry ~ 88342, 88344
Immunodeficiency virus, human ~ see HIV
Immunodeficiency virus type 1 , human ~ see HIV 1
Immunodeficiency virus type 2 , human ~ see HIV 2
Immunodiffusion ~ 86329-86331
Immunoelectrophoresis ~ 86320-86327, 86334-86335
Immunofixation electrophoresis ~ 86334-86335
Immunofluorexcence microscopy
  antibody stain procedure ~ 88346, 88350
  antiserum culture typing ~ 87140
Immunofluorescent study ~ 87140, 88346
Immunogen ~ see antigen

Immunoglobulin ~ 82784-82787
  platelet associated ~ 86023
  thyroid stimulating ~ 84445
Immunoglobulin E ~ 86003-86005
Immunologic skin test ~ see skin, tests
Immunology ~ 86000-86849
Immunotherapies, allergen ~ see allergen immunotherapy
Impedance testing ~ (see also audiologic function tests) 92567
Imperfectly descended testis ~ 54550, 54560
Implantable defibrillator
  subcutaneous implantable defibrillator (SICD)
    device evaluation ~ 93260, 93261, 93287, 93295, 93296, 93644
    insertion
      electrode ~ 33202, 33203, 33271
      pulse generator ~ 33230, 33231, 33240
      system ~ 33270
    relocation of skin pocket ~ 33223
    removal ~ 33241, 33262, 33272
    repair, electrode ~ 33218, 33220
    replacement, pulse generator ~ 33262
    repositioning, electrode ~ 33215, 33273
  substernal implantable cardioverter-defibrillator
    electrophysiological evaluation ~ 0577T
    insertion ~ 0571T, 0572T
    interrogation device evaluation ~ 0576T, 0578T, 0579T
    programming device evaluation ~ 0575T
    removal and replacement of pulse generator ~ 0614T
    removal of electrode ~ 0573T
    removal of pulse generator ~ 0580T
    replacement ~ 0571T
    repositioning of electrode ~ 0574T
  transvenous implantable pacing defibrillator (ICD)
    device evaluation ~ 93282-93284, 93287, 93289, 93295, 93296
    insertion
      electrode ~ 33202, 33203, 33216, 33217, 33224, 33225
      pulse generator ~ 33230, 33231, 33249
      system ~ 33249
    relocation of skin pocket ~ 33223
    removal
      electrode ~ 33243, 33244
      pulse generator ~ 33241, 33262-33264
    replacement of pulse generator ~ 33262-33264
    repositioning, electrode ~ 33215, 33273
Implantation
  abdominal wall, non-biologic or synthetic implant ~ 0437T
  annulus reconstruction device
    mitral valve ~ 0544T
    tricuspic valve ~ 0545T
  aortic valve
    transcatheter ~ 33361-33369
  artificial heart, ~ 33927
  baroreflex activation device ~ 0266T-0268T
  biologic, soft tissue reinforcement ~ 15777
  bone, for external speech processor/cochlear stimulator ~ 69714-69718
  brain, chemotherapy ~ 61517
  drug delivery device ~ 11981, 11983, 61517
  electrode(s)
    brain ~ 61531, 61863, 61864, 61867, 61868
    gastric ~ 43647-43648
    nerve ~ 0312T, 64553-64581
    spinal cord ~ 63650-63655
  ethmoid sinus drug-eluting impllant ~ 0406T, 0407T
  eye
    anterior segment ~ 65920
    aqueous shunt to extraocular placement or replacement of pegs ~ 65125
    corneal ring segments ~ 65785
    posterior segment
      extraocular ~ 67120
      intraocular ~ 67121
    reservoir ~ 66180
    vitreous, drug delivery system ~ 67027
  fallopian tube ~ 58565
  hearing aid hormone pellet(s)
    bone conduction ~ 69710
  hip prosthesis ~ see arthroplasty, hip
  hormone pellet ~ 11980
  interatrial septal shunt device ~ 0613T
  joint ~ see arthroplasty
  left atrial appendage ~ 33340

Implantation ~ *continued*
  mesh ~ 49568
    hernia repair ~ 43333, 43335, 43337, 49568, 49652-49657
    vaginal repair ~ 57267
  nerve
    into bone ~ 64787
    into muscle ~ 64787
  neurostimulators
    gastric ~ 95980-95982
    pulse generator ~ 61885
    receiver ~ 61886
  ovum ~ 58976
  pulmonary valve transcatheter percutaneous ~ 33477
  pulse generator
    brain ~ 61885, 61886
    spinal cord electrode array ~ 63685
  receiver
    brain ~ 61885-61886
    spinal cord ~ 63685
  removal ~ 20670-20680
    elbow/radius ~ 24164
  reservoir vascular access device
    declotting ~ 36593
  retinal electrode array ~ 0100T
  total replacement heart system ~ 33927
  tubouterine ~ 58752
  ventricular assist device ~ 33975-33979
    percutaneousl ~ 33990-33991
Implant removal ~ see specific anatomical site
Impression, maxillofacial
  auricular prosthesis ~ 21086
  definitive obturator prosthesis ~ 21080
  facial prosthesis ~ 21088
  interim obturator ~ 21079
  mandibular resection prosthesis ~ 21081
  nasal prosthesis ~ 21087
  oral surgical splint ~ 21085
  orbital prosthesis ~ 21077
  palatal augmentation prosthesis ~ 21082
  palatal lift prosthesis ~ 21083
  speech aid prosthesis ~ 21084
  surgical obturator ~ 21076
In situ hybridization ~ see nucleic acid probe, cytogenetic studies, morphometric analysis
IM injection ~ see injection, intramuscular
In vitro fertilization ~ 58321-58322
In vivo NMR spectroscopy ~ see magnetic resonance spectroscopy
Incision ~ see also incision and drainage
  abdomen ~ 49000
    exploration ~ 58960
  accessory nerve ~ 63191
  anal
    fistula ~ 46270, 46280
    septum ~ 46070
    sphincter ~ 46080
  ankle ~ 27607
    tendon ~ 27605-27606
  anus ~ see anus, incision
  aortic valve for stenosis ~ 33415
  artery, nose ~ 30915-30920
  atrial septum ~ 33735-33737
  bile duct sphincter ~ 43262, 47460
  bladder
    catheterization ~ 51045
    with destruction ~ 51020-51030
    with radiotracer ~ 51020
  bladder diverticulum ~ 52305
  brachial artery exposure ~ 34834
  brain
    amygdalohippocampectomy ~ 61566
    subpial ~ 61567
  breast capsules ~ 19370
  burn scab ~ 16035-16036
  cataract, secondary
    laser surgery ~ 66821
    stab incision technique ~ 66820
  chest, biopsy ~ 32096-32098

Incision ~ *continued*
  colon
    exploration ~ 44025
    stoma
      creation ~ 44320-44322
      revision ~ 44340-44346
  cornea, for astigmatism ~ 65772
  corpus callosum ~ 61541
  cricothyroid membrane ~ 31605
  duodenum ~ 44010
  ear, inner labyrinth
    transcanal ~ 69801
  elbow ~ 24000
  esophagus ~ 43020, 43045
    muscle ~ 43030
  exploration
    heart ~ 33310-33315
    kidney ~ 50010
  eye
    adhesions ~ 65880
      anterior segment ~ 65860-65865
      anterior synechiae ~ 65870
      corneovitreal ~ 65880
      posterior ~ 65875
    anterior chamber ~ 65820
    trabeculae ~ 65850
  eyelid
    canthus ~ 67715
    sutures ~ 67710
  femoral artery
    exposure ~ 34812-34813
  fibula ~ 27607
  finger
    decompression ~ 26035
    tendon ~ 26060, 26455-26460
    tendon sheath ~ 26055
  foot ~ 28005
    capsule ~ 28260-28264
    fasciotomy ~ 28008
    for infection ~ 28002-28003
    tendon ~ 28230, 28234
  gallbladder ~ 47490
  hand decompression ~ 26035-26037
    tendon ~ 26450, 26460
  heartexploration ~ 33310-33315
  hemorrhoids, external ~ 46083
  hepatic ducts ~ see hepaticostomy
  hip
    denervation ~ 27035
    exploration ~ 27033
    fasciotomy ~ 27025
    joint capsule
      for flexor release ~ 27036
    tendon
      abductor ~ 27006
      adductor ~ 27000-27003
      iliopsoas ~ 27005
  hymen ~ see hymen, incision
  hymenotomy ~ 56442
  hyoid muscle ~ 21685
  iliac artery exposure ~ 34820, 34833
  intercarpal joint dislocation ~ 25670
  interphalangeal joint capsule ~ 26525
  intestines, small ~ 44010
    biopsy ~ 44020
    creation
      pouch ~ 44316
      stoma ~ 44300-44310, 44314
    decompression ~ 44021
    exploration ~ 44020
    incision ~ 44020
    removal foreign body ~ 44020
    revision stoma ~ 44312
  iris ~ 66500-66505
  kidney ~ 50010, 50045
  knee
    capsule ~ 27435
    exploration ~ 27310
    fasciotomy ~ 27305
    removal of foreign body ~ 27310

Incision ~ *continued*
lacrimal punctum ~ 68440
lacrimal sac ~ see dacryocystotomy
leg, lower fasciotomy ~ 27600-27602
leg, upper fasciotomy ~ 27305
   tenotomy ~ 27306-27307, 27390-27392
lip, frenum ~ 40806
liver ~ see hepatotomy
lung
  biopsy ~ 32096-32097
  decortication
    partial ~ 32225
    total ~ 32220
lymphatic channels ~ 38308
mastoid ~ see mastoidotomy
metacarpophalangeal joint capsule ~ 26520
mitral valve ~ 33420-33422
muscle ~ see myotomy
nerve ~ 64575-64580, 64585, 64595, 64702-64772
  foot ~ 28035
  root ~ 63185-63190
  sacral ~ 64581
  vagus ~ 43640-43641
nose ~ see rhinotomy
orbit ~ see orbitotomy
palm fasciotomy ~ 26040-26045
pancreas sphincter ~ 43262
penis
  prepuce ~ 54000-54001
    newborn ~ 54000
pericardium
  with clot removal ~ 33020
  with foreign body removal ~ 33020
pharynx stoma ~ 42955
pleura biopsy ~ 32098
pleural cavity
  empyema ~ 32035-32036
  pneumothorax ~ 32551
prostate
  exposure
    bilateral pelvic lymphadenectomy ~ 55865
    insertion radioactive substance ~ 55860
    lymph node biopsy ~ 55862
    transurethral ~ 52450
pterygomaxillary fossa ~ 31040
pulmonary valve ~ 33470-33474
pyloric sphincter ~ 43520
retina, encircling material ~ 67115
sclera
  fistulization
    sclerectomy with punch or scissors with iridectomy ~ 66160
    thermocauterization with iridectomy ~ 66155
    trabeculectomy ab externo in absence previous surgery ~ 66170
    trephination with iridectomy ~ 66150
seminal vesicle ~ 55600-55605
  complicated ~ 55605
shoulder
  bone ~ 23035
  capsular contracture release ~ 23020
  removal, calcareous deposits ~ 23000
  tenomyotomy ~ 23405-23406
shoulder joint ~ 23040-23044
sinus
  frontal ~ 31070-31087
  maxillary ~ 31020-31032
    endoscopic ~ 31256-31267
  multiple ~ 31090
  sphenoid
    sinusotomy ~ 31050-31051
skin ~ 10040-10180
skull ~ 61316, 62148
  suture ~ 61550-61552
spinal cord ~ 63200
  tract ~ 63170, 63194-63199
stomach
  creation, stoma ~ 43830-43832
  exploration ~ 43500
  pyloric sphincter ~ 43520
synovectomy ~ 26140
temporomandibular joint ~ 21010

Incision ~ *continued*
tendon, arm, upper ~ 24310
thigh, fasciotomy ~ 27025
thorax
  empyema ~ 32035-32036
  pneumothorax ~ 32551
thyroid gland ~ see thyrotomy
tibia ~ 27607
toe
  capsule ~ 28270-28272
  fasciotomy ~ 28008
  tendon ~ 28232-28234
  tenotomy ~ 28010-28011
tongue, frenum ~ 41010
trachea
  emergency ~ 31603-31605
  planned ~ 31600-31601
  with flaps ~ 31610
tympanic membrane ~ 69420
  with anesthesia ~ 69421
ureter ~ 50600
ureterocele ~ 51535
urethra ~ 53000-53010
  meatus ~ 53020-53025
uterus, remove lesion ~ 59100
vagina, exploration ~ 57000
vas deferens ~ 55200
  for X-ray ~ 55300
vestibule of the mouth ~ see mouth, vestibule
vitreous strands
  laser surgery ~ 67031
  pars plana approach ~ 67030
wrist ~ 25100-25105
  capsule ~ 25085
  decompression ~ 25020-25025
  tendon sheath ~ 25000-25001
Incisional hernia repair ~ see hernia, repair, incisional
Incision and drainage ~ see also drainage; incision
abdomen
  fluid ~ 49082-49083
  pancreatitis ~ 48000
abscess
  abdomen ~ 49020, 49040
  anal ~ 46045-46050
  ankle ~ 27603
  appendix ~ 44900
  arm, lower ~ 25028
  arm, upper ~ 23930-23931
  auditory canal, external ~ 69020
  Bartholin's gland ~ 56420
  bladder ~ 51080
  brain ~ 61320-61321
  breast ~ 19020
  ear, external
    complicated ~ 69005
    simple ~ 69000
  elbow ~ 23930
  epididymis ~ 54700
  eyelid ~ 67700
  finger ~ 26010-26011
  gums ~ 41800
  hip ~ 26990
  kidney ~ 50020
  knee ~ 27301
  leg, lower ~ 27603
  leg, upper ~ 27301
  liver ~ 47010
  lung ~ 32200
  lymph node ~ 38300-38305
  mouth ~ 40800-40801, 41005-41009, 41015-41018
  nasal septum ~ 30020
  neck ~ 21501-21502
  nose ~ 30000-30020
  ovary ~ 58820-58822
    abdominal approach ~ 58822
  palate ~ 42000
  paraurethral gland ~ 53060
  parotid gland ~ 42300-42305
  pelvis ~ 26990, 45000
  perineum ~ 56405

Incision and drainage ~ *continued*

peritoneum ~ 49020
prostrate ~ 55720-55725
rectum ~ 45005-45020, 46040, 46050-46060
retroperitoneal ~ 49060
   open ~ 49060
salivary gland ~ 42300-42320
scrotum ~ 54700, 55100
Skene's gland ~ 53060
skin ~ 10060-10061
subdiaphragmatic, percutaneous ~ 49040
sublingual gland ~ 42310-42320
submaxillary gland ~ 42310-42320
subphrenic, percutaneous ~ 49040
testis ~ 54700
thorax ~ 21501-21502
throat ~ 42700-42725
tongue ~ 41000-41006, 41015
tonsil ~ 42700
urethra ~ 53040
uvula ~ 42000
vagina ~ 57010
vulva ~ 56405
wrist ~ 25028
ankle ~ 27610
bile duct ~ 47420-47425
bladder ~ 51040
bulla, skin, puncture aspiration ~ 10160
bursa
   ankle ~ 27604
   arm, lower ~ 25031
   elbow ~ 23931
   foot ~ 28001
   hip ~ 26991
   knee ~ 27301
   leg, lower ~ 27604
   leg, upper ~ 27301
   palm ~ 26025-26030
   pelvis ~ 26991
   wrist ~ 25031
carbuncle
   skin ~ 10060-10061
carpals ~ 25035, 26034
comedones
   skin ~ 10040
cyst
   conjunctiva ~ 68020
   gums ~ 41800
   liver ~ 47010
   lung ~ 32200
   mouth ~ 40800-40801, 41005-41009, 41015-41018
   ovarian ~ 58800-58805
   skin ~ 10040-10061
      pilonidal ~ 10080-10081
      puncture aspiration ~ 10160
      spinal cord ~ 63172-63173
   thyroid gland ~ 60000
   tongue ~ 41000-41006, 41015, 60000
elbow
   abscess ~ 23935
   arthrotomy ~ 24000
femur ~ 27303
fluid collection
   skin ~ 10140
foreign body, skin ~ 10120-10121
furuncle ~ 10060-10061
gallbladder ~ 47480
hematoma
   ankle ~ 27603
   arm, lower ~ 25028
   arm, upper ~ 23930
   brain ~ 61312-61315
   ear, external
      complicated ~ 69005
      simple ~ 69000
   elbow ~ 23930
   epididymis ~ 54700
   gums ~ 41800
   hip ~ 26990

Incision and drainage ~ *continued*

knee ~ 27301
leg, lower ~ 27603
leg, upper ~ 27301
mouth ~ 40800-40801, 41005-41009, 41015-41018
nasal septum ~ 30020
neck ~ 21501-21502
nose ~ 30000-30020
pelvis ~ 26990
scrotum ~ 54700
skin ~ 10140
   puncture aspiration ~ 10160
skull ~ 61312-61315
testis ~ 54700
thorax ~ 21501-21502
tongue ~ 41000-41006, 41015
vagina ~ 57022-57023
wrist ~ 25028
hepatic duct ~ 47400
hip bone ~ 26992, 27030
humerus abscess ~ 23935
interphalangeal joint
   toe ~ 28024
intertarsal joint ~ 28020
kidney ~ 50040, 50125
knee ~ 27303, 27310
lacrimal gland ~ 68400
lacrimal sac ~ 68420
liver
   abscess or cyst ~ 47010
mediastinum ~ 39000-39010
metatarsophalangeal joint ~ 28022
milia, multiple ~ 10040
onychia ~ 10060-10061
orbit ~ 67405, 67440
paronychia ~ 10060-10061
pelvic bone ~ 26992
penis ~ 54015
pericardium ~ 33025
phalanges, finger ~ 26034
pilonidal cyst ~ 10080-10081
pustules, skin ~ 10040
radius ~ 25035
seroma, skin ~ 10140
shoulder
   abscess ~ 23030
   arthrotomy
      acromioclavicular joint ~ 23044
      sternoclavicular joint ~ 23044
   bursa ~ 23031
   hematoma ~ 23030
shoulder joint, arthrotomy, glenohumeral joint ~ 23040
tarsometatarsal joint ~ 28020
tendon sheath
   finger ~ 26020
   palm ~ 26020
thorax
   deep ~ 21510
toe ~ 28024
ulna ~ 25035
ureter ~ 50600
vagina ~ 57020
wound infection, skin ~ 10180
wrist ~ 25028, 25040

Inclusion bodies
fluid ~ 88106
smear ~ 87207-87210

Incomplete abortion ~ see abortion, incomplete
Indicator dilution studies ~ 93561-93562
Induced abortion ~ see abortion
Induced hyperthermia ~ see thermotherapy
Induced hypothermia ~ see hypothermia
Induratio penis plastica ~ see Peyronie disease
Infant, newborn, intensive care ~ see intensive care, neonatal
Infantile paralysis ~ see polio
Infection
actinomyces ~ see actinomycosis
bone ~ see osteomyelitis
diagnosis, group A strep test ~ 3210F
filarioidea ~ see filariasis

Infection ~ continued

immunoassay ~ 86317-86318

postoperative wound ~ see postoperative wound infection

rapid test ~ 86403-86406

treatment, antibiotic prescribed ~ 4045F

wound ~ see wound, infection

Infectious agent

antibody detection

immunoassay, multiple-step

actinomyces ~ 86602

adenovirus ~ 86603

aspergillus ~ 86606

bacterium ~ 86609

bartonella ~ 86611

blastomyces ~ 86612

bordetella ~ 86615

borrelia ~ 86617-86619

brucella ~ 86622

campylobacter ~ 86625

candida ~ 86628

chlamydia ~ 86631, 86632

coccidioides ~ 86635

coronavirus disease (COVID-19) ~ 86769

coxiella burnetii ~ 86638

cryptococcus ~ 86641

cytomegalovirus (CMV) ~ 86644, 86645

delta agent ~ 86692

diphtheria ~ 6648

ehrlichia ~ 86666

encephalitis ~ 86651-86654

enterovirus ~ 86658, 87498

epstein-barr virus ~ 6663-86665

francisella tularensis ~ 86668

fungus, other ~ 86671

giardia lamblia ~ 86674

haemophilus influenzae ~ 86684

helicobacter pylori ~ 86677

helminth ~ 86682

hepatitis, delta agent ~ 86692

hepatitis A (HAAb) ~ 86708, 86709

hepatitis B

core ~ 86704

IgM ~ 86705

surface ~ 86706

hHepatitis Be ~ 86707

hepatitis C ~ 86803, 86804

herpes simplex ~ 86694-86696

histoplasma ~ 86698

HIV ~ 86689, 86701-86703

HIV-1 ~ 86701, 86703, 87389, 87806

HIV-2 ~ 86702, 86703, 87389, 87806

HTLV-I ~ 86687, 86689

HTLV-II ~ 86688

influenza virus ~ 86710

legionella ~ 86713

leishmania ~ 86717

leptospira ~ 86720

listeria monocytogenes ~ 86723

lyme disease ~ 86617

lymphocytic choriomeningitis ~ 86727

malaria ~ 86750

mucormycosis ~ 86732

mumps ~ 86735

mycoplasma ~ 86738

neisseria meningitidis ~ 86741

nocardia ~ 86744

parvovirus ~ 86747

plasmodium ~ 86750

protozoa ~ 86753

respiratory syncytial virus ~ 86756

rickettsia ~ 86757

rotavirus ~ 86759

rubella ~ 86762

rubeola ~ 86765

salmonella ~ 86768

severe acute respiratory syndrome coronavirus 2 (SARS-CoV-2) ~ 86769

Shigella ~ 86771

tetanus ~ 86774

thyroglobulin ~ 86800

Infectious agent ~ continued

toxoplasma ~ 86777, 86778

treponema pallidum ~ 86780

trichinella ~ 86784

tuberculosis ~ 86580

varicella-zoster ~ 86787

virus, other ~ 86790

west nile virus ~ 86788, 86789

yersinia ~ 86793

immunoassay, other antibody, quantitative ~ 86317

immunoassay, single-step

coronavirus disease (COVID-19) ~ 86328

qualitative/semiquantitative ~ 86318

severe acute respiratory syndrome coronavirus 2 (SARS-CoV-2) ~ 86328

antigen detection

direct fluorescence

bordetella ~ 87265

chlamydia trachomatis ~ 87270

cryptosporidium ~ 87272

cytomegalovirus ~ 87271

enterovirus ~ 87267

giardia ~ 87269

influenza A ~ 87276

legionella pneumophila ~ 87278

respiratory syncytial virus ~ 87280

treponema pallidum ~ 87285

varicella-zoster ~ 87290

immunoassay

adenovirus ~ 87301, 87809

aspergillus ~ 87305

chlamydia trachomatis ~ 87320

clostridium difficile ~ 87324

cryptococcus neoformans ~ 87327

cryptosporidium ~ 87328

cytomegalovirus ~ 87332

entamoeba histolytica dispar group ~ 87336

entamoeba histolytica group ~ 87337

escherichia coli 0157 ~ 87335

giardia ~ 87329

helicobacter pylori ~ 87338-87339

hepatitis, delta agent ~ 87380

hepatitis B surface antigen (HBsAg) ~ 87340

hepatitis B surface antigen (HBsAg) neutralization ~ 87341

hepatitis Be antigen (HBeAg) ~ 87350

histoplasma capsulatum ~ 87385

HIV-1 ~ 87390

HIV-2 ~ 87391

influenza A ~ 87400

influenza B ~ 87400

multiple step method ~ 87301-87449, 87451

not otherwise specified ~ 87449, 87451

polyvalent ~ 87451

respiratory syncytial virus ~ 87420

rotavirus ~ 87425

shiga-like toxin ~ 87427

single step method ~ 87450

streptococcus, group A ~ 87430

immunoassay, with direct optical observation

chlamydia trachomatis ~ 87810

clostridium difficile ~ 87803

gonorrhea ~ 87850

HIV-1 ~ 87806

influenza ~ 87804

neisseria gonorrhoeae ~ 87850

not otherwise specified ~ 87899

respiratory syncytial virus ~ 87807

streptococcus, group A ~ 87880

streptococcus, group B ~ 87802

trichomonas vaginalis ~ 87808

immunofluorescence ~ 87260, 87273-87275, 87279, 87281-87283, 87299-87300

adenovirus ~ 87260

herpes simplex ~ 87273-.87274

influenza B ~ 87275

not otherwise specified ~ 87299

parainfluenza virus ~ 87279

pneumocystis carinii ~ 87281

polyvalent ~ 87300

rubeola ~ 87283

Infectious agent ~ _continued_
  nucleic acid probe
    bartonella henselae ~ 87471-87472
    bartonella quintana ~ 87471-87472
    borrelia burgdorferi ~ 87475, 87476
    candida species ~ 87480-87482
    chlamydia pneumoniae ~ 87485-87487
    chlamydia trachomatis ~ 87490-87492
    clostridium difficile ~ 87493
    cytomegalovirus ~ 87495-87497
    enterovirus ~ 87498, 87500
    gardnerella vaginalis ~ 87510-87512
    gastrointestinal pathogen ~ 87505-87507
    gonorrhea ~ 87850
    hepatitis B virus ~ 87516, 87517
    hepatitis C ~ 87520-87522
    hepatitis G ~ 87525-87527
    herpes simplex virus ~ 87528-87530
    herpes virus-6 ~ 87531-87533
    HIV-1 ~ 87534-87536
    HIV-2 ~ 87537-87539
    influenza ~ 87501-87503
    legionella pneumophila ~ 87540-87542
    multiple organisms ~ 87800, 87801
    mycobacteria avium-intracellulare ~ 87560-87562
    mycobacteria species ~ 87550-87552
    mycobacteria tuberculosis ~ 87555-87557
    mycoplasma pneumoniae ~ 87580-87582
    neisseria gonorrhoeae ~ 87590-87592
    not otherwise specified ~ 87797-87799
    papillomavirus, human ~ 0500T, 87623-87625
    respiratory virus ~ 87631-87634
    staphylococcus aureus ~ 87640, 87641
    streptococcus, group A ~ 87650-87652
    streptococcus, group B ~ 87653
    trichomonas vaginalis ~ 87660, 87661
    vancomycin resistance ~ 87500
    zika virus ~ 87662
  concentration ~ 87015
  detection by nucleic acid probe
    central nervous system pathogen ~ 87483
    coronavirus disease (COVID-19) ~ 87635
    severe acute respiratory syndrome coronavirus-2 (SARS-CoV2) ~ 87635
  enzymatic activity ~ 87905
  genotype analysis by nucleic acid
    cytomegalovirus ~ 87910
    hepatitis B virus ~ 87912
    hepatitis C virus ~ 87902
    high-risk HPV types ~ 0500T
    HIV-1 regions ~ 87901, 87906
  phenotype analysis
    by nucleic acid
      HIV-1 drug resistance ~ 87903-87904
  phenotype prediction
    by genetic database ~ 87900
Infectious mononucleosis virus ~ see Epstein-Barr virus
Inflammatory process
  localization
    nuclear medicine ~ 78800-78804, 78830-78832
Inflation
  ear, middle
    eustachian tube ~ 69799
  eustachian tube
    myringotomy ~ 69420
      anesthesia ~ 69424
Influenza A
  antigen detection
    direct fluorescence ~ 87276
    enzyme immunoassay ~ 87400
Influenza B
  antigen detection
    enzyme immunoassay ~ 87400
    immunofluorescence ~ 87275
Influenza vaccine ~ see vaccines
Influenza virus
  antibody ~ 86710
  by immunoassay
    with direct optical observation ~ 87804
  by nucleic acid ~ 87501-87503

Infraorbital nerve
  avulsion ~ 64734
  incision ~ 64734
  transection ~ 64734
Infrared light treatment ~ 97026
Infratentorial craniectomy ~ 61520-61521
Infusion
  amnion, transabdominal ~ 59070
  anesthetic
    paravertebral block (PVB) ~ 64463
  cerebral
    for other than thrombolysis ~ 61650, 61651
    for thrombolysis
      intravenous ~ 37195
      percutaneous ~ 61645
  for thrombolysis
    percutaneous transluminal ~ 61645
    transcatheter therapy ~ 37211-37214
  hydration ~ 96360, 96361
    status documented ~ 2030F, 2031F
  intraosseous ~ 36680
  intravenous, unlisted ~ 96379
    diagnostic/prophylactic/therapeutic ~ 96365-96368, 96379
    hydration ~ 96360, 96361
  radioelement ~ 77750
  subcutaneous ~ 96369-96371
  spinal
    device implantation/replacement ~ 62360-62362
    diagnostic/therapeutic ~ 62324-62327
  transcatheter therapy ~ 37211-37214
Infusion pump
  electronic analysis, spinal cord ~ 62367-62368
  insertion, intra-arterial ~ 36260
  intra-arterial
    removal ~ 36262
    revision ~ 36261
  intravenous
    insertion ~ 36563
    repair ~ 36576
    replacement ~ 36583
  maintenance ~ 95990-95991, 96520-96530
  spinal cord ~ 62361-62362
  ventricular catheter ~ 61215
Infusion therapy ~ 62350-62351, 62360-62362
  arterial catheterization ~ 36640
  chemotherapy ~ 96410-96414, 96422-96425
  home infusion procedures ~ 99601-99602
  intravenous ~ 90780-90781
  pain ~ 62360-62362, 62367-62368
  subcutaneous ~ 96369-96371
Ingestion challenge test ~ 95076, 95079
Inguinal hernia repair ~ see hernia, repair, inguinal
INH ~ see drug assay
Inhalation pentamidine ~ 94642
Inhalation provocation tests ~ see bronchial challenge test
Inhalation treatment ~ (see also pulmonology, therapeutic) 94640, 94644-94645, 94664, 99503
Inhibin A ~ 86336
Inhibition test, hemagglutination ~ see hemagglutination inhibition test
Inhibition, fertilization ~ see contraception
Inhibitor, alpha 1-protease ~ see alpha-1 antitrypsin
Inhibitor, alpha 2-plasmin ~ see alpha-2 antiplasmin
Inhibitory concentration, minimum ~ see minimum inhibitory
  concentration
Initial inpatient consultations ~ see consultation, initial inpatient
Injection ~ see allergen immunotherapy; infusion
  abdomen
    air ~ 49400
    contrast material ~ 49400
  anesthetic agent
    paravertebral block (PVB) ~ 64461, 64462
    sacroiliac joint ~ 27096
    spine
      cervical ~ 62320, 62321, 62324, 62325
      lumbar ~ 62322, 62323, 62326, 62327
      sacral ~ 62322, 62323, 62326, 62327
      thoracic ~ 2320, 62321, 62324, 62325
  angiography, pulmonary ~ 75746
  ankle, radial ~ 27648
  antibiotic ~ see antibiotic administration

Injection ~ *continued*
  antigen (allergen) ~ 95115-95125
  aorta (aortography), radiologic ~ 93567
  aponeurosis ~ 20550
  bile duct, cholangiography ~ 47531, 47532
  bladder, radiologic ~ 51600-51610
  brain canal ~ 61070
  bronchography, segmental ~ 31899
  bursa ~ 20600-20610
  cardiac catheterization ~ 93563-93568
  carpal tunnel, therapeutic ~ 20526
  chemotherapy ~ 96400-96450, 96542
  cistern, medication or other ~ 61055
  contrast, via catheter ~ 49424
  corpora cavernosa ~ 54235
  cyst
    bone ~ 20615
    kidney ~ 50390
    pelvis ~ 50390
    thyroid ~ 60300
  diagnostic, additional sequential, each push ~ 96376
  elbow, arthrography, radiologic ~ 24220
  epidural ~ see epidural, injection
  esophageal varices, endoscopy ~ 43243
  esophagus
    sclerosing agent ~ 43204
    submucosal ~ 43201
  extremity, pseudoaneurysm ~ 36002
  eye
    anterior segment
      air ~ 66020
      medication ~ 66030
    pharmacologic agent ~ 0465T, 67028
    posterior segment
      intravitreal ~ 67028
      suprachoroidal ~ 0465T
  eyelid, subconjunctival ~ 68200
  fluid collection, sclerosant ~ 49185
  foot, nerve ~ 64455
  ganglion, anesthetic ~ 64505, 64510
  ganglion cyst ~ 20612
  gastric varices, endoscopy ~ 43243
  hand, cell therapy for scleroderma ~ 0490T
  heart vessels
    cardiac catheterization ~ 93563-93568
    radiologic ~ 93563
  hemorrhoids, sclerosing solution ~ 46500
  hip, radiologic ~ 27093-27095
  insect venom ~ 95130-95134
  intervertebral disk
    allogenic cellular/tissue-based product ~ 0627T-0630T
    chemonucleolysis agent ~ 62292
    radiological ~ 62290-62291
  intraamniotic ~ 59852
  intra-arterial ~ 96373, 96379
    thrombolytic ~ 37184-37186, 61645
  intradermal, for tattooing ~ 11920-11922
  intralesional, skin ~ 11900-11901
  intramuscular ~ 96372
    therapeutic ~ 96372, 99506
  intravenous ~ 96379
    nuclear diagnostic localization ~ 78808
    thrombolytic ~ 37187-37188
    unlisted ~ 96379
    vascular flow check, graft ~ 15860
  intravenous push ~ 96374-96376
  joint ~ 20600-20610
  kidney
    drugs ~ 50391
    for nephrostogram ~ 50430, 50431
  knee, radiologic ~ 27369
  lacrimal gland, radiologic ~ 68850
  larynx, endoscopic ~ 31570, 31573, 31574
  left heart, radiologic ~ 93565
  lesion, skin ~ 11900-11901
  ligament ~ 20550
  liver ~ 47015
  mammary ductogram/galactogram ~ 19030
  muscle endplate
    facial ~ 64612

Injection ~ *continued*
  nerve
    anesthetic ~ 01991-01992, 64400-64530
    neurolytic agent ~ 64600-64640, 64680-64681
  orbit
    retrobulbar
      alcohol ~ 67505
      medication ~ 67500
    tenon's capsule ~ 67515
  pancreatography ~ 48400
  paravertebral facet joint/nerve ~ 64490-64495
  penis
    for erection ~ 54235
    Peyronie disease ~ 54200
      with surgical exposure of plague ~ 54205
    radiology ~ 54230
    vasoactive drugs ~ 54231
  peritoneal cavity air ~ see pneumoperitoneum
  prophylactic, additional sequential, each push ~ 96376
  radiologic
    breast ~ 19030
    cholangiography ~ 47531, 47532
  rectum, sclerosing solution ~ 45520
  right heart ~ see cardiac catheterization, injection
    radiologic ~ 93566
  sacroiliac joint, for arthrography ~ 27096
  salivary duct ~ 42660
  salivary gland, radiologic ~ 42550
  sclerosing agent
    esophagus ~ 43204
    intravenous ~ 36465, 36466, 36468, 36470, 36471
  sentinel node identification ~ 38792
  shoulder, arthrography, radiologic ~ 23350
  shunt, peritoneal, venous ~ 49427
  sinus tract ~ 20500
    diagnostic ~ 20501
  spider veins, telangiectasia ~ 36468
  spinal artery ~ 62294
  spinal cord
    anesthetic ~ 62320-62327
    blood ~ 62273
    neurolytic agent ~ 62280-62282
    other ~ 62320-62327
    radiological ~ 62284
  steroids
    spine
      cervial ~ 62320, 62321, 62324, 62325
      lumbar ~ 62322, 62323, 62326, 62327
      sacral ~ 62322, 62323, 62326, 62327
      thoracic ~ 62320, 62321, 62324, 62325
    urethral stricture ~ 52283
  subcutaneous ~ 96372
    silicone ~ 11950-11954
    therapeutic ~ 96372
    timed application of on-body injection device ~ 96377
  temporomandibular joint, arthrography ~ 21116
  tendon origin, insertion ~ 20551
  tendon sheath ~ 20550
  therapeutic
    extremity pseudoaneurysm ~ 36002
    lung ~ 32960
    thyroid ~ 60300
    turbinate ~ 30200
  thoracic cavity ~ see pleurodesis, chemical
  trachea ~ 31612
    puncture ~ 31612
  transtracheal, bronchography ~ 31899
  trigger point(s)
    one or two muscles ~ 20552
    two or more muscles ~ 20553
  turbinate ~ 30200
  unlisted services and procedures ~ 90799
  ureter
    drugs ~ 50391
    for ureterogram ~ 50430, 50431
    radiologic ~ 50684
  veins
    sclerosant ~ 36465, 36466, 36468, 36470, 36471
  venography ~ 36005

Injection ~ continued

ventricle
    dye ~ 61120
    medication or other ~ 61026
vitreous ~ 67028
    fluid substitute ~ 67025
vocal cords, therapeutic ~ 31513, 31570-31571
white blood cells, autologous concentrate ~ 0481T
wrist
    carpal tunnel, therapeutic ~ 20526
    radiologic ~ 25246

Inkblot test ~ 96101-96103
Inner ear ~ see ear, inner
Innominate arteries ~ see artery, brachiocephalic
Innominate tumor excision ~ 27077
Inorganic sulfates ~ see sulfate
Insemination, artificial ~ 58321-58322, 89268
Insertion ~ see also implantation; intubation; transplantation

aqueous drainage device
    to extraocular reservoir ~ 66179, 66180
    without extraocular reservoir ~ 0376T, 0449T, 0450T, 66183
balloon, intra-aortic ~ 33967, 33973
breast implants ~ 19340-19342
bronchial valve ~ 31647, 31651
cannula
    arteriovenous ~ 36810-36815
    extra corporeal circulation for regional chemotherapy of extremity ~ 36823
    for on-body injector ~ 96377
    thoracic duct ~ 38794
    vein to vein ~ 36800
catheter
    abdomen ~ 49324, 49419-49421, 49435
    abdominal artery ~ 36245-36248
    aorta ~ 36200
    bladder ~ 51045, 51701-51703
    brachiocephalic artery ~ 36215-36218
    brain ~ 61210, 61770
    breast, for interstitial radioelement application ~ 19296-19298
    bronchi ~ 31717
    bronchus, for intracavitary radioelement application ~ 31643
    cardiac ~ see catheterization, cardiac
        flow directed ~ 93503
    ear, middle ~ 69799
    eustachian tube ~ 69799
    gastrointestinal, upper ~ 43241
    intraperitoneal ~ 49418-49419
    jejunum ~ 44015
    lower extremity artery ~ 36245-36248
    nasotracheal ~ 31720
    pelvic artery ~ 36245-36248
    pericardium ~ 33017-33019
    pleural cavity ~ 32550
    portal vein ~ 36481
    prostate ~ 55875
    pulmonary artery ~ 36013-36015
    right heart ~ 36013, 93451
    skull ~ 61107
    spinal cord ~ 62350-62351
    suprapubic ~ 51102, 51045
    thoracic artery ~ 36215-36218
    tracheobronchial ~ 31725
    urethra ~ 51701-51703
    vena cava ~ 36010
    venous ~ 36011-36012, 36400-36410, 36420-36425, 36500-36510, 36555-36558, 36568-36569
cecostomy tube ~ 49442
cervical dilation ~ 59200
cochlear device ~ 69930
colonic tube ~ 49442
defibrillator system, subcutaneous ~ 33270
distraction device
    interlaminar/interspinous process, lumbar ~ 22867-22870
drug delivery device ~ 20700, 20702, 20704
drug delivery implant ~ 11981, 11983
duodenostomy tube ~ 49441

Insertion ~ continued

electrode
    brain ~ 61531-61533, 61760, 61863, 61864, 61867, 61868
    chest wall, respiratory sensor ~ 0466T
    heart ~ 33202-33203, 33210-33211, 33216-33217, 33224-33225, 33271, 93620-93622
    nerve ~ 64553-64581
    retina ~ 0100T
    sphenoidal ~ 95830
    spinal cord ~ 63650-63655
    stomach
        laparoscopic, neurostimulator ~ 43647
        open, neurostimulator ~ 43881
endotracheal tube ~ 31500
gastrostomy tube
    laparoscopic ~ 43653
    percutaneous ~ 43246, 49440
glucose sensor~ 0446T, 0448T
graft
    aorta ~ 33330-33335
    heart vessel ~ 33330-33335
guide wire
    endoscopy ~ 43248
    esophagoscopy ~ 43248
        with dilation ~ 43226
Heyman capsule, uterus
    for brachytherapy ~ 58346
iliac artery occlusion device ~ 34808
implant, bone
    for external speech processor/cochlear stimulator ~ 69714-69718
infusion pump
    intra-arterial ~ 36260
    intravenous ~ 36563
    spinal cord ~ 62361-62362
intracatheter/needle
    aorta ~ 36160
    dialysis circuit ~ 36901-36903
    intra-arterial ~ 36100-36140
    intravenous ~ 36000
intramedullary lengthening device
    humeral osteotomy ~ 0594T
intraocular lens ~ 66983
    manual or mechanical technique ~ 66982, 66984, 66987, 66988
    not associated with concurrent cataract removal ~ 66985
intrauterine device (IUD) ~ 58300
jejunostomy tube
    endoscopy ~ 44372
    percutaneous ~ 49441
keel, laryngoplasty ~ 31580
laminaria ~ 59200
mesh, pelvic floor ~ 57267
nasobiliary tube, endoscopy ~ 43274
nasopancreatic tube, endoscopy ~ 43274
needle
    bone ~ 36680
    intraosseous ~ 36680
    muscle ~ 20560, 20561
    prostate ~ 55875-55876
needle wire, trachea ~ 31730
neurostimulator
    pulse generator ~ 64590
    receiver ~ 64590
nose, septal prosthesis ~ 30220
obturator, larynx ~ 31527
ocular implant
    with/without conjunctival graft ~ 65150
    with foreign material ~ 65155
    muscles attached ~ 65140
    muscles, not attached ~ 65135
    in scleral shell ~ 65130
orbital transplant ~ 67550
oviduct
    chromotubation ~ 58350
    hydrotubation ~ 58350
ovoid, vagina, for brachytherapy ~ 57155
pacemaker, heart ~ 33206-33208
    pulse generator only ~ 33212-33213, 33221

Insertion ~ *continued*

pacemaker or implantable defibrillator
  leads ~ 33216, 33217, 33224, 33225, 33230, 33231, 33243, 33244, 33249
    pulse generator only ~ 33240
packing, vagina ~ 57180
penile prosthesis, inflatable ~ see penile prosthesis, insertion, inflatable
pessary, vagina ~ 57160
pin, skeletal traction ~ 20650
probe, brain ~ 61770
prostaglandin ~ 59200
prostate, radioactive substance ~ 55860
prosthesis
  knee ~ 27438, 27445
  nasal septal ~ 30220
  palate ~ 42281
  pelvic floor ~ 57267
  penis
    inflatable ~ 54401-54405
    noninflatable ~ 54400
  speech ~ 31611
  testis ~ 54660
  urethral sphincter ~ 53444-53445
radioactive material
  bladder ~ 51020
  cystourethroscopy ~ 52250
receiver
  brain ~ 61885-61886
  spinal cord ~ 63685
reservoir
  brain ~ 61210-61215
  spinal cord ~ 62360
  subcutaneous ~ 49419
sensor, fetal oximetry
  cervix ~ 0021T
  vagina ~ 0021T
shunt ~ 36835
  abdomen
    vein ~ 49425
    venous ~ 49426
  intrahepatic portosystemic ~ 37182
spinal instrument ~ 22849
  spinous process ~ 22841
spinal instrumentation
  anterior ~ 22845-22847
  biomechanical device ~ 22853, 22854, 22859
  internal spinal fixation ~ 22841
  pelvic fixation ~ 22848
  posterior nonsegmental
    Harrington rod technique ~ 22840
  posterior segmental ~ 22842-22844
  stabilization/distraction device ~ 22869, 22870
stent
  bile duct ~ 43274, 47801
  bladder ~ 51045
  conjunctiva ~ 68750
  coronary ~ 92928, 92929
  esophagus ~ 43212
  gastrointestinal, upper ~ 43266
  ileum ~ 44384
  indwelling ~ 50605
  lacrimal duct ~ 68815
  pancreatic duct ~ 43274
  small intestines ~ 44370, 44379
  ureter ~ 50688
  ureter via kidney ~ 50693
  ureteral ~ 50947, 52332
  urethral ~ 52282
tamponade, esophagus ~ 43460
tandem uterus for brachytherapy ~ 57155
tendon graft
  finger ~ 26392
  hand ~ 26392
testicular prosthesis ~ see prosthesis, testicular, insertion
tissue expanders, skin ~ 11960-11971
tube
  bile duct ~ 43268
  esophagus ~ 43510
  gastrointestinal, upper ~ 43241

Insertion ~ *continued*

ileum ~ 44384
pancreatic duct ~ 43268
small intestines ~ 44379
trachea ~ 31730
ureter ~ 50688
ureteral guide wire ~ 52334
urethra
  female intraurethral valve-pump ~ 0596T
valve, bronchial ~ 31647, 31651
vascular pedicle, carpal bone ~ 25430
venous access device
  central ~ 36560-36566
  peripheral ~ 36570-36571
ventilating tube ~ 69433, 0583T
ventricular assist device ~ 33975
wire, skeletal traction ~ 20650

Inspiratory positive pressure breathing ~ see intermittent positive pressure breathing (IPPB)

Instillation

agent for fibrinolysis ~ 32561-32562
agent for pleurodesis ~ 32560
bladder ~ see bladder, instillation
drugs
  bladder ~ 51720
  kidney ~ 50391
  ureter ~ 50391

Instrumentation ~ see application; bone, fixation; spinal instrumentation

spinal
  insertion ~ 22840-22848, 22853, 22854, 22859, 22869, 22870
  reinsertion ~ 22849
  removal ~ 22850, 22852-22855
  with arthrodesis ~ 22586

Insufflation, eustachian tube ~ see eustachian tube, inflation

Insulin ~ 80422, 80432-80435

antibody ~ 86337
blood ~ 83525
free ~ 83527

Insulin C-peptide measurement ~ see C-peptide

Insulin like growth factors ~ see somatomedin

Insurance

basic life and/or disability evaluation services ~ 99450
examination ~ 99450-99456

Integumentary system

ablation
  breast ~ 19105
  photodynamic therapy ~ 96570-96571
biopsy
  lesion
    fine needle aspiration (FNA) ~ 10004-10012, 10021
    incisional ~ 11106, 11107
    punch ~ 11104, 11105
    tangential ~ 11102, 11103
    with imaging of specimen ~ 19081-19086
  breast ~ see Breast
burns ~ 15002-15005, 15100-15121, 16000-16036
debridement ~ 11000-11006, 11010-11047
destruction ~ see also dermatology
  actinotherapy ~ 96900
  benign lesion ~ 17000, 17003-17004, 17110-17111
  chemical exfoliation ~ 17360
  cutaneous vascular proliferative ~ 17106-17108
  cryotherapy ~ 17340
  electrolysis epilation ~ 17380
  malignant lesion ~ 17260-17286
    by photodynamic therapy ~ 96567
  Mohs micrographic surgery ~ 17311-17315
  premalignant lesion ~ 17000, 17003, 17004
    by photodynamic therapy ~ 96567, 96573, 96574
  unlisted services and procedures ~ 17999
drainage, image guided ~ 10030
dressing change, with anesthesia ~ 15851
excision
  benign lesion ~ 11400-11404, 11406, 11420-11424, 11426, 11440-11444, 11446
  lipectomy ~ 15830, 15832-15839
    suction assisted ~ 15771-15774, 15876-15879
  malignant lesion ~ 11600-11604, 11606, 11620-11624, 11626, 11640-11644, 11646
  nail ~ 11750

Integumentary system ~ *continued*
  incision ~ 10040-10181
  introduction
    drug delivery implant ~ 11981, 11983
  nails ~ 11720-11765
  paring ~ 11055-11057
  photography ~ 96904
  pilonidal cyst ~ 10080-10081, 11770-11772
  pressure ulcers ~ 15920-15999
  removal
    contraceptive capsule implant ~ 11976
    drug delivery implant ~ 11982-11983
    foreign body ~ 10120-10121
    sutures with anesthesia ~ 15850-15852
    tissue expander ~ 11970-11971
  repair
    adjacent tissue transfer/rearrangement ~ 14000-14350
    complex ~ 13100-13160
    flaps, other ~ 15740-15776
    free skin grafts ~ 15050-15136, 15200-15261, 15271-15278
    intermediate ~ 12031-12057
    other procedures ~ 15780-15879
    simple ~ 12001-12021
    skin and/or deep tissue ~ 15570-15738
  shaving of epidermal or dermal lesion ~ 11300-11313
  skin replacement surgery and skin substitute grafts
    autograft/tissue cultured autograft ~ 15040-15157
    skin substitute graft ~ 15271-15278
    surgical preparation ~ 15002-15005
  skin tags, removal ~ 11200-11201
Intelligence test ~ 96100
Intensive care
  low birthweight infant, subsequent care ~ 99478-99480
  neonatal, initial ~ 99477
Intercarpal joint
  arthrodesis ~ 25820-25825
  dislocation, closed treatment ~ 25660
  repair ~ 25447
Intercostal nerve
  destruction ~ 64620
  injection
    anesthetic ~ 64420-64421
    neurolytic ~ 64620
Interdental fixation
  device application ~ 21110
  without fracture ~ 21497
  mandibular fracture
    closed treatment ~ 21453
    open treatment ~ 21462
Interdental papilla ~ see gums
Interdental wire fixation
  closed treatment craniofacial separation ~ 21431
Interferometry eye, biometry ~ 92136
Intermediate care facility (ICF) visits ~ 99304-99318
Intermittent positive pressure breathing (IPPB) ~ see continuous positive airway pressure (CPAP); continuous negative pressure breathing (CNPB)
Internal breast prostheses ~ see breast, implants
Internal ear ~ see ear, inner
Internal rigid fixation, reconstruction, mandibular rami ~ 21196
International Normalized Ratio
  patient/caregiver training ~ 93792
  test review ~ 93793
Internet E/M service
  interprofessoinal consultation ~ 99446-99449, 99451, 99452
  online evaluation & management ~ 98970-98972, 99421-99423
Interphalangeal joint
  arthrodesis ~ 26860-26863
  arthroplasty ~ 26535-26536
  arthrotomy ~ 26080, 28054
  biopsy, synovium ~ 26110
  capsule
    excision ~ 26525
    incision ~ 26525
  dislocation
    closed treatment ~ 26770
    with manipulation ~ 26340
    open treatment ~ 26785
    percutaneous fixation ~ 26776
  exploration ~ 26080

Interphalangeal joint ~ *continued*
  fracture
    closed treatment ~ 26740
    with manipulation ~ 26742
    open treatment ~ 26746
  fusion ~ 26860-26863
  great toe
    arthrodesis ~ 28755
      with tendon transfer ~ 28760
    fusion ~ 28755
      with tendon transfer ~ 28760
  removal of foreign body ~ 26080
  repair
    collateral ligament ~ 26545
    volar plate ~ 26548
  synovectomy ~ 26140
  toe ~ 28272
    arthrotomy ~ 28024
    dislocation ~ 28660-28665, 28675
      percutaneous fixation ~ 28666
    excision ~ 28160
    exploration ~ 28024
    removal
      foreign body ~ 28024
      loose body ~ 28024
    synovial biopsy ~ 28054
Interrocation
  of genomic regions
    in acute myelogenous leukemia ~ 0050U
    of chromosome 22q13 ~ 81405
    for copy number variants ~ 81228-81229, 81277, 81445, 81450, 81455
    for isoform expression ~ 81450
    for loss of heterozygosity variants ~ 81277
    for mRNA expression levels ~ 81450
    in non-small cell lunch neoplasia ~ 0022U
    for sequence variants ~ 81445, 81450, 81455
    for simple nucleotide polymorphism (SNP) ~ 81229
    in solid organ neoplasm ~ 0037U, 0048U
Intersex state
  clitoroplasty ~ 56805
  vaginoplasty ~ 57335
Intersex surgery
  female to male ~ 55980
  male to female ~ 55970
Interstitial cell stimulating hormone ~ see luteinizing hormone (LH)
Interstitial cystitides, chronic ~ see cystitis, interstitial
Interstitial cystitis ~ see cystitis, interstitial
Interstitial fluid pressure monitoring ~ 20950
Interstitial cell stimulating hormone ~ see luteinizing hormone (LH)
Interstitial radiation therapy
  radioelement application ~ 77778
    device placement
      breast ~ 19296-19298
      genitalia ~ 55920
      head/neck ~ 41019
      pelvis ~ 55920
      uterus ~ 57155
      vagina ~ 57155, 57156
    heyman capsules insertion ~ 58346
    ultrasonic guidance ~ 76965
Intertarsal joint
  arthrotomy ~ 28020, 28050
  biopsy ~ 28050
  drainage ~ 28020
  exploration ~ 28020
  removal
    foreign body ~ 28020
    loose body ~ 28020
  synovial
    biopsy ~ 28050
    excision ~ 28070
Interthoracoscapular amputation ~ see amputation, interthoracoscapular
Intertrochanteric femur fracture ~ see femur, fracture, intertrochanteric
Intervertebral chemonucleolysis ~ see chemonucleolysis
Intervertebral disc
  annuloplasty ~ 22526-22527
  arthroplasty
    artificial disc ~ 0163T, 22856-22858
      removal ~ 0095T, 0164T, 22864, 22865
      revision ~ 0098T, 0165T, 22861, 22862

Intraocular lens
  exchange ~ 66986
  insertion ~ 66983
    manual or mechanical technique ~ 66982, 66984, 66987, 66988
    not associated with concurrent cataract removal ~ 66985
  intraoperative visual axis identification ~ 0514T
Intratracheal intubation ~ see insertion, endotracheal tube
Intrauterine contraceptive device ~ see intrauterine device (IUD)
Intrauterine device (IUD)
  insertion ~ 58300
  removal ~ 58301
Intravascular stent ~ *see* transcatheter, placement, intravascular stents
Intravascular ultrasound
  intraoperative, noncoronary ~ 37252, 37253
Intravenous infusion
  diagnosis ~ 96365-96368
  hydration ~ 96360-96361
    status documented ~ 2030F-2031F
Intravenous injection ~ see injection, intravenous
Intravenous pyelogram ~ see urography, intravenous
Intravenous therapy ~ (see also injection, chemotherapy) 90780-90781
  pain management ~ 90783-90784
Intravesical instillation ~ see bladder, instillation
Intravitreal injection pharmacologic agent ~ 67028
Intrinsic factor ~ 83528
  antibody ~ 86340
Introduction
  breast
    localization device placement ~ 19081-19086
  drug delivery implant ~ 11981, 11983
  gastrointestinal tube ~ 44500
    with fluoroscopic guidance ~ 74340
  tissue expanders, skin ~ 11960-11971
Intubation ~ *see also* insertion
  duodenal, with aspiration ~ 43756-43757
  endotracheal tube ~ 31500
  eustachian tube ~ see catheterization, eustachian tube
  gastric, with aspiration ~ 43753-43755
Intubation tube ~ see endotracheal tube
Intussusception
  barium enema ~ 74283
  reduction
    laparotomy ~ 44050
Invagination, intestinal ~ see intussusception
Inversion, nipple ~ see nipples, inverted
Iodide test ~ see nuclear medicine, thyroid, uptake
Iodine test ~ see starch granules, feces
Ionization, medical ~ see iontophoresis
Iontophoreses ~ see iontophoresis
Iontophoresis ~ 97033
  sweat collection ~ 89230
IP ~ see allergen immunotherapy
Ipecac administration ~ 99175
IPPB ~ see intermittent positive pressure breathing; pulmonology,
  therapeutic
Iridectomy
  with corneoscleral or corneal section ~ 66600
  by laser surgery ~ 66761
  peripheral for glaucoma ~ 66625
  with sclerectomy with punch or scissors ~ 66160
  with thermocauterization ~ 66155
  with transfixion as for iris bombe ~ 66605
  with trephination ~ 66150
Iridodialysis ~ 66680
Iridoplasty ~ 66762
Iridotomy
  excision
    with corneoscleral or corneal section ~ 66600
    with cyclectomy ~ 66605
    optical ~ 66635
    peripheral ~ 66625
  incision
    stab ~ 66500
    with transfixion as for iris bombe ~ 66505
  by laser surgery ~ 66761
  optical ~ 66635
  peripheral ~ 66625
  sector ~ 66630
    by stab incision ~ 66500

Iris
  cyst, destruction ~ 66770
  excision
    iridectomy
      with corneoscleral or corneal section ~ 66600
      with cyclectomy ~ 66605
      optical ~ 66635
      peripheral ~ 66625
      sector ~ 66630
  incision
    iridotomy
      stab ~ 66500
      with transfixion as for iris bombe ~ 66505
  lesion, destruction ~ 66770
  prosthesis ~ 0616T-0618T
  repair
    with ciliary body ~ 66680
    suture ~ 66682
  revision
    laser surgery ~ 66761
    photocoagulation ~ 66762
  suture, with ciliary body ~ 66682
Iron ~ 83540
  absorption ~ 78162
  chelatable total body iron ~ 78172
  turnover rate ~ 78160
  utilization ~ 78170
Iron binding capacity ~ 83550
Iron hematoxylin stain ~ 88312
Iron stain ~ 85536, 88313
Irradiation blood products ~ 86945
Irrigation
  bladder ~ 51700, 52005, 52010, 53448
  bronchus ~ 31624
  caloric vestibular test ~ 92537, 92538
  catheter, brain ~ 62194, 62225
  corpora cavernosa, priapism ~ 54220
  eye ~ 65815, 68801, 68810
  lung ~ 32997
  penis ~ 54411, 54417
    for priapism ~ 54220
  peritoneal ~ see peritoneal lavage
  shunt
    cerebrospinal fluid ~ 61070
    spinal cord ~ 63744
  sinus
    maxillary ~ 31000
    sphenoid ~ 31002
  ureter, endoscopic ~ 50951, 50970
  vagina ~ 57150
  venous access device ~ 96523
  ventricular catheter ~ 62225
  wrist, arthroscopy ~ 29843
Irving sterilization (ligation, fallopian tube, oviduct) ~ 58600-58611,
  58670
Ischemic stroke
  onset ~ 1065F-1066F
  tissue plasminogen activator (tPA)
    documentation that administration was considered ~ 4077F
Ischial
  bursa excision ~ 27060
  tumor excision ~ 27075, 27078
Ischiectomy ~ 15941
Islands of Langerhans ~ see Islet cell
Island pedicle flaps ~ 15740
Islet cell
  antibody ~ 86341
  transplant ~ 0584T-0586T
Isocitrate dehydrogenase ~ see isocitric dehydrogenase
Isocitric dehydrogenase blood ~ 83570
Isolation sperm ~ 89260-89261
Isomerase, glucose 6 (six) phosphate ~ see phosphohexose isomerase
Isopropanol ~ see isopropyl alcohol
Isopropyl alcohol ~ 84600
Isthmusectomy, thyroid gland ~ 60210-60225
IUD ~ see intrauterine device (IUD)
IV infusion therapy ~ see allergen immunotherapy; chemotherapy;
  infusion; injection, chemotherapy
IV ~ see injection, chemotherapy; intravenous therapy
IVF ~ see artificial insemination; in vitro fertilization
Ivy bleeding time ~ 85002

IV injection ~ see injection, intravenous
IV, coagulation factor ~ see calcium
IX complex, factor ~ see Christmas factor

J

Jaboulay operation ~ 43810, 43850, 43855
Jannetta procedure ~ 61458
Japanese, river fever ~ see scrub typhus
Jatene type procedure ~ 33770-33781
Jaw joint ~ see facial bones; mandible; maxilla
jaws
   muscle reduction ~ 21295-21296
   X-ray for orthodontics ~ 70355
Jejunostomy
   catheterization ~ 44015
   contrast ~ 49465
   insertion
      catheter ~ 44015
      percutaneous ~ 49441
   laparoscopic ~ 44186-44187
   non-tube ~ 44187, 44310
   obstructive material removal ~ 49460
   replacement ~ 49451
   with pancreatic drain ~ 48001
Jejunum
   creation, stoma
      laparoscopic ~ 44201
   transfer
      with microvascular anastomosis free ~ 43496
Johannsen procedure ~ 53400
Johanson operation ~ see reconstruction, urethra
Joint ~ see specific joint
   arthrocentesis ~ 20600-20610
   aspiration ~ 20600-20610
   dislocation ~ see dislocation
   drainage ~ 20600-20610
   finger ~ see intercarpal joint
      fixation (surgical) ~ see arthrodesis
   injection ~ 20600-20610
   nuclear medicine imaging ~ 78300, 78315
   radiology stress views ~ 77071
   replacement
      temporomandibular ~ 21243
      vertebral ~ 0202T, 20931, 20938, 22554, 22556, 22854, 63081, 63085, 63087, 63090
   shoulder ~ see glenohumeral joint
   survey ~ 77077
   wrist ~ see radiocarpal joint
Joint syndrome, temporomandibular ~ see temporomandibular joint (TMJ)
Jones and Cantarow test ~ see blood urea nitrogen; urea nitrogen, clearance
Jones procedure ~ 28760
Jugal bone ~ see cheek bone
Jugular vein ~ see vein, jugular

K

Kader operation ~ see incision, stomach, creation, stoma; incision and drainage
Kala Azar smear ~ 87207
Kallidin I /Kallidin 9 ~ see Bradykinin
Kallikreinogen ~ see Fletcher factor
Kallikrein HK3 ~ see antigen, prostate specific
Kasai procedure ~ 47701
Kedani fever ~ see scrub typhus
Keel, insertion/removal, laryngoplasty ~ 31580
Keen operation (laminectomy) ~ 63600
Kelikian procedure ~ 28280
Keller procedure ~ 28292
Kelly urethral plication ~ 57220
Keratectomy, partial, for lesion ~ 65400
Keratomileusis ~ 65760

Keratophakia ~ 65765
Keratoplasty
   endothelial ~ 65756
      allograft preparation ~ 65757
   lamellar ~ 65710
   penetrating ~ 65730
      in aphakia ~ 65750
      in pseudophakia ~ 65755
Keratoprosthesis ~ 65770
Keratotomy, radial ~ 65771
Ketogenic steroids ~ 83582
Ketone body, acetone ~ 82009-82010
Ketosteroids ~ 83586-83593
Kidner procedure ~ 28238
Kidney
   abscess
      incision and drainage ~ 50020
   anesthesia ~ 00862
   biopsy ~ 50200-50205
      endoscopic ~ 50555-50559, 52354
   catheterization, endoscopic ~ 50572
   cyst
      ablation ~ 50541
      aspiration ~ 50390
      excision ~ 50280-50290
      injection ~ 50390
      X-ray ~ 74470
   destruction
      calculus ~ 50590
      endoscopic ~ 50557, 50576, 52354
   endoscopy
      biopsy ~ 50555, 50574-50576, 52354
      catheterization ~ 50553, 50572
      destruction ~ 50557, 50576, 52354
      dilation
         intra-renal stricture ~ 52343, 52346
         ureter ~ 50553
      excision tumor ~ 52355
      exploration ~ 52351
      lithotripsy ~ 52353
      removal
         calculus ~ 50561, 50580, 52352
         foreign body ~ 50561, 50580
      via incision ~ 50562-50580
      via stoma ~ 50551-50561
   excision
      donor ~ 50300-50320, 50547
      partial ~ 50240
      recipient ~ 50340
      transplantation ~ 50370
      with ureters ~ 50220-50236
   exploration ~ 50010, 50045, 50120
   incision ~ 50010, 50045
   incision and drainage ~ 50040, 50125
   injection
      drugs ~ 50391
      for nephrostogram ~ 50430, 50431
   instillation drugs ~ 50391
   lithotripsy ~ 50590
   manometry pressure ~ 50396
   mass ablation ~ 50542
   needle biopsy ~ 50200
   nuclear medicine
      function study ~ 78725
      imaging ~ 78700
      unlisted services and procedures ~ 78799
   placement, catheter
      nephrostomy ~ 50432
      nephroureteral ~ 50433
   removal
      calculus ~ 50060-50081, 50130, 50561
      foreign body ~ 50561, 50580
   renal function
      glomerular filtration rate (GFR) ~ 06002T-0603T
      manometric studies ~ 50396
   repair
      blood vessels ~ 50100
      fistula ~ 50520-50526
      horseshoe kidney ~ 50540
      renal pelvis ~ 50400-50405
      wound ~ 50500

Kidney ~ *continued*
solitary ~ 50405
suture
fistula ~ 50520-50526
horseshoe kidney ~ 50540
transplantation
anesthesia
donor ~ 00862
recipient ~ 00868
allograft preparation ~ 50323-50329
donor ~ 00862
donor nephrectomy ~ 50300-50320, 50547
implantation of graft ~ 50360
recipient nephrectomy ~ 50340, 50365
reimplantation kidney ~ 50380
removal transplant renal autograft ~ 50370
ultrasound ~ 76770-76776
Kidney stone ~ see calculus, removal, kidney
Killian operation ~ see sinusotomy, frontal
Kinase, creatine ~ see CPK
Kineplasty ~ see cineplasty
Kinetic therapy ~ 97530
Kininase A ~ see angiotensin converting enzyme (ACE)
Kininogen ~ 85293
Kininogen, high molecular weight ~ see Fitzgerald factor
Kleihauer-Betke test ~ 85460
Kloramfenikol ~ see chloramphenicol
Knee ~ see femur; fibula; patella; tibia
abscess ~ 27301
adipose cellular implant for osteoarthritis ~ 0565T, 0566T
arthrocentesis ~ 20610
arthrodesis ~ 27580
arthroplasty ~ 27440-27445, 27447
revision ~ 27486-27487
arthroscopy
diagnostic ~ 29870
surgical ~ 29866-29868, 29871-29889
arthrotomy ~ 27310, 27330-27335, 27403
autograft, osteochondral, open ~ 27416
biopsy ~ 27323-27324, 27330-27331
synovium ~ 27330
bone, drainage ~ 27303
bursa ~ 27301
excision ~ 27340
cyst, excision ~ 27345-27347
disarticulation ~ 27598
dislocation ~ 27550-27552, 27560-27562
open treatment ~ 27556-27558, 27566
drainage ~ 27310
excision
cartilage ~ 27332-27333
ganglion ~ 27347
lesion ~ 27347
synovial lung ~ 27334-27335
exploration ~ 27310, 27331
fasciotomy ~ 27305, 27496-27499
fracture ~ 27520-27524
arthroscopic treatment ~ 29850-29851
fusion ~ 27580
hematoma ~ 27301
incision, capsule ~ 27435
injection, X-ray ~ 27369
magnetic resonance (MRI) ~ 73721-73723
manipulation ~ 27570
meniscectomy ~ 27332-27333
reconstruction ~ 27437-27438
ligament ~ 27427-27429
with prosthesis ~ 27445
removal
foreign body ~ 27310, 27331, 27372
loose body ~ 27331
prosthesis ~ 27488
repair
ligament ~ 27405-27409
collateral ~ 27405
collateral and cruciate ~ 27409
cruciate ~ 27407-27409
meniscus ~ 27403
tendon ~ 27380-27381
replacement ~ 27447

Knee ~ *continued*
retinacular release ~ 27425
strapping ~ 29530
suture tendon ~ 27380-27381
transplantation
chondrocytes ~ 27412
meniscus ~ 29868
osteochondral
allograft ~ 27415-29867
autograft ~ 27412-29866
tumor excision ~ 27327-27329, 27337-27339, 27365
unlisted services and procedures ~ 27599
X-ray ~ 73560-73564
arthrography ~ 73580
bilateral ~ 73565
X-ray with contrast arthrography ~ 73580
Knee cap
excision ~ 27350
repair, instability ~ 27420-27424
Knee joint arthroplasty ~ 27446
Knee prosthesis ~ see prosthesis, knee
Knock-knee repair ~ 27455-27457
Kocher operation ~ 23650-23680
Kocher pylorectomy ~ see gastrectomy, partial
Kock pouch ~ 44316
formation ~ 50825
Kock procedure ~ 44316
Kraske procedure ~ 45116
Krause operation ~ see gasserian ganglion, sensory root, decompression
Kroenlein procedure ~ 67420
Krukenberg procedure ~ 25915
Kuhlmann test ~ 96100
Kyphectomy
more than two segments ~ 22819
up to two segments ~ 22818

L

L-alanine ~ see aminolevulinic acid (ALA)
L ascorbic acid ~ see ascorbic acid
L aspartate 2 oxoglutarate aminotransferase ~ see transaminase, glutamic oxaloacetic
L glutamine ~ see glutamine
L-leucylnaphthylamidase ~ see leucine aminopeptidase
L/S ratio, amniotic fluid ~ 83661
Labial adhesions, lysis ~ 56441
Laboratory panel
ACTH stimulation panel ~ 80400
acute hepatitis panel ~ 80074
basic metabolic panel ~ 80048
comprehensive metabolic panel ~ 80053
corticotropic releasing hormone (CRH) stimulation panel ~ 80412
electrolyte panel ~ 80051
general health panel ~ 80050
glucagon tolerance panel ~ 80422-80424
gonadotropin releasing hormone stimulation panel ~ 80426
growth hormone
stimulation panel ~ 80428
suppression panel ~ 80430
hepatic function panel ~ 80076
insulin
tolerance panel ~ 80434-80435
induced C-peptide suppression panel ~ 80432
lipid panel ~ 80061
metyrapone panel ~ 80436
obstetric panel ~ 80055
renal function ~ 80069
thyrotropin releasing hormone (TRH) stimulation panel ~ 80438-80439, 84146

Laboratory services ~ 8000-8999
  anatomic pathology ~ 88000-88999
  chemistry, unlisted ~ 84999
  consultations, clinical pathology ~ 80500-80502
  cytogenetic studies ~ 88230-88299
  cytopathology ~ 88104-88199
  evocative/suppression testing ~ 80400-80439, 84146
  hematology and coagulation ~ 85002-85999
  immunology ~ 86000-86849
  microbiology ~ 87999
  organ or disease oriented panels ~ 80048-80076
  other pathology and laboratory procedures ~ 89050-89240
  reproductive medicine procedures ~ 89250-89356
  surgical pathology ~ 88300-88399
  therapeutic drug assays ~ 80150-80299
  transcutaneous procedures ~ 88720
  transfusion medicine ~ 86850-86999
  urinalysis ~ 81000-81099
Labyrinth ~ see ear, inner
Labyrinthectomy ~ 69905
  with mastoidectomy ~ 69910
  with skull base surgery ~ 61596
Labyrinthotomy
  transcanal ~ 69801
Laceration repair ~ see specific site **
Lacrimal duct
  canaliculi, repair ~ 68700
  exploration ~ 68810
    with anesthesia ~ 68811
    canaliculi ~ 68840
    stent ~ 68815
  insertion, stent ~ 68815
  removal
    dacryolith ~ 68530
    foreign body ~ 68530
  X-ray with contrast ~ 70170
Lacrimal gland
  biopsy ~ 68510
  close fistula ~ 68770
  excision
    partial ~ 68505
    total ~ 68500
  fistulization ~ 68720
  incision and drainage ~ 68400
  injection, X-ray ~ 68850
  nuclear medicine, tear flow ~ 78660
  removal
    dacryolith ~ 68530
    foreign body ~ 68530
  repair, fistula ~ 68770
  tumor, excision
    without closure ~ 68540
    with osteotomy ~ 68550
Lacrimal punctum
  closure
    by plug ~ 68761
    by thermocauterization, ligation or laser surgery ~ 68760
  dilation ~ 68801
  incision ~ 68440
  repair ~ 68705
Lacrimal sac
  biopsy ~ 68525
  excision ~ 68520
  incision and drainage ~ 68420
Lacrimal system, unlisted services and procedures ~ 68899
Lactase deficiency breath test ~ 91065
Lactate ~ 83605
Lactate dehydrogenase ~ see lactic dehydrogenase
Lactic acid ~ 83605
Lactic acid measurement ~83605
Lactic cytochrome reductase ~ see lactic dehydrogenase
Lactic dehydrogenase ~ 83615-83625
Lactiferous duct
  excision ~ 19112
  exploration ~ 19110
Lactoferrin, fecal ~ 83630
Lactogen, human placental ~ 83632
Lactogenic hormone ~ see prolactin
Lactose, urine ~ 83633
Ladd procedure ~ 44055
Lagophthalmos, repair ~ 67912

Laki Lorand factor ~ see fibrin stabilizing factor
Lamblia intestinalis ~ see giardia lamblia
Lambrinudi operation ~ see arthrodesis, foot joint
Lamellar keratoplasties ~ see keratoplasty, lamellar
Laminaria, insertion ~ 59200
Laminectomy ~ 62351, 63001, 63005-63011, 63015-63044, 63200,
  63265-63290, 63300-63655
  with facetectomy ~ 63045-63048
  lumbar ~ 22630, 63012
  surgical ~ 63170-63172
Laminoplasty, cervical ~ 63050-63051
Langerhans islands ~ see islet cell
Language evaluation
  comprehension and expression ~ 92523
  speech fluency ~ 92521
  speech sound production ~ 92522
  voice resonance ~ 92524
Language therapy ~ 92507-92508
LAP ~ 83670
Laparoscopic appendectomy ~ see appendectomy, laparoscopic
Laparoscopic biopsy of ovary ~ see biopsy, ovary, laparoscopic
Laparoscopy
  abdominal ~ 49320-49327, 49329
  adrenalectomy ~ 50545
  adrenal gland, biopsy or excision ~ 60650
  appendectomy ~ 44970
  aspiration ~ 49322
  biopsy ~ 49321
    lymph nodes ~ 38570
  bladder repair ~ 51990, 51992, 51999
  cecostomy ~ 44188
  cholecystectomy ~ 47562-47564
  cholecystenterostomy ~ 47570
  colectomy
    laparoscopic ~ 44213
    partial ~ 44204-44208, 44213
    total ~ 44210-44212
  colostomy ~ 44188
  destruction, lesion ~ 58662
  ectopic pregnancy ~ 59150
    with salpingectomy and/or oophorectomy ~ 59151
  enterectomy ~ 44202
  enterolysis ~ 44180
  enterostomy, closure ~ 44227
  esophageal lengthening ~ 43283
  esophagus
    esophagogastric fundoplasty ~ 43280
    esophagomyotomy fundoplasty ~ 43279
    hernia repair ~ 43281, 43282
    lengthening ~ 43283
    sphincter augmentation
      device placement ~ 43284
      device removal ~ 43285
  fimbrioplasty ~ 58672
  gastrectomy, longitudinal/sleeve ~ 43775
  gastric
    electrode
      implantation ~ 43647, 43648
      removal ~ 43648
      replacement ~ 43647
      gastric ~ 43648
    restrictive procedures ~ 43644-43645, 43770-43775
  gastrostomy, temporary ~ 43653
  hernia repair
    epigastric
      incarcerated or strangulated ~ 49653
      reducible ~ 49652
    incisional
      incarcerated or strangulated ~ 49655
      reducible ~ 49654
    incisional recurrent
      incarcerated or strangulated ~ 49657
      reducible ~ 49656
    inguinal
      initial ~ 49650
      recurrent ~ 49651
    paraesophageal ~ 43281-43282
    spigelian
      incarcerated or strangulated ~ 49653
      reducible ~ 49652

Laparoscopy ~ continued
umbilical
  incarcerated or strangulated ~ 49653
  reducible ~ 49652
ventral
  incarcerated or strangulated ~ 49653
  reducible ~ 49652
hysterectomy ~ 58541-58544
  radical ~ 58548
  total ~ 58570-58573, 58575
ileostomy ~ 44187
incontinence repair ~ 51990-51992
in vitro fertilization ~ 58976
  retrieve oocyte ~ 58970
  transfer embryo ~ 58974
  transfer gamete ~ 58976
jejunostomy ~ 44186-44187
kidney, ablation ~ 50541-50542
ligation, veins, spermatic ~ 55550
liver ablation, tumor ~ 47370-47371
lymph system
  biopsy ~ 38570
  lymphadenectomy ~ 38571-38573
lysis of adhesions ~ 58660
lysis of intestinal adhesions ~ 44180
nephrectomy ~ 50545-50548
  partial ~ 50543
omentopexy ~ 49326
orchiectomy ~ 54690
orchiopexy ~ 54692
oviduct surgery ~ 58670-58671, 58679
pelvis ~ 49320
proctectomy
  complete ~ 45395
  with creation of colonic reservoir ~ 45397
proctopexy, for prolapse ~ 45400-45402
prostatectomy ~ 55866
pyeloplasty ~ 50544
rectum, resection ~ 45395-45397
  unlisted ~ 45499
removal
  fallopian tubes ~ 58661
  leiomyomata ~ 58545-58546
  ovaries ~ 58661
  spleen ~ 38120
  testis ~ 54690
resection, intestines, with anastomosis ~ 44202-44203
salpingostomy ~ 58673
splenectomy ~ 38120-38129
splenic flexure, mobilization ~ 44213
stomach ~ 43647-43659
  gastric bypass ~ 43644-63645
  gastric restrictive ~ 43770-43775, 43848, 43886-43888
  gastroenterostomy ~ 43644-43645
  gastrostomy, temporary ~ 43653
  neurostimulator electrode
    implantation ~ 0312T, 43647
    removal ~ 0314T, 43648
    replacement ~ 0313T, 43647
    revision ~ 0313T, 43648
  Roux-en-Y ~ 43644
testis
  orchiectomy ~ 54690
  orchiopexy ~ 54692
  unlisted procedure ~ 54699
transplantation, donor allograft preparation, kidney ~ 50325
uterus
  ablation, fibroids ~ 58674
  hysterectomy ~ 58541-58544
    radical ~ 58548
    total ~ 58570-58573, 58575
unlisted services and procedures ~ 38129, 38589, 43289, 43659,
  44238-44239, 44979, 47379, 47579, 49329, 49659, 50549, 50949,
  54699, 55559, 58578-58579, 58679, 59898
ureterolithotomy ~ 50945
ureteroneocystostomy ~ 50947-50948
urethral suspension ~ 51990
vaginal hysterectomy ~ 58550-58554
vaginal suspension ~ 57425
vagus nerves, transection ~ 43651-43652

Laparotomy
with biopsy ~ 49000
exploration ~ 47015, 49000-49002, 58960
hemorrhage control ~ 49002
second look ~ 58960
staging ~ 58960
Laparotomy, exploratory ~ see abdomen, exploration
Lapidus procedure ~ 28297
Large bowel ~ see anus; cecum; rectum
Laroyenne operation ~ see vagina, abscess, incision and drainage, 57010
Laryngeal function study ~ 92520
Laryngeal sensory testing ~ 92614-92617
Laryngectomy ~ 31360-31382
partial ~ 31367-31382
subtotal ~ 31367-31368
Laryngocele, removal ~ 31300
Laryngofissure ~ 31300
Laryngopharyngectomy ~ see excision, larynx, with pharynx, 31390,
  31395
Laryngopharynx ~ see hypopharynx
Laryngoplasty
cricoid split ~ 31587
for fracture
  fixation ~ 31584
  open reduction ~ 31584
for laryngeal stenosis ~ 31551-31554
laryngeal web ~ 31580
medialization ~ 31591
Laryngoscopy
direct ~ 31515-31571
  aspiration ~ 31515
  biopsy ~ 31535, 31536
  diagnostic ~ 31525, 31526
  dilation ~ 31528, 31529
  exploration ~ 31520-31526, 31575
  newborn ~ 31520
flexible ~ 31575-31579
  ablation, lesion ~ 31572
  biopsy ~ 31576
  diagnostic ~ 31575
  injection, vocal cord ~ 31570, 31571, 31573, 31574
  laser destruction, lesion ~ 31572
  removal
    foreign body ~ 31577
    lesion ~ 31578
indirect ~ 31505-31513
  biopsy ~ 31510
  diagnostic ~ 31505
  exploration ~ 31505
  injection, vocal cord ~ 31513
insertion
  obturator ~ 31527
newborn ~ 31520
with stroboscopy ~ 31579
Laryngotomy ~ 31300
Larynx
aspiration, endoscopy ~ 31515
biopsy, endoscopy ~ 31510, 31535-31536, 31576
dilation, endoscopic ~ 31528-31529
endoscopy
  ablation, lesion ~ 31572
  direct ~ 31515-31571
  excision ~ 31545-31546
  exploration ~ 31505, 31520-31526, 31575
  flexible ~ 31575-31579
    with stroboscopy ~ 31579
  indirect ~ 31505-31513
  laser destruction, lesion ~ 31572
  operative ~ 31530-31561
excision
  lesion ~ 31512, 31578
    endoscopic ~ 31545-31546
  partial ~ 31367-31382
  with pharynx ~ 31390-31395
  total ~ 31360-31365
exploration, endoscopic ~ 31505, 31520-31526, 31575
fracture, closed treatment
  with manipulation ~ 31586
  without manipulation ~ 31585
  open treatment ~ 31584

Larynx ~ *continued*
  insertion, obturator ~ 31527
  lesion
    ablation ~ 31572
    laser destruction ~ 31572
    removal ~ 31512, 31578
  medialization ~ 31591
  reconstruction
    cricoid split ~ 31587
    stenosis ~ 31551-31554
    web ~ 31580
  removal
    foreign body, endoscopic ~ 31511, 31530-31531, 31577
    lesion, endoscopic ~ 31512, 31545-31546, 31578
  repair, reinnervation neuromuscular pedicle ~ 31590
  stroboscopy ~ 31579
  tumor excision ~ 31300
    endoscopic ~ 31540-31541
  unlisted services and procedures ~ 31599
  vocal cord(s)
    injection ~ 31513, 31570, 31571, 31573, 31574
    stripping ~ 31540, 31541
  X-ray ~ 70370
Laser surgery
  anal ~ , 46614, 46917
  cautery, esophagus ~ 43227
  fenestration, body surface ~ 0479T, 0480T
  lacrimal punctum ~ 68760
  lens, posterior ~ 66821
  lesion
    larynx ~ 31572
    mouth ~ 40820
    nose ~ 30117-30118
    penis ~ 54057
    skin ~ 17000-17111, 17260-17286
  myocardium ~ 33140-33141
  prostate ~ 52647-52649
  spine, diskectomy ~ 62287
  tumors, urethra and bladder ~ 52234
  urethra and bladder ~ 52214
Laser treatment ~ see destruction ~ 17000-17286, 96920-96922
Lateral epicondylitis ~ see tennis elbow
Latex fixation ~ 86403-86406
LATS ~ see thyrotropin releasing hormone (TRH)
Latzko operation ~ see repair, vagina, fistula; revision
LAV ~ see HIV
LAV-2 (two) ~ see HIV-2 (two)
LAV antibodies ~ see antibody, HIV
Lavage
  colon ~ 44701
  lung
    bronchial ~ 31624
    total ~ 32997
  peritoneal ~ 49084
  stomach ~ 43753
LCM ~ see lymphocytic choriomeningitis
LD ~ lactic dehydrogenase, 83615
LDH ~ 83615-83625
LDL ~ 83721
Lead ~ 83655
Leadbetter procedure ~ 53431
Lecithin-sphingomyelin ratio ~ 83661
Lecithinase C ~ see tissue typing
Lee and White test ~ 85345
Leep procedure ~ 57460
Lefort procedure, vagina ~ 57120
Lefort I procedure
  midface reconstruction ~ 21141-21147, 21155, 21160
  palatal of maxillary fracture ~ 21421-21423
Lefort II procedure
  midface reconstruction ~ 21150-21151
  nasomaxillary complex fracture ~ 21345-21348
Lefort III procedure
  craniofacial separation ~ 21431-21436
  midface reconstruction ~ 21154-21159
Left atrioventricular valve ~ see mitral valve
Left heart cardiac catheterization ~ see cardiac catheterization, left heart

Leg
  cast
    full let ~ 29705
    rigid total contact ~ 29445
  incision
    embolectomy ~ 34201, 34203
    thrombectomy ~ 34201, 34203, 34421, 34451
  injection, sclerosant ~ 36465, 36466, 36468, 36470, 36471
  lower ~ see also ankle; fibula; knee; tibia
    abscess, incision and drainage ~ 27603
    amputation ~ 27598, 27880-27882
      revision ~ 27884-27886
    angiography ~ 73706
    artery, ligation ~ 37618
    biopsy ~ 27613-27614
    bursa, incision and drainage ~ 27604
    bypass graft ~ 35903
    cast ~ 29405-29435, 29450
    CAT scan ~ 73700-73706
    decompression ~ 27600-27602
    exploration, blood vessel ~ 35860
    fasciotomy ~ 27600-27602, 27892-27894
    hematoma, incision and drainage ~ 27603
    lesion, excision ~ 27630
    magnetic resonance imaging (MRI) ~ 73718-73720
    repair
      blood vessel ~ 35226
        with other graft ~ 35286
        with vein graft ~ 35256
      fascia ~ 27656
      tendon ~ 27658-27692
    splint ~ 29515
    strapping ~ 29580
    suture, tendon ~ 27658-27665
    tumor, excision ~ 27615-27619, 27632, 27634
    unlisted services and procedures ~ 27899
    Unna boot ~ 29580
    X-ray ~ 73592
  upper ~ see femur
    abscess ~ 27301
    amputation ~ 27590-27592
      at hip ~ 27290-27295
      revision ~ 27594-27596
    angiography ~ 73706, 75635
    artery, ligation ~ 37618
    biopsy ~ 27323-27324
    bursa ~ 27301
    bypass graft ~ 35903
    cast ~ 29345-29355, 29365, 29450
    cast brace ~ 29358
    CT scan ~ 73700-73706, 75635
    exploration, blood vessel ~ 35860
    fasciotomy ~ 27305, 27496-27499, 27892-27894
    halo application ~ 20663
    hematoma ~ 27301
    magnetic resonance imaging (MRI) ~ 73718-73720
    neurectomy ~ 27325-27326
    removal
      cast ~ 29705
      foreign body ~ 27372
    repair
      blood vessel with other graft ~ 35286
      blood vessel with vein graft ~ 35256
      muscle ~ 27385-27386, 27400, 27430
      tendon ~ 27393-27400
    splint ~ 29505
    strapping ~ 29580
    suture, muscle ~ 27385-27386
    tenotomy ~ 27306-27307, 27390-27392
    tumor, excision ~ 27327-27329, 27337-27339, 27365
    unlisted services and procedures ~ 27599
    Unna boot ~ 29580
    X-ray ~ 73592
  wound exploration, penetrating ~ 20103
Legionella
  antibody ~ 86713
  antigen ~ 87278, 87540-87542
Legionella pneumophila antigen detection, direct fluorescence ~ 87278
Leg length measurement X-ray ~ see scanogram

1175

Leiomyomata, removal ~ 58140, 58545-58546, 58561
Leishmania, antibody ~ 86717
Lengthening, tendon ~ see tendon, lengthening
Lens
    extracapsular ~ 66940
    intracapsular ~ 66920
        dislocated ~ 66930
    intraocular
        exchange ~ 66986
        reposition ~ 66825
    prosthesis, insertion ~ 66983
        manual or mechanical technique ~ 66982, 66984
        not associated with concurrent cataract removal ~ 66985
    removal, lens material
        aspiration technique ~ 66840
        extracapsular ~ 66940
        intracapsular ~ 66920-66930
        pars plana approach ~ 66852
        phacofragmentation technique ~ 66850
Lens material
    aspiration technique ~ 66840
    pars plana approach ~ 66852
    phacofragmentation technique ~ 66850
Leptomeningioma ~ see meningioma
Leptospira, antibody ~ 86720
Leriche operation ~ (thoracolumbar sympathectomy) 64809
Lesion ~ see tumor
    ablation
        endoscopic retrograde cholangio- pancreatography (ERCP) ~ 43278
        stereotactic MRI guided high intensity focused ultrasound (MRgFUS) ~ 0398T
    anal
        destruction ~ 46900-46917, 46924
        excision ~ 45108, 46922
    ankle, tendon sheath ~ 27630
    arm, lower
        tendon sheath
            excision ~ 25110
    auditory canal, external
        excision
            exostosis ~ 69140
            radical with neck dissection ~ 69155
            radical without neck dissection ~ 69150
            soft tissue ~ 69145
    bladder, destruction ~ 51030
    brain
        excision ~ 61534, 61536, 61600-61608, 61615-61616
        radiation treatment ~ 77432
    brainstem, excision ~ 61575-61576
    breast
        detection, mammography ~ 77065-77067
        excision ~ 19120-19126
    carotid body, excision ~ 60600-60605
    chemotherapy ~ 96405-96406
        destruction ~ 67220-67225
    ciliary body, destruction ~ 66770
    colon
        destruction ~ 44401, 45383
        excision ~ 44110-44111
    conjunctiva
        destruction ~ 68135
        excision ~ 68110-68130
            over 1cm ~ 68115
            with adjacent sclera ~ 68130
        expression ~ 68040
    cornea
        destruction ~ 65450
        excision ~ 65400
            of pterygium ~ 65420-65426
    destruction, ureter ~ 52341-52342, 52344-52345, 52354
    ear, middle, excision ~ 69540
    epididymis, excision ~ 54830
    esophagus
        ablation ~ 43229
        excision ~ 43100-43101
        removal ~ 43216
    excision ~ 59100
        bladder ~ 52224
        urethra ~ 52224, 53265
    eye, excision ~ 65900

Lesion ~ *continued*
    eyelid
        destruction ~ 67850
        excision
            under anesthesia ~ 67808
            without closure ~ 67840
        multiple, different lids ~ 67805
        multiple, same lid ~ 67801
        single ~ 67800
    facial, destruction ~ 17000-17004, 17280-17286
    femur, excision ~ 27062
    finger, tendon sheath ~ 26160
    foot, excision ~ 28080, 28090
    gums
        destruction ~ 41850
        excision ~ 41822-41828
    hand tendon sheath ~ 26160
    intestines, excision ~ 44110
    intestines, small
        destruction ~ 44369
        excision ~ 44111
    iris, destruction ~ 66770
    larynx
        ablation ~ 31572
        laser destruction ~ 31572
        removal ~ 31512, 31545, 31546, 31578
    leg, lower, tendon sheath ~ 27630
    lymph node, incision and drainage ~ 38300-38305
    mesentery, excision ~ 44820
    mouth
        destruction ~ 40820
        excision ~ 40810-40816, 41116
        vestibule
            destruction ~ 40820
            repair ~ 40830
    nerve, excision ~ 64774-64792
    nose, intranasal
        external approach ~ 30118
        internal approach ~ 30117
    orbit, excision ~ 61333, 67412
    palate
        destruction ~ 42160
        excision ~ 42104-42120
    pancreas, excision ~ 48120
    pelvis, destruction ~ 58662
    penis
        destruction
            cryosurgery ~ 54056
            electrodesiccation ~ 54055
            extensive ~ 54065
            laser surgery ~ 54057
            simple ~ 54050-54060
            surgical excision ~ 54060
        excision ~ 54060
            penile plaque ~ 54110-54112
    pharynx
        destruction ~ 42808
        excision ~ 42808
    rectum, excision ~ 45108
    removal, larynx ~ 31512, 31578
    resection ~ 52354
    retina
        destruction
            extensive ~ 67227-67228
            localized ~ 67208-67210
        radiation by implantation of source ~ 67218
    sclera, excision ~ 66130
    skin
        abrasion ~ 15786, 15787
        biopsy
            fine needle aspiration (FNA) ~ 10004-10012, 10021
            incisional ~ 11106, 11107
            punch ~ 11104, 11105
            tangential ~ 11102, 11103
            with imaging of specimen ~ 19081-19086
        destruction
            benign ~ 17110, 17111, 17250
            malignant ~ 17260-17286
            premalignant ~ 17000-17004

1176

Lesion ~ *continued*
- excision
  - benign ~ 11400-11471
    - malignant ~ 11600-11646
  - injection ~ 11900-11901
  - paring or curettement ~ 11055-11057
  - reflectance confocal microscopic imaging ~ 96931
  - shaving ~ 11300-11313
  - skin tags, removal ~ 11200, 11201
  - skull, excision ~ 61500, 61600-61608, 61615-61616
  - spermatic cord, excision ~ 55520
  - spinal cord
    - destruction ~ 62280-62282
    - excision ~ 63265-63273
  - stomach, excision ~ 43611
  - testis, excision ~ 54512
  - toe, excision ~ 28092
  - tongue, excision ~ 41110-41114
  - uvula
    - destruction ~ 42145
    - excision ~ 42104-42107
  - vagina, destruction ~ 57061-57065
  - vulva
    - destruction
      - extensive ~ 56515
      - simple ~ 56501
  - wrist tendon, excision ~ 25110

Lesion of sciatic nerve ~ see sciatic nerve, lesion
Leucine aminopeptidase ~ 83670
Leukemia lymphoma virus I (one), adult T cell ~ see HTLV I (one)
Leukemia lymphoma virus II (two) antibodies, human T cell ~ see antibody, HTLV-II (two)
Leukemia lymphoma virus I (one) antibodies, human T cell ~ see antibody, HTLV I (one)
Leukemia virus II (two), hairy cell associated, human T cell ~ see HTLV II (two)
Leukoagglutinins ~ 86021
Leukocyte ~ see also white blood cell
- alkaline phosphatase ~ 85540
- antibody ~ 86021
- count ~ 85032, 85048, 89055
- histamine release test ~ 86343
- phagocytosis ~ 86344
- transfusion ~ 86950

Leu 2 antigens ~ see CD8
Levarterenol ~ see noradrenalin
Levator muscle rep ~ (blepharoptosis, repair) 67901-67909
Leveen shunt
- insertion ~ 49425
- patency test ~ 78291
- revision ~ 49426

Levulose ~ see fructose
LH ~ (luteinizing hormone) 80418, 80426, 83002
LHR ~ (leukocyte histamine release test) 86343
Lid suture ~ (blepharoptosis, repair) 67901-67909
Lidocaine, assay ~ 80176
Lift, face ~ see face lift
Ligament ~ see specific site
- collateral repair, knee with cruciate ligament ~ 27409
- injection ~ 20550
- release
  - coracoacromial ~ 23415
  - transverse carpal ~ 29848
- repair
  - elbow ~ 24343-24346
  - knee joint ~ 27405-27409

Ligation
- artery
  - abdomen ~ 37617
  - carotid ~ 37600-37606
  - chest ~ 37616
  - coronary ~ 33502
  - coronary artery ~ 33502
  - ethmoidal ~ 30915
  - extremity ~ 37618
  - fistula ~ 37607
  - maxillary ~ 30920
  - neck ~ 37615
  - temporal ~ 37609
- esophageal varices ~ 43204, 43400
- fallopian tube, oviduct ~ 58600-58611, 58670

Ligation ~ *continued*
- gastroesophageal ~ 43405
- hemorrhoids ~ 46945, 46946, 46948
- oviducts ~ 59100
- salivary duct ~ 42665
- shunt
  - aorta, pulmonary ~ 33924
  - peritoneal, venous ~ 49428
- thoracic duct ~ 38380
  - abdominal approach ~ 38382
  - thoracic approach ~ 38381
- vein
  - clusters ~ 37785
  - esophagus ~ 43205, 43244, 43400
  - femoral ~ 37650
  - gastric ~ 43244
  - iliac ~ 37660
  - jugular, internal ~ 37565
  - perforate ~ 37500, 37760, 37761
  - saphenous ~ 37700-37735, 37780
  - spermatic ~ 55530, 55535, 55540, 55550
  - vena cava ~ 37619

Ligature strangulation, skin tags ~ 11200-11201
Light coagulation ~ see photocoagulation
Light scattering measurement ~ see nephelometry
Light therapy, UV ~ see actinotherapy
Limb ~ see extremity
Limited lymphadenectomy for staging ~ see lymphadenectomy, limited, for staging
Limited neck dissection, with thyroidectomy ~ 60252
Limited resection mastectomies ~ see breast, excision, lesion
Lindholm operation ~ see tenoplasty
Lingual bone ~ see hyoid bone
Lingual frenectomy ~ see excision, tongue, frenum
Lingual nerve
- avulsion ~ 64740
- incision ~ 64740
- transection ~ 64740

Lingual tonsil ~ see tonsils, lingual
Linton procedure ~ 37760-37761
Lip
- biopsy ~ 40490
- excision ~ 40500-40530
  - frenum ~ 40819
- incision, frenum ~ 40806
- reconstruction ~ 40525-40527
- repair ~ 40650-40654
  - cleft lip ~ 40700-40761
  - fistula ~ 42260
- unlisted services and procedures ~ 40799

Lip, cleft ~ see cleft lip
Lipase ~ 83690
Lipectomies, aspiration ~ see liposuction
Lipectomy ~ 15830-15839
- suction assisted ~ 15876-15879

Lipids, feces ~ 82705-82710
Lipo-lutin ~ see progesterone
Lipolysis, aspiration ~ see liposuction
Lipophosphodiesterase I (one) ~ see tissue typing
Lipoprotein
- (a) ~ 83695
- blood ~ 83695, 83700-83721
- LDL ~ 83700-83704-, 83721
- phospholipase A2 ~ 83698

Lipoprotein, alpha ~ see lipoprotein
Lipoprotein, pre-beta ~ see lipoprotein, blood
Liposuction
- for autologous fat grafting ~ 15771-15774
- lipectomy ~ 15876-15879

Lisfranc operation ~ see amputation, foot; radical resection; replantation
Listeria monocytogenes, antibody ~ 86723
Lithium, assay ~ 80178
Litholapaxy ~ 52317-52318
Lithotripsy ~ see extracorporeal shock wave therapy
- bile duct calculi (stone), endoscopy ~ 43265
- bladder ~ 52353
- kidney ~ 50590, 52353
- pancreatic duct calculi (stone), endoscopy ~ 43265
- ureter ~ 52353
- urethra ~ 52353
- with cystourethroscopy ~ 52353

Lithotrity ~ see litholapaxy
Liver ~ see hepatic duct
  ablation, tumor ~ 47380-47382
    laparoscopic ~ 47370-47371
  abscess
    aspiration ~ 47015
    incision and drainage ~ 47010
    injection ~ 47015
  aspiration ~ 47015
  biopsy ~ 47100
    needle ~ 47000, 47001
    wedge ~ 47100
  cyst
    aspiration ~ 47015
    incision and drainage ~ 47010
  drainage ~ 47400
    image guided fluid collection ~ 49405
  excision
    extensive ~ 47122
    partial ~ 47120, 47125-47130
      donor ~ 47140-47142
    total ~ 47133
  hemorrhage ~ 47350-47362
  injection ~ 47015
  lobectomy ~ 47125-47130
    partial ~ 47120
  needle biopsy ~ 47000-47001
  nuclear medicine
    imaging ~ 78201-78216
  repair
    abscess ~ 47300
    cyst ~ 47300
    wound ~ 47350-47362
  suture, wound ~ 47350-47362
  transplantation ~ 47135
    allograft preparation ~ 47143-47147
  trisegmentectomy ~ 47122
  unlisted services and procedures ~ 47379, 47399
Living activities, daily ~ see activities of daily living
Lobectomy
  brain ~ 61323, 61537-61540
  contralateral subtotal, thyroid gland ~ 60212, 60225
  liver ~ 47120-47130
  lung ~ 32480-32482
    sleeve ~ 32486
  parotid gland ~ 42410-42415
  segmental ~ 32663
  sleeve ~ 32486
  temporal lobe ~ 61537-61538
  thyroid gland partial ~ 60210-60212
    total ~ 60220-60225
  total ~ 32663
Local excision mastectomies ~ see breast, excision, lesion
Local excision of lesion or tissue of femur ~ see excision, lesion, femur
Localization of nodule
  breast, device placement
    with magnetic resonance guidance ~ 19085, 19086, 19287, 19288
    with mammmographic guidance ~ 19281, 19282
    with stereotactic guidance ~ 19081, 19082, 19283, 19284
    with ultrasound guidance ~ 19083, 19084, 19285, 19286
  soft tissue, device placement ~ 10035, 10036
Log hydrogen ion concentration ~ see pH
Lombard test ~ see audiologic function test
Long term care facility visits ~ see nursing facility services
Longmire operation ~ (anastomosis, hepatic duct to intestines) 47765
Long acting thyroid stimulator ~ see thyrotropin releasing hormone (TRH)
Loose body
  removal
    ankle ~ 27620
    carpometacarpal joint ~ 26070
    elbow ~ 24101
    interphalangeal joint ~ 28020
      toe ~ 28024
    knee joint ~ 27331
    metatarsophalangeal joint ~ 28022
    tarsometatarsal joint ~ 28020
    toe ~ 28022
    wrist ~ 25101
Lord procedure ~ (anal sphincter dilation) 45905
Louis Bar syndrome ~ see ataxia telangiectasia

Low birth weight intensive care services ~ 99478-99480
Low density lipoprotein ~ see lipoprotein, LDL
Low frequency ultrasound ~ 97610
Low vision aids ~ see spectacle services
  fitting ~ 92354-92355
  supply ~ 92392
Lower extremities ~ see extremity, lower
Lower GI series ~ see barium enema
LRH ~ (luteinizing releasing hormone) 83727
LTH ~ see prolactin
Lumbar ~ see spine
  aspiration, disk, percutaneous ~ 62287
Lumbar plexus
  decompression ~ 64714
  injection, anesthetic ~ 64449
  neuroplasty ~ 64714
  release ~ 64714
  repair/suture ~ 64862
Lumbar puncture ~ see spinal tap
Lumbar spine fracture ~ see fracture, vertebra, lumbar
Lumbar sympathectomy ~ see sympathectomy, lumbar
Lumbar vertebra ~ see vertebra, lumbar
Lumen dilation ~ 74360
Lumpectomy ~ 19301-19302
Lunate
  arthroplasty, with implant ~ 25444
  dislocation
    closed treatment ~ 25690
    open treatment ~ 25695
Lung
  ablation, tumor ~ 32994, 32998
  abscess
    incision and drainage
      open ~ 32200
      percutaneous ~ 32200
  biopsy ~ 32096-32097
    bronchoscopic ~ 31628, 31629, 31632, 31633
    core needle ~ 32408
    thoracoscopic ~ 32607, 32608
  bullae
    excision ~ 32141
    endoscopic ~ 32655
  cancer screening, thoracic CT scan ~ 71271
  cyst
    incision and drainage
      open ~ 32200
    removal ~ 32140
  decortication
    endoscopic ~ 32651-32652
    partial ~ 32225
    total ~ 32220
    with parietal pleurectomy ~ 32320
  empyema, excision ~ 32540
  excision ~ 32440-32445
    bronchus resection ~ 32486
    completion ~ 32488
    donor
      heart-lung ~ 33930
      lung ~ 32850
    empyema ~ 32540
    lobe ~ 32480-32482
    segment ~ 32484
    tumor ~ 32503-32504
  foreign body, removal ~ 32151
  hemorrhage ~ 32110
  lavage
    bronchial ~ 31624
    total ~ 32997
  lysis, adhesions ~ 32124
  nuclear medicine
    imaging, perfusion ~ 78580, 78597, 78598
    imaging, ventilation ~ 78579, 78582, 78598
    unlisted services and procedures ~ 78599
  placement, interstitial device ~ 32553
  pneumolysis ~ 32652, 32940
  pneumonostomy ~ 32200
  pneumothorax
    repeat ~ 32215
    therapeutic ~ 32960
  pulmonary fluid monitoring system, remote ~ 0607T-0608T

Lung ~ *continued*
  removal ~ 32440-32445
    bilobectomy ~ thoracoscopic ~ 32670
    bronchial valve ~ 31648-31649
    bronchoplasty ~ 32501
    completion pneumonectomy ~ 32488
    extrapleural ~ 32445
    pneumonectomy 32440-32445
      thoracoscopic ~ 32671
    segmentectomy, thoracoscopic ~ 32669
    single lobe ~ 32480
    single segment ~ 32484
    sleeve lobectomy ~ 32486
    sleeve pneumonectomy ~ 32442
    two lobes ~ 32482
    volume reduction ~ 32491
  repair, hernia ~ 32800
  segmentectomy ~ 32484
  tear, repair ~ 32110
  thoracotomy
    biopsy ~ 32096-32097
    cardiac massage ~ 32160
    for post-op complications ~ 32120
    removal
      bullae ~ 32141
      cyst ~ 32140
      intrapleural foreign body ~ 32150
      intrapulmonary foreign body ~ 32151
    repair ~ 32110
  transplantation ~ 32851-32854, 33935
    allograft preparation
      heart/lung ~ 33933
      lung ~ 32855, 32856
      marginal (extended) lung ~ 0494T-0496T
    donor pneumonectomy
      heart-lung ~ 33930
      lung ~ 32850
  unlisted services and procedures ~ 32999
Lung function tests ~ see pulmonology, diagnostic
Lung volume reduction, emphysematous ~ 32491
Lupus anticoagulant assay ~ 85705
Lupus band test ~ see immunofluorescent study
Luteinizing hormone (LH) ~ 80418, 80426, 83002
Luteinizing releasing factor ~ 83727
Luteotropic hormone ~ see prolactin
Luteotropin ~ see prolactin
Luteotropin, placental ~ see lactogen, human placental
Lyme disease ~ 86617-86618
Lyme disease ab ~ see antibody, Lyme disease
Lyme disease vaccine ~ see vaccination
Lymph duct, injection ~ 38790
Lymph nodes
  abscess, incision and drainage ~ 38300-38305
  biopsy ~ 38500, 38510-38530, 38570
    needle ~ 38505
  dissection ~ 38542
  excision ~ 38500, 38510-38530
    abdominal ~ 38747
    aortic ~ 38780
    gastric ~ 38747
    hypogastric ~ 38770, 55845, 55865
    inguinofemoral ~ 38760-38765
    laparoscopic ~ 38571-38573
    limited, for staging
      para-aortic ~ 38562, 38747
    mediastinal ~ 21632, 32674, 38746
    obturator ~ 38770, 55845, 55865
      pelvic ~ 38562
      retroperitoneal ~ 38564
    pelvic ~ 38562, 38770, 38780, 57531
    radical
      axillary ~ 19305-19307, 38740-38745
      cervical ~ 38720-38724
      suprahyoid ~ 38700
    renal ~ 38780
    retroperitoneal transabdominal ~ 38780
    thoracic ~ 38746
  exploration ~ 38542
  gastric, excision ~ 38747

Lymph nodes ~ *continued*
  hilar, sampling
    endobrachial ultrasound (EBUS) guided ~ 31652, 31653
  hygroma, cystic
    axillary/cervical excision ~ 38550-38555
  hypogastric, excision ~ 38770, 55845, 55865
  mediastinal
    excision ~ 21632
      thoracoscopic ~ 32674
      by thoracotomy ~ 38746
  mediastinoscopy ~ 39402
    sampling, endobronchial ultrasound (EBUS) guided ~ 31652, 31653
  nuclear medicine, imaging ~ 78195
  removal
    abdominal ~ 38747
    inguinofemoral ~ 38760-38765
    pelvic ~ 38770
    retroperitoneal transabdominal ~ 38780
    thoracic ~ 38746
  sentinel, mapping ~ 38900
Lymph vessels
  abdomen, lymphangiography ~ 75805-75807
  arm, lymphangiography ~ 75801-75803
  leg, lymphangiography ~ 75801-75803
  nuclear medicine, imaging ~ 78195
  pelvis, lymphangiography ~ 75805-75807
Lymphadenectomy
  abdominal ~ 38747
  bilateral inguinofemoral ~ 54130, 56632, 56637
  bilateral pelvic ~ 51575, 51585, 51595, 54135, 55845, 55865
    total ~ 38571-38573, 57531, 58210
  diaphragmatic assessment ~ 58960
  gastric ~ 38747
  inguinofemoral ~ 38760-38765
  inguinofemoral, iliac and pelvic ~ 56640
  injection, sentinel node ~ 38792
  limited para-aortic, resection of ovarian malignancy ~ 58951, 58954
  limited pelvic ~ 55842, 55862, 58954
  limited, for staging
    para-aortic ~ 38562
    pelvic ~ 38562
    retroperitoneal ~ 38564
  mediastinal ~ 21632
  para-aortic ~ 58958
  pelvic ~ 58958
  peripancreatic ~ 38747
  portal ~ 38747
  radical
    axillary ~ 38740-38745
    cervical ~ 38720-38724
    pelvic ~ 54135, 55845, 58548
    suprahyoid ~ 38700
  regional ~ 50230
  retroperitoneal transabdominal ~ 38780
  thoracic ~ 38746
  unilateral inguinofemoral ~ 56631, 56634
Lymphadenitis, incision and drainage ~ 38300-38305
Lymphadenopathy associated antibodies ~ see antibody, HIV
Lymphadenopathy associated virus ~ see HIV
Lymphangiogram, abdominal ~ see lymphangiography, abdomen
Lymphangiography
  abdomen ~ 75805-75807
  arm ~ 75801-75803
  injection ~ 38790
  leg ~ 75801-75803
  pelvis ~ 75805-75807
Lymphangioma, cystic ~ see hygroma
Lymphangiotomy ~ 38308
Lymphatic channels, incision ~ 38308
Lymphatic cyst ~ see lymphocele
Lymphatic system, unlisted procedure ~ 38999
Lymphatics ~ see specific procedure
Lymphoblast transformation ~ see blastogenesis
Lymphocele
  drainage, laparoscopic ~ 49323
  extraperitoneal, open drainage ~ 49062
Lymphocoele ~ see lymphocele
Lymphocyte
  culture ~ 86821
  toxicity assay ~ 86805-86806
  transformation ~ 86353

Lymphocyte, thymus-dependent ~ see T cells
Lymphocytes, CD4 ~ see CD4
Lymphocytes, CD8 ~ see CD8
Lymphocytic choriomeningitis, antibody ~ 86727
Lymphocytotoxicity ~ 86805-86806
Lymphoma virus, Burkitt ~ see Epstein-Barr virus
Lynch procedure ~ 31075
Lysergide ~ see lysergic acid diethylamide
Lysis
  adhesions
    epidural ~ 62263-62264
    fallopian tube ~ 58740
    foreskin ~ 54450
    intestinal ~ 44005
    labial ~ 56441
    lung ~ 32124
    nose ~ 30560
    ovary ~ 58740
    oviduct ~ 58740
    penile, post-circumcision ~ 54162
    ureter ~ 50715-50725
    urethra ~ 53500
    uterus ~ 58559
  euglobulin ~ 85360
  labial, adhesions ~ 56441
  nose, intranasal synechia ~ 30560
Lysozyme ~ 85549

M

Macewen operation ~ see hernia, repair, inguinal
Machado test ~ (complement, fixation test) 86171
Maclean-De Wesselow test ~ see blood urea nitrogen; urea nitrogen, clearance
Macrodactylia, repair ~ 26590
Madlener operation ~ (tubal ligation) 58600
Magnesium ~ 83735
Magnet operation ~ see eye, removal of foreign body
Magnetic resonance, unlisted services and procedures ~ 76498
Magnetic resonance angiography (MRA)
  abdomen ~ 74185
  arm ~ 73225
  chest ~ 71555
  head ~ 70544-70546
  leg ~ 73725
  neck ~ 70547-70549
  pelvis ~ 72198
  spine ~ 72159
Magnetic resonance imaging (MRI)
  diagnostic
    3-D rendering ~ 76376, 76377
    abdomen ~ 74181-74183
    ankle ~ 73721-73723
    arm ~ 73218-73220, 73221-73223
    bone marrow study ~ 77084
    brain ~ 70551-70555
      intraoperative ~ 70557-70559
    chest ~ 71550-71552
    elbow ~ 73221
    face ~ 70540-70543
    fetal ~ 74712, 74713
    finger joint ~ 73221-73223
    foot ~ 73718-73719
    foot joints ~ 73721-73723
    hand ~ 73218-73220, 73223
    heart ~ 75557-75565
    joint
      lower extremity ~ 73721-73723
      upper extremity ~ 73221-73223
    knee ~ 73721-73723
    leg ~ 73718-73720, 73721-73723
    neck ~ 70540-70543
    obstetrical, maternal pelvis ~ 74712, 74713
    orbit ~ 70540-70543
    pelvis ~ 72195-72197
    spectroscopy ~ 76390

Magnetic resonance imaging (MRI) ~ *continued*
  spine
    cervical ~ 72141, 72142, 72156
    lumbar ~ 72148, 72149, 72158
    thoracic ~ 72146, 72147, 72157
  temporomandibular joint (TMJ) ~ 70336
  toe ~ 73721-73723
  wrist ~ 73221
  guidance
    arthrography, enhanced shoulder injection ~ 23350
    brain
      stereotactic lesion ablation
        MRgFUS ~ 0398T
      stereotactic lesion biopsy ~ 61751
    breast
      with computer aided detection ~ 77048, 77049
      without contrast ~ 77046, 77047
      biopsy ~ 19085, 19086
      lesion localization device placement ~ 19085, 19086, 19287, 19288
      needle placement ~ 77021
      orthopedic procedure, computer -assisted navigation ~ 0055T
      parenchymal tissue ablation ~ 77022
  unlisted procedure ~ 76498
Magnetic resonance spectroscopy
  discogenic pain determination/localization ~ 0609T-0612T
  glycosylated acute phases proteins (GlycA) quantitation ~ 0024U
  lipoprotein particle quantitation ~ 83704
  scan ~ 76390
Magnetic stimulation, transcranial ~ 90867-90868
Magnetoencephalography (MEG) ~ 95965-95967
Magnuson procedure ~ 23450
Magpi operation ~ (hypospadias, repair) 54322
Major vestibular gland ~ see Bartholin's gland
Malar area
  augmentation ~ 21270
  bone graft ~ 21210
  fracture
    with bone graft ~ 21366
    with manipulation ~ 21355
    open treatment ~ 21360-21366
  reconstruction ~ 21270
Malar bone ~ see cheekbone
Malaria antibody ~ 86750
Malaria smear ~ 87207
Malate dehydrogenase ~ 83775
Maldescent, testis ~ see testis, undescended
Male circumcision ~ see circumcision
Male genital system, surgical procedures ~ 54000-55899
Malformation, arteriovenous ~ see arteriovenous malformation
Malic dehydrogenase ~ (malate dehydrogenase) 83775
Malleolus ~ see ankle; fibula; leg, lower; tibia; tibiofibular joint
  metatarsophalangeal joint ~ 27889
Mallet finger repair ~ 26432
Maltose, tolerance test ~ 82951-82952
Malunion repair
  femur
    with graft ~ 27472
    without graft ~ 27470
  metatarsal ~ 28322
  tarsal joint ~ 28320
Mammalian oviduct ~ see fallopian tube
Mammaplasties ~ see breast, reconstruction
Mammary abscess ~ see abscess, breast
Mammary arteries ~ see artery, mammary
Mammary duct
  X-ray with contrast ~ 77053-77054
Mammary ductogram, injection ~ 19030
Mammary stimulating hormone ~ see prolactin
Mammilliplasty ~ see nipples, reconstruction
Mammography ~ 77065-77067
  localization, lesion, device placement ~ 19281, 19282
  magnetic resonance imaging (MRI)
    with computer aided detection ~ 77048, 77049
    without contrast ~ 77046, 77047
  screening mammography ~ 77067
  tomosynthesis ~ 77061-77063
  with computer-aided detection ~ 77065-77067
Mammoplasty
  augmentation ~ 19325
  reduction ~ 19318
Mammotomy ~ see mastotomy

Mammotropic hormone, pituitary ~ see prolactin
Mammotropic hormone, placental ~ see lactogen, human placental
Mammotropin ~ see prolactin
Mandated services, on call services ~ 99027
Mandible ~ see facial bones; maxilla; temporomandibular joint (TMJ)
  abscess, excision ~ 21025
  bone graft ~ 21215
  cyst, excision ~ 21040, 21046-21047
  fracture
    closed treatment
      with interdental fixation ~ 21453
      with manipulation ~ 21451
      without manipulation ~ 21450
    open treatment ~ 21454-21470
      external fixation ~ 21454
      with interdental fixation ~ 21462
      without interdental fixation ~ 21461
    percutaneous treatment ~ 21452
  osteotomy ~ 21198-21199
  reconstruction, with implant ~ 21244-21246, 21248-21249
  removal, foreign body ~ 41806
  torus mandibularis, excision ~ 21031
  tumor, excision ~ 21040-21047
  X-ray ~ 70100-70110
Mandibular body
  augmentation
    with bone graft ~ 21127
    with prosthesis ~ 21125
Mandibular condyle, fracture, open treatment ~ 21465
  reconstruction ~ 21247
Mandibular condylectomy ~ see condylectomy
Mandibular fracture ~ see fracture, mandible
Mandibular rami
  reconstruction
    with bone graft ~ 21194
    without bone graft ~ 21193
    with internal rigid fixation ~ 21196
    without internal rigid fixation ~ 21195
Mandibular resection prosthesis ~ 21081
Mandibular staple bone plate, reconstruction, mandible ~ 21244
Manganese ~ 83785
Manipulation
  chest wall ~ 94667-94668
  chiropractic ~ 98940-98943
  dislocation and/or fracture ~ 25535
    acetabulum ~ 27222
    acromioclavicular ~ 23545
    ankle ~ 27810, 27818, 27860
    carpometacarpal ~ 26670-26676
    clavicular ~ 23505
    elbow ~ 24300, 24640
    femoral ~ 27232, 27502, 27510, 27517
      pertrochanteric ~ 27240
    fibula ~ 27781, 27788
    finger ~ 26725-26727, 26742, 26755
    greater tuberosity, humeral ~ 23625
    hand ~ 26670-26676
    heel ~ 28405-28406
    hip ~ 27257
    hip socket ~ 27222
    humeral ~ 23605, 24505, 24535, 24577
      epicondyle ~ 24565
    hyoid ~ 21494
    intercarpal ~ 25660
    interphalangeal joint ~ 26340, 26770-26776
    larynx ~ 31586
    lunate ~ 25690
    malar area ~ 21355
    mandibular ~ 21451
    metacarpal ~ 26605-26607
    metacarpophalangeal ~ 26700-26706, 26742
    metacarpophlangeal joint ~ 26340
    metatarsal ~ 28475-28476
    nasal bone ~ 21315-21320
    orbit ~ 21401
    phalangeal shaft ~ 26727
      distal, finger or thumb ~ 26755
      phalanges, finger/thumb ~ 26725

Manipulation ~ continued
  phalanges
    finger ~ 26742, 26755, 26770-26776
    finger/thumb ~ 26727
    great toe ~ 28495-28496
    toes ~ 28515
  radial ~ 24655, 25565
  radial shaft ~ 25505
  radiocarpal ~ 25660
  radioulnar ~ 25675
  scapular ~ 23575
  shoulder ~ 23650-23655
    with greater tuberosity ~ 23665
  shoulder dislocation sternoclavicular ~ 23525
    with surgical or anatomical neck fracture ~ 23675
  talus ~ 28435-28436
  tarsal ~ 28455-28456
  thumb ~ 26641-26650
  tibial ~ 27532, 27752
  trans-scaphoperilunar ~ 25680
  ulnar ~ 24675, 25535, 25565
  vertebral ~ 22315
  wrist ~ 25259, 25624, 25635, 25660, 25675, 25680, 25690
  Dupuytren's cord ~ 26341
  foreskin ~ 54450
  globe ~ 92018-92019
  hip ~ 27275
  interphalangeal joint
    finger ~ 26340
    proximal ~ 26742
  knee joint ~ 27570
    adhesions ~ 29884
  lymphatic drainage ~ 97140
  osteopathic ~ 98925-98929
  palmar fascial cord ~ 26341
  shoulder
    adhesions ~ 29825
    application of fixation apparatus ~ 23700
  spine
    with anesthesia ~ 22505
    without anesthesia ~ 97140
  temporomandibular joint(s) (TMJ) ~ 21073
  tibial, distal ~ 27762
Manometric studies
  abdominal voiding pressure ~ 51797
  bladder voiding pressure ~ 51728, 51729
  colon ~ 91117
  cranial pressure ~ 61107, 61210
  duodenal motility ~ 91022
  esophagus ~ 91010, 91013
  gastric motility ~ 91020
  intraocular pressure ~ 0198T, 92100
  kidney, pressure ~ 50396
  rectum/anus ~ 91122
  ureter, pressure ~ 50686
  ureterostomy ~ 50686
  urethra voiding pressure ~ 51727, 51729
Manometry
  anorectal ~ 91122
    with biofeedback training ~ 90912, 90913
  rectum ~ 90911
Mantoux test ~ (TB skin test) 86580
Manual therapy ~ 97140
Maquet procedure ~ 27418
Marcellation operation ~ (vaginal hysterectomy) 58260-58270, 58550
Marrow, bone ~ see bone marrow
Marshall-Marchetti-Krantz procedure ~ 51840-51841, 58152, 58267
Marsupialization ~ 10040
  Bartholin's gland cyst ~ 56440
  cyst, sublingual salivary ~ 42409
  liver, cyst or abscess ~ 47300
  pancreatic cyst ~ 48500
  urethral diverticulum ~ 53240
Mass, kidney, ablation ~ 50542
Massage, cardiac ~ 32160
  therapy ~ 97124
Masseter muscle/bone, reduction ~ 21295-21296
  muscle flap ~ 15733
Mass spectrometry and tandem mass spectrometry
  analyte ~ 83789

Mastectomy
  with axillary lymphadenectomy ~ 19302
  gynecomastia ~ 19300
  intraoperative margin assessment radiofrequency spectroscopy ~ 0546T
  modified radical ~ 19307
  partial ~ 19301-19302
  radical ~ 19305-19306
  simple, complete ~ 19303
Mastectomy, Halsted ~ see radical mastectomy
Mastoid
  excision
    complete ~ 69502
    radical ~ 69511
      modified ~ 69505
      petrous apicectomy ~ 69530
    simple ~ 69501
  obliteration ~ 69670
  repair
    by excision ~ 69601-69603
    fistula ~ 69700
    with tympanoplasty ~ 69604
Mastoid cavity, debridement ~ 69220-69222
Mastoidectomy
  cochlear device implantation ~ 69930
  complete ~ 69502
    revision ~ 69601
  radical ~ 69511
    modified ~ 69505
    revision ~ 69602-69603
  simple ~ 69501
  with labyrinthectomy ~ 69910
  with petrous apicectomy ~ 69530
  with skull base surgery ~ 61590, 61597
    decompression ~ 61595
    facial nerve ~ 61595
  with tympanoplasty ~ 69604, 69641-69646
Mastoidotomy ~ 69635-69637
  with tympanoplasty ~ 69635
    ossicular chain reconstruction ~ 69636
    and synthetic prosthesis ~ 69636
Mastoids
  polytomography ~ 76101-76102
  X-ray ~ 70120-70130
Mastopexy ~ 19316
Mastotomy ~ 19020
Maternity care and delivery ~ see abortion; cesarean delivery; ectopic
  pregnancy; obstetrical care
Maxilla ~ see facial bones; mandible
  bone graft ~ 21210
  CT scan ~ 70486-70488
  cyst, excision ~ 21048-21049
  excision ~ 21030, 21032-21034
  fracture
    closed treatment ~ 21345, 21421
    open treatment ~ 21346-21348, 21422-21423
    with fixation ~ 21345-21347
  osteotomy ~ 21206
  reconstruction, with implant ~ 21245-21246, 21248-21249
  tumor, excision ~ 21048-21049
Maxillary arteries ~ see artery, maxillary
Maxillary sinus ~ see sinus, maxillary
Maxillary torus palatinus, tumor excision ~ 21032
Maxillectomy ~ 31225-31230
Maxillofacial fixation, application, halo type appliance ~ 21100
Maxillofacial impressions
  auricular prosthesis ~ 21086
  definitive obturator prosthesis ~ 21080
  facial prosthesis ~ 21088
  interim obturator prosthesis ~ 21079
  mandibular resection prosthesis ~ 21081
  nasal prosthesis ~ 21087
  oral surgical splint ~ 21085
  orbital prosthesis ~ 21077
  palatal augmentation prosthesis ~ 21082
  palatal lift prosthesis ~ 21083
  speech aid prosthesis ~ 21084
  surgical obturator prosthesis ~ 21076
Maxillofacial procedures, unlisted services and procedures ~ 21299
Maxillofacial prosthesis ~ 21076-21089
  unlisted services and procedures ~ 21089
Maydl operation ~ (colostomy) 45563, 50810

Mayo hernia repair ~ 49580-49587
Mayo operation ~ (varicose vein removal) 37700-37735, 37780, 37785
Mayo procedure ~ 28292
MBC ~ (minimum bactericidal concentration) 87181-87190
McBride procedure ~ 28292
McBurney operation ~ (see also hernia, repair, inguinal) 49495-49500,
  49505
McCannel procedure ~ 66682
McDonald operation ~ (repair, cervix, cerclage, abdominal; revision)
  57700
McIndoe procedure ~ (vagina, construction) 57291
McKissock surgery ~ (breast, reduction) 19318
McVay operation ~ (hernia, repair, inguinal) 49495-49500, 49505
Measles, German ~ see rubella
Measles uncomplicated ~ see rubeola
Measles vaccine ~ see vaccines
Meat fibers, feces ~ 89160
Meatoplasty ~ 69310
Meatotomy ~ 53020-53025
  contact laser vaporization with/without transurethral resection of prostate
    ~ 52648
    with cystourethroscopy ~ 52281
  infant ~ 53025
  non-contact laser coagulation prostate ~ 52647
  transurethral electrosurgical resection, prostate ~ 52601
  ureter ~ 52290
  ureteral, cystourethroscopy ~ 52290-52305
Meckel's diverticulum, excision ~ 44800
  unlisted services and procedures ~ 44899
Median nerve
  decompression ~ 64721
  neuroplasty ~ 64721
  release ~ 64721
  repair/suture, motor ~ 64835
  transposition ~ 64721
Median nerve compression ~ see carpal tunnel syndrome
Mediastinal cyst ~ see cyst, mediastinal
Mediastinoscopy ~ 39401, 39402
Mediastinotomy
  cervical approach ~ 39000
  transthoracic approach ~ 39010
Mediastinum ~ see chest; thorax
  biopsy ~ 32408
  cyst,
    excision ~ 32662
    resection ~ 39200
  drainage, image guided fluid collection ~ 49405
  endoscopy, biopsy ~ 39401, 39402
  excision
    cyst/mass/tumor ~ 32662
    lymph node ~ 21603, 21632, 32674, 38746
    mass ~ 32662
    tumor ~ 32662
  exploration ~ 39000-39010, 60505
  incision and drainage ~ 39000-39010
  lymph node
    biopsy ~ 39402
    lymphadenectomy ~ 21603, 21632, 32674, 38746
    sampling, EBUS guided ~ 31652, 31653
  mass
    biopsy ~ 39401
    excision ~ 32662
  radical dissection ~ 60522
  removal, foreign body ~ 39000-39010
  resection
    cyst ~ 39200
    tumor ~ 39220
  thoracoscopy
    biopsy ~ 32606
    diagnostic ~ 32601
    excision, cyst/mass/tumor ~ 32662
  tumor, excision ~ 32662, 39220
  unlisted procedures ~ 39499
Mediastinum and diaphragm, surgical procedures ~ 39000-39599
Medical disability evaluation services ~ 99455-99456
Medical genetics ~ 96040
Medical nutrition therapy ~ 97802-97804
Medical testimony ~ 99075
Medication management therapy ~ 99605-99607
Medicine, preventive ~ see preventive medicine
Medicine, pulmonary ~ see pulmonology

Medicine services ~ 90281-99602
Meibomian cyst ~ see chalazion
Membrane, mucous ~ see mucosa
Membrane, tympanic ~ see ear, drum
Membrane oxygenation, extracorporeal ~ see extracorporeal membrane
  oxygenation
Meninges
  excision, tumor ~ 61512, 61519
  meningitis, meningococcal
    antibody ~ 86741
    vaccine ~ 90619, 90620, 90621, 90644, 90733, 90734
  repair
    meningocele ~ 63700, 63702
    myelomeningocele ~ 63704, 63706
    pseudomeningocele ~ 63709
Meningioma, excision ~ 61512, 61519
  tumor, excision ~ 61512, 61519
Meningitis, lymphocytic benign ~ see lymphocytic choriomeningitis
Meningocele repair
  meningocele ~ 63700, 63702
  myelomeningocele ~ 63704, 63706
  pseudomeningocele ~ 63709
Meningococcal vaccine ~ see vaccines
Meningococcus ~ see neisseria meningitidis
Meningomyelocele ~ see myelomeningocele
Meniscectomy
  knee joint ~ 27332-27333
  temporomandibular joint ~ 21060
Meniscus
  knee
    excision ~ 27332-27333
    repair ~ 27403
    transplantation ~ 29868
Mental nerve
  avulsion ~ 64736
  incision ~ 64736
  transection ~ 64736
Mercury ~ 83015, 83825
Merskey test ~ see fibrin degradation products
Mesenteric arteries ~ see artery, mesenteric
Mesentery
  lesion, excision ~ 44820
  repair ~ 44850
  suture ~ 44850
  unlisted services and procedures ~ 44899
Mesh
  implantation, hernia ~ 49568
  insertion, pelvic floor ~ 57267
  removal, abdominal infected ~ 11008
Metabisulfite test ~ (red blood cell (RBC), sickling) 85660
Metabolite ~ 80353
  thromboxane ~ 84431
Metacarpal
  amputation ~ 26910
  craterization ~ 26230
  cyst, excision ~ 26200-26205
  diaphysectomy ~ 26230
  fracture
    closed treatment ~ 26605
      with fixation ~ 26607
    open treatment ~ 26615
    percutaneous fixation ~ 26608
    with manipulation ~ 26605-26607
    without manipulation ~ 26600
  ostectomy ~ 26250
  repair
    lengthening ~ 26568
    nonunion ~ 26546
    osteotomy ~ 26565
  saucerization ~ 26230
  tumor
    excision ~ 26200-26205
    radical resection ~ 26250
Metacarpophalangeal joint
  arthrodesis ~ 26850-26852
  arthroplasty ~ 26530-26531
  arthroscopy
    diagnostic ~ 29900
    surgical ~ 29901-29902
  arthrotomy ~ 26075

Metacarpophalangeal joint ~ *continued*
  biopsy, synovium ~ 26105
  capsule
    excision ~ 26520
    incision ~ 26520
  capsulodesis ~ 26516-26518
  dislocation
    closed treatment ~ 26700
    open treatment ~ 26715
    percutaneous fixation ~ 26705-26706
    with manipulation ~ 26340
  exploration ~ 26075
  fracture
    closed treatment ~ 26740
    open treatment ~ 26746
    with manipulation ~ 26742
  fusion ~ 26516-26518, 26850-26852
  removal of foreign body ~ 26075
  repair, collateral ligament ~ 26540-26542
  synovectomy ~ 26135
Metadrenaline ~ see metanephrines
Metals, heavy ~ see heavy metal
Metamfetamine ~ see methamphetamine
Metanephrines ~ 83835
Metatarsal ~ see foot
  amputation ~ 28810
  condyle, excision ~ 28288
  craterization ~ 28122
  cyst, excision ~ 28104-28107
  diaphysectomy ~ 28122
  excision ~ 28110-28114, 28122, 28140
  fracture
    closed treatment
      with manipulation ~ 28475-28476
      without manipulation ~ 28470
    open treatment ~ 28485
    percutaneous fixation ~ 28476
  free osteocutaneous flap with microvascular anastomosis ~ 20972
  repair ~ 28322
    lengthening ~ 28306-28307
    osteotomy ~ 28306-28309
  saucerization ~ 28122
  tumor, excision ~ 28104-28107, 28173
Metatarsectomy ~ 28140
Metatarsophalangeal joint
  amputation ~ 28820
  arthrotomy ~ 28022, 28052
  biopsy ~ 28052
  capsulotomy ~ 28270
  cheilectomy ~ 28289, 28291
  dislocation
    closed treatment ~ 28630-28635
    open treatment ~ 28645
    percutaneous fixation ~ 28636
  drainage ~ 28022
  exploration ~ 28022
  great toe
    arthrodesis ~ 28750
    fusion ~ 28750
  removal
    of foreign body ~ 28022
    of loose body ~ 28022
  repair, hallux rigidus ~ 28289, 28291
  synovial
    biopsy ~ 28052
    excision ~ 28072
  toe ~ 28270
Methaemoglobin ~ see methemoglobin
Methamphetamine, blood or urine ~ 80324-80326
Methanol ~ 84600
Methbipyranone ~ see metyrapone
Methemalbumin ~ 83857
Methemoglobin ~ 83045-83050, 88741
Methenamine silver stain ~ 88312
Methopyrapone ~ see metyrapone
Methoxyhydroxymandelic acid ~ see vanillylmandelic acid
Methylamphetamine ~ see methamphetamine
Methylene bichloride ~ see dichloromethane
Methylfluorprednisolone ~ see dexamethasone
Methylmorphine ~ see codeine
Methyl alcohol ~ (methanol) 84600

Metroplasty ~ see hysteroplasty
Metyrapone ~ 80436
MIC ~ (minimum inhibitory concentration) 87186
Micro-ophthalmia, orbit reconstruction ~ 21256
Microalbumin, urine ~ 82043-82044
Microbiology ~ 0023T, 87999
Microdissection ~ 88380-88381
Microfluorometries, flow ~ see flow cytometry
Microdissection ~ 88380
Microglobulin, beta 2
  blood ~ 82232
  urine ~ 82232
Micrographic surgery, Mohs technique ~ 17311-17315
Micropigmentation, correction ~ 11920-11922
Microscope, surgical ~ see operating microscope
Microscopic evaluation, hair ~ 96902
Microscopies, electron ~ see electron microscopy
Microscopy
  binocular ear exam ~ 92504
  reflectance confocal microscoopy (RCM)
    skin imaging ~ 96931-96936
    lesion ~ 96932
  specular, endothelial cell analysis ~ 92286
Microsomal antibody ~ 86376
Microsomia, hemifacial ~ see hemifacial microsomia
Microsurgery, operating microscope ~ 69990
Microvascular anastomosis
  bone graft
    fibula ~ 20955
    other ~ 20962
  fascial flap, free ~ 15758
  muscle flap, free ~ 15756
  osteocutaneous flap with, ~ 20969-20973
  skin flap, free ~ 15757
Microvite A ~ see vitamin A
Microwave therapy ~ (see also physical medicine/therapy/occupational therapy) 97020
Midbrain ~ see brain; brainstem; mesencephalon; skull base surgery
Midcarpal mediooccipital joint, arthrotomy ~ 25040
Middle cerebral artery velocimetry ~ 76821
Middle ear ~ see ear, middle
Midface
  reconstruction
    with bone graft ~ 21145-21160, 21188
    without bone graft ~ 21141-21143
    forehead advancement ~ 21159-21160
Mile operation ~ see colectomy, total, with proctectomy
Milia, multiple, removal ~ 10040
Miller procedure ~ 28737
Miller-Abbott intubation ~ 44500, 74340
Minerva cast ~ 29035
  removal ~ 29710
Minimum inhibitory concentration (MIC) ~ 87186
Minimum lethal concentration ~ 87187
Minnesota multiphasic personality inventory ~ see MMPI
Miscarriage
  incomplete abortion ~ 59812
  missed abortion
    first trimester ~ 59820
    second trimester ~ 59821
  septic abortion ~ 59830
Missed abortion ~ see abortion; miscarriage, missed abortion
Mitchell procedure ~ 28296
Mitogen blastogenesis ~ 86353
Mitral valve
  annulus transcatheter reconstruction ~ 0544T
  closure, paravalvular leak ~ 93590, 93592
  incision ~ 33420-33422
  occlusion, paravalvular leak ~ 93590, 93592
  repair
    with cardiopulmonary bypass ~ 33425-33427
    transapical ~ 0543T
    transcatheter ~ 33418, 33419, 0345T
  replacement ~ 33430
  transcatheter mitral valve implantation/replacement (TMVI) ~ 0483T, 0484T
Mitrofanoff operation ~ (appendico-vesicostomy) 50845
MMPI ~ (Minnesota multiphasic personality inventory) 96100
MMR shots ~ (measles, mumps and rubella vaccines) 90707

Mobilization
  splenic flexure ~ 44139
  stapes ~ 69650
Modeling, 3D anatomic
  printed from image data set ~ 0559T-0562T
Modified radical mastectomy ~ see mastectomy, modified radical
Mohs micrographic surgery ~ 17311-17315
Molar pregnancy ~ see hydatidiform mole
Mold, culture ~ 87107
Mole, carneous ~ see abortion
Mole, hydatid ~ see hydatidiform mole
Molecular cytogenetics ~ 88271-88275
  interpretation and report ~ 88291
Molecular diagnostics
  reverse transcription and amplified probe
    central nervous system pathogen ~ 87483
    enterovirus ~ 87498
    hepatitis C ~ 87521
    HIV-1 ~ 87535
    HIV-2 ~ 87538
  reverse transcription and quantification
    hepatitis C ~ 87522
    HIV-1 ~ 87536
    HIV-2 ~ 87539
Molecular oxygen saturation ~ see oxygen saturation
Molecular pathology
  ~ (see also Gene analysis) 81200-81383, 81400-81408
Molluscum contagiosum
  destruction ~ 17110-17111, 46900, 46910, 46916-46917, 54050-54065
  excision
    anus ~ 46922
    penis ~ 54060
Molteno procedure ~ 66180
Monilia ~ see candida
Monitoring
  ablation therapy
    incompetent vein ~ 36473-36476, 36478, 36479, 36482, 36483, 0524T
    parenchymal tissue ~ 76940, 77013, 77022
    renal mass ~ 50250, 50542
  ACE/ARB therapy ~ 4188F
  anticonvulsant therapy ~ 4191F
  blood pressure ~ see blood pressure, monitoring
  cardiac
    cardiovascular physiologic monitor system ~ 93290, 93297
    ischemia monitoring system ~ 0525T-0532T
    subcutaneous cardiac rhythm monitoring system ~ 93285, 93291, 93298
  cerebrospinal shunt flow ~ 0639T
  digoxin therapy ~ 4189F
  diuretic therapy ~ 4190F
  ESRD ~ 90951-90959, 90963-90965
  electrocardiogram ~ (see also electrocardiography) 93224-93229
  electroencephalogram ~ 95812-95813
    with drug activation ~ 95954
    with physical activation ~ 95954
    with WADA activation ~ 95958
  fetal
    during labor ~ 59050-59051, 99500
    interpretation only ~ 59051
    magnetic cardiac signal ~ 0475T-0478T
  glucose
    home device ~ 82962
    interstitial fluid ~ 95249-95251
    tolerance test ~ 82951, 82952
  hemodynamic ~ 33289, 93264
  interstitial fluid pressure ~ 20950
  intraocular pressure ~ 0329T
  neurophysiologic, intraoperative ~ 95940, 95941
  pediatric apnea ~ 94774-94777
  physiologic parameters
    remote ~ 99453, 99454
    treatment management services ~ 99457, 99458
  pulmonary fluid monitoring system ~ 0607T-0608T
  retinal disease ~ 92227-92229
  seizure ~ 61531-61533, 61760
  with contrast
    biliary drainage ~ 47533-47540
    catheter ~ 75984, 93503
Monitoring, sleep ~ see polysomnography
Monoethylene glycol ~ see ethylene glycol
Mononuclear cell antigen ~ 86356
Mononucleosis virus, infectious ~ see Epstein-Barr virus

Monophosphate
adenosine ~ (adenosine monophosphate (AMP)) 82030
adenosine cyclic ~ (cyclic AMP) 82030
Monospot test ~ (rapid test for infection) 86308
Monoxide, carbon ~ see carbon monoxide
Monteggia fracture ~ 24620-24635
Monticelli procedure ~ (application, bone fixation device) 20690, 20692
Morbilli ~ see rubeola
Morphine methyl ether ~ see codeine
Morphometric analysis
nerve ~ 88356
skeletal muscle ~ 88355
tumor ~ 88358-88361, 88367-88368
Morton's neuroma, excision ~ 28080
Moschcowitz operation ~ see repair, hernia, femoral; revision
Mosenthal test ~ (urinalysis, routine) 81002
Mother cell ~ see stem cell
Motility study, esophagus ~ 91010
Motion analysis
by video and 3-D kinematics ~ 96000, 96004
computer-based ~ 96000, 96004
Mouth
abscess, incision and drainage ~ 40800-40801, 41005-41009, 41015-41018
biopsy ~ 40808, 41108
cyst, incision and drainage ~ 40800-40801, 41005-41009, 41015-41018
excision, frenum ~ 40819
hematoma, incision and drainage ~ 40800-40801, 41005-41009, 41015-41018
lesion
destruction ~ 40820
excision ~ 40810-40816, 41116
vestibule of
destruction ~ 40820
repair ~ 40830
mucosa, excision ~ 40818
reconstruction ~ 40840-40845
removal, foreign body ~ 40804-40805
repair, laceration ~ 40830-40831
unlisted services, procedures ~ 40899, 41599
vestibule of
excision, destruction ~ 40808-40820
incision ~ 40800-40806
other procedures ~ 40899
removal, foreign body ~ 40804
repair ~ 40830-40845
Move ~ see transfer
finger ~ 26555
toe joint ~ 26556
toe to hand ~ 26551-26554
MPR ~ (multifetal pregnancy reduction) 59866
MRA ~ see magnetic resonance angiography
MRI ~ see magnetic resonance imaging
MSLT ~ (multiple sleep latency testing) 95805
Mucin, synovial fluid ~ 83872
Mucocele sinusotomy, frontal ~ 31075
Mucopolysaccharides ~ 83864
Mucormycoses ~ see mucormycosis
Mucormycosis, antibody ~ 86732
Mucosa
ablation, turbinates ~ 30801, 30802
ectopic gastric imaging ~ 78290
excision of lesion
alveolar, hyperplastic ~ 41828
vestibule of mouth ~ 40810-40818
via esophagoscopy ~ 43229
via small intestinal endoscopy ~ 44369
via upper gi endoscopy ~ 43270
lesion
ablation, vestibule of mouth ~ 40810-40818
phtodynamic therapy ~ 96567, 96573, 96574
periododontal grafting ~ 41870
urethra, mucosal advancement ~ 53450
vaginal biopsy ~ 57100-57105
Mucosa, buccal ~ see mouth, mucosa
Mucous cyst antibody, hand or finger ~ 26160

Mucous membrane ~ see mouth, mucosa
cutaneous
excision
benign lesion ~ 11440-11446
malignant lesion ~ 11640-11646
layer closure, wounds ~ 12051-12057
simple repair, wounds ~ 12011-12018
excision, sphenoid sinus ~ 31288
lid margin
correction of trichiasis ~ 67835
nasal test ~ 95065
ophthalmic test ~ 95060
rectum
proctoplasty for prolapse ~ 45505
MUGA (multiple gated acquisition) ~ 78452, 78454, 78473, 78483
Muller procedure ~ see sleep study
Multianalyte Assays
with Algorithmic Analyses ~ 81500-81599
autoimmune, rheumatoid arthritis ~ 81490
cardiology, heart transplant ~ 81595
coronary artery disease ~ 81493
endocrinology ~ 81506
fetal aneuploidy ~ 81507
fetal congenital abnormalities ~ 81508-81512
infectious disease
bacterial vaginosis ~ 81513
bacterial vaginosis/vaginitis ~ 81514
hepatitis C virus ~ 81596
mycoplasma genitalium ~ 87563
liver disease ~ 0002M, 0003M, 0014M
oncology
adrenal cortical tumor ~ 0015M
bladder cancer ~ 0016M
breast ~ 81518-81521
colon ~ 81525
colorectal ~ 81528
cutaneous melanoma ~ 81529
gastrointestinal neuroendocrine ~ 0007M
gynecologioc ~ 81535, 81536
liver ~ 0006M
lung ~ 81538
ovarian ~ 81500, 81503
prostate ~ 0011M, 81539, 81541, 81542, 81551
thyroid ~ 81546
tissue of origin ~ 81504
tumor of unknown origin ~ 81540
urothelial carcinoma ~ 0012M, 0013M
uveal melanoma ~ 81552
pulmonary disease, idiopathic pulmonary fibrosis (IPF) ~ 81554
scoliosis ~ 0004M
unlisted multianalyte assay with algorithmic analysis ~ 81599
Multifetal pregnancy reduction ~ 59866
Multi-leaf collimator (MLC) device ~ 77338
Multiple sleep latency testing (MSLT) ~ 95805
Multiple valve procedures ~ see valvuloplasty
Mumford operation ~ (partial claviculectomy, arthroscopic) 29824
Mumps
antibody ~ 86735
immunization ~ 90707, 90710
vaccine
MMR ~ 90707
MMRV ~ 90710
Muramidase ~ 85549
Murine typhus ~ 86000
Muscle ~ see specific muscle
biofeedback training, perineal ~ 90912, 90913
biopsy ~ 20200-20206
debridement ~ 11043, 11046
infected ~ 11004-11006
flaps
fasciocutaneous ~ 15733, 15734, 15736, 15738
muscle, free ~ 15842
myocutaneous ~ 15733, 15734, 15736, 15738, 61619
grafts
muscle, free ~ 15841, 25265, 25274
heart ~ see myocardium
neck ~ see neck muscle

Muscle ~ *continued*
incision
esophagus ~ 32665, 43130, 43279, 43330, 43331
hyoid ~ 21685
pharynx ~ 43030, 43130
pylorus ~ 43520
injection ~ 20552, 20553
insertion, needle ~ 20560, 20561
oculomotor ~ see eye muscles
removal, foreign body ~ 20520-20525
repair
extraocular ~ 65290
forearm ~ 25260-25274
wrist ~ 25260-25274
revision, arm, upper ~ 24330-24331
transfer
arm, upper ~ 24301, 24320
elbow ~ 24301
femur ~ 27110
hand ~ 26494
hip ~ 27100-27105, 27111
rotator cuff ~ 23410, 23412
shoulder ~ 23395-23397, 24301, 24320, 23410, 23412
thigh ~ 27400
unlisted extraocular muscle procedure ~ 67399
Muscle compartment syndrome, detection ~ 20950
Muscle denervation ~ see denervation
Muscle division
scalenus anticus ~ 21700-21705
sternocleidomastoid ~ 21720-21725
Muscle flaps ~ 15731-15738
Muscle grafts ~ 15841-15845
Muscle testing
dynamometry, eye ~ 92260
extraocular multiple muscles ~ 92265
ischemic limb ~ 95875
Musculoplasty ~ see muscle, repair
Musculoskeletal system, surgical procedures ~ 20010-29999
Musculotendinous (rotator) cuff, repair ~ 23410-23412
Mustard procedure ~ (repair, great arteries; revision) 33774-33777
Myasthenia gravis, tensilon test ~ 95857-95858
Mycobacteria
culture ~ 87116
identification ~ 87118
detection ~ 87550-87562
sensitivity studies ~ 87190
Mycoplasma
antibody ~ 86738
culture ~ 87109
detection ~ 87580-87582
Mycota ~ see fungus
Myectomy, anorectal ~ see myomectomy, anorectal
Myelencephalon ~ see medulla
Myelin basic protein, cerebrospinal fluid ~ 83873
Myelography
brain ~ 70010
spine
cervical ~ 72240
lumbosacral ~ 72265
thoracic ~ 72255
total ~ 72270
Myelomeningocele, repair ~ 63704-63706
Myeloperoxidase (MPO) ~ 83876
Myelotomy ~ 63170
Myocardial, perfusion imaging ~ 78451-78454
positron emission tomography (PET) ~ 78459
Myocardial imaging
blood flow, absolute quantitation ~ 78434
echocardiography, contrast perfusion ~ 0439T
for strain
speckle-tracking assessment of myocardial mechanics ~ 93356
infarct avid ~ 78466-78469
magnetocardiography ~ 0541T, 0542T
metabolic evaluation, PET ~ 78429, 78432, 78433, 78459
perfusion study
planar ~ 78453, 78454
positron emission tomography (PET) ~ 78430-78433, 78491, 78492
single photon emission computed tomography (SPECT) ~ 78451, 78452
repair, postinfarction ~ 33542
sympathetic innervation ~ 0331T, 0332T

Myocardium
blood flow, absolute quantitation ~ 78434
ischemia assessment
echocardiography ~ 0439T
perfusion imaging ~ 78451-78454
echocardiography ~ 0439T
positron emissin tomography (PET) ~ 78429, 78432, 78433, 78459
resection ~ 33542
revascularization ~ 33140, 33141
Myocutaneous flaps ~ 15731, 15733-15738, 15756
Myofascial pain dysfunction syndrome ~ see temporomandibular joint (TMJ)
Myofibroma ~ see leiomyomata
Myoglobin ~ 83874
Myomectomy
anorectal ~ 45108
uterus ~ 58140-58146, 58545-58546
Myoplasty ~ see muscle, repair
Myotomy
esophagus ~ 43030
hyoid ~ 21685
Myringoplasty ~ 69620
Myringostomy ~ see myringostomy
Myringotomy ~ 69420-69421
Myxoid cyst ~ see ganglion

N

N. meningitidis ~ see Neisseria meningitidis
Naffziger operation ~ (decompression, orbit; section) 61330
Nagel test ~ (color vision examination) 92283
Nail(s)
avulsion ~ 11730-11732
biopsy ~ 11755
debridement ~ 11720-11721
drainage ~ 10060, 10061
evacuation, hematoma, subungual ~ 11740
excision ~ 11750
cyst, pilonidal ~ 11770-11772
KOH examination ~ 87220
reconstruction ~ 11762
removal ~ 11730-11732, 11750
trimming ~ 11719
Nail bed, reconstruction ~ 11762
repair ~ 11760
Nail fold, excision wedge ~ 11765
Nail plate separation ~ see onychia
Narcosynthesis, diagnostic and therapeutic ~ 90865
Nasal abscess ~ see nose, abscess
Nasal area, bone graft ~ 21210
Nasal bleeding ~ see epistaxis
Nasal bone
fracture
closed treatment ~ 21310-21320
open treatment ~ 21325-21335
with manipulation ~ 21315-21320
without manipulation ~ 21310
X-ray ~ 70160
Nasal deformity, repair ~ 40700-40761
Nasal function study ~ 92512
Nasal polyp ~ see nose, polyp
Nasal prosthesis, impression ~ 21087
Nasal septum
abscess, incision and drainage ~ 30020
fracture
closed treatment ~ 21337
open treatment ~ 21336
hematoma, incision and drainage ~ 30020
repair ~ 30630
submucous resection ~ 30520
Nasal sinuses ~ see sinus; sinuses
Nasal smear, eosinophils ~ 89190
Nasal turbinate fracture, therapeutic ~ 30930
Nasal valve
collapse, repair with implant ~ 30468

Nephrotomography ~ 74415
Nephrotomy ~ 50040-50045
  with exploration ~ 50045
Nerve
  see also nerves
  ablation, radiofrequency ~ 64625
  biopsy ~ 64795
  cryoablation ~ 0440T-0442T
  neuroma, excision
    cutaneous ~ 64774
    digital ~ 64776, 64778
    foot, other than digital ~ 64782, 64783
    hand, other than digital ~ 64782, 64783
    peripheral ~ 64784
    sciatic ~ 64786
Nerve block
  paravertebral block (PVB) ~ 64461-64463
  transverse abdominis plant (TAP) ~ 64486-64489
Nerve conduction
  motor nerve ~ 95905, 95907-95913
  preconfigured electrode array ~ 77387
Nerve graft
  additional nerve ~ 64901-64902
  arm or leg ~ 64892-64893, 64897-64898
  foot or hand ~ 64890-64891, 64895-64896
  head or neck ~ 64885-64886
  neurovascular pedicle ~ 15750
  pedicle ~ 64905, 64907
Nerve root ~ see also cauda equina; spinal cord
  decompression ~ 22856, 63020-63048, 63055-63103
  incision ~ 63185-63190
  section ~ 63185-63190
Nerve stimulation, transcutaneous ~ see application, neurostimulation
Nerve teasing ~ 88362
Nerves
  ablation, radiofrequency ~ 64625
  anastomosis
    facial to hypoglossal ~ 64868
    facial to spinal accessory ~ 64866
  avulsion ~ 64732-64772
  biopsy ~ 64795
  cryoablation, percutaneous ~ 0440T-0442T
  decompression ~ 64702-64727
    cranial ~ 61458, 61460
    laminotomy/laminectomy ~ 0274T-0275T
  denervation ~ 27035
  destruction
    by neurolytic agent
      celiac plexus ~ 64680
      genicular ~ 64624
      intercostal ~ 64620
      other peripheral ~ 64640
      paravertebral facet joint ~ 64633-64636
      plantar common digital ~ 64632
      pudendal ~ 64630
      superior hypogastric plexus ~ 64681
      trigeminal ~ 64600, 64605, 64610
  graft ~ 64885-64907
  implantation, electrode ~ 64553-64581
    to bone ~ 64787
    to muscle ~ 64787
  incision ~ 28035, 43640-43641, 64732-64772
  injection
    anesthetic/steroid
      axillary ~ 64417
      brachial plexus ~ 64415
      femoral ~ 64447
      genicular ~ 64454
      greater occipital ~ 64405
      iliohypogastric ~ 64425
      ilioinguinal ` 64425
      intercostal ~ 64420
      for nerve blocks ~ 01991, 01992
      other peripheral ~ 64450
      paracervical (uterine) ~ 64435
      pudendal ~ 64430
      sacroiliac joint ~ 64451
      sciatic ~ 64445
      suprascapular ~ 64418
      trigeminal ~ 64400
      vagus ~ 64408

Nerves ~ *continued*
  diagnostic agent ~ 64493-64495, 0213T
    neurolytic agent ~ 64600-64681
    therapeutic agent ~ 64490-64495, 0213T
  insertion, electrode ~ 64553-64581
  lesion, excision ~ 64774-64792
  neurofibroma, excision ~ 64788-64792
  neurolemmoma, excision ~ 64788-64792
  neurolytic, internal ~ 64727
  neuroma
    destruction ~ 64632
    excision ~ 64774-64786
    injection ~ 64455
  neuroplasty ~ 64702-64721
  removal, electrode ~ 64585
  repair
    allograft ~ 64910, 64912, 64913
    autogenous graft ~ 64911
    microdissection ~ 69990
    suture ~ 64831-64876
  spinal accessory
    incision ~ 63191
    section ~ 63191
  suture ~ 64831-64876
  sympathectomy, excision ~ 64802-64818
  transection ~ 64732-64772
  transposition ~ 64718-64721
  unlisted services and procedures ~ 64999
Nerve V, cranial ~ see trigeminal nerve
Nerve VII, cranial ~ see facial nerve
Nerve X, cranial ~ see vagus nerve
Nerve XI, cranial ~ see accessory nerve
Nerve XII, cranial ~ see hypoglossal nerve
Nervous system
  central nervous system pathogen
    nucleic acid detection ~ 87483
  extracranial, peripheral nerves and autonomic nervous system
    avulsion ~ 64732-64772
    destruction ~ 64600-64681
    excision ~ 64774-64823
    injection ~ 64400-64530
    neurorrhaphy ~ 64831-64911
    neuroplasty ~ 64702-64727
    neurostimulation ~ 64595
    transection ~ 64732-64772
  nuclear medicine
    unlisted services and procedures ~ 78699
  skull, meninges and brain ~ 61000-62258
  spine and spinal cord ~ 62263-63746
  unlisted procedure ~ 64999
Nesidioblast ~ see islet cell
Neural conduction ~ see nerve conduction
Neural ganglion ~ see ganglion
Neurectomy
  foot ~ 28055
  gastrocnemius ~ 27326
  hamstring muscle ~ 27325
  leg, upper ~ 27325
  popliteal ~ 27326
  tympanic ~ 69676
Neuroendoscopy, intracranial ~ 62160-62165
Neurofibroma
  cutaneous nerve, excision ~ 64788
  extensive, excision ~ 64792
  peripheral nerve, excision ~ 64790
Neurolemmoma
  destruction, extensive ~ 0419T, 0420T
  excision
    cutaneous nerve ~ 64788
    extensive ~ 64792
    peripheral nerve ~ 64790
Neurologic system ~ see nervous system
Neurology procedures
  brain cortex magnetic stimulation ~ 90867-90868
  brain mapping ~ 90867, 96020
  brain surface electrode stimulation ~ 95961-95962
  central motor function mapping ~ 64999
  cognitive performance ~ 96125

Neurology procedures ~ *continued*
  diagnostic
    anal sphincter ~ 51785
    autonomic function tests
      heart rate response ~ 95921, 95943
      parasympathetic ~ 95943
      pseudomotor response ~ 95921-95924
      sympathetic function ~ 95921-95924, 95943
      valsalva maneuver ~ 95922, 95943
    brain surface electrode stimulation ~ 95961-95962
    central motor transcranial motor stimulation ~ 95928-95929
    electrocorticogram, intraoperative ~ 95829
    electromyography
      fine wire dynamic ~ 96004
      ischemic limb exercise test ~ 95875
      needle ~ 51785, 95860-95872
      surface dynamic ~ 96002-96004
    evoked potentials
      central motor ~ 95928, 95929, 95939
      somatosensory testing ~ 95925-95927, 95938
      visual ~ 0333T, 0464T, 95930
    higher cerebral function
      aphasia test ~ 96105
      cognitive function tests ~ 96116
      developmental tests ~ 96110-96111
      neurobehavioral status ~ 96116
      neuropsychological testing ~ 96118-96120
    magnetoencephalography (MEG) ~ 95965-95967
    motion analysis
      by video and 3-D kinematics ~ 96000, 96004
      computer-based ~ 96000, 96004
    movement disorder monitoring ~ 0533T-0536T
    nerve conduction
      motor and sensory ~ 95905-95913
    neurofunctional testing ~ 96020
    neuromuscular junction tests ~ 95937
    neurophysiological monitoring, intraoperative ~ 95940-95941
    neuropsychological testing ~ 96118-96120
      cognitive performance ~ 96125
      computer assisted ~ 96120
    plantar pressure measurements, dynamic ~ 96001, 96004
    polysomnography ~ 95782-95783, 95808-95811
    range of motion ~ 95851-95852
    reflex
      blink reflex ~ 95933
    sleep study ~ 96800-95801, 95803-95811
    somatosensory testing ~ 95925-95927, 95938-95939
    tensilon test ~ 95857
    unlisted services and procedures ~ 95999
    urethral sphincter ~ 51785
    visual evoked potential, CNS ~ 95930
Neurolysis
  nerve ~ 64704-64708
    internal ~ 64727
Neuroma
  acoustic ~ see brain, tumor, excision
  excision
    cutaneous nerve ~ 64774
    digital nerve ~ 64776-64778
    foot ~ 28080
    foot nerve ~ 64782-64783
    hand nerve ~ 64782-64783
    interdigital (Morton's) ~ 28080
    peripheral nerve ~ 64784
    sciatic nerve ~ 64786
  injection, anesthetic or steroid ~ 64455
Neuromuscular junction tests ~ 95937
Neuromuscular pedicle reinnervation larynx ~ 31590
Neuromuscular reeducation ~ 97112
Neurophysiologic testing
  autonomic nervous function
    heart rate response ~ 95921-95924
    pseudomotor response ~ 95921-95924
    sympathetic function ~ 95921-95924
  intraoperative ~ 95940-95941
Neuroplasty
  cranial nerve ~ 64716
  digital nerve ~ 64702-64704

Neuroplasty ~ *continued*
  peripheral nerve
    arm ~ 64708
    brachial plexus ~ 64713
    cranial ~ 64716
    lrh ~ 64708
    lumbar plexus ~ 64714
    median at carpal tunnel ~ 64721
    sciatic ~ 64712
    ulnar at elbow ~ 64718
    ulnar at wrist ~ 64719
Neuropsychological testing ~ 96117
Neurorrhaphy ~ 64831-64876
  peripheral nerve
    conduit ~ 64910-64911
    with graft ~ 64885-64907
Neurostimulation, application ~ 64566
Neurostimulators
  brain
    electronic analysis ~ 95970, 95983, 95984
    implantation ~ 61863, 61864, 61867, 61868, 61885, 61886
    removal ~ 61880
    replacement ~ 61885, 61886, 61888
    revision ~ 61880, 61888
  cranial nerve
    electronic analysis ~ 95970, 95977
    implantation ~ 64553, 64568
    removal ~ 64570
    replacement ~ 64569
    revision ~ 64569
  gastric nerve
    electronic analysis ~ 95980-95982
    implantation/replacement ~ 43647, 43881, 64590
    revision/removal ~ 43648, 43882, 64595
  integrated neurostimulation system
    electronic analysis ~ 0589T, 0590T
    implantation ~ 0587T
    programming ~ 0589T, 0590T
    replacement ~ 0587T
    removal ~ 0588T
    revision ~ 0588T
  peripheral nerve
    electronic analysis ~ 95970-95972
    implantation ~ 64555, 64575, 64580
    removal ~ 64585, 64595
    replacement ~ 64590
    revision ~ 64585, 64595
  phrenic nerve system for sleep apnea
    device evaluation ~ 0434T-0436T
    insertion ~ 0424T-0427T
    removal ~ 0428T-0430T
    replacement ~ 0424T-0427T, 0431T
    repositioning ~ 0432T, 0433T
  sacral nerve
    electronic analysis ~ 95970-95972
    implantation ~ 64561, 64581
  spinal cord
    electronic analysis ~ 95970-95972
    implantation ~ 63650, 63655
    removal ~ 63661, 63662, 63688
    replacement ~ 63663, 63664, 63685
    revision ~ 63663, 63664, 63688
  tibia, percutaneous ~ 64566
  vagus nerve system for morbid obesity
    electronic analysis/programming ~ 0317T
    implantation ~ 0312T
    replacement ~ 0313T, 0316T
    removal ~ 0314T, 0315T
    revision ~ 0313T
Neurotomy, sympathetic ~ see gasserian ganglion, sensory root, decompression
Neurovascular pedicle flaps ~ 15750
Neutralization test, virus ~ 86382
New patient
  domiciliary or rest home visit ~ 99324-99328
  emergency department services ~ 99281-99288
  home services ~ 99341-99345
  hospital inpatient services ~ 99221-99239
  hospital observation services ~ 99217-99220

New patient ~ *continued*
   initial office visit ~ 99202-99205
   inpatient consultations ~ 99251-99255
   office and/or other outpatient consultations ~ 99241-99245
Newborn care ~ 99460-99465, 99502
   attendance at delivery ~ 99464
   blood transfusion
      exchange ~ 36450, 36456
      push ~ 36440
   circumcision
      clamp or other device ~ 54150
      surgical excision ~ 54160
   history and examination ~ 99460, 99463
   laryngoscopy ~ 31520
   normal ~ 99460-99463
   prepuce slitting ~ 54000
   preventive, office ~ 99461
   resuscitation ~ 99465
   standby for cesarean delivery ~ 99360
   subsequent hospital care ~ 99462
   umbilical artery catheterization ~ 36660
Next Generation Screening (NGS) and other molecular multianalyte
   assays
   aortic dysfunction or dilation ~ 81410, 81411
   exome ~ 81415-81417
   fetal chromosoma aneuploidy ~ 81420
   genome ~ 81425-81427
   hearing loss ~ 81430, 81431
   hereditary
      breast cancer related disorders ~ 81432, 81433
      colon cancer disorders ~ 81435, 81436
      neuroendoscrine tymor disorders ~ 81437, 81438
      retinal disorders ~ 81434
   noonan spectral disorders ~ 81442
   nuclear encoded mitochondrial genes ~ 81440
   targeted genomic sequence panel ~ 81445, 81450, 81455
   whole mitochondrial genome ~ 81460, 81465
   x-linked intellectual disability (XLID) ~ 81470, 81471
Nickel ~ 83885
Nicolas-Durand-Favre disease ~ see lymphogranuloma venereum
Nicotine ~ 83887
Nidation ~ see implantation
Nipples ~ see breast
   inverted ~ 19355
   reconstruction ~ 19350
Nissen operation ~ see fundoplasty, esophagogastric
Nissen procedure
   laparoscopic ~ 43280
Nitrate reduction test ~ see urinalysis
Nitric Oxide ~ 95012
Nitroblue tetrazolium dye test ~ 86384
Nitrogen, blood urea ~ see blood urea nitrogen
NMR imaging ~ see magnetic resonance imaging (MRI)
NMR spectroscopies ~ see magnetic resonance spectroscopy
No man's land, tendon repair ~ 26356-26358
Noble procedure ~ see repair; suture
Nocardia, antibody ~ 86744
Nocturnal penile rigidity test ~ 54250
Nocturnal penile tumescence test ~ 54250
Node, lymph ~ see lymph nodes
Nodes ~ see lymph nodes
Node dissection, lymph ~ see dissection, lymph nodes
Non-office medical services ~ 99056
Non-stress test, fetal ~ 59025
Nonunion repairS
   femur
      with graft ~ 27472
      without graft ~ 27470
   metatarsal ~ 28322
   tarsal joint ~ 28320
Noradrenalin
   blood ~ 82383-82384
   urine ~ 82384
Norchlorimipramine ~ see imipramine
Norepinephrine ~ see catecholamines
   blood ~ 82383-82384
   urine ~ 82384
Nortriptyline, assay ~ 80335-80337
Norwood procedure ~ 33611-33612, 33619, 33622

Nose
   abscess, incision and drainage ~ 30000-30020
   artery, incision ~ 30915-30920
   biopsy, intranasal ~ 30100
   dermoid cyst, excision
      complex ~ 30125
      simple ~ 30124
   displacement therapy ~ 30210
   endoscopy
      diagnostic ~ 31231-31235
      surgical ~ 31237-31241, 31253-31257, 31259, 31267, 31276, 31287,
         31288, 31290-31298
   excision
      rhinectomy ~ 30150-30160
      turbinate ~ 30140
   fracture
      closed treatment ~ 21345
      open treatment ~ 21325-21336, 21338-21339, 21346-21347
      percutaneous treatment ~ 21340
      with fixation ~ 21330, 21340, 21345-21347
   hematoma, incision and drainage ~ 30000-30020
   hemorrhage, cauterization ~ 30901-30906
   insertion, septal prosthesis ~ 30220
   intranasal lesion
      external approach ~ 30118
      internal approach ~ 30117
   lysis of adhesions ~ 30560
   polyp, excision
      extensive ~ 30115
      simple ~ 30110
   reconstruction
      cleft lip/cleft palate ~ 30460-30462
      dermatoplasty ~ 30620
      primary ~ 30400-30420
      secondary ~ 30430-30450
      septum ~ 30520
   removal
      foreign body ~ 30300
      anesthesia ~ 30310
      lateral rhinotomy ~ 30320
   repair
      adhesions ~ 30560
      cleft lip ~ 40700-40761
      fistula ~ 30580-30600, 42260
      nasal valve collapse ~ 30468
      rhinophyma ~ 30120
      septum ~ 30540-30545, 30630
      synechia ~ 30560
      vestibular stenosis ~ 30465
   skin
      excision ~ 30120
      surgical planing ~ 30120
   submucous resection turbinate
      excision ~ 30140
   turbinate
      excision ~ 30130-30140
      fracture ~ 30930
      injection ~ 30200
   turbinate mucosa, cauterization ~ 30801-30802
   unlisted services and procedures ~ 30999
Nose bleed ~ (hemorrhage, nasal) 30901-30906
NTD ~ (nitroblue tetrazolium dye test) 86384
Nuclear antigen, antibody ~ 86235
Nuclear imaging ~ see nuclear medicine
Nuclear magnetic resonance imaging ~ see magnetic resonance imaging
   (MRI)
Nuclear magnetic resonance spectroscopy ~ see magnetic resonance
   spectroscopy
Nuclear medicine ~ 78012-79999
   adrenal gland imaging ~ 78075
   bladder, residual study ~ 78730
   blood
      flow imaging ~ 78445
      iron
         absorption ~ 78162
         chelatable ~ 78172
         plasma ~ 78160
         red cells ~ 78140
         utilization ~ 78170
      platelet survival ~ 78191

Nuclear medicine ~ *continued*
   red cells ~ 78120-78121
   red cells survival ~ 78130
   unlisted services and procedures ~ 78199
   whole blood volume ~ 78122
  bone
   density study ~ 78350, 78351
   imaging ~ 78300, 78305, 78306, 78315, 78803
   SPECT ~ 78803
   ultrasound ~ 76977
   ultrasound services and procedures ~ 78399
  bone marrow imaging ~ 78102-78104
  brain
   blood flow ~ 78610
   cerebrospinal flow ~ 78630-78650
   imaging ~ 78600-78609
    vascular flow ~ 78610
  endocrine system, unlisted services and procedures ~ 78099
  esophagus
   imaging (motility) ~ 78258
   reflux study ~ 78262
  gastric mucosa imaging ~ 78261
  gastrointestinal
   blood loss study ~ 78278
   protein loss study ~ 78282
   shunt testing ~ 78291
   unlisted services and procedures ~ 78299
  genitourinary system, unlisted services and procedures ~ 78799
  heart
   angiography ~ 78445
   blood flow ~ 78414
   blood pool imaging ~ 78472-78473, 78481-78483, 78494-78496
   myocardial imaging ~ 78459, 78466-78469
   myocardial PET imaging ~ 78429-78434, 78459, 78491, 78492
   myocardial perfusion ~ 78451-78454
   shunt detection ~ 78428
   unlisted services and procedures ~ 78499
   venous thrombosis imaging ~ 78456-78458
  inflammatory process ~ 78800-78804, 78830-78832
  intestines imaging ~ 78290
  kidney
   function study ~ 78725
   imaging ~ 78700-78707
  lacrimal gland, tear flow ~ 78660
  liver
   imaging ~ 78201-78216
  lung
   imaging perfusion ~ 78580, 78597, 78598
   imaging ventilation ~ 78579, 78582, 78598
   unlisted services and procedures ~ 78599
  lymph nodes ~ 78195
  lymphatics ~ 78195
   unlisted services and procedures ~ 78199
  musculoskeletal system, unlisted services and procedures ~ 78399
  nervous system, unlisted services and procedures ~ 78699
  parathyroid gland imaging ~ 78070
  pulmonary perfusion ~ 78580, 78597-78598
  pulmonary ventilation ~ 78579, 78582, 78598
  quantification measurement ~ 78835
  salivary gland function study ~ 78232
   imaging ~ 78230-78231
  spleen
   imaging ~ 78185, 78215-78216
   unlisted services and procedures ~ 78199
  stomach
   blood loss study ~ 78278
   emptying study ~ 78264
   protein loss study ~ 78282
   reflux study ~ 78262
  testes imaging ~ 78761
  therapeutic
   heart ~ 79440
   interstitial ~ 79300
   intra-arterial ~ 79445
   intra-articular ~ 79440
   intracavitary ~ 79200
   intravenous ~ 79101
   intravenous infusion ~ 79403
   oral ~ 79005
   thyroid ~ 79200-79300

Nuclear medicine ~ *continued*
  unlisted services and procedures ~ 79999
  thyroid
   imaging for metastases ~ 78015-78018
   imaging with flow ~ 78013
   metastases uptake ~ 78020
   uptake ~ 78012, 78014
  tumor localization
   by radiopharmaceuticals ~ 78800-78804, 78808, 78830-78832
   by SPECT ~ 78803, 78830-78832
  unlisted services and procedures
   cardiovascular ~ 78499
   endocrine ~ 78099
   gastrointestinal ~ 78299
   genitourinary ~ 78799
   hemopoietic ~ 78199
   lymphatic ~ 78199
   miscellaneous ~ 78399
   nervous system ~ 78699
   respiratory ~ 78599
   reticuloendothelial ~ 78199
  urea breath test ~ 78267-78268
  ureter, reflux study ~ 78740
  vein thrombosis imaging ~ 78455-78458
Nucleases, DNA ~ see DNAse
Nucleic acid probe
  amplified probe detection, infectious agent
   bartonella henselae ~ 87471
   bartonella quintana ~ 87471
   borrelia burgdorferi ~ 87476
   candida species ~ 87481
   central nervous system pathogen ~ 87483
   chlamydia pneumoniae ~ 87486
   chlamydia trachomatis ~ 87491
   cytomegalovirus ~ 87496
   enterovirus ~ 87498, 87500
   gardnerella vaginalis ~ 87511
   hepatitis B virus ~ 87516
   hepatitis C ~ 87521
   hepatitis G ~ 87526
   herpes simplex virus ~ 87529
   herpes virus-6 ~ 87532
   HIV-1 ~ 87535
   HIV-2 ~ 87538
   legionella pneumophila ~ 87541
   multiple organisms ~ 87801
   mycobacteria avium-intracellulare ~ 87561
   mycobacteria species ~ 87551
   mycobacteria tuberculosis ~ 87556
   mycoplasma pneumoniae ~ 87581
   neisseria gonorrheae ~ 87591
   not otherwise specified ~ 87798, 87801
   papillomavirus, human ~ 87623-87625
   staphylococcus aureus ~ 87640-87641
   streptococcus, group A ~ 87651
   streptococcus, group B ~ 87653
   Zika virus ~ 87662
  direct probe detection, infectious agent
   borrelia burgdorferi ~ 87475
   candida species ~ 87480
   chlamydia pneumoniae ~ 87485
   chlamydia trachomatis ~ 87490
   clostridium difficile ~ 87493
   cytomegalovirus ~ 87495
   gardnerella vaginalis ~ 87510
   hepatitis C ~ 87520
   hepatitis G ~ 87525
   herpes simplex virus ~ 87528
   herpes virus-6 ~ 87531
   HIV-1 ~ 87534
   HIV-2 ~ 87537
   legionella pneumophila ~ 87540
   multiple organisms ~ 87800
   mycobacteria avium-intracellulare ~ 87560
   mycobacteria species ~ 87550
   mycobacteria tuberculosis ~ 87555
   mycoplasma pneumoniae ~ 87580
   neisseria gonorrheae ~ 87590
   not otherwise specified ~ 87797
   papillomavirus, human ~ 0500T, 87623-87625

Nucleic acid probe ~ *continued*
streptococcus, group A ~ 87650
trichomonas vaginalis ~ 87660
genotype analysis, infectious agent
HIV-1 ~ 87901, 87906
hepatitis C virus ~ 87902
in situ hybridization ~ 88120-88121, 88365-88368
phenotype analysis, infectious agent
HIV-1 drug resistance ~ 87903-87904
quantification, infectious agent
bartonella henselae ~ 87472
bartonella quintana ~ 87472
candida species ~ 87482
chlamydia pneumoniae ~ 87487
chlamydia trachomatis ~ 87492
cytomegalovirus ~ 87497
gardnerella vaginalis ~ 87512
hepatitis B virus ~ 87517
hepatitis C ~ 87522
hepatitis G ~ 87527
herpes simplex virus ~ 87530
herpes virus-6 ~ 87533
HIV-1 ~ 87536
HIV-2 ~ 87539
legionella pneumophila ~ 87542
mycobacteria avium-intracellulare ~ 87562
mycobacteria species ~ 87552
mycobacteria tuberculosis ~ 87557
mycoplasma pneumoniae ~ 87582
neisseria gonorrheae ~ 87592
not otherwise specified ~ 87799
papillomavirus, human ~ 87623-87625
streptococcus, group A ~ 87652
Nucleolysis, intervertebral disk ~ see chemonucleolysis
Nucleotidase ~ 83915
Nursemaid elbow ~ 24640
Nursing facility discharge services ~ see discharge services, nursing facility
Nursing facility services ~ 99304-99318
annual assessment ~ 99318
care plan oversight services ~ 99379-99380
comprehensive assessments
new or established patient ~ 99301-99303
discharge services ~ 99315-99316, 1110F-1111F
subsequent care ~ 99307-99310
Nuss procedure
with thoracoscopy ~ 21743
without thoracoscopy ~ 21742
Nutrition therapy
group ~ 97804
home infusion ~ 99601-99602
initial assessment ~ 97802
reassessment ~ 97803
Nystagmus tests ~ see vestibular function tests
optokinetic ~ 92534, 92544
positional ~ 92532, 92542
spontaneous ~ 92531, 92540-92541

O

O2 (two) saturation ~ see oxygen saturation
Ober-Yount procedure ~ (fasciotomy, hip) 27025
Obliteration
mastoid ~ 69670
vagina
total ~ 57110
vault ~ 57120
Oblongata, medulla ~ see medulla
Observation ~ (see Evaluation and Management; Hospital Services)
99217-99220, 99224-99225, 99234-99236

Obstetrical care
abortion
induced
by amniocentesis injection ~ 59850-59852
by dilation and curettage ~ 59840
by dilation and evaluation ~ 59841
missed
first trimester ~ 59820
second trimester ~ 59821
spontaneous ~ 59812
therapeutic ~ 59840-59852
antepartum care ~ 59425-59426
cesarean delivery ~ 59618-59622
only ~ 59514
postpartum care ~ 59515
routine ~ 59510
with hysterectomy ~ 59525
curettage, hydatidiform mole ~ 59870
evacuation, hydatidiform mole ~ 59870
external cephalic version ~ 59412
miscarriage, surgical completion ~ 59812-59821
placenta delivery ~ 59414
postpartum care ~ 59430, 59514
septic abortion ~ 59830
total (global) ~ 59400, 59610, 59618
unlisted services and procedures ~ 59898-59899
vaginal, after cesarean ~ 59610-59614
vaginal delivery ~ 59409-59410
delivery after cesarean ~ 59610-59614
Obstruction ~ see occlusion
Obstruction clearance, venous access device ~ 36595-36596
Obstruction colon ~ see colon, obstruction
Obturator nerve
avulsion ~ 64763-64766
incision ~ 64763-64766
transection ~ 64763-64766
Obturator prosthesis ~ 21076
definitive ~ 21080
insertion, larynx ~ 31527
interim ~ 21079
Occipital nerve, greater
avulsion ~ 64744
incision ~ 64744
injection, anesthetic ~ 64405
transection ~ 64744
Occlusion
bronchi, balloon ~ 31634, 31647, 31651
fallopian tube
by biopolymer implant ~ 0567T
by cannulation ~ 58565
by device ~ 58615, 58671
paravalvular leak
aortic valve ~ 93591, 93592
mitral valve ~ 93590, 93592
penis, vein ~ 37790
umbilical cord ~ 59072
ureteral ~ 50705
vascular
arterial, other than hemorrhage or tumor ~ 37242
carotid artery ~ 37605, 61705
dialysis circuit ~ 36909
during endovascular therapy ~ 34820
for hemorrhage ~ 37244
for infarction ~ 37243
for lymphatic extravasation ~ 37244
for organ ischemia ~ 37243
for tumors ~ 37243
nervous system
cranial ~ 61623, 61624, 61626
spinal ~ 61624, 61626, 62294, 63250-63252
placement of occlusive device ~ 34808
venous, other than hemorrhage ~ 37241
with ligation ~ 37606
Occlusive disease of artery ~ see repair, artery; revision
Occult blood ~ 82270
penis, by hemoglobin immunoassay ~ 82274

Occupational therapy
evaluation ~ 97165, 97166, 97167
re-evaluation ~ 97168
Ocular implant ~ see orbital implant
insertion
drug-eluting insert, eyelid ~ 0444T, 0445T
in scleral shell ~ 65130
muscles attached ~ 65140
muscles, not attached ~ 65135
modification ~ 65125
reinsertion ~ 65150
with foreign material ~ 65155
removal ~ 65175
Ocular muscle ~ see eye muscles
Ocular orbit ~ see orbit
Ocular prostheses ~ see prosthesis, ocular
Ocular screening ~ 99174, 99177
retinal polarization scan ~ 0469T
Oculomotor muscle ~ see eye muscles
Oddi sphincter ~ see sphincter of Oddi
Odontoid dislocation
open treatment/reduction ~ 22318
with grafting ~ 22319
Odontoid fracture
open treatment/reduction ~ 22318
with grafting ~ 22319
Odontoid process, excision ~ 22548
Oesophageal neoplasm ~ see tumor, esophagus
Oesophageal varices ~ see esophageal varices
Oesophagus ~ see esophagus
Oestradiol ~ see estradiol
Office and/or other outpatient services
established patient ~ 99211-99215
new patient ~ 99202-99205
normal newborn ~ 99461
office visit
established patient ~ 99211-99215
new patient ~ 99202-99205
outpatient visit
established patient ~ 99211-99215
new patient ~ 99202-99205
prolonged services ~ 99354, 99355, 99415, 99416
Office medical services
after hours ~ 99050
emergency care ~ 99058
extended hours ~ 99051
Office or other outpatient consultations ~ 99241-99245
Olecranon ~ see elbow; humerus; radius; ulna
bursa, arthrocentesis ~ 20605
cyst, excision ~ 24125-24126
tumor
cyst ~ 24120
excision ~ 24125-24126
Olecranon process
craterization ~ 24147
diaphysectomy ~ 24147
excision ~ 24147
abscess ~ 24138
fracture ~ see elbow; humerus; radius
closed treatment ~ 24670-24675
open treatment ~ 24685
osteomyelitis ~ 24138, 24147
saucerization ~ 24147
sequestrectomy ~ 24138
Oligoclonal immunoglobulins ~ 83916
Omentectomy
separate procedure ~ 49255
with laparotomy ~ 58960
with lymph node laparoscopy ~ 38573
with oophorectomy ~ 58943
with tumor debulking ~ 58575, 58950-58954, 58956-58958, 58960
Omentum
excision ~ 49255, 58950-58958
flap ~ 49904-49905
free, with microvascular anastomosis ~ 49906
unlisted services and procedures ~ 49999
Omphalectomy ~ 49250
Omphalocele, repair ~ 49600-49611
Omphalomesenteric duct, excision ~ 44800
Omphalomesenteric duct, persistent ~ see diverticulum, Meckel's

Oncoprotein
des-gamma-carboxyprothrombin (DCP) ~ 83951
HER-2/neu ~ 83950
One stage prothrombin time ~ (see also prothrombin time) 85610-85611
Online medical evaluation
nonphysician ~ 98970-98972
physician ~ 99421-99423
Onychectomy ~ see excision, nails
Onychia, drainage ~ 10060-10061
Oocyte
assisted fertilization, microtechnique ~ 89280-89281
biopsy ~ 89290-89291
culture
extended ~ 89272
less than 4 (four) days ~ 89250
with co-culture ~ 89251
identification, follicular fluid ~ 89254
insemination ~ 89268
retrieval, for in vitro fertilization ~ 58970
storage ~ 89346
thawing ~ 89356
Oophorectomy ~ 58262-58263, 58291-58292, 58552, 58554, 58661, 58940-58943
ectopic pregnancy
laparoscopic treatment ~ 59120
surgical treatment ~ 59120
Oophorectomy, partial ~ see excision, ovary, partial
Oophorocystectomy ~ see cystectomy, ovarian
Open biopsy, adrenal gland ~ see adrenal gland, biopsy
Operating microscope ~ 69990
Operation
Abbe-Estlander ~ 00102, 40527, 40761
Bischof ~ 63170
Blalock-Hanlon ~ 33735-33737
Blalock-Taussig ~ 33750
Bristow ~ 23460
Campbell ~ 27422
Chevron ~ 28296
Cotte ~ 58400-58410
Dunn ~ see arthrodesis, foot joint
Duvries ~ see tenoplasty
Estes ~ see ovary, transposition
Foley y-pyeloplasty ~ 50400-50405
Fontan ~ see repair, heart, anomaly
Gill ~ 63012
Green ~ see scapulopexy
Halsted ~ 49491
Heller ~ 32665
Hibb ~ 22610, 22612, 22614
Jaboulay gastroduodenostomy ~ 43810
Keller ~ 28292
Leriche ~ 64809
Mumford ~ 29824
Nissen ~ 43324
Norwood ~ 33611-33612, 33619
Potts-Smith ~ 33762
Ramstedt ~ see pyloromyotomy
Raskind ~ 33735-33737
Raz ~ 51845
Richardson hysterectomy ~ 53460
Schlatter total gastrectomy ~ 43620-43622
Swanson ~ 28309
Swenson ~ 45120
Takeuchi ~ 33505
Thiersch ~ 15050
Winiwarter ~ 47720-47740
Winter ~ 54435
Operation microscopes ~ see operating microscope
Operculectomy ~ 41821
Operculum ~ see gums
Ophthalmic mucous membrane test ~ (see also allergy tests) 95060
Ophthalmology services ~ 92002-92499
Ophthalmology, diagnostic
color vision exam ~ 92283
computerized scanning ~ 92132-92134
computerized screening ~ 99172, 99174
dark adaptation ~ 92284
electro-oculography ~ 92270
electromyography, needle ~ 92265
electroretinography ~ 92275

Ophthalmology, diagnostic ~ *continued*
  endoscopy ~ 66990
  evoked potentials
    acuity ~ 0333T
    central nervous system ~ 95930
    glaucoma test ~ 0464T
  eye exam
    established patient ~ 92012-92014
    new patient ~ 92002-92004
    with anesthesia ~ 92018-92019
  gonioscopy ~ 92020
  ocular photography
    external ~ 92285
    internal ~ 92286-92287
  photoscreening ~ 99174
  refractive determination ~ 92015
  sensorimotor exam ~ 92060
  tonometry, serial ~ 92100
  ultrasound ~ 76511-76529
  visual acuity screen ~ 99172-99173
  visual field exam ~ 92081-92083
  visual function screen ~ 99172, 99174, 99177
Ophthalmoscopy
  drawing of macula ~ 92202
  drawing of optic nerve ~ 92202
  dynamometry ~ 92260
  fluorescein angiography ~ 92235, 92242
  fluorescein angioscopy ~ 92230
  fundus photography ~ 92250
  indocyanine-green angiography ~ 92240, 92242
  retinal drawing ~ 92201
  retinal imaging ~ 92227-92229
  sceral depression ~ 92201
Opiates ~ 80361-80364
Opinion, second ~ see confirmatory consultations
Optic nerve
  decompression ~ 67570
    with nasal/sinus endoscopy ~ 31294
  head evaluation ~ 2027F
Optical coherence tomography (OCT)
  axillary lympyh node ~ 0351T, 0352T
  breast ~ 0351T-0354T
  intravascular ~ 92978, 92979
  middle ear ~ 0485T, 0486T
  retina, remote ~ 0604T-0606T
  skin lesion ~ 0470T, 0471T
Optical endomicroscopy
  esophageal ~ 43206
  gastrointestinal ~ 43252
  with endoscopic retrograde cholangio- pancreatopgraphy (ERCP) ~ 0397T
Optokinetic nystagmus test ~ see nystagmus tests, optokinetic
Oral lactose tolerance test ~ see glucose, tolerance test ~ 82951
Oral mucosa ~ see mouth, mucosa
Oral surgical splint ~ 21085
Orbit ~ see orbital contents; orbital floor; periorbital region
  biopsy
    exploration ~ 67450
    orbitotomy without bone flap ~ 67400
  CT scan ~ 70480-70482
  decompression ~ 61330
    bone removal ~ 67414, 67445
  exploration ~ 67400, 67450
    lesion, excision ~ 61333
  fracture
    closed treatment
      with manipulation ~ 21401
      without manipulation ~ 21400
    open treatment ~ 21406-21408
      blowout fracture ~ 21385-21395
  incision and drainage ~ 67405, 67440
  injection
    retrobulbar ~ 67500-67505
    tenon's capsule ~ 67515
  insertion, implant ~ 67550
  lesion, excision ~ 67412, 67420
  magnetic resonance imaging (MRI) ~ 70540-70543
  removal
    decompression ~ 67445
    foreign body ~ 67413, 67430
    implant ~ 67560

Orbit ~ *continued*
  sella turcica ~ 70482
  unlisted services and procedures ~ 67599
  X-ray ~ 70190-70200
Orbital contents, aspiration ~ 67415
Orbital floor ~ see orbit; periorbital region
  fracture, blow out ~ 21385-21395
Orbital hypertelorism, osteotomy
  periorbital ~ 21260-21263
Orbital implant ~ see ocular implant
  insertion ~ 67550
  removal ~ 67560
Orbital prosthesis ~ 21077
Orbital rims, reconstruction ~ 21182-21184
Orbital rim and forehead, reconstruction ~ 21172-21180
Orbital transplant ~ 67560
Orbital walls, reconstruction ~ 21182-21184
Orbitocraniofacial reconstruction, secondary ~ 21275
Orbitotomy
  with bone flap
    for exploration ~ 67450
    lateral approach ~ 67420
    with drainage ~ 67440
    with removal foreign body ~ 67430
    with removal of bone for decompression ~ 67445
  without bone flap
    for exploration ~ 67400
    with drainage only ~ 67405
    with removal lesion ~ 67412
  with removal foreign body ~ 67413
  with removal of bone for decompression ~ 67414
Orbit area reconstruction, secondary ~ 21275
Orbit wall decompression with nasal/sinus endoscopy ~ 31292-31293
Orchidectomies ~ see excision, testis
Orchidopexy ~ see orchiopexy
Orchidoplasty ~ see repair, testis
Orchiectomy
  laparoscopic ~ 54690
  partial ~ 54522
  radical
    abdominal exploration ~ 54535
    inguinal approach ~ 54530
  simple ~ 54520
Orchiopexy
  abdominal approach ~ 54650
  inguinal approach ~ 54640
  intra-abdominal testis ~ 54692
Orchioplasty ~ see repair, testis
Organ or disease oriented panels ~ 80048-80076
  electrolyte ~ 80051
  general health panel ~ 80050
  hepatic function panel ~ 80076
  hepatitis panel ~ 80074
  lipid panel ~ 80061
  metabolic
    basic ~ 80047, 80048
    comprehensive ~ 80053
  obstetric panel ~ 80055, 80081
  renal function ~ 80069
Organic acids ~ 83918-83921
Organ grafting ~ see transplantation
Organ system, neurologic ~ see nervous system
Ormond disease ~ see retroperitoneal fibrosis
Orogastric tube placement ~ 43752
Oropharynx, biopsy ~ 42800
Orthodontic cephalogram ~ 70350
Orthomyxoviridae ~ see influenza virus
Orthomyxovirus ~ see influenza virus
Orthopantogram ~ 70355
Orthopedic cast ~ see cast
Orthopedic surgery
  computer assisted navigation ~ 0054T-0055T, 20985
  stereotaxis, computer assisted ~ 20985
Orthoptic training ~ 92065
Orthoroentgenogram ~ 77073
Orthosis ~ see orthotics
Orthotics
  fitting ~ 97760
  management and training ~ 97760, 97763

Osmolality
blood ~ 83930
urine ~ 83935
Osseous survey ~ 77074-77076
Osseous tissue ~ see bone
Ossicles
excision stapes
with footplate drill out ~ 69661
without foreign material ~ 69660-69661
reconstruction ossicular chain
tympanoplasty with antrotomy or mastoidotomy ~ 69636-69637
tympanoplasty with mastoidectomy ~ 69642, 69644, 69646
tympanoplasty without mastoidectomy ~ 69632-69633
release, stapes ~ 69650
replacement, with prosthesis ~ 69633, 69637
Ostectomy
metacarpal ~ 26250
metatarsal ~ 28288
phalanges, finger ~ 26260-26262
pressure ulcer
ischial ~ 15941, 15945
sacral ~ 15933, 15935, 15937
trochanteric ~ 15951, 15953, 15958
scapula ~ 23190
sternum ~ 21620
Osteocalcin ~ 83937
Osteocartilaginous exostoses ~ see exostosis
Osteochondroma ~ see exostosis
Osteocutaneous flap, with microvascular anastomosis ~ 20969-20973
Osteoma sinusotomy, frontal ~ 31075
Osteomyelitis
elbow, incision and drainage ~ 23935
excision
clavicle ~ 23180
facial ~ 21026
humerus, proximal ~ 23184
mandible ~ 21025
scapula ~ 23182
femur/knee, incision and drainage ~ 27303
finger incision ~ 26034
hand incision ~ 26034
hip incision, deep ~ 26992
humerus ~ 24134
incision and drainage ~ 23935
incision
foot ~ 28005
shoulder ~ 23035
thorax ~ 21510
olecranon process ~ 24138, 24147
pelvis incision, deep ~ 26992
radius ~ 24136, 24145
sequestrectomy
clavicle ~ 23170
humeral head ~ 23174
scapula ~ 23172
skull ~ 61501
Osteopathic manipulation ~ 98925-98929
Osteoplasty
carpal bone ~ 25394
facial bones
augmentation ~ 21208
reduction ~ 21209
femoral neck ~ 27179
femur ~ 27179
lengthening ~ 27466-27468
shortening ~ 27465, 27468
fibula, lengthening ~ 27715
humerus ~ 24420
metacarpal ~ 26568
phalanges, finger ~ 26568
radius ~ 25390-25393
tibia, lengthening ~ 27715
ulna ~ 25390-25393
vertebra ~ 72291-72292
lumbar ~ 22521-22522
thoracic ~ 22520-22522

Osteotomy
calcaneus ~ 28300
chin ~ 21121-21123
clavicle ~ 23480-23485
femur ~ 27140, 27151
femoral neck ~ 27161
for slipped epiphysis ~ 27181
with fixation ~ 27165
without fixation ~ 27448-27450
with open reduction of hip ~ 27156
with realignment ~ 27454
fibula ~ 27707-27712
hip ~ 27146-27151
femoral, with open reduction ~ 27156
femur ~ 27151
humerus ~ 0594T, 24410
mandible ~ 21198-21199
extra-oral ~ 21047
intra-oral ~ 21046
maxilla ~ 21206
extra-oral ~ 21049
intra-oral ~ 21048
metacarpal ~ 26565
metatarsal ~ 28306-28309
with bunionectomy ~ 28295, 28296
orbit reconstruction ~ 21256
pelvis ~ 27158
periorbital
orbital hypertelorism ~ 21260-21263
osteotomy with graft ~ 21267-21268
phalanges
finger ~ 26567
toe ~ 28299, 28310-28312
radius
and ulna ~ 25365, 25375
distal third ~ 25350
middle or proximal third ~ 25355
multiple ~ 25370
skull base ~ 61582-61585, 61592
spine
anterior ~ 22220-22226
posterior, posterolateral ~ 22206-22208, 22210-22214
talus ~ 28302
tarsal ~ 28304-28305
tibia ~ 27455-27457, 27705, 27709-27712
ulna ~ 25360
multiple ~ 25370
and radius ~ 25365, 25375
vertebra
additional segment, anterior approach ~ 22226
posterior/posterolateral approach ~ 22216
cervical
anterior approach ~ 22220
posterior/posterolateral approach ~ 22210
lumbar
anterior approach ~ 22224
posterior/posterolateral approach ~ 22214
thoracic
anterior approach ~ 22222
posterior/posterolateral approach ~ 22212
with graft reconstruction periorbital region ~ 21267-21268
with bunionectomy ~ 28295, 28296, 28298, 28299
with graft
reconstruction, periorbital region ~ 21267, 21268
Os calcis fracture ~ see calcaneus, fracture
Otolaryngology, diagnostic exam under anesthesia ~ 92502
Otomy ~ see incision
Otoplasty ~ 69300
Otorhinolaryngology services ~ 92502-92597
Ouchterlony immunodiffusion ~ 86331
Outer ear ~ see ear, outer
Outpatient visit ~ see history and physical; office and/or other outpatient services
Output, cardiac ~ see cardiac output
Ova, smear ~ 87177
Oval window, repair fistula ~ 69666
Oval window fistula ~ see fistula, oval window
Ovarian cyst ~ see cyst, ovarian; ovary, cyst
Ovarian vein syndrome, ureterolysis ~ 50722
Ovariectomies ~ see oophorectomy
Ovariolysis ~ 58740

1195

Ovary
abscess, incision and drainage ~ 58820-58822
    abdominal approach ~ 58822
biopsy ~ 49321, 58900
cyst
    excision ~ 58925
    incision and drainage ~ 58800-58805
excision ~ 58662, 58720
    cyst ~ 58925
    partial
        oophorectomy ~ 58661, 58940
        ovarian malignancy ~ 58943
        peritoneal malignancy ~ 58943
        tubal malignancy ~ 58943
        wedge resection ~ 58920
    total ~ 58940-58943
laparoscopy ~ 58660-58662, 58679
lysis, adhesions ~ 58660, 58740
malignancy
    resection ~ 58950-58952, 58957, 58958
    staging laparotomy ~ 58960
oncology
    biochemical assay
        apolipoprotein A1 ~ 81503
        beta-2 microglobulin ~ 81503
        CA-125 ~ 81500, 81503
        HE4 ~ 81500
        menopausal status ~ 81500
        pre-albumin ~ 81503
        transferrin ~ 81503
    radical resection ~ 58950-58952
removal
    with pelvic exenteration ~ 45126, 58240
    with radical trachelectomy ~ 58531
    with hysterectmy ~ 58150, 58152, 58180, 58200, 58210
    laparoscopic ~ 58542, 58544, 58548, 58554, 58552, 58571, 58573, 58575
    vaginal ~ 58262, 58263, 58291, 58292
transposition ~ 58825
tumor, resection ~ 58950-58958
unlisted services and procedures ~ 58679, 58999
wedge resection ~ 58920
Oviduct
anastomosis ~ 58750
chromotubation ~ 58350
ectopic pregnancy ~ 59120-59121
excision ~ 58700-58720
fulguration, laparoscopic ~ 58670
hysterosalpingography ~ 74740
laparoscopy ~ 58679
ligation ~ 58600-58611
lysis, adhesions ~ 58740
occlusion ~ 58615
    laparoscopic ~ 58671
repair ~ 58752
    anastomosis ~ 58750
    create stoma ~ 58770
unlisted services and procedures ~ 58679, 58999
X-ray with contrast ~ 74740
Ovocyte ~ see oocyte
Ovulation tests ~ 84830
Ovum implantation ~ see implantation
Ovum transfer surgery ~ see gamete intrafallopian transfer (GIT)
Oxalate ~ 83945
Oxidase, ceruloplasmin ~ see ceruloplasmin
Oxidoreductase, alcohol-nad+ ~ see antidiuretic hormone
Oximetry (noninvasive) ~ see pulmonology, diagnostic
blood O2 saturation, ear or pulse ~ 94760-94762
pulse, recording
    car seat/bed testing ~ 94780, 94781
    with pulmonary stess testing ~ 94618
Oxoisomerase ~ see phosphohexose isomerase
Oxosteroids ~ see ketosteroids
Oxygenation, extracorporeal membrane ~ see extracorporeal membrane oxygenation
Oxygen saturation ~ 82805-82810
Oxyproline ~ see hydroxyproline
Oxytocin stress test, fetal ~ 59020

P

P & P ~ (proconvertin) 85230
P-acetamidophenol ~ see acetaminophen
Pacemaker, heart ~ see Cardiac assist devices
Pachymetry, eye ~ 76514
with collagen cross-linking ~ 0402T
Packing
nasal hemorrhage ~ 30901-30906
preperitoneal pelvic hemorrhage ~ 49013, 49014
Pain management
epidural/intrathecal ~ 62350-62351, 62360-62362, 99601-99602
intravenous therapy ~ 90783-90784
Palatal augmentation prosthesis ~ 21082
Palatal lift prosthesis ~ 21083
Palate
abscess, incision and drainage ~ 42000
biopsy ~ 42100
excision ~ 42120, 42145
fracture
    closed treatment ~ 21421
    open treatment ~ 21422-21423
lesion
    destruction ~ 42160
    excision ~ 42104-42120
prosthesis ~ 42280-42281
reconstruction, lengthening ~ 42226-42227
repair
    cleft palate ~ 42200-42225
    laceration ~ 42180-42182
    Vomer flap ~ 42235
unlisted services and procedures ~ 42299
Palate, cleft ~ see cleft palate
Palatoplasty ~ 42200-42225
Palatoschisis ~ see cleft palate
Palm
bursa, incision and drainage ~ 26025-26030
fasciectomy ~ 26121-26125
fasciotomy ~ 26040-26045
tendon, excision ~ 26170
tendon sheath
    excision ~ 26145
    incision and drainage ~ 26020
Palsy, seventh nerve ~ see facial nerve paralysis
Pancreas
anastomosis, with intestines ~ 48520-48540
anesthesia ~ 00794
biopsy ~ 48100
    needle biopsy ~ 48102
cyst
    anastomosis ~ 48520-48540
    repair ~ 48500
debridement, peripancreatic tissue ~ 48105
dilation, ampulla of vater ~ 47542, 43277
excision
    ampulla of vater ~ 48148
    duct ~ 48148
    partial ~ 48140-48146, 48150, 48154, 48160
    peripancreatic tissue ~ 48105
    total ~ 48155-48160
lesion, excision ~ 48120
needle biopsy ~ 48102
placement, drainage ~ 48000-48001
pseudocyst
    drainage ~ 48510
removal, calculi (stone) ~ 48020
removal transplanted allograft ~ 48556
repair, cyst ~ 48500
suture ~ 48545
transplantation ~ 48160, 48550, 48554-48556
    allograft preparation ~ 48550-48552
unlisted services and procedures ~ 48999
X-ray with contrast ~ 74300
    injection procedure ~ 48400
Pancreas, endocrine only ~ see islet cell

Pancreatectomy
  donor ~ 48550
  partial ~ 48140-48146, 48150-48154, 48160
  total ~ 48155-48160
  with transplantation ~ 48160
Pancreaticojejunostomy ~ 48548
Pancreatic DNAse ~ see DNAse
Pancreatic duct
  destruction, calculi (stone) ~ 43265
  dilation, endoscopy ~ 43277
  endoscopic retrograde cholangiopancreatography (ERCP) with optical
      endomicroscopy ~ 0397T
  endoscopy ~ 43273
    collection, specimen ~ 43260
    destruction
      calculi (stone) ~ 43265
      tumor ~ 43272
    dilation ~ 43277
    removal (endoscopic)
      calculi (stone) ~ 43264
      foreign body ~ 43275-43276
      stent ~ 43275-43276
    sphincter pressure ~ 43263
    sphincterotomy ~ 43262
    tube placement ~ 43274
  incision, sphincter ~ 43262
  removal
    calculi (stone) ~ 43264
    foreign body ~ 43275-43276
    stent ~ 43275-43276
  tube placement
    nasopancreatic ~ 43274
    stent ~ 43268
  tumor, destruction ~ 43272
  X-ray
    guide catheter ~ 74329-74330
    injection procedure ~ 47531, 47532, 48400
    intra-operative ~ 74300, 74301
Pancreatic elastase 1 (PEL1) ~ 82656
Pancreatic islet cell ab ~ see antibody, islet cell
Pancreatitis, incision and drainage ~ 48000
Pancreatography
  injection procedure ~ 48400
  intraoperative ~ 74300-74301
  postoperative ~ 47531, 47532
Pancreatojejunostomies ~ see pancreaticojejunostomy
Pancreatorrhaphy ~ 48545
Pancreatotomy ~ see incision, pancreas
Pancreozymin-secretin test ~ 82938
Panel ~ see organ or disease oriented panel
Panniculectomy ~ see lipectomy
Paper chromatographies ~ see chromatography, paper
Papilla, interdental ~ see gums
Pap smears ~ 88141-88155, 88164-88167, 88174-88175
Papillectomy ~ 46220
Papilloma
  destruction ~ 54050-54065
    anus ~ 46900-46924
    penis ~ 54050-54065
PAPP D ~ see lactogen, human placental
Para-tyrosine ~ see tyrosine
Paracentesis
  abdomen ~ 49082-49083
  eye
    with aqueous aspiration ~ 65800
    with aqueous release ~ 65800
    with discission of anterior hyaloid membrane ~ 65810
    with removal
      blood ~ 65815
      vitreous ~ 65810
  thorax ~ 32554-32555
Paracervical nerve
  injection, anesthetic ~ 64435
Paraesophageal hiatal hernia
  repair via
    laparotomy ~ 43332-43333
    thoracoabdominal incision ~ 43336-43337
    thoracotomy ~ 43334-43335
Paraffin bath therapy ~ 97018
Paraganglioma, medullary ~ see pheochromocytoma

Parainfluenza virus antigen detection, immunofluorescence ~ 87279
Paralysis, facial nerve ~ see facial nerve paralysis
Paralysis, infantile ~ see polio
Paranasal sinuses ~ see sinus; sinuses
Parasites
  blood ~ 87207
  examination ~ 87169
  smear ~ 87177
Parasitic worms ~ see helminth
Parathormone ~ 83970
Parathyrin ~ see parathormone
Parathyroidectomy ~ 60500-60505
Parathyroid autotransplantation ~ 60512
Parathyroid gland
  autotransplant ~ 60512
  excision ~ 60500-60502
  exploration ~ 60500-60505
  nuclear medicine, imaging ~ 78070
Parathyroid hormone ~ 83970
Parathyroid hormone measurement ~ see parathormone
Parathyroid transplantation ~ see transplantation, parathyroid
Paraurethral gland
  abscess, incision and drainage ~ 53060
Paravertebral nerve
  destruction ~ 64633-64636
  injection
    anesthetic ~ 64461, 64462, 64490-64495
    neurolytic ~ 64633-64636
  infusion, anesthetic ~ 64463
Parietal cell vagotomies ~ see vagotomy, highly selective
Parietal craniotomy ~ 61556
Paring
  skin lesion, benign hyperkeratotic
    more than four lesions ~ 11057
    single lesion ~ 11055
    two to four lesions ~ 11056
Paronychia, incision and drainage ~ 10060-10061
Parotid duct
  diversion ~ 42507-42510
  reconstruction ~ 42507-42510
Parotid gland
  abscess, incision and drainage ~ 42300-42305
  calculi (stone), excision ~ 42330, 42340
  excision
    partial ~ 42410-42415
    total ~ 42420-42426
  tumor, excision ~ 42410-42426
Parotitides, epidemic ~ see mumps
Pars abdominalis aortae ~ see aorta, abdominal
Partial
  colectomy ~ see colectomy, partial
  cystectomy ~ see cystectomy, partial
  esophagectomy ~ see esophagectomy, partial
  gastrectomy ~ see excision, stomach, partial
  glossectomy ~ see excision, tongue, partial
  hepatectomy ~ see excision, liver, partial
  mastectomies ~ see breast, excision, lesion
  nephrectomy ~ see excision, kidney, partial
  pancreatectomy ~ see pancreatectomy, partial
  splenectomy ~ see splenectomy, partial
  thromboplastin time ~ see thromboplastin, partial, time
  ureterectomy ~ see ureterectomy, partial
Particle agglutination ~ 86403-86406
Parvovirus antibody ~ 86747
Patch allergy tests ~ 95044
Patella
  dislocation ~ 27560-27566
  excision ~ 27350
    with reconstruction ~ 27424
  fracture ~ 27520-27524
  reconstruction ~ 27437-27438
  repair
    chondromalacia ~ 27418
    instability ~ 27420-27424
Patella, chondromalacia ~ see chondromalacia patella
Patellar tendon bearing (PTB) cast ~ 29435
Patellectomy with reconstruction ~ 27424
Paternity testing ~ 86910-86911
Patey's operation ~ see mastectomy, radical
Pathologic dilatation ~ see dilation

Pathology and laboratory

atomic absorption spectroscopy ~ 82190
breath test
    alcohol, ethyl ~ 82075
    Helicobacter pylori ~ 78267-78268, 83013-83014
    hydrogen ~ 91065
    methane ~ 91065
    urea ~ 78267-78268
caffeine ~ 89049
cell count
    body fluid ~ 86152-86153, 89050-89051
        crystal identification ~ 89060
        with immunologic selection ~ 86152-86153
cerebrospinal fluid
    cell count ~ 89050
    immunoelectrophoresis ~ 86325
    myelin basic protein ~ 83873
    protein, total ~ 84157
chemiluminescent assay ~ 82397
chemistry ~ 82009-84999
    acetaminophen ~ 80329-80331
    acetic anhydride ~ 84600
    acetylcholinesterase ~ 82013
    acetylsalicylic acid ~ 80329-80331
    acid, gastric ~ 82930
    adenosine ~ 82030
    adrenalin
        blood ~ 82383
        urine ~ 82382, 82384
    adrenocorticotropic hormone (ACTH) ~ 80400-80406, 80412, 80418, 82024
    albumin ~ 82040-82045
    alcohol
        breath ~ 82075
        urine ~ 80320-80322
    aldosterone ~ 82088
        suppression evaluation ~ 80408
    alpha-1 antitrypsin ~ 82103, 82104
    alpha-fetoprotein (AFP)
        amniotic fluid ~ 82106
        serum ~ 82105, 82107
    aluminum, blood ~ 82108
    amino acids ~ 82127-82139
    aminolevulinic acid (ALA) ~ 82135
    ammonia, blood ~ 82140
    amniotic fluid ~ 82143
    amobarbital ~ 80345
    amphetamine ~ 80324-80326
    amylase ~ 82150
    androsterone ~ 82160
    arsenic ~ 82175, 83015, 83018
    ascorbic acid ~ 82180
    aspirin ~ 80329-80331
    barbiturates ~ 80345
    barium ~ 83015, 83018
    beta glucosidase ~ 82963
    bicarbonate ~ 82374
    bile ~ 82239
    bilirubin
        blood ~ 82247, 82248
        feces ~ 82252
        total ~ 82247, 82248
    blood gases
        CO2 ~ 82803
        oxygen saturation ~ 82805, 82810
        pH ~ 82800, 82803, 82930
        pO2 ~ 82803, 82820
    blood, occult ~ 82270-82274
    calcium ~ 82310, 82330, 82331, 82340
    carbon dioxid ~ 82374, 82803
    cholesterol
        HDL ~ 83718
        LDL ~ 83721, 83722
        seium or whole blood ~ 82465
    chorionic gonadotropin (hCG) ~ 84702-84704
    cocaine, screen ~ 80305-80307
    cortisol
        free ~ 82530
        total ~ 82533
    creatinine ~ 82565, 82570, 82575

Pathology and laboratory ~ *continued*

cyanide ~ 82600
dopamine ~ 82383, 82384
epinephrine ~ 82382-82384
estradiol
    free ~ 82681
    total ~ 82670
estriol ~ 82677
estrogen receptor assay ~ 84233
estrogens ~ 82671, 82672
estrone ~ 82679
ethanol
    any source, except breath ~ 80320-80322
    any source, except breath and urine ~ 82077
    breath ~ 82075
ethyl alcohol ~ 80320, 82075
fluoride ~ 82735
flurazepam ~ 80346, 80347
folic acid ~ 82746, 82747
follicle stimulating hormone (FSH) ~ 83001
fructose ~ 82757, 84375
gammaglobulin IgA ~ 82784, 82787
gammaglobulin IgE ~ 82785, 82787
    allergen specific ~ 86003, 86005, 86008
gammaglobulin IgG ~ 82784, 82787
gammaglobulin IgM ~ 82784, 82787
glucose
    blood ~ 82947, 82948
    home monitoring device ~ 82962
    other than blood ~ 82945
    tolerance ~ 82951, 82952
heroin ~ 80305-80307, 80356
histamine ~ 83088
homocysteine83090
human growth hormone (HGH) ~ 83003
IgA ~ 82784
IgE ~ 82785, 82787, 86003, 86005, 86008
IgG ~ 82784, 82787
IgM ~ 82784, 82787
iron ~ 83540
ketone body ~ 82009, 82010
lactate ~ 83605
lactate dehydrogenase ~ 83615, 83625
lactic acid ~ 83605
lead ~ 83655
lipase ~ 83690
magnesium ~ 83735
marijuana ~ 80305-80307
mercury ~ 83018, 83825
methadone ~ 80358
methamphetamine ~ 80324-80326
nickel ~ 83885
nicotine ~ 80323
opiates ~ 80361-80364
oral lactose tolerance test ~ 82951, 82952
pancreatic elastase 1 (PE1) ~ 82656
pancreosymin-secretin test ~ 82938
PKU ~ 84030
potassium ~ 84132, 84133
prealbumin ~ 84134
pregnancy test ~ 81025, 84702-84704
progesterone ~ 84144
progesterone receptors ~ 84234
proinsulin ~ 84206
prolactin ~ 84146
pyruvate ~ 84210
pyruvate kinase ~ 84220
quinine ~ 84228
receptor assay
    estrogen ~ 84233
    non-endocrine ~ 84238
    progesterone ~ 84234
    unspecified hormone ~ 84235
riboflavin ~ 84252
salicylates ~ 80329-80331
selenium ~ 84255
serotonin ~ 84260
sickle hemoglobin ~ 85660
sodium, blood ~ 84295
specific gravity, urine ~ 81000-81003

Pathology and laboratory ~ *continued*

   sugars ~ 84375-84379
   sweat test ~ 82435
   T-3 ~ 84479-84482
   T-4 ~ 84436, 84437, 84439, 84479
   testosterone ~ 84402, 84403, 84410
   thiamine ~ 84425
   thyroid stimulating hormone (TSH) ~ 84443
   thyroxine ~ 84436, 84437, 84439
   tobramycin ~ 80200
   triglycerides ~ 84478
   tyrosine ~ 84510
   urea nitrogen ~ 84520, 84525
   valproic acid ~ 80164, 80165
   volatiles ~ 84600
   xylose absorption ~ 84620
   zinc ~ 84630
  cholesterol
   HDL ~ 83718
   LDL ~ 83721
   lipid panel ~ 80061
   serum ~ 82465
   VLDL ~ 83719
  chronic gonadotropin ~ 84702-84704
   stimulation panel ~ 80414-80415
  cryopreservation
   cells ~ 88240, 88241
   oocyte(s) ~ 89337
   testicular ~ 89335
  cytogenic studies ~ 88230-88299
  cytopathology ~ 88104-88140
  cytotoxicity assay, cancer stem cells (CSCs) ~ 0564T
  evocative/suppression testing
   agent administration ~ 96360, 96361, 96372-96375
   suppression panel
    dexamethasone ~ 80420
    growth hormone ~ 80430
    insulin-induced C-peptide ~ 80432
   tolerance panel
    glucagon ~ 80422, 80424
    insulin ~ 80434, 80435
  gene analysis
   chimerism analysis ~ 81267, 81268
   comparative analysis using short tandem repeat (STR) markers ~ 81265, 81266
   cytogenomic microarray analysis ~ 81406
   HLA class I and II typing, low resolution ~ 81370, 81371
   HLA class I typing, low resolution ~ 81372-81374
   HLA class II typing, low resolution ~ 81375-81377
   HLA class I and II typing, high resolution ~ 81378
   HLA class I typing, high resolution ~ 81379-81381
   HLA class II typing, high resolution ~ 81382, 81383
   human platelet antigen genotyping ~ 81105-81112
   microsatellite instability analysis ~ 81301
  hematology and coagulation ~ 85002-85999
   blood typing ~ 86920-86923
  infectious agent
   immunoassay detection ~ 86317, 86318, 87449-87451, 87802-87804, 87806-87810, 87850, 87880, 87899
  in vivo procedures ~ 88720-88749
  microbiology ~ 87003-87999
  molecular pathology ~ 81200-81099
  multianalyte assays with algorithmic analyses
   adoponectin ~ 81506
   apolipoprotein A1 ~ 81503
   AFP ~ 81510-81512
   beta-2 microglobulin ~ 81503
   CA-125 ~ 81500, 81503
   DIA ~ 81509, 81511, 81512
   ferritin ~ 81506
   glucose ~ 81506
   HbA1c ~ 81506
   hCG ~ 81508-81512
   HE4 ~ 81500
   hs-CRP ~ 81506
   insulin ~ 81506
   interleukin 2-receptor alpha ~ 81506
   mRNA ~ 81519-81521
   oncological gene profiling ~ 81504
   PAPP-A ~ 81508, 81509

Pathology and laboratory ~ *continued*

   prealbumin ~ 81503
   trisomy 21, 18, and 13 ~ 81507
   transferrin ~ 81503
   uE3 ~ 81510-81512
   unlisted ~ 81599
  optical endomicroscopy ~ 88375
  ovulation tests ~ 84830
  particle agglutination ~ 86403-86406
  paternity testing ~ 86910-86911
  postmortem ~ 88000-88099
  radioimmunoassay ~ 82009-84999
  reticulocyte count ~ 85044-85046
  reproductive medine ~ 89250-89398
  spectroscopy
   atomic absorption ~ 82190
   bioimpedance spectoscopy (BIS) ~ 93702
   fluorescent AGE ~ 88749
   infrared ~ 82365
   magnetic resonance ~ 76390
  surgical pathology ~ 88300-88399
   antibody stain procedure immunofluorescence ~ 88346, 88350
   archived tissue examination ~ 88363
   consultation ~ 88321-88325
    intraoperative ~ 88329-88334
   decalcification procedure ~ 88311
   electron microscopy ~ 88348
   gross and micro exam
    level II ~ 88302
    level III ~ 88304
    level IV (four) ~ 88305
    level V (five) ~ 88307
    level VI (six) ~ 88309
   gross exam, level I ~ 88300
   histochemistry ~ 88313-88319
   immunocytochemistry ~ 88313, 88342
   immunofluorescent study ~ 88346, 88350
   nerve teasing ~ 88362
   special stain ~ 88312-88314, 88319
   tissue hybridization ~ 88365
   unlisted procedures ~ 88399, 89240
  toxicology screen ~ 80305-80307
  transfusion medicine
   antibody ~ 86850, 86860, 86870
   blood processing
    autologous ~ 86890-86891
    frozen ~ 86927, 86930-86932
    irradiation ~ 86945
    pooling ~ 86965
    pretreatment ~ 86970-86972, 86975-86978
    splitting ~ 86985
    volume reduction ~ 86960
   leukocyte transfusion ~ 86950
   unlisted procedure ~ 86999
  Western blot
   HIV ~ 86689
   protein ~ 84181-84182
   tissue analysis ~ 88371-88372
  white blood cell
   alkaline phosphatase ~ 85540
   antibody ~ 86021
   count ~ 85032, 85048, 89055
   differential ~ 85004-85007, 85009
   histamine release test ~ 86343
   phagocytosis ~ 86344
   transfusion ~ 86950

Patterson's test ~ see blood urea nitrogen
Paul-Bunnell test ~ see antibody; antibody identification; microsomal antibody
P B antibodies ~ see antibody, heterophile
PBG ~ see porphobilinogen
PCP ~ (phencyclidine) 83992
Pean's operation ~ (amputation, upper leg, at hip) 27290
Pectoral cavity ~ see chest cavity
Pectus carinatum
  reconstructive repair ~ 21740-21742
   with thoracoscopy ~ 21743
Pectus excavatum
  reconstructive repair ~ 21740-21742
   with thoracoscopy ~ 21743

Pediatric critical care ~ 99471-99472
Pediatric intensive care ~ 99478
Pedicle fixation insertion ~ 22842-22844
Pedicle flap
  abbe-estlander type ~ 40761
  for breast reconstrucion
    double ~ 19369
    sincle ~ 19367
  for cerebrospinal fluid leak ~ 61619
  for eyelid repair ~ 67961
  for lip repair ~ 40761
  for vaginal lengthening ~ 46748
  formation ~ 15570-15576
  island ~ 15740
  neurovascular ~ 15750
  transfer ~ 15650
  vascular ~ 15730, 15731, 15733
  sygomaticofacial flap ~ 15730
PEEP ~ see pressure breathing, positive
Peet operation ~ see nerves, sympathectomy, excision
Pelvi-ureteroplasty ~ see pyeloplasty
Pelvic adhesions ~ see adhesions, pelvic
Pelvic exam ~ 57410
Pelvic exenteration ~ 51597
Pelvic fixation insertion ~ 22848
Pelvic lymphadenectomy ~ 58240
Pelvimetry ~ 74710
Pelviolithotomy ~ 50130
Pelvis ~ see also hip
  abscess, incision and drainage ~ 26990, 45000
  angiography ~ 72191
  biopsy ~ 27040-27041
  bone, drainage ~ 26992
  brace application ~ 20662
  bursa, incision and drainage ~ 26991
  CT scan ~ 72191-72194, 74176-74178
  cyst
    aspiration ~ 50390
    injection ~ 50390
  destruction, lesion ~ 58662
  endoscopy
    destruction of lesion ~ 58662
    lysis of adhesions ~ 58660
    oviduct surgery ~ 58670-58671
  exclusion, small intestine ~ 44700
  exenteration ~ 45126, 58240
  fasciotomy, decompression ~ 27027
    with debridement ~ 27057
  halo ~ 20662
  hematoma, incision and drainage ~ 26990
  lysis, adhesions ~ 58660
  magnetic resonance angiography ~ 72198
  magnetic resonance imaging (MRI) ~ 72195-72197
    obstetric MRI ~ 74712, 74713
  removal, foreign body ~ 27086-27087
  repair
    osteotomy ~ 27158
    tendon ~ 27098
  ring dislocation/fracture
    closed treatment ~ 27197, 27198
      with manipulation ~ 27198
      without manipulation ~ 27197
    open treatment ~ 27217, 27218
      with internal fixation ~ 27217, 27218
    percutaneous skeletal fixation ~ 27216
  tumor
    excision ~ 27043-27048
    radical resectin ~ 27049, 27059
  ultrasound ~ 76856, 76857
  unlisted services and procedures for hips and hip joint ~ 27299
  wound ~ 49013, 49014
  X-ray ~ 72170-72190
    with hip(s) ~ 73501-73503, 73521-73523
    manometry ~ 74710
Pemberton osteotomy of pelvis ~ see osteotomy, pelvis
Penectomy ~ see amputation, penis
Penetration keratoplasties ~ see keratoplasty, penetrating
Penile induration ~ see Peyronie disease

Penile prosthesis
  insertion
    inflatable ~ 54401-54405
    noninflatable ~ 54400
  removal
    inflatable ~ 54406, 54410-54417
    semi-rigid ~ 54415-54417
  repair, inflatable ~ 54408
  replacement
    inflatable ~ 54410-54411, 54416-54417
    semi-rigid ~ 54416-54417
Penile rigidity test ~ 54250
Penile tumescence test ~ 54250
Penis
  amputation
    partial ~ 54120
    radical ~ 54130-54135
    replanted ~ 54438
    total ~ 54125
  biopsy ~ 54100-54105
  circumcision
    with clamp or other device ~ 54150
      newborn ~ 54150
    repair ~ 54163
    surgical excision, newborn ~ 54160
  excision
    partial ~ 54120
    prepuce ~ 54150-54161, 54163
    total ~ 54125-54135
  frenulum, excision ~ 54164
  incision, prepuce ~ 54000-54001
  incision and drainage ~ 54015
  injection
    for erection ~ 54235
    peyronie disease ~ 54200
      surgical exposure plague ~ 54205
    vasoactive drugs ~ 54231
    X-ray ~ 54230
  insertion, prosthesis
    inflatable ~ 54401-54405
    noninflatable ~ 54400
  irrigation, priapism ~ 54220
  lesion
    destruction
      cryosurgery ~ 54056
      electrodesiccation ~ 54055
      extensive ~ 54065
      laser surgery ~ 54057
      simple ~ 54050-54060
      surgical excision ~ 54060
    excision ~ 54060
      penile plague ~ 54110-54112
  nocturnal penile tumescence test ~ 54250
  occlusion, vein ~ 37790
  plaque, excision ~ 54110-54112
  plethysmography ~ 54240
  prepuce, stretch ~ 54450
  reconstruction
    angulation ~ 54360
    chordee ~ 54300-54304, 54328
    complications ~ 54340-54348
    epispadias ~ 54380-54390
    hypospadias ~ 54328-54352
    injury ~ 54440
  removal
    foreign body ~ 54115
    prosthesis
      inflatable ~ 54406, 54410-54417
      semi-rigid ~ 54415-54417
  repair
    corporeal tear(s) ~ 54437
    fistulization ~ 54435
    priapism with shunt ~ 54420-54430
    prosthesis, inflatable ~ 54408
  replacement, prosthesis
    inflatable ~ 54410-54411, 54416-54417
    semi-rigid ~ 54416-54417
  replantation ~ 54438
  revascularization ~ 37788

Penis ~ *continued*
  rigidity test ~ 54250
  test erection ~ 54250
  unlisted services and procedures ~ 55899
  venous studies ~ 93980-93981
Penis adhesions
  lysis, post-circumcision ~ 54162
Penis prostheses ~ see penile prosthesis
Pentagastrin test ~ see gastric analysis test
Pentamidine ~ see inhalation treatment
Peptidase P ~ see angiotensin converting enzyme (ACE)
Peptidase S ~ see leucine aminopeptidase
Peptide, connecting ~ see C-peptide
Peptide, vasoactive intestinal ~ see vasoactive intestinal peptide
Peptidyl dipeptidase A ~ see angiotensin converting enzyme (ACE)
Percutaneous abdominal paracentesis ~ see abdomen, drainage
Percutaneous atherectomies ~ see artery, atherectomy
Percutaneous biopsy, gallbladder/bile ducts ~ see bile duct, biopsy
Percutaneous discectomies ~ see diskectomy, percutaneous
Percutaneous electric nerve stimulation ~ see application, neurostimulation
Percutaneous fixation ~ 25671
Percutaneous insertion, ventricular assist device
  arterial access ~ 33990, 33991
  venous access ~ 33991, 33995
Percutaneous lumbar diskectomy ~ see aspiration, nucleus of disk, lumbar
Percutaneous lysis ~ 62263-62264
Percutaneous nephrostomies ~ see nephrostomy, percutaneous
Percutaneous transluminal angioplasty
  artery
    aortic ~ 37246, 37247
    brachiocephalic ~ 37246, 37247
    coronary ~ 92920, 92921
    pulmonary ~ 92997, 92998
    renal ~ 37246, 37247
    visceral ~ 37246, 37247
  vein ~ 36902, 36905, 36907, 37248, 37249
Percutaneous transluminal coronary angioplasty ~ see percutaneous transluminal angioplasty
Pereyra procedure ~ 51845, 57289, 58267
Performance measures
  acute bronchitis, interventions
    antibiotics prescribed ~ 4120F-4124F
  acute otitis externa/media with effusion
    hearing test ~ 3230F
    history auricular/periauricular pain ~ 1116F
    interventions
      antimicrobial therapy ~ 4131F-4132F
      effusion antihistamines/decongestants ~ 4133F-4134F
      systemic steroids ~ 4135F-4136F
      topical therapy ~ 4130F
    physical exam, membrane motility ~ 2035F
  advance care plan ~ 1157F-1158F
  age-related eye disease study (AREDS) ~ 4177F
  anginal symptom assessment ~ 1002F
  aortic aneurysm ~ 9001F-9004F
  antiplatelet therapy ~ 4011F
  asthma
    followup, discharge plan ~ 5250F
    history
      intermittent ~ 1039F
      persistent ~ 1038F
    interventions ~ 4140F, 4144F
    pharmacologic therapy ~ 4015F
  atrial fibrillation/flutter
    diagnostic screening processes ~ 3555F
    thromboembolism risk ~ 1180F, 3550F-3552F
    warfarin therapy ~ 4300F-4301F
  back pain ~ 3330F, 3331F
  care for older adults
    advance care plan ~ 1157F-1158F
    function status assessment ~ 1170F
    medication review ~ 1111F, 1159F-1160F
  carotid stenosis ~ 9005F-9007F
  chronic kidney disease
    diagnostic screening processes
      blood pressure, diastolic ~ 3078F-3080F
      blood pressure, systolic ~ 3074F-3079F
      hemoglobin ~ 3279F-3281F

Performance measures ~ *continued*
    serum levels ~ 3278F
  interventions
    ESA therapy ~ 4171F-4172F
    patient management ~ 0513F, 0514F
  chronic obstructive pulmonary disease
    diagnostic screening processes
      functional expiratory volume ~ 3040F-3042F
      oxygen saturation ~ 3035F
      spirometry ~ 3023F, 3025F
    history
      dyspnea ~ 0535F, 1018F-1019F
      pneumococcus immunization ~ 1022F
      smokeless tobacco use ~ 1035F
      symptom assessment ~ 1015F
      tobacco use ~ 1000F
      tobacco smoker ~ 1034F
      tobacco non-use ~ 1036F
    intervention
      bronchodilator prescription ~ 4025F
      counseling ~ 4000F
      influenza immunization ~ 4035, 4037F
      oxygen therapy ~ 4030F
      pharmacologic therapy ~ 4001F
      pneumococcus immunization ~ 4040F
      pulmonary rehabilitation ~ 4033F
    test results
      chest X-ray ~ 3006F
      functional expiratory volume ~ 3040F
      oxygen saturation ~ 3035F
      spirometry ~ 3023F, 3025F
  community acquired bacterial pneumonia
    care level ~ 6005F
    examination
      hydration status ~ 2018F
      mental status ~ 2014F
      vital signs ~ 2010F
    history
      co-morbid conditions ~ 1026F
      influenza immunization ~ 1030F
      pneumococcus immunization ~ 1022F
      pneumonia assessment ~ 0012F
      smokeless tobacco use ~ 1035F
      tobacco use ~ 1000F
      tobacco smoker ~ 1034F
      tobacco non-use ~ 1036F
    intervention
      antibiotic prescription ~ 4045F
      counseling ~ 4000F
      pharmacologic therapy ~ 4001F
    test results
      oxygen saturation ~ 3028F
  composite measures
    heart failure assessment ~ 0001F
    osteoarthritis assessment ~ 0005F
  coronary artery bypass graft intervention
    mammary artery graft ~ 4110F, 4115F
  coronary artery disease
    examination, blood pressure ~ 2000F
    history
      angina and activity ~ 1002F
      smokeless tobacco use ~ 1035F
      tobacco use ~ 1000F
      tobacco smoker ~ 1034F
      tobacco non-use ~ 1036F
    interventions
      ACE/ARB ~ 4010F
      anti-hypertensive agent ~ 4145F
      aspirin or clopidrogel ~ 4086F-4087F
      antiplatelet ~ 4011F
      beta-blocker ~ 4008F
      cardiac rehab program ~ 4500F, 4510F
      counseling ~ 4000F
      pharmacologic ~ 4001F
      statin ~ 4013F
      tobacco cessation
        counseling ~ 4000F, 4004F
        pharmacologic therapy ~ 4001F, 4004F

Performance measures ~ *continued*

patient management
    anginal symptoms plan of care ~ 0557F
    lipid control plan of care ~ 0556F
test results
    left ventricular ejection fraction ~ 3021F-3022F
    lipid panel ~ 3011F
diabetes
    examination
        eye ~ 2022F, 2024F, 2026F
        foot ~ 2028F
    history
        smokeless tobacco use ~ 1035F
        tobacco smoker ~ 1034F
        tobacco non-use ~ 1036F
    intervention
        counseling ~ 4001F
        pharmacologic therapy ~ 4001F, 4004F
    physical examination
        dilated retinal exam ~ 2022F, 2023F
        foot exam ~ 2028F
        stereoscopic retinal photos ~ 2024F-2026F, 2033F
    test results
        blood results
            diastolic ~ 3078F-3080F
            systolic ~ 3077F
        hemoglobin
            A1c ~ 3044F, 3045F,
            lipid ~ 3048F-3050F
            macroalbuminuria ~ 3060F-3062F
            nephropathy treatment ~ 3066F
            retinopathy risk ~ 3072F
            urine protein ~ 3060F-3062F
diagnostic/screening processes or results
    ABO and Rh typing ~ 3293F
    alcohol use ~ 3016F
    barium swallow test ~ 3142F, 3200F
    body mass index (BMI) ~ 3008F
    breast cancer ~ 3370F-3380F
    carotid image study ~ 3100F
    cervical cancer screening ~ 3015F
    chest x-ray ~ 3006F
    colon cancer ~ 3382F-3390F
    colorectal cancer screening ~ 3017F
    corneal power ~ 3073F
    CT/MRI hemorrhage detection ~ 3110F
    CT/MRI brain ~ 3111F-3112F
    cytogenetic testing ~ 3155F
    depression ~ 1220F, 3088F-3093F
    DEXA ~ 3095F-3096F
    diastolic blood pressure ~ 3078F-3080F
    dyspnea ~ 3450F-3452F
    ECG ~ 3120F
    epilepsy
        EEG ~ 3650F
        MRI/CT scan 3324F
    erythropoietin ~ 3160F
    esophageal biopsy ~ 3150F
    flow cytometry ~ 3170F
    functional expiratory volume ~ 3040F, 3042F
    group B Streptococcus (GBS) ~ 3294F
    hemoglobin A1c ~ 3044F-3046F
    HIV ~ 3490F-3515F
    Kt/V measurement ~ 3082F-3084F
    LDL cholestorel ~ 3048F-3050F
    left ventricular ejection fraction ~ 3021F, 3022F
    left ventricular function ~ 3020F
    lipid panel ~ 3011F
    macroalbuminuria test ~ 3062F
    melanoma ~ 3321F-3322F
    microalbuminuria test 3060F-3061F
    nephropathy treatment ~ 3066F
    oxygen saturation ~ 3028F, 3035F-3037F
    pulmonary function test ~ 3038F
    retinopathy screening ~ 3072F
    rheumatoid arthritis ~ 3470F-3476F
    screening mammography ~ 3014F
    spirometry ~ 3023F-3027F
    Strep A testing ~ 3210F
    suicide risk ~ 3085F

Performance measures ~ *continued*

    systolic blood pressure ~ 3074F, 3075F-3077F
    TB ~ 3455F
    thromboembolism ~ 3550F-3552F
    tumor node and metastases staging (TNM) ~3323F
    upper GI endoscopy ~ 3130F, 3132F, 3140F-3142F
    urine protein ~ 3060F-3062F
end-stage renal disease
    dialysis plan of care ~ 0505F, 0507F
    intervention, AV fistula ~ 4051F-4055F
    test results, Kt/V measurement ~ 3082F-3084F
epilepsy
    diagnostic screening
        electroencephalogram (EEG) ~ 3650F
        MRI/CT scan ~ 3324F
    follow-up or other outcomes
        surgical therapy considered ~ 5200F
    history
        etiology reviewed, documented ~ 1205F
        seizure type/frequency documented ~ 1200F
    interventions
        childbearing counseling ~ 4340F
        safety counseling ~ 4330F
    patient safety
        anti-epileptic drug (AED) side effects counseling ~ 6070F
follow up
    exam communicated ~ 5010F
    fracture documentation ~ 5015F
    mole examination ~ 5005F
    osteoporosis ~ 5015F
gastro-esophageal reflux disease (GERD)
    history, alarm symptoms ~ 1070F-1071F
    test results
        upper endoscopy ~ 3130F, 3132F
        biopsy for Barrett's esophagus ~ 3140F-3142F, 3150F, 3200F
        barium swallow ~ 3140F-3142F, 3150F, 3200F
geriatrics (GER)
    fall screening ~ 1100F-1101F
    history
        advance care plan ~ 1123F, 1124F
        medication reconciliation ~ 1110F-1111F
        urinary incontinence ~ 1090F-1091F
    patient management
        urinary incontinence plan ~ 0509F
heart failure
    assessment ~ 0001F
    examination ~ 2000F-2002F
    history ~ 1003F-1004F
    intervention
        ACE/ARB ~ 4010F, 4480F-4481F
        beta-blocker ~ 4008F
    test results ~ 3020F-3022F
hematology
    intervention ~ 4090F, 4095F, 4100F
    test results ~ 3155F, 3160F, 3170F
hepatitis
    intervention
        antiviral therapy ~ 4150F, 4153F
        counseling ~ 4158F, 4159F
        education, alcohol ~ 4158F
        education, contraception ~ 4159F
        hepatitis A vaccination ~ 4148F, 4155F
        hepatitis B vaccination ~ 4149F, 4157F
        peginterferon & ribavirin therapy ~ 4153F
        RNA testing ~ 4150F-4151F
    test results
        genotype testing ~ 3266F
        hepatitis A immunity ~ 3215F
        hepatitis B immunity ~ 3216F
        RNA testing ~ 3218F, 3220F, 3265F
hydration ~ 2030F-2031F
hypertension
    blood pressure measurement ~ 2000F
    intervention plan of care ~ 4050F
    test results, plan of care ~ 3074F-3075F, 3077F-3080F
major despressive disorder
    diagnostic/screening
        depression ~ 3351F-3354F
        severity classification ~ 3088F-3093F
        suicide risk ~ 3085F, 3092F

Performance measures ~ *continued*

history, diagnostic status ~ 1040F
intervention
counseling ~ 4000F
electroconvulsive therapy ~ 4066F-4067F
medication management ~ 4064F-4065F
pharmacologic ~ 4001F
psychotherapy ~ 4060F-4062F
patient management, follow-up care documented ~ 0545F
severity classification ~ 3088F-3093F
suicide risk assessment ~ 3085F
melanoma
diagnostic/screening processes
cancer stage ~ 3321F-3322F
imaging studies ~ 3319F, 3320F
history, moles ~ 1050F
outcomes, counseling ~ 5005F
skin exam ~ 2029F
osteoarthritis
assessment ~ 0005F
examination, involved joint ~ 2004F
history
anti-inflammatory risk ~ 1008F
assessment ~ 1006F
medication use ~ 1007F
intervention
anti-inflammatory/analgesic ~ 4016F
GI prophylaxis ~ 4017F
therapeutic exercise ~ 4018F
osteoporosis
care coordination ~ 5015F
counseling ~ 4019F
fracture management/screening ~ 3095F-3096F
pharmacologic intervention ~ 4005F
Parkinson's disease
diagnosis/screening
cognitive impairment assessed ~ 3720F
psychiatric disorders assessed ~ 3700F
interventions
autonomic dysfunction symptoms ~ 4326F
medication-related complications ~ 4324F
rehabilitation options discussed with patient ~ 4400F
sleep disturbances ~ 4328F
treatment options reviewed ~ 4325F
patient history
diagnosis reviewed ~ 1400F
patient safety
falls incidence ~ 6080F
stage-specific safety counseling ~ 6090F
patient history
activity level assessment ~ 1003F
advance care plan ~ 1123F, 1124F
anti-inflammatory or analgesic ~ 1007F
atrial fibrillation ~ 1060F-1061F
asthma assessment ~ 1005F
COPD assessment ~ 1015F
co-morbid conditions assessment ~ 1026F
community-acquired bacterial pneumonia assessment ~ 0012F
current smokeless tobacco user ~ 1035F
current tobacco non-user ~ 1036F
dyspnea assessment ~ 1018F-1019F
fall history ~ 1100F-1101F
facility discharge ~ 1110F
functional status assessed ~ 1170F
gastroesophageal reflux ~ 1070F-1071F
influenza immunization status ~ 1030F
intermittent asthma ~ 1039F
major depresive disorder ~ 1040F
medication reconsiliation ~ 1111F
moles ~ 1050F
non-steroidal anti-inflammatory drug (NSAID) ~ 1008F
osteoarthritis ~ 1006F
persistent asthma ~ 1038F
pneumococcus immunization assessment ~ 1022F
risk of death ~ 1150F-1151F
seizure type/frequency documented ~ 1200F
stroke symptom ~ 1065F-1066F
urinary incontinence ~ 1090F-1091F
visual function ~ 1055F

Performance measures ~ *continued*

patient management
colonoscopy follow-up ~ 0528F-0529F
dyspnea management plan ~ 0535F
glucorticoid management plan ~ 0540F
HIV RNA control plan ~ 0575F
major depressive disorder plan of follow-up care ~ 0545F
postpartum care visit ~ 0503F
prenatal care visit, initial ~ 0500F
prenatal care visit, subsequent ~ 0502F
prenatal flow sheet ~ 0501F
urinary incontinence plan of care ~ 0509F
patient safety
anti-epileptic drug counseling ~ 6070F
dysphagea screening ~ 6010F
falls incidence queried with patient ~ 6080F
level of care rationale ~ 6005F
Parkinson's disease stage-specific safety counseling ~ 6090F
pediatric
acute gastroenteritis
examination
hydration status ~ 2030F-2031F
oral rehydration ~ 2030F-2031F
weight measurement ~ 2001F
intervention
education ~ 4058F
oral rehydration ~ 4056F
pharyngitis
intervention, testing ~ 4120F, 4124F
test results, appropriate testing ~ 3210F
perioperative care, intervention
discontinuation, prophylactics ~ 4042F-4043F, 4046F, 4049F
selection, prophylactics ~ 4041F
timing, prophylactics ~ 4047F-4048F
venous thromboembolism ~ 4044F
physical examination
dilated retinal eye exam ~ 2022F
eye imaging ~ 2026F
field stereoscopic photos ~ 2024F
foot ~ 2028F
fundus ~ 2020F-2021F
hydration status ~ 2018F, 2030F-2031F
macular ~ 2019F, 2021F
major depressive disorder clinical interview ~ 2060F
mental status ~ 2014F, 2044F
optic nerve ~ 2027F
osteoarthritis assessment ~ 2004F
skin ~ 2029F
vital signs ~ 2010F
volume overload assessment ~ 2002F
weight ~ 2001F
prenatal-postpartum care
diagnosis/screening
ABO and Rh typing ~ 3293F
D Rh typing ~ 3290F-3291F
HIV status ~ 3292F
patient management ~ 0500F-0503F
preventive care & screening
history
tobacco use ~ 1000F, 1034F-1036F
intervention
pharmacologic therapy ~ 4001F
influenza immunization ~ 4037F
tobacco use counseling ~ 4000F, 4004F
test results
screening mammography ~ 3014F
colorectal screening ~ 3017F
statin therapy ~ 4013F
stroke and stroke rehabilitation
history
anticoagulant therapy ~ 1060F-1061F
tissue plasminogen ~ 1065F-1066F
intervention
anticoagulant therapy ~ 4075F
antiplatelet therapy ~ 4073F
rehabilitation services ~ 4079F
thrombosis prophylaxis ~ 4070F
tissue plasminogen ~ 4077F

Performance measures ~ *continued*
  test results
    carotid imaging ~ 3100F
    lesion screening ~ 3110F-3112F
  patient safety
    dysphagia screening ~ 6010F
    swallowing eligibility ~ 6015F
    NPO order ~ 6020F
  therapeutic, preventive or other interventions
    anesthesia ~ 4255F-4256F
    anti-inflammatory/analgesic ~ 4016F
    antibiotic agent ~ 4045F, 4048F, 4049F, 4120F, 4124F
    anticoagulant therapy ~ 4075F
    antiplatelet therapy ~ 4073F
    arterio-venous fistula ~ 4051F
    aspirin ~ 4084F
    asthma medication ~ 4015F
    beta blocker ~ 4115F
    bisphosphonate therapy ~ 4100F
    dialysis ~ 4052F-4055F
    electroconvulsive therapy ~ 4066F-4067F
    erythropoietin therapy ~ 4090F-4095F
    gastroenteritis education ~ 4058F
    gastrointestinal prophylaxis for NSAID use ~ 4017F
    heart failure education ~ 4003F
    hepatitis vaccination ~ 4148F-4149F, 4275F
    hypertension care plan ~ 4050F
    influenza immunization ~ 4035F-4037F
    inhaled bronchodilator ~ 4025F
    internal mammary artery graft ~ 4110F
    oxygen therapy, long term ~ 4030F
    pharmacologic therapy ~ 4005F, 4063F-4065F
    pneumococcal immunization ~ 4040F
    psychotherapy services ~ 4060F, 4062F
    pulmonary rehabilitation ~ 4033F
    rehabilitation services ~ 4089F
    rehydration solution ~ 4056F
    statin therapy ~ 4013F
    therapeutic exercise ~ 4018F
    thrombosis prophylaxis ~ 4070F
    tissue plasminogen administration ~ 4077F
    warfarin therapy ~ 4012F
  tobacco use
    assessment ~ 1000F
    counseling ~ 4000F
    pharmacologic therapy ~ 4001
  vital signs, documented and reviewed ~ 2010F
Performance test ~ see physical medicine/therapy/occupational therapy
  performance test, physical therapy ~ 97750
  psychological test ~ 96100
Perfusion
  imaging
    brain
      CT Scan ~ 0042T
      PET Scan ~ 78609
    myocardial ~ 78451-78454
      PET Scan ~ 78430-78433, 78491, 78492
    pulmonary ~ 78580, 78582, 78597, 78598
  for esophageal motility study ~ 91013
  test, esophageal acid 91030
  therapeutic
    hemoperfusion, dialysis ~ 90997
    vestibuloactive drugs ~ 69801
Perfusion, intracranial arterial thrombolysis ~ 61624
Perfusion pump ~ see infusion pump
Pericardectomies ~ see excision, pericardium
Pericardial cyst ~ see cyst, pericardial
Pericardial sac drainage ~ 32659
Pericardial window for drainage ~ 33025
Pericardial window technic ~ see pericardiostomy
Pericardiectomy
  complete ~ 33030-33031
  subtotal ~ 33030-33031
Pericardiocentesis ~ 33016
Pericardiotomy
  removal
    clot ~ 33020
    foreign body ~ 33020

Pericardium
  biopsy, endoscopic ~ 32604
  cyst, excision/resection ~ 32661, 33050
  diagnostic thoracoscopy ~ 32601
  drainage
    insertion of indwelling catheter ~ 33017-33019
    window or partial resection ~ 32659, 33025
  excision ~ 32659, 33025, 33030-33031
  incision
    removal
      clot ~ 33020
      foreign body ~ 33020
  incision and drainage ~ 33025
  puncture aspiration ~ 33016
  removal
    clot, endoscopic ~ 32658
    foreign body, endoscopic ~ 32658
  tumor, excision ~ 32661, 33050
Peridural anesthesia
  infusion ~ 62324-62327
  injection ~ 62320-62323
Peridural injection ~ see epidural, injection
Perineal prostatectomy ~ see prostatectomy, perineal
Perineoplasty ~ 56810
Perineorrhaphy
  repair, rectocele ~ 57250
Perineum
  abscess, incision and drainage ~ 56405
  colposcopy ~ 99170
  debridement, infected ~ 11004, 11006
  removal, prosthesis ~ 53442
  repair ~ 56810
  X-ray with contrast ~ 74775
Perionychia ~ see paronychia
Periorbital region
  reconstruction, osteotomy with graft ~ 21267-21268
  repair, osteotomy ~ 21260-21263
Peripheral artery disease (PAD) rehabilitation ~ 93668
Peripheral nerve repair/suture, major ~ 64856, 64859
Periprosthetic capsulectomy breast ~ 19371
Peristaltic pumps ~ see infusion pump
Peritoneal dialysis ~ 90945-90947, 4055F
  Kt/V level ~ 3082F-3084F
Peritoneal free air ~ see pneumoperitoneum
Peritoneal lavage ~ 49084
Peritoneoscopy ~ see endoscopy, peritoneum
Peritoneum
  abscess, incision and drainage ~ 49020
  endoscopy
    drainage, lymphocele ~ 49323
  exchange, drainage catheter ~ 49423
  injection, contrast, via catheter ~ 49424
  ligation, shunt ~ 49428
  removal
    cannula/catheter ~ 49422
    foreign body ~ 49402
    shunt ~ 49429
  tumor, resection ~ 58950-58956
  unlisted services and procedures ~ 49999
  venous shunt, injection ~ 49427
  X-ray ~ 74190
Persistent, omphalomesenteric duct ~ see diverticulum, Meckel's
Persistent truncus arteriosus ~ see truncus arteriosus
Personal care ~ see self care
Pessary insertion ~ 57160
Pesticides chlorinated hydrocarbons ~ 82441
PET ~ see positron emission tomography
Petrous temporal excision, Apex ~ 69530
Peyronie disease
  with graft ~ 54110-54112
  injection ~ 54200
  surgical exposure ~ 54205
pH ~ *see also* blood
  exhaled breath ~ 83987
  other fluid ~ 83986
  urine ~ 83986
Phacoemulsification
  removal
    extracapsular cataract ~ 66982, 66984
    secondary membranous cataract ~ 66850

Phagocytosis, white blood cells ~ 86344
Phalangectomy
  toe ~ 28150
    partial ~ 28160
Phalanges (hand)) ~ see finger, bone
Phalanx, finger
  craterization ~ 26235-26236
  cyst, excision ~ 26210-26215
  diaphysectomy ~ 26235-26236
  excision ~ 26235-26236
    radical, for tumor ~ 26260-26262
  fracture
    articular
      closed treatment ~ 26740
      with manipulation ~ 26742
      open treatment ~ 26746
    distal ~ 26755-26756
      closed treatment ~ 26750
      open treatment ~ 26765
      percutaneous fixation ~ 26756
    open treatment ~ 26735
      distal ~ 26765
    shaft ~ 26720-26727
      open treatment ~ 26735
  incision and drainage ~ 26034
  ostectomy, radical, for tumor ~ 26260-26262
  repair
    lengthening ~ 26568
    nonunion ~ 26546
    osteotomy ~ 26567
  saucerization ~ 26235-26236
  thumb fracture, shaft ~ 26720-26727
  tumor, excision ~ 26210-26215
Phalanx, great toe ~ see also phalanx, toe
  fracture ~ 28490
    with manipulation ~ 28495-28496
    open treatment ~ 28505
    without manipulation ~ 28490
    percutaneous fixation ~ 28496
Phalanx, toe
  condyle, excision ~ 28126
  craterization ~ 28124
  cyst, excision ~ 28108
  diaphysectomy ~ 28124
  excision ~ 28124, 28150-28160
  fracture
    with manipulation ~ 28515
    without manipulation ~ 28510
    open treatment ~ 28525
  repair, osteotomy ~ 28310-28312
  saucerization ~ 28124
  tumor, excision ~ 28108, 28175
Pharmaceutic preparations ~ see drug
Pharmacotherapies ~ see chemotherapy
Pharyngeal tonsil ~ see adenoids
Pharyngectomy partial ~ 42890
Pharyngolaryngectomy ~ 31390-31395
Pharyngoplasty ~ 42950
Pharyngorrhaphy ~ see suture, pharynx
Pharyngostomy ~ 42955
Pharyngotomy ~ see incision, pharynx
Pharyngotympanic tube ~ see eustachian tube
Pharynx ~ see also nasopharynx; throat
  biopsy ~ 42800-42806
  cineradiography ~ 70371, 74230
  creation, stoma ~ 42955
  excision ~ 42145
    with larynx ~ 31390-31395
    partial ~ 42890
    resection ~ 42892-42894
  hemorrhage ~ 42960-42962
  lesion
    destruction ~ 42808
    excision ~ 42808
  reconstruction ~ 42950
  removal, foreign body ~ 42809
  repair, with esophagus ~ 42953
  unlisted services and procedures ~ 42999
  video study ~ 70371, 74230
  X-ray ~ 70370, 74210

Phencyclidine ~ 80305-80307, 83992
Phenobarbital ~ 80345
  assay ~ 80184
Phenothiazine ~ 80342-80344
Phenotype
Phenotype Analysis
  Alpha-1-antitrypsin ~ 82104
  by Genotypic Bioinformatics ~ 87900
  by Nucleic Acid ~ 87901-87904, 87906
    Infectious Agent
      HIV-1 Drug Resistance ~ 87903, 87904, 87906
Phenotype Prediction
  by Genetic Database
    HIV-1 Drug Susceptibility ~ 87900
Phenylalanine ~ 84030
Phenylalanine-tyrosine ratio ~ 84030
Phenylketones ~ 84035
Phenylketonuria ~ see phenylalanine
Phenytoin assay ~ 80185-80186
Pheochromocytoma ~ 80424
Pheresis ~ see apheresis
Phlebectasia ~ see varicose vein
Phlebectomy varicose veins ~ 37765-37766
Phlebographies ~ see venography
Phleborrhaphy ~ see suture, vein
Phlebotomy therapeutic ~ 99195
Phoria ~ see strabismus
Phosphatase
  alkaline ~ 84075, 84080
  blood ~ 84078
Phosphatase acid ~ 84060
  blood ~ 84066
Phosphate, pyridoxal ~ see pyridoxal phosphate
Phosphatidylcholine cholinephosphohydrolase ~ see tissue typing
Phosphatidylglycerol ~ 84081
Phosphatidyl glycerol ~ see phosphatidylglycerol
Phosphocreatine phosphotransferase, ADP ~ see CPK
Phosphogluconate-6 dehydrogenase ~ 84085
Phosphoglycerides, glycerol ~ see phosphatidylglycerol
Phosphohexose isomerase ~ 84087
Phosphohydrolases ~ see phosphatase
Phosphokinase, creatine ~ see CPK
Phospholipase C ~ see tissue typing
Phospholipid antibody ~ 86147
Phosphomonoesterase ~ see phosphatase
Phosphoric monoester hydrolases ~ see phosphatase
Phosphorus ~ 84100
  urine ~ 84105
Phosphotransferase, ADP phosphocreatine ~ see CPK
Photo patch allergy test ~ see allergy tests ~ 95052
Photochemotherapies, extracorporeal ~ see photopheresis
Photochemotherapy ~ see dermatology ~ 96910-96913
  endoscopic light ~ 96570-96571
Photocoagulation
  endolaser panretinal, vitrectomy ~ 67040
  focal endolaser, vitrectomy ~ 67040
  iridoplasty ~ 66762
  lesion
    cornea ~ 65450
    retina ~ 67210, 67227-67228
  retinal detachment
    prophylaxis ~ 67145
    repair ~ 67105
Photodynamic therapy
  for lesion ~ 67221, 67225, 96567, 96573, 96574
  for tissue ablation ~ 96570, 96571
Photography skin, diagnostic ~ 96904
Photography, ocular ~ see ophthalmoscopy, diagnostic
Photopheresis extracorporeal ~ 36522
Photophoresis ~ see actinotherapy; photochemotherapy
Photoradiation therapies ~ see actinotherapy
Photoscreen ocular ~ 99174
Photosensitivity testing ~ see allergy tests ~ 95056
Phototherapies ~ see actinotherapy
Phototherapy, ultraviolet ~ see actinotherapy
Phrenic nerve
  anastomosis ~ 61711
  avulsion ~ 64746
  incision ~ 64746

Phrenic nerve ~ continued
  neurostimulator system for sleep apnea
    device evaluation ~ 0434T-0436T
    insertion ~ 0424T-0427T
    removal ~ 0428T-0430T
    replacement ~ 0424T-0427T, 0431T
    repositioning ~ 0432T-0433T
  transection ~ 64746
Physical medicine/therapy/occupational therapy
  activities of daily living ~ 97535, 99509
  aquatic therapy, with exercises ~ 97113
  athletic training
    evaluation ~ 97169-97171
    re-evaluation ~ 97172
    orthotic/prosthetic ~ 97763
  cognitive skills development ~ 97129, 97130
  community/work reintegration ~ 97537
  evaluation
    athletic training ~ 97169-97171
      re-evaluation ~ 97172
    occupational therapy ~ 97165-97167
      re-evaluation ~ 97168
    physical therapy ~ 97161-97163
      re-evaluation ~ 97164
  kinetic therapy ~ 97530
  manual therapy ~ 97140
  modalities
    contrast baths ~ 97034
    diathermy treatment ~ 97024
    electric simulation
      unattended ~ 97014
      attended, manual ~ 97032
    hot or cold pack ~ 97010
    hydrotherapy (Hubbard tank) ~ 97036
    infrared light treatment ~ 97026
    iontophoresis ~ 97033
    microwave therapy ~ 97024
    paraffin bath ~ 97018
    traction ~ 97012
    ultrasound ~ 97035
    ultraviolet light ~ 97028
    unlisted services and procedures ~ 97039
    vasopneumatic device ~ 97016
    whirlpool therapy ~ 97022
  orthotics training ~ 97760, 97763
  osteopathic manipulation ~ 98925-98929
  procedures
    aquatic therapy ~ 97113
    gait training ~ 97116
    group therapeutic ~ 97150
    massage therapy ~ 97124
    neuromuscular reeducation ~ 97112
    physical performance test ~ 97750
    therapeutic exercises ~ 97110
    traction therapy ~ 97140
    work hardening ~ 97545-97546
  prosthetic training ~ 97761
  sensory integration ~ 97533
  therapeutic activities ~ 97530
  unlisted services and procedures ~ 97139, 97799
  wheelchair management/propulsion ~ 97542
  work reintegration ~ 97537
Physical therapy
  evaluation ~ 97161-97163
  re-evaluation ~ 97164
Physician services
  care management
    behavioral health conditions ~ 99484
    psychiatric collaborative care ~ 99492-99494
  care planning
    cognitive impairment ~ 99483
  care plan oversight services
    domiciliary facility ~ 99339, 99340
    home health agency care ~ 99374, 99375
    home or rest home care ~ 99339, 99340
    hospice ~ 99377, 99378
    nursing facility ~ 99379, 99380
  case management services ~ 99366-99368
  consultation, interprofessional telephone/ internet discussion ~
    99446-99449

Physician services ~ continued
  direction, advanced life support ~ 99288
  online ~ 99421-99423
  prolonged
    with direct patient contact
      inpatient ~ 99356, 99357
      outpatient/office ~ 99354, 99355, 99417
    without direct patient contact ~ 99358, 99359
  standby ~ 99360
  supervision, care plan oversight services ~ 99339, 99340, 99374-99380
  team conference ~ 99367
  telephone ~ 99441-99443
Piercing of ear lobe ~ 69090
Piles ~ see hemorrhoids
Pilonidal cyst
  excision ~ 11770-11772
  incision and drainage ~ 10080-10081
Pin ~ see also wire
  insertion/removal, skeletal traction ~ 20650
  prophylactic treatment
    femur ~ 27187
    humerus ~ 24498
    shoulder ~ 23490-23491
Pinch graft ~ 15050
Pinna ~ see ear, external
Pinworms examination ~ 87172
Pirogoff procedure ~ 27888
Pituitary epidermoid tumor ~ see craniopharyngioma
Pituitary gland
  excision ~ 61546-61548
  tumor, excision ~ 61546-61548, 62165
Pituitary growth hormone ~ see growth hormone
Pituitary lactogenic hormone ~ see prolactin
Pituitectomy ~ see excision, pituitary gland
PKU ~ see phenylalanine
Placement
  adjustable gastric restrictive device ~ 43770
  artificial chordae tendineae ~ 0543T
  balloon continence device ~ 0548T, 0549T
  biodegradable material, peri-prostatic ~ 55874
  catheter
    breast, for interstitial radioelement application ~ 19296-19298
    bronchus, for intracavitary radioelement application (see also
      catheterization) ~ 31643
    kidney
      nephrostomy ~ 50432
      Nephroureteral ~ 50433
    prostate ~ 55875
    renal artery
      selective ~ 36251, 36252
      superselective ~ 36253, 36254
    reter via kidney ~ 50695
  catheter, cardiac (see also catheterization, cardiac) ~ 93503
  dosimeter, prostate ~ 55876
  drainage, pancreas ~ 48001
  drug-eluting ocular insert, eyelid ~ 0444T, 0445T
  duodenostomy tube ~ 49441
  endovascular prosthesis
    aorta ~ 33883-33886, 34709-34711
    iliac artery ~ 34709-34711
  enterostomy tube ~ 44300
  esophageal sphincter augmentation device ~ 43284
  guidance
    catheter
      abscess ~ 75989
      specimen ~ 75989
    prosthesis
      thoracic aorta ~ 75958-75959
  interstitial device
    abdomen ~ 49411-49412
    lungs ~ 32553
    omentum ~ 49411-49412
    pelvis ~ 49411-49412
    pleura ~ 32553
    peritoneum ~ 49411-49412
    prostate ~ 55876
    retroperitoneum ~ 49411-49412
  intravascular stent
    coronary ~ 92980-92981
    intracranial ~ 61635

Polyp
- antrochoanal, removal ~ 31032
- esophagus, ablation ~ 43229
- nose, excision
  - endoscopic ~ 31237-31240
  - extensive ~ 30115
  - simple ~ 30110
- sphenoid sinus, removal ~ 31051
- urethra, excision ~ 53260

Polypectomy
- nose, endoscopic ~ 31237
- uterus ~ 58558

Polypeptide, vasoactive intestinal ~ see vasoactive intestinal peptide
Polysomnography ~ 95808-95811
Polyuria test ~ see water load test
Pomeroy's operation ~ (tubal ligation) 58600
Pooling blood products ~ 86965
Popliteal arteries ~ see artery, popliteal
Popliteal synovial cyst ~ see Baker's cyst
Poradenitistras ~ see lymphogranuloma venereum
PORP (partial ossicular replacement prosthesis) ~ 69633, 69637
Porphobilinogen urine ~ 84106-84110
Porphyrin precursors ~ 82135

Porphyrins
- feces ~ 84126
- urine ~ 84119-84120

Portal vein ~ see vein, hepatic portal
Porter-Silber test ~ see corticosteroid, blood
Portoenterostomies, hepatic ~ see hepaticoenterostomy
Port film ~ 77417
Portoenterostomy ~ 47701
Posadas-Wernicke disease ~ see coccidioidomycosis
Positional nystagmus test ~ see nystagmus tests, positional
Positive-pressure breathing, inspiratory ~ see intermittent positive
  - pressure breathing (IPPB)
Positive end expiratory pressure ~ see pressure breathing, positive

Positron emission tomography (PET)
- brain ~ 78608, 78609
- chest ~ 78811
- head/neck ~ 78811
- heart ~ 78429-78434, 78459, 78491, 78492
- myocardial imaging
  - blood flow absolute quantitation ~ 78434
  - metabolic evaluation study ~ 78429, 78432, 78433, 78459
  - perfusion study ~ 78430-78433, 78491, 78492
- skull base to mid-thigh ~ 78812
- whole body ~ 78813
- with computed tomography (CT) ~ 78814, 78815

Post-op visit ~ 99024
Postauricular fistula ~ see fistula, postauricular
Postcaval ureter ~ see retrocaval ureter
Postmortem ~ see autopsy
Postoperative wound infection incision and drainage ~ 10180
Postop vas reconstruction ~ see vasovasorrhaphy

Postpartum care
- cesarean delivery ~ 59515
  - after attempted vaginal delivery ~ 59622
  - previous ~ 59610, 59614-59618, 59622
- vaginal delivery ~ 59430
  - after previous cesarean delivery ~ 59614

Potassium ~ 84132
- urine ~ 84133

Potential, auditory evoked ~ see auditory evoked potentials
Potential, evoked ~ see evoked potential
Potts-Smith procedure ~ 33762
Pouch, Kock ~ see Kock pouch
PPP ~ see fibrin degradation products
PRA ~ see cytotoxic screen
Prealbumin ~ 84134
Prebeta lipoproteins ~ see lipoprotein, blood
Pregl's test ~ (cystourethroscopy, catheterization, urethral) 52005

Pregnancy
- abortion
  - induced ~ 59855-59857
    - by amniocentesis injection ~ 59850-59852
    - by dilation and curettage ~ 59840
    - by dilation and evaluation ~ 59841
  - septic ~ 59830

Pregnancy ~ continued
- therapeutic
  - by dilation and curettage ~ 59851
  - by hysterectomy ~ 59852
  - by saline ~ 59850
- cesarean delivery ~ 59618-59622
  - with hysterectomy ~ 59525
  - only ~ 59514
  - postpartum care ~ 59514-59515
  - routine care ~ 59510
  - vaginal birth after ~ 59610-59614
- ectopic
  - abdominal ~ 59130
  - cervix ~ 59140
  - interstitial
    - partial resection uterus ~ 59136
    - total hysterectomy ~ 59135
  - laparoscopy
    - with salpingectomy and/or oophorectomy ~ 59151
    - without salpingectomy and/or oophorectomy ~ 59150
  - tubal ~ 59121
    - with salpingectomy and/or oophorectomy ~ 59120
- miscarriage
  - surgical completion
    - any trimester ~ 59812
    - first trimester ~ 59820
    - second trimester ~ 59821
  - molar ~ see also hydatidiform mole
- multifetal reduction ~ 59866
- placenta delivery ~ 59414
- test ~ 84702-84703
  - urinalysis ~ 81025
- vaginal delivery ~ 59409-59410
  - antepartum care ~ 59425-59426
  - after cesarean delivery ~ 59610-59614
  - postpartum care ~ 59430
  - total obstetrical care ~ 59400, 59610, 59618

Pregnanediol ~ 84135
Pregnanetriol ~ 84138
Pregnenolone ~ 84140
Prekallikrein ~ see Fletcher factor
Prekallikrein factor ~ 85292
Premature, closure, cranial suture ~ see craniosynostosis
Prenatal procedure ~ 59897
- amnioinfusion, transabdominal ~ 59070
- drainage, fluid ~ 59074
- occlusion, umbilical cord ~ 59072
- stunt ~ 59076

Prenatal testing
- amniocentesis ~ 59000
  - with amniotic fluid reduction ~ 59001
- chorionic villus sampling ~ 59015
- cordocentesis ~ 59012
- fetal blood sample ~ 59030
- fetal monitoring ~ 59050
  - interpretation only ~ 59051
- magnetic resonance imaging (MRI) ~ 74712, 74713
- non-stress test, fetal ~ 59025, 99500
- oxytocin stress test ~ 59020
- stress test, oxytocin ~ 59020
- ultrasound ~ 76801-76817
  - fetal biophysical profile ~ 76818-76819
  - fetal heart ~ 76825

Prentiss operation ~ see orchiopexy, inguinal approach
Preparation
- for transfer, embryo ~ 89255
- thawing
  - embryo, cryopreserved ~ 89352
  - oocytes, cryopreserved ~ 89356
  - reproductive tissue, cryopreserved ~ 89354
  - sperm, cryopreserved ~ 89353

Presacral sympathectomy ~ see sympathectomy, presacral
Prescription
- contact lens (see also contact lens services) ~ 92310-92317
- ocular prosthesis (see also prosthesis, ocular) ~ 92330-92335

Pressure, blood ~ see blood pressure
Pressure, venous ~ see blood pressure, venous
Pressure breathing ~ (see also pulmonology, therapeutic)
- negative, continuous (CNP) ~ 94662
- positive, continuous (CPAP) ~ 94660

Pressure measurement of sphincter of Oddi ~ see sphincter of Oddi, pressure measurement
Pressure ulcer (decubitus) ~ see debridement; skin graft and flap
Pressure ulcers excision ~ 15920-15999
Pretreatment
  red blood cell
    antibody identification ~ 86970-86972
  serum
    antibody identification ~ 86975-86978
Prevention & control ~ see prophylaxis
Preventive medicine
  behavior change intervention
    group
      diabetes prevention ~ 0403T
      risk factor reduction ~ 99411, 99412
    individual
      diabetes prevention ~ 0488T
      substance abuse other than tobacco ~ 99408, 99409
      tobacco use cessation ~ 99406, 99407
  comprehensive
    established patient ~ 99382-99397
    new patient ~ 99381-99387
  counseling
    behavior change, individual ~ 99406-99408
    exercise ~ 4019F
    group ~ 99411, 99412
    self exam for moles ~ 5005F
  fluoride varnish application ~ 99188
  health risk assessment ~ 96160, 96161
  health and well-being coaching ~ 0591T-0593T
  newborn care ~ 99461
  self-exam for moles ~ 5005F
  unlisted services and procedures ~ 99429
Priapism
  repair
    fistulization ~ 54435
    with shunt ~ 54420-54430
Primidone assay ~ 80188
PRL ~ see prolactin
Pro-insulin C peptide ~ see C-peptide
Proalbumin ~ see prealbumin
Probes, DNA ~ see nucleic acid probe
Probes, nucleic acid ~ see nucleic acid probe
Procainamide assay ~ 80190-80192
Procalcitonin (PCT) ~ 84145
Procedure, Fontan ~ see repair, heart, anomaly
Procedure, maxillofacial ~ see maxillofacial procedures
Process, odontoid ~ see odontoid process
Procidentia
  rectum
    excision ~ 45130-45135
    repair ~ 45900
Procoagulant activity, glomerular ~ see thromboplastin
Proconvertin ~ 85230
Proctectasis ~ see dilation, rectum
Proctectomy
  partial ~ 45111, 45113-45116, 45123
  total ~ 45110, 45112, 45119-45120
    with colon ~ 45121
    with colectomy ~ 44157-44158
    with ileostomy ~ 44212
Proctocele ~ see rectocele
Proctopexy ~ 45540-45541
  with sigmoid resection ~ 45550
Proctoplasty ~ 45500-45505
Proctorrhaphy ~ see rectum, suture
Proctoscopies ~ see anoscopy
Proctosigmoidoscopy
  ablation, polyp or lesion ~ 45320
  biopsy ~ 45305
  destruction, tumor ~ 45320
  dilation ~ 45303
  exploration ~ 45300
  hemorrhage control ~ 45317
  placement, stent ~ 45327
  removal
    foreign body ~ 45307
    polyp ~ 45308-45315
    tumor ~ 45315
  volvulus repair ~ 45321
Products, gene ~ see protein

Proetz therapy nose ~ 30210
Profibrinolysin ~ see plasminogen
Progenitor cell ~ see stem cell
Progesterone ~ 84144
Progesterone receptors ~ 84234
Progestin receptors ~ see progesterone receptors
Proinsulin ~ 84206
Projective test ~ 96100
Prokallikrein ~ see Fletcher factor
Prokallikrein, plasma ~ see Fletcher factor
Prokinogenase ~ see Fletcher factor
Prolactin ~ 80418, 84146
Prolapse ~ see procidentia
Prolapse, rectal ~ see procidentia, rectum
Prolastin ~ see alpha-1 antitrypsin
Prolonged services
  with direct patient contact
    inpatient ~ 99356, 99357
    outpatient/office ~ 99354, 99355, 99417
      clinical staff with physician supervision ~ 99415, 99416
  without direct patient contact ~ 99358-99359, 99417
Prophylactic treatment
  antibiotic ~ 4045F, 4047F-4049F
  antimicrobial ~ 4046F
    cefazolin or cefuroxime ~ 4041F-4043F
  femoral neck or proximal femur
    nailing, pinning or wiring ~ 27187
  femur
    nailing, pinning or wiring ~ 27495
  humerus
    pinning, wiring ~ 24498
  radius
    nailing, pinning, plating or wiring ~ 25490, 25492
  shoulder
    clavicle ~ 23490
    humerus ~ 23491
  tibia ~ 27745
  ulna
    nailing, pinning, plating or wiring ~ 25491-25492
  venous thromboembolism (VTE) ~ 4044F
Prophylaxis
  anticoagulant therapy ~ 4075F
  deep vein thrombosis (DVT) ~ 4070F
  retina detachment
    cryotherapy, diathermy ~ 67141
    photocoagulation ~ 67145
Proprietary laboratory analyses (PLAs)
  acute myeloid leukemia
    myelodysplastic syndrome ~ 0171U
    myeloproliferative neoplasms ~ 0171U
  ataxia telangiectasia mutated (ATM) mRNA sequence analysis ~ 0136U
  autoimmune disease
    deoxyribonucleic acid (DNA) antibody, high avidity ~ 0039U
    inflammatory bowel disease, gene expression profiling ~ 0203U
    systemic lupus erythematosus ~ 0062U
  cardiology
    ceramide quantification ~ 0119U
    heart transplant ~ 0055U, 0087U
  chemistry
    glycosylated acute phase proteins ~ 0024U
    tenofovir ~ 0025U
    vitamin D, 25 hydroxy D2 and D3 ~ 0038U
  chromosomal abnormalities
    cytogenomic constitutional analysis ~ 0209U
  clostridium difficile toxin(s) antigen detection ~ 0107U
  drug assay
    multiple reaction monitoring (MRM) ~ 0143U-0150U
  drug testing
    drug metabolism ~ 0029U, 0030U
    drug test, presumptive ~ 0007U
    interactions ~ 0082U
    opioid-use disorder ~ 0078U
    prescription drug monitoring ~ 0011U, 0051U, 0054U, 0093U, 0110U
    prescription drug-to-drug interactions ~ 0116U
  fetal aneuploidy ~ 0168U
  gastroenterology
    barrett's esophagus ~ 0108U, 0114U
    gastric emptying rate ~ 0106U
    irritable bowel syndrome (IBS)
      anti-CdtB and anti-vinculin antibodies ~ 0164U

Proprietary laboratory analyses (PLAs) ~ *continued*

    cytolethal distending toxin B (CdtB and vinculin IgG antibodies ~ 0176U

  gene analysis

    APC (APC regulator of WNT signaling pathway) ~ 0157U

    MLH1 (mutL homolog 1) ~ 0158U

    MSH2 (mutS homolog 2) ~ 0159U

    MSH6 (mutS homolog 6) ~ 0160U

    NUDT15 (nudix hydrolase 15) and TPMT (thiopurine S-methyltransferase) ~ 0169U

    PMS2 (PMS1 homolog 2, mismatch repair system component) ~ 0161U

  genome rapid sequence analysis ~ 0094U

  genomic copy number sequence analysis ~ 0156U

  germline disorders

    COMT (catechol-O-methyltransferase) ~ 0032U

    CYP1A2 (cytochrome P450 family 1, subfamily A, member 2) ~ 0031U

    CYP2D6 (cytochrome P450, family 2, subfamily D, polypeptide 6) ~ 0070U-0076U

    exome (somatic mutations) ~ 0036U

    FLT3 (fms-related tyrosine kinase 3) ~ 0046U

    gene rearrangement detection ~ 0012U

    HTR2A (5-hydroxytryptamine receptor 2A) ~ 0033U

    JAK2 (janus kinase 2) ~ 0027U

    NPM1 (nucleophosmin) ~ 0049U

    TPMT (thiopurine S-methyltransferase) ~ 0034U

  gonadotropin, chorionic (hCG) ~ 0167U

  hematology

    ctHb1, ctHb2, ctHbO2, ctHbR, StO2 ~ 0061U

    hematolymphoid neoplasia ~ 0014U

    RBC antigen typing ~ 0001U, 0084U

    RBC mechanical fragility profiling ~ 0123U

    red cell antigen genotyping ~ 0180U-0201U, 0221U, 0222U

  infectious agent

    human immunodeficiency virus antiviral drug susceptibility prediction ~ 0219U

  infectious disease

    agent detection and identification ~ 0112U

    aspergillus species detection ~ 0109U

    bacteria and fungi identification ~ 0141U, 0142U

    bacterial, strain typing ~ 0010U

    borrelia burgdorferi, antibody detection ~ 0041U-0044U

    fungal pathogen identification ~ 0140U

    gastrointestinal pathogen ~ 0097U

    human papillomavirus (HPV) ~ 0096U

    microbial organism detection ~ 0152U

    organism identification ~ 0086U

    respiratory pathogen ~ 0098U-0100U, 0115U

    respiratory tract infection ~ 0151U

      pathogen detection including SARS-CoV-2 ~ 0202U

    syphilis, non-treponemal antibody ~ 0065U, 0210U

    treponema pallidum antibody ~ 0064U

  inflammation

    eosinophilic esophagitis ~ 0095U

  lipoprotein ~ 0052U

  liver disease ~ 0166U

  microbiology

    candida species panel ~ 0068U

    helicobacter pylori detection ~ 0008U

    specimen identity dna analysis ~ 0079U

  nephrology

    chronic kidney disease rapid kidney function decline (RKFD) probability ~ 0105U

  neurology

    alzheimer disease

      cell aggregation ~ 0206U

      quantitative imaging of phosphorylated ERK1 and ERK2 ~ 0207U

    autism ~ 0063U

    autism spectrum disorder (ASD) ~ 0139U, 0170U

    inherited ataxias

      identification/categorization of genetic variants ~ 0216U, 0217U

    muscular dystrophy DMD gene sequence analysis ~ 0218U

    prion disease ~ 0035U

  oncology

    acute myelogenous leukemia ~ 0023U, 0050U, 0056U

    B-cell lymphoma classification by mRNA gene expression profiling ~ 0120U

    BRCA1 and BRCA2

      homologous recombination deficiency pathways ~ 0172U

Proprietary laboratory analyses (PLAs) ~ *continued*

    mRNA sequence analysis ~ 0138U

    somatic mutation analysis ~ 0172U

  breast cancer

    breast ductal carcinoma in situ profiling ~ 0045U

    ERBB2 analysis ~ 0009U

    hereditary disorders ~ 0102U, 0129U, 0131U

    histologic and immunohistochemical features assessment ~ 0220U

    immunohistochemistry ~ 0067U

    PIK3CA gene mutation status ~ 0155U, 0177U

    triple negative subtype identification ~ 0153U

  colon cancer

    hereditary disorders ~ 0130U

    KRAS and NRAS gene analysis ~ 0111U

  colorectal cancer ~ 0002U, 0069U, 0091U

    CRC/advanced adenoma likelihood ~ 0163U

  gynecological cancer

    hereditary gene analysis ~ 0135U

  hematolymphoid neoplasia ~ 0016U

  hematolymphoidneoplasia ~ 0017U

  hereditary gene analysis

    colon cancer (lynch syndrome) ~ 0162U

    gynecological cancer ~ 0135U

    ovarian cancer ~ 0103U

    pan cancer ~ 0134U

  immunoglobulin paraprotein (M-protein) ~ 0077U

  leukemia BCR/ABL1 analysis ~ 0040U

  lung cancer

    malignancy probability ~ 0080U, 0092U

    non-small cell lung neoplasia treatment ~ 0022U

  medullary thyroid carcinoma gene expression analysis ~ 0208U

  merkel cell carcinoma ~ 0058U, 0059U

  non-small cell lung cancer genetic mutations analysis ~ 0179U

  ovarian cancer

    hereditary gene analysis ~ 0103U, 0132U

    likelihood score ~ 0003U

  PALB2 mRNA sequence analysis ~ 0137U

  pan tumor

    gene analysis with therapy association ~ 0211U

  prostate cancer

    hereditary related disorders ~ 0133U

    higher-grade probability ~ 0053U

    risk score ~ 0005U, 0021U, 0047U, 0113U

  response to chemotherapy drugs ~ 0083U

  RNA ~ 0019U

  solid organ neoplasm ~ 0037U, 0048U

  solid tumor targeted oncology agents ~ 0174U

  thyroid ~ 0018U, 0026U

  thyroid cancer gene expression analysis ~ 0204U

  urothelial cancer FGFR gene alteration status ~ 0154U

  ophthalmology

    age-related macular degeneration risk associated with zinc supplements ~ 0205U

  pain management ~ 0117U

  peanut allergy

    clinical reaction threshold ~ 0178U

    probability ~ 0165U

  placental alpha-micro globulin-1 (PAMG-1) ~ 0066U

  psychiatry

    anxiety, depression genomic analysis panel ~ 0173U, 0175U

  rare diseases (constitutional/heritable disorders)

    exome and mitochondrial DNA sequence analysis ~ 0214U, 0215U

    genome and mitochondrial DNA sequence analysis ~ 0212U, 0213U

    sickle cell disease microfluidic flow adhesion analysis ~ 0121U, 0122U

  transplantation medicine

    donor-derived cell-free DNA ~ 0118U

    kidney allograft rejection ~ 0088U

  twin zygosity ~ 0060U

Prostaglandin ~ 84150

  insertion ~ 59200

Prostanoids ~ see prostaglandin

Prostate

  ablation

    cryosurgery ~ 55873

    transurethral water vapor thermotherapy ~ 0582T

    waterjet ~ 0421T

  abscess, drainage ~ 52700

    incision and drainage ~ 55720-55725

Prosthesis ~ continued
  testicular, insertion ~ 54660
  training ~ 97520
  urethral sphincter
    insertion ~ 53444-53445
    removal ~ 53446-53447
    repair ~ 53449
    replacement ~ 53448
  urethral voiding valve-pump
    insertion ~ 0596T
    replacement ~ 0597T
  vagina
    insertion ~ 57267
    removal/revision ~ 57295, 57296, 57426
  wrist, removal ~ 25250-25251
Protease F ~ see plasmin
Protein
  C-reactive ~ 86140-86141
  glycated ~ 82985
  myelin basic ~ 83873
  osteocalcin ~ 83937
  prealbumin ~ 84134
  serum ~ 84155, 84165
  total ~ 84155-84160
  urine ~ 84156
  western blot ~ 84181-84182, 88372
Protein analysis, tissue western blot ~ 88371
Protein C activator ~ 85337
Protein C antigen ~ 85302
Protein C assay ~ 85303
Protein C resistance assay ~ 85307
Protein S
  assay ~ 85306
  total ~ 85305
Prothrombase ~ see thrombokinase
Prothrombin ~ 85210
Prothrombinase ~ see thromboplastin
Prothrombin time ~ 85610-85611
Prothrombokinase ~ 85230
Protime ~ see prothrombin time
Proton treatment delivery
  complex ~ 77525
  intermediate ~ 77523
  simple ~ 77520-77522
Protoporphyrin ~ 84202-84203
Protozoa antibody ~ 86753
Provitamin A ~ see vitamin, A
Prower factor ~ see Stuart-Prower factor
PSA ~ see prostate specific antigen
Pseudocyst, pancreas ~ see pancreas, pseudocyst
PSG ~ see polysomnography
Psoriasis treatment ~ (see also dermatology; photochemotherapy)
  96910-96922
Psychiatric diagnosis
  assessment
    brief emotional/behavioral ~ 96127
    behavior identification ~ 0362T, 97151, 97152
  evaluation of records or reports ~ 90885
  evaluation ~ 90791
    with medical services ~ 90792
  interactive complexity ~ 90785
  major depressive disorder (MDD) ~ 3088F-3093F
  psychological testing ~ 96101-96103, 96125
    computer assisted ~ 96103
  suicide risk assessment ~ 3085F
  unlisted services and procedures ~ 90899
Psychiatric treatment
  biofeedback training ~ 90875-90876
  consultation with family ~ 90887
  drug management ~ 90863
  electroconvulsive therapy ~ 90870, 4066F
    referral documented ~ 4067F
  environmental intervention ~ 90882
  family ~ 90846-90849, 99510
  group ~ 90853
  hypnotherapy ~ 90880
  narcosynthesis analysis ~ 90865

Psychiatric treatment ~ continued
  pharmacotherapy
    antidepressant ~ 4063F-4064F
    antipsychotic ~ 4065F
    drug management ~ 90863
  psychoanalysis ~ 90845
  report preparation ~ 90889
  suicide risk assessment ~ 3085F
  transcranial magnetic stimulation ~ 90867-90869
  unlisted services and procedures ~ 90899
Psychoanalysis ~ 90845
Psychophysiologic feedback ~ see biofeedback
Psychotherapy
  family of patient ~ 90846-90847
  for crisis ~ 90839-90840
  group other than multifamily ~ 90853
  individual patient/family member ~ 90832-90834, 90836-90838
  interactive complexity ~ 90785
  major depressive disorder ~ 4060F-4062F
  multifamily ~ 90849
  referral, documented ~ 4062F
  with pharmacologic management ~ 90863
PTA (clotting factor XI (eleven)) ~ 85270
PTB (patellar tendon bearing) cast ~ 29435
PTC (clotting factor IX (nine); Christmas factor) ~ 85250
PTC ~ see percutaneous transluminal coronary angioplasty
Pteroylglutamic acid ~ see folic acid
Pterygium
  excision ~ 65420
    with graft ~ 65426
Pterygomaxillary fossa incision ~ 31040
Pterygopalatine ganglion ~ see sphenopalatine ganglion
PTH ~ see parathormone
Ptosis ~ see blepharoptosis; procidentia
PTT ~ see thromboplastin, partial, time
Ptyalectasis ~ see dilation, salivary duct
Pubic symphysis ~ 27282
Pubis
  craterization ~ 27070
  cyst, excision ~ 27065-27067
  excision ~ 27070
  saucerization ~ 27070
  tumor, excision ~ 27065-27067
Pudendal nerve
  destruction ~ 64630
  injection
    anesthetic ~ 64430
    neurolytic ~ 64630
Puestow procedure ~ 48548
Pulled elbow ~ see nursemaid elbow
Pulmonary artery ~ 33690
  banding ~ 33620
  catheterization ~ see also catheterization, pulmonary artery
  embolism ~ 33910-33916
    excision ~ 33910-33916
  nerves, ultrasound ablation ~ 0632T
  percutaneous transluminal angioplasty ~ 92997-92998
  reimplantation ~ 33788
  repair ~ 33620, 33690, 33917-33920
    reimplantation ~ 33788
  shunt
    from aorta ~ 33755-33762, 33924
    subclavian ~ 33750
    from vena cava ~ 33766-33767
  transection ~ 33922
Pulmonary function test ~ see pulmonology, diagnostic
Pulmonary hemorrhage ~ see hemorrhage, lung
Pulmonary medical services ~ 94010-94799
Pulmonary perfusion imaging ~ 78580, 78597, 78598
Pulmonary valve
  implantation, prosthesis, transcatheter ~ 33477
  incision ~ 33470, 33471, 33474
  repair ~ 33470, 33471, 33474
  replacement ~ 33475
Pulmonary vein
  repair
    complete ~ 33730
    partial ~ 33724
    stenosis ~ 33726
  stenosis
    repair ~ 33726

Pulmonology
diagnostic
  airway closing volume ~ 94727
  apnea monitoring, pediatric ~ 94774-94777
  bronchodilation ~ 94664
  bed testing, neonate ~ 94780-94781
  car seat testing, neonate ~ 94780-94781
  carbon monoxide diffusion capacity ~ 94729
  expired gas analysis
    NO ~ 95012
    O2 and CO2 ~ 94681
    O2 update, direct ~ 94680
    O2 uptake, indirect ~ 94690
  flow-volume loop ~ 94375
  hemoglobin O2 affinity ~ 82820
  high altitutde simulation test (HAST) ~ 94452-9444-53
  hypoxia response curve ~ 94450
  inhalation treatment ~ 94640
  maximum breathing capacity ~ 94200
  maximal voluntary ventilation ~ 94200
  membrane diffusion capacity ~ 94729
  oximetry, ear or pulse ~ 94760-94762
  pediatric pneumogram ~ 94772
  plethysmograph ~ 94726
  pulmonary fluid monitoring system, remote ~ 0607T-0608T
  resistance to airflow ~ 94726, 94728
  spirometry ~ 94010-94070
    evaluation ~ 94010-94070
    patient initiated with bronchospasm ~ 94014-94016
  sputum mobilization with inhalants ~ 94664
  stress test, pulmonary ~ 94618
  vital capacity ~ 94150
  wheeze rate ~ 94799
therapeutic
  inhalation, pentamidine ~ 94642
  inhalation treatment ~ 94640, 94644-94645, 94664, 99503
  intrapulmonary surfactant admin ~ 94610
  manipulation of chest wall ~ 94667-94668
  pressure ventilation
    negative CNPB ~ 94662
    positive CPAP ~ 94660
  unlisted services and procedures ~ 94799
  ventilation assist ~ 94002-94005, 99504
unlisted services and procedures ~ 94799

Pulse generator
baroreflex activation device
  implantation/replacement ~ 0268T
  revision/removal ~ 0271T
implantable defibrillator
  insertion ~ 33230, 33231, 33240
  removal ~ 33241
  removal with replacement ~ 33262-33264
neurostimulator
  insertion ~ 61885, 61886, 64568, 64590
  removal/revision ~ 61888, 64595, 64570
pacemaker
  insertion ~ 33212, 33213, 33221
  removal ~ 33233
  replacement ~ 33227-33229
respiratory Sensor Electrode/Electrode Array
  insertion ~ 0466T
  removal ~ 0468T
  replacement ~ 0467T
  revision ~ 0467T
substernal implantable cardioverter-defibrillator
  removal ~ 0580T
  removal and replacement ~ 0614T

Pulse rate increased ~ see tachycardia
Pump ~ see chemotherapy, pump services; infusion pump
Pump, infusion ~ see infusion pump
Pump services oxygenator/heat exchanger ~ 99190-99192
Punch graft ~ 15775-15776
Puncture
artery ~ 36600
chest, drainage ~ 32554-32555
cisternal ~ see cisternal puncture
lumbar ~ see spinal tap
pericardium ~ 33016
pleural cavity, drainage ~ 32554-32555

Puncture ~ *continued*
skull, drain fluid ~ 61000-61020
  cistern ~ 61050
  inject cistern ~ 61055
  inject ventricle ~ 61026
  shunt
    drain fluid ~ 61070
    injection ~ 61070
spinal cord
  diagnostic ~ 62270, 62328
  drain fluid ~ 62272, 62329
  lumbar ~ 62270, 62328
tracheal, aspiration and/or injection ~ 31612

Puncture aspiration
abscess, skin ~ 10160
bulla ~ 10160
cyst
  breast ~ 19000-19001
  skin ~ 10160
hematoma ~ 10160

Pure-tone audiometry ~ 92552, 92553
Pustules removal ~ 10040
PUVA ~ (dermatology; photochemotherapy; ultraviolet light therapy) 96912
Pyelogram ~ see urography, intravenous; urography, retrograde
Pyelography ~ 74400, 74425
Pyelolithotomy ~ 50130
anatrophic ~ 50075
coagulum ~ 50130
Pyeloplasty ~ 50400-50405, 50544
repair, horseshoe kidney ~ 50540
secondary ~ 50405
Pyeloscopy
with cystourethroscopy ~ 52351
  biopsy ~ 52354
  destruction ~ 52354
  lithotripsy ~ 52353
  removal, calculus ~ 52352
  tumor excision ~ 52355
Pyelostolithotomy percutaneous ~ 50080-50081
Pyelostomy
with drainage ~ 50125
with pyeloplasty ~ 50400, 50405
change tube ~ 50435
Pyelotomy
complicated ~ 50135
with drainage ~ 50125
endoscopic ~ 50570
exploration ~ 50120
with removal calculus ~ 50130
Pyeloureteroplasty ~ see pyeloplasty
Pyloric sphincter
incision ~ 43520
reconstruction ~ 43800
Pyloromyotomy ~ 43520
with gastrectomy ~ 43639
Pyloroplasty ~ 43800
with gastrectomy ~ 43639
with vagotomy ~ 43640
Pyothorax ~ see abscess, thorax
Pyridoxal phosphate ~ 84207
Pyrophosphate, adenosine ~ see adenosine diphosphate
Pyrophosphorylase, Udp galactose ~ (galactose-one-phosphate, uridyl transferase) 82775, 82776
Pyruvate ~ 84210-84220

Q

Q fever ~ 86000, 86638
Q fever ab ~ see antibody, coxiella burnetii
Quadriceps repair ~ 27430
Quantitative sudomotor axon reflex test (QSART) ~ 95923
Quick test ~ prothrombin time 85610, 85611
Quinidine assay ~ 80194
Quinine ~ 84228

R

Rabies Immune Globulin (RIg)
　human ~ 90375
　human, heat- and solvent-treated (RIg-HT S/D) ~ 90377
　human, heat-treated (RIg-HT) ~ 90376
Rabies vaccine ~ 90675-90676
Rachicentesis ~ see spinal tap
Radial head, subluxation ~ see nursemaid elbow
Radial keratotomy ~ 65771
Radiation ~ see irradiation
Radiation physics
　consultation ~ 77336-77370
　unlisted services and procedures ~ 77399
Radiation therapy
　CT scan guidance ~ 77014
　consultation, radiation physics ~ 77336-77370
　dose plan ~ 77300, 77301, 77306, 77307, 77331
　　brachytherapy ~ 0394T, 0395T, 77316-77318
　　intensity modulation IMRT ~ 77338
　　teletherapy ~ 77306, 77307, 77321
　field set-up ~ 77280, 77285, 77290
　guidance
　　CT ~ 77014
　　for localization of target volume ~ 77387
　　interstitial device placement ~ 49411-49412
　intraoperative radiation therapy
　　breast, preparation of tumor cavity ~ 19294
　planning ~ 77261-77263, 77299
　port image(s) ~ 77417
　radiosurgery ~ 77317-77373
　special ~ 77470
　stereotactic
　　body ~ 77373
　　cerebral lesions ~ 77371-77372
　treatment delivery ~ 77401, 77402, 77407, 77412
　　high energy neutron radiation ~ 77423
　　intensity modulation ~ 77385, 77386
　　intraoperative ~ 77424, 77425
　　localization ~ 77387
　　proton beam ~ 77520-77525
　　stereotactic ~ 77371-77373
　　superficial ~ 77401
　　tracking ~ 77387
　treatment device ~ 77332-77334
　treatment management
　　1 or 2 fractions only ~ 77431
　　intraoperative ~ 77469
　　unlisted services and procedures ~ 77499
　　weekly ~ 77427
Radical excision of lymph nodes ~ see excision, lymph nodes, radical
Radical mastectomies, modified ~ see mastectomy, modified radical
Radical neck dissection
　with auditory canal surgery ~ 69155
　laryngectomy ~ 31365-31368
　pharyngolaryngectomy ~ 31390-31395
　with thyroidectomy ~ 60254
　with tongue excision ~ 41135, 41145, 41153-41155
Radical resection ~ see also resection, radical
　abdomen ~ 51597
　acetabulum ~ 27076
　ankle ~ 27615, 27616
　arm, lower ~ 25077
　calcaneus ~ 27647
　elbow, capsule, soft tissue,
　　bone with contracture release ~ 24149
　face ~ 21015
　fibula ~ 27646
　finger ~ 26117
　foot ~ 28046, 28047
　forearm ~ 25077
　hand ~ 26115
　hip
　　soft tissue ~ 27049
　　tumor or infection ~ 27075-27076
　humerus ~ 23220
　innominate ~ 27077

Radical resection ~ *continued*
　ischial ~ 27078
　knee ~ 27329
　leg
　　lower ~ 27615
　　upper ~ 27329
　metacarpal ~ 26250
　metatarsal ~ 28173
　mouth, with tongue excision ~ 41150, 41155
　ovarian tumor
　　bilateral
　　　salpingo-oophorectomy-omentectomy ~ 58950-58954
　　　with radical dissection for debulking ~ 58952-58954
　　　with total abdominal hysterectomy ~ 58951, 58953-58954
　pelvis, soft tissue ~ 27049
　peritoneal tumor
　　bilateral
　　　salpingo-oophorectomy-omentectomy ~ 58952-58954
　　　with radical dissection for debulking ~ 58952-58954
　phalanges
　　fingers ~ 26260-26262
　　toe ~ 28175
　radius ~ 25170
　scalp ~ 21015
　scapula ~ 23210
　shoulder ~ 23077
　sternum ~ 21630-21632
　talus, tumor ~ 27647
　tarsal ~ 28171
　tibia ~ 27645
　tonsil ~ 42842-42845
　tumor
　　back/flank ~ 21935, 21936
　　femur ~ 27365
　　knee ~ 27329, 27365
　　leg, upper ~ 27329
　　neck ~ 21557, 21558
　　thorax ~ 21557, 21558
　ulna ~ 25170
　wrist ~ 25077
Radical vulvectomy ~ see vulvectomy, radical
Radio-cobalt B12 Schilling test ~ see vitamin, B-12, absorption study
Radioactive colloid therapy ~ 79200-79300
Radioactive substance
　insertion
　　kidney ~ 50578
　　prostate ~ 55860
　　ureteral endoscopic ~ 50978
　　urethral endoscopic ~ 50959
Radiocarpal joint
　arthrotomy ~ 25040
　dislocation, closed treatment ~ 25660
Radiocinematographies ~ see cineradiography
Radioelement
　application ~ 77761-77763, 77767, 77768, 77770-77772, 77778, 77789
　handling ~ 77790
　infusion ~ 77750
Radioelement device placement
　breast ~ 19296-19298
　genitalia ~ 55920
　head ~ 41019
　intracavitary ~ 31643
　muscle ~ 20555
　neck ~ 41019
　pelvis ~ 55920
　prostate ~ 55875
　soft tissue ~ 20555
　ultrasound guidance ~ 76965
　uterus ~ 57155
　vagina ~ 57155, 57156
Radioelement substance
　catheter placement
　　breast ~ 19296-19298
　　bronchus ~ 31643
　　muscle or soft tissue ~ 20555
　　pelvic organ ~ 55920
　　prostate ~ 55875
　　soft tissue ~ 20555

Radioelement substance ~ *continued*
  needle placement
    head/neck ~ 41019
    muscle ~ 20555
    prostate ~ 55875-55876
    soft tissue ~ 20555
Radiography ~ see radiology, diagnostic; X-ray
Radioimmunosorbent test ~ see gammaglobulin, blood
Radioisotope brachytherapy ~ see brachytherapy
Radioisotope scan ~ see nuclear medicine
Radiological marker, preoperative placement, excision of breast lesion ~ 19125-19126
Radiology
  bone/joint studies
    computed tomography ~ 77078
    dual energy X-ray absorptiometry (DXA) ~ 77080, 77081, 77085, 77086
    radiography ~ 77071-77077
  diagnostic imaging
    abdomen ~ 74018, 74019, 74021
    abscess, fistula or sinus tract, study ~ 76080
    chest ~ 71045-71048
    computed tomography follow-up study ~ 76380
    fluoroscopy ~ 76000, 76496
    gastrointestinal tract ~ 74210-74363
    gynecological and obstetrical ~ 74710-74775
    head and neck ~ 70010-70559
    lower extremities ~ 73501-73725
    magnetic resonance spectroscopy ~ 76390
    spine and pelvis ~ 72020-72295
    3D rendering, tomographic ~ 76376, 76377
    upper extremities ~ 73000-73225
    urinary tract ~ 74018-74485
    vascular procedures
      aorta and arteries ~ 36901-36906, 75600-75774
      transcatheter procedures ~ 75894-75989
      veins and lymphatics ~ 75801-75893
  radiologic guidance
    computed tomography ~ 77011-77014
    fluoroscopy ~ 77001-77003
    magnetic resonance ~ 77021, 77022
Radionuclide CT scan ~ see emission computerized tomography
Radionuclide imaging ~ see nuclear medicine
Radionuclide therapy
  intra-articular ~ 79440
  intravascular ~ 79420
  intravenous infusion ~ 79403
  leukemia ~ 79100
  other ~ 79400
  polycythemia vera ~ 79100
  thyroid gland ~ 79000-79035
  unlisted services and procedures ~ 79999
Radionuclide tomography, single photon emission- computed ~ see SPECT
Radiopharmaceutical localization
  of inflammatory process ~ 78800-78804, 78830-78832
  injection for ~ 78808
  of radiopharmaceutical agent ~ 78800-78804, 78830-78832
  of tumor ~ 78800-78804, 78830-78832
Radiopharmaceutical therapy
  heart ~ 79440
  interstitial ~ 79300
  intra-arterial ~ 79445
  intra-articular ~ 79440
  intracavitary ~ 79200
  intravenous ~ 79101, 79403
  leukemia ~ 79100
  oral ~ 79005
  other ~ 79400
  polycythemia vera ~ 79100
  thyroid gland ~ 79020-79035
  unlisted services and procedures ~ 79999
Radiotherapeutic ~ see radiation therapy
Radiotherapies ~ see irradiation
Radiotherapy, surface ~ see application, radioelement, surface
Radioulnar joint
  arthrodesis, with resection of ulna ~ 25830
  dislocation
    closed treatment ~ 25675
    open treatment ~ 25676

Radius ~ see also also arm, lower; elbow; ulna
  arthroplasty ~ 24365
    with implant ~ 24366, 25441
  craterization ~ 24145, 25151
  cyst, excision ~ 24125-24126, 25120-25126
  diaphysectomy ~ 24145, 25151
  dislocation
    with fracture
      closed treatment ~ 24620
      open treatment ~ 24635
    partial ~ 24640
    subluxate ~ 24640
  excision ~ 24130, 24136, 24145, 24152
    epiphyseal bar ~ 20150
    partial ~ 25145
    styloid process ~ 25230
  fracture ~ 25605
    closed treatment ~ 25500-25505, 25520, 25600-25605
      with manipulation ~ 25605
      without manipulation ~ 25600
    distal ~ 25600-25609
      open treatment ~ 25607-25609
    head/neck
      closed treatment ~ 24650-24655
      open treatment ~ 24665-24666
    open treatment ~ 25515, 25525-25526, 25574
    percutaneous fixation ~ 25606
    shaft ~ 25500-25526
      open treatment ~ 25574
    with ulna ~ 25560-25565
      open treatment ~ 25575
  implant, removal ~ 24164
  incision and drainage ~ 25035
  osteomyelitis ~ 24136, 24145
  osteoplasty ~ 25390-25393
  prophylactic treatment ~ 25490, 25492
  repair
    epiphyseal arrest ~ 25450-25455
    epiphyseal separation
      closed ~ 25600
      closed with manipulation ~ 25605
      open treatment ~ 25607-25609
      percutaneous fixation ~ 25606
    with graft ~ 25405, 25420-25426
    malunion or nonunion ~ 25400, 25415
    osteotomy ~ 25350-25355, 25370-25375
      and ulna ~ 25365
  saucerization ~ 24145, 25151
  sequestrectomy ~ 24136, 25145
  tumor, cyst ~ 24120
    excision ~ 24125-24126, 25120-25126, 25170
Ramstedt operation ~ see pyloromyotomy
Ramus anterior, nervus thoracicus ~ see intercostal nerve
Range of motion test
  extremities or trunk ~ 95851
  eye ~ 92018-92019
  hand ~ 95852
Rapid heart rate ~ see tachycardia
Rapid plasma reagin test ~ 86592-86593
Rapid test for infection ~ 86308, 86403-86406
  monospot test ~ 86308
Rapoport test ~ 52005
Raskind procedure ~ 33735-33737
Rathke pouch tumor ~ see craniopharyngioma
Rat typhus ~ (Murine typhus) 86000
Rays, roentgen ~ see X-ray
Raz procedure ~ (repair, bladder, neck) 51845
RBC ~ see red blood cell (RBC)
RBC ab ~ see antibody, red blood cell
Reaction lip without reconstruction ~ 40530
Reaction, polymerase chain ~ see polymerase chain reaction (PCR)
Realignment
  femur with osteotomy ~ 27454
  knee extensor ~ 27422
Receptor ~ see CD4; estrogen, receptor; FC receptor; progesterone receptors
Receptor assay
  hormone ~ 84233-84235
  non hormone ~ 84238

Recession gastrocnemius leg, lower ~ 27687
Reconstruction ~ see revision
  abdominal wall
    omental flap ~ 49905
  acetabulum ~ 27120-27122
  anal
    congenital absence ~ 46730-46740
    fistula ~ 46742
    graft ~ 46753
    sphincter ~ 46750-46751, 46760
  ankle ~ 27700-27703
  apical-aortic conduit ~ 33404
  atrial
    endoscopic ~ 33265-33266
    open ~ 33254-33256
  auditory canal, external ~ 69310-69320
  bile duct, anastomosis ~ 47800
  bladder
    from colon ~ 50810
    from intestines ~ 50820, 51960
    and urethra ~ 51800-51820
  breast ~ 19357-19369
    augmentation ~ 19325
    with free flap ~ 19364
    with latissimus dorsi flap ~ 19361
    mammoplasty ~ 19318-19325
    nipple ~ 19350-19355
    revision ~ 19380
    with tissue expander ~ 19357
    transverse rectus abdominis myocutaneous flap ~ 19367-19369
  bronchi ~ 32501
    graft repair ~ 31770
    stenosis ~ 31775
  canthus ~ 67950
  cardiac anomoly, complex ~ 33622
  carpal ~ 25443
  carpal bone ~ 25394, 25430
  cheekbone ~ 21270
  chest wall, omental flap ~ 49904
    trauma ~ 32820
  cleft palate ~ 42200-42225
  conduit, apical-aortic ~ 33404
  conjunctiva ~ 68320-68335
    with flap
      bridge or partial ~ 68360
      total ~ 68362
  cranial bone, extracranial ~ 21181-21184
  ear, middle
    tympanoplasty with antrotomy or mastoidotomy
      with ossicular chain reconstruction ~ 69636-69637
    tympanoplasty with mastoidectomy ~ 69641
      with intact or reconstructed wall ~ 69643-69644
      with ossicular chain reconstruction ~ 69642
      radical or complete ~ 69644-69645
    tympanoplasty without mastoidectomy ~ 69631
      with ossicular chain reconstruction ~ 69632-69633
  elbow ~ 24360
    with implant ~ 24361-24362
    total replacement ~ 24363
  esophagus ~ 43300, 43310, 43313
    creation, stoma ~ 43352
    esophagostomy ~ 43351, 43352
    fistula ~ 43305, 43312, 43314
    gastrointestinal ~ 43360-43361
  eye
    graft
      conjunctiva ~ 65782
      stem cell ~ 65781
    transplantation
      amniotic membrane ~ 65780
  eyelid
    canthus ~ 67950
    second stage ~ 67975
    total ~ 67973-67975
    total eyelid
      lower, one stage ~ 67973
      upper, one stage ~ 67974
    transfer tarsoconjunctival flap from opposing eyelid ~ 67971
  facial bones, secondary ~ 21275
  fallopian tube ~ see repair

Reconstruction ~ *continued*
  femur
    lengthening ~ 27466-27468
    shortening ~ 27465, 27468
  fibula, lengthening ~ 27715
  finger, polydactylous ~ 26587
  foot, cleft ~ 28360
  forehead ~ 21172-21180, 21182-21184
  glenoid fossa ~ 21255
  gums
    alveolus ~ 41874
    gingiva ~ 41872
  hand
    tendon pulley ~ 26390, 26500-26502
    toe to finger transfer ~ 26551-26556
  heart
    atrial ~ 33253
      endoscopic ~ 33265-33266
      open ~ 33254-33256
    atrial septum ~ 33735-33737
    pulmonary artery shunt ~ 33924
    vena cava ~ 34502
  hip
    replacement ~ 27130-27132
    secondary ~ 27134-27138
  hip joint, with prosthesis ~ 27125
  interphalangeal joint ~ 26535-26536
    collateral ligament ~ 26545
  intestines, small, anastomosis ~ 44130
  knee ~ 27437-27438
    femur ~ 27442-27443, 27446
    ligament ~ 27427-27429
    prosthesis ~ 27438, 27445
    replacement ~ 27447
    revision ~ 27486-27487
    tibia ~ 27440-27443, 27446
  kneecap, instability ~ 27420-27424
  larynx
    cricoid split ~ 31587
    medialization ~ 31591
    stenosis ~ 31551-31554
    web ~ 31580
  lip ~ 40525-40527, 40761
  lunate ~ 25444
  malar augmentation,
    prosthetic material ~ 21270
    with bone graft ~ 21210
  mandible, with implant ~ 21244-21246, 21248-21249
  mandibular condyle ~ 21247
  mandibular rami
    with bone graft ~ 21194
    without bone graft ~ 21193
    with internal rigid fixation ~ 21196
    without internal rigid fixation ~ 21195
  maxilla, with implant ~ 21245-21246, 21248-21249
  metacarpophalangeal joint ~ 26530-26531
  midface
    with bone graft ~ 21145-21160, 21188
    without bone graft ~ 21141-21143
    forehead advancement ~ 21159-21160
  mouth ~ 40840-40845
  nail bed ~ 11762
  nasoethmoid complex ~ 21182-21184
  navicular ~ 25443
  nose
    cleft lip/cleft palate ~ 30460-30462
    dermatoplasty ~ 30620
    primary ~ 30400-30420
    secondary ~ 30430-30450
    septum ~ 30520
  orbit ~ 21256
  orbit area, secondary ~ 21275
  orbit with bone grafting ~ 21182-21184
  orbital rim ~ 21172-21180
  orbital rims ~ 21182-21184
  orbital walls ~ 21182-21184
  orbitocraniofacial, secondary revision ~ 21275
  oviduct, fimbrioplasty ~ 58760

Reconstruction ~ _continued_
palate
  cleft palate ~ 42200-42225
  lengthening ~ 42226-42227
parotid duct, diversion ~ 42507-42510
patella ~ 27437-27438
  instability ~ 27420-27424
penis
  angulation ~ 54360
  chordee ~ 54300-54304
  complications ~ 54340-54348
  epispadias ~ 54380-54390
  hypospadias ~ 54332, 54352
    one stage distal with urethroplasty ~ 54324-54328
    one stage perineal ~ 54336
periorbital region, osteotomy with graft ~ 21267-21268
pharynx ~ 42950
pyloric sphincter ~ 43800
radius ~ 24365, 25390-25393, 25441
  arthroplasty, with implant ~ 24366
shoulder joint, with implant ~ 23470-23472
skull ~ 21172-21180
  defect ~ 62140-62141, 62145
sternum ~ 21740-21742
  with thoracoscopy ~ 21743
stomach
  with duodenum ~ 43810, 43850-43855, 43865
  gastric bypass ~ 43846
  with jejunum ~ 43820-43825, 43860
  for obesity ~ 43846-43848
  Roux-en-Y ~ 43846
superior-lateral orbital rim and forehead ~ 21172-21175
supraorbital rim and forehead ~ 21179-21180
symblepharon ~ 68335
temporomandibular joint, arthroplasty ~ 21240-21243
throat ~ 42950
thumb
  from finger ~ 26550
  opponensplasty ~ 26490-26496
tibia
  lengthening ~ 27715
  tubercle ~ 27418
toe
  angle deformity ~ 28313
  extra toes ~ 28344
  hammertoe ~ 28285-28286
  macrodactyly ~ 28340-28341
  polydactylous ~ 26587
  syndactyly ~ 28345
  webbed toe ~ 28345
tongue, frenum ~ 41520
trachea
  carina ~ 31766
  cervical ~ 31750
  fistula ~ 31755
  intrathoracic ~ 31760
trapezium ~ 25445
tympanic membrane ~ 69620
ulna ~ 25390-25393, 25442
  radioulnar ~ 25337
ureter ~ 50700
  with intestines ~ 50840
urethra ~ 53410-53440, 53445
  complications ~ 54340-54348
  hypospadias
    one stage distal with meatal advancement ~ 54322
    one stage distal with urethroplasty ~ 54324-54328
    suture to bladder ~ 51840-51841
    urethroplasty for second stage ~ 54308-54316
    urethroplasty for third stage ~ 54318
uterus ~ 58540
vas deferens ~ see vasovasorrhaphy
vena cava ~ 34502
  with resection ~ 37799
wound repair ~ 13100-13160
wrist ~ 25332
  capsulectomy ~ 25320
  capsulorrhaphy ~ 25320
  realign ~ 25335
zygomatic arch ~ 21255
Rectal bleeding ~ see hemorrhage, rectum

Rectal prolapse ~ see procidentia, rectum
Rectal sphincter dilation ~ 45910
Rectocele repair ~ 45560
Rectopexy ~ see proctopexy
Rectoplasty ~ see proctoplasty
Rectorrhaphy ~ see rectum, suture
Rectovaginal fistula ~ see fistula, rectovaginal
Rectovaginal hernia ~ see rectocele
Rectum ~ see also anus
abscess, incision and drainage ~ 45005-45020, 46040, 46060
advancement flap ~ 46288
biopsy ~ 45100
dilation, endoscopy ~ 45303
endoscopy
  biopsy ~ 45305
  destruction, tumor ~ 45320
  dilation ~ 45303, 45910
  exploration ~ 45300
  hemorrhage ~ 45317
  removal
    foreign body ~ 45307
    polyp ~ 45308-45315
    tumor ~ 45308-45315
  volvulus ~ 45321
excision
  with colon ~ 45121
  partial ~ 45111, 45113-45116, 45123
  total ~ 45110, 45112, 45119-45120
exploration, endoscopic ~ 45300
hemorrhage, endoscopic ~ 45317
incontinence, graft ~ 46753
injection, sclerosing solution ~ 45520
laparoscopy ~ 45499
lesion, excision ~ 45108
manometry ~ 91122
mucosectomy ~ 44157-44158, 44211, 45113
prolapse, excision ~ 45130-45135
removal
  fecal impaction ~ 45915
  foreign body ~ 45307, 45915
repair
  fistula ~ 45800-45825, 46707
  incontinence ~ 46753
  injury ~ 45562-45563
  prolapse ~ 45505-45541, 45900
  rectocele ~ 45560
  stenosis ~ 45500
  with sigmoid excision ~ 45550
sensation, tone and compliance test ~ 91120
stricture, excision ~ 45150
suture
  fistula ~ 45800-45825
  prolapse ~ 45540-45541
tumor
  destruction ~ 45190, 45320
  excision ~ 45160-45172
    transanal endoscopic ~ 0184T
unlisted services and procedures ~ 45999
Red blood cell (RBC)
antibody ~ 86850-86870
  pretreatment ~ 86970-86972
count ~ 85032-85041
fragility
  mechanical ~ 85547
  osmotic ~ 85555-85557
hematocrit ~ 85014
iron utilization ~ 78170
morphology ~ 85007
platelet estimation ~ 85007
sedimentation rate
  automated ~ 85652
  manual ~ 85651
sequestration ~ 78140
sickling ~ 85660
survival test ~ 78130
volume determination ~ 78120-78121
Red blood cell ab ~ see antibody, red blood cell

Reductase, glutathione ~ see glutathione reductase
Reductase, lactic cytochrome ~ see lactic dehydrogenase
Reduction
  amniotic fluid ~ 59001
  breast ~ 19318
  collateral ligament, ulnar ~ 29902
  craniomegalic skull ~ 62115, 62117
  ear, protruding ~ 69300
  for fracture
    laryngeal ~ 31584
    odontoid ~ 22318, 22319
    tracheal ~ 31630
    vertebral ~ 22325-22328
  forehead ~ 21137-21139
  internal hernia, mesentary ~ 44050
  lung volume ~ 32491
  mammaplasty ~ 19318
  masseter muscle/bone ~ 21295-21296
  osteoplasty, facial bones ~ 21209
  overcorrection of ptosis ~ 67909
  pregnancy, multi-fetal ~ 59866
  skull, craniomegalic ~ 62115-62117
  tissue ~ 30801
  torsion, testis ~ 54600
  tumor
    bone, ablation therapy ~ 20982, 20983
    pulmonary ~ 32994, 32998
  volume
    blood products ~ 86960
    lung ~ 32491
  volvulus ~ 44050, 44055
  with reconstruction
    hip ~ 27147, 27156
    radioulnar joint ~ 25337
    wrist ~ 25230
Reflex test
  blink reflex ~ 95933
Reflux study ~ 78262
Refraction ~ 92015
Rehabilitation
  artery, occlusive disease ~ 93668
  auditory
    post-lingual hearing loss ~ 92633
    pre-lingual hearing loss ~ 92630
    status evaluation ~ 92626-92627
  cardiac ~ 93797-93798
  services considered, documentation ~ 4079F
Rehabilitative ~ see rehabilitation
Rehfuss test ~ see gastroenterology diagnostic, stomach
Reichstein's substances ~ see deoxycortisol
Reimplantation
  arteries
    aorta prosthesis ~ 35697
    carotid ~ 35691, 35694-35695
    subclavian ~ 35693-35695
    vertebral ~ 35691-35693
    visceral ~ 35697
  kidney ~ 50380
  ovary ~ 58825
  pulmonary artery ~ 33788
  ureters ~ 51565
  ureter, to bladder ~ 50780-50785
Reinnervation larynx, neuromuscular pedicle ~ 31590
Reinsch test ~ 83015
Reinsertion
  drug delivery implant ~ 11983
  spinal fixation device ~ 22849
Relative density ~ see specific gravity
Release
  capsule
    ankle ~ 27612
    elbow ~ 24149
    foot ~ 28260
    knee ~ 27435
    metatarsophalangeal joint ~ 28289, 28291
    shoulder ~ 23020
  carpal tunnel ~ 64721
  elbow contracture, with radical release of capsule ~ 24149
  flexor muscles, hip ~ 27036
  muscle, knee ~ 27422

Release ~ *continued*
  nerve ~ 64702-64726
    neurolytic ~ 64727
  retina, encircling material ~ 67115
  spinal cord ~ 63200
  stapes ~ 69650
  tarsal tunnel ~ 28035
  tendon ~ 24332, 25295
Release-inhibiting hormone, somatotropin ~ see somatostatin
Removal
  adjustable gastric restrictive device ~ 43772-43774
  allograft, intestinal ~ 44137
  artificial heart ~ 33929
  artificial intervertebral disc
    cervical interspace ~ 0095T, 22864
    lumbar interspace ~ 22865, 0164T
  balloon, intra-aortic ~ 33974
  balloon assist device, intra-aortic ~ 33968, 33971
  blood clot, eye ~ 65930
  blood component, apheresis ~ 36511-36516
  breast
    capsules ~ 19371
    implants ~ 19328-19330
    modified radical ~ 19307
    partial ~ 19300-19302
    radical ~ 19305-19306
    simple, complete ~ 19303
  calcareous deposit, subdeltoid ~ 23000
  calculi (stone)
    bile duct ~ 43264, 47420-47425
      percutaneous ~ 47554
    bladder ~ 51050, 52310-52318, 52352
    gallbladder ~ 47480
    hepatic duct ~ 47400
    kidney ~ 50060-50081, 50130, 50561, 50580, 52352
    pancreas ~ 48020
    pancreatic duct ~ 43264
    salivary gland ~ 42330-42340
    ureter ~ 50610-50630, 50961, 50980, 51060-51065, 52320-52330, 52352
    urethra ~ 52310-52315, 52352
  cast ~ 29700
  cataract
    dilated fundus evaluation ~ 2021F
    with replacement
      not associated with concurrent ~ 66983
      extracapsular ~ 66982, 66984
      intracapsular ~ 66983
  catheter
    central venous ~ 36589
    fractured ~ 37197
    peritoneum ~ 49422
    pleural cavity ~ 32552
    spinal cord ~ 62355
  cerclage, cervix ~ 59871
  cerumen, auditory canal, external ~ 69209, 69210
  clot pericardium ~ 33020
    endoscopic ~ 32658
  comedones ~ 10040
  contraceptive capsules ~ 11976
  cranial tongs ~ 20665
  cyst ~ 10040
  dacryolith
    lacrimal duct ~ 68530
    lacrimal gland ~ 68530
  defibrillator
    heart ~ 33244
      pulse generator only ~ 33241
      via thoracotomy ~ 33243
  drug delivery implant ~ 11982-11983
  ear wax, auditory canal, external ~ 69209, 69210
  electrode
    brain ~ 61535, 61880
    chest wall, respiratory sensor ~ 0468T
    heart ~ 33238
    nerve ~ 64585
    spinal cord ~ 63661-63664
    stomach ~ 43648, 43882
  esophageal sphincter augmentation device ~ 43285
  external fixation system ~ 20694

Removal ~ continued
  sleeve pneumonectomy ~ 32442
  two lobes ~ 32482
  volume reduction ~ 32491
 lymph nodes
  abdominal ~ 38747
  inguinofemoral ~ 38760-38765
  pelvic ~ 38770
  retroperitoneal, transabdominal ~ 38780
  thoracic ~ 38746
 mammary implant ~ 19328-19330
 mastoid, air cells ~ 69670
 mesh, abdominal wall ~ 11008
 milia, multiple ~ 10040
 nails ~ 11730-11732, 11750
 neurostimulators
  pulse generator ~ 64595
  receiver ~ 64595
 ocular implant ~ 65175, 65920
 orbital implant ~ 67560
 ovaries, laparoscopy ~ 58661
 pacemaker, heart ~ 33233-33237
 patella, complete ~ 27424
 plate, skull ~ 62142
 polyp
  anal ~ 46610, 46612
  antrochoanal ~ 31032
  colon ~ 44392, 45385
  colon-sigmoid ~ 45333
  endoscopy ~ 44364-44365, 44394
  esophagus ~ 43217, 43250
  gastrointestinal, upper ~ 43250-43251
  rectum ~ 45315
  sphenoid sinus ~ 31051
 prosthesis
  abdomen ~ 49606
  abdominal wall ~ 11008
  hip ~ 27090-27091
  knee ~ 27488
  penis ~ 54406, 54410-54417
  perineum ~ 53442
  skull ~ 62142
  urethral sphincter ~ 53446-53447
  wrist ~ 25250-25251
 pulse generator
  brain ~ 61888
  spinal cord ~ 63688
 pustules ~ 10040
 receiver, brain ~ 61888
  spinal cord ~ 63688
 reservoir, spinal cord ~ 62365
 seton, anal ~ 46030
 shoulder joint, foreign or loose body ~ 23107
 shunt
  brain ~ 62256-62258
  heart ~ 33924
  peritoneum ~ 49429
  spinal cord ~ 63746
 skin tags ~ 11200-11201
 sling
  urethra ~ 53442
  vagina ~ 57287
 spinal instrumentation
  anterior ~ 22855
  posterior nonsegmental
   Harrington rod ~ 22850
  posterior segmental ~ 22852
 stent
  bile duct ~ 43275-43276
  pancreatic duct ~ 43275-43276
 suture
  anal ~ 46754
  anesthesia ~ 15850-15851
 thrombus ~ see thrombectomy
 tissue expanders ~ 11971
 total replacement heart system ~ 33929
 transplant intestines ~ 44137
 transplant kidney ~ 50370

Removal ~ continued
 tube
  ear, middle ~ 69424
  finger ~ 26392, 26416
  hand ~ 26392, 26416
 tumor
  larynx ~ 31578
  small intestine ~ 43250
  temporal bone ~ 69970
 ureter, ligature ~ 50940
 urethral stent
  bladder ~ 52310-52315
  urethra ~ 52310-52315
 vein
  clusters ~ 37785
  perforation ~ 37760-37761
  saphenous ~ 37720-37735, 37780
  varicose ~ 37765-37766
 venous access device ~ 36590
  obstruction ~ 75901-75902
 ventilating tube, ear, middle ~ 69424
 ventricular assist device ~ 33977-33978
  extracorporeal ~ 33990-33993
  intracorporeal ~ 33980
 vitreous, anterior approach ~ 67005-67010
 wire, anal ~ 46754
Renal ~ (see also kidney)
 abscess ~ see abscess, kidney
 arteries ~ see artery, renal
 autotransplantation ~ see autotransplantation, renal
 calculus ~ see calculus, removal, kidney
 cyst ~ see cyst, kidney
 dialyses ~ see hemodialysis
 disease services ~ see dialysis
 transplantation ~ see kidney, transplantation
Renin ~ 80408, 80416, 84244
 peripheral vein ~ 80417
Renin-converting enzyme ~ 82164
Reoperation
 carotid thromboendarterectomy ~ 35390
 coronary artery bypass
  valve procedure ~ 33530
 distal vessel bypass ~ 35700
Repair ~ see also revision
 abdomen ~ 49900
  hernia ~ 49491-49525, 49565, 49570, 49582-49590
  omphalocele ~ 49600-49611
  suture ~ 49900
 abdominal wall ~ 15830, 15847
 anal
  anomaly ~ 46744-46748
  fistula ~ 46288, 46706, 46715-46716
  stricture ~ 46700-46705
 aneurysm
  aorta
   abdominal ~ 34845-34848
   infrarenal ~ 34830-34832
   thoracic ~ 33877-33886
  intracranial artery ~ 61697-61708
 ankle
  ligament ~ 27695-27698
  tendon ~ 27612, 27650-27654, 27680-27687
 aorta ~ 33320-33322, 33802-33803
  coarctation ~ 33840-33851
  graft ~ 337858, 33859, 33877
  infrarenal abdominal endovascular ~ 34701-34706, 34845-34848
  sinus of valsalva ~ 33702-33720
  thoracic ~ 75956-75959
   endovascular ~ 33880-33891
  visceral
   endovascular ~ 34841-34848
   physician planning ~ 34839
 anorectum fistula ~ 46707
 aortic arch
  with cardiopulmonary bypass ~ 33853
  without cardiopulmonary bypass ~ 33852
 aortic valve ~ 33390, 33391
  obstruction, outflow tract ~ 33414
  septic hypertrophy ~ 33416
  stenosis ~ 33415

Repair ~ *continued*
  arm
    lower ~ 25260-25263, 25270
      fasciotomy ~ 24495
      secondary ~ 25265, 25272-25274
      tendon ~ 25290
      tendon sheath ~ 25275
    muscle ~ 24341
    tendon ~ 24332, 24341, 25280, 25295, 25310-25316
    upper
      muscle revision ~ 24330-24331
      muscle transfer ~ 24301, 24320
      tendon lengthening ~ 24305
      tendon revision ~ 24320
      tendon transfer ~ 24301
      tenotomy ~ 24310
  arteriovenous aneurysm ~ 36832
  arteriovenous fistula
    abdomen ~ 35182
      acquired or traumatic ~ 35189
    head ~ 35180
      acquired or traumatic ~ 35188
    lower extremity ~ 35184
      acquired or traumatic ~ 35190
    neck ~ 35180
      acquired or traumatic ~ 35188
    thorax ~ 35182
      acquired or traumatic ~ 35189
    upper extremity ~ 35184
      acquired or traumatic ~ 35190
  arteriovenous malformation
    intracranial ~ 61680-61692
    intracranial artery ~ 61705-61708
    spinal artery ~ 62294
    spinal cord ~ 63250-63252
  artery
    angioplasty
      aorta ~ 37246-37247
      axillary ~ 37246-37247
      brachiocephalic ~ 37246-37247
    bypass graft ~ 35501-35571, 35601-35683, 35691-35695, 35700
    bypass in-situ ~ 35582-35587
    bypass venous graft ~ 33510-33516, 35510-35525
    femoral ~ 35456
    iliac ~ 37220-37222, 37227
    occlusive disease ~ 35001, 35005-35021, 35045-35081, 35091, 35102,
      35111, 35121, 35131, 35141, 35151, 35161
    popliteal ~ 37224
    pulmonary ~ 33690
    renal ~ 37246, 37247
    renal or visceral ~ 37246, 37247
    subclavian ~ 37246-37247
    thromboendarterectomy ~ 35301-35321, 35341-35390
    tibioperoneal ~ 37228-37235
    viscera ~ 37246, 37247
  arytenoid cartilage ~ 31400
  bile duct ~ 47701
    with intestines ~ 47760, 47780-47785
    wound ~ 47900
  bladder
    exstrophy ~ 51940
    fistula ~ 44660-44661, 45800-45805, 51880-51925
    neck ~ 51845
    resection ~ 52500
    wound ~ 51860-51865
  blepharoptosis, frontalis muscle technique with fascial sling ~ 67902
  blood vessel
    abdomen ~ 35221
      with other graft ~ 35281
      with vein graft ~ 35251
    chest ~ 35211-35216
      with other graft ~ 35271-35276
      with vein graft ~ 35241-35246
    finger ~ 35207
    graft defect ~ 35870
    hand ~ 35207
    kidney ~ 50100
    lower extremity ~ 35226
      with other graft ~ 35286
      with vein graft ~ 35256

Repair ~ *continued*
  neck ~ 35201
    with other graft ~ 35261
    with vein graft ~ 35231
  upper extremity ~ 35206
    with other graft ~ 35266
    with vein graft ~ 35236
  body cast ~ 29720
  brain, wound ~ 61571
  breast, suspension ~ 19316
  bronchi, fistula ~ 32815
  brow pyrosis ~ 67900
  bunion ~ 28292, 28295-28299
  bypass graft ~ 35901-35907
    fistula ~ 35870
  calcaneus, osteotomy ~ 28300
  cannula ~ 36860-36861
  carpal ~ 25440
  carpal bone ~ 25431
  cervix
    cerclage ~ 57700
      abdominal ~ 59320-59325
    suture ~ 57720
  chest wall ~ 32905
    closure ~ 32810
    fistula ~ 32906
  chin
    augmentation ~ 21120, 21123
    osteotomy ~ 21121-21123
  clavicle, osteotomy ~ 23480-23485
  cleft hand ~ 26580
  cleft lip ~ 40525-40527, 40700-40761
    nasal deformity ~ 40700-40701, 40720-40761
  cleft palate ~ see cleft palate, repair
  colon
    fistula ~ 44650-44661
    hernia ~ 44050
    malrotation ~ 44055
    obstruction ~ 44050
  cornea ~ see cornea, repair
  coronary chamber fistula ~ 33500-33501
  cyst
    Bartholin's gland ~ 56440
    liver ~ 47300
  diaphragm
    for eventration ~ 39545
    hernia ~ 39503-39541
    laceration ~ 39501
  ductus arteriosus ~ 33820-33824
  ear, middle
    oval window fistula ~ 69666
    round window fistula ~ 69667
  elbow
    hemiepiphyseal arrest ~ 24470
    ligament ~ 24343-24346
    muscle ~ 24341
    muscle transfer ~ 24301
    tendon ~ 24340-24342
      each ~ 24341
    tendon lengthening ~ 24305
    tendon transfer ~ 24301
    tennis elbow ~ 24357-24359
  encephalocele ~ 62121
  enterocele
    hysterectomy ~ 58270, 58294
  epididymis ~ 54900-54901
  epispadias ~ 54380-54390
  esophagus ~ 43300, 43310, 43313
    esophagogastrostomy ~ 43320
    esophagojejunostomy ~ 43340-43341
    fistula ~ 43305, 43312, 43314, 43420-43425
    fundoplasty ~ 43210, 43325
    muscles ~ 43330-43331
    pre-existing perforation ~ 43405
    wound ~ 43410-43415
  eye
    ciliary body ~ 66680
      suture ~ 66682
    conjunctiva ~ 65270-65273
      wound ~ 65270-65273

Repair ~ *continued*

cornea ~ 65275
 astigmatism ~ 65772-65775
 with glue ~ 65286
 wound ~ 65275-65285
fistula, lacrimal gland ~ 68770
iris
 with ciliary body ~ 66680
 suture ~ 66682
lacrimal duct, canaliculi ~ 68700
lacrimal punctum ~ 68705
retina, detachment ~ 67101-67113
sclera
 with glue ~ 65286
 with graft ~ 66225
 reinforcement ~ 67250-67255
 staphyloma ~ 66225
 wound ~ 65286, 66250
strabismus, chemodenervation ~ 67345
symblepharon
 division ~ 68340
 with graft ~ 68335
 without graft ~ 68330
trabeculae ~ 65855
eye muscles
strabismus
 adjustable sutures ~ 67335
 one horizontal muscle ~ 67311
 one vertical muscle ~ 67314
 posterior fixation suture technique ~ 67334-67335
 previous surgery, not involving extraocular muscles ~ 67331
 release extensive scar tissue ~ 67343
 superior oblique muscle ~ 67318
 two horizontal muscles ~ 67312
 two or more vertical muscles ~ 67316
wound, extraocular muscle ~ 65290
eyebrow, ptosis ~ 67900
eyelashes
epilation
 by forceps ~ 67820
 by other than forceps ~ 67825
incision of lid margin ~ 67830
 with free mucous membrane graft ~ 67835
eyelid ~ 21280-21282
ectropion ~ 67916-67917
 suture ~ 67914
 thermocauterization ~ 67915
entropion ~ 67924
 excision tarsal wedge ~ 67923
 suture ~ 67921-67924
 thermocauterization ~ 67922
excisional ~ 67961-67966
lagophthalmos ~ 67912
ptosis, conjunctivo-tarso-Muller's muscle-levator resection ~ 67908
 frontalis muscle technique ~ 67901-67902
 levator resection ~ 67903-67904
reduction of overcorrection ~ 67909
 superior rectus technique ~ 67906
retraction ~ 67911
wound, suture ~ 67930-67935
facial bones ~ 21208-21209
facial nerve
paralysis ~ 15840-15845
suture, intratemporal, lateral to geniculate ganglion ~ 69740
 intratemporal, medial to geniculate ganglion ~ 69745
fallopian tube ~ 58752
anastomosis ~ 58750
create stoma ~ 58770
fascial defect ~ 50728
femur ~ 27470-27472
epiphysis ~ 27475-27485, 27742
 arrest ~ 27185
 open treatment ~ 27177-27178
 osteoplasty ~ 27179
 osteotomy ~ 27181
 by pinning ~ 27176
 by traction ~ 27175
with graft ~ 27170
muscle transfer ~ 27110

Repair ~ *continued*

osteotomy ~ 27140, 27151, 27450-27454
 femoral neck ~ 27161
 with fixation ~ 27165
 with open reduction ~ 27156
fibula
epiphysis ~ 27477-27485, 27730-27742
nonunion or malunion ~ 27726
osteotomy ~ 27707-27712
finger
claw finger ~ 26499
macrodactylia ~ 26590
polydactylous ~ 26587
syndactyly ~ 26560-26562
tendon
 extensor ~ 26415-26434, 26445-26449
 flexor ~ 26356-26358, 26440-26442
 joint stabilization ~ 26474
 pip joint ~ 26471
toe transfer ~ 26551-26556
trigger ~ 26055
volar plate ~ 26548
web finger ~ 26560-26562
fistula
carotid-cavernous ~ 61710
mastoid ~ 69700
rectovaginal ~ 57308
foot
fascia ~ 28250
muscle ~ 28250
tendon ~ 28200-28226, 28238
gallbladder
with gastroenterostomy ~ 47741
with intestines ~ 47720-47740
great arteries ~ 33770-33781
great vessel ~ 33320-33322
hallux valgus ~ 28292, 28295-28299
hamstring ~ 27097
hand
cleft hand ~ 26580
muscle ~ 26591-26593
tendon
 extensor ~ 26410-26416, 26426-26428, 26433-26437
 flexor ~ 26350-26358, 26440
 profundus ~ 26370-26373
hearing aid, bone conduction ~ 69711
heart
anomaly ~ 33600-33617
aortic sinus ~ 33702-33722
artificial heart ~ 33928
atrioventricular canal ~ 33660-33665
 complete ~ 33670
atrioventricular valve ~ 33660-33665
blood vessel ~ 33320-33322
cor triatriatum ~ 33732
infundibular ~ 33476-33478
mitral valve
 with cardiopulmonary bypass ~ 33425-33427
 transapical ~ 0543T
 transcatheter ~ 33418, 33419, 0345T, 0544T
myocardium ~ 33542
outflow tract ~ 33476-33478
postinfarction ~ 33542-33545
prosthetic valve ~ 33670, 33852-33853
prosthetic valve dysfunction ~ 33496
pulmonary artery shunt ~ 33924
pulmonary valve ~ 33470-33474
septal defect ~ 33545, 33608-33610, 33681-33688, 33692-33697
 atrial and ventricular ~ 33647
 atrium ~ 33641
sinus of valsalva ~ 33702-33722
sinus venosus ~ 33645
tetralogy of Fallot ~ 33692-33697
total replacement heart system ~ 33927-33929
tricuspid valve ~ 33465
ventricle ~ 33611-33612
 obstruction ~ 33619
ventricular tunnel ~ 33722
wound ~ 33300-33305

Repair ~ *continued*
  hepatic duct, with intestines ~ 47765, 47802
  hernia
    abdomen ~ 49565, 49590
      incisional ~ 49560
    epigastric ~ 49570
      incarcerated ~ 49572
    epigelian
      incarcerated or strangulated ~ 49653
      reducible ~ 49652
    femoral ~ 49550
      incarcerated ~ 49553
      recurrent ~ 49555
      recurrent incarcerated ~ 49557
      reducible recurrent ~ 49555
    hiatal ~ 43332-43337
    incisional
      incarcerated or strangulated ~ 49561, 49655
      recurrent incarcerated ~ 49566, 49657
      recurrent reducible ~ 49656
      reducible ~ 49564
    inguinal ~ 49491-49521
      initial ~ 49650
      recurrent ~ 49651
      sliding ~ 49525
    intestinal ~ 44025-44050
    lumbar ~ 49540
    lung ~ 32800
    orchiopexy ~ 54640
    paraesophageal ~ 43332-43337
    reducible ~ 49565, 49570
      femoral ~ 49550
      incisional ~ 49560
      inguinal ~ 49500, 49505
      recurrent ~ 49520
    sliding ~ 49525
    spigelian ~ 49590
      incarcerated or strangulated ~ 49653
      reducible ~ 49652
    umbilical ~ 49580, 49585
      incarcerated ~ 49582, 49587, 49653
      reducible ~ 49580, 49652
    ventral
      incarcerated or strangulated ~ 49653
      reducible ~ 49652
    with spermatic cord ~ 54640
  hip
    muscle transfer ~ 27100-27105, 27111
    osteotomy ~ 27146-27156
    tendon ~ 27097
  humerus ~ 24420-24430
    with graft ~ 24435
    osteotomy ~ 24400-24410
  ileostomy ~ see ileostomy, repair
  interphalangeal joint, volar plate ~ 26548
  intestines
    enterocele
      abdominal approach ~ 57270
      vaginal approach ~ 57268
    obstruction ~ 44615
  intestines, large
    closure enterostomy ~ 44620-44626
    diverticula ~ 44605
    ulcer ~ 44605
    wound ~ 44605
  intestines, small
    closure enterostomy ~ 44620-44626
    diverticula ~ 44602-44603
    fistula ~ 44640-44661
    hernia ~ 44050
    malrotation ~ 44055
    obstruction ~ 44025-44050
    ulcer ~ 44602-44603
    wound ~ 44602-44603
  introitus, vagina ~ 56800
  iris, ciliary body ~ 66680
  jejunum
    free transfer, with microvascular anastomosis ~ 43496

Repair ~ *continued*
  kidney
    fistula ~ 50520-50526
    horseshoe ~ 50540
    renal pelvis ~ 50400-50405
    wound ~ 50500
  knee
    cartilage ~ 27403
    instability ~ 27420
    ligament ~ 27405-27409
      collateral ~ 27405
      collateral and cruciate ~ 27409
      cruciate ~ 27407-27409
    meniscus ~ 27403
    tendon ~ 27380-27381
  larynx
    fracture ~ 31584-31586
    reinnervation, neuromuscular pedicle ~ 31590
  leg
    lower
      fascia ~ 27656
      tendon ~ 27658-27692
    upper
      muscle ~ 27385-27386, 27400, 27430
      tendon ~ 27393-27400
  ligament ~ see ligament, repair
  lip ~ 40650-40654
    cleft lip ~ 40700-40761
    fistula ~ 42260
  liver, abscess ~ 47300
    cyst ~ 47300
    wound ~ 47350-47361
  lung
    hernia ~ 32800
    pneumolysis ~ 32940
    tear ~ 32110
  mastoidectomy
    complete ~ 69601
    modified radical ~ 69602
    radical ~ 69603
    with tympanoplasty ~ 69604
  maxilla, osteotomy ~ 21206
  mesentery ~ 44850
  metacarpal
    lengthening ~ 26568
    nonunion ~ 26546
    osteotomy ~ 26565
  metacarpophalangeal joint
    capsulodesis ~ 26516-26518
    collateral ligament ~ 26540-26542
    fusion ~ 26516-26518
  metatarsal ~ 28322
    osteotomy ~ 28306-28309
  microsurgery ~ 69990
  mitral valve ~ 33420-33427
  mouth
    laceration ~ 40830-40831
    vestibule of ~ 40830-40845
  musculotendinous cuff ~ 23410-23412
  nail bed ~ 11760
  nasal deformity, cleft lip ~ 40700-40761
  nasal septum ~ 30630
  nasal valve collapse ~ 30468
  navicular ~ 25440
  neck muscles
    scalenus anticus ~ 21700-21705
    sternocleidomastoid ~ 21720-21725
  nerve ~ 64876
    graft ~ 64885-64907
    microrepair ~ 69990
    suture ~ 64831-64876
  nose
    adhesions ~ 30560
    fistula ~ 30580-30600, 42260
    rhinophyma ~ 30120
    septum ~ 30540-30545, 30630
    synechia ~ 30560
    vestibular stenosis ~ 30465

Repair ~ *continued*

- omphalocele ~ 49600-49611
- osteotomy
  - femoral neck ~ 27161
  - radius, and ulna ~ 25365
  - ulna, and radius ~ 25365
  - vertebra
    - additional segment ~ 22216, 22226
    - cervical ~ 22210, 22220
    - lumbar ~ 22214, 22224
    - thoracic ~ 22212, 22222
- oviduct ~ 58752
  - create stoma ~ 58770
- pacemaker, heart
  - electrode ~ 33218-33220
- palate
  - laceration ~ 42180-42182
  - vomer flap ~ 42235
- pancreas
  - cyst ~ 48500
  - pseudocyst ~ 48510
- paravaginal defect ~ 57284-57285, 57423
- pectus carinatum ~ 21740-21742
  - with thoracoscopy ~ 21743
- pectus excavatum ~ 21740-21742
  - with thoracoscopy ~ 21743
- pelvic floor, prosthetic insertion ~ 57267
- pelvis
  - osteotomy ~ 27158
  - tendon ~ 27098
- penis
  - corporeal tear ~ 54437
  - fistulization ~ 54435
  - injury ~ 54440
  - priapism ~ 54420-54435
  - shunt ~ 54420-54430
- perineum ~ 56810
- periorbital region, osteotomy ~ 21260-21263
- phalanx
  - finger
    - lengthening ~ 26568
    - osteotomy ~ 26567
  - nonunion ~ 26546
  - toe, osteotomy ~ 28310-28312
- pharynx, with esophagus ~ 42953
- pleura ~ 32215
- prosthesis, penis ~ 54408
- pulmonary artery ~ 33917-33920
  - reimplantation ~ 33788
- pulmonary valve ~ 33470-33474
- quadriceps ~ see quadriceps, repair
- radius
  - epiphyseal ~ 25450-25455
  - malunion or nonunion ~ 25400, 25415
  - osteotomy ~ 25350-25355, 25370-25375
  - with graft ~ 25405, 25420-25426
- rectocele ~ see rectocele, repair
- rectovaginal fistula ~ 57308
- rectum
  - fistula ~ 45800-45825
  - injury ~ 45562-45563
  - prolapse ~ 45505-45541, 45900
  - rectocele ~ 45560
  - stenosis ~ 45500
  - with sigmoid excision ~ 45550
- retinal detachment with diathermy ~ see diathermy, retinal detachment, repair
- rotator cuff ~ see rotator cuff, repair
- salivary duct ~ 42500-42505
  - fistula ~ 42600
- scapula
  - fixation ~ 23400
  - scapulopexy ~ 23400
- sclera ~ see sclera, repair
- scrotum ~ 55175-55180
- septal defect ~ 33813-33814
- shoulder, capsule ~ 23450-23466
  - cuff ~ 23410-23412
  - ligament release ~ 23415

Repair ~ *continued*

- muscle transfer ~ 23395-23397
- musculotendinous rotator cuff ~ 23415-23420
- tendon ~ 23410-23412, 23430-23440
- tenomyotomy ~ 23405-23406
- simple, integumentary system ~ see integumentary system, repair, simple
- sinus
  - ethmoid, cerebrospinal fluid leak ~ 31290
  - sphenoid, cerebrospinal fluid leak ~ 31291
- sinus of valsalva ~ 33702-33722
- skin, wound
  - complex ~ 13100-13160
  - intermediate ~ 12031-12057
  - simple ~ 12020-12021
- skull
  - cerebrospinal fluid leak ~ 62100
  - encephalocele ~ 62120
- spica cast ~ 29720
- spinal cord ~ 63700
  - cerebrospinal fluid leak ~ 63707-63709
  - meningocele ~ 63700-63702
  - myelomeningocele ~ 63704-63706
- spinal meningocele ~ see meningocele, repair
- spine, osteotomy ~ 22210-22226
- spleen ~ 38115
- stomach
  - esophagogastrostomy ~ 43320
  - fistula ~ 43880
  - fundoplasty ~ 43325, 43327-43328
  - laceration ~ 43501-43502
  - stoma ~ 43870
  - ulcer ~ 43501
- talus, osteotomy ~ 28302
- tarsal ~ 28320
  - osteotomy ~ 28304-28305
- testis
  - injury ~ 54670
  - suspension ~ 54620-54640
  - torsion ~ 54600
- throat
  - pharyngoesophageal ~ 42953
  - wound ~ 42900
- thumb
  - muscle ~ 26508
  - tendon ~ 26510
- tibia ~ 27720-27725
  - epiphysis ~ 27477-27485, 27730-27742
  - osteotomy ~ 27455-27457, 27705, 27709-27712
  - pseudoarthrosis ~ 27727
- toe
  - bunion ~ 28292, 28295-28299
  - muscle ~ 28240
  - tendon ~ 28240
  - webbing ~ 28280, 28345
- toes
  - macrodactylia ~ 26590
  - polydactylous ~ 26587
- tongue ~ 41250-41252
  - laceration ~ 41250-41252
  - suture ~ 41510
- trachea, fistula ~ 31755
  - stenosis ~ 31780-31781
  - stoma ~ 31613-31614
    - scar ~ 31830
      - with plastic repair ~ 31825
      - without plastic repair ~ 31820
    - with plastic repair ~ 31825
    - without plastic repair ~ 31820
  - wound
    - cervical ~ 31800
    - intrathoracic ~ 31805
- tricuspid valve ~ 33463-33465
  - transcatheter tricuspid valve repair (TTVr) ~ 0569T, 0570T
- truncus arteriosus, Rastelli type ~ 33786
- tunica vaginalis, hydrocele ~ 55060
- tympanic membrane ~ 69450, 69610
- ulna
  - epiphyseal ~ 25450-25455
  - malunion or nonunion ~ 25400, 25415

Repair ~ *continued*
   osteotomy ~ 25360, 25370-25375, 25425-25426
   with graft ~ 25405, 25420
  umbilicus, omphalocele ~ 49600-49611
  ureter
   anastomosis ~ 50740-50825
   continent diversion ~ 50825
   deligation ~ 50940
   fistula ~ 50920-50930
   lysis adhesions ~ 50715-50725
   suture ~ 50900
   urinary undiversion ~ 50830
  ureterocele ~ 51535
  urethra
   artificial sphincter ~ 53449
   diverticulum ~ 53240, 53400-53405
   fistula ~ 45820-45825, 53400-53405, 53520
   stoma ~ 53520
   stricture ~ 53400-53405
   urethrocele ~ 57230
   with replantation of penis ~ 54438
   wound ~ 53502-53515
  urethral sphincter ~ 57220
  urinary incontinence ~ 53431-53440, 57284
  uterus
   fistula ~ 51920-51925
   rupture ~ 58520, 59350
   suspension ~ 58400-58410
  vagina
   anterior ~ see colporrhaphy, anterior
   cystocele ~ 57240, 57260
   enterocele ~ 57265
   fistula ~ 46715-46716, 51900
    rectovaginal ~ 57300-57307
    transvesical and vaginal approach ~ 57330
    urethrovaginal ~ 57310-57311
    vesicovaginal ~ 57320-57330
   hysterectomy ~ 58267
   incontinence ~ 57284, 57288
   pereyra procedure ~ 57289
   postpartum ~ 59300
   prolapse ~ 57282-57284
   rectocele ~ 57250-57260
   suspension ~ 57280, 57284
    laparoscopic ~ 57425
   wound ~ 57200-57210
  vaginal wall prolapse ~ see colporrhaphy
  vas deferens, suture ~ 55400
  vein
   angioplasty ~ 37248, 37249
   femoral ~ 34501
   graft ~ 34520
   pulmonary ~ 33730
   transposition ~ 34510
  vulva, postpartum ~ 59300
  wound
   complex ~ 13100-13160
   intermediate ~ 12031-12057
   simple ~ 12001-12021
  wound dehiscence
   complex ~ 13160
   simple ~ 12020-12021
  wrist ~ 25260-25263, 25270, 25447
   bone ~ 25440
   carpal bone ~ 25431
   cartilage ~ 25107
   removal, implant ~ 25449
   secondary ~ 25265, 25272-25274
   tendon ~ 25280-25316
   tendon sheath ~ 25275
   total replacement ~ 25446
Repeat surgeries ~ see reoperation
Replacement
  aortic valve ~ 33405-33413
  artificial heart, intracorporeal ~ 33928
  cerebrospinal fluid shunt ~ 62160, 62194, 62225-62230
  contact lens ~ see contact lens services
  elbow, total ~ 24363

Replacement ~ *continued*
  electrode
   heart ~ 33210-33211, 33216-33217
   stomach ~ 43647
  eye, drug delivery system ~ 67121
  hearing aid, bone conduction ~ 69710
  hip ~ 27130-27132
   revision ~ 27134-27138
  implant, bone, for external speech processor/cochlear stimulator ~ 69717-69718
  knee, total ~ 27447
  mitral valve ~ 33430
  nerve ~ 64726
  neurostimulator
   pulse generator/receiver
    intracranial ~ 61885
    peripheral nerve ~ 64590
    spinal ~ 63685
  ossicles, with prosthesis ~ 69633, 69637
  ossicular replacement ~ see TORP (total ossicular replacement prosthesis)
  pacemaker ~ 33206-33208
   catheter ~ 33210
   electrode ~ 33210-33211, 33216-33217
  pacing cardioverter-defibrillator
   leads ~ 33243-33244
  pulse generator only ~ 33241
  penile, prosthesis ~ 54410-54411, 54416-54417
  prosthesis, skull ~ 62143
   urethral sphincter ~ 53448
  pulmonary valve ~ 33475
  pulse generator
   brain ~ 61885
   peripheral nerve ~ 64590
   spinal cord ~ 63685
  receiver
   brain ~ 61885
   peripheral nerve ~ 64590
   spinal cord ~ 63685
  skull plate ~ 62143
  spinal cord, reservoir ~ 62360
  tissue expanders, skin ~ 11970
  total replacement ~ see hip, total replacement
  total replacement heart system, intracorporeal ~ 33928
  tricuspid valve ~ 33465
  ureter, with intestines ~ 50840
  venous access device ~ 36582-36583, 36585
   catheter ~ 36578
  venous catheter, central ~ 36580-36581, 36584
  ventricular assist device ~ 33981-33983
Replantation
  arm, upper ~ 20802
  digit ~ 20816-20822
  foot ~ 20838
  forearm ~ 20805
  hand ~ 20808
  penis ~ 54438
  thumb ~ 20824-20827
Report preparation
  extended, medical ~ 99080
  psychiatric ~ 90889
Reposition toe to hand ~ 26551-26556
Repositioning
  baroreflex activation device ~ 0266T-0271T
  central venous catheter ~ 36597
  electrode
   cardiac contractility modulation ~ 0415T
   heart ~ 33215, 33226
  gastrostomy tube ~ 43761
  heart, defibrillator leads ~ 33215-33216, 33226, 33249
  intraocular lens ~ 66825
  tricuspid valve ~ 33468
Reproductive tissue
  cryopreservation
   embryo(s) ~ 89258
   sperm ~ 89259
   testicular tissue ~ 89335
  thawing of cryopreserved
   embryo(s) ~ 89352
   oocytes, each aliquot ~ 89356
   sperm/semen ~ 89353
   testicular/ovarian tissue ~ 89354

Reproductive tissue ~ *continued*
storage
oocyte(s) ~ 89346
sperm/semen ~ 89343
testicular/ovarian ~ 89344
Reprogramming, shunt, brain ~ 62252
Reptilase test ~ 85635
Repilase time ~ see thrombin time
Resection
aortic valve, stenosis ~ 33415
bladder diverticulum ~ 52305
bladder neck, transurethral ~ 52500
brain lobe ~ see lobectomy, brain
chest wall ~ 21601-21603
clavicle, tumor ~ 23200
cricotracheal ~ 31592
diaphragm ~ 39560-39561
endaural ~ see ear, inner, excision
humeral head ~ 23195
intestines, small, laparoscopic ~ 44202-44203
lung ~ 32520-32525
mouth, with tongue excision ~ 41153
myocardium
aneurysm ~ 33542
septal defect ~ 33545
nasal septum submucous ~ see nasal septum, submucous resection
nose
septum ~ 30520
ovary, wedge ~ see ovary, wedge resection
palate ~ 42120
phalangeal head, toe ~ 28153
prostate transurethral ~ see prostatectomy, transurethral
radical
arm, upper ~ 24077, 24079
elbow ~ 24077, 24079
with contracture release ~ 24149
foot ~ 28046-28047
humerus ~ 24150
radius ~ 24152
tumor
ankle ~ 27615-27616
calcaneus or talus ~ 27647
clavicle ~ 23200
femur ~ 27329, 27364-27365
fibula ~ 27646
humerus ~ 23220
knee ~ 27329, 27364-27365
leg, lower ~ 27615-27616
leg, upper ~ 27329, 27364-27365
metatarsal ~ 28173
scapula ~ 23210
shoulder 23077-23078
tarsal ~ 28171
tibia ~ 27645
wrist ~ 25077-25078
temporal bone ~ 69535
trachea, cricotracheal ~ 31592
tumor
fallopian tube ~ 58957-58958
ovary ~ 58957-58958
peritoneum ~ 58957-58958
ulna, arthrodesis radioulnar joint ~ 25830
ureterocele
ectopic ~ 52301
orthotopic ~ 52300
vena cava, with reconstruction ~ 37799
Resonance spectroscopy, magnetic ~ see magnetic resonance spectroscopy
Respiration, positive-pressure ~ see pressure breathing, positive
Respiratory pattern recording, preventive, infant ~ 94772
Respiratory system, surgical procedures ~ 30000-32999
Respiratory syncytial virus (RSV)
antibody ~ 86756
antigen detection
direct fluorescence ~ 87280
direct optical observation ~ 87807
enzyme immunoassay ~ 87420
nucleic acid ~ 87631-87634
Response, auditory evoked ~ see auditory evoked potentials
Rest home visit ~ see domiciliary services

Resuscitation
cardiac ~ see cardiac massage
cardio-pulmonary ~ see cardio-pulmonary resuscitation (CPR)
newborn ~ 99465
Reticulocyte count ~ 85044-85045
Retina
diagnostic imaging
computerized scanning ~ 92134
electroretinography ~ 0509T, 92273, 92274
fluorescein angiography ~ 92235, 92242
ophthalmoscopy ~ 92201
imaging ~ 92227-92229
incision, encircling material ~ 67115
intr-ocular retinal electrode array
device evaluation ~ 0472T, 0473T
initial programming ~ 0472T
interrogation ~ 0472T, 0473T
lesion
extensive, destruction ~ 67227-67228
localized, destruction ~ 67208-67218
macular/fundus exam, dilated ~ 2019F-2021F
findings communicated for diabetes management ~ 5010F
optical coherence tomography (OCT), remote ~ 0604T-0606T
prophylaxis, retial detachment ~ 67141, 67145
prosthesis ~ 0100T
release, encircling material ~ 67115
removal, implanted material ~ 67120
repair
detachment ~ 67113
cryotherapy or diathermy ~ 67101
injection of air ~ 67110
photocoagulation ~ 67105
scleral dissection ~ 67107
with vitrectomy ~ 67108
prophylaxis, detachment ~ 67141-67145
retinopathy
destruction
cryotherapy, diathermy ~ 67227
detection ~ 92201
treatment
photocoagulation ~ 67228, 67229
Retinacular knee release ~ 27425
Retinopathy
destruction
cryotherapy, diathermy ~ 67227
detection ~ 92201, 92227-92229
macular degeneration ~ 2019F
monitoring ~ 92227-92229
treatment
photocoagulation, cryotherapy ~ 67228, 67229
Retraction, clot ~ see clot retraction
Retrieval transcatheter foreign body ~ 37197
Retrocaval ureter ureterolysis ~ 50725
Retrograde cholangiopancreatographies, endoscopic ~ see cholangiopancreatography
Retrograde cystourethrogram ~ see urethrocystography, retrograde
Retrograde pyelogram ~ see urography, retrograde
Retroperitoneal area
abscess, incision and drainage ~ 49060
biopsy ~ 49010
cyst, destruction/excision ~ 49203-49205, 58957, 58958
endometriomas, destruction/excision ~ 49203-49205, 58957, 58958
exploration ~ 49010
needle biopsy, mass ~ 49180
tumor, destruction/excision ~ 49203-49205, 58957, 58958
Retroperitoneal fibrosis ureterolysis ~ 50715
Retropubic prostatectomies ~ see prostatectomy, retropubic
Revascularization
distal upper extremity with interval ligation ~ 36838
endovascular
femoral ~ 37224-37227
iliac ~ 37220-37223
peroneal ~ 37228-37235
popliteal ~ 37224-37227
tibeal ~ 37228-37235
interval ligation distal upper extremity ~ 36838
penis ~ 37788
transmyocardial ~ 33140-33141
Reversal, vasectomy ~ see vasovasorrhaphy
Reverse T3 ~ see triiodothyronine, reverse
Reverse triiodothyronine ~ see triiodothyronine, reverse

Revision ~ see reconstruction
  aorta ~ 33404
  blepharoplasty ~ 15820-15823
  bronchial stent ~ 31638
  bronchus ~ 32501
  bypass graft, vein patch ~ 35685
  cervicoplasty ~ 15819
  colostomy ~ see colostomy, revision
  cornea
    prosthesis ~ 65770
    reshaping
      epikeratoplasty ~ 65767
      keratomileusis ~ 65760
      keratophakia ~ 65765
  defibrillator site, chest ~ 33223
  ear, middle ~ 69662
  external fixation system ~ 20693
  eye, aqueous shunt ~ 66185
  gastrostomy tube ~ 44373
  hip replacement ~ see replacement, hip, revision
  hymenal ring ~ 56700
  ileostomy ~ see ileostomy, revision
  infusion pump
    intra-arterial ~ 36261
    intravenous ~ 36576-36578, 36582-36583
  iris
    iridoplasty ~ 66762
    iridotomy ~ 66761
  jejunostomy tube ~ 44373
  lower extremity arterial bypass ~ 35879-35881
  pacemaker site, chest ~ 33222
  rhytidectomy ~ 15824-15829
  semicircular canal, fenestration ~ 69840
  shunt, intrahepatic portosystemic ~ 37183
  sling ~ 53442
  stapedectomy ~ see stapedectomy, revision
  stomach, for obesity ~ 43848
  tracheostomy, scar ~ 31830
  urinary-cutaneous anastomosis ~ 50727-50728
  vagina
    prosthetic graft ~ 57295-57296
    sling
      stress incontinence ~ 57287
  venous access device ~ 36576-36578, 36582-36583, 36585
  ventricle
    ventriculomyectomy ~ 33416
    ventriculomyotomy ~ 33416
Rheumatoid factor ~ 86430-86431
Rhinectomy
  partial ~ 30150
  total ~ 30160
Rhinomanometry ~ 92512
Rhinopharynx ~ see nasopharynx
Rhinophyma repair ~ 30120
Rhinoplasty
  cleft lip/cleft palate ~ 30460-30462
  primary ~ 30400-30420
  secondary ~ 30430-30450
Rhinoscopy ~ see endoscopy, nose
Rhinotomy lateral ~ 30118, 30320
Rhizotomy ~ 63185-63190
Rho variant du ~ 86905
Rhytidectomy ~ 15824-15829
Rhytidoplasties ~ see face lift
Rh (D) ~ see blood typing
Rh immune globulin ~ see immune globulins, Rho (D)
Rib
  cartilage, graft to face ~ 21230
  excision ~ 21600-21616, 32900
  fracture
    with internal fixation ~ 21811-21813
  resection ~ 21601-21603, 32900
  X-ray ~ 71100-71111
Riboflavin ~ 84252
Richardson operation hysterectomy ~ see hysterectomy, abdominal, total
Richardson procedure ~ 53460
Rickettsia antibody ~ 86757
Ridell operation ~ see sinusotomy, frontal
Ridge, alveolar ~ see alveolar ridge
Right atrioventricular valve ~ see tricuspid valve

Right heart cardiac catheterization ~ see cardiac catheterization, right heart
Ripstein operation ~ see proctopexy
Risk factor reduction intervention
  group ~ 99411, 99412
    diabetes prevention ~ 0403T
  individual ~ 99401-99404
    diabetes prevention ~ 0488T
Risser jacket ~ 29010-29015
  removal ~ 29710
Rocky mountain spotted fever ~ 86000
Roentgenographic ~ see X-ray
Roentgenography ~ see radiology, diagnostic
Roentgen rays ~ see X-ray
Ropes test ~ 83872
Rorschach test ~ 96100
Ross procedure ~ 33413
Rotation flap ~ see skin, adjacent tissue transfer
Rotator cuff repair ~ 23410-23420
Rotavirus
  antibody ~ 86759
  antigen detection, enzyme immunoassay ~ 87425
Rotavirus vaccine ~ 90680
Round window repair fistula ~ 69667
Round window fistula ~ see fistula, round window
Roux-en-y procedure ~ 43621, 43633-43634, 43644, 43846, 47740-47741, 47780-47785, 48540
Rpr ~ 86592-86593
RSV (respiratory syncytial virus)
  antibody ~ 86756
  antigen detection
    by direct fluorescence ~ 87280
    by direct optical observation ~ 87807
    by enzyme immunoassay ~ 87420
  immune globulins ~ 90378
RT3 ~ see triiodothyronine, reverse
Rubbing alcohol ~ see isopropyl alcohol
Rubella
  antibody ~ 86762
Rubella/mumps ~ see vaccines
Rubella HI test ~ see hemagglutination inhibition test
Rubeola
  antibody ~ 86765
  antigen detection, immunofluorescence ~ 87283
Rubeolla ~ see rubeola
Russell viper venom time ~ 85612-85613

S

Sac, endolymphatic ~ see endolymphatic sac
Saccomanno technique ~ 88108
Sacral nerve
  implantation, electrode ~ 64561, 64581
  insertion, electrode ~ 64561, 64581
Sacroiliac joint
  arthrodesis
    open ~ 27280
    percutaneous ~ 27279
  arthrotomy ~ 27050
  biopsy ~ 27050
  dislocation, open treatment ~ 27218
  fusion ~ 27280
  injection, anesthetic/steroid
    for arthrography ~ 27096
    nerves ~ 64451
  X-ray ~ 72200-72202
Sacrum
  augmentation
    percutaneous ~ 0200T-0201T
    with CT guidance ~ 72292
    with fluoroscopic guidance ~ 72291
  sacroplasty, percutaneous ~ 0200T-0201T
  tumor, excision ~ 49215
  X-ray ~ 72220
Salabrasion ~ 15810-15811
Salicylate assay ~ 80329-80331
Saline-solution abortion ~ see abortion, induced, by saline

Salivary duct
 catheterization ~ 42660
 dilation ~ 42650-42660
 ligation ~ 42665
 repair ~ 42500-42505
 fistula ~ 42600
Salivary gland virus ~ see Cytomegalovirus
Salivary glands
 abscess, incision and drainage ~ 42310-42320
 biopsy ~ 42405
 calculi (stone), excision ~ 42330-42340
 cyst
  creation, fistula ~ 42325-42326
  drainage ~ 42409
  excision ~ 42408
 injection, X-ray ~ 42550
 needle biopsy ~ 42400
 nuclear medicine
  function study ~ 78232
  imaging ~ 78230-78231
 parotid, abscess ~ 42300-42305
 unlisted services and procedures ~ 42699
 X-ray ~ 70380-70390
  with contrast ~ 70390
Salmonella antibody ~ 86768
Salpingectomy ~ 58262-58263, 58291-58292, 58552, 58554, 58661, 58700
 ectopic pregnancy
  laparoscopic treatment ~ 59151
  surgical treatment ~ 59120
 oophorectomy ~ 58943
Salpingo-oophorectomy ~ 58720
 laparoscopic ~ 58571, 58573, 58575
 resection ovarian malignancy ~ 58950-58956
 resection peritoneal malignancy ~ 58950-58956
 resection tubal malignancy ~ 58950-58956
Salpingohysterostomy ~ see implantation, tubouterine
Salpingolysis ~ 58740
Salpingoneostomy ~ 58673, 58770
Salplingoplasty ~ see fallopian tube, repair
Salpingostomy ~ 58673, 58770
 laparoscopic ~ 58673
Salter osteotomy of the pelvis ~ see osteotomy, pelvis
Sampling ~ see also biopsy; brush biopsy; needle biopsy
 blood
  arteial ~ 36620
  fetal scalp ~ 59030
  ocular ~ 0198T
  organ ~ 36500
  plasma ~ 78110, 78111
  red cell ~ 78120, 78121
  venous ~ 75893
 chorionic villus ~ 59015, 76945
 endometrium ~ 58100, 58558
 lymph node
  EBUS guided hilar ~ 31652, 31653
  para-aortic ~ 57109, 57531, 58200, 58210, 58548
  pelvic ~ 58200
  periaortic ~ 38572, 38573
  retroperitoneal ~ 38570
 stereotactic template guided ~ 55706
Sang-Park procedure ~ 33735-33737
Sao Paulo typhus ~ see Rocky Mountain spotted fever
SARS-CoV-2 (Severe Acute Respiratory Syndrome Coronavirus 2)
 antibody detection
  immunoassay, multiple-step ~ 86769
  immunoassay, single-step ~ 86328
 infectious agent detection, nucleic acid probe ~ 87635
 pathogen detection, pathogen-specific nucleic acid ~ 0202U
Saucerization
 calcaneus ~ 28120
 clavicle ~ 23180
 femur ~ 27070, 27360
 fibula ~ 27360, 27641
 hip ~ 27070
 humerus ~ 23184, 24140
 ileum ~ 27070
 metacarpal ~ 26230
 metatarsal ~ 28122
 olecranon process ~ 24147

Saucerization ~ *continued*
 phalanges, finger ~ 26235-26236
  toe ~ 28124
 pubis ~ 27070
 radius ~ 24145, 25151
 scapula ~ 23182
 talus ~ 28120
 tarsal ~ 28122
 tibia ~ 27360, 27640
 ulna ~ 24147, 25150
Saundby test ~ see blood, feces
Scabies ~ see tissue, examination for ectoparasites
Scalenotomy ~ see muscle division, scalenus anticus
Scalenus anticus division ~ 21700-21705
Scaling ~ see exfoliation
Scalp tumor resection, radical ~ 21015
Scalp blood sampling ~ 59030
Scan ~ see specific site, nuclear medicine
 abdomen ~ see abdomen, CT scan
 CT ~ see CT scan
 MRI ~ see magnetic resonance imaging
 PET ~ see positron emission tomography
 radionuclide ~ see emission computerized tomography
Scanning, radioisotope ~ see nuclear medicine
Scanogram ~ 77073
Scaphoid fracture
 closed treatment ~ 25622
 open treatment ~ 25628
 with manipulation ~ 25624
Scapula
 craterization ~ 23182
 cyst excision ~ 23140
  with allograft ~ 23146
  with autograft ~ 23145
 diaphysectomy ~ 23182
 excision ~ 23172, 23190
  partial ~ 23182
 fracture
  closed treatment
   with manipulation ~ 23575
   without manipulation ~ 23570
  open treatment ~ 23585
 ostectomy ~ 23190
 repair
  fixation ~ 23400
  scapulopexy ~ 23400
 saucerization ~ 23182
 sequestrectomy ~ 23172
 tumor
  excision ~ 23140, 23210
   with allograft ~ 23146
   with autograft ~ 23145
  radical resection ~ 23210
 X-ray ~ 73010
Scapulopexy ~ 23400
Scarification pleural ~ 32215
Scarification of pleura ~ see pleurodesis
Schanz operation ~ see femur, osteotomy
Schauta operation ~ see hysterectomy, vaginal, radical
Schede procedure ~ 32905-32906
Scheie procedure ~ see iridectomy
Schlatter operation total gastrectomy ~ see excision, stomach, total
Schlicter test ~ (bactericidal titer, serum) 87197
Schocket procedure ~ (aqueous shunt) 66180
Schonbein test ~ see blood, feces
Schuchard procedure osteotomy, maxilla ~ 21206
Schwannoma, acoustic ~ see brain, tumor, excision
Sciatic nerve
 decompression ~ 64712
 injection, anesthetic ~ 64445-64446
 lesion, excision ~ 64786
 neuroma, excision ~ 64786
 neuroplasty ~ 64712
 release ~ 64712
 repair/suture ~ 64858
Scintigraphy ~ see nuclear medicine
 computed tomographic ~ see emission computerized tomography
Scissoring skin tags ~ 11200-11201

Sclera
aqueous drainage device
to extraocular reservoir ~ 66179, 66180
without extraocular reservoir ~ 66183, 0376T
diagnostic imaging
ophthalmoscopy ~ 92201
excision, sclerectomy with punch or scissors ~ 66160
fistulization
sclerectomy with punch or scissors with iridectomy ~ 66160
thermocauterization with iridectomy ~ 66155
trabeculectomy ab externo in absence of previous surgery ~ 66170
trephination with iridectomy ~ 66150
incision, fistulization
sclerectomy with punch or scissors with iridectomy ~ 66160
thermocauterization with iridectomy ~ 66155
trabeculectomy ab externo in absence of previous surgery ~ 66170
trephination with iridectomy ~ 66150
lesion, excision ~ 66130
repair
reinforcement
with graft ~ 67255
without graft ~ 67250
staphyloma ~ 66225
with glue ~ 65286
wound
operative ~ 66250
tissue glue ~ 65286
Scleral buckling operation ~ see retina, repair, detachment
Scleral ectasia ~ see staphyloma, sclera
Sclerectomy ~ 66160
Sclerotherapy
esophageal varices ~ 43204, 43243
fluid collection ~ 49185
gastric varices ~ 43243
hemorrhoids ~ 46500
perirectal ~ 45520
venous ~ 36465, 36466, 36468, 36470, 36471
Sclerotomy ~ see incision, sclera
Screening
for abdominal aortic aneurysm (AAA) ultrasound ~ 76706
alcohol and/or substance abuse ~ 99408, 99409
audiology
Bekesy audiometry ~ 92560
evoked otoacoustic emissions ~ 92558
colonography CT ~ 74263
development tests ~ 96110
drug ~ see drug screen
ocular ~ 99174, 99177
oncology
colorectal DNA testing ~ 81528
for lung cancer, CT scan ~ 71271
ophthalamology, suprathreshold ~ 92082
visual acuity ~ 99173
visual function ~ 99173
Scribner cannulization ~ 36810
Scrotal varices ~ see varicocele
Scrotoplasty ~ 55175-55180
Scrotum
abscess, incision and drainage ~ 54700, 55100
excision ~ 55150
exploration ~ 55110
hematoma, incision and drainage ~ 54700
removal, foreign body ~ 55120
repair ~ 55175-55180
ultrasound ~ 76870
unlisted services and procedures ~ 55899
Scrub typhus ~ 86000
Second look surgery ~ see reoperation
Second opinion ~ see confirmatory consultations
Section ~ see also decompression
cesarean ~ see cesarean delivery
cranial nerve ~ 61460
spinal access ~ 63191
gasserian ganglion, sensory root ~ 61450
medullary tract ~ 61470
nerve root ~ 63185-63190
spinal accessory nerve ~ 63191
spinal cord tract ~ 63194-63199
vestibular nerve
transcranial approach ~ 69950
translabyrinthine approach ~ 69915

Sedation
moderate ~ 99151-99153, 99155-99157
with independent observation ~ 99151-99153
Seddon-Brookes procedure ~ 24320
Sedimentation rate
blood cell
automated ~ 85652
manual ~ 85651
Segmentectomy
breast ~ 19301-19302
lung ~ 32484
Seidlitz powder test ~ see X-ray, with contrast
Selective cellular enhancement technique ~ 88112
Selenium ~ 84255
Self care ~ see physical medicine/therapy/occupational therapy
training ~ 97535, 99509
Sella turcica
CT scan ~ 70480-70482
X-ray ~ 70240
Semen ~ see sperm
Semen analysis ~ 89300-89322
sperm analysis ~ 89331
antibodies ~ 89325
with sperm isolation ~ 89260-89261
Semenogelase ~ see antigen, prostate specific
Semilunar bone ~ see lunate
ganglion ~ see gasserian ganglion
Seminal vesicle(s)
cyst, excision ~ 55680
excision ~ 55650
incision ~ 55600-55605
mullerian duct, excision ~ 55680
unlisted services and procedures ~ 55899
vesiculography ~ 74440
X-ray with contrast ~ 74440
Seminin ~ see antigen, prostate specific
Semiquantitative ~ 81005
Sengstaaken tamponade esophagus ~ 43460
Senning procedure ~ (repair/revision, great arteries) 33774-33777
Senning type ~ 33774-33777
Sensitivity study
antibiotic
agar ~ 87181
disc ~ 87184
enzyme detection ~ 87185
macrobroth ~ 87188
MIC (minimum inhibitory concentration) ~ 87186
microtiter ~ 87186
MLC (minimum lethal concentration) ~ 87187
mycobacteria ~ 87190
antiviral drugs, HIV-1, tissue culture ~ 87904
Sensor, fetal oximetry
cervix ~ 0021T
vagina ~ 0021T
Sensorimotor exam ~ 92060
Sensory nerve common, repair/suture ~ 64834
Sentinel node injection procedure ~ 38792
Separation, craniofacial
closed treatment ~ 21431
open treatment ~ 21432-21436
Septal defect
repair ~ 33813-33814
ventricular
closure ~ 33675-33688
open ~ 33675-33688
Septectomy
atrial ~ 33735-33737
closed ~ see septostomy, atrial
submucous nasal ~ see nasal septum, submucous resection
Septic abortion ~ see abortion, septic
Septoplasty ~ 30520
Septostomy, atrial
balloon (Rashkind type) ~ 33741
blade method (Park) ~ 33741
Blalock-Hanlon type ~ 33735
open heart ~ 33736, 33737
transcatheter, for congenital anomaly ~ 33741
Septum, nasal ~ see nasal septum

Sequestrectomy
  carpal ~ 25145
  clavicle ~ 23170
  humeral head ~ 23174
  humerus ~ 24134
  olecranon process ~ 24138
  radius ~ 24136, 25145
  scapula ~ 23172
  skull ~ 61501
  ulna ~ 24138, 25145
Serialography aorta ~ 75625
Serodiagnosis, syphilis ~ see serologic test for syphilis
Serologic test for syphilis ~ 86592-86593
Seroma incision and drainage, skin ~ 10140
Serotonin ~ 84260
Serum
  albumin ~ see albumin, serum
  antibody identification, pretreatment ~ 86975-86978
  CPK ~ see creatine kinase, total
  serum immune globulin ~ 90281-90283
Sesamoid bone
  finger, excision ~ 26185
  foot
    excision ~ 28292, 28295-28299
    fracture ~ 28530-28531
  thumb, excision ~ 26185
  toe, excision ~ 28315
Sesamoidectomy
  finger ~ 26185
  foot ~ 28292, 28295-28299
  thumb ~ 26185
  toe ~ 28315
Sever procedure ~ see contracture, palm, release
Severe Acute Respiratory Syndrome Coronavirus 2 (SARS-CoV-2)
  antibody detection
    immunoassay, multiple-step ~ 86769
    immunoassay, single-step ~ 86328
  infectious agent detection, nucleic acid probe ~ 87635
  pathogen detection, pathogen-specific nucleic acid ~ 0202U
Severing of blepharorrhaphy ~ see tarsorrhaphy, severing
Sex change operation
  female to male ~ 55980
  male to female ~ 55970
Sex chromatin identification ~ 88130-88140
Sex hormone binding globulin ~ 84270
Sex-linked ichthyoses ~ see syphilis test
SGOT ~ 84450
SGPT ~ 84460
Shaving skin lesion ~ 11300-11313
SHBG (sex hormone binding globulin) ~ 84270
Shelf procedure ~ (see also osteotomy, hip) 27146-27151
Shiga-like toxin antigen detection, enzyme immunoassay ~ 87427
Shigella antibody ~ 86771
Shirodkar operation ~ (repair, cervix, cerclage, abdominal) 57700
Shock wave (extracorporeal) therapy ~ 0020T
Shock wave, lithotripsy ~ 50590
Shock wave, ultrasonic ~ see ultrasound
Shop typhus of Malaya ~ see Murine typhus
Shoulder ~ see also clavicle; scapula
  abscess, drainage ~ 23030
  amputation ~ 23900-23921
  arthrocentesis ~ 20610
  arthrodesis ~ 23800
    with autogenous graft ~ 23802
  arthrography, injection, radiologic ~ 23350
  arthroscopy
    diagnostic ~ 29805
    surgical ~ 29806-29828
      biceps tenodesis ~ 29828
  arthrotomy, with removal loose or foreign body ~ 23107
  biopsy
    deep ~ 23066
    soft tissue ~ 23065
  blade ~ see scapula
  bone
    excision
      acromion ~ 23130
      clavicle ~ 23120-23125
    incision ~ 23035
    tumor, excision ~ 23140-23146

Shoulder ~ *continued*
  bursa, drainage ~ 23031
  capsular contracture release ~ 23020
  cast
    figure eight ~ 29049
    removal ~ 29710
    spica ~ 29055
    velpeau ~ 29058
  disarticulation ~ 23920-23921
  dislocation, closed treatment, with manipulation ~ 23650-23655
  exploration ~ 23107
  hematoma, drainage ~ 23030
  manipulation, application of fixation apparatus ~ 23700
  prophylactic treatment ~ 23490-23491
  radical resection ~ 23077
  removal
    calcareous deposits ~ 23000
    cast ~ 29710
    foreign body
      intramuscular ~ 23333
      subcutaneous ~ 23330
    foreign or loose body ~ 23107
  repair
    capsule ~ 23450-23466
    ligament release ~ 23415
    muscle transfer ~ 23395-23397
    rotator cuff ~ 23410-23420
    tendon ~ 23410-23412, 23430-23440
    tenomyotomy ~ 23405-23406
  strapping ~ 29240
  surgery, unlisted services and procedures ~ 23929
  tumor, excision ~ 23071-23078
  unlisted services and procedures ~ 23929
  X-ray ~ 73020-73030
  X-ray with contrast ~ 73040
Shoulder joint ~ see also clavicle; scapula
  arthroplasty, with implant ~ 23470-23472
  arthrotomy
    with biopsy ~ 23100-23101
    with synovectomy ~ 23105-23106
  dislocation
    with greater tuberosity fracture
      closed treatment ~ 23665
      open treatment ~ 23670
    open treatment ~ 23660
    with surgical or anatomical neck fracture
      closed treatment with manipulation ~ 23675
      open treatment ~ 23680
  excision, torn cartilage ~ 23101
  exploration ~ 23040-23044
  incision and drainage ~ 23040-23044
  removal, foreign body ~ 23040-23044
  X-ray ~ 73050
Shunt(s)
  aqueous
    to extraocular reservoir ~ 66179, 66180
      revision ~ 66184, 66185
    without extraocular reservoir ~ 0376T, 66183
  arteriovenous ~ see arteriovenous shunt
  atria, interatrial septal shunt device ~ 0613T
  brain
    creation ~ 62180-62223
    removal ~ 62256-62258
    replacement ~ 62160, 62194, 62225-62230, 62258
    reprogramming ~ 62252
  cerebrospinal fluid ~ see cerebrospinal fluid shunt
  creation
    arteriovenous
      direct ~ 36821
      Thomas shunt ~ 36835
      transposition ~ 36818-36820
      with bypass graft ~ 35686
      with graft ~ 36825-36830
    cerebrospinal fluid ~ 62200
    Thomas shunt ~ 36835
    transcatheter intracardiac shunt (TIS) ~ 33745, 33746
  fetal ~ 59076

Shunt(s) ~ *continued*
  great vessel
    aorta to pulmonary artery, ascending ~ 33755
      descending ~ 33762
    central ~ 33764
    subclavian pulmonary artery ~ 33750
    systemic to pulmonary ~ 33924
    vena cava to pulmonary artery ~ 33766-33767
  intra-atrial ~ 33735-33737
  Levenn
    insertion ~ 49425
    patency test ~ 78291
    revision ~ 49426
  nonvascular, X-ray ~ 75809
  peritoneal, venous
    injection ~ 49427
    ligation ~ 49428
    removal ~ 49429
  peritoneal X-ray ~ 75809
  pulmonary artery
    from aorta ~ 33755-33762, 33924
    subclavian ~ 33750
    from vena cava ~ 33766-33767
  revision, arteriovenous ~ 36832
  spinal cord
    creation ~ 63740-63741
    irrigation ~ 63744
    removal ~ 63746
    replacement ~ 63744
  superior mesenteric-caval ~ see anastomosis, caval to mesenteric
  ureter to colon ~ 50815
  ventriculocisternal with valve ~ (ventriculocisternostomy) 62180, 62200, 62201
Shuntogram ~ 75809
Sialic acid ~ 84275
Sialodochoplasty ~ 42500-42505
Sialogram ~ see sialography
Sialography ~ 70390
Sickling electrophoresis ~ 83020
Siderocytes ~ 85536
Siderophilin ~ see transferrin
Sigmoid ~ see colon-sigmoid
Sigmoid bladder cystectomy ~ 51590
Sigmoidoscopy
  ablation
    polyp ~ 45346
    tumor ~ 45346
  biopsy ~ 45331
  collection, specimen ~ 45331
  exploration ~ 45330, 45335
  hemorrhage control ~ 45334
  injection, submucosal ~ 45335
  needle biopsy ~ 45342
  placement, stent ~ 45347
  removal
    foreign body ~ 45332
    polyp ~ 45333, 45338
    tumor ~ 45333, 45338
  repair, volvulus ~ 45337
  ultrasound ~ 45341-45342
Signal-averaged electrocardiography ~ see electrocardiogram
Silica ~ 84285
Silicon dioxide ~ see silica
Silicone contouring injections ~ 11950-11954
Silver operation ~ see Keller procedure
Simple mastectomies ~ see mastectomy
Single photon absorptiometry ~ see absorptiometry, single photon
Single photon emission computed tomography (SPECT) ~ *see also*
  emission computed tomography
  bone ~ 78803
  brain imaging ~ 78803
  cerebrospinal fluid ~ 78803
  heart
    blood pool imaging ~ 78494
    myocardial imaging ~ 78469, 0332T
    perfusion imaging ~ 78451-78454
  kidney ~ 78803
  liver ~ 78803
  tumor localization ~ 78803

Sinus
  ethmoidectomy, excision ~ 31254
  pilonidal ~ see cyst, pilonidal
Sinus of valsalva repair ~ 33702-33722
Sinus venosus repair ~ 33645
Sinusectomy, ethmoid ~ see ethmoidectomy
Sinuses
  cranial
    decompression ~ 61595
    excision of lesion ~ 61607
    ligation ~ 61598
    resection ~ 61591
  dilation ~ 31295-31297
  endoscopy, nasal
    biopsy ~ 31237
    debridement ~ 31237
    decompression ~ 31292-31294
    diagnostic ~ 31231, 31233, 31235
    dilation ~ 31295-31297
    exploration ~ 31276
    hemorrhage control ~ 31238
    polypectomy ~ 31237
    surgical ~ 31237-31241, 31253-31257, 31259, 31267, 31276, 31287, 31288, 31290-31298
  ethmoid
    drug-eluting implant placement ~ 0406T, 0407T
    excision ~ 31200-31205
      with nasal/sinus endoscopy ~ 31254-31255
    repair of cerebrospinal leak ~ 31290
  frontal
    destruction ~ 31080-31085
    exploration ~ 31070-31075
      with nasal/sinus endoscopy ~ 31276
    fracture, open treatment ~ 21343-21344
    incision ~ 31070-31087
  injection ~ 20500
    diagnostic ~ 20501
  maxillary
    antrostomy ~ 31256-31267
    excision ~ 31225-31230
    exploration ~ 31020-31032
      with nasal/sinus endoscopy ~ 31233
    incision ~ 31020-31032, 31256-31267
    irrigation ~ 31000
    skull base ~ 61581
    surgery ~ 61581
  multiple
    incision ~ 31090
    paranasal, incision ~ 31090
  nasal endoscopy
    diagnostic ~ 31231, 31233, 31235
    surgical ~ 31237-31241, 31253-31257, 31259, 31267, 31276, 31287, 31288, 31290-31298
  sphenoid
    biopsy ~ 31050, 31051
    dilation ~ 31295-31298
    exploration ~ 31050, 31051
      with nasal/sinus endoscopy ~ 31235, 31253
    incision ~ 31050, 31051
      with nasal/sinus endoscopy ~ 31257, 31259, 31287, 31288
    irrigation ~ 31002
    repair of cerebrospinal leak ~ 31291
    sinusotomy ~ 31050-31051
    skull base surgery ~ 61580-61581
  unlisted services and procedures ~ 31299
  X-ray ~ 70210-70220
Sinusoidal rotational testing ~ see ear, nose and throat
Sinusoscopy
  maxillary sinus ~ 31233
  sphenoid sinus ~ 31235
Sinusotomy ~ see also sinus, multiple
  combined ~ 31090
  frontal sinus
    exploratory ~ 31070-31075
    nonobliterative ~ 31086-31087
    obliterative ~ 31080-31085
  maxillary ~ 31020-31032
  multiple, paranasal ~ 31090
  sphenoid sinus ~ 31050-31051
Sisi test ~ 92564
Sistrunk operation ~ see cyst, thyroid gland, excision

Six-minute walk test ~ 94618
Size reduction, breast ~ see breast, reduction
Skeletal fixation humeral epicondyle, percutaneous ~ 24566
Skeletal traction, insertion/removal pin/wire ~ 20650
Skene's gland abscess
  destruction ~ 53270
  excision ~ 53270
  incision and drainage ~ 53060
Skilled nursing facilities (SNF) services
  initial care ~ 99304-99306
  discharge services ~ 99315-99316
  other services ~ 99318
  subsequent care ~ 99307-99310
Skin
  abrasion ~ 15786-15787
    chemical peel ~ 15788-15793
    dermabrasion ~ 15780-15783
    salabrasion ~ 15810-15811
  abscess ~ see abscess, skin
  adjacent tissue transfer ~ 14000-14350
  autograft ~ see autograft, skin
  chemical exfoliation ~ 17360
  complete physical examination ~ 2029F
  cyst ~ see cyst, skin
  debridement ~ 11000-11006, 11010-11047
    eczematous ~ 11000-11001
    infected ~ 11000-11006
    subcutaneous tissue ~ 11042, 11045
      infected ~ 11004-11006
    with open fracture and/or dislocation ~ 11010-11012
  decubitus ulcer(s) ~ see pressure ulcer (decubitus)
  desquamation ~ see exfoliation
  destruction
    benign lesions
      fifteen or more lesions ~ 17004
      first lesion ~ 17000
      two-fourteen lesions ~ 17003
    flat warts ~ 17110-17111
    lesions ~ 17106-17108
    malignant lesions ~ 17260-17286
      by photodynamic therapy ~ 96567
    premalignant lesions
      by photodynamic therapy ~ 96567, 96573, 96574
      fifteen or more lesions ~ 17004
      first lesion ~ 17000
      two-fourteen lesions ~ 17003
  excision
    debridement ~ 11000-11006, 11010-11047
    excess skin ~ 15830-15839, 15847
    hemangioma ~ 11400-11446
    lesion
      benign ~ 11400-11446
      malignant ~ 11600-11646
  expanders
    breast ~ 19357
    removal ~ 11971
    replacement with implant ~ 11970
  fasciocutaneous flaps ~ 15730, 15731, 15733, 15734, 15736, 15738
  grafts
    free ~ 15050-15157, 15200-15261, 15757
    harvesting, for tissue culture ~ 15040
    skin substitute graft ~ 15271-15278
  homografts ~ see homograft, skin
  incision and drainage ~ see incision, skin ~ 10040-10180
  lesion ~ see lesion; tumor
    verrucous ~ see warts
  muscle flaps ~ 15731-15738
  myocutaneous flaps ~ 15731-15738
  nevi
    history ~ 1050F
    patient self-examination counseling ~ 5005F
  nose, surgical planing ~ 30120
  paring ~ 11055-11057
  photography, diagnostic ~ 96904
  removal, skin tags ~ 11200-11201
  revision
    blepharoplasty ~ 15820-15823
    cervicoplasty ~ 15819
    rhytidectomy ~ 15824-15829
  shaving ~ 11300-11313

Skin ~ *continued*
  tags, removal ~ 11200-11201
  tests ~ see allergy tests
    candida ~ 86485
    coccidioidomycosis ~ 86490
    histoplasmosis ~ 86510
    other antigen ~ 86486
    tuberculosis ~ 86580
  unlisted services and procedures ~ 17999
  wound repair
    complex ~ 13100-13160
    intermediate ~ 12031-12057
    simple ~ 12001-12021
Skin graft and flap
  composite graft ~ 15760-15770
  cross finger flap ~ 15574
  delay ~ 15600-15630
  delay of flap ~ 15600-15630
  derma-fat-fascia ~ 15570
  dermal autograft ~ 15130-15136
  epidermal autograft ~ 15110-15116
  fascial, free ~ 15758
  fasciocutaneous ~ 15733, 15734, 15736, 15738
  fillet flap, finger or toe ~ 14350
  formation ~ 15570-15576
  free, microvascular anastomosis ~ 15756-15758
  free skin graft, full thickness ~ 15200-15261
  island pedicle flap ~ 15740
  muscle ~ 15733, 15734, 15736, 15738, 15842
    free ~ 15756
  myocutaneous ~ 15731, 15733, 15734, 15736, 15756
  pedicle flap
    formation ~ 15570-15576
    island ~ 15740
    neurovascular ~ 15750
    transfer ~ 15650
  pinch graft ~ 15050
  platysmal ~ 15825
  punch graft ~ 15775-15776
  punch graft for hair transplant ~ 15775-15776
  recipient site preparation ~ 15002-15005
  skin
    autograft ~ 15150-15157, 15769
    free ~ 15757
    substitute graft ~ 15271-15278
  split graft ~ 15100-15101, 15120-15121
  superficial musculoaponeurotic system ~ 15829
  tissue transfer ~ 14000-14350
  tissue-cultured ~ 15040, 15150-15157
  transfer ~ 15650
  vascular flow check ~ 15860
  zygomaticofacial flap ~ 15730
Skull
  burr hole
    biopsy brain ~ 61140
    drainage
      abscess ~ 61150-61151
      cyst ~ 61150-61151
      hematoma ~ 61154-61156
    exploration
      infratentorial ~ 61253
      supratentorial ~ 61250
    insertion
      catheter ~ 61210
      EEG electrode ~ 61210
      reservoir ~ 61210
    intracranial, biopsy ~ 61140
    with injection ~ 61120
  decompression ~ 61322-61323, 61340-61345
    orbit ~ 61330
  drill hole
    catheter ~ 61107
    drainage hematoma ~ 61108
    exploration ~ 61105
  excision ~ 61501
  exploration, drill hole ~ 61105
  fracture ~ 62000-62010
  ematoma, drainage ~ 61108
  incision, suture ~ 61550-61552
  insertion, catheter ~ 61107

Skull ~ *continued*
  lesion, excision ~ 61500, 61600-61608, 61615-61616
  orbit
    excision, lesion ~ 61333
  puncture
    cervical ~ 61050
    cisternal ~ 61050
    drain fluid ~ 61070
    injection ~ 61070
    subdural ~ 61000-61001
    ventricular fluid ~ 61020
  reconstruction ~ 21172-21180
    defect ~ 62140-62141, 62145
  reduction, craniomegalic ~ 62115-62117
  removal
    plate ~ 62142
    prosthesis ~ 62142
  repair
    cerebrospinal fluid leak ~ 62100
    encephalocele ~ 62120
  replacement
    plate ~ 62143
    prosthesis ~ 62143
  stereotactic navigational procedure ~ 61781-61783
  tumor, excision ~ 61500
  X-ray ~ 70250-70260
Skull base surgery
  anterior cranial fossa
    bicoronal approach ~ 61586
    craniofacial approach ~ 61580-61583
    extradural ~ 61600-61601
    Lefort 1 osteotomy approach ~ 61586
    orbitocranial approach ~ 61584-61585
    transzygomatic approach ~ 61586
  carotid aneurysm ~ 61613
  carotid artery
    transection/ligation ~ 61611
  craniotomy ~ 62121
  dura, repair of cerebrospinal fluid leak ~ 61618-61619
  middle cranial fossa
    extradural ~ 61605, 61607
    infratemporal approach ~ 61590-61591
    intradural ~ 61606, 61608
  orbitocranial zygomatic approach ~ 61592
  posterior cranial fossa
    extradural ~ 61615
    intradural ~ 61616
    transcondylar approach ~ 61596-61597
    transpetrosal approach ~ 61598
    transtemporal approach ~ 61595
Sleep study ~ 95800-95801, 95806-95807
  actigraphy ~ 95803
  latency testing ~ 95805
  polysomnography ~ 95808-95811
Sliding inlay graft, tibia ~ see ankle; tibia, repair
Sling operation
  incontinence ~ 53440
    removal ~ 53442
  stress incontinence ~ 51992, 57287
  vagina ~ 57287-57288
Small bowel ~ see intestines, small
  neoplasm ~ see tumor, intestines, small
Smas flap ~ 15829
Smear cervical ~ see cervical smears
  Papanicolaou ~ see Pap smears
Smear and stain ~ see also cytopathology, smears
  cornea ~ 65430
  fluorescent ~ 87206
  gram or giesma ~ 87205
  ova, parasites ~ 87177
  parasites ~ 87207
  wet mount ~ 87210
Smith fracture ~ 25600-25605
Smith-Robinson operation ~ see arthrodesis, vertebra
Smithwick operation ~ see excision, nerve, sympathetic
SO4 ~ see sulfate
Soave procedure ~ 45120
Sodium ~ 84295, 84302
  urine ~ 84300

Sodium glycinate, theophylline ~ see theophylline
Sofield procedure ~ 24410
Soft tissue ~ see tissue, soft
Solar plexus ~ see celiac plexus
Solitary cyst ~ see bone, cyst
Somatomammotropin, chorionic ~ 83632
Somatomedin ~ 84305
Somatosensory testing
  lower limbs ~ 95926
  trunk or head ~ 95927
  upper limbs ~ 95925
Somatostatin ~ 84307
Somatotropin ~ 83003
Somatotropin release inhibiting hormone ~ see somatostatin
Somatropin ~ see growth hormone, human
Somnographies ~ see polysomnography
Somophyllin T ~ see theophylline
Sonography ~ see echography
Sonohysterography ~ 76831
  saline infusion, injection procedure ~ 58340
Sore, bed ~ see pressure ulcer (decubitus)
Spasm eyelid ~ see blepharospasm
Special services, procedures and reports ~ 99000-99091
  after hours medical services ~ 99050
  analysis, remote physiologic data ~ 99091
  computer data analysis ~ 99090
  device handling ~ 99002
  emergency care in office ~ 99058
  emergency care out of office ~ 99060
  extended hours, medical services ~ 99051-99053
  group education ~ 99078
    self-management ~ 98961-98962
  hyperbaric oxygen ~ 99183
  individual education, self management ~ 98960
  medical testimony ~ 99075
  non-office medical services ~ 99056
  on call services ~ 99026-99027
  phlebotomy ~ 99199
  post-op visit ~ 99024
  pump services ~ 99190-99192
  reports and forms
    medical, extended ~ 99080
    psychiatric ~ 90889
  specimen handling ~ 99000-99001
  supply of materials ~ 99070
    educational ~ 99071
  unlisted services and procedures ~ 99199
  unusual travel ~ 99082
Specific gravity body fluid ~ 84315
Specimen concentration ~ 87015
Specimen handling ~ 99000-99001
SPECT
  bone ~ 78803
  brain imaging ~ 78803
  cerebrospinal fluid ~ 78803
  heart
    blood pool imaging ~ 78494
    myocardial imaging ~ 78469
      sympathetic innervation ~ 0332T
    perfusion imaging ~ 78451, 78452
      multiple ~ 78452, 78454
      single ~ 78451, 78453
  kidney ~ 78803
  liver ~ 78803
  localization
    inflammatory process ~ 78803
    parathyroid gland ~78072
    tumor ~ 78803
  parathyroid gland ~ 78071, 78072
  tumor localization ~ 78803
Spectacle services
  fitting
    low vision aid ~ 92354-92355
    spectacle prosthesis ~ 92352-92353
    spectacles ~ 92340-92342
  repair ~ 92370-92371
Spectrometry, mass
  analyte ~ 83789
Spectrophotometry ~ 84311
  atomic absorption ~ see atomic absorption spectroscopy

Spectroscopy
atomic absorption ~ 82190
bioimpedance spectroscopy (BIS) ~ 93702
fluorescent
advanced glycation endproducts (AGE) ~ 88749
real-time spectral analysis, prostate tissue ~ 0443T
infrared ~ 82365
magnetic resonance ~ 76390
lipoprotein ~ 83704
near infrared wound study ~ 0493T
radiofrequency, intraoperative ~ 0546T
Spectrum analyses ~ see spectrophotometry
Speech evaluation
behavioral and qualitative analysis ~ 92524
cine ~ 70371
comprehension ~ 92523
expression ~ 92523
fluency ~ 92521
for prosthesis ~ 92597, 92607-92608
sound production ~ 92522, 92523
video ~ 70371
Speech prosthesis ~ 21084, 92609
creation ~ 31611
evaluation for speech ~ 92597, 92607-92608
insertion ~ 31611
Speech therapy ~ 92507-92508
Sperm
cryopreservation ~ 89259
evaluation ~ 89329-89331
storage ~ 89343
thawing ~ 89353
washing ~ 58323
Sperm analysis
antibodies ~ 89325
cervical mucus penetration test ~ 89330
count ~ 89310, 89320, 89322
forensic ~ 88125
hamster penetration test ~ 89329
hyaluron binding assay ~ 89398
identification, aspiration ~ 89257
from testis tissue ~ 89264
isolation ~ 89260-89261
motility ~ 89300, 89310, 89320-89322
Sperm evaluation, cervical mucus penetration test ~ see Huhner test
Spermatic cord
hydrocele, excision ~ 55500
laparoscopy ~ 55559
lesion, excision ~ 55520
repair, veins ~ 55530-55540
abdominal approach ~ 55535
with hernia repair ~ 55540
varicocele, excision ~ 55530-55540
Spermatic veins
excision ~ 55530-55540
ligation ~ 55550
Spermatocele excision ~ 54840
Spermatocystectomy ~ (spermatocele excision) 54840
Sphenoid sinus ~ see sinuses, sphenoid
Sphenoidotomy excision, with nasal/sinus endoscopy ~ 31287-31288
Sphenopalatine ganglion injection, anesthetic ~ 64505
Sphincter ~ see specific sphincter
anal ~ see anal sphincter
artificial genitourinary ~ see prosthesis, urethral sphincter
pyloric ~ see pyloric sphincter
Sphincter of Oddi
dilation ~ 47542
excision ~ 43262
pressure measurement, endoscopy ~ 43263
Sphincteroplasty
ampulla of vater ~ 47542
anal ~ 46750-46751, 46760-46761
bile duct ~ 47460
bladder neck ~ see bladder, repair, neck
Sphincterotomy ~ 52277
anal ~ 46080
bile duct ~ 47460
Spica cast
hip ~ 29305-29325
repair ~ 29720
shoulder ~ 29055

Spinal accessory nerve
anastomosis to facial nerve ~ 64866
incision ~ 63191
section ~ 63191
Spinal column ~ see spine
Spinal cord ~ see also cauda equina; nerve root
biopsy ~ 63275-63290
cyst
aspiration ~ 62268
incision and drainage ~ 63172-63173
decompression ~ 63001-63003, 63055-63057, 63064, 63066, 63101-63103, 62380, 0274T, 0275T
with cervical laminoplasty ~ 63050, 63051
with craniectomy ~ 61343
with discectomy ~ 62380
with facetectomy ~ 62380
with foreaminotomy ~ 0202T, 62380
with laminotomy ~ 62380
drain fluid ~ 62272
exploration ~ 63001-63044
graft, dura ~ 63710
implantation
electrode ~ 63650-63655
pulse generator ~ 63685
receiver ~ 63685
incision ~ 63200
tract ~ 63170, 63194-63199
injection
anesthetic ~ 62320-62327
blood ~ 62273
CT scan ~ 62284
neurolytic agent ~ 62280-62282
other ~ 62320-62327
X-ray ~ 62284
insertion
electrode ~ 63650-63655
pulse generator ~ 63685
receiver ~ 63685
lesion
destruction ~ 62280-62282
excision ~ 63265-63273, 63300-63308
needle biopsy ~ 62269
neoplasm, excision ~ 63275-63290
neurostimulator pulse generator system, electronic analysis ~ 95972
puncture (tap)
diagnostic ~ 62270, 62328
drain fluid ~ 62272, 62329
lumbar ~ 62270, 62328
release ~ 63200
reconstruction, dorsal spine elements ~ 63295
removal
catheter ~ 62355
electrode ~ 63661-63664
pulse generator ~ 63688
pump ~ 62365
receiver ~ 63688
reservoir ~ 62365
repair
cerebrospinal fluid leak ~ 63707-63709
meningocele ~ 63700-63702
myelomeningocele ~ 63704-63706
section
tract ~ 63194-63199
shunt
create ~ 63740-63741
irrigation ~ 63744
removal ~ 63746
replacement ~ 63744
stereotaxis
creation lesion ~ 63600
stimulation ~ 63610
syrinx, aspiration ~ 62268
tumor, excision ~ 63275-63290
Spinal fluid ~ see cerebrospinal fluid
Spinal fracture ~ see fracture, vertebra
Spinal instrumentation
anterior ~ 22845-22847
removal ~ 22855
biomechanical device ~ 22853, 22854, 22859
Harrington rod technique ~ 22840, 22850

Spinal instrumentation ~ *continued*
  internal fixation ~ 22841
  pelvic fixation ~ 22848
  posterior nonsegmental ~ 22840
    removal ~ 22850
  posterior segmental ~ 22842-22844
    removal ~ 22852
  reinsertion of spinal fixation device ~ 22849
Spinal manipulation ~ see manipulation, chiropractic
Spinal nerve
  avulsion ~ 64772
  decompression, root ~ 62380
  transection ~ 64772
Spinal tap ~ see cervical puncture; cisternal puncture; subdural tap;
    ventricular puncture
  drainage fluid ~ 62272, 62329
  lumbar ~ 62270, 62328
Spine ~ see also spinal cord; vertebra; vertebral body; vertebral process
  allograft
    morselized ~ 20930
    structural ~ 20931
  arthroplasty, lumbar ~ 22856-22865
  aspiration ~ 62267
  autograft
    bone marrow aspiration ~ 20939
    local ~ 20936
    morselized ~ 20937
    structural ~ 20938
  biopsy ~ 20250-20251
  chemotherapy administration ~ (see also chemotherapy) 96450
  CT scan
    cervical ~ 72125-72127
    lumbar ~ 72131-72133
    thoracic ~ 72128-72130
  decompression ~ 62287, 62380, 0274T, 0275T
  deformity
    arthrodesis ~ 22800-22812
    exposure ~ 22818, 22819
    scoliosis x-ray study ~ 72081-72084
  discogenic pain determination/localization
    magnetic resonance spectroscopy ~ 0609T-0612T
  fixation ~ 22842
  fusion
    anterior ~ 22808-22812
    anterior approach ~ 22548-22585, 22812
    exploration ~ 22830
    lateral extracavitary ~ 22532-22534
    posterior approach ~ 22590-22802
  injection
    allogenic cellular/tissue-based product lumbar ~ 0627T-0630T
    cervical ~ 62320, 62321, 62324, 62325
    lumbar ~ 62322, 62323, 62326, 62327
    sacral ~ 62322, 62323, 62326, 62327
    thoracic ~ 62320, 62321, 62324, 62325
    with fluoroscopic guidance ~ 77003
  insertion, instrumentation ~ 22840-22848, 22853, 22854, 22859
  kyphectomy ~ 22818-22819
  magnetic resonance angiography ~ 72159
  magnetic resonance imaging
    cervical ~ 72141-72142, 72156-72158
    lumbar ~ 72148-72158
    thoracic ~ 72146-72147, 72156-72158
  manipulation, with anesthesia ~ 22505
  myelography
    cervical ~ 72240
    lumbosacral ~ 72265
    thoracic ~ 72255
    total ~ 72270
  reconstruction, dorsal spine elements ~ 63295
  reinsertion, instrumentation ~ 22849
  removal, instrumentation ~ 22850, 22852-22855
  repair, osteotomy
    anterior ~ 22220-22226
    posterior ~ 22210-22214
      cervical laminoplasty ~ 63050-63051
      posterolateral ~ 22216
  ultrasound ~ 76800
  unlisted services and procedures, surgery ~ 22899

Spine ~ *continued*
  X-ray ~ 72020
    absorptiometry ~ 77080, 77081, 77085, 77086
    cervical ~ 72040, 72050, 72052
    lumbosacral ~ 72100, 72110, 72114, 72120
    scoliosis study ~ 72081-72084
    thoracic ~ 72070, 72072, 72074
    thoracolumbar ~ 72080
    total ~ 72081-72084
    with contrast
      cervical ~ 72240
      lumbosacral ~ 72265
      thoracic ~ 72255
      total ~ 72270
Spirometry ~ (see also pulmonology, diagnostic) 94010-94070
  patient initiated ~ 94014-94016
Splanchnicectomy ~ see nerves, sympathectomy, excision
Spleen
  excision ~ 38100-38102
    laparoscopic ~ 38120
  injection, radiologic ~ 38200
  nuclear medicine, imaging ~ 78185, 78215-78216
  repair ~ 38115
Splenectomy
  laparoscopic ~ 38120
  partial ~ 38101
  partial with repair, ruptured spleen ~ 38115
  total ~ 38100
    en bloc ~ 38102
Splenoplasty ~ see repair, spleen
Splenoportography ~ 75810
  injection procedures ~ 38200
Splenorrhaphy ~ 38115
Splint ~ see casting; strapping
  arm
    long ~ 29105
    short ~ 29125-29126
  finger ~ 29130-29131
  leg
    long ~ 29505
    short ~ 29515
  oral surgical ~ 21085
  ureteral ~ see ureteral splinting
Split grafts ~ 15100-15121
Split renal function test ~ see cystourethroscopy, catheterization, ureteral
Splitting blood products ~ 86985
Spontaneous abortion ~ see abortion
Sprengel's deformity ~ 23400
Spring water cyst ~ see cyst, pericardial
Spur, bone ~ see exostosis
  calcaneal ~ see heel spur
Sputum analysis ~ 89220
SRH ~ (somatostatin) 84307
Ssabanejew-Frank operation ~ (incision, stomach, creation, stoma)
    43830-43832
Stabilizing factor, fibrin ~ see fibrin stabilizing factor
Stable factor ~ 85230
Stallard procedure ~ see conjunctivorhinostomy
Stamey procedure ~ (repair, bladder, neck) 51845
Standby services physician ~ 99360
Stanford-Binet test ~ see psychiatric diagnosis
Stanftan ~ (Binet test) 96101-96103
Stapedectomy
  revision ~ 69662
  with footplate drill out ~ 69661
  without foreign material ~ 69660
Stapedotomy
  revision ~ 69662
  with footplate drill out ~ 69661
  without foreign material ~ 69660
Stapes
  excision
    with footplate drill out ~ 69661
    without foreign material ~ 69660
  release ~ 69650
  revision ~ 69662
Staphyloma
  sclera repair ~ 66225
State operation ~ see proctectomy
Statin therapy ~ see performance measures
Statistics/biometry ~ see biometry

Steindler stripping ~ 28250
Stellate ganglion injection, anesthetic ~ 64510
Stem cell
  concentration ~ 38215
  count ~ 86587
  cryopreservation ~ 38207, 88240
  donor search ~ 38204
  harvesting ~ 38205-38206
  limbal, allograft ~ 65781
  plasma depletion ~ 38214
  platelet depletion ~ 38213
  red blood cell depletion ~ 38212
  T-cell depletion ~ 38210
  thawing ~ 38208-38209, 88241
  transplantation ~ 38240-38242
  tumor cell depletion ~ 38211
  washing ~ 38209
Stem, brain ~ see brainstem
Stenger test ~ (audiologic function test; ear, nose and throat) ~ 92565, 92577
Stenosis
  aortic ~ see aortic stenosis
  auditory canal, external reconstruction ~ 69310
  bronchi ~ 96570, 96571
    reconstruction ~ 31775
    relief ~ 31641
  laryngeal repair ~ 31551-31554
  nasal repair ~ 30465
  pulmonary artery repair ~ 33782, 33917
  pulmonary vein repair ~ 33726
  reconstruction, auditory canal, external ~ 69310
  tracheal excision ~ 31780, 31781
  urethral ~ see urethral stenosis
  ventricular resection ~ 33476
Stensen duct ~ see parotid duct
Stent
  exchange
    biliary duct ~ 43276
    pancreatic duct ~ 43276
  for revascularization, intracoronary ~ 92937-92938, 92941, 92943-92944
  indwelling insertion, ureter ~ 50605, 52282, 52356, 53855
  placement
    bronchoscopy ~ 31631, 31636-31637
    cardiac ~ 33621
    colonoscopy ~ 45397
    endoscopy
      bile duct ~ 43274
      gastrointestinal, upper ~ 43266
      intestinal ~ 44379
      pancreatic ~ 43274
    enteroscopy ~ 44370
    esophagoscopy ~ 43212
    ileoscopy ~ 44384
    larynx ~ 31553, 31554, 31580
    proctosigmoidoscopy ~ 45327
    sigmoidoscopy ~ 45347
    tracheal ~ 31631
    for transcatheter intracardiac shunt ~ 33745, 33746
    ureteroneocystomy ~ 50947-50948
    for venous arterialization ~ 0620T
  removal/replacement, ureteral ~ 50382-50387
  revision, bronchoscopy ~ 31638
  transcatheter, intravascular, intracranial ~ 61635
  transluminal placement, arterial ~ 37221, 37223, 37226-37227, 37230-37231, 37234-37235
  urethra ~ 52282
Stent, intravascular ~ see transcatheter, placement, intravascular stents
Stents, tracheal ~ see tracheal stent
Stereotactic frame application/removal ~ 20660
Stereotaxis
  aspiration
    brain lesion ~ 61750
      with CT scan and/or MRI ~ 61751
  biopsy
    aspiration, brain lesion ~ 61750
    brain ~ 61750
      with CT scan and/or MRI ~ 61751
    prostate ~ 55706
  catheter placement, brain
    radiation source ~ 61770

Stereotaxis ~ *continued*
  computer assisted
    cranial ~ 61781-61782
    orthopedic surgery ~ 0054T-0055T, 20985
    spinal ~ 61783
  creation lesion
    brain
      deep ~ 61720-61735
      percutaneous ~ 61790
    gasserian ganglion ~ 61790
    spinal cord ~ 63600
    trigeminal tract ~ 61791
  CT scan
    aspiration ~ 61751
    biopsy ~ 61751
  excision lesion
    brain ~ 61750
  focus beam, radiosurgery ~ 77371-77373
    cranial ~ 61796-61799
    spinal ~ 63620-63621
    stereotactic frame application ~ 20660, 61800
  lesion ablation, intracranial
    MRgFUS-guided ~ 0398T
  radiation therapy ~ 77421, 77432-77435
  stimulation, spinal cord ~ 63610
  target volume guidance ~ 77421
Sterile coverings ~ see dressings
Sternal fracture ~ see fracture, sternum
Sternoclavicular joint
  arthrotomy ~ 23044
    with biopsy ~ 23101
    with synovectomy ~ 23106
  dislocation
    closed treatment
      with manipulation ~ 23525
      without manipulation ~ 23520
    open treatment ~ 23530-23532
      with fascial graft ~ 23532
Sternocleidomastoid division ~ 21720-21725
Sternotomy closure ~ 21750
Sternum
  debridement ~ 21627
  excision ~ 21620, 21630-21632
  fracture
    closed treatment ~ 21820
    open treatment ~ 21825
  ostectomy ~ 21620
  radical resection ~ 21630-21632
  reconstruction ~ 21740-21742, 21750
    with thoracoscopy ~ 21743
  X-ray ~ 71120-71130
Steroid-binding protein, sex ~ see globulin, sex hormone binding
Steroids
  anabolic ~ see androstenedione
  injection, urethral stricture ~ 52283
  ketogenic, urine ~ 83582
STH (somatotropic hormone) ~ see growth hormone
Stimulating antibody, thyroid ~ see immunoglobulin, thyroid stimulating
Stimulation
  electric ~ see electrical stimulation
  lymphocyte ~ see blastogenesis
  spinal cord, stereotaxis ~ 63610
  transcutaneous electric ~ see application, neurostimulation
Stimulator, long-acting thyroid ~ see thyrotropin releasing hormone (TRH)
Stimulators, cardiac ~ see heart, pacemaker
Stimulus evoked response ~ 51792
Stoffel operation ~ (rhizotomy) 63185, 63190
Stoma
  creation
    bladder ~ 51980
    kidney ~ 50551-50561
    stomach, neonatal ~ 43831
      temporary ~ 43830-43831
    ureter ~ 50860
  ureter, endoscopy via ~ 50951-50961
Stomach
  anastomosis
    with duodenum ~ 43810, 43850-43855
    with jejunum ~ 43820-43825, 43860-43865

Stomach ~ _continued_
  biopsy ~ 43605
  creation
    stoma
      temporary ~ 43830-43831
      laparoscopic ~ 43653
  electrogastrography ~ 91132-91133
  excision
    partial ~ 43631-43639, 43845
    total ~ 43620-43622
  exploration ~ 43500
  gastric bypass ~ 43644-43645, 43846
    revision ~ 43848
  incision ~ 43830-43832
    exploration ~ 43500
    pyloric sphincter ~ 43520
    removal, foreign body ~ 43500
  nuclear medicine
    blood loss study ~ 78278
    emptying study ~ 78264
      with small bowel transit ~ 78265
      with small bowel and colon transit ~ 78266
    imaging ~ 78261
    protein loss study ~ 78282
    reflux study ~ 78262
  reconstruction
    for obesity ~ 43644-43645, 43842-43847
    Roux-en-Y ~ 43644, 43846
  removal, foreign body ~ 43500
  repair ~ 48547
    fistula ~ 43880
    fundoplasty ~ 43325
      laparoscopic ~ 43279-43282
    laceration ~ 43501-43502
    stoma ~ 43870
    ulcer ~ 43501
  suture
    fistula ~ 43880
    for obesity ~ 43842-43843
    stoma ~ 43870
    ulcer ~ 43840
    wound ~ 43840
  tumor, excision ~ 43610-43611
  ulcer, excision ~ 43610
  unlisted services and procedures ~ 43659, 43999
Stomatoplasty ~ see mouth, repair
Stone, kidney ~ see calculus, removal, kidney
Stookey-Scarff procedure ~ (ventriculocisternostomy) 62200
Stool blood ~ see blood, feces
Storage
  embryo ~ 89342
  oocyte ~ 89346
  reproductive tissue ~ 89344
  sperm ~ 89343
Strabismus
  chemodenervation ~ 67345
  repair
    adjustable sutures ~ 67335
    extraocular muscles ~ 67340
    one horizontal muscle ~ 67311
    one vertical muscle ~ 67314
    posterior fixation suture technique ~ 67334-67335
    previous surgery, not involving extraocular muscles ~ 67331
    release extensive scar tissue ~ 67343
    superior oblique muscle ~ 67318
    transposition ~ 67320
    two horizontal muscles ~ 67312
    two or more vertical muscles ~ 67316
Strapping ~ see cast; splint
  ankle ~ 29540
  back ~ 29799
  chest ~ 29200
  elbow ~ 29260
  finger ~ 29280
  foot ~ 29540
  hand ~ 29280
  hip ~ 29520
  knee ~ 29530
  shoulder ~ 29240
  thorax ~ 29200

Strapping ~ _continued_
  toes ~ 29550
  unlisted services and procedures ~ 29799
  Unna boot ~ 29580
  wrist ~ 29260
Strassman procedure ~ 58540
Strayer procedure leg, lower ~ 27687
Streptococcus pneumoniae vaccine ~ see vaccines
Streptococcus
  group A
    antigen detection
      enzyme immunoassay ~ 87430
      nucleic acid ~ 87650-87652
    direct optical observation ~ 87880
  group B
    antigen detection by immunoassay with direct optical observation ~ 87802
    prenatal screening ~ 3294F
Streptokinase, antibody ~ 86590
Stress tests
  cardiovascular ~ 93015-93024
  multiple gated acquisition (MUGA) ~ 78472-78473
  myocardial perfusion imaging ~ 78451-78454
  pulmonary ~ 94618
Stricture
  dilation
    gastric/duodenal ~ 43245
    ureteral
      balloon ~ 50706
      endoscopy ~ 50553, 50572, 50575, 50953, 50972
        with cystourethroscopy ~ 52341-52343
        with ureteroscopy ~ 52344-52346
  repair, urethra ~ 53400-53405
Stricturoplasty intestines ~ 44615
Stroboscopy larynx ~ 31579
STS ~ (syphilis test) 86592-86593
Stuart-Prower factor ~ 85260
Study, color vision ~ see color vision examination
Sturmdorf procedure ~ 57520
Styloid process radial, excision ~ 25230
Styloidectomy radial ~ 25230
Stypven time ~ see Russell viper venom time
Subacromial bursa arthrocentesis ~ 20610
Subclavian arteries ~ see artery, subclavian
Subcutaneous injection ~ see injection, subcutaneous
Subcutaneous mastectomies ~ see mastectomy, subcutaneous
Subcutaneous tissue excision ~ 15830-15839, 15847
Subdiaphragmatic abscess ~ see abscess, subdiaphragmatic
Subdural electrode
  insertion ~ 61531-61533
  removal ~ 61535
Subdural hematoma ~ see hematoma, subdural
Subdural puncture ~ 61105-61108
Subdural tap ~ 61000-61001
Sublingual gland
  abscess, incision and drainage ~ 42310-42320
  calculi (stone), excision ~ 42330
  cyst
    drainage ~ 42409
    excision ~ 42408
  excision ~ 42450
Subluxation elbow ~ 24640
Submandibular gland
  calculi (stone), excision ~ 42330-42335
  excision ~ 42440
Submaxillary gland abscess, incision and drainage ~ 42310-42320
Submucous resection of nasal septum ~ see nasal septum, submucous resection
Subperiosteal implant reconstruction
  mandible ~ 21245-21246
  maxilla ~ 21245-21246
Subphrenic abscess ~ see abscess, subdiaphragmatic
Substance S, Reichstein's ~ see deoxycortisol
Subtrochanteric fracture ~ see femur, fracture, subtrochanteric
Sucrose hemolysis test ~ see red blood cell (RBC), fragility, osmotic
Suction lipectomies ~ see liposuction
Sudiferous gland ~ see sweat gland
Sugar water test ~ see red blood cell (RBC), fragility, osmotic
Sugars ~ 84375-84379
Sugiura procedure ~ see esophagus, repair, varices

Sulfate
    chondroitin ~ see chondroitin sulfate
    DHA ~ see dehydroepiandrosterone sulfate
    urine ~ 84392
Sulfation factor ~ see somatomedin
Sulphates ~ see sulfate
Sumatran mite fever ~ see scrub typhus
Superficial musculoaponeurotic system (SMAS) flap rhytidectomy ~ 15829
Supernumerary digit
    reconstruction ~ 26587
    repair ~ 26587
Supply
    chemotherapeutic agent ~ (see also chemotherapy) 96545
    contact lenses ~ 92391, 92396
    educational materials ~ 99071
    low vision aids ~ (see also spectacle services) 92392
    materials ~ 99070
    ocular prosthesis ~ 92393
    prosthesis, breast ~ 19396
    spectacle prosthesis ~ 92395
    spectacles ~ 92390
Suppositories, vaginal ~ see pessary
Suppression ~ 80400-80408
Suppression/testing ~ see evocative/suppression test
Suppressor T lymphocyte marker ~ see CD8
Suppurative hidradenitides ~ see hidradenitis, suppurative
Suprahyoid lymphadenectomy ~ 38700
Supraorbital nerve
    avulsion ~ 64732
    incision ~ 64732
    transection ~ 64732
Supraorbital rim and forehead reconstruction ~ 21179-21180
Suprapubic prostatectomies ~ see prostatectomy, suprapubic
Suprarenal
    gland ~ see adrenal gland
    vein ~ see vein, adrenal
Suprascapular nerve injection, anesthetic ~ 64418
Suprasellar cyst ~ see craniopharyngioma
Surface CD4 receptor ~ see CD4
Surface radiotherapy ~ see application, radioelement, surface
Surgeries
    breast-conserving ~ see breast, excision, lesion
    conventional ~ see celiotomy
    laser ~ see laser surgery
    Mohs ~ see Mohs micrographic surgery
    repeat ~ see reoperation
Surgery services ~ 10000-69999
    auditory system ~ 69000-69979
    cardiovascular system ~ 33000-37799
    digestive system ~ 40490-49999
    endocrine system ~ 60000-60699
    eye and ocular adnexa ~ 65091-68899
    female genital system ~ 56405-58999
    hemic and lymphatic systems ~ 38100-38999
    integumentary system ~ 10000-19999
    intersex surgery ~ 55970-55980
    male genital system ~ 54000-55899
    maternity care and delivery ~ 59000-59899
    mediastinum and diaphragm ~ 39000-39599
    musculoskeletal system ~ 20010-29999
    nervous system ~ 61000-64999
    respiratory system ~ 30000-32999
    urinary system ~ 50010-53899
Surgical
    avulsion ~ see avulsion
    cataract removal ~ see cataract, excision
    collapse therapy; thoracoplasty ~ see thoracoplasty
    diathermy ~ see electrocautery
    galvanism ~ see electrolysis
    incision ~ see incision
    microscopes ~ see operating microscope
    pathology ~ 88300-88309
    planing, nose, skin ~ 30120
    pneumoperitoneum ~ see pneumoperitoneum
    removal, eye ~ see enucleation, eye
    revision ~ see reoperation
    services, post-op visit ~ 99024
Surveillance ~ see monitoring

Suspension
    aorta ~ 33800
    kidney ~ see nephropexy
    muscle, hyoid ~ 21865
    vagina ~ see colpopexy
Suture ~ see repair
    abdomen ~ 49900
    aorta ~ 33320-33322
    bile duct, wound ~ 47900
    bladder
        fistulization ~ 44660-44661, 45800-45805, 51880-51925
            vesicouterine ~ 51920-51925
            vesicovaginal ~ 51900
        wound ~ 51860-51865
    cervix ~ 57720
    colon
        diverticula ~ 44604-44605
        fistula ~ 44650-44661
        plication ~ 44680
        stoma ~ 44620-44625
        ulcer ~ 44604-44605
        wound ~ 44604-44605
    esophagus, wound ~ 43410-43415
    eyelid ~ 67880
        closure of ~ 67875
        with transposition of tarsal plate ~ 67882
        wound
            full thickness ~ 67935
            partial thickness ~ 67930
    facial nerve, intratemporal
        lateral to geniculate ganglion ~ 69740
        medial to geniculate ganglion ~ 69745
    foot, tendon ~ 28200-28210
    gastroesophageal ~ 43405
    great vessel ~ 33320-33322
    hemorrhoids ~ 46945, 46946, 46848
    hepatic duct ~ see hepatic duct, repair
    intestine, large
        diverticula ~ 44605
        ulcer ~ 44605
        wound ~ 44605
    intestines
        large
            diverticula ~ 44604
            ulcer ~ 44604
            wound ~ 44604
        small
            diverticula ~ 44602-44603
            fistula ~ 44640-44661
            plication ~ 44680
            ulcer ~ 44602-44603
            wound ~ 44602-44603
        stoma ~ 44620-44625
    iris, with ciliary body ~ 66682
    kidney
        fistula ~ 50520-50526
        horseshoe ~ 50540
        wound ~ 50500
    leg, lower, tendon ~ 27658-27665
    leg, upper, muscle ~ 27385-27386
    liver, wound ~ 47350-47361
    mesentery ~ 44850
    nerve ~ 64831-64876
    pancreas ~ 48545
    pharynx, wound ~ 42900
    rectum
        fistula ~ 45800-45825
        prolapse ~ 45540-45541
    removal, anesthesia ~ 15850-15851
    spleen ~ see splenorrhaphy
    stomach
        fistula ~ 43880
        laceration ~ 43501-43502
        stoma ~ 43870
        ulcer ~ 43501, 43840
        wound ~ 43840
    tendon
        foot ~ 28200-28210
        knee ~ 27380-27381

Suture ~ *continued*
  testis
    injury ~ 54670
    suspension ~ 54620-54640
  thoracic duct
    abdominal approach ~ 38382
    cervical approach ~ 38380
    thoracic approach ~ 38381
  throat, wound ~ 42900
  tongue
    base suspension ~ 41512
    to lip ~ 41510
  trachea
    fistula
      with plastic repair ~ 31825
      without plastic repair ~ 31820
    stoma
      with plastic repair ~ 31825
      without plastic repair ~ 31820
    wound
      cervical ~ 31800
      intrathoracic ~ 31805
  ulcer ~ 44604-44605
  ureter ~ 50900
    deligation ~ 50940
    fistula ~ 50920-50930
  urethra
    fistula ~ 45820-45825, 53520
    stoma ~ 53520
    to bladder ~ 51840-51841
    wound ~ 53502-53515
  uterus
    fistula ~ 51920-51925
    rupture ~ 58520, 59350
    suspension ~ 58400-58410
  vagina
    cystocele ~ 57240, 57260
    enterocele ~ 57265
    fistula
      rectovaginal ~ 57300-57307
      transvesical and vaginal approach ~ 57330
      urethrovaginal ~ 57310-57311
      vesicovaginal ~ 51900, 57320-57330
    rectocele ~ 57250-57260
    suspension ~ 57280, 57283
    wound ~ 57200-57210
  vas deferens ~ 55400
  vein, femoral ~ 37650
    iliac ~ 37660
  wound ~ 44604-44605
Swallowing evaluation ~ 92526, 92610-92613, 92616-92617
  cine ~ 74230
  treatment ~ 92526
  video ~ 74230
Swanson procedure ~ 28309
Sweat collection iontophoresis ~ 89230
Sweat glands, excision
  axillary ~ 11450-11451
  inguinal ~ 11462-11463
  perianal ~ 11470-11471
  perineal ~ 11470-11471
  umbilical ~ 11470-11471
Sweat test ~ (chloride, blood) 82435
Swenson procedure ~ 45120
Syme procedure ~ 27888
Sympathectomy
  artery
    digital ~ 64820
    radial ~ 64821
    superficial palmar arch ~ 64823
    ulnar ~ 64822
  cervical ~ 64802
  cervicothoracic ~ 64804
  digital artery, with magnification ~ 64820
  lumbar ~ 64818
  presacral ~ 58410
  thoracic ~ 32664
  thoracolumbar ~ 64809
  with rib excision ~ 21616

Sympathetic nerve
  excision ~ 64802-64818
  injection, anesthetic ~ 64520-64530
Sympathins ~ see catecholamines
Symphysiotomy horseshoe kidney ~ 50540
Symphysis, pubic ~ see pubic symphysis
Syncytial virus, respiratory ~ see respiratory syncytial virus
Syndactylism, toes ~ see webbed, toe
Syndactyly repair ~ 26560-26562
Syndesmotomy ~ see ligament, release
Syndrome
  andrenogenital ~ see adrenogenital syndrome
  ataxia-telangiectasia ~ see ataxia telangiectasia
  Bloom ~ see Bloom syndrome
  carpal tunnel ~ see carpal tunnel syndrome
  Costen's ~ see temporomandibular joint (TMJ)
  Eerb-Goldflam ~ see myasthenia gravis
  ovarian vein ~ see ovarian vein syndrome
  synechiae, intrauterine ~ see adhesions, intrauterine
  Treacher Collins ~ see Treacher-Collins syndrome
  urethral ~ see urethral syndrome
Syngesterone ~ see progesterone
Synostosis (cranial) ~ see craniosynostosis
Synovectomy
  arthrotomy with, glenohumeral joint ~ 23105
    sternoclavicular joint ~ 23106
  elbow ~ 24102
  excision
    carpometacarpal joint ~ 26130
    finger joint ~ 26135-26140
    hip joint ~ 27054
    interphalangeal joint ~ 26140
    knee joint ~ 27334-27335
    metacarpophalangeal joint ~ 26135
    palm ~ 26145
  wrist ~ 25105, 25118-25119
    radical ~ 25115-25116
Synovial
  bursa ~ see bursa
  cyst ~ see ganglion
  membrane ~ see synovium
  popliteal space ~ see baker's cyst
Synovium
  biopsy
    carpometacarpal joint ~ 26100
    interphalangeal joint ~ 26110
    knee joint ~ 27330
    metacarpophalangeal joint, with synovial biopsy ~ 26105
  excision
    carpometacarpal joint ~ 26130
    finger joint ~ 26135-26140
    hip joint ~ 27054
    interphalangeal joint ~ 26140
    knee joint ~ 27334-27335
Syphilis ab ~ see antibody, Treponema pallidum
Syphilis test ~ 86592-86593
Syrinx spinal cord, aspiration ~ 62268
System
  endocrine ~ see endocrine system
  hemic ~ see hemic system
  lymphatic ~ see lymphatic system
  musculoskeletal ~ see musculoskeletal system
  nervous ~ see nervous system

T

T cell leukemia virus I antibodies, adult ~ 86687, 86689
T cell leukemia virus, I, human ~ 86687, 86689
T cell leukemia virus II antibodies, human ~ 86688
T cell leukemia virus II , human ~ 86688
T cells
  CD4, absolute ~ 86361
  count ~ 86359
  gene rearrangement ~ 81340-81342
  ratio ~ 86360
T lymphotropic virus type III antibodies, human ~ 86689, 86701-86703
T-3 ~ see triiodothyronine

T-4 ~ 84436-84439, 86360
T-7 index ~ 84436
T-8 ~ 86360
T-cells CD4, absolute ~ 86361
  count ~ 86359
  ratio ~ 86360
T- cell T8 antigens ~ 86360
T- phyl ~ 80198
T3 free ~ 84481
T4 molecule ~ 86360
T4 total ~ 84436
Taarnhoj Procedure ~ see section ~ 61450
Tachycardia heart, recording ~ 93609
Tacrolimus drug assay ~ 80197
Tag, skin ~ see skin, tags
Tail bone
  excision ~ 27080
  fracture ~ 27200-27202
Takeuchi Procedure ~ 33505
Talectomy ~ see astragalectomy
Talotarsal joint dislocation ~ 28570-28575, 28585
  percutaneous fixation ~ 28576
Talus
  arthrodesis
    pantalar ~ 28705
    subtalar ~ 28725
    triple ~ 28715
  arthroscopy
    surgical ~ 29891-29892
    subtalar ~ 29904-29907, 29915-29916
  autograft, osteochondral ~ 28446
  craterization ~ 28120
  cyst, excision ~ 28100-28103
  diaphysectomy ~ 28120
  excision ~ 28120, 28130
  fracture
    open treatment ~ 28445
    percutaneous fixation ~ 28436
    with manipulation ~ 28435-28436
    without manipulation ~ 28430
  repair
    osteochondritis dissecans ~ 29892
    osteotomy ~ 28302
  saucerization ~ 28120
  tumor, excision ~ 27647, 28100-28103
Tap
  cisternal ~ see cisternal puncture
  lumbar diagnostic ~ see spinal tap
Tarsal fracture
  percutaneous fixation ~ 28456
Tarsal bone ~ see ankle bone
Tarsal joint ~ see foot
  arthrodesis ~ 28730-28735, 28740
    with advancement ~ 28737
    with lengthening ~ 28737
  craterization ~ 28122
  cyst, excision ~ 28104-28107
  diaphysectomy ~ 28122
  dislocation ~ 28540-28545, 28555
    percutaneous fixation ~ 28545-28546
  excision ~ 28116, 28122
  fracture
    open treatment ~ 28465
    with manipulation ~ 28455-28456
    without manipulation ~ 28450
  fusion ~ 28730-28735, 28740
    with advancement ~ 28737
    with lengthening ~ 28737
  repair ~ 28320
    osteotomy ~ 28304-28305
  saucerization ~ 28122
  tumor, excision ~ 28104-28107, 28171
Tarsal strip procedure ~ 67917-67924
Tarsal tunnel release ~ 28035
Tarsal wedge procedure ~ 67916-67923
Tarsometatarsal joint
  arthrodesis ~ 28730-28735, 28740
  arthrotomy ~ 28020, 28050
  dislocation ~ 28600-28605, 28615
    percutaneous fixation ~ 28606

Tarsometatarsal joint ~ continued
  exploration ~ 28020
  fusion ~ 28730-28735, 28740
  removal
    foreign body ~ 28020
    loose body ~ 28020
  synovial
    biopsy ~ 28050
    excision ~ 28070
Tarsorrhaphy ~ 67875
  median ~ 67880
  severing ~ 67710
    with transposition of tarsal plate ~ 67882
Tattoo
  cornea ~ 65600
  skin ~ 11920-11922
TB test, antigen response ~ 0010T
  skin test ~ 86580-86585
TBG ~ see thyroxine binding globulin
TBS ~ see Bethesda system
TCT ~ see thrombin time
TD shots ~ see tetanus immunization; vaccines
Team conference case management services ~ 99366-99368
Tear duct ~ see lacrimal duct
Tear gland ~ see lacrimal gland
Technique
  pericardial window ~ see pericardiostomy
  projective ~ see projective test
Teeth X-ray ~ 70300-70320
Telangiectasia
  chromosome analysis ~ 88248
  injection ~ 36468
Telangiectasia
  chromosome analysis ~ 88248
  sclerotherapy ~ 36465, 36466, 36468, 36470, 36471
Telephone
  evaluation and management services
    non-physician ~ 98966-98968
    physician ~ 99441-99443
  pacemaker analysis ~ 93293
Teletherapy dose plan ~ 77306, 77307
Temperature gradient studies ~ 93740
Temporal arteries ~ 37609
Temporal bone
  electromagnetic bone conduction hearing device
    implantation/replacement ~ 69710
    removal/repair ~ 69711
  excision ~ 69535
  resection ~ 69535
  tumor, removal ~ 69970
  unlisted services and procedures ~ 69979
Temporal, petrous
  excision, apex ~ 69530
Temporomandibular joint (TMJ)
  arthrocentesis ~ 20605
  arthrography ~ 70328-70332
    injection ~ 21116
  arthroplasty ~ 21240-21243
  arthroscopy
    diagnostic ~ 29800
    surgical ~ 29804
  arthrotomy ~ 21010
  cartilage, excision ~ 21060
  condylectomy ~ 21050
  coronoidectomy ~ 21070
  dislocation
    closed treatment ~ 21480-21485
    open treatment ~ 21490
  injection, radiologic ~ 21116
  magnetic resonance imaging (MRI) ~ 70336
  manipulation ~ 21073
  meniscectomy ~ 21060
  prosthesis ~ see prosthesis, temporomandibular joint
  reconstruction ~ see reconstruction, temporomandibular joint
  X-ray with contrast ~ 70328-70332
Tenago Procedure ~ 53431
Tendinosuture ~ see suture, tendon

Tendon
 Achilles ~ see Achilles tendon
 arm, upper, revision ~ 24320
 excision
  forearm ~ 25109
  finger, excision ~ 26180
  forearm, repair ~ 25260-25274
  graft, harvesting ~ 20924
  insertion, biceps tendon ~ 24342
 lengthening
  ankle ~ 27685-27686
  arm, upper ~ 24305
  elbow ~ 24305
  finger ~ 26476, 26478
  forearm ~ 25280
  hand ~ 26476, 26478
  leg, lower ~ 27685-27686
  leg, upper ~ 27393-27395
  toe ~ 28240
  wrist ~ 25280
 palm, excision ~ 26170
 release
  arm, lower ~ 25295
  arm, upper ~ 24332
  wrist ~ 25295
 shortening
  ankle ~ 27685-27686
  finger ~ 26477, 26479
  hand ~ 26477, 26479
  leg, lower ~ 27685-27686
 transfer
  arm, lower ~ 25310-25312, 25316
  arm, upper ~ 24301
  elbow ~ 24301
  finger ~ 26497-26498
  hand ~ 26480-26489
  leg, lower ~ 27690-27692
  leg, upper ~ 27400
  pelvis ~ 27098
  thumb ~ 26490-26492, 26510
  wrist ~ 25310-25312, 25316
 transplant, leg, upper ~ 27396-27397
 wrist, repair ~ 25260-25274
Tendon origin insertion, injection ~ 20551
Tendon pulley reconstruction of hand ~ see hand, reconstruction, tendon pulley
Tendon sheath
 arm, lower, repair ~ 25275
 finger
  incision ~ 26055
  incision and drainage ~ 26020
  lesion ~ 26160
 foot, excision ~ 28086-28088
 hand lesion ~ 26160
 injection ~ 20550
 palm, incision and drainage ~ 26020
 removal, foreign body ~ 20520-20525
 wrist
  excision, radical ~ 25115-25116
  incision ~ 25000-25001
  repair ~ 25275
Tenectomy, tendon sheath ~ 25110
Tennis elbow repair ~ 24357-24359
Tenodesis
 biceps tendon
  arthroscopic ~ 29828
  at elbow ~ 24340
  shoulder ~ 23430
 finger ~ 26471-26474
 wrist ~ 25300-25301
Tenolysis
 ankle ~ 27680-27681
 arm, lower ~ 25295
 arm, upper ~ 24332
 finger
  extensor ~ 26445-26449
  flexor ~ 26440-26442
 foot ~ 28220-28226
 hand extensor ~ 26445-26449
  flexor ~ 26440-26442

Tenolysis ~ *continued*
 leg, lower ~ 27680-27681
 wrist ~ 25295
Tenomyotomy, shoulder ~ 23405-23406
Tenon's capsule injection ~ 67515
Tenoplasty anesthesia ~ 01714
Tenorrhaphy ~ see suture, tendon
Tenosuspension ~ see tenodesis
Tenosuture ~ see suture, tendon
Tenotomy
 Achilles tendon ~ 27605-27606
 ankle ~ 27605-27606
 arm, lower ~ 25290
 arm, upper ~ 24310
 finger ~ 26060, 26455-26460
 foot ~ 28230, 28234
 hand ~ 26450, 26460
 hip, iliopsoas tendon ~ 27005
 hip, abductor ~ 27006
 hip, adductor ~ 27000-27003
 leg, upper ~ 27306-27307, 27390-27392
 toe ~ 28010-28011, 28232-28234, 28240
 wrist ~ 25290
TENS ~ see physical medicine/therapy/ occupational therapy
Tensilon test ~ 95857-95858
Tension, ocular ~ see glaucoma
Terman-Merrill test ~ 96100
Termination, pregnancy ~ see abortion
Test
 antiglobulin ~ 86880
 aphasia ~ 96105
 Bender visual-motor Gestalt ~ 96101-96103
 Binet ~ 96101-96103
 blood ~ see blood tests
 blood coagulation ~ see coagulation
 bone quality by microindentation ~ 0547T
 breath ~ see breath test
 cervical mucus penetration ~ 89330
 clinical chemistry ~ 84999
 complement fixation ~ 86171
 exercise ~ 93015-93018
 fern ~ 87210
 fetal, nonstress ~ 59025
 function, vestibular ~ see vestibular function tests
 gel diffusion ~ 86329-86331
 glucose tolerance ~ 82951-82952
 hearing ~ see audiologic function tests
 hemagglutination inhibition ~ 86280
 ink blot ~ see inkblot test
 intelligence ~ 96101-96102
 lung function ~ see pulmonology, diagnostic
 neutralization ~ 86382
 Papanicolaou ~ 88141-88155, 88164-88167, 88174-88175
 pregnancy ~ 84702-84703
 quick ~ 85610-85611
 radioimmunosorbent ~ 82784-82787
 Rorschach ~ 96101
 skin ~ see skin, tests
 Stanford-Binet ~ see psychiatric diagnosis
 tuberculin ~ 86580
Test tube fertilization ~ 58321-58322
Tester, color vision ~ 92283
Testes
 cryopreservation ~ 89335
 nuclear medicine
  imaging ~ 78761
 undescended ~ 54550-54560
Testicular vein ~ 55530-55540
Testimony, medical ~ 99075
Testing, histocompatibility ~ see tissue typing
Testing, neurophysiologic intraoperative ~ 95940-95941
Testing, neuropsychological ~ 96117
Testing, range of motion ~ see range of motion test
Testis
 abscess, incision and drainage ~ 54700
 biopsy ~ 54500-54505
 excision
  laparoscopic ~ 54690
  partial ~ 54522
  radical ~ 54530-54535
  simple ~ 54520

Testis ~ *continued*
  hematoma, incision and drainage ~ 54700
  insertion, prosthesis ~ 54660
  lesion, excision ~ 54512
  needle biopsy ~ 54500
  repair
    injury ~ 54670
    suspension ~ 54620-54640
    torsion ~ 54600
  suture
    injury ~ 54670
    suspension ~ 54620-54640
  transplantation, to thigh ~ 54680
  tumor, excision ~ 54530-54535
  undescended, exploration ~ 54550-54560
  unlisted services and procedures ~ 54699, 55899
Testosterone ~ 84402
  response ~ 80414
    stimulation ~ 80414-80415
  total ~ 84403
Testosterone estradiol binding globulin ~ 84270
Tetanus ~ 86280
  antibody ~ 86774
  immunoglobulin ~ 90389
Tetrachloride, carbon ~ 84600
Tetralogy of Fallot ~ 33692-33697, 33924
Thal-Nissen Procedure ~ 43325
Thawing ~ 86930-86932
  cryopreserved
    embryo ~ 89352
    oocytes ~ 89356
    reproductive tissue ~ 89354
    sperm ~ 89353
  previously frozen cells ~ 38208-38209
Thawing and expansion of frozen cell ~ 88241
THBR ~ 84479
Theleplasty ~ 19350
Theophylline assay ~ 80198
Therapeutic
  abortion ~ 59850-59852
  apheresis ~ 36511-36516
  mobilization ~ see mobilization
  photopheresis ~ 36522
  radiology ~ see radiology, therapeutic
Therapeutic Drug Assays
  acetaminophen ~ 80143
  adalimumab ~ 80145
  amikacin ~ 80150
  amiodarone ~ 80151
  amitriptyline ~ 80335-80337
  benzodiazepine ~ 80346, 80347
  caffeine ~ 80155
  carbamazepine, 10,11-epoxide ~ 80161
  carbamazepine ~ 80156-80157
  clozapine ~ 80159
  cyclosporine ~ 80158
  desipramine ~ 80335-80337
  digoxin ~ 80162, 80163
  dipropylacetic acid ~ 80164, 80165
  doxepin ~ 80335-80337
  ethosuximide ~ 80168
  everolimus ~ 80169
  felbamate ~ 80167
  flecainide ~ 80181
  gabapentin ~ 80171
  gentamicin ~ 80170
  gold ~ 80375
  haloperidol ~ 80173
  imipramine ~ 80335-80337
  infliximab ~ 80230
  itraconazole ~ 80189
  lacosamide ~ 80235
  lamotrigine ~ 80175
  leflunomide ~ 80193
  levetiracetam ~ 80177
  lidocaine ~ 80176
  lithium ~ 80178
  methotrexate ~ 80204
  nortriptyline ~ 80335-80337
  oxcarbazepine ~ 80183

Therapeutic Drug Assays ~ *continued*
  phenobarbital ~ 80184
  phenytoin ~ 80185-80186
  posaconazole ~ 80187
  primidone ~ 80188
  procainamide ~ 80190-80192
  quantitative, other ~ 80299
  quinidine ~ 80194
  rufinamide ~ 80210
  salicylate ~ 80179
  sirolimus ~ 80195
  tacrolimus ~ 80197
  theophylline ~ 80198
  tiagabine ~ 80199
  tobramycin ~ 80200
  topiramate ~ 80201
  vancomycin ~ 80202
  vedolizumab ~ 80280
  voriconazole ~ 80285
  zonisamide ~ 80203
Therapies
  cold ~ see cryotherapy
  exercise ~ 97110-97113
  family ~ 90846-90849, 99510
  language ~ 92507-92508
  milieu ~ 90882
  occupational ~ 97165-97168
  photodynamic ~ 96910-96913
  photoradiation ~ 96900
  physical ~ see physical medicine/therapy/occupational therapy
  speech ~ 92507-92508
  tocolytic ~ 59412
  ultraviolet ~ 96900
Therapy
  CAR-T cell ~ 0537T-0540T
  radiation, brachytherapy ~ 77767, 77768, 77770-77772, 0394T, 0395T
Thermocauterization
  ectropion, repair ~ 67922
  lesion, cornea ~ 65450
Thermocoagulation ~ 17000-17286
Thermotherapy
  prostate ~ 53850-53852
    microwave ~ 53850
    radiofrequency ~ 53852
Thiamine ~ 84425
Thiersch Operation ~ 15050
Thiersch Procedure ~ 46753
Thigh fasciotomy ~ see femur; leg, upper ~ 27025
Thiocyanate ~ 84430
Third disease ~ 86762
Third opinion ~ see confirmatory consultations
Thompson Procedure ~ 27430
Thompson test ~ see smear and stain, routine
Thoracectomy ~ 32905
Thoracentesis ~ 32554-32555
Thoracic
  anterior ramus ~ see intercostal nerve
  arteries ~ 36215-36218
  cavity ~ see chest cavity
  duct ~ see lymphatics
    cannulation ~ 38794
    ligation ~ 38380
      abdominal approach ~ 38382
      thoracic approach ~ 38381
    suture
      abdominal approach ~ 38382
      cervical approach ~ 38380
      thoracic approach ~ 38381
  empyema ~ 21501-21502
  surgery, video-assisted ~ see thoracoscopy
  vertebra ~ 22101, 22112
  wall ~ see chest wall
Thoracocentesis ~ 32554-32555
Thoracoplasty ~ 32905
  with closure bronchopleural fistula ~ 32906
Thoracoscopy
  diagnostic
    with biopsy ~ 32604, 32606, 32607-32609
    without biopsy ~ 32601

Thoracoscopy ~ *continued*
surgical ~ 32650-32674
  with control traumatic hemorrhage ~ 32654
  with creation pericardial window ~ 32659
  with diagnostic wedge resection ~ 32668
  with esophagomyotomy ~ 32665
  with excision mediastinal cyst, tumor and/or mass ~ 32662
  with excision pericardial cyst, tumor and/or mass ~ 32661
  with lobectomy ~ 32663
  with mediastinal lymphadenectomy ~ 32674
  with parietal pleurectomy ~ 32656
  with partial pulmonary decortication ~ 32651
  with pleurodesis ~ 32650
  with regional lymphadenectomy ~ 32674
  with removal intrapleural foreign body ~ 32653
  with removal of clot/foreign body ~ 32658
  with resection of thymus ~ 32673
  with resection/plication of bullae ~ 32655
  with sternum reconstruction ~ 21743
  with therapeutic wedge resection ~ 32666, 32667
  with thoracic sympathectomy ~ 32664
  with total pulmonary decortication ~ 32652

Thoracostomy empyema ~ 32035-32036
tube, with/without water seal ~ 32551

Thoracotomy
cardiac massage ~ 32160
for post-op complications ~ 32120
hemorrhage ~ 32110
lymphadenectomy, thoracic ~ 38746
removal
  bullae ~ 32141
  cyst ~ 32140
  defibrillator ~ 33243
  electrodes ~ 33238
  foreign body
    intrapleural ~ 32150
    intrapulmonary ~ 32151
  pacemaker ~ 33236-33237
resection
  diagnostic wedge ~ 32507
  therapeutic wedge ~ 32505-32506
revascularization ~ 33140-33141
transmyocardial laser
  with biopsy ~ 32096-32097
  with lung repair ~ 32110
  with open intrapleural pneumolysis ~ 32124
  with resection-plication of bullae ~ 32141

Thorax ~ see chest; chest cavity; mediastinum
angiography ~ 71275
bioimpedance ~ 93701
biopsy ~ 21550
CT scan ~ 71250-71275
incision, empyema ~ 32035-32036
  pneumothorax ~ 32551
incision and drainage
  abscess ~ 21501-21502
  deep ~ 21510
  hematoma ~ 21501-21502
strapping ~ 29200
tumor
  excision ~ 21552-21558
  excision/resection ~ 21557, 21558
unlisted services and procedures, surgery ~ 21899

Three glass test ~ 81020
Three-day measles ~ 86762
Throat ~ see pharynx
abscess, incision and drainage ~ 42700-42725
biopsy ~ 42800-42806
hemorrhage ~ 42960-42962
reconstruction ~ 42950
removal, foreign body ~ 42809
repair
  pharyngoesophageal ~ 42953
  wound ~ 42900
suture, wound ~ 42900
unlisted services and procedures ~ 42999

Thrombectomy
aortoiliac artery ~ 34151-34201
arteriovenous fistula, graft ~ 36830-36833
axillary artery ~ 34101
axillary vein ~ 34490
brachial artery ~ 34101
bypass graft, other than hemodialysis graft or fistula ~ 35875-35876
carotid artery ~ 34001
celiac artery ~ 34151
dialysis graft ~ 36831, 36833
femoral ~ 34201
femoropopliteal vein ~ 34421-34451
iliac ~ 34151-34201
iliac vein ~ 34401-34451
innominate artery ~ 34001-34101
mesenteric artery ~ 34151
percutaneous
  coronary artery ~ 92973
  dialysis circuit ~ 36904-36906
  intracranial artery ~ 61645
  mechanical arterial ~ 37184-37186
  mechanical venous ~ 37187-37188
peroneal artery ~ 34203
popliteal artery ~ 34201-34203
radial artery ~ 34111
renal artery ~ 34151
subclavian artery ~ 34001-34101
subclavian vein ~ 34471-34490
tibial artery ~ 34203
ulnar artery ~ 34111
vena cava ~ 34401-34451
vena caval ~ 50230

Thrombin inhibitor I ~ 85300-85301
Thrombin time ~ 85670-85675
Thrombocyte (platelet) ~ see blood, platelet
Thrombocyte AB ~ 86022-86023
Thromboendarterectomy ~ see thrombectomy
aorta, abdominal ~ 35331
aortoiliofemoral artery ~ 35363
axillary artery ~ 35321
brachial artery ~ 35321
carotid artery ~ 35301, 35390
celiac artery ~ 35341
femoral artery ~ 35302, 35371-35372
iliac artery ~ 35351, 35361-35363
iliofemoral artery ~ 35355, 35363
innominate artery ~ 35311
mesenteric artery ~ 35341
peroneal artery ~ 35305-35306
popliteal artery ~ 35303
renal artery ~ 35341
subclavian artery ~ 35301-35311
superficial femoral artery ~ 35302
tibial artery ~ 35305-35306
tibioperoneal trunk artery ~ 35304
vertebral artery ~ 35301

Thrombokinase ~ 85260
Thrombolysin ~ 85400
Thrombolysis
arterial
  intracranial
    transcatheter infusion ~ 37211, 37195
    percutaneous ~ 61645
  other than coronary
    transcatheter infusion ~ 37211, 37213
cerebral, intravenous infusion ~ 37195
coronary vessels ~ 92975, 92977
cranial vessels ~ 37195
infusion, arterial ~ 37211-37214, 37195
transcatheter therapy ~ 37211-37214

Thrombolysis biopsy intracranial arterial perfusion ~ 61624
Thrombolysis intracranial ~ see ciliary body; cornea; eye, removal, foreign body; iris; lens; retina; sclera; vitreous ~ 65205
Thrombomodulin ~ 85337
Thromboplastin
inhibition ~ 85705
inhibition test ~ 85347
partial time ~ 85730-85732

Thromboplastin antecedent, plasma ~ 85270
Thromboplastinogen ~ 85210-85293
Thromboplastinogen B ~ 85250
Thromboxane, urine ~ 84431
Thumb ~ 26720-26727
  amputation ~ 26910, 26952
  arthrodesis, carpometacarpal joint ~ 26841-26842
  dislocation
    with fracture ~ 26645-26650
      open treatment ~ 26665
    with manipulation ~ 26641
  fracture
    with dislocation ~ 26645-26650
      open treatment ~ 26665
  fusion, in opposition ~ 26820
  reconstruction
    from finger ~ 26550
    opponensplasty ~ 26490-26496
  repair
    muscle ~ 26508
    muscle transfer ~ 26494
    tendon transfer ~ 26510
  replantation ~ 20824-20827
  sesamoidectomy ~ 26185
  unlisted services and procedures ~ 26989
Thymectomy ~ 60520-60521
  sternal split/transthoracic approach ~ 60521-60522
  transcervical approach ~ 60520
Thymotaxin ~ 82232
Thymus gland ~ 60520
  excision ~ 60520-60521
Thyramine ~ 80324-80326
Thyrocalcitonin ~ 80410, 82308
Thyroglobulin ~ 84432
  antibody ~ 86800
Thyroglossal duct cyst, excision ~ 60280-60281
Thyroid gland
  cyst
    aspiration ~ 60300
    excision ~ 60200
    incision and drainage ~ 60000
    injection ~ 60300
  excision
    for malignancy
      limited neck dissection ~ 60252
      radical neck dissection ~ 60254
    partial ~ 60210-60225
    secondary ~ 60260
    total ~ 60240, 60271
      cervical approach ~ 60271
      removal all thyroid tissue ~ 60260
      sternal split/transthoracic approach ~ 60270
      transcervical approach ~ 60520
  metastatic cancer, nuclear imaging ~ 78015-78018
  needle biopsy ~ 60100
  nuclear medicine
    imaging for metastases ~ 78015-78018
    imaging with flow ~ 78013
    metastases uptake ~ 78020
    uptake ~ 78012, 78014
  tumor, excision ~ 60200
Thyroid hormone binding ratio ~ 84479
Thyroid hormone uptake ~ 84479
Thyroid stimulating hormone (TSH) ~ 80418, 80438-80439, 84443
Thyroid stimulating hormone receptor AB ~ 80438-80439
Thyroid stimulating immune globulins ~ 84445
Thyroid stimulator, long acting ~ 80438-80439
Thyroid suppression test ~ 78012, 78014
Thyroidectomy
  partial ~ 60210-60225
  secondary ~ 60260
  total ~ 60240, 60271
    cervical approach ~ 60271
    for malignancy
      limited neck dissection ~ 60252
      radical neck dissection ~ 60254
    removal all thyroid tissue ~ 60260
    sternal split/transthoracic approach ~ 60270

Thyrolingual cyst ~ 60000, 60280-60281
Thyrotomy ~ 31300
Thyrotropin receptor AB ~ 80438-80439
Thyrotropin releasing hormone (TRH) ~ 80438-80439
Thyroxine
  free ~ 84439
  neonatal ~ 84437
  total ~ 84436
  true ~ 84436
Thyroxine binding globulin ~ 84442
Tibia ~ see ankle
  arthroscopy surgical ~ 29891-29892
  artery
    thrombectomy ~ 34203
    thromboendarterectomy ~ 35305, 35306
  axial bone density, pulse-echo ultrasound ~ 0508T
  bone quality testing by microindentation ~ 0547T
  craterization ~ 27360, 27640
  cyst, excision ~ 27635-27638
  diaphysectomy ~ 27360, 27640
  excision ~ 27360, 27640
    epiphyseal bar ~ 20150
  fracture ~ 27759
  fracture
    arthroscopic treatment ~ 29855-29856
      plafond ~ 29892
    closed treatment ~ 27824-27825
    distal ~ 27824-27828
    intercondylar ~ 27538-27540
    malleolus ~ 27760-27766, 27808-27814
    open treatment ~ 27535-27536, 27758-27759, 27826-27828
    plateau ~ 29855-29856
      closed treatment ~ 27530-27536
    shaft ~ 27752-27759
    with manipulation ~ 27825
    without manipulation ~ 27824
  incision ~ 27607
  osteoplasty, lengthening ~ 27715
  prophylactic treatment ~ 27745
  reconstruction ~ 27418
    at knee ~ 27440-27443, 27446
  repair ~ 27720-27725
    epiphysis ~ 27477-27485, 27730-27742
    osteochondritis dissecans arthroscopy ~ 29892
    osteotomy ~ 27455-27457, 27705, 27709-27712
    pseudoarthrosis ~ 27727
  saucerization ~ 27360, 27640
  tumor, excision ~ 27635-27638, 27645
  X-ray ~ 73590
Tibial
  arteries ~ see artery, tibial
  nerve
    neurostimulation ~ 64566
    repair/suture, posterior ~ 64840
Tibiofibular joint
  arthrodesis ~ 27871
  dislocation ~ 27830-27832
  disruption, open treatment ~ 27829
  fusion ~ 27871
TIG ~ see immune globulins, tetanus
Time
  bleeding ~ 85002
  prothrombin ~ 85610-85611
  reptilase ~ 85670-85675
Tinnitus assessment ~ 92625
Tissue
  culture
    chromosome analysis ~ 88230-88239
    homogenization ~ 87176
    non-neoplastic disorder ~ 88230, 88237
    skin grafts ~ 15100-15121, 15342-15343
    solid tumor ~ 88239
    toxin/antitoxin ~ 87230
    virus ~ 87252-87253
  dissection, macroscopic ~ 88387-88388
  enzyme activity ~ 82657
  examination
    for ectoparasites ~ 87220
    for fungi ~ 87220
    macroscopic ~ 88387-88388

Tissue ~ *continued*
  expander
    breast reconstruction with ~ 19357
    insertion, skin ~ 11960
    removal, skin ~ 11971
    replacement, skin ~ 11970
  granulation ~ 17250
  homogenization ~ 87176
  hybridization in situ ~ 88365-88368
  mucosal ~ see mucosa
  preparation
    macroscopic ~ 88387-88388
  skin harvest for culture ~ 15040
  transfer
    adjacent
      eyelids ~ 67961
      skin ~ 14000-14350
    facial muscles ~ 15845
    finger flap ~ 14350
    toe flap ~ 14350
  typing
    culture ~ 87140-87158
    HLA antibodies ~ 86812-86817
    HLA crossmatch ~ 86825-86826
    lymphocyte culture ~ 86821
Tissue factor ~ see thromboplastin
TLC
  screen ~ 84375
TMJ ~ see temporomandibular joint (TMJ)
  prostheses ~ 21243
Tobramycin assay ~ 80200
Tocolysis ~ 59412
Tocopherol ~ 84446
Toe ~ see phalanx ~ 28270, 28272
  amputation ~ 28810-28825
  capsulotomy ~ 28270-28272
  fasciotomy ~ 28008
  fracture ~ see fracture, phalanges, toe
  lesion, excision ~ 28092
  reconstruction
    angle deformity ~ 28313
    extra toes ~ 28344
    hammer toe ~ 28285-28286
    macrodactyly ~ 28340-28341
    syndactyly ~ 28345
    webbed toe ~ 28345
  repair
    bunion ~ 28292, 28295-28299
    muscle ~ 28240
    tendon ~ 28232-28234, 28240
    webbed ~ 28280
    webbed toe ~ 28345
  tenotomy ~ 28010-28011, 28232-28234
  unlisted services and procedures ~ 28899
Toe flap tissue transfer ~ 14350
Toes
  arthrocentesis ~ 20600
  dislocation ~ see specific joint**
  magnetic resonance imaging (MRI) ~ 73721-73723
  reconstruction, extra digit ~ 26587
  repair
    extra digit ~ 26587
    macrodactylia ~ 26590
  reposition to hand ~ 26551-26556
  strapping ~ 29550
  X-ray ~ 73660
Tolerance test
  glucagon ~ 82946
  glucose ~ 82951-82952
  heparin-protamine ~ 85530
  insulin ~ 80434-80435
  maltose ~ 82951-82952
Tomodensitometries ~ see CT scan
Tomographic spect myocardial imaging ~ 78469
Tomographies, computed X-ray ~ see CT scan
Tomography, computerized axial abdomen ~ 74150-74175, 75635
  head ~ 70450-70470, 70496
Tomography, emission computed ~ see positron emission tomography
Tompkins metroplasty ~ 58540

Tongue
  ablation, submucosal tongue base ~ 41530
  abscess, incision and drainage ~ 41000-41006, 41015
  base suspension ~ 41512
  biopsy ~ 41100-41105
  cyst, incision and drainage ~ 41000-41006, 41015, 60000
  excision
    complete ~ 41140-41155
    frenum ~ 41115
    partial ~ 41120-41135
    with mouth resection ~ 41150-41153
    with radical neck ~ 41135, 41145, 41153-41155
  hematoma, incision and drainage ~ 41000-41006, 41015
  incision, frenum ~ 41010
  lesion, excision ~ 41110-41114
  reconstruction, frenum ~ 41520
  repair ~ 41250-41252
    laceration ~ 41250-41252
    suture ~ 41510
  suture ~ 41510
  unlisted services and procedures ~ 41599
Tonometry, serial ~ 92100
Tonsil, pharyngeal ~ see adenoids
Tonsillectomy ~ 42820-42826
Tonsils
  abscess, incision and drainage ~ 42700
  excision ~ 42825-42826
    lingual ~ 42870
    radical ~ 42842-42845
    tag ~ 42860
    with adenoids ~ 42820-42821
  lingual, destruction ~ 42870
  unlisted services and procedures ~ 42999
Topiramate assay ~ 80201
Torek Procedure ~ see orchiopexy
Torkildsen Procedure ~ 62180
TORP (total ossicular replacement prosthesis) ~ 69633, 69637
Torsion swing test ~ 92546
Torula ~ see cryptococcus
Torus mandibularis tumor excision ~ 21031
Total
  abdominal hysterectomy ~ 58150, 58200, 58956
  bilirubin level ~ 82247-82248, 88720
  catecholamines ~ 82382
  cystectomy ~ 51570, 51580, 51590-51597
  dacryoadenectomy ~ 68500
  elbow replacement ~ 24363
  esophagectomy ~ 43107-43113, 43124
  gastrectomy ~ 43620-43622
  hemolytic complement ~ 86162
  hip arthroplasty ~ 27130-27132
  knee arthroplasty ~ 27438, 27445
  mastectomies ~ see mastectomy
  ostectomy of patella ~ 27424
  splenectomy ~ 38100
Touroff Operation ~ 37615
Toxicology screen ~ 80305-80307
Toxin assay ~ 87230
Toxin, botulinum ~ see chemodenervation
Toxoplasma antibody ~ 86777-86778
Trabeculectomies ~ 65855
Trabeculectomy ab externo
  in absence of previous surgery ~ 66170
  with scarring previous surgery ~ 66172
Trabeculoplasty by laser surgery ~ 65855
Trabeculostomy ab interno
  laser ~ 0621T, 0622T
Trabeculotomy
  ab Externo ~ 65850
  goniotomy ~ 65820
Trachea
  aspiration ~ 31720
  catheter ~ 31720-31725
  dilation ~ 31630-31631, 31636-31638
  endoscopy, via tracheostomy ~ 31615
  excision, stenosis ~ 31780-31781
  fistula
    with plastic repair ~ 31825
    without plastic repair ~ 31820
  fracture, endoscopy ~ 31630

Trachea ~ *continued*
  incision
    emergency ~ 31603-31605
    planned ~ 31600-31601
    with flaps ~ 31610
  introduction, needle wire ~ 31730
  puncture, aspiration and/or injection ~ 31612
  reconstruction
    carina ~ 31766
    cervical ~ 31750
    fistula ~ 31755
    intrathoracic ~ 31760
  repair
    cervical ~ 31750
    fistula ~ 31755
    intrathoracic ~ 31760
    stoma ~ 31613-31614
  resection, cricotracheal ~ 31592
  revision, stoma, scars ~ 31830
  scar, revision ~ 31830
  stenosis
    excision ~ 31780-31781
    repair ~ 31780-31781
  stoma
    repair
      with plastic repair ~ 31825
      without plastic repair ~ 31820
    revision, scars ~ 31830
  tumor
    excision
      cervical ~ 31785
      thoracic ~ 31786
  unlisted services and procedures, bronchi ~ 31899
  wound, suture
    cervical ~ 31800
    intrathoracic ~ 31805
Tracheal stent, placement ~ 31631
  tubes ~ 31500
Trachelectomy ~ 57530
  radical ~ 57531
Tracheloplasty ~ 15819
Trachelorrhaphy ~ 57720
Tracheo-esophageal fistula ~ see fistula, tracheoesophageal
Tracheobronchoscopy through tracheostomy ~ 31615
Tracheoplasty
  cervical ~ 31750
  intrathoracic ~ 31760
  tracheopharyngeal fistulization ~ 31755
Tracheostoma revision ~ 31613-31614
Tracheostomy
  emergency ~ 31603-31605
  planned ~ 31600-31601
  revision, scar ~ 31830
  surgical closure
    with plastic repair ~ 31825
    without plastic repair ~ 31820
  tracheobronchoscopy through ~ 31615
  with flaps ~ 31610
Tracheotomy tube change ~ 31502
Tracking tests (ocular) ~ 92545
Tract, urinary ~ 74400-74425
Traction therapy ~ 97140
  manual ~ 97140
  mechanical ~ 97012
Training
  activities of daily living ~ 97535, 99509
  biofeedback ~ 90875, 90901-90913
  cognitive skills ~ 97129, 97130
  community/work reintegration ~ 97537
  compensatory ~ 97129, 97130, 97535
  home management ~ 97535, 99509
  orthoptic/pleoptic ~ 92065
  orthotics ~ 97760, 97763
  prosthetics ~ 97761
  self care ~ 97535, 98960-98962, 99509
  sensory integration ~ 97533
  walking (physical therapy) ~ 97116
  wheelchair management ~ 97542
Tram flap
  breast reconstruction ~ 19367-19369

Trans-scaphoperilunar fracture/dislocation
  closed treatment ~ 25680
  open treatment ~ 25685
Transaminase
  glutamic oxaloacetic ~ 84450
  glutamic pyruvic ~ 84460
Transcatheter
  aortic valve replacement
    open axillary artery approach ~ 33363
    open femoral artery approach ~ 33362
    open iliac artery approach ~ 33364
    percutaneous femoral artery approach ~ 33361
    transaortic approach ~ 33365
    transapical approach ~ 33366
    with cardiopulmonary bypass support ~ 33367-33369
  arterialization, venous
    peroneal vein ~ 0620T
    tibial vein ~ 0620T
  biopsy ~ 37200
  closure
    percutaneous
      ductus arteriosus ~ 93582
      heart ~ 93580-93582
    transmyocardial
      cranial ~ 61624-61626
  denervation, renal sympathetic ~ 0338T, 0339T
  embolization
    cranial ~ 61624-61626
    vascular ~ 37241-37244
  insertion, leadless pacemaker system ~ 33274
  interatrial septal shunt device implantation ~ 0613T
  mitral valve implantation/replacement (TMVI) ~ 0483T, 0484T
  mitral valve repair ~ 33418, 33419, 0345T
  occlusion, cranial ~ 61624-61626
  paravalvular leak
    aortic valve ~ 93591, 93592
    mitral valve ~ 93590, 93592
    vascular ~ 37241-37244
  placement
    arteriovenous anastomosis implant ~ 0553T
    intravascular stent ~ 37215-37218, 37236-37239, 92928, 92929, 0075T, 0076T, 0505T
    central dialysis segment ~ 36908
    peripheral dialysis segment ~ 36906
    stent for intracardiac shunt ~ 33745, 33746
  removal, leadless pacemaker system ~ 0388T
  replacement, leadless pacemaker system ~ 0387T
  therapy
    embolization ~ 75894, 75898
    infusion (arterial or venous) ~ 37211-37214, 61650, 61651
    perfusion, cranial ~ 61624-61626
    septal reduction ~ 93583
  transcatheter tricuspid valve repair (TTVr) ~ 0569T, 0570T
Transcatheter Aortic Valve Replacement (TAVR/TAVI)
  axillary artery approach ~ 33363
  femoral artery approach ~ 33361-33362
  iliac artery approach ~ 33364
  transaortic approach ~ 33365
  transapical approach ~ 33366
  with cardiopulmonary bypass support ~ 33367-33369
  with arterial./venous cannulation ~ 33367-33369
Transcatheter foreign body retrieval ~ 37197
Transcortin ~ 84449
Transcranial Doppler study (TCP) ~ 93886-93893
  stimulation, motor ~ 95928-95929
Transcutaneous electric nerve stimulation (TENS) ~ 97014
Transcutaneous electrical modulation pain reprocessing ~ 0278T
Transcutaneous measurement
  visible light hyperspectral imaging (VLHI) ~ 0631T
Transection
  artery, carotid ~ 61611
  blood vessel, kidney ~ 50100
  brain, subpial ~ 61567
  nerve ~ 64732-64772
    vagus ~ 43640-43641
  pulmonary artery ~ 33922
Transesophageal Doppler echocardiography ~ 93312-93318

Transfer
blastocyst ~ 58974-58976
gamete intrafallopian ~ see GIFT
jejunum, with microvascular anastomosis, free ~ 43496
preparation, embryo ~ 89255
cryopreserved ~ 89352
surgical ~ see transposition
tendon ~ see tendon, transfer
toe to hand ~ 26551-26556
Transferase
aspartate amino ~ 84450
glutamic oxaloacetic ~ 84450
Transferrin ~ 84466
Transformation lymphocyte ~ 86353
Transfusion
blood ~ 36430
exchange ~ 36455
newborn ~ 36450, 36456
fetal ~ 36460
push, infant ~ 36440
blood parts, exchange ~ 36511-36516
unlisted services and procedures ~ 86999
white blood cells ~ 86950
Transfusion medicine ~ 86850-86999
Transluminal
angioplasty, arterial
radiological supervision ~ 37246, 37247
Transmyocardial laser revascularization ~ 33140-33141
Transosteal bone plate reconstruction, mandible ~ 21244
Transpeptidase, gamma-glutamyl ~ 82977
Transplant ~ see graft
bone ~ see bone graft
hair ~ see hair, transplant
islet cells ~ 0584T-0586T
Transplantation ~ see graft
autologous ~ see autograft
bone marrow ~ 38240-38242
cartilage, knee
allograft ~ 27415, 29867
autograft ~ 27412, 29866
chondrocytes, knee ~ 27412
conjunctiva ~ 65782
cornea
autograft/homograft
allograft preparation ~ 65757
endothelials ~ 65756
lamellar ~ 65710
penetrating ~ 65730-65755
for aphakia ~ 65750
eye
amniotic membrane ~ 65780
conjunctiva ~ 65782
stem cell ~ 65781
hair
punch graft ~ 15775-15776
strip ~ 15220-15221
heart ~ 33945
allograft preparation ~ 33933, 33944
heart-lung ~ 33935
intestines
allograft preparation ~ 44715-44721
allotransplantation ~ 44135-44136
donor enterectomy ~ 44132-44133
removal of allograft ~ 44137
liver ~ 47135
allograft preparation ~ 47143-47147
lung
allograft preparation ~ 0494T, 32855-32856, 33933
anesthesia ~ 00580
donor pneumonectomy ~ 32850
double, with cardiopulmonary bypass ~ 32854
double, without cardiopulmonary bypass ~ 32853
initiation and monitoring, cadaver ~ 0495T-0496T
single, with cardiopulmonary bypass ~ 32852
single, without cardiopulmonary bypass ~ 32851
meniscus, knee ~ 29868
pancreas ~ 48160, 48550, 48554-48556
allograft preparation ~ 48551-48552
parathyroid ~ 60512

Transplantation ~ *continued*
renal
allograft preparation ~ 50323-50329
allotransplantation ~ 50360
with recipient nephrectomy ~ 50365
autotransplantation ~ 50380
donor nephrectomy ~ 50300-50320, 50547
recipient nephrectomy ~ 50340
removal transplanted renal allograft ~ 50370
skin ~ see dermatology
stem cells ~ 38240-38241
cell concentration ~ 38215
cryopreservation ~ 38207
harvesting ~ 38205-38206
plasma depletion ~ 38214
platelet depletion ~ 38213
red blood cell depletion ~ 38212
T-cell depletion ~ 38210
thawing ~ 38208
tumor cell depletion ~ 38211
washing ~ 38209
testis ~ 38208
to thigh ~ 54680
Transposition
arteries
carotid ~ 0037T, 35691, 35694-35695
subclavian ~ 0037T, 35693-35695
vertebral ~ 35691-35693
cranial nerve ~ 64716
eye muscles ~ 67320
great arteries, repair ~ 33770-33781
nerve ~ 64718-64721
ovary ~ 58825
peripheral nerve
major ~ 64856
vein valve ~ 34510
Transthoracic echocardiography ~ 93303-93318, 93350
Transthyretin ~ 84134
Transureteroureterostomy ~ 50770
Transurethral procedure ~ see specific procedure**
prostate
incision ~ 52450
resection ~ 52630
thermotherapy ~ 53850-53852
microwave ~ 53850
radiofrequency ~ 53852
Trapezium arthroplasty with implant ~ 25445
Travel, unusual ~ 99082
Treacher-Collins syndrome midface reconstruction ~ 21150-21151
Treatment, tocolytic ~ 59412
Trendelenburg Operation ~ 37785
Trephine procedure sinusotomy, frontal ~ 31070
Treponema pallidum
antibody, confirmation test ~ 86780
antigen detection, direct fluorescence ~ 87285
TRH ~ see thyrotropin releasing hormone (TRH)
Triacylglycerol ~ 84478
Triacylglycerol hydrolase ~ 83690
Tributyrinase ~ 83690
Trichiasis repair ~ 67825
epilation, by forceps ~ 67820
epilation, by other than forceps ~ 67825
incision of lid margin ~ 67830
with free mucous membrane graft ~ 67835
Trichina ~ 86784, 96902
Trichinella
antibody ~ 86784
trichogram ~ 96902
Trichomonas vaginalis
antigen detection
nucleic acid ~ 87660
by immunoassay with direct optical observation ~ 87808
Trichrome stain ~ 88313
Tricuspid valve
annulus reconstruction ~ 0545T
excision ~ 33460
repair ~ 33463-33465, 0569T, 0570T
replacement ~ 33465
repositioning ~ 33468
Tridymite ~ 84285
Trigeminal ganglia ~ see Gasserian ganglion

1247

Trigeminal nerve
　destruction ~ 64600-64610
　injection
　　anesthetic ~ 64400
　　neurolytic ~ 64600-64610
Trigeminal tract stereotactic, create lesion ~ 61791
Trigger finger repair ~ 26055
Trigger point injection
　one or two muscles ~ 20552
　two or more muscles ~ 20553
Triglyceridase ~ 83690
Triglyceride lipase ~ 83690
Triglycerides ~ 84478
Trigonocephaly ~ 21175
Triiodothyronine
　free ~ 84481
　reverse ~ 84482
　total ~ 84480
　true ~ 84480
Triolean hydrolase ~ 83690
Trioxopurine ~ 84550, 84560
Tripcellim ~ 84485, 84488-84490
Trisegmentectomy ~ 47122
Trocar biopsy bone marrow ~ 38221
Trochanteric femur fracture ~ 27246, 27248
Trophoblastic tumor GTT ~ 59100, 59870
Troponin ~ 84484
　qualitative ~ 84512
　quantitative ~ 84484
Truncal vagotomies ~ 43640
Truncus arteriosus repair ~ 33786
Truncus brachiocephalicus ~ see artery, brachiocephalic
Trunk, brachiocephalic ~ see artery, brachiocephalic
Trypanosomiases ~ 86171, 86280
Trypanosomiasis ~ 86171, 86280
Trypsin
　duodenum ~ 84485
　feces ~ 84488-84490
Trypsin inhibitor, alpha 1-antirypsin ~ see alpha-1 antitrypsin
Trypure ~ 84485, 84488-84490
Tsalicylate intoxication ~ 80329-80331
TSH ~ see thyroid stimulating hormone
TSI ~ see thyroid stimulating immunoglobulin
Tsutsugamushi disease ~ 86000
TT ~ see thrombin time
TT-3 ~ see triiodothyronine, true
TT-4 ~ see thyroxine, true
Tuba auditoria (auditiva) ~ see eustachian tube
Tubal embryo stage transfer ~ see embryo transfer
Tubal ligation ~ 58600
　laparoscopic ~ 58670
　with cesarean section ~ 58611
Tubal occlusion ~ 58615
　with cesarean delivery ~ see occlusion ~ 58615
　　creat lesion ~ 58565, 58615
Tubal pregnancy ~ 59121
　with salpingectomy and/or oophorectomy ~ 59120
Tube change
　colonic ~ 49450
　duodenostomy ~ 49451
　gastro-jejunostomy ~ 49452
　gastrostomy ~ 49446
　jejunostomy ~ 49451
　tracheotomy ~ 31502
Tube placement
　cecostomy tube ~ 44300, 49442
　duodenostomy tube ~ 49441
　endoscopic
　　bile duct, pancreatic duct ~ 43268
　　jejunostomy tube, percutaneous ~ 49441
　　nasobiliary, nasopancreatic
　　　for drainage ~ 43274
　enterostomy tube ~ 44300
　gastrostomy tube ~ 43246, 49440
　nasogastric tube ~ 43752
　orogastric tube ~ 43752
Tube, fallopian ~ see fallopian tube
Tubectomy ~ 58700, 58720
Tubed pedicle flap formation ~ 15570-15576
Tubercle bacilli culture ~ 87116
Tubercleplasty tibia, anterior ~ 27418

Tuberculin test ~ 85480
Tuberculosis
　antigen response test ~ 86480
　culture ~ 87116
　skin test ~ 86580
Tuberculosis vaccine (BCG) ~ 90585-90586
Tubes
　endotracheal ~ 31500
　gastrostomy ~ 43246, 43761
Tudor "rabbit ear" ~ see urethra, repair
Tuffier vaginal hysterectomy ~ 58260-58270, 58290-58294, 58550-58554
Tumor
　abdomen, destruction/excision ~ 49203-49205, 58957, 58958
　abdominal wall, excision ~ 22900-22905
　ablation, electroporation ~ 0600T-0601T
　acetabulum, excision ~ 27076
　ankle ~ 27615-27619, 27632, 27634
　arm, lower ~ 25071-25078
　arm, upper, excision ~ 24071-24079
　back/flank
　　excision ~ 21930-21936
　　radical resection ~ 21935, 21936
　bile duct
　　destruction ~ 43272
　　extrahepatic ~ 47711
　　intrahepatic ~ 47712
　bladder ~ 52234-52240
　　excision ~ 51530, 52355
　bone, ablation ~ 20982
　brain ~ 61510
　　excision ~ 61518, 61520-61521, 61526-61530, 61545, 62164
　breast
　　ablation ~ 0581T
　　excision ~ 19120-19126
　　intraoperative radiation therapy (IORT), preparation of tumor cavity ~ 19294
　bronchi, excision ~ 31640
　calcaneus ~ 28100-28103
　　excision ~ 27647
　carpal ~ 25130-25136
　cheekbone ~ 21030, 21034
　chest wall
　　cryoablation ~ 32994
　　excision ~ 21601-21603
　clavicle excision ~ 23140, 23200
　　with allograft ~ 23146
　　with autograft ~ 23145
　coccyx ~ 49215
　colon, destruction ~ 44401, 45383
　cranial bone, reconstruction ~ 21181-21184
　destruction
　　chemosurgery ~ 17311-17315
　　urethra ~ 53220
　ear, middle
　　extended ~ 69554
　　transcanal ~ 69550
　　transmastoid ~ 69552
　elbow, excision ~ 24071-24079
　esophagus, ablation ~ 43229
　excision, femur ~ 27355-27358
　face or scalp
　　excision ~ 21011-21014
　　radical resection ~ 21015-21016
　facial bone ~ 21029-21030, 21034
　fallopian tube, resection ~ 58950, 58952-58958
　femoral ~ 27355-27358
　femur ~ 27065-27067
　　excision ~ 27365
　fibroid ~ 58140, 58545-58546, 58561
　fibula ~ 27635-27638
　　excision ~ 27646
　finger, excision ~ 26111-26118
　foot ~ 28039-28047
　forearm, radical resection ~ 25077
　gastrostomy ~ see lesion
　gums, excision ~ 41825-41827
　hand, excision ~ 26111-26118
　heart, excision ~ 33120-33130
　hip ~ 27043-27045, 27049, 27059, 27065-27067
　　excision ~ 27075-27076

Tumor ~ *continued*

humerus excision ~ 23150, 23220, 24110
  with allograft ~ 23156, 24116
  with autograft ~ 23155, 24115
ileum ~ 27065-27067
immunoassay for antigen ~ 86294, 86316
  CA 125 ~ 86304
  CA 15-3 ~ 86300
  CA 19-9 ~ 86301
innominate, excision ~ 27077
intestines, small, destruction ~ 44369
ischial, excision ~ 27078
kidney, excision ~ 50562, 52355
knee, excision ~ 27327-27329, 27337-27339, 27365
lacrimal gland, excision
  frontal approach ~ 68540
  with osteotomy ~ 68550
larynx
  excision ~ 31300
    endoscopic ~ 31540-31541, 31578
  incision ~ 31300
leg, lower ~ 27615-27619, 27632, 27634
leg, upper, excision ~ 27327-27329, 27337-27339, 27365
localization, nuclear medicine ~ 78800-78804, 78830-78832
mandible ~ 21044-21047
maxilla ~ 21030, 21034, 21048-21049
maxillary torus palatinus ~ 21032
mediastinal, excision ~ 39220
mediastinum ~ 32662
meningioma ~ 61512
  excision ~ 61519
metacarpal ~ 26200-26205, 26250
metatarsal ~ 28104-28107
  excision ~ 28173
neck
  excision ~ 21552-21558
  radical resection ~ 21557, 21558
olecranon, excision ~ 24120
olecranon process
  with allograft, excision ~ 24126
  with autograft, excision ~ 24125
ovary, resection ~ 58950-58958
pancreatic duct, destruction ~ 43272
parotid gland, excision ~ 42410-42426
pelvis ~ 27043-27045, 27049, 27059
pericardial
  endoscopic ~ 32661
  excision ~ 33050
peritoneum
  excision ~ 49203-49205
  debulking ~ 58575, 58950-58958
phalanges
  finger ~ 26210-26215, 26260-26262
  toe ~ 28108
    excision ~ 28175
pituitary gland, excision ~ 61546-61548, 62165
pleura, cryoablation ~ 32994
positron emission tomography (PET) ~ 78811-78816
pubis ~ 27065-27067
pulmonary ablation
  cryoablation ~ 32994
  radiofrequency ~ 32998
radiation therapy ~ 77295
radius ~ 25120-25126, 25170
  excision ~ 24120
  with allograft, excision ~ 24126
  with autograft, excision ~ 24125
rectum
  destruction ~ 45190, 45320, 46937-46938
  excision ~ 45160-45172
resection
  face ~ 21015
  scalp ~ 21015
  with cystourethroscopy ~ 52355
retroperitoneal, destruction/excision ~ 49203-49205, 58957, 58958
sacrum ~ 49215
scapula
  excision ~ 23140, 23210
    with allograft ~ 23146
    with autograft ~ 23145

Tumor ~ *continued*

shoulder, excision ~ 23071-23078
skull, excision ~ 61500
soft tissue
  elbow, excision ~ 24071-24079
  finger, excision ~ 26115
  forearm, radical resection ~ 25077
  hand, excision ~ 26115
  wrist
    excision ~ 25071-25078
    radical resection ~ 25077, 25078
spinal cord, excision ~ 63275-63290
stomach, excision ~ 43610-43611
talus ~ 28100-28103
  excision ~ 27647
tarsal ~ 28104-28107
  excision ~ 28171
temporal bone, removal ~ 69970
testis, excision ~ 54530-54535
thorax
  excision ~ 21552-21558
  radical resection ~ 21557, 21558
thyroid, excision ~ 60200
tibia ~ 27365, 27635-27638
  excision ~ 27645
torus mandibularis ~ 21031
trachea, excision
  cervical ~ 31785
  thoracic ~ 31786
ulna ~ 25120-25126, 25170
  excision ~ 24120
  with allograft, excision ~ 24126
  with autograft, excision ~ 24125
ureter, excision ~ 52355
urethra ~ 52234-52240, 53220
  excision ~ 52355
uterus
  excision ~ 58140-58146
  resection ~ 58950-58958
vagina, excision ~ 57135
vertebra, additional segment
  excision ~ 22116
  cervical, excision ~ 22100
  lumbar ~ 22102
  thoracic, excision ~ 22101
wrist ~ 25071-25078, 25135-25136
  radical resection ~ 25077

Tunica vaginalis hydrocele
  aspiration ~ 55000
  excision ~ 55040-55041
  repair ~ 55060

Turbinate
  excision ~ 30130-30140
  fracture, therapeutic ~ 30930
  injection ~ 30200
  submucous resection, nose excision ~ 30140

Turbinate mucosa cauterization ~ 30801-30802

Turcica, sella ~ 70240, 70480-70482

TURP ~ 52630

Tylectomy ~ *see* breast, excision, lesion

Tylenol urine ~ 80329-80331

Tympanic membrane
  create stoma ~ 69433, 69436, 0583T
    myringoplasty ~ 69620
    myringotomy ~ 69421
    neurectomy ~ 69676
    repair ~ 69610
    tympanolysis ~ 69450
    tympanostomy ~ 69433, 69436, 0583T
  incision ~ 69420-69421
  reconstruction ~ 69620
  repair ~ 69450, 69610

Tympanic nerve excision ~ 69676

Tympanolysis ~ 69450

Tympanomastoidectomy ~ *see* tympanoplasty

Tympanometry ~ *see* audiologic function tests ~ 92550, 92567, 92570

Tympanoplasty

radical or complete ~ 69645
  with ossicular chain reconstruction ~ 69646
with antrotomy or mastoidotomy ~ 69635
  with ossicular chain reconstruction ~ 69636
    and synthetic prosthesis ~ 69637
with mastoidectomy ~ 69641
  with intact or reconstructed wall ~ 69643
    and ossicular chain reconstruction ~ 69644
  with ossicular chain reconstruction ~ 69642
without mastoidectomy ~ 69631
  with ossicular chain reconstruction ~ 69632
    and synthetic prosthesis ~ 69633

Tympanostomy

with automatied tube delivery system ~ 0583T
with general anesthesia ~ 69436
with lontophoresis anesthesia ~ 0583T
with local anesthesia ~ 69433, 0583T
removal of tube ~ 69424

Tympanotomy ~ 69420-69421
Typhoid vaccine ~ 90690

oral ~ 90690
polysaccharide ~ 90691

Typhus

endemic ~ 86000
mite-bone ~ 86000
Sno Paulo ~ 86000
tropical ~ 86000

Typing, blood ~ see blood typing
Typing, HLA ~ 86812-86817
Typing, tissue ~ see tissue typing
Tyrosine ~ 84510
Tzank smear ~ 87207

U

Uchida Procedure ~ 58600
UDP galactose pyrophosphorylase ~ 82775-82776
UFR ~ 51736-51741
Ulcer

anal ~ 46200, 46940-46942
decubitus ~ see debridement; skin graft and flap ~ 15920-15999
pinch graft ~ 15050
pressure ~ 15920-15999
stomach, excision ~ 43610

Ulcerative, cystitis ~ 52260-52265
Ulna ~ see arm, lower; elbow; humerus; radius

arthrodesis, radioulnar joint, with resection ~ 25830
arthroplasty, with implant ~ 25442
centralization or wrist ~ 25335
craterization ~ 24147, 25150-25151
cyst, excision ~ 24125-24126, 25120-25126
diaphysectomy ~ 24147, 25150-25151
excision ~ 24147
  abscess ~ 24138
  complete ~ 25240
  epiphyseal bar ~ 20150
  partial ~ 25145..2515, 1, 25240
fracture
  closed treatment ~ 25530-25535
  olecranon ~ 24670-24675
    open treatment ~ 24685
  open treatment ~ 25545
  shaft ~ 25530-25545
    open treatment ~ 25574
  styloid
    closed treatment ~ 25650
    open treatment ~ 25652
    percutaneous fixation ~ 25651
    with dislocation
      closed treatment ~ 24620
      open treatment ~ 24635
  with manipulation ~ 25535
  with radius ~ 25560-25565
    open treatment ~ 25575
  without manipulation ~ 25530

Ulna ~ *continued*

incision and drainage ~ 25035
osteoplasty ~ 25390-25393
prophylactic treatment ~ 25491-25492
reconstruction, radioulnar ~ 25337
repair
  epiphyseal arrest ~ 25450-25455
  malunion or nonunion ~ 25400, 25415
  osteotomy ~ 25360, 25370-25375
    and radius ~ 25365
  with graft ~ 25405, 25420-25426
saucerization ~ 24147, 25150-25151
sequestrectomy ~ 24138, 25145
tumor
  cyst ~ 24120
  excision ~ 24125-24126, 25120-25126, 25170

Ulnar arteries ~ see artery, ulnar
Ulnar nerve

decompression ~ 64718
neuroplasty ~ 64718-64719
reconstruction ~ 64718-64719
release ~ 64718-64719
repair/suture, motor ~ 64836
transposition ~ 64718-64719

Ultrasonic ~ see ultrasound
Ultrasonic cardiography ~ see echocardiography
Ultrasonic procedure ~ 52325
Ultrasonography ~ see echography
Ultrasound ~ see echocardiography; echography

abdomen ~ 76700-76706
aortic aneurysm screening ~ 76706
artery
  intracranial ~ 93886-93893
  middle cerebral ~ 76821
  umbilical ~ 76820
bladder ~ 51798
bone density study ~ 76977
breast ~ 76641, 76642
bronchi
  endobronchial ultrasound (EBUS)~ 31652-31654
chest ~ 76604
colon, endoscopic ~ 45391-45392
colon-sigmoid, endoscopic ~ 45341-45342
drainage, abscess ~ 75989
echoencephalography ~ 76506
esophagus, endoscopy ~ 43231-43232
extremity(s) ~ 76881-76882
eye ~ 76510-76513
  biometry ~ 76516-76519
  foreign body ~ 76529
  pachymetry ~ 76514
fallopian tube ~ 0568T
fetus ~ 76818-76828
for physical therapy ~ 97035
gastrointestinal ~ 76975
gastrointestinal, upper, endoscopic ~ 43237-43238, 43242, 43259
guidance
  amniocentesis ~ 59001, 76946
  amnioinfusion ~ 59070
  arteriovenous fistulae ~ 76936
  chorionic villus sampling ~ 76945
  cryosurgery ~ 55873
  drainage, fetal fluid ~ 59074
  endometrial ablation ~ 58356
  fetal cordocentesis ~ 76941
  fetal transfusion ~ 76941
  heart biopsy ~ 76932
  needle biopsy ~ 43232, 43238, 43242, 45342, 45392, 76942
  occlusion, umbilical cord ~ 59072
  ova retrieval ~ 76948
  pericardiocentesis ~ 33016
  pseudoaneurysm ~ 76936
  radiation therapy ~ 77387
  radioelement ~ 76965
  shunt placement, fetal ~ 59076
  thoracentesis ~ 76942
  tissue ablation ~ 76490
  uterine fibroid ablation ~ 58674
  vascular access ~ 76937

Ultrasound ~ *continued*
head ~ 76506, 76536
heart, fetal ~ 76825
hips, infant ~ 76885-76886
hysteronsonography ~ 76831
intraoperative ~ 76998
intravascular, noncoronary ~ 37252, 37253
kidney ~ 76770-76776
liver, elastography, shear wave ~ 91200
MRI-guided high intensity focused ultrasound (MRgFUS) ~ 0398T
 stereotactic lesion ablation ~ 0398T
neck ~ 76536
non-coronary, intravascular ~ 37252, 37253
pelvis ~ 76856-76857
pregnant uterus ~ 76801-76817
prostate ~ 76873
rectal ~ 76872-76873
retroperitoneal ~ 76770-76775
scrotum ~ 76870
sonohysterography ~ 76831
sonosalpingography ~ 0568T
spine ~ 76800
stimulation to aid bone healing ~ 20979
umbilical artery ~ 76820
unlisted services and procedures ~ 76999
uterus, tumor ablation ~ 0071T-0072T
vagina ~ 76830
Ultraviolet light therapy dermatology
ultraviolet A ~ 96912
ultraviolet B ~ 96910
for dermatology ~ 96900
for physical medicine ~ 97028
Umbilectomy ~ 49250
Umbilical
artery ultrasound ~ 76820
hernia ~ 49600-49611
vein catheterization ~ 36510
Umbilical cord occlusion ~ 59072
Umbilicus
excision ~ 49250
repair
 hernia ~ 49580-49587
 omphalocele ~ 49600-49611
Undescended testicle ~ 54550-54560
Unfertilized egg ~ 87177
Unguis ~ see nails
Unilateral simple mastectomy ~ see mastectomy
Unlisted services and procedures ~ 99499, 99600
abdomen ~ 22999, 49329, 49999
allergy/immunology ~ 95199
anal ~ 46999
anesthesia ~ 01999
arm ~ 25999
arthroscopy ~ 29999
autopsy ~ 88099
bile duct ~ 47999
brachytherapy ~ 77799
breast ~ 19499
bronchi ~ 31899
cardiac ~ 33999
cardiovascular studies ~ 93799
casting ~ 29799
cervix ~ 58999
chemistry procedure ~ 84999
chemotherapy ~ 96549
chest ~ 32999
coagulation ~ 85999
colon ~ 44799
conjunctiva surgery ~ 68399
craniofacial ~ 21299
CT scan ~ 76497
cytogenetic study ~ 88299
cytopathology ~ 88199
pdermatology ~ 96999
dialysis ~ 90999
diaphragm ~ 39599
ear, external ~ 69399
 inner ~ 69949
 middle ~ 69799
endocrine system ~ 60699

Unlisted services and procedures ~ *continued*
epididymis ~ 55899
esophagus ~ 43289, 43499
evaluation and management services ~ 99499
eye muscle ~ 67399
eye surgery
 anterior segment ~ 66999
 posterior segment ~ 67299
eyelid ~ 67999
fluoroscopy ~ 76496
forearm ~ 25999
gallbladder ~ 47999
gastroenterology test ~ 91299
gum ~ 41899
hand ~ 26989
hemic system ~ 38999
hepatic duct ~ 47999
hip joint ~ 27299
home services ~ 99600
hysteroscopy ~ 58579
immunization ~ 90749
immunology ~ 86849
injection ~ 90799
injection of medication ~ 90799
intestine ~ 44238, 44799
kidney ~ 53899
lacrimal system ~ 68899
laparoscopy ~ 38129, 38589, 43289, 43659, 44238-44239, 44979, 47379, 47579, 49329, 49659, 50549, 50949, 54699, 55559, 58578, 58679, 59898, 60659
larynx ~ 31599
lip ~ 40799
liver ~ 47379, 47399
lungs ~ 32999
lymphatic system ~ 38999
magnetic resonance ~ 76498
maxillofacial ~ 21299
maxillofacial prosthetics ~ 21089
Meckel's diverticulum ~ 44899
mediastinum ~ 39499
mesentery surgery ~ 44899
microbiology ~ 87999
mouth ~ 40899, 41599
musculoskeletal ~ 25999, 26989
musculoskeletal surgery, abdominal wall ~ 22999
 neck ~ 21899
 spine ~ 22899
 thorax ~ 21899
musculoskeletal system ~ 20999
 ankle ~ 27899
 arm, upper ~ 24999
 elbow ~ 24999
 head ~ 21499
 knee ~ 27599
 leg, lower ~ 27899
 leg, upper ~ 27599
necropsy ~ 88099
nervous system surgery ~ 64999
neurology/neuromuscular testing ~ 95999
nose ~ 30999
nuclear medicine ~ 78999
 blood ~ 78199
 bone ~ 78399
 endocrine system ~ 78099
 genitourinary system ~ 78799
 heart ~ 78499
 hematopoietic system ~ 78199
 lymphatic system ~ 78199
 musculoskeletal system ~ 78399
 nervous system ~ 78699
 therapeutic ~ 79999
obstetrical care ~ 59898-59899
omentum ~ 49329, 49999
ophthalmology ~ 92499
orbit ~ 67599
otorhinolaryngology ~ 92700
ovary ~ 58679, 58999
oviduct ~ 58679, 58999
palate ~ 42299
pancreas surgery ~ 48999

Unlisted services and procedures ~ *continued*
  pathology ~ 89240
  pelvis ~ 27299
  penis ~ 55899
  peritoneum ~ 49329, 49999
  pharynx ~ 42999
  physical therapy ~ 97039, 97139, 97799
  pleura ~ 32999
  pressure ulcer ~ 15999
  preventive medicine ~ 99429
  prostate ~ 55899
  psychiatric ~ 90899
  pulmonology ~ 94799
  radiation physics ~ 77399
  radiation therapy ~ 77499
    planning ~ 77299
  radiology, diagnostic ~ 76499
  radionuclide therapy ~ 79999
  radiopharmaceutical therapy ~ 79999
  rectum ~ 44239, 45999
  reproductive medicine, lab procedure ~ 89398
  salivary gland ~ 42699
  scrotum ~ 55899
  seminal vesicle ~ 55899
  shoulder surgery ~ 23929
  sinuses ~ 31299
  skin ~ 17999
  special services and reports ~ 99199
  spine ~ 22899
  stomach ~ 43659, 43999
  strapping ~ 29799
  surgical pathology ~ 88399
  temporal bone ~ 69979
  testis ~ 54699, 55899
  throat ~ 42999
  tongue ~ 41599
  tonsil/adenoid ~ 42999
  trachea ~ 31899
  transfusion ~ 86999
  ultrasound ~ 76999
  ureter ~ 50949
  urinary system ~ 53899
  uterus ~ 58578-58579, 58999
  uvula ~ 42299
  vagina ~ 58999
  vas deferens ~ 55899
  vascular ~ 37799
  vascular endoscopy ~ 37501
  vascular injection ~ 36299
  vascular studies ~ 93799
  wrist ~ 25999
Unna paste boot ~ 29580
  removal ~ 29700
UPP ~ 51727, 51729
Upper
  digestive system endoscopy ~ see endoscopy, gastrointestinal, upper
  extremity ~ see arm, upper; elbow; humerus
  gastrointestinal bleeding ~ 43255
  gastrointestinal endoscopy, biopsy ~ 43239
    planning ~ 43239
  GI tract ~ 43249
Urachal cyst ~ 51500
Urea breath test ~ 78267-78268, 83014
Urea nitrogen ~ 84520-84525
  clearance ~ 84545
  quantitative ~ 84520
  semiquantitative ~ 84525
  urine ~ 84540
Urea nitrogen, blood ~ 84520-84525
Urecholine supersensitivity test ~ 51725-51726
Ureter
  anastomosis
    to bladder ~ 50780-50785
    to colon ~ 50810-50815
    to intestine ~ 50800, 50820-50825
    to kidney ~ 50740-50750
    to ureter ~ 50760-50770
  biopsy
    endoluminal, non-endoscopic ~ 50606
    endoscopic ~ 50955, 50957, 50974, 50976, 52007

Ureter ~ *continued*
  catheterization ~ 52005
    construction ~ 50840
    via kidney ~ 50693
  continent diversion ~ 50825
  creation, stoma ~ 50860
  destruction
    endoscopic ~ 50957, 50976
  dilation ~ 52341-52342, 52344-52345
    balloon ~ 50706
    endoscopic ~ 50553, 50572, 50953, 50972
  drainage ~ 50600
  embolization ~ 50705
  endoscopy
    biopsy ~ 50955-50957, 50974-50976, 52007, 52354
    catheterization ~ 50953, 50972, 52005
    destruction ~ 50957, 50976, 52354
    dilation ~ 52341-52342, 52344-52345
    excision, tumor ~ 52355
    exploration ~ 52351
    injection of implant material ~ 52327
    insertion, stent ~ 50947, 52332-52334
    lithotripsy ~ 52353
    tmanipulation of ureteral calculus ~ 52330
    removal
      calculus ~ 50961, 50980, 52320-52325, 52352
      foreign body ~ 50961, 50980
    resection ~ 52355
    via incision ~ 50970-50980
    via stoma ~ 50951-50961
  exploration ~ 50600
  incision and drainage ~ 50600
  injection
    drugs ~ 50391
    radiologic ~ 50430, 50431, 50684, 50690
  insertion
    stent ~ 50688, 50693, 50695, 50947, 52332
    tube ~ 50688
  instillation, drugs ~ 50391
  lesion, destruction ~ 52354
  lithotripsy ~ 52353
  lysis, adhesions ~ 50715-50725
  manometric studies, pressure ~ 50686
  meatotomy ~ 52290
  nuclear medicine, reflux study ~ 78740
  occlusion ~ 50705
  postcaval ~ 50725
  reconstruction ~ 50700
    with intestines ~ 50840
  reflux study ~ 78740
  reimplantation ~ 51565
  removal
    anastomosis ~ 50830
    calculus ~ 50610-50630, 50961, 51060-51065, 52320-52325
    foreign body ~ 50961
    stent ~ 50382-50387
  repair ~ 50900
    anastomosis ~ 50740-50825
    continent diversion ~ 50825
    deligation ~ 50940
    fistula ~ 50920-50930
    lysis adhesions ~ 50715-50725
    ureterocele ~ 51535
      ectopic ~ 52301
      orthotopic ~ 52300
    urinary undiversion ~ 50830
  replacement
    stent ~ 50382, 50387
    with intestines ~ 50840
  resection ~ 52355
  revision, anastomosis ~ 50727-50728
  stent
    change ~ 50688
    insertion ~ 50688
    placement
      with nephrostogram ~ 50693-50695
      with ureterogram ~ 50693-50695
  suture ~ 50900
    deligation ~ 50940
    fistula ~ 50920-50930

Ureter ~ *continued*
tube
change ~ 50688
insertion ~ 50688
tumor resection ~ 52355
unlisted services and procedures ~ 50949, 53899
X-ray with contrast
guide dilation ~ 74485
Ureteral
catheterization ~ see catheterization, ureter
guide wire insertion ~ 52334
meatotomy ~ 52290
splinting ~ 50400-50405
stent insertion ~ 52332
Ureterectomy ~ 50650-50660
partial ~ 50220, 50546
total ~ 50548
Ureterocalycostomy ~ 50750
Ureterocele
excision ~ 51535
fulguration
ectopic ~ 52301
orthotopic ~ 52300
incision ~ 51535
repair ~ 51535
resection, ectopic ~ 52301
orthotopic ~ 52300
Ureterocolon conduit ~ 50815
Ureteroenterostomy ~ 50800
revision ~ 50830
Ureterography
injection procedure ~ 50430, 50431, 50684
with catheter conversion, nephrostomy to nephroureteral ~ 50434
with nephrostomy catheter exchange ~ 50435
with pacement of ureteral stent ~ 50693-50695
Ureteroileal conduit ~ 50820
cystectomy ~ 51590
removal ~ 50830
Ureterolithotomy ~ 50610-50630
laparoscopy ~ 50945
transvesical ~ 51060
Ureterolysis
for ovarian vein syndrome ~ 50722
for retrocaval ureter ~ 50725
for retroperitoneal fibrosis ~ 50715
Ureteroneocystostomy ~ 50780-50785, 50830, 51565
laparoscopic ~ 50947-50948
Ureteroplasty ~ 50700
Ureteropyelography ~ 50951, 52005
injection procedure ~ 50684, 50690
Ureteropyelostomy ~ 50740
Ureteroscopy
dilation
intra-renal stricture ~ 52346
ureter ~ 52344-52345
third stage with cystourethroscopy ~ 52351
biopsy ~ 52354
destruction ~ 52354
lithotripsy ~ 52353
removal, calculus ~ 52352
tumor excision ~ 52355
Ureterosigmoidostomy ~ 50810
revision ~ 50830
Ureterostomy ~ 50860, 50951
injection procedure ~ 50684
manometric studies ~ 50686
Ureterostomy tube change ~ 50688
Ureterotomy ~ 50600
insertion indwelling stent ~ 50605
Ureteroureterostomy ~ 50760-50770, 50830
Urethra
abscess, incision and drainage ~ 53040
adhesions, lysis ~ 53500
artificial sphincter, repair ~ 53449
balloon continence device
placement ~ 0548T, 0549T
removal ~ 0550T
volume adjustment ~ 0551T
biopsy ~ 52204, 53200
cystourethroscopy ~ 52204-52315

Urethra ~ *continued*
destruction ~ 52214-52224
dilation ~ 52260-52265, 53600-53621
general ~ 53665
suppository and/or instillation ~ 53660-53661
diverticulum ~ 53240
drainage, extravasation ~ 53080-53085
endoscopy ~ 52000
biopsy ~ 52204, 52354
catheterization ~ 52010
destruction ~ 52354, 52400
evacuation, clot ~ 52001
excision, tumor ~ 52355
exploration ~ 52351
incision, ejaculatory duct ~ 52402
injection of implant material ~ 51715
lithotripsy ~ 52353
removal, calculus ~ 52352
resection, ejaculatory duct ~ 52402
vasectomy ~ 52402
vasotomy ~ 52402
excision
diverticulum ~ 53230-53235
total
female ~ 53210
male ~ 53215
incision ~ 53000-53010
meatus ~ 53020-53025
incision and drainage ~ 53060
insertion
female intraurethral valve-pump ~ 0596T
stent ~ 52282
lesion
destruction ~ 53265
excision ~ 53260
paraurethral gland, incision and drainage ~ 53060
polyp
destruction ~ 53260
excision ~ 53260
pressure profile ~ 51727, 51729
prolapse
destruction ~ 53275
excision ~ 53275
repair ~ 53275
proximal, micro-remodeling ~ 53860
radiotracer ~ 52250
reconstruction ~ 53410-53440, 53445
and bladder ~ 51800-51820
complications ~ 54340-54348
hypospadias
one stage ~ 54322-54328
second stage ~ 54308-54316
third stage ~ 54318
meatus ~ 53450-53460
removal
calculus ~ 52310-52315
foreign body ~ 52310-52315
sling ~ 53442
urethral stent ~ 52310-52315
repair
diverticulum ~ 53240, 53400-53405
fistula ~ 45820-45825, 53400-53405, 53520
sphincter ~ 57220
stricture ~ 53400-53405
urethrocele ~ 57230
with replantation of penis ~ 54438
wound ~ 53502-53515
Skene's gland, incision and drainage ~ 53060
sphincter ~ 57277
electromyography ~ 51784-51785
needle ~ 51785
insertion, prosthesis ~ 53444
reconstruction ~ 53445
removal, prosthesis ~ 53446-53447
repair, prosthesis ~ 53449
replacement, prosthesis ~ 53448
stent
insertion
premanent ~ 52282
temporary ~ 53855

Urethra ~ *continued*
  suture
    fistula ~ 45820-45825, 53520
    to bladder ~ 51840-51841
    wound ~ 53502-53515
  tumor
    destruction ~ 53220
    excision ~ 53220
  unlisted services and procedures ~ 53899
  urethrocystography ~ 74450-74455
  urethrotomy ~ 52270-52276
  X-ray with contrast ~ 74450-74455
Urethral
  diverticulum
    marsupialization ~ 53240
    meatus, dorsal ~ see epispadias
  sphincter
    biofeedback training ~ 90912, 90913
    insertion, prosthesis ~ 53444
    removal, prosthesis ~ 53446-53447
    replacement, prosthesis ~ 53448
  stenosis, dilation ~ 52281
  stent
    insertion ~ 0084T, 52282
    removal
      bladder ~ 52310-52315
      urethra ~ 52310-52315
  stricture
    dilation ~ 52281, 53600-53621
    injection, steroids ~ 52283
  syndrome, cystourethroscopy ~ 52285
Urethrectomy total
  female ~ 53210
  male ~ 53215
Urethrocele ~ 53275
Urethrocystography ~ 74450-74455
  contrast and/or chain ~ 51605
  retrograde ~ 51610
  voiding ~ 51600
Urethrocystopexy ~ 51840-51841
Urethromeatoplasty ~ 53450-53460
Urethropexy ~ 51840-51841
Urethroplasty ~ 46744-46746
  first stage ~ 53400
  one stage, hypospadias ~ 54322-54328
  reconstruction
    female urethra ~ 53430
    male anterior urethra ~ 53410
    prostatic/membranous urethra
      first stage ~ 53420
      one stage ~ 53415
      second stage ~ 53425
  second stage ~ 53405
    hypospadias ~ 54308-54316
  third stage, hypospadias ~ 54318
Urethrorrhaphy ~ 53502-53515
Urethroscopy ~ 52000
Urethrostomy ~ 53000-53010
Urethrotomy ~ 53000-53010
  direct vision, with cystourethroscopy ~ 52276
  internal ~ 52601, 52647-52648
  with cystourethroscopy
    female ~ 52270
    male ~ 52275
Uric acid
  blood ~ 84550
  other source ~ 84560
  urine ~ 84560
Uridyltransferase
  galactose-1-phosphate ~ 82775-82776
  galactosephosphate ~ 82775-82776
Urinalysis ~ 81000-81099
  automated ~ 81001, 81003
  glass test ~ 81020
  microalbumin ~ 82043-82044
  microscopic ~ 81015
  pregnancy test ~ 81025
  qualitative ~ 81005
  routine ~ 81002
  screen ~ 81007

Urinalysis ~ *continued*
  semiquantitative ~ 81005
  unlisted services and procedures ~ 81099
  volume measurement ~ 81050
  without microscopy ~ 81002
Urinary bladder ~ see bladder
Urinary catheter irrigation ~ 62194, 62225
Urinary sphincter, artificial ~ 53444-53449
Urinary system, surgical procedures ~ 50010-53899
Urinary tract X-ray w contrast ~ 74400-74425
Urine
  albumin ~ 82042-82044
  blood ~ 83491
  colony count ~ 87086
  pregnancy test ~ 81025
  tests ~ 81001
Urobilinogen
  feces ~ 84577
  urine ~ 84578-84583
Urodynamic tests
  bladder capacity, ultrasound ~ 51798
  cystometrogram ~ 51725-51729
  electromyography studies, needle ~ 51785
  residual urine, ultrasound ~ 51798
  stimulus evoked response ~ 51792
  urethra pressure profile ~ 51727, 51729
  uroflowmetry ~ 51736-51741
  voiding pressure studies
    bladder ~ 51728, 51729
    intra-abdominal ~ 51797
Uroflowmetry ~ 51736-51741
Urography
  antegrade ~ 74425
  infusion ~ 74410-74415
  intravenous ~ 74400-74415
  retrograde ~ 74420
Uroporphyrin ~ 84120
Urothromboplastin ~ see thromboplastin
Uterine
  adhesion ~ 58559
  cervix ~ see cervix
  endoscopies ~ see endoscopy, uterus
  haemorrhage ~ 59160
Uterus
  ablation
    endometrium ~ 58353-58356
    fibroid
      laparoscopic ~ 58674
      radiofrequency ~ 0404T
    tumor, ultrasound, focused ~ 0071T-0072T
  biopsy
    endometrium ~ 58100-58110
    endoscopic ~ 58558
  catheterization, X-ray ~ 58340
  chromotubation ~ 58350
  curettage ~ 58356
    postpartum ~ 59160
  dilation and curettage ~ 58120
    postpartum ~ 59160
  ectopic pregnancy
    interstitial
      partial resection uterus ~ 59136
      total hysterectomy ~ 59135
  endoscopy
    endometrial ablation ~ 58563
    exploration ~ 58555
    surgery ~ 58558-58565
    treatment ~ 58558-58565
  excision
    laparoscopic ~ 58541-58544, 58550
      with removal of ovaries ~ 58262-58263, 58291, 58552, 58554, 58575
      total ~ 58570-58573, 58575
    partial ~ 58180
    radical
      laparoscopic ~ 58548
      open ~ 58210, 58285
    removal of tubes and/or ovaries ~ 58262-58263, 58291, 58552, 58554
    total ~ 58150-58152, 58200, 58570-58573, 58575, 58953-58956

Vagina ~ *continued*

excision

closure ~ 57120

complete

with removal of paravaginal tissue ~ 57111

with removal of vaginal wall ~ 57110

partial

with removal of paravaginal tissue ~ 57107

with removal of paravaginal tissue with lymphadenectomy ~ 57109

with removal of vaginal wall ~ 57106

total ~ 57110

with hysterectomy ~ 58275-58280

with repair of enterocele ~ 58280

exploration

endocervical ~ 57452

incision ~ 57000

hematoma, incision and drainage ~ 57022-57023

hemorrhage ~ 57180

hysterectomy ~ 58290, 58550-58554

incision and drainage ~ 57020

insertion

ovoid, for brachytherapy ~ 57155

packing for bleeding ~ 57180

pessary ~ 57160

radiation afterloading appliance ~ 57156

sensor, fetal oximetry ~ 0021T

irrigation ~ 57150

lesion

destruction ~ 57061-57065

extensive ~ 57065

simple ~ 57061

prolapse, sacrospinous ligament fixation ~ 57282

removal

foreign body ~ 57415

prosthetic graft ~ 57295-57296, 57426

sling, stress incontinence ~ 57287

repair ~ 56800

cystocele ~ 57240, 57260

combined anteroposterior ~ 57260-57265

posterior ~ 57240

enterocele ~ 57265

fistula ~ 51900

rectovaginal ~ 57300-57308

transvesical and vaginal approach ~ 57330

urethrovaginal ~ 57310-57311

vesicovaginal ~ 51900, 57320-57330

hysterectomy ~ 58267

incontinence ~ 57284, 57288

obstetric ~ 59300

paravaginal defect ~ 57284-57285, 57423

Pereyra Procedure ~ 57289

prolapse ~ 57282-57284, 57423

prosthesis insertion ~ 57267

rectocele

combined anteroposterior ~ 57260-57265

posterior ~ 57250

suspension ~ 57280-57283

laparoscopic ~ 57425

urethral sphincter ~ 57220

wound ~ 57200-57210

colpoperineorrhaphy ~ 57210

colporrhaphy ~ 57200

revision

prosthetic graft ~ 57295-57296, 57426

sling, stress incontinence ~ 57287

septum, excision ~ 57130

suspension ~ 57280-57283

laparoscopic ~ 57425

suture

cystocele ~ 57240, 57260

enterocele ~ 57265

fistula ~ 51900, 57300-57330

rectocele ~ 57250-57260

wound ~ 57200-57210

Vagina ~ *continued*

tumor, excision ~ 57135

ultrasound ~ 76830

unlisted services and procedures ~ 58999

X-ray with contrast ~ 74775

Vaginal delivery ~ 59400, 59610-59614

after previous cesarean delivery ~ 59610-59612

attempted ~ 59618-59622

antepartum care ~ 59400

cesarean delivery after attempted ~ 59618

delivery only ~ 59620

postpartum care ~ 59622

delivery after previous, vaginal delivery only, postpartum care ~ 59614

delivery only ~ 59409

external cephalic version ~ 59412

placenta ~ 59414

postpartum care ~ 59410

routine care ~ 59400

Vaginal hysterectomy ~ 58552-58554

Vaginal smear ~ 88141-88155, 88164-88167, 88174-88175

Vaginal suppositories

induced abortion ~ 59855

with dilation and curettage ~ 59856

with hysterectomy ~ 59857

Vaginectomy ~ see colpectomy

Vaginoplasty intersex state ~ 57335

Vaginorrhaphy ~ see colporrhaphy

Vaginoscopy

biopsy ~ 57454

exploration ~ 57452

Vaginotomy ~ see colpotomy

Vagotomy

abdominal ~ 64760

highly selective ~ 43641

parietal cell ~ 43641, 64755

selective ~ 43640

truncal ~ 43640

with gastroduodenostomy revision, reconstruction ~ 43855

with gastrojejunostomy revision, reconstruction ~ 43865

with partial distal gastrectomy ~ 43635

Vagus nerve

avulsion

abdominal ~ 64760

selective ~ 64755

incision ~ 43640-43641

abdominal ~ 64760

implantation ~ 64568

selective ~ 64755

injection, anesthetic ~ 64408

removal, neurostimulator ~ 64570

revision or replacement ~ 64569

transection ~ 43640-43641

abdominal ~ 64760

selective ~ 43652, 64755

truncal ~ 43651

Valentine's test ~ 81020

Valproic acid ~ 80164

Valproic acid measurement ~ 80164

Valsalva sinus ~ 33702-33722

Valva atrioventricularis sinistra (valva mitralis) ~ see mitral valve

Valve

aortic ~ 33405-33414

bicuspid ~ see mitral valve

mitral ~ see mitral valve

pulmonary ~ 33470-33475

tricuspid ~ 33460, 33463-33465, 33468

Valve stenoses, aortic ~ 33415, 33417

Valvectomy tricuspid valve ~ 33460

Valvotomy

mitral valve ~ 33420-33422

pulmonary valve ~ 33470-33474

reoperation ~ 33530

Valvuloplasty

aortic valve ~ 33390, 33391

femoral vein ~ 34501

mitral valve ~ 33425-33427

percutaneous balloon

aortic valve ~ 92986

mitral valve ~ 92987

pulmonary valve ~ 92990

Valvuloplasty ~ continued
  prosthetic valve ~ 33496
  reoperation ~ 33530
  transcatheter tricuspid valve repair ~ 0569T, 0570T
  tricuspid valve ~ 33463-33465
Van Deen test ~ 82270, 82272
Van Den Bergh test ~ 82247-82248
Vancomycin assay ~ 80202
Vanillylmandelic acid urine ~ 84585
Vanilmandelic acid ~ 84585
Varicella (chicken pox) ~ 90716
Varicella-zoster
  antibody ~ 86787
  antigen detection, direct fluorescence ~ 87290
Varices esophageal ~ 43205, 43400
Varicocele spermatic cord, excision ~ 55530-55540
Varicose vein
  ablation
    chemical adhesive ~ 36482, 36483
    laser ~ 36478, 36479
    mechanochemical ~ 36473, 36474
    radiofrequency ~ 36475, 36476
  removal ~ 37765-37785
  secondary varicosity ~ 37785
  with tissue excision ~ 37735-37761
Vas deferens
  anastomosis
    to epididymis ~ 54900, 54901
  excision ~ 55250
  incision ~ 55200
    for X-ray ~ 55300
  repair, suture ~ 55400
  unlisted services and procedures ~ 55899
  vasography ~ 74440
  X-ray with contrast ~ 74440
Vascular flow check, graft ~ 15860
Vascular injection unlisted services and procedures ~ 36299
Vascular lesion
  cranial, excision ~ 61600-61608, 61615-61616
  cutaneous, destruction ~ 17106-17108
Vascular malformation
  cerebral
    obliteration ~ 61613
    repair ~ 61680, 61682, 61684, 61686, 61690, 61692, 61705, 61708, 61710
  finger, excision ~ 26111-26116
  hand, excision ~ 26111-26116
  spine, occlusion ~ 62294, 63250-63252
Vascular procedure(s)
  angioscopy, non-coronary vessels ~ 35400
  brachytherapy, intracoronary artery ~ 92974
  embolization ~ 37241-37244
  endoscopy, surgical ~ 37500
  harvest, lower extremity vein ~ 35572
  intravascular ultrasound
    coronary vessels ~ 92978-92979
    non-coronary vessels ~ 37252, 37253
  ligation, vena cava ~ 37619
  occlusion ~ 37241-37244
  stent, intracoronary ~ 92928-92929
  thrombolysis
    cerebral ~ 37195
    coronary vessels ~ 92975-92977
    intracranial ~ 61645
    noncoronary ~ 37211-37214
Vascular rehabilitation ~ 93668
Vascular studies ~ see Doppler scan, Duplex, Plethysmography
  angioscopy, non-coronary vessels ~ 35400
  aorta ~ 93978-93979
  arterial studies (non-invasive)
    extracranial ~ 93880-93882
    extremities ~ 93922-93924
    intracranial ~ 93886-93890
    lower extremity ~ 93925-93926
    middle cerebral artery, fetal ~ 76821
    umbilical artery, fetal ~ 76820
  artery studies, upper extremity ~ 93930-93931
  bioimpedance cardiovascular analysis ~ 93701
  blood pressure monitoring, 24 hour ~ 93784-93790

Vascular studies ~ continued
  cardiac catheterization, imaging ~ 93452-93461
  hemodialysis access ~ 93985, 93986, 93990
  kidney
    multiple study, with pharmacological intervention ~ 78709
    single study, with pharmacological intervention ~ 78708
  penile vessels ~ 93980-93981
  temperature gradient ~ 93740
  unlisted services and procedures ~ 93799
  venous studies
    extremity ~ 93970, 93971
    venous pressure ~ 93770
  visceral studies ~ 93975-93979
Vascular surgery
  arm, upper, anesthesia ~ 01770-01782
  elbow, anesthesia ~ 01770-01782
  endoscopy ~ 37500
  unlisted services and procedures ~ 37799
Vasectomy ~ 55250
  contact laser vaporization with/without transurethral resection, of prostate ~ 52648
  non-contact laser coagulation of prostate ~ 52647
  reversal ~ 55400
  transurethral, cystourethroscopic ~ 52402
  transurethral electrosurgical resection of prostate ~ 52601, 52648
Vasoactive drugs injection, penis ~ 54231
Vasoactive intestinal peptide ~ 84586
Vasogram ~ 74440
Vasography ~ 74440
Vasointestinal peptide ~ 84586
Vasopneumatic device therapy ~ see physical medicine/therapy/occupational therapy ~ 97016
Vasopressin ~ 84588
Vasotomy ~ 55200, 55300
  transurethral, cystourethroscopic ~ 52402
Vasovasorrhaphy ~ 55400
Vasovasostomy ~ 55400
VATS ~ see thoracoscopy
VDRL ~ 86592-86593
Vein
  ablation, endovenous ~ 36473-36479, 36482, 36483
  adrenal, venography ~ 75840-75842
  anastomosis
    caval to mesenteric ~ 37160
    intrahepatic portosystemic ~ 37182-37183
    portocaval ~ 37140
    reniportal ~ 37145
    saphenopopliteal ~ 34530
    splenorenal ~ 37180-37181
    to vein ~ 37140-37160, 37182-37183
  angioplasty
    transluminal ~ 37248, 37249
  arm
    harvest of vein for bypass graft ~ 35500
    venography ~ 75820-75822
  arterialization
    transcatheter stent placement ~ 0620T
  axillary, thrombectomy ~ 34490
  biopsy, transcatheter ~ 75970
  cannulization
    to artery ~ 36810-36815
    to vein ~ 36800
  catheterization
    central insertion ~ 36555-36558
    organ blood ~ 36500
    peripheral insertion ~ 36568-36569
    removal ~ 36589
    repair ~ 36575
    replacement ~ 36578-36581, 36584
    umbilical ~ 36510
  endoscopic harvest, for bypass graft ~ 33508
  external cannula, declotting ~ 36860-36861
  extremity, non-invasive studies ~ 93970, 93971
  femoral, repair ~ 34501
  femoropopliteal, thrombectomy ~ 34421-34451
  guidance
    fluoroscopic ~ 77001
    ultrasound ~ 76937

Vein ~ continued
hepatic portal
  splenoportography ~ 75810
  venography ~ 75885-75887
iliac, thrombectomy ~ 34401-34451
injection, sclerosing agent ~ 36465, 36466, 36468, 36470, 36471
interrupt
  femoral ~ 37650
  iliac ~ 37660
jugular, venography ~ 75860
leg
  harvest for vascular reconstruction ~ 35572
  venography ~ 75820-75822
ligation
  clusters ~ 37785
  esophagus ~ 43205
  jugular ~ 37565
  perforation ~ 37760-37761
  saphenous ~ 37700-37735, 37780
  secondary ~ 37785
liver, venography ~ 75889-75891
neck, venography ~ 75860
nuclear medicine, thrombosis imaging ~ 78455-78458
orbit, venography ~ 75880
portal, catheterization ~ 36481
pulmonary, repair ~ 33730
removal
  clusters ~ 37785
  saphenous ~ 37720-37735, 37780
  varicose ~ 37765-37766
renal, venography ~ 75831-75833
repair
  angioplasty ~ 37248, 37249
  graft ~ 34520
sampling, venography ~ 75893
sinus, venography ~ 75870
skull, venography ~ 75870-75872
spermatic
  excision ~ 55530-55540
  ligation ~ 55550
splenic, splenoportography ~ 75810
stripping, saphenous ~ 37720-37735
subclavian, thrombectomy ~ 34471-34490
thrombectomy, other than hemodialysis graft or fistula ~ 35875-35876
unlisted services and procedures ~ 37799
valve transposition ~ 34510
vena cava
  thrombectomy ~ 34401-34451
  venography ~ 75825-75827
Velpeau cast ~ 29058
VEMP (vestibular evoked myogenic potential) testing
cervical (cVEMP) ~ 92517, 92519
ocular (oVEMP) ~ 92518, 92519
Vena cava
catheterization ~ 36010
filter
  insertion ~ 37191
  repositioning ~ 37192
  retreival ~ 37193
ligation ~ 37619
reconstruction ~ 34502
resection with reconstruction ~ 37799
Vena caval thrombectomy ~ 50230
Venereal disease research laboratory ~ see VDRL
Venesection ~ 99195
Venipuncture ~ see catheterization ~ 36821
child/adult
  cutdown ~ 36425
  percutaneous ~ 36410
infant
  cutdown ~ 36420
  percutaneous ~ 36400-36406
routine ~ 36415
Venography
adrenal ~ 75840-75842
arm ~ 75820-75822
epidural ~ 75872
hepatic portal ~ 75885-75887
injection ~ 36005
jugular ~ 75860

Venography ~ continued
leg ~ 75820-75822
liver ~ 75889-75891
neck ~ 75860
nuclear medicine ~ 78445, 78457-78458
orbit ~ 75880
renal ~ 75831-75833
sagittal sinus ~ 75870
vena cava ~ 75825-75827
venous sampling ~ 75893
Venorrhaphy ~ see suture, vein
Venotomy ~ 99195
Venous access device
blood collection ~ 36591-36592
declotting ~ 36593
fluoroscopic guidance ~ 77001
insertion
  central ~ 36560-36566
  peripheral ~ 36570-36571
irrigation ~ 96523
obstruction clearance ~ 36595-36596
  guidance ~ 75901-75902
removal ~ 36590
repair ~ 36576
replacement ~ 36582-36583, 36585
  catheter only ~ 36578
Venous arterialization
transcatheter stent placement ~ 0620T
Venous blood pressure ~ 93770
Venovenostomy ~ 34530
Ventilating tube
insertion ~ 69433, 69436, 0583T
removal ~ 69424
Ventilation assist ~ 94002-94005, 99504
Ventricular assist device (VAD)
implantable counterpulsation aortic system
  insertion ~ 0451T-0454T
  interrogation device evaluation ~ 0463T
  programming device evaluation ~ 0462T
  relocation ~ 0459T
  removal ~ 0455T-0458T
  repositioning ~ 0460T, 0461T
  replacement ~ 0451T-0454T
insertion
  extracorporeal ~ 33975, 33976, 33978
  implantable ~ 33979
  percutaneous ~ 33990, 33991, 33995
removal ~ 33977, 33980, 33992, 33997
replacement ~ 33981, 33982
repositioning ~ 33993
Ventricular puncture ~ 61020-61026, 61105-61120
Ventriculocisternostomy ~ 62180, 62200-62201
Ventriculography
anesthesia
  brain ~ 00214
  cardiac ~ 01920
nuclear imaging ~ 78635
Ventriculomyectomy ~ 33416
Ventriculomyotomy ~ 33416
Vermiform appendix ~ see appendix
Vermilionectomy ~ 40500
Verruca plana ~ 17110-17111
Verruca(e) ~ 17110-17111
Version, cephalic ~ 59412
Vertebra ~ see spinal cord; spine; vertebral body ~ 22315
additional segment, excision ~ 22103, 22116
arthrodesis
  anterior ~ 22548-22585
  exploration ~ 22830
  lateral extracavitary ~ 22532-22534
  posterior ~ 22590-22802
  spinal deformity
    anterior approach ~ 22808-22812
    posterior approach ~ 22800-22804
cervical, excision, for tumor ~ 22100, 22110
  fracture ~ 23675-23680
decompression ~ 62287
  laminotomy/laminectomy ~ 0274T, 0275T
excision, partial ~ 22100-22103, 22110, 22110, 22112, 22114, 22116
facetectomy, partial ~ 62380, 63020

Vitreous
  aspiration ~ 67015
  excision
    pars planta approach ~ 67036
    with epiretinal membrane stripping ~ 67041-67043
    with focal endolaser photocoagulation ~ 67039
  implantation, drug delivery system ~ 67027
  incision, strands ~ 67030-67031
  injection
    fluid substitute ~ 67025
    pharmacologic agent ~ 67028
  removal
    anterior approach ~ 67005
    subtotal ~ 67010
  replacement, drug delivery system ~ 67027
  strands
    discission ~ 67030
    severing ~ 67031
  subtotal ~ 67010
VLDL ~ 83695-83721
VMA ~ 84585
Vocal cords
  injection, endoscopy ~ 31513
    augmentiva ~ 31574
    therapeutic ~ 31570-31571, 31573
  laryngeal medialization ~ 31591
Voice box ~ see larynx
Voice button ~ 31611
Voiding pressure studies
  abdominal ~ 51797
  bladder ~ 51728, 51729
  rectum ~ 51797
Volatiles ~ 84600
Volkman contracture ~ 25315-25316
Volume reduction, lung ~ 32491
Von Kraske proctectomy ~ 45111, 45113-45116, 45123
VP ~ see voiding pressure studies
Vulva
  abscess, incision and drainage ~ 56405
  colposcopy ~ 56820
    biopsy ~ 56821
  excision
    complete ~ 56625, 56633-56640
    partial ~ 56620, 56630-56632
    radical ~ 56630-56631, 56633-56640
      complete ~ 56633-56640
      partial ~ 56630-56632
    simple
      complete ~ 56625
      partial ~ 56620
  lesion, destruction ~ 56501-56515
  perineum
    biopsy ~ 56605-56606
    incision and drainage ~ 56405
  repair, obstetric ~ 59300
Vulvectomy
  complete ~ 56625, 56633-56640
  partial ~ 56620, 56630-56632
  radical ~ 56630-56631, 56633-56640
    complete
      with bilateral inguinofemoral lymphadenectomy ~ 56637
      with inguinofemoral, iliac, and pelvic lymphadenectomy ~ 56640
      with unilateral inguinofemoral lymphadenectomy ~ 56634
    partial
      with bilateral inguinofemoral lymphadenectomy ~ 56632
      with unilateral inguinofemoral lymphadenectomy ~ 56631
  simple, complete ~ 56625
    partial ~ 56620
VZIG ~ 90396

W

W-plasty ~ see skin, adjacent tissue transfer
WADA activation test ~ 95958
WAIS-R ~ 96100
Waldius Procedure ~ 27445
Wall, abdominal ~ see abdominal wall

Walsh modified radical prostatectomy ~ 52601
Warts, flat, destruction ~ 17110-17111
Washing sperm ~ 58323
Wasserman test ~ 86592-86593
Wassmund Procedure osteotomy, maxilla ~ 21206
Water wart ~ 17110-17111, 54050-54065
Waterston Procedure ~ 33755
Watson-Jones Procedure ~ 27695-27698
Wave, ultrasonic shock ~ see ultrasound
WBC ~ see white blood cell
Webbed toe, repair ~ 28280
Wedge excision osteotomy ~ 21122
Wedge resection ovary ~ 58920
Well-baby care ~ 99381, 99391, 99461
Wellness behavior ~ see evaluation and management, health behavior
Wernicke-posadas disease ~ 86490
West Nile virus ~ 86788-86789
Westergren test ~ 85651-85652
Western blot
  HIV ~ 86689
  protein ~ 84181-84182
  tissue analysis ~ 88371-88372
Wheelchair management/propulsion ~ 97542
  training ~ 97542
Wheeler knife procedure ~ 66820-66821
Wheeler Procedure ~ 15820-15823
  discission secondary membranous cataract ~ 66820
Whipple Procedure ~ 48150
Whirlpool therapy ~ 97022
White blood cell
  alkaline phosphatase ~ 85540
  antibody ~ 86021
  count ~ 85032, 85048, 89055
  differential ~ 85004-85007, 85009
  histamine release test ~ 86343
  injection, autologous concentrate ~ 0481T
  phagocytosis ~ 86344
  transfusion ~ 86950
Whitemead Operation ~ 46260
Whitman astragalectomy ~ 28120, 28130
Whitman Procedure ~ 27120
Wick catheter technique ~ 20950
Widal serum test ~ 86000
Window
  oval ~ 69666
  round ~ 69667
Windpipe ~ see trachea
Winiwarter Operation ~ 47720-47740
Winter Procedure ~ 54435
Wintrobe test ~ 85651-85652
Wire ~ see pin
  insertion/removal, skeletal traction ~ 20650
  interdental, without fracture ~ 21497
Wiring prophylactic treatment, humerus ~ 24498
Wirsung duct ~ see pancreatic duct
Witzel Operation ~ see incision, stomach, creation, stoma; incision and
  drainage ~ 43500, 43520, 43830-43832
Womb ~ see uterus
Wood alcohol ~ 84600
Work hardening ~ see physical medicine/therapy/occupational therapy ~
  97545-97546
Work related evaluation services ~ 99455-99456
Worm ~ 86682
Wound
  debridement
    non-selective ~ 97602
    selective ~ 97597-97598
  dehiscence, repair ~ 12020-12021, 13160
  exploration
    penetrating
      abdomen/flank/back ~ 20102
      chest ~ 20101
      extremity ~ 20103
      neck ~ 20100
      penetrating trauma ~ 20100-20103
  imaging
    fluorescent imaging for bacteria ~ 0598T-0599T
  infection, incision and drainage, postoperative ~ 10180
  negative pressure therapy ~ 97605-97606

Wound ~ *continued*
packing
preperitoneal pelvis ~ 49013, 49014
repair
complex ~ 13100-13160
intermediate ~ 12031-12057
simple ~ 12001-12021
urethra ~ 53502-53515
suture
bladder ~ 51860-51865
kidney ~ 50500
trachea
cervical ~ 31800
intrathoracic ~ 31805
urethra ~ 53502-53515
vagina repair ~ 57200-57210
Wrist ~ see arm, lower; carpal bone
abscess ~ 25028
arthrocentesis ~ 20605
arthrodesis ~ 25800
with graft ~ 25810
with sliding graft ~ 25805
arthrography ~ 73115
arthroplasty ~ 25332, 25443, 25447
revision ~ 25449
total replacement ~ 25446
with implant ~ 25441-25442, 25444-25445
arthroscopy, diagnostic ~ 29840
surgical ~ 29843-29848
arthrotomy ~ 25040, 25100-25105
for repair ~ 25107
biopsy ~ 25065-25066, 25100-25101
bursa
excision ~ 25115-25116
incision and drainage ~ 25031
capsule, incision ~ 25085
cast ~ 29085
cyst ~ 25130-25136
decompression ~ 25020-25025
disarticulation ~ 25920
reamputation ~ 25924
revision ~ 25922
dislocation
closed treatment ~ 25660
intercarpal ~ 25660
open treatment ~ 25670
open treatment ~ 25670, 25676
percutaneous fixation ~ 25671
radiocarpal ~ 25660
open treatment ~ 25670
radioulnar
closed treatment ~ 25675
percutaneous fixation ~ 25671
with fracture
closed treatment ~ 25680
open treatment ~ 25685
with manipulation ~ 25259, 25660, 25675
excision
carpal ~ 25210-25215
cartilage ~ 25107
exploration ~ 25040, 25101
fasciotomy ~ 25020-25025
fracture ~ 25645
closed treatment ~ 25622, 25630
open treatment ~ 25628
with dislocation ~ 25680-25685
with manipulation ~ 25259, 25624, 25635
ganglion cyst, excision ~ 25111-25112
hematoma ~ 25028
incision ~ 25040, 25100-25105
tendon sheath ~ 25000-25001
injection
carpal tunnel, therapeutic ~ 20526
X-ray ~ 25246
joint ~ 25040, 25660
lesion, tendon sheath, excision ~ 25110
magnetic resonance imaging (MRI) ~ 73221

Wrist ~ *continued*
reconstruction
capsulectomy ~ 25320
capsulorrhaphy ~ 25320
carpal bone ~ 25394, 25430
realign ~ 25335
removal
foreign body ~ 25040, 25101, 25248
implant ~ 25449
loose body ~ 25101
prosthesis ~ 25250-25251
repair ~ 25447
bone ~ 25440
carpal bone ~ 25431
muscle ~ 25260, 25270
secondary ~ 25263-25265, 25272-25274
tendon ~ 25260, 25270, 25280-25316
secondary ~ 25263-25265, 25272-25274
tendon sheath ~ 25275
strapping ~ 29260
synovium, excision ~ 25105, 25115-25119
tendon sheath, excision ~ 25115-25116
tenodesis ~ 25300-25301
tenotomy ~ 25290
tumor ~ 25130-25136
excision ~ 25071-25078
unlisted services and procedures ~ 25999
X-ray ~ 73100-73110
with contrast ~ 73115

X

X, coagulation factor ~ 85260
X, cranial nerve ~ see vagus nerve
X-linked ichthyoses ~ 86592-86593
X-ray
abdomen ~ 74018, 74019, 74021, 74022
abscess ~ 76080
acromioclavicular joint ~ 73050
ankle ~ 73600-73610
arm, lower ~ 73090
arm, upper ~ 73092
auditory meatus ~ 70134
barium swallow test ~ 3142F, 3200F
bile duct, guide dilation ~ 74360
body section ~ 76100
motion ~ 76101-76102
bone
age study ~ 77072
dual energy absorptiometry ~ 77080-77081
length study ~ 77073
osseous survey ~ 77074-77077
ultrasound ~ 76977
breast ~ 77065-77067
tomosynthesis ~ 77061-77063
with computer-aided detection ~ 77065-77067
calcaneus ~ 73650
chest ~ 71045-71048
with computer-aided detection ~ 0174T, 0175T
clavicle ~ 73000
coccyx ~ 72220
consultation ~ 76140
elbow ~ 73070-73080
esophagus ~ 74220, 74221
eye ~ 70030
facial bones ~ 70140-70150
fallopian tube ~ 74742
femur ~ 73551, 73552
radiostereometric analysis (RSA) ~ 0350T
fibula ~ 73590
finger ~ 73140
fistula ~ 76080
foot ~ 73620-73630
gastrointestinal tract ~ 74246
guide dilation ~ 74360
guide intubation ~ 74340
upper ~ 3142F, 3200F

X-ray ~ *continued*
  hand ~ 73120-73130
  head ~ 70350
  heel ~ 73650
  hip
    bilateral ~ 73521-73523
    unilateral ~ 73501-73503
    radiostereometric analysis (RSA) ~ 0350T
  humerus ~ 73060
  intestines, small ~ 74248, 74250, 74251
    guide intubation ~ 74355
  jaws ~ 70355
  joint, stress views ~ 77071
  knee ~ 73560-73564, 73580
    bilateral ~ 73565
  larynx ~ 70370
  leg ~ 73592
  lumen dilator ~ 74360
  mandible ~ 70100-70110
  mastoids ~ 70120-70130
  nasal bone ~ 70160
  neck ~ 70360
  nose to rectum, foreign body ~ 76010
  orbit ~ 70190-70200
  pelvis ~ 72170-72190
    with hips ~ 73501-73503, 73521-73523
    manometry ~ 74710
  peritoneum ~ 74190
  pharynx ~ 70370, 74210
  ribs ~ 71100-71111
  sacroiliac joint ~ 72200-72202
  sacrum ~ 72220
  salivary gland ~ 70380
  scapula ~ 73010
  sella turcica ~ 70240
  shoulder ~ 73020-73030, 73050
  sinus tract ~ 76080
  sinuses ~ 70210-70220
  skull ~ 70250, 70260
    with spine ~ 72081-72084
  specimen/surgical ~ 76098
  spine ~ 72020
    cervical ~ 72040, 72050, 72052, 72081-72084
    lumbosacral ~ 72100-72120, 72081-72084
    thoracic ~ 72070-72074, 72081-72084
    thoracolumbar ~ 72080, 72081-72084
    total ~ 72081-72084
  standing
    radiostereometric analysis (RSA) ~ 0348T
  sternum ~ 71120-71130
  teeth ~ 70300-70320
  tibia ~ 73590
  toe ~ 73660
  total body, foreign body ~ 76010
  unlisted services and procedures ~ 76120-76125
  upper GI series ~ 3142F, 3200F
  with contrast
    ankle ~ 73615
    aorta ~ 75600-75630
    artery
      abdominal ~ 75726
      additional vessels ~ 75774
      adrenal ~ 75731-75733
      arm ~ 75710-75716
      head and neck ~ 36221-36226
      leg ~ 75710-75716
      mammary ~ 75756
      pelvic ~ 75736
      pulmonary ~ 75741-75746
      renal ~ 36251-36254
      spine ~ 75705
      transcatheter therapy ~ 75894-75898
    bile duct ~ 47531, 47532, 74300, 74301
      catheterization ~ 75984
      drainage ~ 47533-47540
      guide catheter ~ 74328, 74330
    bladder ~ 74430, 74450-74455
    brain ~ 70010-70015
    bronchi ~ 76499
    colon, barium enema ~ 74270-74280

X-ray ~ *continued*
    corpora cavernosa ~ 74445
    elbow ~ 73085
    epididymis ~ 74440
    gallbladder ~ 74290-74291
    gastrointestinal tract ~ 74246-74249
    hip ~ 73525
    iliofemoral artery ~ 75630
    intervertebral disk
      cervical ~ 72285
      lumbar ~ 72295
      thoracic ~ 72285
    joint, stress views ~ 77071
    kidney
      cyst ~ 74470
    knee ~ 73560-73564, 73580
    lacrimal duct ~ 70170
    lymph vessel
      abdomen ~ 75805-75807
      arm ~ 75801-75803
      leg ~ 75801-75803
    nasolacrimal duct ~ 70170
      guide dilation ~ 74485
    oviduct ~ 74740
    pancreas ~ 47531, 74300, 74301
    pancreatic duct, guide catheter ~ 74329, 74330
    perineum ~ 74775
    peritoneum ~ 74190
    salivary gland ~ 70390
    seminal vesicles ~ 74440
    shoulder ~ 73040
    spine
      cervical ~ 72240
      lumbosacral ~ 72265
      thoracic ~ 72255
      total ~ 72270
    temporomandibular joint (TMJ) ~ 70328-70332
    ureter
      guide dilation ~ 74485
    urethra ~ 74450-74455
    urinary tract ~ 74400-74425
    uterus ~ 74740
    vas deferens ~ 74440
    vein
      adrenal ~ 75840-75842
      arm ~ 75820-75822
      hepatic portal ~ 75810, 75885-75887
      jugular ~ 75860
      leg ~ 75820-75822
      liver ~ 75889-75891
      neck ~ 75860
      orbit ~ 75880
      renal ~ 75831-75833
      sampling ~ 75893
      sinus ~ 75870
      skull ~ 75870-75872
      splenic ~ 75810
      vena cava ~ 75825-75827
    wrist ~ 73115
  wrist ~ 73100-73110
X-ray tomography, computed ~ see CT scan
XA, coagulation factor ~ 85260
Xenoantibodies ~ 86308-86310
XI, coagulation factor ~ 85270
XI, cranial nerve ~ see accessory nerve
XII, coagulation factor ~ 85280
XII, cranial nerve ~ see hypoglossal nerve
XIII, coagulation factor ~ 85290-85291
Xylose absorption test
  blood ~ 84620
  urine ~ 84620

Y

Yeast culture ~ 87106
Yellow fever vaccine ~ 90717
Yersinia antibody ~ 86793

Z

Ziegler Procedure discission secondary membranous cataract ~ 66820
Zinc ~ 84630
Zinc manganese leucine aminopeptidase ~ 83670
Zonisamide
  drug assay ~ 80203
Zygoma ~ see cheekbone
Zygomatic arch fracture
  open treatment ~ 21356-21366
  with manipulation ~ 21355